# MECHANICAL VENTILATION:
## CLINICAL APPLICATIONS AND PATHOPHYSIOLOGY

# CONTENTS ·····

Mechanical ventilation has become the most commonly used mode of life support in medicine today. It is widely used in management of acutely ill surgical and ICU patients; it is also used in the chronic support of patients with a wide spectrum of chronic diseases that can cause respiratory failure. For many years the impact of this commonly preformed procedure was not fully understood, either in how it modulated lung function or how it affected other organ function. In recent years researchers have made great strides in understanding how respiratory failure and mechanical ventilation affect the complex interaction of gas exchange, cytokine release and cellular immunity. We have made a great effort to assemble the leaders of the field to review all aspects of mechanical ventilation. Our contributors span the globe and constitute a renowned group of experts who have contributed much to our basic knowledge and patient care. Through many years of researching, writing, lecturing and caring for patients they have created the framework for this book.

The primary aim of this text is to cover the breadth of the topic in a practical yet organized fashion. We hope its primary use will be as a practical everyday reference, but it will also be a useful foundation for further reading and research. We begin with chapters that review the myriad diseases and conditions that lead to respiratory failure, including common restrictive and obstructive diseases. We also review current knowledge on acute lung injury and ventilator-induced lung injury. All important aspects of the anatomy and ventilation mechanics are reviewed to allow the reader to better understand their importance patient care. New aspects of acid–base balance are discussed to give us the ability to better recognize derangements of cellular function due to failure to deliver oxygen and remove waste products. Various interactions between the pulmonary system and other organ systems are presented in such a way to reinforce the elegant concept of cell–cell interaction.

The many modalities of monitoring and diagnosing respiratory failure are necessary to rapidly observe changes in disease states and provide benchmarks and endpoints in the care of those patients. The book reviews all modes of ventilatory support currently used in all age groups, but it also introduces computer-guided therapies and other cutting-edge technologies. We took special care to review the many unique environments in which patients are supported, from prehospital sites to specialized units of the tertiary medical centers.

Information on adjunctive therapy, both pharmacologic and special device therapy, is integrated throughout to provide a complete information package that it intended to reduce complications and decrease time on ventilatory support. New aspects and guidelines for use of antibiotics are presented to educate clinicians on the latest in bacterial resistance that plagues the modern ICUs. The importance of sedation and neuromuscular blockade in titrating mechanical ventilation is emphasized to provide bedside clinicians with further cost- and time-effective tools to develop protocols and guidelines. Case reports and discussions are used to illustrate and reinforce the multiple topics covered. We hope that they will also serve as a basis for training in the care of common disease states.

Economic and ethical aspects of mechanical ventilation are important core topics. The high cost of ICU patient care greatly affects individual hospital budgets as well as broader health care budgets. The ability to provide cost-effective care is key to both the developed and developing world as the information highway leads to rapid sharing of techniques and care plans. The care provided at the end of life has become a cornerstone of ethical care.

The editors hope that their twenty-year collaboration between Rotterdam and Rochester will serve to illustrate how investigators and clinicians look for common ground to increase their understanding of pulmonary pathophysiology and apply this knowledge at the bedside. Researchers and bedside clinicians should work together to provide patient care supported by strong scientific evidence. All levels of readers can learn from this group of authors and their impressive knowledge of the many diverse aspects of this ever-growing field.

Peter J. Papadakos, MD, FCCM
Burkhard Lachmann, MD, PhD

# CONTRIBUTORS ·····

**Michael J. Apostolakos,** MD
Associate Professor of Medicine, Director, Adult Critical Care, University of Rochester Medical Center, Rochester, New York

**Joan R. Badia,** MD
Intensive Care Unit, Pulmonary Medicine Service, Clinical Institute for Pulmonary Medicine and Thoracic Surgery; Respiratory Care and Allergy Service, Hospital Clinic, Barcelona, Spain

**Sean M. Bagshaw,** MD, MSc, FRCPC
Division of Critical Care Medicine, Faculty of Medicine and Dentistry, University of Alberta Hospital, University of Alberta, Edmonton, Canada

**David J. Baker,** DM, FRCA
Staff Anesthesiologist, Department of Anesthesiology, Necker Hospital for Sick Children, Paris, France

**Rinaldo Bellomo,** MD, FRACP, FCCP, FJFICM
Professor, University of Melbourne; Honorary Professor of Medicine, Monash University; Director of Research, Department of Intensive Care, Austin Hospital, Melbourne, Australia

**Sven Bercker,** MD
Department of Anesthesiology and Intensive Care Medicine, University of Leipzig Medical Faculty, Leipzig, Germany

**Zaida D. Bisbal,** MD
Research Associate, Dorrington Medical Associates, Houston, Texas

**Anthony F. T. Brown,** MBChB, FRCP, FRCS, FACEM, FCEM
Senior Staff Specialist, Department of Emergency Medicine, Royal Brisbane and Women's Hospital, Brisbane; Associate Professor of Anesthesiology and Critical Care, School of Medicine, University of Queensland, Australia

**Gustavo Buchele,** MD
Department of Intensive Care Medicine, Erasme University Hospital, Brussels, Belgium

**Thilo Busch,** PhD
Department of Anesthesiology and Intensive Care Medicine, University of Leipzig Medical Faculty, Leipzig, Germany

**Enrico Calzia,** MD
Pathophysiology Section, Department of Anesthesiology, University of Ulm, Ulm, Germany

**Annalisa Carlucci,** MD
Respiratory Intensive Care Unit, Salvatore Maugeri Foundation, IRCCS, Scientific Institute of Pavia, Pavia, Italy

**Jean Chastre,** MD
Intensive Care Unit, Division of Cardiology, Pitié–Salpêtrière Hospital, Pierre and Marie Curie University, Paris, France

**Sanjeev V. Chhangani,** MBA, MD, FCCM
Medical Director, Surgical Intensive Care Unit, Rochester General Hospital; Associate Professor, Department of Anesthesiology and Critical Care, University of Rochester School of Medicine and Dentistry, Rochester, New York

**Davide Chiumello,** MD
Department of Anesthesia and Intensive Care Medicine, IRCCS Foundation, Ospedale Maggiore Policlinico, Mangiagalli e Regina Elena, University of Milan, Milan, Italy

**Alain Combes,** MD, PhD
Intensive Care Unit, Division of Cardiology, Pitié–Salpêtrière Hospital, Pierre and Marie Curie University, Paris, France

**Edgardo D'Angelo,** MD
Professor of Physiology, Institute of Human Physiology, University of Milan, Milan, Italy

**Gary Dudek,** MD
Assistant Professor of Medicine, Pulmonary and Critical Care Division, University of Rochester Medical Center, Rochester, New York

**Michael Ebsen,** MD
Director, Institute of Pathology, Städtisches Krankenhaus Kiel, Kiel, Germany

**Brigitte Fauroux,** MD, PhD
Pediatric Pulmonary Department and Research Unit, INSERM, Armand Trousseau Children's Hospital, Paris, France

**Terence R. Flotte,** MD
Dean and Deputy Executive Chancellor, University of Massachusetts Medical School, Worcester, Massachusetts

**Saskia Gischler,** MD
Pediatric Surgical Intensive Care Unit, Erasmus Medical Center, Sophia Children's Hospital, Rotterdam, The Netherlands

**Diederik Gommers,** MD
Department of Anesthesiology, Erasmus Medical Center, Rotterdam, The Netherlands

**Hérve Guénard,** MD, PhD
Department of Physiology, University Hospital of Bordeaux, Victor Segalen University, Bordeaux, France

**Claude Guérin,** MD
Division of Intensive Care Medicine, Croix Rousse Hospital, University of Lyon, Lyon, France

**Jack J. Haitsma,** MD, PhD
Interpartmental Division of Critical Care, University of Toronto; Keenan Research Centre, Li Ka Shing Knowledge Institute, St. Michael's Hospital, Toronto, Ontario, Canada

**Robert-Jan Houmes,** MD
Pediatric Surgical Intensive Care Unit, Erasmus Medical Center, Sophia Children's Hospital, Rotterdam, The Netherlands

**Yuh-Chin T. Huang,** MD, MHS, FCCP
Professor of Medicine, Division of Pulmonary, Allergy and Critical Care Medicine, Duke University Medical Center, Durham, North Carolina

**Shazia M. Jamil, MD, FCCP**
Division of Chest/Critical Care Medicine, Scripps Clinic and Scripps Green Hospital; Assistant Clinical Professor, Department of Medicine, University of California–San Diego School of Medicine, San Diego, California

**Jens Ingemann Jensen,** MD, PhD, DSc, FCCP
Associate Clinical Professor, Department of Anesthesiology, University of Rochester Medical Center, Rochester, New York

**Keith E. Johnson,** MD
Resident, Department of Anesthesiology, New York Methodist Hospital, Brooklyn, New York

**Gavin M. Joynt,** MBBCh, FFA, FHKCA(IC), FJFICM, FCCP
Professor, Department of Anesthesia and Intensive Care, The Chinese University of Hong Kong; Intensive Care Unit, Prince of Wales Hospital, Hong Kong, People's Republic of China

**Udo Kaisers,** MD, PhD
Department of Anesthesiology and Intensive Care Medicine, University of Leipzig Faculty of Medicine, Leipzig, Germany

**George E. Karras, Jr.,** MD, FCCM
Medical Director, Critical Care Unit and Respiratory Care Services, Mercy Medical Center, Springfield, Massachusetts

**Hans-Ulrich Kauczor,** MD
Director of Radiology, German Cancer Research Center, Heidelberg, Germany

**John A. Kellum,** MD, FCCP, FACP, FCCM
Departments of Critical Care Medicine, Anesthesiology and Medicine, University of Pittsburgh Medical Center, Pittsburgh, Pennsylvania

**Nick H. Kim,** MD
Assistant Clinical Professor of Medicine, Department of Medicine, University of California–San Diego, San Diego, California

**Younsuck Koh,** MD, PhD, FCCM
Professor, Division of Pulmonary and Critical Care Medicine, Department of Internal Medicine, Asan Medical Center, Ulsan University College of Medicine, Seoul, Korea

**Antonia Koutsoukou,** MD
Assistant Professor, Department of Critical Care and Pulmonary Medicine, University of Athens Medical School, Evangelismos Hospital, Athens, Greece

**Werner Kuckelt,** MD
Director, Division of Surgical and General Intensive Care Medicine, Department of Anesthesiology, Central Hospital Links der Weser, Bremen, Germany

**Burkhard Lachmann,** MD, PhD
Professor of Experimental Anesthesiology, Department of Anesthesiology, Erasmus University, Rotterdam, The Netherlands

**Chae-Man Lim,** MD, PhD
Professor, Division of Pulmonary and Critical Care Medicine, Department of Internal Medicine, Asan Medical Center, Ulsan University College of Medicine, Seoul, Korea

**Jeffrey Lipman,** MBBCh, DA, FFA, FJFICM, MD
Professor and Head, Department of Anesthesiology and Critical Care, University of Queensland; Director, Intensive Care Unit, Royal Brisbane and Women's Hospital, Brisbane, Queensland, Australia

**Frédéric Lofaso,** MD, PhD
Department of Physiology, Raymond Poincaré Hospital, Garches, France

**Charles-Edouard Luyt,** MD, PhD
Intensive Care Unit, Division of Cardiology, Pitié–Salpêtrière Hospital, Pierre and Marie Curie University, Paris, France

**Paul E. Marik,** MD, FCCP, FCCM
Chief of Pulmonary and Critical Care Medicine, Jefferson Medical College of Thomas Jefferson University, Philadelphia, Pennsylvania

**Klaus Markstaller,** MD
Department of Anesthesiology, Inselspital, University of Bern, Bern, Switzerland

**Jürgen P. Meinhardt,** MD
Departments of Anesthesiology and Intensive Care Medicine and Radiology, University Hospital of Mannheim, Faculty of Clinical Medicine Mannheim, University of Heidelberg, Mannheim, Germany

**Joseph Milic-Emili,** MD
Professor Emeritus, Departments of Physiology and Medicine, McGill University, Montreal, Quebec, Canada

**Konrad Morgenroth,** MD
Professor, Department of Pathology, Ruhr University Bochum, Bochum, Germany

**Iqbal Mustafa,** MD, PhD (deceased)
Formerly, Professor and Founder of Critical Care Medicine, Harapan Kita National Cardiac Center, Jakarta, Indonesia

**Claus-Martin Muth,** MD
Pathophysiology Section, Department of Anesthesiology, University of Ulm, Ulm, Germany

**Rahul Nanchal,** MD
Assistant Professor of Medicine, Medical College of Wisconsin, Milwaukee, Wisconsin

**Stefano Nava,** MD
Respiratory Intensive Care Unit, Salvatore Maugeri Foundation, IRCCS, Scientific Institute of Pavia, Pavia, Italy

**Michael S. Niederman,** MD
Professor and Vice-Chairman, Department of Medicine, SUNY Stony Brook; Chairman, Department of Medicine, Winthrop University Hospital, Mineola, New York

**Gustavo A. Ospina-Tascón,** MD
Department of Intensive Care Medicine, Erasme University Hospital, Brussels, Belgium

**Jaideep J. Pandit,** DPhil, FRCA
Consultant Anaesthetist, Nuffield Department of Anaesthetics, John Radcliffe Hospital, Oxford University, Oxford, United Kingdom

**Peter J. Papadakos,** MD, FCCM
Professor of Anesthesiology, Surgery and Neurosurgery, University of Rochester; Director, Division of Critical Care Medicine, Department of Medicine, University of Rochester Medical Center, Rochester, New York

**Paolo Pelosi,** MD, PhD
Department of Anesthesia and Intensive Care Medicine, University of Insubria, Varese-Circolo and Fondazione Macchi Hospital, Varese, Italy

**Irene Perillo,** MD
Department of Medicine, School of Medicine and Dentistry, University of Rochester, Rochester, New York

**Michael R. Pinsky,** MD, CM, Dr hc, FCCP, FCCM
Professor of Critical Care Medicine, Bioengineering and Anesthesiology, Department of Critical Care Medicine, University of Pittsburgh School of Medicine, Pittsburgh, Pennsylvania

**Christian Putensen,** MD
Professor and Director, Division of Intensive Care Medicine, Department of Anesthesiology and Intensive Care Medicine, University of Bonn, Bonn, Germany

**Michael Quintel,** MD
Department of Anesthesiology and Intensive Care Medicine, Georg-August University Hospital, Göttingen, Germany

**Milena Racagni,** MD
Department of Anesthesia and Intensive Care Medicine, IRCCS Foundation, Ospedale Maggiore Policlinico, Mangiagalli e Regina Elena, University of Milan, Milan, Italy

**Peter Radermacher,** MD
Pathophysiology Section, Department of Anesthesiology, University of Ulm, Ulm, Germany

**Jayashree Raikhelkar,** MD
Assistant Professor, Department of Anesthesiology, Mount Sinai School of Medicine, New York, New York

**Miranda D. Reis,** MD
Department of Anesthesiology, Erasmus Medical Center, Rotterdam, The Netherlands

**Irwin Reiss,** MD
Pediatric Surgical Intensive Care Unit, Erasmus Medical Center, Sophia Children's Hospital, Rotterdam, The Netherlands

**Andreas Reske,** MD
Department of Anesthesiology and Intensive Care Medicine, University Hospital Leipzig, Leipzig, Germany

**Hans Ulrich Rothen,** MD, PhD
Division of Intensive Care Medicine, Departments of Anesthesiology and Emergency Medicine, University Hospital Bern, Bern, Switzerland

**Charis Roussos,** MD, MSc, PhD, MRS, FRCP(C)
Department of Critical Care and Pulmonary Services, University of Athens Medical School, Evangelismos Hospital, Athens, Greece

**Dierk Schreiter,** MD
Surgical Intensive Care Unit and Division of Traumatology, Department of Surgery, University of Leipzig, Leipzig, Germany

**Marcus J. Schultz,** MD, PhD
Department of Intensive Care, Laboratory of Experimental Intensive Care and Anesthesiology, Academic Medical Center, University of Amsterdam, Amsterdam, The Netherlands; The Interdepartmental Division of Critical Care, St. Michael's Hospital, Toronto, Ontario, Canada

**Thomas P. Shanley,** MD
Janette Ferrantino Professor of Pediatrics and Communicable Diseases; Director, Pediatric Critical Care Medicine, C.S. Mott Children's Hospital, The University of Michigan Medical School, Ann Arbor, Michigan

**Ioanna Sigala,** MD
Department of Critical Care and Pulmonary Services, University of Athens Medical School, Evangelismos Hospital, Athens, Greece

**Indra Singh,** MD
Department of Critical Care Medicine, University of Pittsburgh School of Medicine, Pittsburgh, Pennsylvania

**Jaspal Singh,** MD, MHS
Assistant Professor of Medicine, Division of Pulmonary, Allergy and Critical Care Medicine, Duke University Medical Center, Durham, North Carolina

**Arthur S. Slutsky,** MD
Professor of Medicine, Surgery and Biomedical Engineering, Interdepartmental Division of Critical Care, University of Toronto; Vice President for Research, St. Michael's Hospital, Toronto; Keenan Research Centre, Li Ka Shing Knowledge Institute, St. Michael's Hospital, Toronto, Ontario, Canada

**Pejman Soheili,** MD
Pulmonary and Critical Care Division, Department of Medicine, University of Rochester Medical Center, Rochester, New York

**Roger G. Spragg,** MD
Professor of Medicine Emeritus, Department of Medicine, University of California–San Diego, San Diego, California

**Robert W. Taylor,** MD, FCCM, FCCP
ICU-USA, St. Louis, Missouri

**Per A.J. Thorborg,** MD, PhD
Department of Anesthesiology and Perioperative Medicine, Oregon Health Sciences University, Portland, Oregon

**Dick Tibboel,** MD
Pediatric Surgical Intensive Care Unit, Erasmus Medical Center and Sophia Children's Hospital, Rotterdam, The Netherlands

**Antonio Torres,** MD, PhD, FACS
Pulmonary Medicine and Respiratory Care Service, Hospital Clinic of Barcelona, Barcelona, Spain

**Mark J. Utell,** MD
Professor of Medicine and Environmental Medicine, University of Rochester Medical Center; Pulmonary and Critical Care Division, Department of Medicine, Rochester, New York

**Robert A. van Hulst,** MD, PhD
Department of Anesthesiology, Erasmus Medical Center; Diving Medical Center, Royal Netherlands Navy, Rotterdam, The Netherlands

**A.H.L.C. van Kaam,** MD, PhD
Department of Neonatology, Emma Children's Hospital, Amsterdam, The Netherlands

**Joseph Varon,** MD, FACP, FCCP, FCCM
Professor, The University of Texas Health Science Center, St. Luke's Episcopal Hospital, Houston, Texas

**Theodoros Vassilakopoulos,** MD
Department of Critical Care and Pulmonary Services, University of Athens Medical School, Evangelismos Hospital, Athens, Greece

**Bala Venkatesh,** MBBS, MD (Int. Med), FRCA, FFARCSI, MD (UK), EDICM, FJFICM
Senior Specialist in Intensive Care, Princess Alexandra Hospital; Deputy Director of Intensive Care, Wesley Hospital; Professor, Division of Anesthesiology and Critical Care, University of Queensland, Queensland, Australia

**Jean-Louis Vincent,** MD
Professor of Intensive Care Medicine, University of Brussels; Department of Intensive Care Medicine, Erasme University Hospital, Brussels, Belgium

**Denham S. Ward,** MD, PhD
Professor of Anesthesiology and Biomedical Engineering, Associate Dean for Faculty Development, Department of Medical Education, University of Rochester, Rochester, New York

**Helmar Wauer,** MD
Department of Anesthesiology and Critical Care, Charite University Hospital, Humboldt University of Berlin, Berlin, Germany

**Steffen Wolf,** MD
Department of Anesthesiology and Critical Care, Charite University Hospital, Humboldt University of Berlin, Berlin, Germany

**Hector R. Wong,** MD
Department of Pediatrics, University of Cincinnati College of Medicine, Division of Critical Care Medicine, Cincinnati Children's Hospital Medical Center and the Children's Hospital Research Foundation, Cincinnati, Ohio

# SECTION 1

# CAUSES OF RESPIRATORY FAILURE REQUIRING VENTILATORY SUPPORT

# CHAPTER 1

# Restrictive Diseases

Joseph Varon, Paul E. Marik, and Zaida D. Bisbal

The restrictive lung diseases (RLDs) are a group of pulmonary disorders with parenchymal "infiltrates" that result in disruption of the distal lung parenchyma. RLDs can be classified as fibrotic, traumatic, or infectious diseases that cause parenchymal disruption. The common features of RLDs include the reduction of lung volumes secondary to an alteration in lung parenchyma or a disease of the pleura, chest wall, or neuromuscular apparatus.[1] In most RLDs, the total lung capacity, vital capacity, and the resting lung volume are significantly compromised.[2] Mechanical ventilation for patients with RLDs may be a difficult challenge. This chapter presents some of the common RLDs as well as some ventilatory strategies for these patients.

## PATHOPHYSIOLOGY AND BASIC EPIDEMIOLOGIC FEATURES

The lung interstitium corresponds to an anatomic space interposed between alveolar membranes of the alveolar epithelial lining cells and the endothelial cells of the interstitial capillaries. Most patients with RLDs have alterations of this anatomic space. In the United States, the prevalence of RLDs has been estimated at five cases per 100,000 people. The prevalence in persons between the ages of 35 and 44 years is 2.7 cases per 100,000 persons. In people more than 75 years of age, the prevalence is higher than 175 cases per 100,000 persons.

Most RLDs are diseases of the lung interstitium.[3] Of the common interstitial lung diseases (ILDs) that cause RLDs, the most common include idiopathic pulmonary fibrosis, sarcoidosis, and some of the pneumoconioses.[4]

Occupational and environmental exposures to organic and inorganic dusts are important causes of ILDs.[5]

## MANAGEMENT OF ACUTE RESPIRATORY FAILURE IN PATIENTS WITH RESTRICTIVE LUNG DISEASES

The precipitating events leading to progressive respiratory failure in patients with ILD include upper and lower respiratory tract infections (bacterial or viral), pulmonary embolism, arrhythmias, myocardial ischemia, and biventricular cardiac failure. All attempts should be made to avoid endotracheal intubation and mechanical ventilation with aggressive medical treatment. The limited potential benefit of mechanical ventilation in a patient with end-stage ILD should be discussed with both the patient and his or her family. These discussions are best held with the patient and his or her primary care physician or pulmonologist before an acute crisis occurs, to determine the patient's preferences for end-of-life medical care and limitations of therapy. Mechanical ventilation is not curative and may serve only to prolong the dying process. The increased right ventricular afterload consequent to positive pressure ventilation (PPV) may precipitate acute or chronic cor pulmonale with hemodynamic embarrassment. Although available data on the role of noninvasive PPV (NIPPV) in patients with ILD are limited, this ventilatory modality may relieve dyspnea and improve patient comfort. NIPPV should therefore be considered in alert and cooperative patients. Mechanical ventilation should be considered in patients with a treatable precipitating cause who are likely to survive their hospital stay.

The ventilatory management of these patients is, however, quite challenging. The goal of mechanical ventilation is to improve dyspnea without aiming to normalize the blood gas profile. The ventilatory strategy should include measures to minimize the risk of barotrauma, principally by using reduced tidal volumes to maintain the plateau inspiratory pressures at less than 35 cm $H_2O$.[6] Anzueto and colleagues reported a 10% incidence of barotrauma in patients with chronic ILD who required mechanical ventilation.[7] "Physiologic positive end-expiratory pressure (PEEP)" of 5 cm $H_2O$ is suggested to minimize the risk of atelectasis, although evidence to support this practice is lacking. A trial of higher PEEP should be considered in patients with refractory hypoxemia. Once the patient has been intubated and stabilized, an early trial of pressure support ventilation may be warranted. Early extubation may minimize the morbidity associated with mechanical ventilation. To facilitate this goal, the use of sedative agents should be minimized, and invasive forms of ventilation should be avoided (controlled mechanical ventilation/pressure controlled ventilation).

## Idiopathic Pulmonary Fibrosis

Idiopathic pulmonary fibrosis (IPF), also known as cryptogenic fibrosing alveolitis, is a chronic, progressive inflammatory disorder of the lower respiratory tract of unknown origin. It is characterized by an atypical proliferation of mesenchymal cells, overproduction and disorganized deposition of collagen, and impaired gas exchange.[8,9] These pathologic processes, in turn, lead to decreased lung compliance, with a progressive increase in the work of breathing.[10]

The exact incidence and prevalence of IPF are unknown; however, the prevalence in the United States has been estimated to be between three and six cases per 100,000 of the population.[5,11] The usual age at diagnosis is between the fourth and sixth decade. This disorder does not have predilection for race or ethnicity. Approximately two thirds of patients with IPF are more than 60 years old at the time of presentation, with a mean age at diagnosis of 66 years.[5,12] The prognosis of IPF is poor; almost all patients die of respiratory failure. The survival range is approximately 4 to 5 years.[10,13]

From a pathophysiologic standpoint, IPF is initiated by an alveolar epithelial microinjury, followed by the production of fibroblastic foci leading to an excessive deposition of extracellular matrix and destruction of the lung parenchymal architecture.[14,15] The initial mechanism includes interactions of cytokines and other mediators with cells resident in the lung.[16]

Polypeptide mediators, including proinflammatory cytokines and chemokines such as tumor necrosis factor-α (TNF-α), interleukin-1β (IL-1β), and monocyte chemoattractant protein-1 (MCP-1) are released by inflammatory cells, most notably alveolar macrophages. The resident epithelial cells, fibroblasts, and endothelial cells within the lungs also produce a multitude of cytokines and growth factors that activate fibroblast proliferation and matrix synthesis. Tissue injury with fibrosis is believed to result from an imbalance between proinflammatory and anti-inflammatory cytokines, fibrogenic and antifibrogenic polypeptides, and angiogenic and angiostatic molecules.[17,18]

The most common clinical presentation of IPF is that of insidious progressive shortness of breath, dyspnea on exertion, and a nonproductive cough. Almost 50% of patients have constitutional symptoms such as fatigue and weight loss.[10,19] On auscultation, there are fine inspiratory crackles, heard best in midinspiration to end inspiration. With more severe disease, increased right-sided heart pressures and right ventricular failure may be evident, with signs of cor pulmonale, digital clubbing, and cyanosis. In fewer than 10% of patients with severe IPF, left ventricular dysfunction is present, the result of coexisting right-sided heart failure with ventricular interdependence.

In the diagnostic workup of patients with suspected IPF, a detailed medical history is required that should include a review of symptoms associated with systemic disorders, exposure to occupational and environmental agents, and the use of medications and drugs. Almost all patients with IPF have an abnormal chest radiograph.[20] Retrospectively, basal reticular opacities are often evident on previous chest radiographs for several years before the development of symptoms. A normal chest radiograph cannot be used to exclude IPF. High-resolution computed tomographic (HRCT) scans are likely to show evidence of interstitial disease in most patient with a normal chest radiograph or ill-defined opacities.[21–23] Pulmonary function tests demonstrate a restrictive pattern (reduced vital capacity often with an increased ration of forced expiratory volume in 1 second to forced vital capacity) which becomes more severe with time. The diffusing capacity is decreased with evidence of impaired gas exchange (decreased partial pressure of arterial oxygen and increased alveolar-arterial pressure of oxygen) initially with exercise and then at rest.

## Sarcoidosis

Sarcoidosis is a common ILD that leads to RLD. This disorder is a multisystem inflammatory disorder of unknown origin that primarily affects the lung and lymphatic systems. It is distinguished by the presence of discrete, compact, noncaseating epithelioid granulomas in any organ system. The noncaseating epithelioid granulomas are characterized by highly differentiated mononuclear phagocytes and lymphocytes. These granulomas are responsible for the development of fibrotic changes that commonly begin at the periphery of the granuloma and extend centrally, resulting in complete fibrosis and hyalinization.[24]

The incidence rates of sarcoidosis in one population-based study in the United States were 5.9 per 100,000 person-years for men and 6.3 per 100,000 person-years for woman.[25] This disorder affects people of all races and all ages, but African Americans have a higher risk for sarcoidosis than any other race. Sarcoidosis normally affects young adults between 25 and 35 years of age and has a worldwide distribution. The illness can be self-limited or chronic, with episodic recrudescence and remissions.

Sarcoidosis almost always affects the lungs and thoracic lymph nodes. Patients usually present with acute or insidious respiratory problems with bilateral hilar lymphadenopathy or pulmonary infiltrates and variable symptoms associated with involvement of the skin, muscle, eyes, liver, heart, or central nervous system.[26–28]

T cells are considered to play a central role in the pathogenesis of sarcoidosis, which is associated with an exaggerated cellular immune reaction to unknown antigens (exogenous or autoantigens).[29] The inflammatory response is distinguished by a large number of activated macrophages and CD4 helper T (Th) lymphocytes. Sarcoidosis is characterized by a Th1-type immune response with IL-2 release, accumulation of CD4 cells, an inverted CD4/CD8 ratio, and the release of Th1 cytokines including interferon and TNF.[30–32] Finally, there is significant immunoglobulin production secondary to B-cell hyperreactivity.[33]

In some patients, sarcoidosis can be asymptomatic or have mild nonspecific symptoms. However, most patients present with systemic complaints including fever, anorexia, and arthralgias. Almost 50% of patients present with dyspnea and dry cough, one third present with chest pain; clubbing and crackles rarely occur.[34–36] Hemoptysis is rare. Löfgren's syndrome is characterized by fever, bilateral hilar lymphadenopathy, and polyarthralgias. Because pulmonary sarcoidosis affects the alveoli, blood vessels, and bronchioles, pulmonary function abnormalities include a restricted lung pattern and abnormalities in gas exchange. Given that the conducting airways are usually involved, limitation of air flow is a common finding.

The diagnosis of sarcoidosis can be difficult and usually requires histologic confirmation of granulomatous inflammation, exclusion of other noncaseating granulomatous diseases, and clinical evidence of involvement in more than one organ. An extensive history and physical examination are imperative and should include historical information regarding occupational and environmental exposure to potential pulmonary pathogens.[37] The diagnosis of sarcoidosis is best established by histology, to exclude infectious or malignant conditions. Biopsy specimens should be collected from the most accessible organ and by the least invasive method. The diagnosis of pulmonary sarcoidosis depends on three findings: the presence of granulomas and a rim of lymphocytes and fibroblasts in the outer margin of granulomas, perilymphatic interstitial distribution of granulomas, and the exclusion of another cause.[38,39]

Three stages of pulmonary sarcoidosis have been described. The first stage is characterized by bilateral hilar adenopathy without parenchymal infiltrates on chest radiograph. The second stage is characterized by bilateral hilar adenopathy with pulmonary infiltration. The third stage is pulmonary infiltration or fibrosis. The final stage is characterized for infiltrates without adenopathy and shows evidence of bullae, cysts, and emphysematous changes.[40]

The treatment of sarcoidosis remains problematic, with no known curative therapy. Multiple therapeutic modalities have been investigated.[41] Treatment depends on the patient's symptoms, stage of disease, and degree of organ involvement.

## Asbestosis

Asbestosis is an important occupational lung disease and a common cause of pulmonary fibrosis. Asbestos is a group of naturally occurring, heat-resistant fibrous silicates.[42,43] The most common type of asbestos is chrysotile fiber.[44] In the United States, millions of workers have had occupational exposure to asbestos throughout the last century; asbestos has been used in industrial and nonindustrial environments. Asbestos has been used in textiles, cement, insulation and construction material, and friction materials.

Asbestosis is characterized by slowly progressive diffuse interstitial fibrosis of the lung parenchyma caused by inhalation of asbestos fibers. The condition has been recognized for more than a century. It occurs when there is exposure to high levels of asbestos, as was common among asbestos workers of last century. In addition, asbestos exposure can produce non–small cell and small cell carcinoma of the lung and mesothelioma of the pleura and peritoneum.[45–47]

People who smoke have an increased risk for the development of bronchogenic carcinoma because tobacco smoke and asbestos have synergistic carcinogenicity.[48] People who smoke and have been exposed to asbestos are 90 times more susceptible to developing lung carcinoma than people who either smoke or have been exposed to asbestos.[49]

In asbestosis, the alveolar bifurcation is the predominant site of inflammation and is related to the influx of alveolar macrophages. Asbestos-activated macrophages generate growth factors including fibronectin, platelet-derived growth factor, insulin-like growth factor, and fibroblast growth factor, which interact to induce fibroblast proliferation. Oxygen-free radicals that are released by macrophages damage proteins and lipid membranes, thereby maintaining the inflammatory process. A plasminogen activator causes further damage of the interstitium of the lung by degrading matrix glycoproteins.[50–52]

Asbestosis is usually asymptomatic for at least 20 to 30 years after the initial exposure. The time can be shorter with intense exposure.[53] The most common symptom is dyspnea on exertion; a productive cough denotes concomitant bronchitis or a respiratory infection. Chest discomfort is present particularly in advanced cases. Persistent rales are a common clinical finding. They are best auscultated at the base of the lungs posteriorly and in the lower lateral areas. Rales can be heard in the end-inspiratory phase at the beginning of the disease, but in advanced disease, rales may be heard during the whole inspiratory phase. Finger clubbing is present in 25% to 50% of cases. In advanced stages, patients may develop cor pulmonale with peripheral edema, jugular venous distention, hepatojugular reflux, and right ventricular gallop.[54]

A history of remote exposure to asbestos is required to make the diagnosis. The presence of pleural plaques is practically pathognomonic of previous exposure. Common findings on chest radiographs include small bilateral parenchymal opacities with diffuse reticulonodular pattern, notably at the lung bases. In addition, bilateral midlung zone plaques on the parietal pleura can be seen.[55–57] The diffuse lung infiltrates cause the appearance of shaggy heart borders and bilateral pleural thickening. Pleural involvement is the most characteristic finding of asbestos exposure. Almost 50% of patients exposed to asbestos develop pleural plaques. CT scanning has good sensitivity and is very useful in the assessment of pleural abnormalities and in the delineation of a parenchymal density that could be related to bronchogenic carcinoma. An HRCT scan allows better definition of interstitial infiltrates and may be helpful in diagnosing early stages of asbestosis.[58] The early physiologic manifestations include air trapping, as demonstrated by an increased ratio of residual volume to total lung capacity, and small airway obstruction.[59] With disease progression, there is a reduction of lung volumes.

## Silicosis

Silicosis is a debilitating and often fatal coal worker's occupational lung disease caused by the prolonged exposure and inhalation of free crystalline silica dust (quartz, tridyrnite, and cristobalite).[60,61] Silica is the most abundant mineral on the earth. Silicosis presents as varying degrees of fibronodular lung disease, depending on dose and period since onset of exposure. Patients with a history of silicosis are at a high risk of developing tuberculosis. In the United States, more than one million people have been exposed to crystalline silica and are at risk of developing silicosis.[62–64]

There are three clinical types of silicosis. The first is chronic silicosis, which is the most common form of the disease. It appears after contact with low concentrations of silica and with a period of at least 10 years of exposure;

the disease can be either simple silicosis or complicated silicosis, known as progressive massive fibrosis. The difference between simple and complicated silicosis is based in the chest radiographic findings. The second type of silicosis is called accelerated silicosis, which develops after 5 to 10 years of exposure to high concentrations of silica. In these cases, the lesions appear earlier, and progression is faster. In acute silicosis, symptoms develop within the first weeks to 5 years after exposure to very high concentrations of silica.[65]

Large silica particles are deposited in the upper airways and are cleared by local defense mechanisms. Smaller particles are deposited distally in the alveoli, where they lead to pulmonary fibrosis. These particles activate silicon-based radicals, which, in turn generate hydroxyl, hydrogen peroxide, and other radicals.[66] These radicals produce an injury to the cell membranes by lipid peroxidation and inactivate essential cell proteins. Alveolar macrophages phagocytose the silica particles and become activated, releasing cytokines and chemokines such as TNF, IL-1, IL-8, and leukotriene $B_4$, which enlist other inflammatory cells. Transforming growth factor-$\alpha$ induces proliferation of type 2 pneumocytes, and several cytokines stimulate fibroblasts to generate collagen with resulting fibrosis. Silica particles survive attempts of digestion by the alveolar macrophages, thus perpetuating the cycle of injury.

Patients in early stages of silicosis present with shortness of breath and a nonproductive cough. Patients with advanced silicosis may have chest pain. Patients with silicosis are at high risk for developing tuberculosis. In general, tachypnea, expiratory prolongation, rhonchi, and rales may be present. Digital clubbing is uncommon. Advanced stages of complicated silicosis results in cor pulmonale. The progression of silicosis in complicated cases leads to respiratory failure, which may cause death.[67] Symptoms in acute silicosis include severe dyspnea, fever, cough, and weight loss.

An occupational history and chest radiographs are usually sufficient for the diagnosis of uncomplicated silicosis. Radiographically, silicosis is characterized by small, nodular pulmonary opacifications and by eggshell calcification of hilar nodes.[68] In simple chronic silicosis, the opacities are less than 1 cm in diameter, mostly in the upper lung fields, whereas in complicated silicosis, the opacities are greater than 1 cm in diameter. Initial changes in acute silicosis include a diffuse haze in the lower lung fields; subsequently, ground-glass opacities and coarse linear or rounded opacities occur. A miliary picture with very small, round opacities may also occur in the lower lung fields.[69]

## Traumatic Diseases

Trauma is the leading cause of death in persons less than 44 years of age and is the fourth leading cause of death overall.[70] Approximately 140,000 traumatic deaths occur in the United States annually. Chest trauma is the cause of death in up to one fourth of patients with multiple system trauma. Injury may occur to the chest wall, lung, great vessels, and mediastinal viscera. Traumatic injuries to the chest may result in restrictive pulmonary complications including tension pneumothorax, open pneumothorax, and flail chest with pulmonary contusion. Each of these conditions requires different management and ventilatory strategies. However, most injuries are initially managed with supplementary oxygen, chest tube insertion, and volume resuscitation. The indications for thoracotomy in a chest trauma victim include cardiac tamponade, massive hemothorax; pulmonary air leak larger than 15 to 20 L/minute, and aortic arch, esophageal, tracheal, or major bronchial disruption.

### Chest Wall Trauma

Rib fractures are the most common chest wall injury. Rib fractures are an important indicator of underlying injury. Fractures of the first to third ribs are associated with injury to the great vessel and with bronchial injury, whereas lower rib fractures are associated with kidney, liver, and splenic lacerations. Flail chest occurs when three or more ribs are fractured in two places or in multiple fractures associated with sternal fracture. The clinical significance of flail chest varies, depending on the size and location of the flail segment and the extent of the underlying pulmonary contusion. Patients with severe hypoxemia require endotracheal intubation and PPV.[71,72] Indeed, correction of flail chest occurs with the application of PPV. However, the clinician must observe for late development of pneumothorax, especially tension pneumothorax, in the mechanically ventilated patient.[73]

Sternal fractures can occur in the trauma patient and are associated with myocardial contusion, cardiac rupture and tamponade, and pulmonary contusion.[74] Early surgical fixation is often necessary; urgent surgery may be indicated when costosternal dislocations compromise the trachea or the neurovascular structures at the thoracic inlet.

### Pneumothorax

Pneumothoraces result from penetrating trauma or blunt trauma with rib fractures. Pneumothorax may be caused by PPV (barotrauma). The presence of pneumothorax in a mechanically ventilated patient requires chest tube insertion.[75]

Open pneumothorax requires covering of chest wall injury with an airtight dressing and insertion of a chest tube. Tension pneumothorax requires immediate needle decompression and chest tube insertion.[76] Clinical findings include unilateral absence of breath sounds, severe dyspnea, tracheal shift, jugular venous distention, and cyanosis.

### Hemothorax

Initial treatment of hemothorax requires insertion of chest tube to evacuate the hemothorax, reexpand the lung, and monitor the rate of bleeding. Indications for thoracotomy include initial chest tube drainage of greater than 1500 mL or continued bleeding of more than 300 mL/hour for more than 2 to 3 hours.[77]

### Major Vessel Injury and Cardiac Tamponade

Major vessel injury and cardiac tamponade are common causes of death in major trauma. Major vascular bleeding or cardiac injury can compress the heart and lungs and physiologically can behave like an RLD. Radiographic evidence includes a widened mediastinum, aortic knob obliteration, and tracheal or nasogastric tube deviation. Arteriography or CT scanning is required for the diagnosis. Cardiac tamponade requires thoracotomy and pericardial decompression. Pericardiocentesis may be performed if the diagnosis is uncertain or as a temporizing measure during preparation for thoracotomy.[78,79]

### Pulmonary Contusion

Pulmonary contusion is a common complication of chest trauma. Ventilatory management consists of supplemental oxygen administration and mechanical ventilation with the addition of PEEP, if indicated in patients with worsening hypoxemia.

## Infectious Diseases

Numerous infectious processes can compromise the elastic properties of the lungs. Common restrictive situations arise from infections that lead to the acute respiratory distress syndrome (ARDS) and thoracic empyema.

### Pulmonary Infections and Acute Respiratory Distress Syndrome

The basic abnormality in ARDS is the disruption of the normal alveolar-capillary barrier. Moreover, it is now evident that ARDS is not simply a form of pulmonary edema caused by increased microvascular permeability, but rather is a manifestation of a more generalized permeability defect.[80] Research in recent years has been focused on possible mediators of lung injury in ARDS such as free radicals, proteinases, and soluble agents including cytokines, arachidonic acid metabolites, and charged proteins.[81]

The pathophysiologic consequences of lung edema in ARDS include decreases in lung volumes and compliance and large intrapulmonary shunts (blood perfusing unventilated segments of the lung). A fall in the residual volume is uniformly present and contributes to ventilation-perfusion inequality. It has been hypothesized that a defective surfactant may be partially responsible for the small lung volumes and that it may worsen edema accumulation in ARDS (because increases in alveolar surface tension have been shown to increase lung water content by lowering interstitial hydrostatic pressure).[82,83] The decrease in lung compliance is secondary to the increased lung recoil pressure of the edematous lung, which clinically increases the work of breathing and leads to respiratory muscle fatigue.

The pulmonary vasculature is prominently affected in ARDS. Pulmonary hypertension not related to hypoxemia is a very common finding in patients with ARDS. Indeed, this condition is caused by a three- to five-fold increase in pulmonary vascular resistance and is associated with an increase in right ventricular work.[84] Pulmonary angiography studies performed within 48 hours of the onset of ARDS have shown that 48% of patients have demonstrable filling defects (intravascular thrombi) in vessels larger than 1 mm in diameter.[85] Patients who die of respiratory failure usually show a progressive decrease in lung compliance, worsening hypoxemia, and a progressive increase in dead space with hypercapnia. Pathologic examination of the lungs in these patients reveals extensive interstitial and alveolar fibrosis.[86]

To date, there are no specific pharmacologic interventions of proven value for the treatment of ARDS. Although corticosteroids and prostaglandin E$_1$ have been widely used clinically, studies have failed to show any benefit in outcome, lung compliance, pulmonary shunts, chest radiograph, severity score, or survival.[87-90]

The mainstay therapy of ARDS is the management of the underlying disorder. Unfortunately, this is not always possible (as is the case in aspiration of gastric contents, smoke inhalation, or trauma). Treatable causes of ARDS include sepsis, respiratory infections, and shock. The ventilatory management of patients with ARDS is extensively reviewed elsewhere (see Chapter 4).

## Empyema

Any respiratory tract infection that leads to complicated pleural effusion and empyema has the potential to cause RLD. This restrictive process may be transitory or permanent, depending on how soon the clinician can achieve drainage of the infectious process.

## REFERENCES

1. Hsia CC: Cardiopulmonary limitations to exercise in restrictive lung disease. Med Sci Sports Exerc 1999;31(Suppl):S28–S32.
2. Green FH: Overview of pulmonary fibrosis. Chest 2002;122(Suppl):S334–S339.
3. Raghu G, Nyberg F, Morgan G: The epidemiology of interstitial lung disease and its association with lung cancer. Br J Cancer 2004;91(Suppl 2):S3–S10.
4. Thomeer MJ, Vansteenkiste J, Verbeken EK, Demedts M: Interstitial lung diseases: Characteristics at diagnosis and mortality risk assessment. Respir Med 2004;98:567–573.
5. Coultas DB, Zumwalt RE, Black WC, Sobonya RE: The epidemiology of interstitial lung diseases. Am J Respir Crit Care Med 1994;150:967–972.
6. Boussarsar M, Thierry G, Jaber S, et al: Relationship between ventilatory settings and barotrauma in the acute respiratory distress syndrome. Intensive Care Med 2002;28:406–413.
7. Anzueto A, Frutos-Vivar F, Esteban A, et al: Incidence, risk factors and outcome of barotrauma in mechanically ventilated patients. Intensive Care Med 2004;30:612–619.
8. Gross TJ, Hunninghake GW: Idiopathic pulmonary fibrosis. N Engl J Med 2001;345:517–525.
9. Ryu JH, Colby TV, Hartman TE: Idiopathic pulmonary fibrosis: Current concepts. Mayo Clin Proc 1998;73:1085–1101.
10. American Thoracic Society: Idiopathic pulmonary fibrosis: Diagnosis and treatment. International consensus statement. American Thoracic Society (ATS) and the European Respiratory Society (ERS). Am J Respir Crit Care Med 2000;161:646–664.
11. Hougardy JM, Ocmant A, Place S, et al: Usual interstitial pneumonia. Rev Med Brux 2004;25:178–183.
12. Scott J, Johnston I, Britton J: What causes cryptogenic fibrosing alveolitis? A case-control study of environmental exposure to dust. BMJ 1990;301:1015–1017.
13. Schwartz DA, Helmers RA, Galvin JR, et al: Determinants of survival in idiopathic pulmonary fibrosis. Am J Respir Crit Care Med 1994;149:450–454.
14. White ES, Lazar MH, Thannickal VJ: Pathogenetic mechanisms in usual interstitial pneumonia/idiopathic pulmonary fibrosis. J Pathol 2003;201:343–354.
15. Khalil N, O'Connor R: Idiopathic pulmonary fibrosis: Current understanding of the pathogenesis and the status of treatment. CMAJ 2004;171:153–160.
16. Selman M, King TE, Pardo A, et al: Idiopathic pulmonary fibrosis: Prevailing and evolving hypotheses about its pathogenesis and implications for therapy. Ann Intern Med 2001;134:136–151.
17. Center DM, Berman JS, Kornfeld H, et al: Mechanisms of lymphocyte accumulation in pulmonary disease. Chest 1993;103(Suppl):S88–S91.
18. Brody AR: Occupational lung disease and the role of peptide growth factors. Curr Opin Pulm Med 1997;3:203–208.
19. Johnston ID, Prescott RJ, Chalmers JC, Rudd RM: British Thoracic Society study of cryptogenic fibrosing alveolitis: Current presentation and initial management. Fibrosing Alveolitis Subcommittee of the Research Committee of the British Thoracic Society. Thorax 1997;52:38–44.
20. Petrova E, Petkov D, Shoshkov P, Nachev C: The diagnostic value of conventional X-ray examination of the lungs in comparison with high-resolution computed tomography (HRCT), isotope perfusion scintigraphy and the diffusion capacity in patients with pneumoconiosis. Int J Occup Med Environ Health 1995;8:231–238.
21. Raghu G, Mageto YN, Lockhart D, et al: The accuracy of the clinical diagnosis of new-onset idiopathic pulmonary fibrosis and other interstitial lung disease: A prospective study. Chest 1999;116:1168–1174.
22. Epler GR, McLoud TC, Gaensler EA, et al: Normal chest roentgenograms in chronic diffuse infiltrative lung disease. N Engl J Med 1978;298:934–939.
23. Orens JB, Kazerooni EA, Martinez FJ, et al: The sensitivity of high-resolution CT in detecting idiopathic pulmonary fibrosis proved by open lung biopsy: A prospective study. Chest 1995;108:109–115.

24. Rosen Y: Sarcoidosis. In Dail DH, Hammer SP (eds): Pulmonary Pathology. New York: Springer-Verlag, 1994, pp 615–645.

25. Henke CE, Henke G, Elveback LR, et al: The epidemiology of sarcoidosis in Rochester, Minnesota: A population-based study of incidence and survival. Am J Epidemiol 1986;123:840–845.

26. Chapelon-Abric C: Epidemiology of sarcoidosis and its genetic and environmental risk factors. Rev Med Interne 2004;25:494–500.

27. Borchers AT, So C, Naguwa SM, et al: Clinical and immunologic components of sarcoidosis. Clin Rev Allergy Immunol 2003;25:289–303.

28. Bub E: Heart failure, skin manifestations, enlarged hilar lymph nodes: Is it sarcoidosis? MMW Fortschr Med 2003;145:36–38.

29. Katchar K, Eklund A, Grunewald J: Expression of Th1 markers by lung accumulated T cells in pulmonary sarcoidosis. J Intern Med 2003;254:564–571.

30. Kataria YP, Holter JF: Immunology of sarcoidosis. Clin Chest Med 1997;18:719–739.

31. Hunninghake GW, Crystal RG: Pulmonary sarcoidosis: A disorder mediated by excess helper T-lymphocyte activity at sites of disease activity. N Engl J Med 1981;305:429–434.

32. Konishi K, Moller DR, Saltini C, et al: Spontaneous expression of the interleukin 2 receptor gene and presence of functional interleukin 2 receptors on T lymphocytes in the blood of individuals with active pulmonary sarcoidosis. J Clin Invest 1988;82:775–781.

33. Agostini C, Trentin L, Zambello R, et al: CD8 alveolitis in sarcoidosis: Incidence, phenotypic characteristics, and clinical features. Am J Med 1993;95:466–472.

34. Harrison BD, Shaylor JM, Stokes TC, Wilkes AR: Airflow limitation in sarcoidosis: A study of pulmonary function in 107 patients with newly diagnosed disease. Respir Med 1991;85:59–64.

35. Highland KB, Retalis P, Coppage L, et al: Is there an anatomic explanation for chest pain in patients with pulmonary sarcoidosis? South Med J 1997;90:911–914.

36. Liesching T, O'Brien A: Dyspnea, chest pain, and cough: The lurking culprit. Nitrofurantoin-induced pulmonary toxicity. Postgrad Med 1924;112:19–20.

37. American Thoracic Society/European Respiratory Society/World Association of Sarcoidosis and Other Granulomatous Disorders: ATS/ERS/WASOG statement on sarcoidosis. Sarcoidosis Vasc Diffuse Lung Dis 1999;16:149–173.

38. Gilman MJ, Wang KP: Transbronchial lung biopsy in sarcoidosis: An approach to determine the optimal number of biopsies. Am Rev Respir Dis 1980;122:721–724.

39. Kitaichi M: Pathology of pulmonary sarcoidosis. Clin Dermatol 1986;4:108–115.

40. World Association of Sarcoidosis and Other Granulomatous Disorders (WASOG): Consensus conference: Activity of sarcoidosis. Third WASOG meeting, Los Angeles, USA, 1993. Eur Respir J 1994;7:624–627.

41. Kerdel FA, Moschella SL: Sarcoidosis: An updated review. J Am Acad Dermatol 1984;11:1–19.

42. Peterson MW, Kirschbaum J: Asbestos-induced lung epithelial permeability: Potential role of nonoxidant pathways. Am J Physiol 1998;275:L262–L268.

43. Churg A: The diagnosis of asbestosis. Hum Pathol 1989;20:97–99.

44. Green FH, Harley R, Vallyathan V, et al: Exposure and mineralogical correlates of pulmonary fibrosis in chrysotile asbestos workers. Occup Environ Med 1997;54:549–559.

45. Upton AC, Shaikh RA: Asbestos exposures in public and commercial buildings. Am J Indust Med 1995;27:433–437.

46. Wang NS: Pleural mesothelioma: An approach to diagnostic problems. Respirology 1996;1:259–271.

47. Gaensler EA: Asbestos exposure in buildings. Clin Chest Med 1992;13:231–242.

48. Guidotti TL: Apportionment in asbestos-related disease for purposes of compensation. Ind Health 2002;40:295–311.

49. Churg A, Warnock ML: Asbestos fibers in the general population. Am Rev Respir Dis 1980;122:669–678.

50. Robledo R, Mossman B: Cellular and molecular mechanisms of asbestos-induced fibrosis. J Cell Physiol 1999;180:158–166.

51. Branchaud RM, Garant LJ, Kane AB: Pathogenesis of mesothelial reactions to asbestos fibers: Monocyte recruitment and macrophage activation. Pathobiology 1993;61:154–163.

52. Smith DD: What is asbestosis? Chest 1990;98:963–964.

53. Beckett WS: Diagnosis of asbestosis: Primum non nocere. Chest 1997;111:1427–1428.

54. Fraser RG, Pare JA, Pare PD, et al: Pleuropulmonary disease caused by inhalation of inorganic dust (pneumoconiosis). In Fraser RS, Pare PD (eds): Diagnosis of Diseases of the Chest. Philadelphia: WB Saunders, 1990, pp 2276–2381.

55. Kuku O, Parker DL: Diagnosis and management of asbestosis. Minn Med 2000;83:47–49.

56. Valeyre D, Letourneux M. Asbestosis. Rev Mal Respir 1999;16:1294–1307.

57. Jones RN, Diem JE, Hughes JM, et al: Progression of asbestos effects: A prospective longitudinal study of chest radiographs and lung function. Br J Indust Med 1989;46:97–105.

58. Aberle DR, Gamsu G, Ray CS, Feuerstein IM: Asbestos-related pleural and parenchymal fibrosis: Detection with high-resolution CT. Radiology 1988;166:729–734.

59. Kilburn KH, Warshaw RH: Airways obstruction from asbestos exposure and asbestosis revisited. Chest 1995;107:1730–1731.

60. Maxim DL, Venturin D, Allshouse JN: Respirable crystalline silica exposure associated with the installation and removal of RCF and conventional silica-containing refractories in industrial furnaces. Regul Toxicol Pharmacol 1999;29:44–63.

61. Altree-Williams S, Clapp R: Specific toxicity and crystallinity of alpha-quartz in respirable dust samples. AIHA J 2002;63:348–353.

62. Rosenman KD, Reilly MJ, Kalinowski DJ, Watt FC: Silicosis in the 1990s. Chest 1997;111:779–786.

63. Banks DE, Wang ML, Parker JE: Asbestos exposure, asbestosis, and lung cancer. Chest 1999;115:320–322.

64. American Thoracic Society Committee of the Scientific Assembly on Environmental and Occupational Health: Adverse effects of crystalline silica exposure. Am J Respir Crit Care Med 1997;155:761–768.

65. Seaton A: Silicosis. In Morgan WK, Seaton A (eds): Occupational Lung Diseases. Philadelphia: WB Saunders, 1998, pp 222–267.

66. Fubini B, Hubbard A: Reactive oxygen species (ROS) and reactive nitrogen species (RNS) generation by silica in inflammation and fibrosis. Free Radic Biol Med 2003;34:1507–1516.

67. Duchange L, Brichet A, Lamblin C, et al: Acute silicosis: Clinical, radiologic, functional, and cytologic characteristics of the broncho-alveolar fluids. Observations of 6 cases. Rev Mal Respir 1998;15:527–534.

68. Baldwin DR, Lambert L, Pantin CF, et al: Silicosis presenting as bilateral hilar lymphadenopathy. Thorax 1996;51:1165–1167.

69. Ziskind M, Jones RN, Weill H: Silicosis. Am Rev Respir Dis 1976;113:643–665.

70. Centers for Disease Control and Prevention: Medical expenditures attributable to injuries: United States, 2000. MMWR Morb Mortal Wkly Rep 2004;53:1–4.

71. Bianchi M, Cataldi M: Closed thoracic trauma: Considerations on surgical treatment of flail chest. Minerva Chir 2000;55: 861–868.

72. Ahmed Z, Mohyuddin Z: Management of flail chest injury: Internal fixation versus endotracheal intubation and ventilation. J Thorac Cardiovasc Surg 1995;110:1676–1680.

73. Kallel N, Beloeil H, Geffroy A, et al: Post-traumatic tension pneumothorax and pneumopericardium in spontaneous ventilation. Ann Fr Anesth Reanim 2004;23:364–366.

74. Roy-Shapira A, Levi I, Khoda J: Sternal fractures: A red flag or a red herring? J Trauma 1994;37:59–61.

75. American College of Chest Physicians: Management of spontaneous Pneumothorax: An American College of Chest Physicians Delphi Consensus statement. Chest 2001;119: 590–602.

76. Heiner M: Pneumothorax. Aust Fam Physician 1991;20: 1275–1281.

77. Gambazzi F, Schirren J: Thoracic drainage: What is evidence based? Chirurg 2003;74:99–107.

78. Moores DW, Dziuban SW Jr: Pericardial drainage procedures. Chest Surg Clin North Am 1995;5:359–373.

79. Campione A, Cacchiarelli M, Ghiribelli C, et al: Which treatment in pericardial effusion? J Cardiovasc Surg 2002;43: 735–739.

80. Kreuzfelder E, Joka T, Keinecke HO, et al: Adult respiratory distress syndrome as a specific manifestation of a general permeability defect in trauma patients. Am Rev Respir Dis 1988;137:95–99.

81. Dal Nogare AR: Adult respiratory distress syndrome. Am J Med Sci 1989;298:413–430.

82. Hallman M, Spragg R, Harrell JH, et al: Evidence of lung surfactant abnormality in respiratory failure: Study of bronchoalveolar lavage phospholipids, surface activity, phospholipase activity, and plasma myoinositol. J Clin Invest 1982;70:673–683.

83. Petty TL, Silvers GW, Paul GW, Stanford RE: Abnormalities in lung elastic properties and surfactant function in adult respiratory distress syndrome. Chest 1979;75:571–574.

84. Zapol WM, Snider MT: Pulmonary hypertension in severe acute respiratory failure. N Engl J Med 1977;296:476–480.

85. Greene R, Zapol WM, Snider MT, et al: Early bedside detection of pulmonary vascular occlusion during acute respiratory failure. Am Rev Respir Dis 1981;124:593–601.

86. Zapol WM, Trelstad RL, Coffey JW, et al: Pulmonary fibrosis in severe acute respiratory failure. Am Rev Respir Dis 1979;119: 547–554.

87. Luce JM, Montgomery AB, Marks JD, et al: Ineffectiveness of high-dose methylprednisolone in preventing parenchymal lung injury and improving mortality in patients with septic shock. Am Rev Respir Dis 1988;138:62–68.

88. Bernard GR, Luce JM, Sprung CL, et al: High-dose corticosteroids in patients with the adult respiratory distress syndrome. N Engl J Med 1987;317:1565–1570.

89. Chatterjee K: Congestive heart failure: Advances in treatment. Hemodynamic studies: Their uses and limitations. Am J Cardiol 1989;63:3D–7D.

90. Melot C, Lejeune P, Leeman M, et al: Prostaglandin E1 in the adult respiratory distress syndrome: Benefit for pulmonary hypertension and cost for pulmonary gas exchange. Am Rev Respir Dis 1989;139:106–110.

# CHAPTER 2

# Chronic Obstructive Pulmonary Disease

Keith E. Johnson

Chronic obstructive pulmonary disease (COPD) is one of the most common pulmonary disorders seen by physicians in the world. In the United States, it is estimated that more than 16 million Americans are affected by this disease. COPD is a term that describes a collection of diseases that result in chronic obstruction of airflow within the lungs and to the external environment and are generally not fully reversible. COPD is a disease that is strongly associated with smoking, typically is more common in men, and often is either asymptomatic or only mildly symptomatic. Traditionally, it has been subdivided into several entities, including chronic bronchitis and emphysema. Additionally, asthma is also included in the group of obstructive diseases in many paradigms.

## CHRONIC BRONCHITIS

Chronic bronchitis is a medical condition describing excessive tracheobronchial mucus production that results in obstruction of the small airways. This mucus production is sufficient to cause a cough with expectoration for at least 3 months out of every year for a period of 2 successive years. It is important to delineate this condition from acute bronchitis, a self-limited condition of the bronchi most often caused by viral infections in association with an upper respiratory infection.

### Pathology

Chronic bronchitis results from hypertrophy of the submucosal glands that line the large cartilaginous airways. This hypertrophy leads to airflow obstruction in the small airways. This condition is characterized by hyperplasia of the goblet cells and proliferation of the inflammatory cells of the mucosa and submucosa that lead to edema, peribronchial fibrosis, and mucus plugging of these airways, as well as hypertrophy of the surrounding smooth muscles.

The pathogenesis of this disorder is based in the alveolar epithelial layer. The inflammation associated with bronchitis is neutrophilic. It results from the actions of interleukin-8 and other chemotactic and proinflammatory cytokines, as well as colony-stimulating factors, that are released by these airway epithelial cells in response to stimuli.

### Epidemiology

The pathogenesis of bronchitis and emphysema has several contributors, perhaps the largest of which is smoking. In addition, air pollution, occupation, and genetic factors all play a role in the formation of this disease.

Smoking has been shown in repeated studies to inhibit the ciliary motion responsible for "sweeping" the airways clean. This inhibits the function of alveolar macrophages and directly leads to mucosal cell hypertrophy. Inhaled cigarette smoke produces an increase in pulmonary resistance secondary to smooth muscle contraction. The risk of death from emphysema or chronic bronchitis is more than 30 times higher for smokers consuming at least 30 cigarettes/day.

Air pollution has been shown to be another factor in the development of emphysema and bronchitis. Heavy pollution with sulfur dioxide has been shown to exacerbate bronchitis. In industrialized areas, emphysema and bronchitis exacerbations are shown to increase in times of high sulfur dioxide levels, such as happens with warm weather inversions over the cities of southern California.

An individual's occupation can also encourage the formation of bronchitis. Chronic bronchitis is more common among workers whose employment exposes them to dusts or noxious gases. Reviewing epidemiologic studies, one can see an accelerated decline in lung function in plastic plant workers and cotton carding mill workers.

In reviewing bronchitis, there is evidence of a familial tendency to the disease. Children of parents who smoke are more likely to experience severe respiratory illnesses and have a higher incidence of chronic respiratory symptoms.

A predominant feature of the progression of COPD is progressive airflow obstruction, leading to decreased forced expiratory volume in 1 second ($FEV_1$). Respiratory infections have not been found to influence the overall course of the disease. By the time chronic airflow obstruction is present, the $FEV_1$ has decreased well below the normal range. Smoking cessation will not reverse the changes to this point, but it will slow the rate of the progressive loss of lung function.

## Clinical Features

The primary symptom of this disease is sputum production. Dyspnea does not usually appear until bronchitis is fairly advanced. Patients generally have a long history of sputum production and cough, lasting many years, with a modest history of smoking. Generally, the cough begins in the winter months, and it progresses through the rest of the year. Often, the patient is overweight and cyanotic. There is usually no respiratory distress at rest.

These patients are often described as "blue bloaters," secondary to chronically elevated partial arterial pressure of carbon dioxide ($PaCO_2$) and lowered partial arterial pressure of oxygen ($PaO_2$). The cough and sputum production are usually accompanied by frequent respiratory tract infections and recurrent episodes of cor pulmonale.

The total lung capacity (TLC) is often normal, and there is a moderate elevation in residual volume (RV) (Fig. 2.1). The increase in RV is secondary to the slowing of expiratory airflow, in combination with the resulting gas trapping behind the prematurely closed airways. The advantages of the increase in the RV and functional residual capacity (FRC) for the patient are an enlarged airway diameter and an increase in elastic recoil on expiration. The disadvantage is that the work of breathing dramatically increases at the higher lung volumes. The vital capacity (VC) is diminished, and the maximal expiratory flow rates are low, because a decreased ratio of $FEV_1$ to forced VC (FVC) is noted. The best tests to determine these values are the forced expiratory flow between 25% and 75% VC ($FEF_{25-75}$) and the maximal midexpiratory flow (MMEF). Normally, $FEV_1 / FVC$ is 80%. In the presence of mild COPD, this ratio decreases to 60% to 50%.

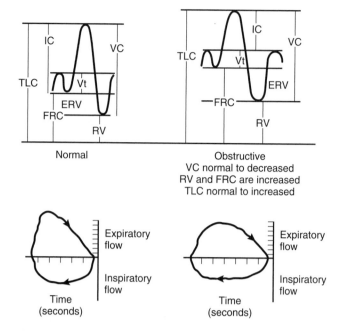

**Figure 2.1** Top: Lung Volumes and Capacities: Normal (left) vs. Obstructive (right) diseases. Bottom: Flow Volume Loops: Normal (left) vs. Obstructive (right) diseases.

In moderate COPD, the ratio is 40% to 60%, and less than 40% is considered severe COPD.

On chest radiography, chronic bronchitis is rarely identified. The two most commonly encountered findings associated with chronic bronchitis are thickened bronchial walls identified by tubular shadows and a generalized increase in bronchovascular markings. These patients are commonly described as "blue bloaters" because they have more severe hypoxia, with an elevated $PaCO_2$. Arterial blood gas determinations show a $PaO_2$ generally less than 65 mm Hg and a $PaCO_2$ chronically increased to greater than 45 mm Hg. As a result of the chronic retention of carbon dioxide, these patients develop a compensatory metabolic alkalosis as seen in their arterial blood gas values. The hypoxic and hypercarbic combination of the blood gas leads to pulmonary hypertension (arterial hypoxemia and the ensuing respiratory acidosis result in pulmonary vasoconstriction) and to indirect erythrocytosis caused by the chronic arterial hypoxemia. The chronic pulmonary hypertension leads to cor pulmonale and right ventricular hypertrophy, evidenced by right axis deviation on the electrocardiogram (ECG). Right ventricular failure often results, leading to systemic hypertension of the venous circulation, distended jugular veins, peripheral edema, hepatomegaly secondary to passive venous congestion, and, occasionally, ascites. Pleural effusions also can develop if left ventricular failure occurs.

## EMPHYSEMA

Emphysema is a medical condition that results from the permanent, abnormal distention of the distal air spaces of the terminal bronchioles, with destruction of the alveolar septa. It is estimated that of the 16 million Americans with COPD, 3 million of them have emphysema. Emphysema is characterized by a loss of elasticity in the walls of the alveolar pathways that results in an increase in lung compliance. Eventually, the smaller alveoli stretch and break, thus creating larger air spaces that are less efficient in handling the $O_2$ and $CO_2$ exchange. As a result, there is airway collapse on exhalation that leads to an increase in airway resistance. This obstruction also can cause bullae formation, with compression of adjacent lung tissue.

Although smoking is the major predisposing factor in emphysema, an imbalance between antiprotease and protease enzymes results in degradation of pulmonary interstitial fibers. This degradation is caused by the elastase enzyme, as well as by the absence of $\alpha_1$-antitrypsin. The absence of the $\alpha_1$-antitrypsin gene is found in about 0.1% of the population, but 80% of these individuals develop emphysema. The tendency to develop emphysema is variable, but smokers develop disabling emphysema 15 to 20 years before those who do not smoke. In addition, 5% to 10% of persons with this deficiency develop liver disease, most often cirrhosis. Those who are heterozygotes for $\alpha_1$-antitrypsin and who have 50% or more of the enzymatic activity seem to be protected against the development of emphysema. Although most smokers have normal levels of $\alpha_1$-antitrypsin, long-term inhalation of cigarette smoke increases elastase activity and inactivates $\alpha_1$-antitrypsin in the lungs.

### Clinical Features

The major symptom of emphysema is severe dyspnea, often exertional. Patients describe a minimal cough that is frequently nonproductive. As the $FEV_1$ decreases to less than 40% of normal, the patient will begin to experience dyspnea during activities of daily living. The patient's body build shows evidence of weight loss secondary to increased energy expenditure for breathing, with less caloric intake. The patient is generally distressed, with obvious use of accessory muscles to lift the sternum with each inspiration. These patients are often described as "pink puffers" because they have mild hypoxia with normal $PaCO_2$. They are also free of signs of right-sided heart failure.

Chest radiography demonstrates overinflation of the lungs, with flattened low diaphragms. Often, the lung fields are hyperlucent secondary to the arterial vascular deficiency in the lung periphery. If bullae are noted as well, then the diagnosis of emphysema is almost a certainty. However, only a few patients with emphysema have bullae. Another finding associated with emphysema is the loss of the normal, domed appearance of the cardiac silhouette; instead, it shifts to a vertically oriented appearance. If the $FEV_1/FVC$ is less than or equal to 50% or the $PaCO_2$ is greater than or equal to 50 to 55, the risk of respiratory failure following surgery is increased and post-operative mechanical ventilation should be expected.

### Diagnosis

Pulmonary function tests are relatively insensitive to obstruction of small, peripheral airways. These tests show increased TLC with decreased VC and a decrease in maximal expiratory flow rates, such as $FEV_1/FVC$. RV is also increased, reflecting the larger TLC with decreased VC. The decrease in the $FEF_{25-75}$ is even greater. The best tests to determine this are the $FEF_{25-75}$ and the MMEF. Normally, $FEV_1/FVC$ is 80%. In the presence of mild COPD, this ratio decreases to 60% to 50%. In moderate COPD, the ratio is 40% to 60%, and less than 40% is considered severe COPD.

Patients with emphysema are often described as "pink puffers." This description is secondary to the increase in $PaO_2$, which is found on an arterial blood gas determination to be greater than 65 mm Hg, and the normal (40 mm Hg) or slightly decreased $PaCO_2$. Emphysematous lung destruction leads to a loss of pulmonary capillaries as a result of destruction of the alveoli walls. The ensuing loss of pulmonary capillary bed area causes the loss of diffusion capacity, although $PaO_2$ is found to be only mildly depressed, resulting in minimal pulmonary vasoconstriction. Unlike in chronic bronchitis, erythrocytosis does not occur, nor does one see cor pulmonale.

## TREATMENT OF CHRONIC BRONCHITIS AND EMPHYSEMA

The goals of treatment of COPD are relatively simple. The treatment plan is designed to relieve the existing symptoms of COPD while slowing the progressive decline in pulmonary function that is associated with this disease. There are two types of therapies attempted in COPD. The first revolves around the cessation of smoking and the addition of supplemental $O_2$ for the patient with COPD. These are the only two therapeutic interventions that have been proven to alter the natural progression of COPD favorably. In addition, drug therapies are available to assist in reducing the symptoms of COPD.

First, cessation of smoking is critical. Smoking cessation diminishes the symptoms of chronic bronchitis. It also eliminates the accelerated loss of lung function observed in persons who continue to smoke. In addition, long-term $O_2$ administration, also known as home $O_2$, is usually recommended to patients whose $PaO_2$ is less than 55 mm Hg or whose hematocrit is greater than 55%. In addition, if there is evidence of cor pulmonale, the addition of home $O_2$ is often implemented. Supplemental $O_2$ administration should allow the $PaO_2$ to increase to between 55 and 80 mm Hg. This is often accomplished through the use of a nasal cannula, flowing at 2 L/minute. However, the flow rate often must be titrated to each individual patient, based on the arterial blood gas measurements. Relief of arterial hypoxemia has been proven to be more effective than any current drug therapy in reducing pulmonary vascular resistance and in reducing excessive erythrocytosis with corresponding increases in blood viscosity (Table 2.1).

In addition, drug therapy is often prescribed to patients with COPD. Bronchodilators are the main agents for treatment of these diseases. These drugs cause only a limited increase in the $FEV_1$ in these patients, but more importantly, they eliminate symptoms by decreasing hyperinflation of the lungs and reducing the dyspneic feeling, and they often improve exercise tolerance. Surprisingly, with the subjective improvement in the patient's symptoms, one finds little improvement in the spirometric measurements.

$\beta_2$-Agonists also have been suggested to provide a decrease in lung infections. This benefit is postulated to be a result of the decrease in the adhesion of bacteria such as *Haemophilus influenzae* to the airway epithelial cells.

| Table 2-1 | Chronic Obstructive Pulmonary Disease: Differentiating Emphysema and Bronchitis | |
|---|---|---|
| **Characteristic** | **Emphysema** | **Bronchitis** |
| Age at time of diagnosis (yr) | 60+/− | 50+/− |
| Dyspnea | Severe | Mild |
| Cough | After dyspnea begins | Before dyspnea |
| Sputum | Scant, mucoid | Copious, purulent |
| Chest film | Hyperinflated, bullous changes, reduced cardiac size | Increased bronchovascular markings in the lung fields, cardiomegaly |
| Chronic $Paco_2$ (mm Hg) | 35–40 | 50–60 |
| Chronic $Pao_2$ (mm Hg) | 65–75 | 45–60 |
| Hematocrit (%) | 35–45 | 50–55 |
| Pulmonary hypertension: Rest Exercise | None to mild Moderate | Moderate to severe Worsens |
| Cor pulmonale | Rare, except in terminal disease | Common |
| Elastic recoil | Severely decreased | Normal |
| Resistance | Normal to slightly increased | High |
| Diffusing capacity | Decreased | Normal to slightly decreased |

$Paco_2$, partial arterial pressure of carbon dioxide; $Pao_2$, partial arterial pressure of oxygen.

However, COPD is more effectively treated by anticholinergics than by $\beta_2$-agonists, unlike in asthma. Inhaled corticosteroids are an important part of the drug arsenal as well. In addition, broad-spectrum antibiotics, such as ampicillin or erythromycin, are prescribed for acute episodes of worsening clinical symptoms, associated with increased sputum production, increased dyspnea, or purulence of sputum. Annual vaccinations against pneumococcal infection and influenza are also likely to be of help.

In patients with cor pulmonale secondary to bronchitis, drug-induced diuresis may be necessary. This approach is considered in patients with cor pulmonale and signs of right ventricular failure. A common sign of these conditions is increasing peripheral edema. However, side effects, such as diuretic-induced chloride depletion, can result in metabolic alkalosis, especially important in these patients because it decreases the respiratory drive and can result in chronic retention of $CO_2$. A newer surgical modality to ameliorate the respiratory dysfunction caused by severe emphysema is lung volume reduction surgery. Generally, surgical excision of the most diseased portion of the lung results in a greater amount of functional lung tissue afterwards. It is only found to be effective in those patients having emphysema in the upper lobes of the lung. It is not effective for emphysema confined to the lower lobes of the lung, or those who have emphysema throughout the lungs. Surgical excision of 20-30% of the most diseased portion of the lung results in an approximately 50% reduction in the work of breathing within 24 hours after surgery. Secondly, dynamic compliance is found to be abnormally low in patients with severe emphysema. This compliance value dramatically normalizes with surgical excision. Thirdly, severe emphysema is characterized by intrinsic PEEP (positive end-expiratory pressure) due to air trapping distal to those airways which collapse upon exhalation. After excision of 20-30% of the most diseased portion of the lung, intrinsic peer is reduced by 80% immediately after surgery, and this reduction is seen months after surgery. Lastly residual volume, generally seen as increased secondary to this air trapping, also is found to decrease with lung reduction surgery.

## ASTHMA

Asthma is another common obstructive disease seen by physicians. It is estimated that 17 million Americans, nearly 5% of the population and including 5 million children, have asthma. Recently, the number of asthmatic patients, and the mortality rate associated with this disease have both been increasing. Risk factors associated with increased mortality include: black race, adolescence, history of any previous life-threatening epidoses, hospitalization within the last year, poor long-term medical care, medication non-compliance, and psychological or social problems. Asthma is a disease characterized by reversible expiratory airway obstruction secondary to airway narrowing in response to stimuli, airway hyperresponsiveness, and airway inflammation. In contrast to bronchitis and emphysema, in asthma the airway obstruction is not fixed, but rather it can vary widely over time and change in a period of minutes or in days to weeks. Although reversibility of expiratory airflow is an important characteristic of asthma, irreversible airflow obstruction can develop in some patients.

### Epidemiology

The features of asthma have several possible explanations. These include an allergen-induced immunologic response and an abnormality in the parasympathetic-sympathetic regulation of the autonomic nervous system.

One of the most accepted explanations for asthma is that it is immunologic. In atopic persons, repeated exposure to antigens leads to a synthesis of specific immunoglobulin E (IgE) antibodies. Patients are frequently found to have increased levels of IgE in the serum. When an antigen attaches to this IgE, they form a cross-link, attach to a mast cell, and cause the mast cell to release histamine, eosinophilic chemotactic factor, interleukin, tumor necrosis factor, leukotrienes, prostaglandins, platelet-aggregating factor, and bradykinin. The substances cause a decrease of cyclic adenosine monophosphate (cAMP) in the bronchial smooth muscle cells that leads to bronchospasm and edema secondary to increased capillary permeability. In addition, these substances cause the eosinophilic infiltration of the airways in the hours following the allergen exposure.

Another theory related to the features characteristic of asthma is associated with central nervous system autoregulation. This hypothesis is supported by the observation that nonselective $\beta$-agonists, such as propranolol, result in increased airway obstruction. The hypothesis suggests a neural imbalance between the parasympathetic bronchoconstricting system and the inhibitory, bronchodilatory sympathetic system. It is postulated that chemical mediators released from mast cell degranulation interact with the autonomic nervous system. For example, chemical mediators can stimulate receptors in the airway to trigger reflex bronchoconstriction. In contrast, other mediators can sensitize smooth muscle bronchial cells to the effects of acetylcholine. In addition, stimulation of muscarinic receptors encourages mast cell release, thus providing a reinforcement of inflammation and bronchoconstriction.

## Clinical Features

Typically, there is a family history of asthma. Asthma is associated with numerous predisposing factors. These include airborne allergens, aspirin, environmental and occupational factors, exercise, stress, and infection.

Asthma usually results in an attack, leading to an episode of wheezing, cough, and dyspnea. During the time before the attack, patients have periods of normal or near-normal pulmonary function, and no physical finding suggests asthma. As obstruction severity increases, wheezing becomes more audible and progresses earlier in the expiration phase. The absence of wheezing often suggests full airway obstruction. The cough of asthma is characteristic and can be associated with the production of copious sputum, typically mucoid and tenacious. Eosinophils often cause a yellowish tint to the sputum. Occasionally, cough is the only manifestation of asthma. The degree of dyspnea tends to vary greatly with time and is directly related to the severity of obstruction. In severe obstruction, the patient may experience "air hunger" as the foremost symptom. Patients often insist on sitting up to ease their breathing. In addition, patients often report chest tightness and discomfort relating to a sensation of not being able to inhale fully.

In mild asthma, $PaO_2$ and $PaCO_2$ are generally normal. The tachypnea and hyperventilation observed often result from pulmonary neural reflexes rather than from arterial hypoxia. The most common finding on the arterial blood gas determination during a severe asthmatic attack is hypoxemia. Hypercarbia or $CO_2$ retention is relatively uncommon because the diffusing capacity of $CO_2$ is 20 times greater than with $O_2$. $CO_2$ retention is found only late and only in severely affected patients. These patients typically hyperventilate, resulting in respiratory alkalosis.

In addition, during this attack, the $FEV_1/FVC$ ratio is markedly reduced, as are the MMEF and the maximum breathing capacity. These measurements directly relate to the severity of expiratory airflow obstruction. They provide the ability to assess and monitor the severity of an asthmatic exacerbation. Typically, a patient presenting for hospitalization for treatment of an asthma attack has an $FEV_1$ of less than 35% of normal and an MMEF that is 20% of normal or lower. In addition, in moderate to severe attacks, the FRC increases by 1 to 2 L, whereas TLC remains normal. There is no change in the diffusing capacity of carbon monoxide. Flow volume looping shows a characteristic downward "scoop" of the expiratory limb (Fig. 2.2), reflecting the decreased expiratory volume overtime.

Status asthmaticus, an unrelenting asthma attack is the most severe episode of asthma and can be life-threatening. Most episodes of status asthmaticus respond to emergency management with oxygen, nebulized or inhaled β-agonists, anticholinergics, and IV steroids. Occasionally, however, a few patients fail to respond to this treatment.

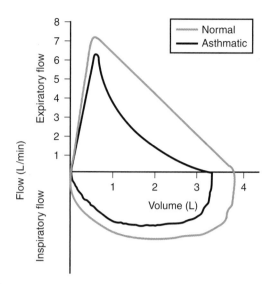

**Figure 2.2** Flow Volume Loop of Normal vs. Asthmatic patients.

They develop signs of impending respiratory failure, which include tachypnea, tachycardia, marked sternal retractions reflecting accessory muscle usage, nasal flaring, anxiety, or alteration of mental. There is moderate to severe hypoxemia, and $PaCO_2$ can either remain normal or elevated. Along with conservative therapy already in place, an IV terbutaline infusion is the drug of choice, titrating to a clinical endpoint of respiratory improvement, or tachycardia, with heart rate exceeding 180 beats/minute. Intubation of the trachea, with mechanical ventilation are done as a last resort, and is avoided because the endotracheal tube can itself serve as an airway irritant, thereby worsening the ongoing bronchoconstriction.

Chest radiography is not specific for asthma. One may see hyperinflation of the lungs. Generally, the use of chest radiography is better to rule out pneumonia or congestive heart failure, diagnoses often confused with asthma.

No single laboratory test can serve to confirm the diagnosis of asthma. However, a test for the response to bronchodilators often provides supportive evidence for clinical suspicions of asthma. The ECG can also be helpful by demonstrating evidence of acute right-sided heart failure and ventricular irritability during an acute asthma attack.

Other disorders with various causes are also classified as asthma. These include allergen-induced immunologic, exercise-induced, nocturnal, aspirin-induced, occupational, and infectious asthma. The first variant, allergen-induced asthma, is IgE mediated, and it is the most common form of reversible expiratory obstruction. Patients with this form commonly manifest other atopic manifestations, such as allergic rhinitis or dermatitis. A genetic predisposition is often identified by a presence of a family history. Peripheral blood eosinophilia and increased plasma IgE suggest this variant.

Exercise-induced asthma describes a patient in whom vigorous physical activity triggers acute airway narrowing and expiratory obstruction. This disorder is generally viewed as thermally induced asthma, thus identifying the association with fluctuation of heat and water that develops in the tracheal bronchial tree with warming and humidifying large air volumes during exercise.

Nocturnal asthma, a third variant, is said to reflect changes in airway tone, circadian variation in circulating catecholamine concentration, and gastroesophageal reflux related to the supine position associated with sleep. The incidence of asthma-related deaths has been shown to increase between midnight and morning.

Aspirin-induced asthma is a variant in which asthma and most nonsteroidal anti-inflammatory drugs cause acute bronchospasm. This condition occurs in approximately 10% to 15% of adult patients with asthma. It occurs anywhere from 15 minutes to 4 hours after drug ingestion. Although nasal polyps are associated with aspirin sensitivity, they are often present in the absence of this condition. It is thought that aspirin triggers bronchoconstriction in susceptible patients with asthma by blocking the cyclooxygenase mediation of arachidonic acid to prostaglandins. This would shunt the arachidonic acid toward the production of leukotrienes, a potent bronchoconstrictor.

Occupational asthma is the most common occupational lung disease. It is estimated to affect 5% to 10% of the world's population. Treatment for this disorder involves removing the individual from the work environment. More than 250 identified agents can cause occupational asthma; isocyanates are the leader and are responsible for 10% of cases. Chlorine and ammonia are two other common causes of occupational asthma.

Finally, the infectious asthma variant is one associated with an acute inflammatory disease of the bronchi. These cases may be caused by bacteria, viruses, or *Mycoplasma*. The treatment for this variant is eradication of the infection.

## Treatment

The treatment of asthma is accomplished through a multimodal medical approach. Anti-inflammatory agents interrupt the development of inflammation, a central feature of asthma. These agents include oral corticosteroid drugs, inhaled corticosteroid therapy, and cromolyn sodium.

Corticosteroids have been found to be the most effective pharmacologic treatment for the control of chronic symptoms of asthma, as well as for preventing exacerbations, in patients with mild or severe asthma. These agents are generally given as inhaled drugs because the systemic side effects are less than with oral administration. Because the inhaled corticosteroids are highly lipophilic, they quickly access the airway cells and inhibit the genetic transcription of cytokine synthesizing genes. By reducing cytokine transcription, the corticosteroids

serve to decrease airway inflammation and reduce airway hyperresponsiveness.

Cromolyn sodium, another anti-inflammatory agent, acts directly on the mast cell by stabilizing the cell membrane. It thereby limits the release of mast cell inflammatory mediators. Like the corticosteroids, this drug is administered as a metered dose inhalation. Although cromolyn sodium is an anti-inflammatory agent, it will not relieve bronchospasm once the condition is present.

A second modality is the use of bronchodilators that serve to relax the bronchiole smooth muscle. They include the $\beta_2$-agonist family, which serve as the optimal treatment for acute exacerbations. The $\beta_2$-agonists stimulate $\beta_2$-receptors on the bronchial smooth muscle, thereby activating adenylate cyclase and increasing intracellular cAMP concentrations. In addition, the methylxanthines are used, an example of which is theophylline, which results in mild bronchodilation with a long period of activity. Although theophylline reduces respiratory muscle fatigue and has a long duration of action, it is considered a third-line treatment because of its numerous significant side effects, such as nausea, vomiting, seizures, and tachyarrhythmia.

A third medical modality is the use of anticholinergic medications. These medications produce bronchodilation by decreasing the vagal tone through blocking the muscarinic receptors. Ipratropium, a derivative of atropine, has revived interest in this approach to treating asthma. Administered by metered dose inhaler, it is slower and less effective than the $\beta$-agonists such as albuterol. It causes bronchodilation by the blocking of cyclic guanosine monophosphate, and it has the advantage of not changing heart rate or intraocular pressure.

## SUGGESTED READINGS

Asthma: United States, 1982–1992. MMWR Morb Mortal Wkly Rep 1995;43:952–959.

Barnes PJ: Chronic obstructive pulmonary disease. N Engl J Med 2003;343:269–280.

Barnes PJ: Inhaled glucocorticoids for asthma. N Engl J Med 1995;332:868–875.

Busse WW, Lemanske RF: Asthma. N Engl J Med 2001;344:350–362.

Chan-Yeung M, Malo J-L: Occupational asthma. N Engl J Med 1995;333:107–112.

Ferguson GT, Cherniack RM: Management of chronic obstructive pulmonary disease. N Engl J Med 1993;328:1017.

McFadden ER, Gilbert IA: Exercise-induced asthma. N Engl J Med 1994;330:1362–1367.

Power I: Aspirin-Induced Asthma. Br J Anaesth 1993; 71:619–620.

Tarpy SP, Celli B: Long-term oxygen therapy. N Engl J Med 1995; 333:710–714.

Wulfsberg EA, Hoffmann DE, Cohen MM: Alpha-1 antitrypsin deficiency: Impact of genetic discovery on medicine and society. JAMA 1994;271:217–222.

CHAPTER 3

# Acute Lung Injury: Injury from Drugs

Nick H. Kim and Roger G. Spragg

The clinical presentation of drug-induced lung disease (DILD) can vary from acute to delayed, mild to severe, and reversible to permanent injury. For some drugs, the incidence of DILD is relatively high, whereas with the majority of drugs, the incidence remains rare and unpredictable. The drugs implicated in DILD can be found in all major therapeutic classes, and the number of drugs associated with pulmonary toxicity is likely to rise as new agents are introduced and as additional experience is gained with current agents. The evidence linking individual drugs to lung injury is largely based on case reports. These reports provide evidence that many drugs are capable of producing a range of host responses and types of lung injury. Such pathologic and clinical heterogeneity underscores the importance of maintaining DILD in the differential diagnosis in patients presenting with acute lung injury (ALI). The diagnosis remains one of exclusion. Early recognition and cessation of the offending drug are critical to provide the best chance for a favorable outcome.

## PATHOPHYSIOLOGY

The lung has limited ways of responding to injury. The histopathologic features of DILD are nonspecific and can be seen with other lung diseases. The clinical manifestations of DILD fall under a spectrum of pulmonary syndromes, including, but not limited to, the following: interstitial pneumonitis with or without pulmonary fibrosis, ALI (including acute respiratory distress syndrome [ARDS]), hypersensitivity pneumonitis, bronchiolitis obliterans with organizing pneumonia (BOOP), noncardiogenic pulmonary edema, and diffuse alveolar hemorrhage.

Although a drug may usually be associated with a particular syndrome, many of these drugs have the potential for causing a variety of syndromes.

Most of the implicated drugs appear to cause an idiosyncratic reaction, although several drugs have recognized dose-related toxicities. Certain drugs also have known risk factors for the development of DILD. The pathogenesis of DILD, however, remains largely speculative or extrapolated from animal models. The proposed mechanisms of lung injury from drugs can be broadly divided into two categories: direct and indirect (Table 3.1). Direct mechanisms include enhanced production of reactive oxygen species and direct toxicity from drug or drug metabolites. Indirect mechanisms include immune or inflammatory responses and coagulation- or fibrin-mediated injury. These indirect mechanisms, however, are not unique to DILD and have been proposed as causes of other acute and chronic lung injuries.[1,2]

Lung injury mediated by reactive oxygen species has been implicated in DILD as well as in other causes of ALI.[3] Bleomycin, nitrofurantoin, oxygen, and paraquat are examples of agents believed to cause lung injury mediated by reactive oxygen species.[4] Reactive oxygen and nitrogen species are generated principally from phagocytic leukocytes, but they can also be produced by fibroblasts, smooth muscle cells, endothelium, and epithelium.[5] These reactive species are normally neutralized by glutathione, catalase, superoxide dismutase, and other naturally present antioxidants. Bronchoalveolar lavage analyses from patients with ARDS have shown an imbalance, with evidence of excess production of reactive oxygen species and diminished levels of glutathione.[3,5] Excess production of reactive oxygen species can induce cellular damage through several pathways, including

**Table 3-1    Proposed Pathogenic Mechanisms of Drug-Induced Lung Injury**

| Mechanism of Injury | Evidence Sources | Example(s) |
|---|---|---|
| Direct: Reactive oxygen species/ oxidative stress | Bronchoalveolar lavage analyses, animal models, investigations of the role of iron | Bleomycin, other cytotoxic drugs, oxygen |
| Direct: drug/ metabolite(s) | Bronchoalveolar lavage analyses, observations on dose dependency | Amiodarone, narcotics, salicylate |
| Indirect: acute immune | Type I hypersensitivity reactions, bronchoalveolar lavage analyses | Nitrofurantoin, methotrexate |
| Indirect: delayed immune | Bronchoalveolar lavage analyses, observations on drug induced-systemic lupus erythematosus | Bleomycin, isoniazid |
| Indirect: fibrin deposition | Animal models | Bleomycin |

oxidation of DNA with resultant cleavage of nucleic acids; peroxidation and alteration of membrane lipids, alteration of protein function by oxidative changes, and release of arachidonic acid and its inflammatory products with resulting secondary injury.[6] Given the evidence for the contribution of reactive oxygen species to the pathogenesis of ALI, treatment with antioxidants seems rational. However, randomized placebo-controlled trials with the antioxidant N-acetylcysteine in the setting of ALI showed no evidence of outcome benefit.[7–10]

The case for immune-mediated DILD has been bolstered by analysis of bronchoalveolar lavage fluid, histopathologic observations, reports of response to anti-inflammatory treatment, and extensive data from investigations of animal models. Animals with bleomycin-induced lung injury have pulmonary sequestration of leukocytes and activation of cytokines and growth factors as plausible mechanisms for lung injury.[11] Bronchoalveolar lavage samples analyzed from human patients with DILD often reveal an abundance of leukocytes, typically lymphocytes.[12] Furthermore, withdrawal of a causative drug has been associated with normalization of bronchoalveolar lavage cellularity, and reintroduction of the drug has resulted in the reappearance of lymphocytes in that fluid.[13] Hypersensitivity reactions with peripheral eosinophilia have been described with nitrofurantoin, methotrexate, non-steroidal anti-inflammatory drugs (NSAIDs), and gold,

among others.[14] Although pneumonitis remains a less common manifestation than pleural reactions in drug-induced systemic lupus erythematosus, numerous agents including isoniazid, methyldopa, and hydralazine have been linked with drug-induced lupus.[15]

An additional mechanism for indirect lung injury associated with bleomycin has been proposed. Treatment with aerosolized heparin or urokinase inhibited bleomycin-induced pulmonary fibrosis in rabbits,[16] and inhibition of thrombin activity abrogated lung collagen accumulation in bleomycin-induced pulmonary fibrosis in rats.[17] Transgenic mice with increased plasminogen activator also were shown to be less susceptible to bleomycin-induced lung injury.[18] Taken together, these findings suggest that fibroblast proliferation secondary to activation of the coagulation system may be a relevant mechanism in bleomycin-induced pulmonary fibrosis.

## CLINICAL PRESENTATION

### General Features

The temporal relation between drug exposure and clinical presentation can vary depending on the drug, type of pulmonary reaction, and degree of host response. DILDs have clinically distinct presentations that range from an acute febrile illness temporally related to administration of the new drug to an insidious presentation that may occur even after drug discontinuation. Although broad generalizations regarding presentation in DILD have obvious limitations, there are some common features.

Patients exposed to antineoplastic therapies appear particularly susceptible to DILD, and they represent the majority of cases. Dyspnea and dry cough are the most frequent complaints in patients with parenchymal toxicity. Examination may reveal tachypnea, hypoxia, or crackles. Standard laboratory studies are often unremarkable, but they may demonstrate eosinophilia or a widened alveolar-arterial oxygen gradient. The chest radiograph often reveals opacities that are most often bilateral or diffuse, often favoring the lower lung zones. However, radiographic findings are generally nonspecific.[19]

Risk factors for developing DILD have been identified for several drugs. Dose-related toxicity has been observed for bleomycin, busulfan, carmustine (BCNU), and amiodarone. Cumulative doses of bleomycin higher than 400 U, busulfan doses greater than 500 mg, and BCNU doses higher than 1500 mg/m² have been associated with increased risk of DILD.[14] Lung injury from amiodarone has been more common when daily doses exceed 400 mg.[20]

## Specific Agents

Although the selection of agents for discussion is somewhat arbitrary, it is useful to focus on agents in the following categories: (1) drugs estimated to cause DILD in more than 1% of exposed individuals, (2) drugs for which there are credible data regarding the potential pathogenesis and risk factors, and (3) drugs that, although associated with an incidence of DILD in fewer than 1% of exposed individuals, are in common use and are thus responsible for a substantial fraction of DILD cases.

### Bleomycin

Bleomycin has been the most thoroughly studied of all drugs associated with DILD. This cytotoxic antibiotic comes from *Streptomyces verticillus* and continues to have wide application in treatment of a variety of malignant diseases. Well recognized for its pulmonary toxicity, bleomycin reportedly causes DILD in 2% to 40% of exposed individuals.[21] This wide range may result from factors such as differences in diagnostic criteria and recognition of risk factors leading to treatment modifications. In addition to cumulative dose, other risk factors for bleomycin-induced lung injury include advanced age, renal insufficiency, concomitant multidrug regimen or

radiation therapy, and high inspired oxygen concentration.[22] The additional risk posed by supplemental oxygen is unknown, but the use of supplemental oxygen is generally discouraged. Estimates of the incidence of DILD from bleomycin have been in the range of 10%. The mortality from bleomycin-induced lung injury depends on the type and degree of injury and on the presence of risk factors such as advanced age and renal insufficiency.[22,23] For pulmonary fibrosis related to bleomycin, mortality estimates have ranged from 2% to 60%.[23]

Bleomycin is cleared from the body through inactivation by bleomycin hydrolase or through urinary excretion. Inactivity of bleomycin hydrolase in the lung may predispose this organ to toxicity.[24] Direct cellular damage from bleomycin is believed to occur through an interaction of the drug with iron that results in production of reactive oxygen species. Hamsters made iron deficient through phlebotomy and diet have been shown to acquire resistance to bleomycin-induced lung injury.[25] Conversely, a study testing multiple iron chelating agents in hamsters found no protective effect from bleomycin.[26]

The most common lung injury seen with bleomycin is interstitial pneumonitis progressing to pulmonary fibrosis. BOOP (cryptogenic organizing pneumonia) occurs less commonly and can manifest as asymptomatic, poorly defined nodules detected on thoracic computed tomography[19] (Fig. 3.1). Patients with bleomycin-induced DILD typically present 1 to 6 months after initiation of therapy. Lung toxicity can also manifest several months to years following the last bleomycin exposure and may be triggered by administration of a high fraction of inspired oxygen.[27,28] Insidious nonproductive cough and dyspnea are the most common presenting complaints. Chest pain and fevers have also been reported. Radiographic studies typically reveal bibasilar infiltrates; however, focal or unilateral defects do not rule out bleomycin-induced lung injury.[22] Bronchoalveolar lavage findings of lymphocytosis and pathology findings of diffuse alveolar damage are often seen, but they are nonspecific for bleomycin-associated injury.[29] Although some investigators have reported that carbon monoxide diffusing capacity (DLCO) is a sensitive screening test for lung toxicity from bleomycin,[30] others have disputed the reliability of this measure in DILD.[31,32]

### Mitomycin

Mitomycin is also an antibiotic with cytotoxic activity; it has applications in a variety of malignant diseases including lung, gastrointestinal, gynecologic, and breast carcinomas. The reported incidence of lung toxicity ranges from 3% to 12%.[33] The incidence may be higher with multidrug regimens and doses exceeding 30 mg/m².[34,35] The usual presentation consists of a nonproductive cough and dyspnea associated with interstitial pneumonitis or fibrosis approximately 2 to 4 months into therapy.[34] Subsets of patients treated with mitomycin

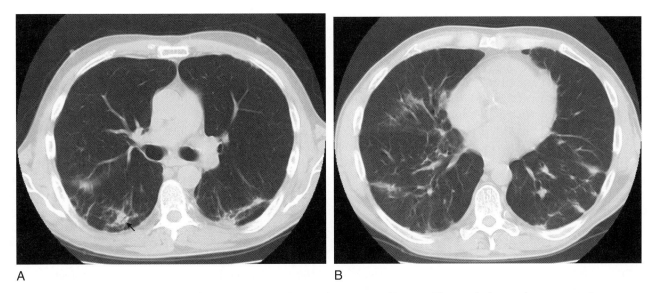

**Figure 3.1** Computed tomography scan of the thorax of a 50-year-old man with a testicular seminoma treated with three cycles of chemotherapy including cisplatin, etoposide, and bleomycin (total bleomycin of 270 U). New findings of focal poorly defined opacities with air bronchograms were seen throughout the lungs 3 months after initiation of therapy. *A*, Several poorly defined nodular opacities with air bronchograms (*arrow*). *B*, Both nodular and diffuse opacities. Discontinuation of bleomycin therapy was followed by marked clearing of the parenchymal opacities.

may also present with noncardiogenic pulmonary edema associated with the hemolytic-uremic syndrome.[23] As with other cases of DILD, there is no pathognomonic radiographic, pulmonary function, or histopathologic pattern in mitomycin-induced lung toxicity.

## Carmustine

The incidence of pulmonary fibrosis from BCNU has been reported to be as high as 30%.[36] The risk has been associated with a cumulative dose greater than 1200 mg/m², with the highest risk occurring when the dose exceeds 1500 mg/m².[34] Although presentations with ARDS have been reported with BCNU, as with other agents causing primarily pulmonary fibrosis, the usual presentation is insidious and often delayed. The resultant fibrosis from BCNU has been described histologically as bland; granulomatous lesions have also been reported. BCNU has been shown to reduce pulmonary glutathione levels and to alter glutathione reductase activity. These observations suggest that oxidative stress may contribute to toxicity.[37]

## Busulfan

Busulfan, the first cytotoxic agent associated with pulmonary toxicity, is an alkylating agent used primarily in the treatment of hematologic malignant diseases.[38] Pulmonary fibrosis is the usual manifestation of busulfan-associated DILD, and it has been detected in 46% of asymptomatic, treated patients.[39] Symptomatic fibrosis

from busulfan occurs in fewer than 10% of exposed patients. A cumulative dose exceeding 500 mg has been associated with a higher incidence of the disorder.[40] Unique features of busulfan-induced lung injury include the potential for considerable delay in onset of symptoms following exposure (range, 6 weeks to 10 years; mean, 4 years) and characteristically bizarre (but nonpathognomonic), dysplastic pneumocytes on cytologic examination of bronchoalveolar lavage cells or on tissue pathologic examination. The mechanism of lung injury is unknown.

## Cyclophosphamide

Although the incidence of pulmonary toxicity from cyclophosphamide is considered rare (<1%), the drug is widely used for both malignant and nonmalignant conditions. Cyclophosphamide is generally associated with pulmonary fibrosis, usually manifesting within weeks of treatment.[34] Both clinical and preclinical investigations suggest that an increased risk of lung injury occurs with exposure to either a high inspired fraction of oxygen or radiation therapy; injury from the latter exposure may be from drug sensitizing the lung to radiation. Proposed pathogenic mechanisms of lung injury have included alteration of glutathione stores by drug metabolites[41] and indirect injury from immunomodulation.[33]

## Methotrexate

Methotrexate has also seen wide application in both malignant and nonmalignant conditions, in particular rheumatoid arthritis. The incidence of pulmonary toxicity is roughly 7%.[33,42] Unlike the previous drugs, methotrexate is more commonly associated with a subacute presentation and hypersensitivity pneumonitis.[34] Patients typically complain of fever, malaise, and headache, along with cough and dyspnea, usually within weeks of initiating therapy. Peripheral eosinophilia is common, reported in 40% to 50% of patients; skin eruptions have been described in 17%.[42,43] Bronchoalveolar lavage data also support an immune-mediated process.[44] The prognosis is relatively favorable; pneumonitis often clears with either cessation of the drug or the addition of steroids to the regimen.[45,46]

## Cytarabine

Cytarabine (formerly cytosine arabinoside), an inhibitor of DNA synthesis, is primarily used in the treatment of leukemia. Patients with cytarabine-induced lung injury typically present with fever, cough, dyspnea, hypoxia, and evidence of pulmonary edema. In one series with high-dose cytarabine (3 g/m$^2$ every 12 hours for 4 days), 22% of treated patients developed noncardiogenic pulmonary edema within 6 days (median value) after treatment initiation.[47] In this cohort, patients receiving fewer than six doses only had a 7% incidence of the disorder, a finding suggesting dose-dependent toxicity. An autopsy review of patients who received cytarabine within 30 days of death reported that 67% had evidence of unexplained, significant pulmonary edema.[48] In survivors, pulmonary edema tends to clear within several days. The mechanism of lung injury is unknown.

## All-*Trans*-Retinoic Acid

All-*trans*-retinoic acid (ATRA), through its myeloid differentiation and maturation effects, remains an important and often effective therapy in acute promyelocytic leukemia. However, retinoic acid syndrome is a recognized, potentially fatal complication during induction treatment with ATRA.[49–51] Retinoic acid syndrome is a clinical diagnosis, suspected with the development of fever, respiratory distress, and pulmonary infiltrates. Additional clinical findings may include rising peripheral leukocytosis, weight gain, pleural or pericardial effusions, hypotension, and renal failure. In two case series (total, 108 cases), the incidence of retinoic acid syndrome was 15% and 26%, with a median onset of 7 and 11 days, respectively, following ATRA initiation.[49,51] Mortality associated with retinoic acid syndrome has ranged from 7% to 28%.[52] Although the pathogenesis of retinoic acid syndrome is not entirely known, ALI induced by ATRA may involve adhesion and infiltration of leukocytes. Early recognition, discontinuation of ATRA, and initiation of dexamethasone (10 mg every 12 hours intravenously for at least 3 days) remain the main treatments for retinoic acid syndrome. In one study of 306 patients with acute promyelocytic leukemia, concomitant chemotherapy was shown to decrease the incidence of retinoic acid syndrome from 18% for patients treated with ATRA alone to 9% for patients treated with ATRA, daunorubicin, and cytarabine.[52]

## Amiodarone

Ever since the first report of lung toxicity in 1980,[53] DILD associated with amiodarone has been a major concern, both because of the continued wide application of amiodarone for the effective control of various arrhythmias and because of the drug's potential for causing severe pulmonary toxicity. Before dosage was recognized as a risk factor for DILD, the incidence of pulmonary toxicity from amiodarone was reported to be as high as 27%.[54] None of the patients in the reported cohort treated with less than 400 mg/day developed pulmonary toxicity. A meta-analysis of four randomized, double-blind, placebo-controlled trials with 1465 patients treated with low-dose amiodarone (defined as less than 400 mg/day; mean dose ranged from 152 to 330 mg) revealed a statistically insignificant twofold greater incidence of lung injury when patients were treated with amiodarone.[55] The overall incidence of DILD in these four trials was 1.9%.

The most common form of amiodarone-induced lung injury is interstitial pneumonitis presenting with subacute or indolent symptoms. Although DILD associated with amiodarone can manifest at any time, most patients present within a year of initiating amiodarone therapy.[23] Pulmonary toxicity occurs even after drug discontinuation and may be related to the uniquely long systemic half-life of amiodarone of 45 to 60 days.[56,57] ARDS, BOOP, and solitary pulmonary nodules have also been reported but occur much less frequently. Presentation with ARDS from amiodarone has been associated with surgery and critical illness, in particular cardiothoracic surgery;[58] exposure to high oxygen concentrations and mechanical or circulatory factors (e.g., lung manipulation and bypass) have been theorized as potential triggers of the acute pulmonary syndrome. Pleural effusions, which are generally less common manifestations of DILD except in cases of drug-induced lupus, are rare but have been reported with amiodarone use.

Patients with amiodarone-related interstitial pneumonitis typically present with cough and dyspnea; chest pain, fever, and malaise can be present but are less common.[59] Leukocytosis and elevations of sedimentation rate and serum lactate dehydrogenase are common. Serum markers such as KL-6 have limitations and are discussed later. Reduction in DLCO occurs frequently with treatment and does not necessarily denote disease; however, lack of change in DLCO from baseline values has a high negative predictive value for amiodarone-associated pneumonitis.[60,61] Gallium-67 lung scintigraphy may be sensitive but lacks specificity for amiodarone-associated pneumonitis.[59,62]

Furthermore, the relatively high radiation dose and cost, together with the lengthy duration (48 to 72 hours) of the test, have detracted from the utility of gallium scintigraphy in evaluating DILD.[59] Abnormally high attenuation of lung parenchyma and pleura by computed tomography has been associated with amiodarone-related lung disease.[63,64] The clinical significance of these high-attenuation findings remains inconclusive, because data in asymptomatic patients treated with amiodarone are lacking. In addition, high-attenuation changes in the liver have been recognized in association with amiodarone treatment without clinical correlation.[65] Examination of bronchoalveolar lavage and lung biopsy specimens, as in other cases of DILD, cannot make the specific diagnosis of amiodarone-induced lung injury.[66,67]

Amiodarone belongs to a class of drugs associated with phospholipidosis, causing cellular accumulation of lipids that produces a characteristic foamy appearance (Fig. 3.2). Although implicated in the pathogenesis, the contribution of phospholipidosis to amiodarone-induced lung injury remains uncertain, and thus the finding of foamy lipid-laden macrophages in bronchoalveolar lavage fluid may indicate a drug effect rather than disease.[68] The long systemic half-life and accumulation of the drug in lung parenchyma (≤10,000-fold serum levels) may be contributing factors predisposing patients to lung toxicity.[57]

## Nitrofurantoin

Despite the occurrence of lung injury in less than 1% of exposed patients, nitrofurantoin has been considered the drug most commonly associated with human DILD.[29]

Although the use of nitrofurantoin has diminished with the advent of newer antibiotics, nitrofurantoin remains an effective agent against both acute and chronic urinary tract infections. Lung toxicity occurs most commonly in elderly patients and in women, perhaps reflecting populations at risk for such infections. The presenting lung injury in nearly 90% of individuals is acute hypersensitivity pneumonitis.[69] The typical presentation is an acute febrile illness with cough and dyspnea within days of drug exposure. Chest pain, myalgias, and rash have also been reported. The acuity of symptoms can be confused with myocardial infarction or pulmonary embolism.[23] In a Swedish report of 447 cases of nitrofurantoin-associated lung injury, 83% had greater than 5% peripheral eosinophils. The erythrocyte sedimentation rate may also be elevated.[14] The degree of eosinophilia in lung tissue and in blood is less than that seen in eosinophilic pneumonia.[29] A type I hypersensitivity mechanism has been postulated, with sensitization from prior exposure increasing the chance of an acute reaction.[29,70] The remainder of patients present with insidious symptoms of chronic interstitial pneumonitis. Eosinophilia in these patients is less common.[70] The primary treatment is withdrawal of the drug. Although deaths have occurred, particularly in patients with the chronic form of lung injury, the overall prognosis is good. The role of corticosteroids remains undefined.

## Salicylates

Excessive intake of aspirin has been associated with noncardiogenic pulmonary edema. The typical presentation is an elderly patient with a history of long-term aspirin

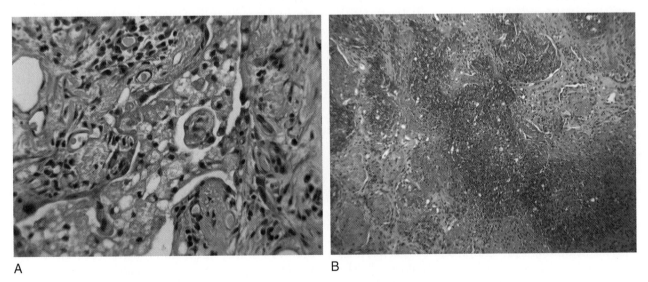

A

B

**Figure 3.2** Examination of pulmonary tissue from a patient with amiodarone pulmonary toxicity. *A,* Foamy macrophages with alveolar spaces that are consistent with amiodarone therapy but are not necessarily indicative of toxicity (hematoxylin and eosin; magnification × 63). *B,* Areas of tissues necrosis, moderate interstitial inflammation, and areas in which polyploid plugs of connective tissue fill alveolar spaces, consistent with amiodarone pulmonary toxicity (hematoxylin and eosin; magnification × 25).

use and with altered mental status. Serum salicylate levels are usually greater than 40 mg/dL[71]; however, some patients, particularly younger ones, with high serum levels fail to develop pulmonary edema.[71,72] Additional laboratory studies may reveal lactic acidosis and proteinuria. The latter finding may be related to a generalized capillary permeability defect.[14,71] Reported mortality rates have ranged from 0.3% to 15%.[73,74] In addition to supportive care, hemodialysis may be warranted in some cases.[73]

## Nonsteroidal Anti-inflammatory Drugs

Along with aspirin, NSAIDs have been commonly associated with bronchospasm, especially in patients with asthma.[46] Although comparatively rare, an important pulmonary toxicity induced by NSAIDs as a class is hypersensitivity pneumonitis. Implicated NSAIDs have included ibuprofen, naproxen, nabumetone, diclofenac, sulindac, and piroxicam.[29,46] Patients typically present with acute onset of cough, dyspnea, and fever after brief drug exposure. Leukocytosis, peripheral and sputum eosinophilia, and diffuse interstitial infiltrates can be present. Recovery after drug cessation is usually rapid;[46] however, fatalities have been reported.[75]

## Narcotics

Noncardiogenic pulmonary edema can occur with both illicit and therapeutic uses of numerous narcotics.[76] Although intravenous heroin overdose is associated with the highest risk and incidence, pulmonary edema has been reported with codeine, methadone, morphine, and even the opioid antagonists naloxone and nalbuphine.[29] Depressed mental status, although common, is not required to make this diagnosis. The mechanism may be an alteration in permeability.[77] Neurogenic and immunologic mechanisms have also been proposed.[76] Treatment is supportive. In the absence of superimposed infection or significant aspiration (which can be common), clinical recovery occurs within 48 hours.[14]

## Cocaine

Cocaine has been associated with numerous pulmonary complications that are typically acute and that include, but are not limited to, ARDS, pulmonary hemorrhage, eosinophilic pneumonia, and barotrauma.[78] Although all routes of drug use have been associated with pulmonary toxicity, the highest risk may be with smoking "freebase" or "crack" cocaine, the alkaline derivative of cocaine.[76] Chronic lung disease from cocaine has also been reported; in these case reports, pathologic examination suggested concomitant exposure to silica or cellulose-like particles causing chronic changes including granulomas.[29] The pathogenesis of ALI remains uncertain; from the heterogeneity of the pathologic manifestations, multiple mechanisms are likely. Treatment remains supportive, and the role of corticosteroids is unknown. In rare cases of fleeting infiltrates and eosinophilia (Löffler's syndrome), treatment with corticosteroids has been suggested.[78,79]

## DIAGNOSIS

**The Diagnosis Is One of Exclusion**    The task can be particularly challenging in patients treated with multiple drugs or in patients with a compromised immune system who have other underlying processes that can mimic lung injury (e.g., malignant disease or collagen vascular disease) or who are susceptible to numerous pulmonary infections. There is no current consensus on the diagnostic criteria for DILD. However, the following have been proposed as prerequisites: (1) history of using the drug, (2) exclusion of other causes, (3) prior observations associating the drug with lung injury, (4) clinical improvement following discontinuation of the drug, and (5) recurrence of the lung disorder with reintroduction of the drug.[23]

**The Diagnosis Is Clinical**    There is no pathognomonic finding from an array of available investigative tests to make the diagnosis of DILD. Pulmonary function tests (with DLCO), radiographic modalities (including chest radiograph, computed tomography, and nuclear scintigraphy), cytologic examination, and histopathologic examination all have their individual and sometimes vital role (e.g., ruling out infection) in the evaluation of patients suspected of having DILD, but they all have limitations.[13,31,32,62,67,80–82] Serum KL-6 and surfactant protein D are markers of pneumocyte activity and are increased in amiodarone lung toxicity.[82,83] Serum KL-6 is also increased in patients with diffuse alveolar damage or chronic interstitial pneumonitis associated with other drug exposures.[84] However, these markers are nonspecific and can be elevated in other causes of lung injury.[85]

## TREATMENT

Universally, the most important intervention in DILD is discontinuation of the offending drug. There exist innumerable conflicting reports, invariably anecdotal and with small sample sizes, on the efficacy of systemic corticosteroids. One plausible explanation for the mixed responses may be in the timing of corticosteroid therapy. More consistent observations have been made with amiodarone-associated pneumonitis and retinoic acid syndrome, in which administration of systemic corticosteroids appears to afford benefit. Accordingly, despite the lack of prospective, randomized data, the addition of systemic corticosteroids to drug cessation in the treatment of amiodarone-associated pneumonitis or retinoic acid syndrome is recommended. In all other cases of DILD, however, the absence of conclusive data should heavily influence the decision whether to treat with systemic corticosteroids; such a decision should be made on case-by-case basis, with recognition of the potential risks and benefits and of the uncertainty of treatment duration and outcome.

The preventive potential of inhaled steroids (fluticasone propionate, 880 µg twice daily) was reported in a prospective, nonrandomized, historically controlled study of 63 patients with breast cancer who were receiving high-dose chemotherapy (with cyclophosphamide, cisplatin, and BCNU), followed by autologous stem cell transplantation.[86] Compared with a 73% incidence in the historical control group, the treatment group had a 35% incidence of predefined pulmonary toxicity based on DLCO and symptom criteria. Currently, however, no randomized controlled trials address the efficacy of either pharmacologic prevention or treatment of DILD.

Additional novel targets for the treatment and prevention of DILD have been identified through study of animal models of bleomycin-induced lung disease. Bosentan, a dual endothelin-1 (ET-1) receptor antagonist approved for the treatment of pulmonary arterial hypertension, has been shown to protect rats from bleomycin-induced lung injury.[87] ET-1 up-regulates fibroblast activity and has been implicated in the pathogenesis of idiopathic pulmonary fibrosis.[88] Currently, a clinical trial is ongoing to investigate the effect of bosentan in idiopathic pulmonary fibrosis. Bleomycin has also been shown to up-regulate the angiotensin II type 1 receptor (AT1), a receptor involved in cardiac and renal fibrosis. Treatment with an AT1 receptor antagonist (candesartan) in a rat bleomycin model resulted in significant attenuation of transforming growth factor-$\beta_1$ expression and decreased lung injury.[89] An in vitro study of rat cardiac fibroblasts described the roles of reactive oxygen species and antioxidants in the regulation of ET-1 expression through angiotensin II;[90] this may represent yet another pathway through which reactive oxygen species mediate lung injury. Günther and associates treated rabbits exposed to bleomycin with aerosolized heparin or urokinase and demonstrated attenuation of lung injury.[16] Accordingly, alveolar fibrin deposition may represent an additional pathogenic target for the treatment of DILD and other causes of ALI.

Antioxidants have been studied for their potential role in restoring the oxidant imbalance and thereby obviating a proinflammatory trigger.[3,5] Clinical trials of N-acetylcysteine for treatment of ARDS have failed to show benefit.[7-10] The case for N-acetylcysteine may have been further worsened by a report of increased mortality (61%; n = 41) in the treated group compared with the placebo-treated control group (32%; n = 45) in newly admitted critically ill patients at risk for multisystem organ failure.[91] Another antioxidant that has received attention in lung injury has been α-tocopherol (vitamin E). Mice treated with α-tocopherol developed significantly less lung fibrosis after exposure to bleomycin.[92] In summary, the effect and impact of agents to relieve oxidative stress in DILD remain unanswered.

## CONCLUSION

Although uncertainty remains regarding the pathogenesis, diagnostic criteria, and role of adjunctive treatment, DILD is an important clinical syndrome. Considering the countless number of patients at risk, awareness is required. This diagnosis must be considered in patients with ALI. Recognition and early withdrawal of the causative drug are the most important and effective interventions.

## REFERENCES

1. Goodman RB, Pugin J, Lee JS, et al: Cytokine-mediated inflammation in acute lung injury. Cytokine Growth Factor Rev 2003;14:523–535.
2. Matthay MA, Zimmerman GA, Esmon C, et al: Future research directions in acute lung injury: Summary of a National Heart, Lung, and Blood Institute working group. Am J Respir Crit Care Med 2003;167:1027–1035.
3. Lang JD, McArdle PJ, O'Reilly PJ, et al: Oxidant-antioxidant balance in acute lung injury. Chest 2002;122:S314–S320.
4. Martin WJ, Gadek JE, Hunninghake GW, et al: Oxidant injury of lung parenchymal cells. J Clin Invest 1981;68:1277–1288.
5. Chow CW, Herrera AM, Suzuki T, et al: Oxidative stress and acute lung injury. Am J Respir Cell Mol Biol 2003;29:427–431.
6. Ryrfeldt A: Drug-induced inflammatory responses to the lung. Toxicol Lett 2000;112–113:171–166.
7. Bernard GR, Wheeler AP, Arons MM, et al: A trial of antioxidants N-acetylcysteine and procysteine in ARDS: The Antioxidant in ARDS Study Group. Chest 1997;112:164–172.
8. Domenighetti G, Suter PM, Schaller MD, et al: Treatment with N-acetylcysteine during acute respiratory distress syndrome: A randomized, double-blind, placebo-controlled clinical study. J Crit Care 1997;12:177–182.
9. Jepsen S, Herlevsen P, Knudsen P, et al: Antioxidant treatment with N-acetylcysteine during adult respiratory distress syndrome: A prospective, randomized, placebo-controlled study. Crit Care Med 1992;20:918–923.
10. Suter PM, Domenighetti G, Schaller MD, et al: N-acetylcysteine enhances recovery from acute lung injury in man: A randomized, double-blind, placebo-controlled clinical study. Chest 1994;105: 190–194.
11. Chandler DB: Possible mechanisms of bleomycin-induced fibrosis. Clin Chest Med 1990;11:21–30.
12. Costabel U, Uzaslan E, Guzman J: Bronchoalveolar lavage in drug-induced lung disease. Clin Chest Med 2004;25:25–35.
13. Akoun GM, Cadranel JL, Milleron BJ, et al: Bronchoalveolar lavage cell data in 19 patients with drug-associated pneumonitis (except amiodarone). Chest 1991;99:98–104.

14. Oldham SAA: Drug-induced diseases of the thorax and reaction to radiation therapy. In Freunlich IM, Bragg DG (eds): A Radiologic Approach to Diseases of the Chest, 2nd ed. Baltimore: Williams & Wilkins, 1997, p 675.

15. Ozkan M, Dweik RA, Ahmad M: Drug-induced lung disease. Cleve Clin J Med 2001;68:782–795.

16. Günther A, Lubke N, Ermert M, et al: Prevention of bleomycin-induced lung fibrosis by aerosolization of heparin or urokinase in rabbits. Am J Respir Crit Care Med 2003;168:1358–1365.

17. Howell DC, Laurent GJ, Chambers RC: Role of thrombin and its major cellular receptor, protease-activated receptor-1, in pulmonary fibrosis. Biochem Soc Trans 2002;30:211–216.

18. Sisson TH, Hattori N, Xu Y, et al: Treatment of bleomycin-induced pulmonary fibrosis by transfer of urokinase-type plasminogen activator genes. Hum Gene Ther 1999;10: 2315–2323.

19. Rossi SE, Erasmus JJ, McAdams HP, et al: Pulmonary drug toxicity: Radiologic and pathologic manifestations. Radiographics 2000;20:1245–1259.

20. Dusman RE, Stanton MS, Miles WM, et al: Clinical features of amiodarone-induced pulmonary toxicity. Circulation 1990;82:51–59.

21. Jules-Elysee K, White DA: Bleomycin-induced pulmonary toxicity. Clin Chest Med 1990;11:1–20.

22. Sleijfer S: Bleomycin-induced pneumonitis. Chest 2001;120: 617–624.

23. Camus P: Drug induced infiltrative lung diseases. In Schwartz MI, King TE (eds): Interstitial Lung Disease. Hamilton, Ontario, Canada: Decker, 2003, p 485.

24. Schwartz DR, Homanics GE, Hoyt DG, et al: The neutral cysteine protease bleomycin hydrolase is essential for epidermal integrity and bleomycin resistance. Proc Natl Acad Sci U S A 1999;96:4680–4685.

25. Chandler DB, Barton JC, Briggs DD, et al: Effect of iron deficiency on bleomycin-induced lung fibrosis in the hamster. Am Rev Respir Dis 1988;137:85–89.

26. Tryka AF: ICRF 187 and polyhydroxyphenyl derivatives fail to protect against bleomycin induced lung injury. Toxicology 1989;59:127–138.

27. Gilson AJ, Sahn SA: Reactivation of bleomycin lung toxicity following oxygen administration: A second response to corticosteroids. Chest 1985;88:304–306.

28. White DA, Stover DE: Severe bleomycin-induced pneumonitis: Clinical features and response to corticosteroids. Chest 1984;86:723–728.

29. Myers JL: Pathology of drug-induced lung disease. In Katzenstein AA (ed): Katzenstein and Askin's Surgical Pathology of Non-Neoplastic Lung Disease, 3rd ed. Philadelphia: WB Saunders, 1997, p 81.

30. Comis RL: Bleomycin pulmonary toxicity: Current status and future directions. Semin Oncol 1992;19:64–70.

31. Lewis BM, Izbicki R: Routine pulmonary function tests during bleomycin therapy: Tests may be ineffective and potentially misleading. JAMA 1980;243:347–351.

32. McKeage MJ, Evans BD, Atkinson C, et al: Carbon monoxide diffusing capacity is a poor predictor of clinically significant bleomycin lung: New Zealand Clinical Oncology Group. J Clin Oncol 1990;8:779–783.

33. Cooper JAJ, White DA, Matthay RA: Drug-induced pulmonary disease. Part 1: Cytotoxic drugs. Am Rev Respir Dis 1986;133:321–340.

34. Twohig KJ, Matthay RA: Pulmonary effects of cytotoxic agents other than bleomycin. Clin Chest Med 1990;11:31–54.

35. Verweij J, van Zanten T, Souren T, et al: Prospective study on the dose relationship of mitomycin C-induced interstitial pneumonitis. Cancer 1987;60:756–761.

36. Selker RG, Jacobs SA, Moore PB, et al: 1,3-Bis(2-chloroethyl)-1-nitrosourea (BCNU)-induced pulmonary fibrosis. Neurosurgery 1980;7:560–565.

37. Smith AC, Boyd MR: Preferential effects of 1,3-bis (2-chloroethyl)-1-nitrosourea (BCNU) on pulmonary glutathione reductase and glutathione/glutathione disulfide ratios: Possible implications for lung toxicity. J Pharmacol Exp Ther 1984;229:658–663.

38. Oliner H, Schwartz R, Rubio F, et al: Interstitial pulmonary fibrosis following busulfan therapy. Am J Med 1961;31: 134–349.

39. Heard BE, Cooke RA: Busulphan lung. Thorax 1968;23: 187–193.

40. Ginsberg SJ, Comis RL: The pulmonary toxicity of antineoplastic agents. Semin Oncol 1982;9:34–51.

41. Gurtoo HL, Hipkens JH, Sharma SD: Role of glutathione in the metabolism-dependent toxicity and chemotherapy of cyclophosphamide. Cancer Res 1981;41:3584–3591.

42. Sostman HD, Matthay RA, Putman CE, et al: Methotrexate-induced pneumonitis. Medicine (Baltimore) 1976;55:371–388.

43. Carson CW, Cannon GW, Egger MJ, et al: Pulmonary disease during the treatment of rheumatoid arthritis with low dose pulse methotrexate. Semin Arthritis Rheum 1987;16:186–195.

44. White DA, Rankin JA, Stover DE, et al: Methotrexate pneumonitis: Bronchoalveolar lavage findings suggest an immunologic disorder. Am Rev Respir Dis 1989;139:18–21.

45. Imokawa S, Colby TV, Leslie KO, et al: Methotrexate pneumonitis: Review of the literature and histopathological findings in nine patients. Eur Respir J 2000;15:373–381.

46. Zitnik RJ, Cooper JAJ: Pulmonary disease due to antirheumatic agents. Clin Chest Med 1990;11:139–150.

47. Andersson BS, Cogan BM, Keating MJ, et al: Subacute pulmonary failure complicating therapy with high-dose Ara-C in acute leukemia. Cancer 1985;56:2181–2184.

48. Haupt HM, Hutchins GM, Moore GW: Ara-C lung: Noncardiogenic pulmonary edema complicating cytosine arabinoside therapy of leukemia. Am J Med 1981;70: 256–261.

49. de Botton S, Dombret H, Sanz M, et al: Incidence, clinical features, and outcome of all trans-retinoic acid syndrome in 413 cases of newly diagnosed acute promyelocytic leukemia: The European APL Group. Blood 1998;92:2712–2718.

50. Frankel SR, Eardley A, Lauwers G, et al: The "retinoic acid syndrome" in acute promyelocytic leukemia. Ann Intern Med 1992;117:292–296.

51. Tallman MS, Andersen JW, Schiffer CA, et al: Clinical description of 44 patients with acute promyelocytic leukemia who developed the retinoic acid syndrome. Blood 2000;95:90–95.

52. de Botton S, Chevret S, Coiteux V, et al: Early onset of chemotherapy can reduce the incidence of ATRA syndrome in newly diagnosed acute promyelocytic leukemia (APL) with low white blood cell counts: Results from APL 93 trial. Leukemia 2003;17:339–342.

53. Rotmensch HH, Liron M, Tupilski M, et al: Possible association of pneumonitis with amiodarone therapy. Am Heart J 1980;100:412–413.

54. Adams GD, Kehoe R, Lesch M, et al: Amiodarone-induced pneumonitis: Assessment of risk factors and possible risk reduction. Chest 1988;93:254–263.

55. Vorperian VR, Havighurst TC, Miller S, et al: Adverse effects of low dose amiodarone: A meta-analysis. J Am Coll Cardiol 1997;30:791–798.

56. Parra O, Ruiz J, Ojanguren I, et al: Amiodarone toxicity: Recurrence of interstitial pneumonitis after withdrawal of the drug. Eur Respir J 1989;2:905–907.

57. Martin WJ 2nd: Mechanisms of amiodarone pulmonary toxicity. Clin Chest Med 1990;11:131–138.

58. Ashrafian H, Davey P: Is amiodarone an underrecognized cause of acute respiratory failure in the ICU? Chest 2001;120:275–282.

59. Kennedy JI: Clinical aspects of amiodarone pulmonary toxicity. Clin Chest Med 1990;11:119–129.

60. Gleadhill IC, Wise RA, Schonfeld SA, et al: Serial lung function testing in patients treated with amiodarone: A prospective study. Am J Med 1989;86:4–10.

61. Magro SA, Lawrence EC, Wheeler SH, et al: Amiodarone pulmonary toxicity: Prospective evaluation of serial pulmonary function tests. J Am Coll Cardiol 1988;12:781–788.

62. Dirlik A, Erinc R, Ozcan Z, et al: Technetium-99m-DTPA aerosol scintigraphy in amiodarone induced pulmonary toxicity in comparison with Ga-67 scintigraphy. Ann Nucl Med 2002;16:477–481.

63. Kuhlman JE, Teigen C, Ren H, et al: Amiodarone pulmonary toxicity: CT findings in symptomatic patients. Radiology 1990;177:121–125.

64. Siniakowicz RM, Narula D, Suster B, et al: Diagnosis of amiodarone pulmonary toxicity with high-resolution computerized tomographic scan. J Cardiovasc Electrophysiol 2001;12:431–436.

65. Shenasa M, Vaisman U, Wojciechowski M, et al: Abnormal abdominal computerized tomography with amiodarone therapy and clinical significance. Am Heart J 1984;107:929–933.

66. Coudert B, Bailly F, Lombard JN, et al: Amiodarone pneumonitis: Bronchoalveolar lavage findings in 15 patients and review of the literature. Chest 1992;102:1005–1012.

67. Ohar JA, Jackson F, Dettenmeier PA, et al: Bronchoalveolar lavage cell count and differential are not reliable indicators of amiodarone-induced pneumonitis. Chest 1992;102:999–1004.

68. Bedrossian CW, Warren CJ, Ohar J, et al: Amiodarone pulmonary toxicity: Cytopathology, ultrastructure, and immunocytochemistry. Ann Diagn Pathol 1997;1:47–56.

69. Holmberg L, Boman G: Pulmonary reactions to nitrofurantoin: 447 cases reported to the Swedish Adverse Drug Reaction Committee 1966–1976. Eur J Respir Dis 1981;62:180–189.

70. Holmberg L, Boman G, Bottiger LE, et al: Adverse reactions to nitrofurantoin: Analysis of 921 reports. Am J Med 1980;69:733–738.

71. Heffner JE, Sahn SA: Salicylate-induced pulmonary edema: Clinical features and prognosis. Ann Intern Med 1981;95:405–409.

72. Fisher CJJ, Albertson TE, Foulke GE: Salicylate-induced pulmonary edema: Clinical characteristics in children. Am J Emerg Med 1985;3:33–37.

73. Chapman BJ, Proudfoot AT: Adult salicylate poisoning: Deaths and outcome in patients with high plasma salicylate concentrations. Q J Med 1989;72:699–707.

74. Thisted B, Krantz T, Stroom J, et al: Acute salicylate self-poisoning in 177 consecutive patients treated in ICU. Acta Anaesthesiol Scand 1987;31:312–316.

75. Weber JC, Essigman WK: Pulmonary alveolitis and NSAIDs: Fact or fiction? Br J Rheumatol 1986;25:5–6.

76. Heffner JE, Harley RA, Schabel SI: Pulmonary reactions from illicit substance abuse. Clin Chest Med 1990;11:151–162.

77. Katz S, Aberman A, Frand UI, et al: Heroin pulmonary edema: Evidence for increased pulmonary capillary permeability. Am Rev Respir Dis 1972;106:472–474.

78. Haim DY, Lippmann ML, Goldberg SK, et al: The pulmonary complications of crack cocaine: A comprehensive review. Chest 1995;107:233–240.

79. Nadeem S, Nasir N, Israel RH: Loffler's syndrome secondary to crack cocaine. Chest 1994;105:1599–1600.

80. Castro M, Veeder MH, Mailliard JA, et al: A prospective study of pulmonary function in patients receiving mitomycin. Chest 1996;109:939–944.

81. Cleverley JR, Screaton NJ, Hiorns MP, et al: Drug-induced lung disease: High-resolution CT and histological findings. Clin Radiol 2002;57:292–299.

82. Smith GJ: The histopathology of pulmonary reactions to drugs. Clin Chest Med 1990;11:95–117.

83. Ohnishi H, Yokoyama A, Yasuhara Y, et al: Circulating KL-6 levels in patients with drug induced pneumonitis. Thorax 2003;58:872–875.

84. Umetani K, Abe M, Kawabata K, et al: SP-D as a marker of amiodarone-induced pulmonary toxicity. Intern Med 2002;41:709–712.

85. Ohnishi H, Yokoyama A, Kondo K, et al: Comparative study of KL-6, surfactant protein-A, surfactant protein-D, and monocyte chemoattractant protein-1 as serum markers for interstitial lung diseases. Am J Respir Crit Care Med 2002;165:378–381.

86. McGaughey DS, Nikcevich DA, Long GD, et al: Inhaled steroids as prophylaxis for delayed pulmonary toxicity syndrome in breast cancer patients undergoing high-dose chemotherapy and autologous stem cell transplantation. Biol Blood Marrow Transplant 2001;7:274–278.

87. Park SH, Saleh D, Giaid A, et al: Increased endothelin-1 in bleomycin-induced pulmonary fibrosis and the effect of an endothelin receptor antagonist. Am J Respir Crit Care Med 1997;156:600–608.

88. Giaid A, Michel RP, Stewart DJ, et al: Expression of endothelin-1 in lungs of patients with cryptogenic fibrosing alveolitis. Lancet 1993;341:1550–1554.

89. Otsuka M, Takahashi H, Shiratori M, et al: Reduction of bleomycin induced lung fibrosis by candesartan cilexetil, an angiotensin II type 1 receptor antagonist. Thorax 2004;59:31–38.

90. Cheng TH, Cheng PY, Shih NL, et al: Involvement of reactive oxygen species in angiotensin II–induced endothelin-1 gene expression in rat cardiac fibroblasts. J Am Coll Cardiol 2003;42:1845–1854.

91. Molnar Z, Shearer E, Lowe D: N-Acetylcysteine treatment to prevent the progression of multisystem organ failure: A prospective, randomized, placebo-controlled study. Crit Care Med 1999;27:1100–1104.

92. Kilinc C, Ozcan O, Karaoz E, et al: Vitamin E reduces bleomycin-induced lung fibrosis in mice: Biochemical and morphological studies. J Basic Clin Physiol Pharmacol 1993;4:249–269.

# CHAPTER 4

# Acute Lung Injury: Acute Respiratory Distress Syndrome

Shazia M. Jamil and Roger G. Spragg

The acute respiratory distress syndrome (ARDS), first described in the medical literature in 1967,[1] consists of the symptom constellation of acute respiratory distress, cyanosis refractory to oxygen administration, decreased lung compliance, and diffuse opacities on the chest radiograph not explained by hydrostatic causes. Although initially called the adult respiratory distress syndrome because of clinical experience with adult patients,[2] it is now termed the *acute respiratory distress syndrome* and is recognized in the pediatric population.

Confusion over the natural history, incidence, and outcome of this syndrome secondary, in part, to lack of a uniform definition was addressed in 1994 by the American-European Consensus Conference (AECC), which provided operational definitions.[3] The Committee recognized apparent variation in the severity of this disorder and recommended criteria for acute lung injury (ALI) and for ARDS as a more severe subset of ALI. Both ALI and ARDS were recognized as belonging to the same clinical spectrum, with acute onset, bilateral infiltrates on the chest radiograph, and absence of evidence of elevated left atrial pressure. However, the term ALI was used to describe disease in which the $PaO_2/FiO_2$ ratio (partial pressure of arterial oxygen/fraction of inspired oxygen) is 300 mm Hg or less, whereas ARDS was considered to be present if this ratio was 200 Hg mm or less. Although these criteria are simple to use and are recommended for description of patient groups, they have several weaknesses. They do not specify the cause of the disorder; the description of

bilateral pulmonary infiltrates is nonspecific and difficult to implement reproducibly,[4] and response to positive end-expiratory pressure (PEEP) is not considered. Finally, it has become apparent that mortality outcome is not different between patients with only ALI and patients with ARDS.[5]

## ETIOLOGY

### Predispositions

Critical care physicians frequently observe that patients respond differently to similar predisposing causes of ALI/ARDS and also respond differently to similar treatments. These observations suggest the presence of underlying genetic predispositions to the development of ALI. Two different approaches, namely, candidate gene and genome-wide analysis, may provide new insight. Leikauf and colleagues, studying gene-environment interactions in inbred mouse strains, examined the relative susceptibility to ALI induced by a variety of environmental agents.[6,7] These investigators found a varied response among different strains and concluded that susceptibility to ALI is heritable. Using complementary DNA (cDNA) microarray analysis to identify clusters of coregulated genes, they found altered expression of relatively few genes that control the complex responses of lung injury and repair. These findings suggest candidate genes that may contribute to individual susceptibility to the development of ARDS.

Several genetic polymorphisms may predispose patients to the clinical development of ALI. Asp299Gly and Thr399Ile mutations affecting the extracellular domain of the toll-like receptor 4 (TLR-4) are associated with a blunted response to inhaled lipopolysaccharide in humans.[8] The Asp299Gly mutation occurred in 5.5% of patients with septic shock (a recognized predisposition to development of ALI), as opposed to 0% of 73 healthy blood donors. For patients in whom exposure to lipopolysaccharide is a critical determinant of the development of ALI, the presence of the Asp299Gly mutation may be a predisposing factor.

The human angiotensin-converting enzyme (ACE) gene contains a restriction fragment length polymorphism consisting of the presence (insertion, I) or absence (deletion, D) of a 287 base pair alu repeat sequence in intron 16.[9] This (I/D) polymorphism, in a healthy population, accounted for 47% of the variance in observed plasma ACE levels, and it was highest in those with the DD genotype.[10] The ACE DD genotype is reported to be present with markedly increased frequency in patients with ARDS compared with patients in intensive care units (ICUs), patients undergoing coronary artery bypass grafting, or healthy populations.[11] Further, the DD genotype is significantly associated with mortality in the ARDS group. These data suggest a role for the renin-angiotensin systems in the pathogenesis of ARDS and further implicate the DD genotype as a predisposing genetic factor.

Additional genetic predispositions for ALI may be presence of polymorphisms in the SP-B gene. Lin and associates described the C/T (1580) polymorphism that results in an amino acid change (Thr131Ile) that may affect protein glycosylation, and they reported increased frequency of the C allele in patients with idiopathic ARDS compared with patients with ARDS secondary to systemic disease or compared with healthy persons.[12] In addition, the frequency of an I/D variant in SP-B intron 4 was reported to be 46.6% among 15 patients with ARDS in contrast to 4.3% among control subjects. Gong and colleagues attempted to reproduce this latter observation and found a significant association between the variant polymorphism and ARDS only in women.[13]

ARDS was described in four children with a functional defect in a mitochondrial enzyme involved in β-oxidation of long-chain fatty acids.[14] Three of the patients shared a common mutation in the enzyme. The authors theorized that accumulating fatty acid metabolites in patients with 3-hydroxylacyl-coenzyme A dehydrogenase and mitochondrial trifunctional protein defects may alter the phospholipid component of surfactant and may impair its function.

These genetic studies are still in their infancy and require confirmation in larger populations with ARDS.

Identification of genes associated with increased susceptibility to ALI should lead to greater understanding of relevant disease mechanisms and to the development of targeted therapy.

## Clinical Associations

ALI/ARDS is thought to be the uniform expression of a diffuse and overwhelming inflammatory reaction of the pulmonary parenchyma to either a direct injury to the lung (pulmonary ALI/ARDS) or an indirect lung injury related to a systemic process (extrapulmonary ALI/ARDS) (Table 4.1).[15–18] The most frequent causes include sepsis, severe pneumonia, peritonitis, and multiple trauma.[15,19] However, among these, sepsis is associated with the highest risk, because approximately 40% of septic patients develop ALI or ARDS.[17,20] The presence of multiple predisposing disorders substantially increases the risk of developing ARDS,[20] as does the presence of chronic alcohol abuse.[21] Moss and colleagues showed that the incidence of ARDS in patients with chronic alcohol abuse was 70% compared with 31% in individuals without this history,[22] and using a multivariable logistic regression, these investigators concluded that chronic alcohol abuse is an independent risk factor in this disorder.[23] Using animal models of chronic ethanol ingestion, investigators identified alcohol-mediated

**Table 4-1** Examples of Causes and Clinical Disorders Associated with Acute Lung Injury/Acute Respiratory Distress Syndrome

| Direct Lung Injury | Indirect Lung Injury |
|---|---|
| Pneumonia | Sepsis and septic shock |
| Aspiration of acid/gastric contents | Multiple trauma |
| Air or fat emboli | Acute pancreatitis |
| Inhalational injury | Cardiopulmonary bypass |
| Near drowning | Transfusion-related acute lung injury (TRALI) |
| Pulmonary contusion | Drugs |
| Reperfusion pulmonary edema (post-thrombectomy, post-transplantation) | Neurogenic pulmonary edema |
| Severe acute respiratory syndrome (SARS) | |

alterations in epithelial and endothelial function, surfactant synthesis and secretion, and alveolar-capillary barrier function.[24]

Severe acute respiratory syndrome (SARS) deserves special mention. This disease, thought to be caused by a novel coronavirus (SARS CoV), appeared in November of 2002 and was first described in March of 2003.[25] In a retrospective study of a cohort of patients with SARS who were admitted to ICUs in Asia, there was a 25% incidence of progression to ALI/ARDS, 37% mortality at 28 days, and 52.5% overall ICU mortality after 13 weeks.[26] One third of the patients with SARS and ALI/ARDS recovered within 14 days of illness; however, most patients underwent a protracted course, with high mortality despite maximum supportive therapy. ARDS has been described as the most common complication of this disease.[27]

## Ventilator-Induced Lung Injury

ALI that is directly induced by mechanical ventilation is recognized both in animal models and clinically and is designated ventilator-induced lung injury (VILI).[28-30] VILI is indistinguishable morphologically, physiologically, and radiologically from diffuse alveolar damage resulting from other causes of ALI.[31] The contributions of increased pressure and volume to the development of ALI were first studied systematically by Webb and Tierney,[28] who found that increases in rat lung volume were predominantly responsible for development of acute high permeability lung injury or VILI. Subsequently, Dreyfuss and colleagues were able to dissociate the influence of pressure and volume and confirmed, in animal studies, both the central role of volume in the pathogenesis of VILI and the protective effect of PEEP.[30]

Mechanical factors can lead to lung injury through a variety of mechanisms.[32] Tremblay and associates found a three- to sixfold increase in lung cytokines in ex vivo isolated rat lungs ventilated with high tidal volumes with no PEEP or PEEP of 10 cm $H_2O$, respectively.[33] The increase in lung cytokines was also associated with an increase in c-fos messenger RNA, an early response gene. Alveolar overdistention coupled with the repeated collapse and reopening of alveoli has also been shown to initiate a cascade of proinflammatory cytokines.[34] Additional mechanisms by which repetitive opening and closing of lung units may result in damage to alveolar cells may include activation of complex intracellular signaling pathways, stimulation of paracrine stimulation of pathways, and disruption of alveolar cell plasma membranes.[35] However, the concept of repetitive opening and closing of distal lung units has been called into question, and the alternative concept of the filling of dependent lung regions with edema fluid and foam has been proposed.[36] The mechanisms associated with development of VILI are reviewed in depth in Chapter 5.

A large body of evidence indicates that ventilation at low lung volumes may also contribute to lung injury. In 1984, Robertson proposed that repeated opening and closing of lung units during tidal breathing of infants with respiratory distress syndrome could result in lung injury.[37] Robertson suggested that in an atelectatic lung, the air-liquid interface may be found proximally in the terminal conducting airways, rather than in the alveoli. Opening of these airways would require relatively higher forces, and the shear stresses produced could cause epithelial disruption. Other investigators have shown evidence for lung injury from low lung volume ventilation using various species, lung injury models, PEEP strategies, and modes of ventilation.[38-42]

In patients with ALI/ARDS, ventilation at traditional tidal volumes (10 to 15 mL/kg of predicted body weight) may overdistend uninjured alveoli, promote further lung injury, and contribute to multiorgan failure.[34] Clinical trials have examined the benefit of protective ventilatory strategies that reduce alveolar overdistention and increase the recruitment of atelectatic alveoli. A National Institutes of Health (NIH) National Heart, Lung and Blood Institute (NHLBI) trial showed that the use of a tidal volume of 6 mL/kg ideal body weight resulted in a 22% decrease in mortality compared with ventilation with 12 mL/kg ideal body weight in patients with ALI/ARDS.[43] The excess mortality associated with large tidal volume ventilation may be related to cytokine response and the development of multisystem organ failure.[34,44,45] Ranieri and colleagues found that both the pulmonary and the systemic cytokine responses were reduced in patients with ARDS who were treated with low tidal volume ventilation.[44]

## PATHOPHYSIOLOGY

The acute or exudative phase of ALI/ARDS is characterized by increased permeability of the alveolar-capillary barrier leading to the influx of protein-rich edema fluid and inflammatory cells into distal airways and alveoli.[46] The alveolar-capillary barrier is formed of two separate barriers, the alveolar epithelium and the vascular endothelium. The importance of endothelial injury leading to increased vascular permeability and formation of pulmonary edema is well established, and a critical role of epithelial injury in ALI/ARDS has also been recognized.[47] The alveolar epithelium is composed of type I and type II cells, occupying 90% and 10% of the alveolar surface area, respectively. The loss of epithelial integrity and injury to type II cells disrupt normal epithelial fluid transport and impair the removal of edema fluid from the alveolar space in animal models of ALI,[48,49] as well as in the majority of patients with ARDS/ALI.[50] Injury to type II cells also reduces the production and turnover of surfactant.[51]

The pathogenesis and mechanisms of lung injury have been extensively reviewed.[51–53] In response to an inciting event, the pulmonary macrophages and endothelium become activated; surface expression of adhesion molecules is increased, and this leads to neutrophil migration to the alveoli. Activated neutrophils produce a variety of inflammatory mediators, including reactive oxygen species, nitric oxide (NO), leukotrienes, cytokines, chemokines, proteases, platelet-activating factor, and cationic proteins. Other cells, including pulmonary macrophages and alveolar endothelial and epithelial cells, also produce inflammatory mediators. Alveolar macrophages are able to secrete cytokines including interleukin (IL)-1, IL-6, IL-8, IL-10, and tumor necrosis factor-α (TNF-α). Apart from these proinflammatory mediators, a host of endogenous anti-inflammatory mediators can simultaneously be present, including IL-1 receptor antagonist, soluble TNF receptor, autoantibodies against IL-8, and anti-inflammatory cytokines such as IL-10 and IL-11.[54] In fact, imbalance between proinflammatory and anti-inflammatory mediators may play an important role in the pathogenesis of lung injury. The end result of this vicious cycle is alveoli filled with protein-rich edema fluid, cells, cellular debris, red blood cells, and fibrin-rich hyaline membranes on the denuded basement membrane.

Extravascular fibrin deposition, and the abnormalities in the coagulation and fibrinolytic pathways that promote it, may be important in the pathogenesis of ALI.[55] Procoagulant activity is increased in bronchoalveolar lavage (BAL) samples from patients with ALI/ARDS, whereas fibrinolytic activity is markedly decreased or undetectable. This procoagulant response is mainly attributable to tissue factor associated with factor VII,[55] whereas the decrement in fibrinolytic response is attributable to inhibition of urokinase plasminogen activator by plasminogen activators or inhibition of plasmin by antiplasmins.[55,56] The concurrent changes in procoagulant and fibrinolytic activity would be expected to promote pulmonary fibrin deposition and are likely to account for the persistence of alveolar fibrin in ALI.

The acute exudative phase of ALI/ARDS may lead either to rapid resolution of the disorder[57,58] or to progression to a late fibroproliferative phase that may start as early as 5 to 7 days after the onset of injury.[59] At this latter stage, the alveolar space becomes filled with mesenchymal cells, and there is extensive proliferation of myofibroblasts in the lung interstitium.[60] Patients who die during this stage have increased fibronectin and collagen in lung autopsy specimens.[61] This stage of ALI/ARDS may be promoted by early proinflammatory mediators, including IL-1, that stimulate production by fibroblasts of extracellular matrix components including procollagen III peptide.[62–64] The findings of alveolar fibrosis and the appearance of procollagen III in the alveolar space correlate with an increased risk of death.[65,66]

## CLINICAL PRESENTATION AND DIAGNOSIS

Symptoms of ALI/ARDS can be nonspecific and consist of dyspnea and dry cough. After the inciting event, tachypnea and tachycardia usually develop within the first 12 to 24 hours, followed by a dramatic increase in work of breathing and a rapid decrease in oxygenation, manifested as cyanosis. Lung examination may reveal bilateral, high-pitched, end-expiratory crackles, although often only bronchial breath sounds are heard, and lung compliance is decreased. The patient may initially be agitated; however, lethargy and obtundation may ensue, with worsening respiratory failure. Clinical and chest radiographic findings may lag behind hypoxemia, and therefore early measurement of arterial blood gases in patients at risk of developing this syndrome is warranted.

Early laboratory abnormalities include hypoxemia, widening of the alveolar-arterial oxygen gradient, and respiratory alkalosis. The hypoxia is attributable to ventilation-perfusion mismatch, intrapulmonary shunting, oxygen diffusion impairment, and hypoventilation.[67,68] As the disease progresses, sometimes rapidly, the patient develops severe hypoxemia unresponsive to oxygen (secondary to increased intrapulmonary shunting) and respiratory acidosis resulting from respiratory muscle failure and increased pulmonary dead space. The clinical, radiographic, and laboratory findings can be indistinguishable from those of cardiogenic pulmonary edema, and therefore measurement of pulmonary arterial wedge pressure is sometimes considered necessary to differentiate between the two conditions.

### Chest Radiography

In the first 12 to 24 hours after lung injury, the chest radiograph is often normal; however, when ARDS has followed direct lung injury such as massive aspiration of gastric contents or pneumonia, the chest radiograph is likely to be abnormal at the outset. In the next 36 hours, with greater exudation of fluid in alveolar spaces, a characteristic bilateral diffuse interstitial infiltrate may progress to ground-glass opacification and frank consolidation, as illustrated in Figure 4.1*A*.[69] As shown in Figure 4.2, the patient may also develop pleural effusions, and their presence should not sway the physician from making the diagnosis of ARDS. This progression is typical but not pathognomonic of ARDS.

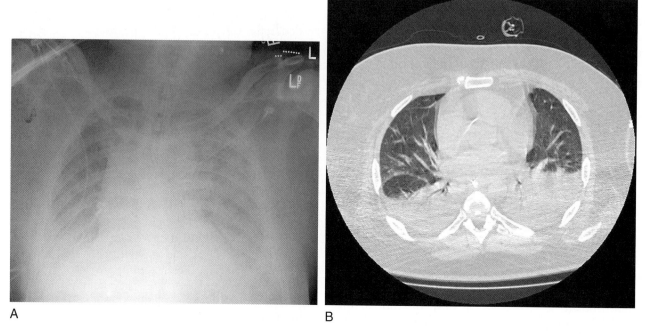

**Figure 4.1** *A,* The chest radiograph of a 54-year-old man with acute respiratory distress syndrome of unknown cause demonstrates diffuse opacification of all quadrants. *B,* A computed tomography scan demonstrates marked heterogeneity of parenchymal involvement, with dense consolidation posteriorly, and with air bronchograms evident. The anterior lung areas are relatively spared.

Radiographic findings may resolve rapidly in patients with near drowning, opiate-related ALI/ARDS, or uncomplicated viral pneumonia. However, in most cases, the radiographic findings resolve over weeks. During this time, the development of new focal areas of air space opacities may indicate the development of nosocomial pneumonia.[70] In addition, ARDS may be complicated by pneumothorax and pneumomediastinum secondary to the disease itself or as a complication of mechanical ventilation. With the complete resolution of the disease, the chest radiograph may either revert to normal or reveal coarse reticular opacities, diffuse interstitial fibrosis, and cysts, likely as a consequence of the effects of both lung repair and barotrauma.[71–74] The radiographic criterion of bilateral diffuse infiltrates in the AECC definition of ALI/ARDS shows high interobserver variability when applied by investigators expert in the fields of mechanical ventilation and ARDS.[4]

## Computed Tomography Patterns

Computed tomography (CT) scans in patients with ALI/ARDS have revealed that lung disease in ALI/ARDS is not a homogeneous process and that the scan pattern may vary with cause, time, mechanical ventilation, and prone positioning. The most striking CT finding in the early phase of disease is the heterogeneous nature of detectable lung injury (see Figs. 4.1 and 4.2).

Three areas of lung are easily recognized: (1) normal or almost normal lung regions, most frequently located in nondependent lung; (2) ground-glass opacification, defined as a hazy increase in lung attenuation, with preservation of bronchial and vascular margins, in the midlung area; and (3) consolidation in the most dependent lung.[75,76] During the late or fibroproliferative phase of the disease, fluid is reabsorbed, leading to a decrease in CT density of the lung. There is also an increase in subpleural cysts or bullae.[77] In patients who survive ALI/ARDS, a reticular pattern is described in the nondependent normal lung regions; this pattern has been correlated with the length of mechanical ventilation and the use of inverse ratio ventilation.[78]

Differences in CT findings in patients with direct as opposed to indirect ALI/ARDS were described by Goodman and colleagues. Abnormalities in patients with direct ARDS tended to be a mixture of consolidation and ground-glass opacification, whereas patients with indirect ARDS had predominantly symmetric ground-glass opacification. In both groups, pleural effusions and air bronchograms were common.[79]

Puybasset and associates found differences between these groups to be less distinct.[80] These investigators showed that in patients with ARDS, the cardiorespiratory effects of PEEP were affected predominantly by lung morphology rather than by the presence of a direct or

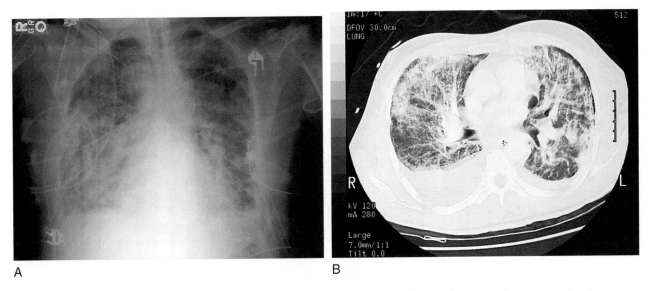

**Figure 4.2** *A,* The chest radiograph of a 64-year-old man with acute respiratory distress syndrome secondary to bacterial pneumonia demonstrates patchy involvement of all quadrants. B, A computed tomography scan demonstrates diffuse heterogeneous involvement of all lung fields and the presence of bilateral pleural effusions.

indirect ARDS. In their study, PEEP induced marked alveolar recruitment without overdistention in patients with diffuse CT attenuations, whereas in patients with lobar attenuation, PEEP induced mild alveolar recruitment associated with overdistention of previously aerated lung regions.

Study of the relationship between CT data and lung mechanics in patients with ALI/ARDS showed that respiratory compliance was not related to the amount of nonaerated or poorly aerated tissue, but rather was closely related to the amount of normally aerated tissue. Thus, the respiratory compliance in early ALI/ARDS appears to be a direct measure of normally aerated tissue, a finding suggesting that in ALI/ARDS the aerated lung is not stiff, but rather small.[81] The value of the information gained from CT scans must be balanced against the potential risk of transporting critically ill patients, the additional costs, and the additional radiation dose. Therefore, CT scanning of the lungs of patients with ALI/ARDS is most clearly indicated for solving clinical dilemmas, such as detecting occult complications in patients who are deteriorating or not improving at the expected rate, or for formal research protocols.

### Respiratory Mechanics

Patients with ALI/ARDS are frequently found to have smaller tidal volumes and higher peak airway and plateau pressures than physiologically normal subjects. Gattinoni and colleagues found a markedly higher static lung elastance in patients with pulmonary ARDS and a high static elastance of the chest wall in patients with extrapulmonary ARDS.[82] Increasing PEEP to 15 cm $H_2O$ caused an increase in static elastance of the total respiratory system in patients with pulmonary ARDS. These investigators proposed that this difference in respiratory mechanics and response to PEEP is consistent with a prevalence of consolidation in pulmonary ARDS, as opposed to the presence of predominantly edema and alveolar collapse in extrapulmonary ARDS. Patients with ARDS also have increased resistance to airflow,[83] and this is substantially reduced by inhalation of a β-agonist.[84]

## TREATMENT

Hypoxic and hypercapnic respiratory failure is a common component of ALI/ARDS, and it requires mechanical ventilation to reduce the work of breathing and to ensure adequate gas exchange. The support provided by mechanical ventilation allows time for antibiotics (in infected patients), innate immunity, and endogenous reparative processes to overcome the acute inflammatory state. As a result, approximately 60% or more of patients with ALI survive to hospital discharge.[52]

### Lung Protective Ventilation Strategies

Historically, there was a great disparity in physicians' approach to mechanical ventilation of patients with

ALI/ARDS, largely because of a lack of clear guidance from clinical studies and the absence of standards for initiating, monitoring, and adjusting ventilator settings. For example, in a survey of ventilation practices, critical care physicians reported using a broad range of tidal volumes (5 to 17 mL/kg) in patients with ALI.[85] In the 1990s, several clinical trials were conducted to guide clinicians in the choice of tidal volumes.[43,86–89] Amato and colleagues evaluated the effects of a lung protective ventilation strategy on pulmonary complications and mortality at 28 days in patients with ARDS.[86] Patients were randomized to either a conventional study group or a lung protective ventilation group. Patients in the conventional group received tidal volumes of approximately 12 mL/kg of body weight and a mean PEEP of approximately 8 cm $H_2O$ during the first 7 days of treatment, whereas those in the lung protective strategy group received tidal volumes of approximately 6 mL/kg and a mean PEEP level of 16.4 cm $H_2O$ during the first 36 hours of treatment. The tidal volumes in this latter group were further decreased if inspiratory airway pressures exceeded 40 cm $H_2O$. The results showed that patient survival, frequency of barotrauma, and rate of weaning from mechanical ventilation were all improved in the group receiving lower tidal volumes and higher PEEP. In this small study, it was unclear whether the improvement in outcome was attributable to the lower tidal volumes, the inspiratory pressure limits, or the higher PEEP. There have been four subsequent randomized clinical trials to investigate the role of different tidal volume ventilation strategies in patients with ALI or at risk of developing ALI.[43,87–89] In three of these trials, the volume- and pressure-limited approach was not associated with improved clinical outcome.[87–89] However, a trial[43] by the NHLBI's Acute Respiratory Distress Syndrome Network (ARDS Network) was stopped after enrollment of 861 patients because the mortality was significantly lower in the group treated with lower tidal volumes than in the group treated with traditional tidal volumes (31% versus 39.8%). Further, the lower tidal volume group had more ventilator-free and end-organ failure–free days during the first 28 days and a greater reduction in plasma IL-6 levels compared with patients treated with larger tidal volumes and higher pressures. Results of the ARDS Network ALVEOLI study showed no survival benefit when a low tidal volume ventilation strategy was used in conjunction with a higher, as opposed to lower, PEEP value.[90]

Application of a lung protective strategy is associated with reduction in BAL concentrations of polymorphonuclear cells, TNF-α, IL-1β, soluble TNF-α receptor 55, and IL-8. In both plasma and BAL, concentrations of IL-6, soluble TNF-α receptor 75, and IL-1 receptor antagonist are reduced.[44] Reduction in the circulating levels of proinflammatory mediators is associated with

reduction in the development of multiorgan failure, the major cause of mortality in patients with ARDS.[91]

## Open Lung Approach

The low tidal volume ventilation strategy endorsed by the NHLBI study results in a modest decrement in gas exchange over the first several days of treatment, as compared with the higher tidal volume ventilation strategy. A contrasting "open lung" strategy is to adjust tidal volume and PEEP based on gas exchange and airway pressure measurements (see Chapter 25). Although use of the open lung strategy is effective in animal models of ALI,[92,93] the effect was short-lived in patients with ALI/ARDS who were treated with a low tidal volume strategy and 30-second applications of continuous positive airway pressure of 35 to 40 cm $H_2O$.[94,95]

## High-Frequency Oscillatory Ventilation

During high-frequency oscillatory ventilation (HFOV) use in adults, tidal volumes approaching 150 to 260 mL can be delivered when respiratory rates are set between 3 and 5 cps, mean distending airway pressures are set between 25 and 45 cm $H_2O$, and pressure amplitudes are set between 60 and 90 cm $H_2O$. Frequent small breaths augment diffusive exchange of respiratory gases. Use of HFOV theoretically avoids the high peak airway pressure common with conventional ventilation, prevents alveolar overdistention, and maintains a higher peak end-expiratory pressure, thus possibly avoiding lung injury resulting from repetitive recruitment and derecruitment of alveoli. Derdak and associates reported on a multicenter, randomized, controlled trial of oscillatory ventilation for ARDS.[96] Although this trial was not powered to evaluate mortality differences, a trend toward overall improved mortality was observed in the HFOV-treated group (37%) versus the group treated with conventional mechanical ventilation (52%). However, the group treated with conventional mechanical ventilation was not ventilated with a lung protective ventilation approach, because the tidal volumes in this group were approximately 10 mL/kg.

In summary, HFOV is an alternative method of mechanical ventilation for patients with severe adult ARDS, and it may be considered in those who require high mean airway pressures (≥20 cm $H_2O$) with conventional ventilation, especially if the $Fio_2$ requirement exceeds 0.60 and the inspiratory plateau pressure cannot be maintained at less than 30 cm $H_2O$.

## Avoidance of Oxygen Toxicity

Both laboratory data and clinical experience suggest that exposure of humans to elevated levels of inspired oxygen results in lung injury.[97,98] This injury, which may occur as a result of increased generation in the lung of reactive oxygen species, may be mitigated by the presence of antioxidants. Levels of critical components of the antioxidant defense system are induced during exposure to modest levels of inspired oxygen, and thus the patient who requires high levels of inspired oxygen may be at somewhat less risk of lung injury than the patient with a sudden requirement for sustained high levels of inspired oxygen. Thus, a high $FiO_2$ may be used for brief periods as a temporizing measure; however, it is recommended that aggressive steps be taken to reduce the $FiO_2$ whenever it exceeds 0.65. These measures include increasing mean airway pressure, improving cardiovascular function, inducing diuresis, or accepting somewhat lower values for hemoglobin oxygen saturation.

## Use of Sedation and Paralysis

Deep sedation is frequently used in severely affected patients who are undergoing mechanical ventilation when oxygen consumption demands must be minimized to relieve hypoxemia. Sedation may occasionally be supplemented by nondepolarizing muscle relaxants when an uncomfortable or poorly tolerated ventilatory pattern, such as inverse ratio ventilation, is needed. Any use of a paralytic agent should be brief, with frequent reassessment of depth and continued need, because such use may be associated with the development of neuromuscular dysfunction.[99]

## Prone Positioning

Use of the prone position may improve oxygenation in patients with ARDS. Mechanisms that may account for this effect include an increase in end-expiratory lung volume, better ventilation-perfusion matching, and regional changes in ventilation associated with alterations in chest wall mechanics.[100–103] In addition, this modality has also been shown in animal models to lessen VILI.[104] Gattinoni and colleagues conducted a multicenter randomized trial to evaluate use of the prone position for 7 hours per day for up to 10 days in the treatment of ventilated patients with ALI or ARDS.[105] The study showed a significant improvement in oxygenation with prone positioning, no effect on complication rate and no effect on mortality. Post hoc analysis suggested a survival benefit when prone positioning was used for patients with the most severe disease.

## Glucocorticoids

Glucocorticoids exert their effects through binding to cytoplasmic glucocorticoid receptors. These receptors, in turn, modulate the transcription rates of many inflammatory response elements, including augmenting synthesis of I-κB that binds and thus limits the proinflammatory action of nuclear factor-κB.[106] Glucocorticoids thus act as natural inhibitors of proinflammatory cytokine production.[107] Glucocorticoids also inhibit fibroblast proliferation and collagen deposition, stimulate T-cell, eosinophil, and monocyte apoptosis, and inhibit neutrophil activation. Glucocorticoid treatment in ARDS/ALI is controversial. Short courses of high-dose glucocorticoids were shown to be ineffective, and possibly harmful, in clinical trials of ARDS prevention in patients with severe sepsis and in patients with established ARDS.[108–111] A small randomized placebo-controlled trial suggested a beneficial effect of prolonged use of glucocorticoids in late ARDS.[112] However, the NIH ARDS Network conducted a larger study of methylprednisolone for patients with ARDS of 7 to 28 days' duration that suggests no outcome benefit.[113] Though use of glucocorticoids improved the cardiopulmonary physiology and increased the number of ventilator-free days, ICU-free days, and shock-free days during the first 28 days, it failed to reduce hospital stay or improve the in-hospital mortality and was associated with an increased incidence of neuromyopathy. In fact, initiation of glucocorticoids two or more weeks after the onset of ARDS was associated with an increased mortality rate when compared with the placebo group. The ARDS Network investigators concluded that their results did "not provide support for the routine use of methylprednisolone in patients with persistent ARDS and suggest that methylprednisolone therapy may be harmful when initiated more than two weeks after the onset of ARDS."[113]

## Catheter and Fluid Management

ARDS Network investigators have also shown that the routine use of a pulmonary artery catheter (PAC) to guide fluid therapy in ARDS/ALI patients neither decreases mortality nor reduces the incidence or the duration of organ failure. Such use is associated with higher complications such as atrial and ventricular arrhythmias when compared with central venous catheter (CVC)-guided therapy in patients with ARDS.[114]

The optimal fluid management of ALI and ARDS has long been controversial. The ARDS Network has reported results of a large clinical trial comparing a conservative and liberal fluid management strategy in patients with ALI. Although, there was no difference in mortality between the two groups, those in the conservative strategy group had significantly improved lung function and central nervous system function, and a decreased need for sedation, mechanical ventilation, and intensive care, without an increase in nonpulmonary organ failures or shock.

## Surfactant Therapy

Pulmonary surfactant is found at the air-liquid interface of the alveoli and functions to reduce the surface tension, particularly at low lung volumes. It is composed of approximately 90% lipids and 10% surfactant proteins (SP-A, SP-B, SP-C, and SP-D). Analysis of BAL fluid samples obtained from patients with ARDS and from various animal models of lung injury demonstrated changes in the endogenous surfactant system. Specifically, decreased amounts of dipalmitoylphosphatidylcholine and phosphatidylglycerol and decreased amounts of the surfactant-associated proteins were documented in patients with ARDS compared with control subjects.[116]

Several randomized controlled clinical trials have evaluated exogenous surfactant treatment in patients with ARDS. Anzueto and colleagues showed no difference between patients receiving very small doses of the exogenous synthetic surfactant Exosurf by aerosol and control subjects with respect to physiology, ventilator-free days, and mortality rates.[117] A trial in which the modified natural surfactant Survanta was instilled directly into the airways of patients with ARDS evaluated eight doses of 50 mg/kg, four doses of 100 mg/kg, and eight doses of 100 mg/kg over a 28-day period. The middle-dose group had the best outcome, with a mortality of 18.8% compared with 43.8% in the control group.[118] Spragg and colleagues performed a phase I/II randomized clinical trial of a short course of a recombinant surfactant protein C–based surfactant (Venticute) as treatment for ARDS.[119] The results showed no benefit, but they established safety of the intervention. In subsequent phase III studies, treatment with the same surfactant was associated with improvement in oxygenation and with a suggestion of benefit in the subgroup of patients with direct lung injury.[120]

## Liquid Ventilation

Tidal liquid ventilation is a technique of respiratory support during which gaseous functional residual capacity (FRC) and tidal volume are replaced with a perfluorocarbon (PFC) liquid.[121] Liquid ventilation has been shown to improve lung mechanics and ventilation-perfusion matching effectively, decrease intrapulmonary shunt, and thereby support pulmonary gas exchange and cardiovascular stability in animal models of ALI/ARDS.[122-124] Moreover, studies have demonstrated that partial liquid ventilation (during which the lung FRC is partially or completely filled with PFC, and gaseous tidal breaths are delivered) and tidal liquid ventilation are associated with a decrease in oxidative lung damage in animal models of ARDS/ALI.[125,126] A prospective randomized controlled trial of partial liquid ventilation compared with conventional mechanical ventilation in adult patients with ARDS/ALI failed to show a significant improvement in the number of ventilator-free days or in mortality in patients treated with partial liquid ventilation.[127] In addition, transient and self-limited episodes of bradycardia, hypoxia, and respiratory acidosis occurred more frequently in the group treated with partial liquid ventilation. In summary, although liquid ventilation may be more effective than conventional mechanical ventilation in selected laboratory models, this advantage has not been shown in clinical studies.

## Extracorporeal Membrane Oxygenation

Extracorporeal membrane oxygenation (ECMO) is a technique of providing life support in the treatment of failing lungs that are unable to maintain blood oxygenation. Several terms have been used to describe the variety of techniques that have been designed to oxygenate blood and remove carbon dioxide extracorporeally. These include ECMO, extracorporeal carbon dioxide removal (ECCO2-R) and extracorporeal life support (ECLS). In the typical ECMO setting, a femoral-jugular venovenous bypass is established with oxygenation of the circulating blood by the membrane oxygenator. ECMO was introduced into the treatment of ARDS in the 1970s. In adults with ARDS, two randomized controlled trials failed to show an advantage of ECMO over conventional ventilation.[128,129] However, both these trials were performed before the development of modern heparinized tubings and membrane oxygenators, which may reduce the complications of this modality.

ECMO may be a useful adjunct to the lung protective ventilation strategy in severe ARDS. In profoundly ill patients, use of low tidal volumes and airway pressures may not result in sufficient levels of hemoglobin saturation to sustain life. In such settings, ECMO is able to support gas exchange to the extent that ventilator settings (tidal volume, PEEP, respiratory rate, peak inspiratory pressure, fractional inspired oxygen) may be adjusted to avoid inducing VILI.[130]

## Treatment of Pulmonary Hypertension by Inhaled Nitric Oxide

Early in the evolution of ARDS, pulmonary vasoconstriction, thromboembolism, and interstitial edema contribute to the development of pulmonary hypertension. Inhaled NO (iNO) selectively vasodilates the pulmonary vasculature with few systemic effects. Randomized controlled trials comparing iNO treatment with conventional therapy in adult patients with ARDS showed acute improvement in oxygenation and hemodynamics.[131,132] However, because no reduction in mortality has been demonstrated, iNO has an unproven role in the treatment of patients with ALI/ARDS.

## OUTCOME

Numerous factors influence the risk of death for a patient with established ARDS. Since publication of the 1992 AECC criteria, most clinical series have reported mortality rates for patients with ARDS that range from 25% to 70%. Differences in the application of ALI/ARDS definitions, associated risk factors and comorbidities, and the time period during which mortality is recorded are likely to contribute to this variation. The mortality rate from ARDS appears to have decreased since the mid- to late 1990s.[5,133131,132 136]

Although the annual age-adjusted mortality, as observed by Moss and colleagues, may have increased from 1979 (5.0 deaths per 100,000 individuals) to 1993 (8.1 deaths per 100,000 individuals), a decrease in mortality was observed from 1993 to 1996 (7.4 deaths per 100,000 individuals). Reasons for the decline in ARDS-associated mortality are varied. In a 9-year retrospective review of surgical and trauma patients, Rocco and colleagues found, predominantly in trauma patients, a declining death rate from ARDS largely resulting from the use of lung protective ventilation strategies.[137] The predictors of death in this study at the onset of ARDS were advanced age, a Multiple Organ Dysfunction Score of 8 or more, and a Lung Injury Score of 2.76 or more. In a similar study, the decrease in mortality of patients with ARDS was attributed mostly to a decreased incidence of nonpulmonary organ failure.[138] Consistent with this view, Page and associates found that, for patients with ARDS who were managed with a lung protective ventilation strategy, the strongest predictor of death was not the degree of pulmonary failure, but rather the presence and severity of circulatory failure.[139] The dominant influence on mortality of comorbidities was noted by Estenssoro and associates, who prospectively studied all patients who developed ARDS in four ICUs for 1 year.[140] Hospital mortality was reported to be 58%, and the main causes of mortality were multiple organ dysfunction syndrome, sepsis, and septic shock. In this study, independent predictors of death included organ dysfunction and $PaO_2/FiO_2$. A decrease in pulmonary dead space fraction has also been identified as a separate risk factor.[141] The influence of comorbidities was also observed by Davidson and colleagues, who, in a prospective cohort study of 127 patients with ARDS associated with trauma or sepsis, found no difference in the long-term mortality rate for the patients with ARDS compared with 127 control subjects matched for age, risk factors for ARDS, comorbidity, and severity of illness.[142]

It is unclear whether patients with mild ALI (those with $PaO_2$ between 200 and 300 mm Hg) have a mortality that differs from that of patients with ARDS. In a study of patients in Scandinavian ICUs, Luhr and associates found a similar mortality of approximately 40% in both groups.[5] However, in a study of patients in 78 ICUs in Europe, Brun-Buisson and colleagues found ICU and hospital mortality to be 49.4% and 57.9%, respectively, for patients who developed ARDS and 22.6% and 32.7%, respectively, for patients with ALI.[143] Mortality was associated with age, immunocompetence, physiologic measures of injury, organ dysfunction, and early air leak.

The long-term health consequences in ARDS survivors are significant. Herridge and associates studied 1-year outcomes in 109 survivors of the ARDS.[144] Muscle weakness and fatigue were the major reasons for the functional limitation observed after 1 year, whereas normalization of lung volumes and spirometric measurements were seen by 6 months. Other studies found residual obstructive or restrictive defects to persist for a year or more in a subset of patients.[145,146] All three of the foregoing studies, however, found diffusing capacity to remain low on long-term follow-up. Orme and colleagues found no significant differences in pulmonary function between surviving patients treated with a low or high tidal volume strategy.[146]

Direct measures of the quality of life in patients who survive ARDS indicate impairment in general physical health, mental health, and neuropsychological function.[147,148] Hopkins and associates stressed the significant cognitive impairments in memory, attention, concentration, or mental processing speed exhibited by 78% of the 55 ARDS survivors they evaluated at 1 year after the onset of ARDS.[149] Decrements in quality of life and functional status appear to stabilize by 6 months. An unresolved issue is the extent to which the decrement in quality of life is the result of ARDS or of other factors such as prior health status or other elements of the acute illness. Further research is needed to characterize patients' recovery from ARDS and ALI and the extent to which recovery may be influenced by treatment in the ICU and during rehabilitation.

## REFERENCES

1. Ashbaugh DG, Bigelow DB, Petty TL, Levine BE: Acute respiratory distress in adults. Lancet 1967;2:319–323.
2. Petty TL, Ashbaugh DG: The adult respiratory distress syndrome: Clinical features, factors influencing prognosis and principles of management. Chest 1971;60:233–239.
3. Bernard GR, Artigas A, Brigham KL, et al: The American-European Consensus Conference on ARDS: Definitions, mechanisms, relevant outcomes, and clinical trial coordination. Am J Respir Crit Care Med 1994;149:818–824.
4. Rubenfeld GD, Caldwell E, Granton J, et al: Interobserver variability in applying a radiographic definition for ARDS. Chest 1999;116:1347–1353.
5. Luhr OR, Antonsen K, Karlsson M, et al: Incidence and mortality after acute respiratory failure and acute respiratory

distress syndrome in Sweden, Denmark, and Iceland: The ARF Study Group. Am J Respir Crit Care Med 1999;159: 1849–1861.

6. Leikauf GD, McDowell SA, Bachurski CJ, et al: Functional genomics of oxidant-induced lung injury. Adv Exp Med Biol 2001;500:479–487.

7. Leikauf GD, McDowell SA, Wesselkamper SC, et al: Acute lung injury: Functional genomics and genetic susceptibility. Chest 2002;121(Suppl):S70–S75.

8. Arbour NC, Lorenz E, Schutte BC, et al: TLR4 mutations are associated with endotoxin hyporesponsiveness in humans. Nat Genet 2000;25:187–191.

9. Tiret L, Rigat B, Visvikis S, et al: Evidence, from combined segregation and linkage analysis, that a variant of the angiotensin I–converting enzyme (ACE) gene controls plasma ACE levels. Am J Hum Genet 1992;51:197–205.

10. Rigat B, Hubert C, Alhenc-Gelas F, et al: An insertion/deletion polymorphism in the angiotensin I–converting enzyme gene accounting for half the variance of serum enzyme levels. J Clin Invest 1990;86:1343–1346.

11. Marshall RP, Webb S, Bellingan GJ, et al: Angiotensin converting enzyme insertion/deletion polymorphism is associated with susceptibility and outcome in acute respiratory distress syndrome. Am J Respir Crit Care Med 2002;166: 646–650.

12. Lin Z, Pearson C, Chinchilli V, et al: Polymorphisms of human SP-A, SP-B, and SP-D genes: Association of SP-B Thr131Ile with ARDS. Clin Genet 2000;58:181–191.

13. Gong MN, Wei Z, Xu LL, et al: Polymorphism in the surfactant protein-B gene, gender, and the risk of direct pulmonary injury and ARDS. Chest 2004;125:203–211.

14. Lundy CT, Shield JP, Kvittingen EA, et al: Acute respiratory distress syndrome in long-chain 3-hydroxyacyl-CoA dehydrogenase and mitochondrial trifunctional protein deficiencies. J Inherit Metab Dis 2003;26:537–541.

15. Sloane PJ, Gee MH, Gottlieb GE, et al: A multicenter registry of patients with acute respiratory distress syndrome: Physiology and outcome. Am Rev Respir Dis 1992;146:419–426.

16. Doyle RL, Szaflarski N, Modin GW, et al: Identification of patients with acute lung injury: Predictors of mortality. Am J Respir Crit Care Med 1995;152:1818–1824.

17. Hudson LD, Milberg JA, Anardi D, Maunder RJ: Clinical risks for development of the acute respiratory distress syndrome. Am J Respir Crit Care Med 1995;151:293–301.

18. Flick M, Matthay M: Pulmonary edema and acute lung injury. In Murray JF, Nadel JA (eds): Textbook of Respiratory Medicine. Philadelphia: WB Saunders, 2000, pp 1575–1629.

19. Knaus WA, Sun X, Hakim RB, et al: Evaluation of definitions of adult respiratory distress syndrome. Am J Respir Crit Care Med 1994;150:311–317.

20. Pepe PE, Potkin RT, Reus DH, et al: Clinical predictors of the adult respiratory distress syndrome. Am J Surg 1982;144: 124–130.

21. Moss M, Bucher B, Moore FA, et al: The role of chronic alcohol abuse in the development of acute respiratory distress syndrome in adults. JAMA 1996;275:50–54.

22. Moss M, Burnham E: Chronic alcohol abuse, acute respiratory distress syndrome, and multiple organ dysfunction. Crit Care Med 2003;31(Suppl):S207–S212.

23. Moss M, Parsons PE, Steinberg KP, et al: Chronic alcohol abuse is associated with an increased incidence of acute respiratory distress syndrome and severity of multiple organ dysfunction in patients with septic shock. Crit Care Med 2003;31:869–877.

24. Guidot DM, Roman J: Chronic ethanol ingestion increases susceptibility to acute lung injury: Role of oxidative stress and tissue remodeling. Chest 2002;122(Suppl):S309–S314.

25. Rota PA, Oberste MS, Monroe SS, et al: Characterization of a novel coronavirus associated with severe acute respiratory syndrome. Science 2003;300:1394–1399.

26. Lew TW, Kwek TK, Tai D, et al: Acute respiratory distress syndrome in critically ill patients with severe acute respiratory syndrome. JAMA 2003;290:374–380.

27. Li XW, Jiang RM, Guo JZ, Wang QY: [Clinical analysis of SARS: 27 cases report]. Zhonghua Yi Xue Za Zhi 2003;83:910–912.

28. Webb HH, Tierney DF: Experimental pulmonary edema due to intermittent positive pressure ventilation with high inflation pressures: Protection by positive end-expiratory pressure. Am Rev Respir Dis 1974;110:556–565.

29. Dreyfuss D, Basset G, Soler P, Saumon G: Intermittent positive-pressure hyperventilation with high inflation pressures produces pulmonary microvascular injury in rats. Am Rev Respir Dis 1985;132:880–884.

30. Dreyfuss D, Soler P, Basset G, Saumon G: High inflation pressure pulmonary edema: Respective effects of high airway pressure, high tidal volume, and positive end-expiratory pressure. Am Rev Respir Dis 1988;137:1159–1164.

31. Slutsky AS: Lung injury caused by mechanical ventilation. Chest 1999;116(Suppl):S9–S15.

32. Tremblay LN, Slutsky AS: Ventilator-induced injury: From barotrauma to biotrauma. Proc Assoc Am Physicians 1998;110:482–488.

33. Tremblay L, Valenza F, Ribeiro SP, Slutsky AS: Injurious ventilatory strategies increase cytokines and c-fos m-RNA expression in an isolated rat lung model. J Clin Invest 1997;99:944–952.

34. Slutsky AS, Tremblay LN: Multiple system organ failure: Is mechanical ventilation a contributing factor? Am J Respir Crit Care Med 1998;157:1721–1725.

35. Vlahakis NE, Hubmayr RD: Response of alveolar cells to mechanical stress. Curr Opin Crit Care 2003;9:2–8.

36. Hubmayr RD: Perspective on lung injury and recruitment: A skeptical look at the opening and collapse story. Am J Respir Crit Care Med 2002;165:1647–1653.

37. Robertson B: Pulmonary Surfactant. Amsterdam: Elsevier, 1984.

38. Hamilton PP, Onayemi A, Smyth JA, et al: Comparison of conventional and high-frequency ventilation: Oxygenation and lung pathology. J Appl Physiol 1983;55:131–138.

39. McCulloch PR, Forkert PG, Froese AB: Lung volume maintenance prevents lung injury during high frequency oscillatory ventilation in surfactant-deficient rabbits. Am Rev Respir Dis 1988;137:1185–1192.

40. Sandhar BK, Niblett DJ, Argiras EP, et al: Effects of positive end-expiratory pressure on hyaline membrane formation in a rabbit model of the neonatal respiratory distress syndrome. Intensive Care Med 1988;14:538–546.

41. Corbridge T, Wood L, Crawford G: Adverse effects of large tidal volume and low PEEP in canine acid aspiration. Am Rev Respir Dis 1990;142:311–315.

42. Muscedere JG, Mullen JB, Gan K, Slutsky AS: Tidal ventilation at low airway pressures can augment lung injury. Am J Respir Crit Care Med 1994;149:1327–1334.

43. Acute Respiratory Distress Syndrome Network: Ventilation with lower tidal volumes as compared with traditional tidal volumes for acute lung injury and the acute respiratory distress syndrome. N Engl J Med 2000;342:1301–1308.

44. Ranieri VM, Suter PM, Tortorella C, et al: Effect of mechanical ventilation on inflammatory mediators in patients with acute respiratory distress syndrome: A randomized controlled trial. JAMA 1999;282:54–61.

45. Imai Y, Parodo J, Kajikawa O, et al: Injurious mechanical ventilation and end-organ epithelial cell apoptosis and organ

dysfunction in an experimental model of acute respiratory distress syndrome. JAMA 2003;289:2104–2112.

46. Pugin J, Verghese G, Widmer MC, Matthay MA: The alveolar space is the site of intense inflammatory and profibrotic reactions in the early phase of acute respiratory distress syndrome. Crit Care Med 1999;27:304–312.

47. Wiener-Kronish JP, Albertine KH, Matthay MA: Differential responses of the endothelial and epithelial barriers of the lung in sheep to *Escherichia coli* endotoxin. J Clin Invest 1991;88: 864–875.

48. Modelska K, Pittet JF, Folkesson HG, et al: Acid-induced lung injury: Protective effect of anti-interleukin-8 pretreatment on alveolar epithelial barrier function in rabbits. Am J Respir Crit Care Med 1999;160:1450–1456.

49. Sznajder JI: Strategies to increase alveolar epithelial fluid removal in the injured lung. Am J Respir Crit Care Med 1999;160: 1441–1442.

50. Ware LB, Matthay MA: Alveolar fluid clearance is impaired in the majority of patients with acute lung injury and the acute respiratory distress syndrome. Am J Respir Crit Care Med 2001;163:1376–1383.

51. Greene KE, Wright JR, Steinberg KP, et al: Serial changes in surfactant-associated proteins in lung and serum before and after onset of ARDS. Am J Respir Crit Care Med 1999;160: 1843–1850.

52. Ware LB, Matthay MA: The acute respiratory distress syndrome. N Engl J Med 2000;342:1334–1349.

53. Chow CW, Herrera Abreu MT, Suzuki T, Downey GP: Oxidative stress and acute lung injury. Am J Respir Cell Mol Biol 2003;29:427–431.

54. Pittet JF, Mackersie RC, Martin TR, Matthay MA: Biological markers of acute lung injury: Prognostic and pathogenetic significance. Am J Respir Crit Care Med 1997;155: 1187–1205.

55. Idell S: Coagulation, fibrinolysis, and fibrin deposition in acute lung injury. Crit Care Med 2003;31(Suppl):S213–S220.

56. Idell S: Extravascular coagulation and fibrin deposition in acute lung injury. New Horiz 1994;2:566–574.

57. Matthay MA, Wiener-Kronish JP: Intact epithelial barrier function is critical for the resolution of alveolar edema in humans. Am Rev Respir Dis 1990;142:1250–1257.

58. Ware LB, Golden JA, Finkbeiner WE, Matthay MA: Alveolar epithelial fluid transport capacity in reperfusion lung injury after lung transplantation. Am J Respir Crit Care Med 1999;159: 980–988.

59. Bachofen M, Weibel ER: Structural alterations of lung parenchyma in the adult respiratory distress syndrome. Clin Chest Med 1982;3:35–56.

60. Fukuda Y, Ishizaki M, Masuda Y, et al: The role of intraalveolar fibrosis in the process of pulmonary structural remodeling in patients with diffuse alveolar damage. Am J Pathol 1987;126: 171–182.

61. Zapol WM, Trelstad RL, Coffey JW, et al: Pulmonary fibrosis in severe acute respiratory failure. Am Rev Respir Dis 1979;119: 547–554.

62. Lindroos PM, Coin PG, Osornio-Vargas AR, Bonner JC: Interleukin 1 beta (IL-1 beta) and the IL-1 beta-alpha 2-macroglobulin complex upregulate the platelet-derived growth factor alpha-receptor on rat pulmonary fibroblasts. Am J Respir Cell Mol Biol 1995;13:455–465.

63. Martinet Y, Menard O, Vaillant P, et al: Cytokines in human lung fibrosis. Arch Toxicol Suppl 1996;18:127–139.

64. Chesnutt AN, Matthay MA, Tibayan FA, et al: Early detection of type III pro-collagen peptide in acute lung injury: Pathogenetic and prognostic significance. Am Rev Respir Dis 1997;156: 840–845.

65. Martin C, Papazian L, Payan MJ, et al: Pulmonary fibrosis correlates with outcome in adult respiratory distress syndrome: A study in mechanically ventilated patients. Chest 1995;107: 196–200.

66. Clark JG, Milberg JA, Steinberg KP, Hudson LD: Type III procollagen peptide in the adult respiratory distress syndrome: Association of increased peptide levels in bronchoalveolar lavage fluid with increased risk for death. Ann Intern Med 1995;122: 17–23.

67. Kuckelt W, Dauberschmidt R, Bender V, et al: Gas exchange, pulmonary mechanics and hemodynamics in adult respiratory distress syndrome: Experimental results in Lewe miniature pigs. Resuscitation 1979;7:13–33.

68. Neumann P, Hedenstierna G: Ventilation-perfusion distributions in different porcine lung injury models. Acta Anaesthesiol Scand 2001;45:78–86.

69. Milne EN, Pistolesi M, Miniati M, Giuntini C: The radiologic distinction of cardiogenic and noncardiogenic edema. AJR Am J Roentgenol 1985;144:879–894.

70. Winer-Muram HT, Rubin SA, Ellis JV, et al: Pneumonia and ARDS in patients receiving mechanical ventilation: Diagnostic accuracy of chest radiography. Radiology 1993;188: 479–485.

71. Albelda SM, Gefter WB, Kelley MA, et al: Ventilator-induced subpleural air cysts: Clinical, radiographic, and pathologic significance. Am Rev Respir Dis 1983;127:360–365.

72. Pingleton SK: Complications of acute respiratory failure. Am Rev Respir Dis 1988;137:1463–1493.

73. Elliott CG: Pulmonary sequelae in survivors of the adult respiratory distress syndrome. Clin Chest Med 1990;11: 789–800.

74. Rouby JJ, Lherm T, Martin de Lassale E, et al: Histologic aspects of pulmonary barotrauma in critically ill patients with acute respiratory failure. Intensive Care Med 1993;19: 383–389.

75. Gattinoni L, Mascheroni D, Torresin A, et al: Morphological response to positive end expiratory pressure in acute respiratory failure: Computerized tomography study. Intensive Care Med 1986;12:137–142.

76. Maunder RJ, Shuman WP, McHugh JW, et al: Preservation of normal lung regions in the adult respiratory distress syndrome: Analysis by computed tomography. JAMA 1986;255: 2463–2465.

77. Goodman LR: Congestive heart failure and adult respiratory distress syndrome: New insights using computed tomography. Radiol Clin North Am 1996;34:33–46.

78. Desai SR, Wells AU, Rubens MB, et al: Acute respiratory distress syndrome: CT abnormalities at long-term follow-up. Radiology 1999;210:29–35.

79. Goodman LR, Fumagalli R, Tagliabue P, et al: Adult respiratory distress syndrome due to pulmonary and extrapulmonary causes: CT, clinical, and functional correlations. Radiology 1999;213: 545–552.

80. Puybasset L, Gusman P, Muller JC, et al: Regional distribution of gas and tissue in acute respiratory distress syndrome. III. Consequences for the effects of positive end-expiratory pressure: CT Scan ARDS Study Group. Adult Respiratory Distress Syndrome. Intensive Care Med 2000;26:1215–1227.

81. Gattinoni L, Pesenti A, Avalli L, et al: Pressure-volume curve of total respiratory system in acute respiratory failure: Computed tomographic scan study. Am Rev Respir Dis 1987;136:730–736.

82. Gattinoni L, Pelosi P, Suter PM, et al: Acute respiratory distress syndrome caused by pulmonary and extrapulmonary disease: Different syndromes? Am J Respir Crit Care Med 1998;158: 3–11.

83. Wright PE, Bernard GR: The role of airflow resistance in patients with the adult respiratory distress syndrome. Am Rev Respir Dis 1989;139:1169–1174.

84. Wright PE, Carmichael LC, Bernard GR: Effect of bronchodilators on lung mechanics in the acute respiratory distress syndrome (ARDS). Chest 1994;106:1517–1523.

85. Carmichael LC, Dorinsky PM, Higgins SB, et al: Diagnosis and therapy of acute respiratory distress syndrome in adults: An international survey. J Crit Care 1996;11:9–18.

86. Amato MB, Barbas CS, Medeiros DM, et al: Effect of a protective-ventilation strategy on mortality in the acute respiratory distress syndrome. N Engl J Med 1998;338:347–354.

87. Brochard L, Roudot-Thoraval F, Roupie E, et al: Tidal volume reduction for prevention of ventilator-induced lung injury in acute respiratory distress syndrome: The Multicenter Trial Group on Tidal Volume reduction in ARDS. Am J Respir Crit Care Med 1998;158:1831–1838.

88. Stewart TE, Meade MO, Cook DJ, et al: Evaluation of a ventilation strategy to prevent barotrauma in patients at high risk for acute respiratory distress syndrome: Pressure- and Volume-Limited Ventilation Strategy Group. N Engl J Med 1998;338:355–361.

89. Brower RG, Shanholtz CB, Fessler HE, et al: Prospective, randomized, controlled clinical trial comparing traditional versus reduced tidal volume ventilation in acute respiratory distress syndrome patients. Crit Care Med 1999;27:1492–1498.

90. Brower RG, Lanken PN, MacIntyre N, et al: Higher versus lower positive end-expiratory pressures in patients with the acute respiratory distress syndrome. N Engl J Med 2004;351:327–336.

91. Ranieri VM, Giunta F, Suter PM, Slutsky AS: Mechanical ventilation as a mediator of multisystem organ failure in acute respiratory distress syndrome. JAMA 2000;284:43–44.

92. Rimensberger PC, Cox PN, Frndova H, Bryan AC: The open lung during small tidal volume ventilation: Concepts of recruitment and "optimal" positive end-expiratory pressure. Crit Care Med 1999;27:1946–1952.

93. Rimensberger PC, Pristine G, Mullen BM, et al: Lung recruitment during small tidal volume ventilation allows minimal positive end-expiratory pressure without augmenting lung injury. Crit Care Med 1999;27:1940–1945.

94. Villagra A, Ochagavia A, Vatua S, et al: Recruitment maneuvers during lung protective ventilation in acute respiratory distress syndrome. Am J Respir Crit Care Med 2002;165:165–170.

95. Brower RG, Morris A, MacIntyre N, et al: Effects of recruitment maneuvers in patients with acute lung injury and acute respiratory distress syndrome ventilated with high positive end-expiratory pressure. Crit Care Med 2003;31:2592–2597.

96. Derdak S, Mehta S, Stewart TE, et al: High-frequency oscillatory ventilation for acute respiratory distress syndrome in adults: A randomized, controlled trial. Am J Respir Crit Care Med 2002;166:801–808.

97. Hyde RW, Rawson AJ: Unintentional iatrogenic oxygen pneumonitis: Response to therapy. Ann Intern Med 1969;71:517–531.

98. Pagano A, Barazzone-Argiroffo C: Alveolar cell death in hyperoxia-induced lung injury. Ann N Y Acad Sci 2003;1010:405–416.

99. De Jonghe B, Sharshar T, Lefaucheur JP, et al: Paresis acquired in the intensive care unit. JAMA 2002;288:2859–2867.

100. Douglas WW, Rehder K, Beynen FM, et al: Improved oxygenation in patients with acute respiratory failure: The prone position. Am Rev Respir Dis 1977;115:559–566.

101. Albert RK, Leasa D, Sanderson M, et al: The prone position improves arterial oxygenation and reduces shunt in oleic-acid–induced acute lung injury. Am Rev Respir Dis 1987;135:628–633.

102. Pappert D, Rossaint R, Slama K, et al: Influence of positioning on ventilation-perfusion relationships in severe adult respiratory distress syndrome. Chest 1994;106:1511–1516.

103. Pelosi P, Tubiolo D, Mascheroni D, et al: Effects of the prone position on respiratory mechanics and gas exchange during acute lung injury. Am J Respir Crit Care Med 1998;157:387–393.

104. Broccard A, Shapiro RS, Schmitz LL, et al: Prone positioning attenuates and redistributes ventilator-induced lung injury in dogs. Crit Care Med 2000;28:295–303.

105. Gattinoni L, Tognoni G, Pesenti A, et al: Effect of prone positioning on the survival of patients with acute respiratory failure. N Engl J Med 2001;345:568–573.

106. Scheinman RI, Cogswell PC, Lofquist AK, Baldwin AS Jr: Role of transcriptional activation of I kappa B alpha in mediation of immunosuppression by glucocorticoids. Science 1995;270:283–286.

107. Newton R: Molecular mechanisms of glucocorticoid action: What is important? Thorax 2000;55:603–613.

108. Sprung CL, Caralis PV, Marcial EH, et al: The effects of high-dose corticosteroids in patients with septic shock: A prospective, controlled study. N Engl J Med 1984;311:1137–1143.

109. Weigelt JA, Norcross JF, Borman KR, Snyder WH 3rd: Early steroid therapy for respiratory failure. Arch Surg 1985;120:536–540.

110. Bernard GR, Luce JM, Sprung CL, et al: High-dose corticosteroids in patients with the adult respiratory distress syndrome. N Engl J Med 1987;317:1565–1570.

111. Luce JM, Montgomery AB, et al: Ineffectiveness of high-dose methylprednisolone in preventing parenchymal lung injury and improving mortality in patients with septic shock. Am Rev Respir Dis 1988;138:62–68.

112. Meduri GU, Chinn AJ, Leeper KV, et al: Corticosteroid rescue treatment of progressive fibroproliferation in late ARDS: Patterns of response and predictors of outcome. Chest 1994;105:1516–1527.

113. Steinberg KP, Hudson LD, Goodman RB, Hough CL, Kanken PN, Hyzy R, Thompson BT, Ancukiewicz M. Efficacy and safety of corticosteroids for persistent acute respiratory distress syndrome. New Engl J Med 2006;354:1671–1684.

114. Wheeler AP, Bernard GR, Thompson BT, Schoenfeld DA, Wiedemann HP, deBoisblanc BP, Connors Jr. AF, Hite RD, Harabin AL. Pulmonary-artery versus central venous catheter to guide treatment of acute lung injury. New Engl J Med 2006;354:2213–2224.

115. Wiedemann HP, Wheeler AP, Bernard GR, Thompson BT, Hayden D, deBiosblanc BP, Connors Jr AF, Hite RD, Harabin AL. Comparison of two fluid-management strategies in acute lung injury. New Engl J Med 2006;354:2564–2575.

116. Spragg RG, Lewis JF: Surfactant therapy in the acute respiratory distress syndrome. In Matthay MA (ed): Acute Respiratory Distress Syndrome. New York: Marcel Dekker, 2003, pp 533–562.

117. Anzueto A, Baughman RP, Guntupalli KK, et al: Aerosolized surfactant in adults with sepsis-induced acute respiratory distress syndrome: Exosurf Acute Respiratory Distress Syndrome Sepsis Study Group. N Engl J Med 1996;334:1417–1421.

118. Gregory TJ, Steinberg KP, Spragg R, et al: Bovine surfactant therapy for patients with acute respiratory distress syndrome. Am J Respir Crit Care Med 1997;155:1309–1315.

119. Spragg RG, Lewis JF, Wurst W, et al: Treatment of acute respiratory distress syndrome with recombinant surfactant protein C surfactant. Am J Respir Crit Care Med 2003;167: 1562–1566.

120. Spragg RG, Lewis JF, Rathgeb F, et al: Intratracheal instillation of rSP-C surfactant improves oxygenation in patients with ARDS. Am J Respir Crit Care Med 2002;165:A22.

121. Shaffer TH: A brief review: Liquid ventilation. Undersea Biomed Res 1987;14:169–179.

122. Shaffer TH, Douglas PR, Lowe CA, Bhutani VK: The effects of liquid ventilation on cardiopulmonary function in preterm lambs. Pediatr Res 1983;17:303–306.

123. Wolfson MR, Greenspan JS, Deoras KS, et al: Comparison of gas and liquid ventilation: Clinical, physiological, and histological correlates. J Appl Physiol 1992;72:1024–1031.

124. Hirschl RB, Parent A, Tooley R, et al: Liquid ventilation improves pulmonary function, gas exchange, and lung injury in a model of respiratory failure. Ann Surg 1995;221:79–88.

125. Hirschl RB, Tooley R, Parent AC, et al: Improvement of gas exchange, pulmonary function, and lung injury with partial liquid ventilation: A study model in a setting of severe respiratory failure. Chest 1995;108:500–508.

126. Dani C, Costantino ML, Martelli E, et al: Perfluorocarbons attenuate oxidative lung damage. Pediatr Pulmonol 2003;36:322–329.

127. Hirschl RB, Croce M, Gore D, et al: Prospective, randomized, controlled pilot study of partial liquid ventilation in adult acute respiratory distress syndrome. Am J Respir Crit Care Med 2002;165:781–787.

128. Zapol WM, Snider MT, Hill JD, et al: Extracorporeal membrane oxygenation in severe acute respiratory failure: A randomized prospective study. JAMA 1979;242:2193–2196.

129. Morris AH, Wallace CJ, Menlove RL, et al: Randomized clinical trial of pressure-controlled inverse ratio ventilation and extracorporeal $CO_2$ removal for adult respiratory distress syndrome. Am J Respir Crit Care Med 1994;149:295–305.

130. Lewandowski K: Extracorporeal membrane oxygenation for severe acute respiratory failure. Crit Care 2000;4:156–168.

131. Dellinger RP, Zimmerman JL, Taylor RW, et al: Effects of inhaled nitric oxide in patients with acute respiratory distress syndrome: Results of a randomized phase II trial. Inhaled Nitric Oxide in ARDS Study Group. Crit Care Med 1998;26:15–23.

132. Lundin S, Mang H, Smithies M, et al: Inhalation of nitric oxide in acute lung injury: Results of a European multicentre study. The European Study Group of Inhaled Nitric Oxide. Intensive Care Med 1999;25:911–919.

133. Schuster DP: What is acute lung injury? What is ARDS? Chest 1995;107:1721–1726.

134. Lewandowski K, Rossaint R, Pappert D, et al: High survival rate in 122 ARDS patients managed according to a clinical algorithm including extracorporeal membrane oxygenation. Intensive Care Med 1997;23:819–835.

135. Abel SJ, Finney SJ, Brett SJ, et al: Reduced mortality in association with the acute respiratory distress syndrome (ARDS). Thorax 1998;53:292–294.

136. Jardin F, Fellahi JL, Beauchet A, et al: Improved prognosis of acute respiratory distress syndrome 15 years on. Intensive Care Med 1999;25:936–941.

137. Rocco T, Reinert S, Cioffi W, et al: A 9-year, single institution, retrospective review of death rate and prognostic factors in adult respiratory distress syndrome. Ann Surg 2001;233:414–422.

138. Suchyta MR, Orme JF Jr, Morris AH: The changing face of organ failure in ARDS. Chest 2003;124:1871–1879.

139. Page B, Vieillard-Baron A, Beauchet A, et al: Low stretch ventilation strategy in acute respiratory distress syndrome: Eight years of clinical experience in a single center. Crit Care Med 2003;31:765–769.

140. Estenssoro E, Dubin A, Laffaire E, et al: Incidence, clinical course, and outcome in 217 patients with acute respiratory distress syndrome. Crit Care Med 2002;30:2450–2456.

141. Nuckton TJ, Alonso JA, Kallet RH, et al: Pulmonary dead-space fraction as a risk factor for death in the acute respiratory distress syndrome. N Engl J Med 2002;346: 1281–1286.

142. Davidson T, Rubenfeld G, Caldwell E, et al: The effect of acute respiratory distress syndrome on long-term survival. Am J Respir Crit Care Med 1999;160:1838–1842.

143. Brun-Buisson C, Minelli C, Bertolini G, et al: Epidemiology and outcome of acute lung injury in European intensive care units: Results from the ALIVE study. Intensive Care Med 2004;30:51–61.

144. Herridge MS, Cheung AM, Tansey CM, et al: One-year outcomes in survivors of the acute respiratory distress syndrome. N Engl J Med 2003;348:683–693.

145. Neff TA, Stocker R, Frey HR, et al: Long-term assessment of lung function in survivors of severe ARDS. Chest 2003;123: 845–853.

146. Orme J Jr, Romney JS, Hopkins RO, et al: Pulmonary function and health-related quality of life in survivors of acute respiratory distress syndrome. Am J Respir Crit Care Med 2003;167: 690–694.

147. McHugh LG, Milberg JA, Whitcomb ME, et al: Recovery of function in survivors of the acute respiratory distress syndrome. Am J Respir Crit Care Med 1994;150:90–94.

148. Angus DC, Musthafa AA, Clermont G, et al: Quality-adjusted survival in the first year after the acute respiratory distress syndrome. Am J Respir Crit Care Med 2001;163:1389–1394.

149. Hopkins R, Weaver L, Pope D, et al: Neuropsychological sequelae and impaired health status in survivors of severe acute respiratory distress syndrome. Am J Respir Crit Care Med 1999;160:50–56.

# CHAPTER 5

# Ventilator-Induced Lung Injury

Jack J. Haitsma and Arthur S. Slutsky

At the dawn of the new millennium, the National Institutes of Health–sponsored Acute Respiratory Distress Syndrome (ARDS) Network showed unequivocally that the specific ventilatory strategy used influences patient outcome.[1] This group compared two ventilation strategies: the first strategy used traditional tidal volume ($V_T$; 12 mL/kg predicted body weight [PBW], corresponding to about 10 mL/kg body weight [BW]) and a plateau pressure of 50 cm $H_2O$, and the second strategy used reduced $V_T$ (6 mL/kg PBW, corresponding to about 5 mL/kg BW), and plateau pressures were limited to 30 cm $H_2O$, deemed to be protective (Fig. 5.1). Using the protective strategy, the ARDS Network reduced mortality to 31% compared with 40% in the traditionally ventilated group.[1]

This study of 861 patients demonstrated that ventilator-induced lung injury (VILI) has an attributable mortality of at least 9%. So what is VILI, how does it happen, and what can we do to minimize it?

## ACUTE RESPIRATORY DISTRESS SYNDROME, ACUTE LUNG INJURY, VENTILATOR-INDUCED LUNG INJURY, AND VENTILATOR-ASSOCIATED LUNG INJURY

Every year, millions of patients worldwide receive ventilator support for numerous indications including respiratory failure, as well as during surgery procedures. Mechanical ventilation has become an important therapeutic modality in the treatment of patients with impaired pulmonary function and particularly in patients suffering from ARDS. Several terms need

defining (Table 5.1). The criteria for acute lung injury (ALI), according to the American-European Consensus Conference on ALI/ARDS, are as follows: acute onset, a ratio of arterial partial pressure of oxygen to fraction of inspired oxygen ($PaO_2/FiO_2$) lower than 300 mm Hg, bilateral infiltrates seen on a frontal chest radiograph, and pulmonary artery wedge pressure less than 18 mm Hg or

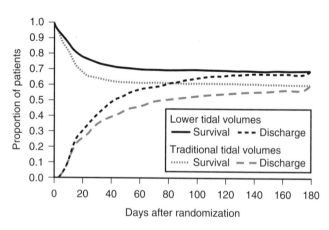

**Figure 5.1**   Plot from the Acute Respiratory Distress Syndrome (ARDS) Network trial showing the probability of survival and of being discharged home and breathing without assistance during the first 180 days after randomization in patients with acute lung injury (ALI) and ARDS. Patients were randomized to either traditional tidal volume (12 mL/kg predicted body weight [PBW]) and a plateau pressure lower than 50 cm of $H_2O$ or lower tidal volume (6 mL/kg PBW) and plateau pressures limited to 30 cm $H_2O$. (From Acute Respiratory Distress Syndrome Network: Ventilation with lower tidal volumes as compared with traditional tidal volumes for acute lung injury and the acute respiratory distress syndrome. N Engl J Med 2000;342:1301–1308.)

**Table 5-1** Definition of Acute Lung Injury, Acute Respiratory Distress Syndrome, Ventilator-Induced Lung Injury, and Ventilator-Associated Lung Injury

| | |
|---|---|
| Acute lung injury (ALI)* | Acute onset<br>$Pao_2/Fio_2$ <300 mm Hg<br>Bilateral infiltrates seen on a frontal chest radiograph<br>Pulmonary artery wedge pressure <18 mm Hg or no clinical evidence of left atrial hypertension |
| Acute respiratory distress syndrome (ARDS)* | Acute onset<br>$Pao_2/Fio_2$ <200 mm Hg<br>Bilateral infiltrates seen on a frontal chest radiograph<br>Pulmonary artery wedge pressure <18 mm Hg or no clinical evidence of left atrial hypertension |
| Ventilator-induced lung injury (VILI)† | Acute lung injury directly induced by mechanical ventilation in animal models |
| Ventilator-associated lung injury (VALI)† | Acute lung injury that resembles ARDS in patients receiving mechanical ventilation<br>VALI possibly associated with preexisting lung disease such as ARDS<br>VALI associated only with mechanical ventilation |

*Data from Bernard GR, Artigas A, Brigham KL, et al: Report of the American-European Consensus Conference on Acute Respiratory Distress Syndrome: Definitions, mechanisms, relevant outcomes, and clinical trial coordination. Consensus Committee. J Crit Care 1994;9:72–81.
†Data from International Consensus Conferences in Intensive Care Medicine: Ventilator-associated lung injury in ARDS. Am J Respir Crit Care Med 1999;160:2118–2124.

no clinical evidence of left atrial hypertension.[2] ARDS is simply ALI with greater hypoxemia; the criteria are the same except that $Pao_2/Fio_2$ is less than 200 mm Hg. VILI was defined by the International Consensus Conference on Ventilator-Associated Lung Injury (VALI) in ARDS as ALI directly induced by mechanical ventilation in animal models.[3] Because VILI is usually indistinguishable morphologically, physiologically, and radiologically from the diffuse alveolar damage of ALI, it can be discerned definitively only in animal models. VALI is defined as lung injury that resembles ARDS and is thought to result from mechanical ventilation. VALI may be associated with preexisting lung disease such as ARDS. However, unlike in VILI, one cannot be sure that VALI is caused by mechanical ventilation. Barotrauma, defined as extra-alveolar air, most often results from overdistension of alveoli and rupture of their walls down a pressure gradient from an air space into a bronchovascular sheath.[4]

ARDS is caused by multiple factors and is characterized by respiratory dysfunction including hypoxemia and decreased lung compliance.[2] It is known that the decrease in lung distensibility is caused, in part, by a disturbed surfactant system resulting in elevated surface tension. This increase in surface tension leads to instability of alveoli at end expiration and subsequent collapse,[4] as well as an increase in right-to-left shunt and a decrease in $Pao_2$.

Mechanical ventilation can maintain arterial oxygenation and allow ventilation of atelectatic areas by generating high enough airway pressures to overcome the opening pressures needed to open up these alveoli. However, mechanical ventilation can also cause adverse effects.

## Acute Respiratory Distress Syndrome

The propensity to injury is partly related to the inhomogeneity in distensibility of the injured lung.[5,6] The open and thus relatively healthy lung parts are prone to over-inflation, whereas the injured lung areas are not inflated. Progression of the injury to the lung results in atelectatic lung areas and patches of still open lung tissue. When this lung is ventilated, even with small $V_T$s, air will go preferentially to these open, still compliant parts. This phenomenon was described by Gattinoni as a "baby lung," and subsequent ventilation even with small $V_T$s results in overdistention.[3,5] Depending on the amount of collapsed lung tissue, these small $V_T$s increase the actual $V_T$ delivered to the open lung areas severalfold.

## Atelectrauma

These potentially pathogenic forces include repetitive (cyclic) strain (stretch) from overdistention and interdependence, as well as shear stress to the epithelial cells as lung units collapse and reopen, so-called atelectrauma.[7] Pioneering work of Mead and colleagues demonstrated that, because of the pulmonary interdependence of the alveoli, the forces acting on the fragile lung tissue in nonuniformly expanded lungs are not only the applied transpulmonary pressures, but also the shear forces that are present in the interstitium between open and closed alveoli.[8] Based on a theoretical analysis, these investigators predicted that a transpulmonary pressure of 30 cm $H_2O$ could result in shear forces of 140 cm $H_2O$.[8] Shear forces, rather than end-inspiratory overstretching, may well be the major reason for epithelial disruption and the loss of barrier function of the alveolar epithelium. In an ARDS-affected lung, alveoli are subjected to opening and closing during ventilation.[3,8,9] Using in vivo video microscopy, Steinberg and colleagues directly assessed alveolar stability in normal and surfactant-deactivated lungs and elegantly showed alveolar instability (atelectrauma) during ventilation.[9]

Important evidence for this mechanism comes from the finding that ventilation, even at low lung volumes, can augment lung injury.[10,11] Muscedere and colleagues ventilated isolated, nonperfused, lavaged rat lungs with physiologic VTs (5 to 6 mL/kg) at different end-expiratory pressures (higher and lower than the pinf Inflection Point (Pinf)).[10] Lung injury was significantly greater in the groups ventilated with a positive end-expiratory pressure (PEEP) lower than Pinf, and in these groups the site of injury was dependent on the level of PEEP (Fig. 5.2) Thus, in addition to high airway pressures, end-expiratory lung volume is an important determinant of the degree and site of lung injury during positive pressure ventilation. Therefore, preventing repeated collapse by stabilizing lung tissue at end expiration with PEEP can reduce lung injury.[3,12–14]

## Volutrauma

In a classical paper published in 1974, Webb and Tierney demonstrated the critical role that PEEP plays in preventing or reducing lung injury.[14] In rats ventilated with 10 cm $H_2O$ of PEEP and a peak pressure of 45 cm $H_2O$, little lung injury was present, but when the same peak pressure was used with zero PEEP, the animals developed severe pulmonary edema within 20 minutes.[14] Dreyfuss and colleagues further explored the role of VT and peak inspiratory pressures on lung injury (Fig. 5.3).[15] In an animal model, these investigators applied high inspiratory pressures in combination with high volumes, and the result was increased alveolar permeability.[15] In a second group, low pressures were combined with high volume (iron lung ventilation), again resulting in increased alveolar permeability.[15] In the third group, the effect of high pressures combined with low volume was studied, by strapping the chest wall to reduce chest excursions; the permeability of this group (high-pressure low-volume group) did not differ from that of the control group.[15] Thus, large-VT ventilation increases alveolar permeability, whereas peak inspiratory pressures do not influence the development of this type of lung injury. Dreyfuss and Saumon called this injury volutrauma to indicate that it is not the pressure at the airway opening, but rather the distention of the lung that is important in causing lung injury.[16]

Similar observations were made in rabbits ventilated with high peak pressures in which thorax excursions were limited by a plaster cast.[17] In injured lungs, the effect of higher volumes only aggravated the permeability, as demonstrated in animals in which the surfactant system was inactivated and that were subsequently ventilated with high VTs.[18,19] High transpulmonary pressure has also been demonstrated to lead to much more subtle injury. Ultrastructural abnormalities such as endothelial cell detachment, intracapillary blebs, and disrupted or damaged type I pneumocytes with areas of denuded basement membrane have been described as evidence of volutrauma secondary to alveolar overdistension.[12,20]

## Biotrauma

Research has focused on how mechanical stresses caused by mechanical ventilation can affect cellular and molecular processes in the lung, a mechanism that we have called biotrauma.[21] It has become clear that, during VILI,

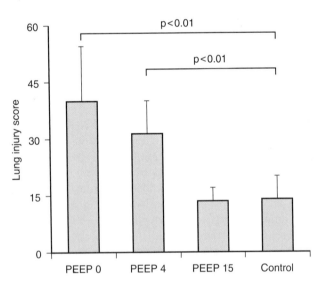

**Figure 5.2** Lung injury scores obtained from isolated nonperfused rat lungs ventilated with identical tidal volumes of 5 to 6 mL/kg body weight (BW), but with different levels of end-expiratory pressures. Lung injury score is a composite of alveolar duct, respiratory bronchiole, and membranous bronchiole injury scored by a pathologist blinded for the samples. (Adapted from Muscedere JG, Mullen JB, Gan K, et al: Tidal ventilation at low airway pressures can augment lung injury. Am J Respir Crit Care Med 1994;149:1327–1334.)

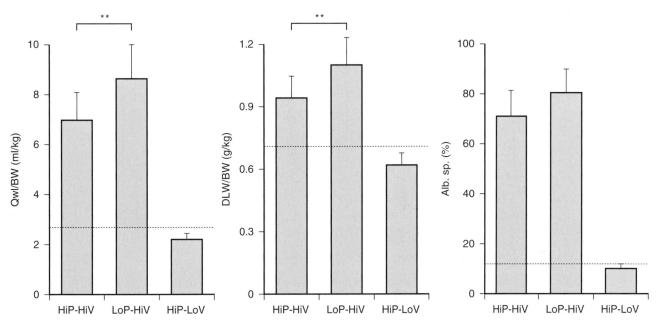

**Figure 5.3** Comparisons of the effects of high-pressure–high-volume (HiP-HiV) ventilation with those of negative inspiratory airway pressure high-tidal volume ventilation (iron lung ventilation = LoP-HiV) and of HiP–low-volume (LoV) ventilation (thoracoabdominal strapping = HiP-LoV). Pulmonary edema was assessed by measuring the extravascular lung water content (Qwl/BW) and changes in permeability by determining the bloodless dry lung weight (DLW/BW) and the distribution space of iodine-125–labeled albumin (Alb. Sp) in lungs. Permeability edema occurred in both groups receiving high-tidal volume ventilation. Animals ventilated with a high peak pressure and a normal tidal volume had no edema. (From Dreyfuss D, Soler P, Basset G, et al: High inflation pressure pulmonary edema: Respective effects of high airway pressure, high tidal volume, and positive end-expiratory pressure. Am Rev Respir Dis 1988;137:1159–1164.)

mechanical ventilation can trigger an inflammatory reaction in the lung and that the degree of inflammation depends on the ventilation strategy.[22,23] Furthermore, this inflammatory reaction may not be limited to the lungs but may also initiate and propagate a systemic inflammatory response, possibly contributing to the onset of multiorgan failure.[24,25] The biotrauma hypothesis proposes that biophysical forces alter normal cellular physiology in the lung and lead to increases in local mediator levels and changes in pulmonary repair, remodeling, and apoptotic mechanisms.[24–26]

Mechanical ventilation generates pressures on lung tissue and especially on lung cells. Depending on the extent of the physical forces applied, this stress may lead to activation of pulmonary cells through mechanotransduction[27] or to rupture of membranes and tissue destruction.[28] We have demonstrated that VILI can result in loss of the compartmentalized inflammatory response, thereby leading to increased serum levels of inflammatory mediators.[29] In the early stage of inflammation in the lung, the response may be compartmentalized, as observed in community-acquired pneumonia.[30] Steinberg and associates employed in vivo video microscopy to assess alveolar stability directly in normal and surfactant-deactivated lungs and showed that alveolar instability (atelectrauma) causes mechanical injury that initiates an inflammatory response and finally leads to secondary neutrophil-mediated proteolytic injury.[9] These data suggest that a key inciting event leading to biotrauma is cyclic stretch-induced lung injury (atelectrauma).

## CYTOKINES AND INFLAMMATORY MEDIATORS

Tremblay and colleagues demonstrated that VILI could induce cytokine release.[22] Using an isolated nonperfused rat lung model, these investigators demonstrated that ventilation with high volumes (40 mL/kg BW) and no PEEP resulted in increased levels of tumor necrosis factor-α (TNF-α), interleukin (IL)-1β, IL-6, macrophage inflammatory protein-2, interferon-γ, and IL-10.[22] Zero PEEP in combination with high-volume ventilation (HVZP) had a synergistic effect on cytokine levels (e.g., a 56-fold increase of TNF-α versus controls) (Fig. 5.4). Ventilation with equal or higher peak airway

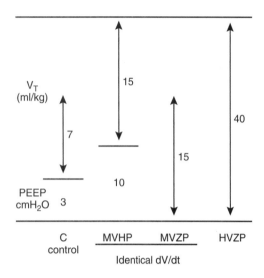
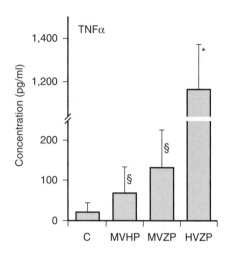

**Figure 5.4** *Left,* Schematic diagram of tidal volume and positive end-expiratory pressure (PEEP) levels used in the ex vivo ventilated lung model. *Right,* The values of tumor necrosis factor-α (TNF-α) versus the four different ventilatory strategies shown on the *left.* Note the break in the axis at the TNF-α value of approximately 250 pg/mL. C, control; HVZP, high volume, zero PEEP; MVZP, medium volume, zero PEEP. (From Tremblay L, Valenza F, Ribeiro SP, et al: Injurious ventilatory strategies increase cytokines and c-fos m-RNA expression in an isolated rat lung model. J Clin Invest 1997;99:944–952.)

pressures but with a PEEP of 10 cm $H_2O$ reduced (MVHP) resulted in only a threefold increase in TNF-α.[22] Ventilation with a lower volume (15 mL/kg BW; similar to MVHP) but now without PEEP (MVZP) produced a sixfold increase in lavage TNF-α, a finding again highlighting the importance of atelectrauma.[22] In Chapter 19, we further explore the pathways and effects of cytokine release during mechanical ventilation.

## Ventilator-Induced Lung Injury in Clinical Trials

The observations that mechanical ventilation influences mediator levels are supported by data from clinical trials. Ranieri and colleagues randomized patients with ARDS to either a traditional ventilatory strategy or a lung protective strategy (low $V_T$; high PEEP). The latter resulted in lower levels of inflammatory mediators (Fig. 5.5),[31] which correlated with lower levels of multiorgan failure and improved patient outcome.[32]

In 1990, Hickling and colleagues demonstrated that mechanical ventilation could influence mortality in patients with ARDS.[33] In a retrospective analysis, these investigators demonstrated that 50 patients with ARDS who were ventilated with a low $V_T$ and who had permissive hypercapnia had decreased mortality compared with historical controls.[33] The outcome of this study sparked renewed interest in lowering $V_T$ in patients with ARDS. Three subsequent controlled trials using low-$V_T$ strategies were simultaneously started, but all failed to demonstrate improved patient outcomes.[34–36] These studies used a $V_T$ of approximately 7 mL/kg in their low-$V_T$

arms and a $V_T$ of 10 mL/kg in their control arms.[34–36] In contrast, using a $V_T$ of 6 mL/kg in their treatment arm and a $V_T$ of 12 mL/kg in their control arm ($V_T$ calculated by using PBW), the ARDS Network was able to reduce mortality.[1] In the ARDS Network study, PBW was approximately 20% lower than measured BW, and the result was a $V_T$ of approximately 10 mL/kg measured BW for the control arm.[37]

The explanation given by the ARDS Network trial for the beneficial effect on mortality was the greater difference in $V_T$ between the two arms of the study, the power of the study (ARDS Network studied 861 patients, whereas the other three trials studied a maximum of 120 patients), and the aggressive treatment and prevention of acidosis.[1] Other studies performed since then have demonstrated that higher $V_T$ increases VILI and leads to the development of ALI.[38,39]

The only other randomized controlled trial to show a reduction of mortality in patients with ARDS had been published 2 years earlier. Amato and colleagues reported that mortality in 53 patients was significantly reduced by applying a protective ventilation strategy.[40] In their study, $V_T$ was also reduced to less than 6 mL/kg in the low-$V_T$ group compared with 12 mL/kg $V_T$ in the control arm. In contrast to the three negative studies,[34–36] the PEEP level in the low-$V_T$ group of Amato and colleagues[40] was significantly higher (i.e., almost 17 cm $H_2O$ compared with 8 to 10 cm $H_2O$ PEEP in the studies by Brochard and associates,[34] Brower and colleagues,[35] and Stewart and associates[36]). Experimental data have shown that ventilation with low $V_Ts$ by itself

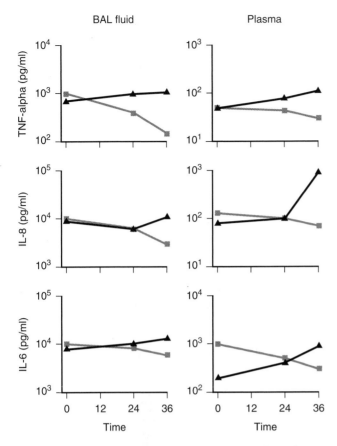

**Figure 5.5** Mean levels of tumor necrosis factor-α (TNF-α), interleukin (IL)-8, and IL-6 in bronchoalveolar lavage fluid and plasma in patients receiving either lung protective ventilation (squares; tidal volume [VT], 8 mL/kg; positive end-expiratory pressure [PEEP], 15 cm $H_2O$) or control ventilation (triangles; VT, 11 mL/kg; PEEP, 7 cm $H_2O$). Time 0 indicates study entry, time 24 is the sample between 24 and 30 hours after study entry, and time 36 is between 36 and 40 hours after study entry. (Adapted from Ranieri VM, Suter PM, Tortorella C, et al: Effect of mechanical ventilation on inflammatory mediators in patients with acute respiratory distress syndrome: A randomized controlled trial. JAMA 1999;282:54–61.)

would decrease mortality.[43] Mean PEEP values on days 1 through 4 were 8.3 cm $H_2O$ in the lower-PEEP group and 13.2 cm $H_2O$ in the higher-PEEP group. Although in this study no benefit in outcome was observed between the patient groups (the study was stopped early after enrollment of 549 patients), the mortality rate in both study arms was relatively low (24.9%, lower PEEP; and 27.5%, higher PEEP),[43] thus providing supportive data that adjusting the ventilatory settings decreases mortality in patients with ARDS/ALI. Unfortunately, patients randomized to the higher-PEEP group also had at baseline more characteristics that predict a higher mortality; adjustment for these differences in baseline covariates did not alter the final outcome but did favor the higher-PEEP group.[43]

A major problem in improving patient care in patients with ARDS is the heterogeneity of the patient population. Recent studies have demonstrated that different populations exist within patients with ARDS.[44] Ferguson and colleagues showed that patients who had "transient ARDS" (improved oxygenation >200 mm Hg, under standard ventilatory settings, within 30 minutes) had a significant lower mortality of 12.5% versus 52.9% in persistent ARDS.[44] Further stratification of patient populations with ARDS should help in improving the power of studies and thus help to identify improved ventilation techniques.

## Role of Ventilator-Induced Lung Injury in Patient Outcome

Although ARDS is defined by the $Pao_2/Fio_2$ ratio in the American-European Consensus Conference on ARDS,[2] patients do not usually die of hypoxemia but rather of multiorgan failure.[45,46] Tremblay and Slutsky hypothesized that mediators released in the lung could be translocated into the systemic circulation and could lead to the development of multiorgan failure.[21] Ranieri and co-workers demonstrated a linkage between increased levels of serum inflammatory mediators and organ failure in patients suffering from ARDS.[32] These increased serum levels of inflammatory mediators were observed in patients ventilated with conventional ventilation, compared with a lung protective ventilation strategy (high PEEP, low VT) that minimized the inflammatory response and subsequently was associated with a lower incidence of organ failure (Fig. 5.6).[31,32] As discussed earlier, ventilation can induce mediator release. Increased levels of cytokines in the serum were also observed in the ARDS Network trial, in which higher levels of IL-6 were observed after 3 days of ventilation in the control arm compared with the reduced VT.[1] An analysis performed later also demonstrated that IL-6, IL-8, and IL-10 correlated with patient outcome.[47] Similarly, the number of days without nonpulmonary

does not prevent lung injury and may even worsen lung injury when atelectrauma is not prevented.[10] In the ARDS Network trial, the low-VT group had a slightly higher set PEEP of 9 cm $H_2O$ compared with a set PEEP of 8 cm $H_2O$ in the control group.[1] However, the increased respiratory rate (to help prevent acidosis) used in the low-VT group may have resulted in intrinsic PEEP that contributed to a higher total PEEP (16 cm $H_2O$) in this group,[41,42] compared with 12 cm $H_2O$ in the group with traditional VTs. This higher total PEEP could help explain the decrease in mortality observed in this group, although the data addressing this issue are somewhat contradictory.

In 2004, the ARDS Network published their follow-up study, investigating whether increased PEEP levels

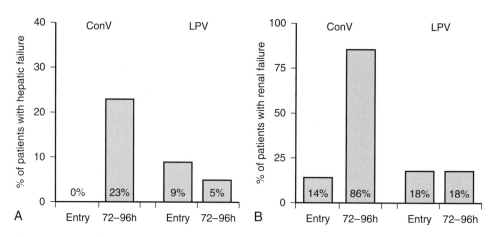

**Figure 5.6** Percentage of hepatic and renal failure in patients receiving either lung protective ventilation (LPV; tidal volume [Vт], 8 mL/kg; positive end-expiratory pressure [PEEP], 15 cm H₂O) or control ventilation (ConV; Vт, 11 mL/kg, PEEP, 7 cm H₂O) at the time of entry (start of randomization) and 76 to 92 hours after entry. (Adapted from Ranieri VM, Giunta F, Suter PM, et al: Mechanical ventilation as a mediator of multisystem organ failure in acute respiratory distress syndrome. JAMA 2000;284:43–44.)

organ or system failure (circulatory, coagulation, and renal failure) was significantly higher in the group treated with lower Vтs.[1]

The final outcome of patients with ARDS correlates with the magnitude and duration of the host inflammatory response in the serum and is independent of the precipitating cause of ARDS or the occurrence of infections.[48] Similar observations were made in patients with multiple trauma in whom high concentrations of cytokines correlated with the development of ARDS and finally multiorgan failure.[49]

Adjusting ventilation to reduce VILI can dramatically reduce cytokine release.[50] Stüber and associates demonstrated that the time course of cytokine release resulting from VILI can be extremely rapid (Fig. 5.7).[50] Patients with ARDS were ventilated with a lung protective strategy; subsequently, the strategy was changed to a less protective approach using higher Vтs and zero PEEP for a few hours. An increase in measurable levels of inflammatory cytokines was observed within an hour of changing the ventilatory strategy.[50] A decrease in cytokine levels was detected within an hour of reversal of the ventilatory strategy back to a protective mode using low Vтs. This elegant study demonstrated that VILI is reversible and that mechanical ventilation has an immediate effect on cytokine release.

Thus, in ARDS, there is an inflamed lung with increased levels of proinflammatory mediators, and ventilation itself can increase the amount of inflammatory mediators produced by the lung. When the barrier function of the alveolar-capillary membrane is disrupted by the underlying disease process or by mechanical ventilation, there may be leakage of mediators into the circulation (decompartmentalization). The subsequent increased levels of these mediators in the circulation correlate with

multiorgan failure and finally mortality. Prevention of VILI by the use of lung protective ventilation in both experimental and clinical studies has demonstrated that a reduction in atelectrauma and biotrauma reduces organ failure and mortality.

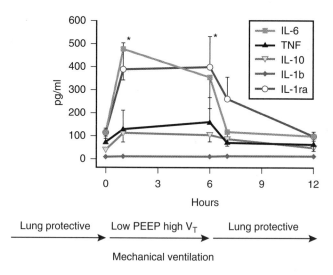

**Figure 5.7** Plot of cytokine levels on the Y axis versus time on the X axis. Patients were ventilated initially with a lung protective strategy, then a low-positive end-expiratory pressure (PEEP)/high-tidal volume (high-Vт) strategy, and then with a lung protective strategy again. When the strategy was changed to the low-PEEP/ high-Vт strategy, the levels of most cytokines increased. Similarly, when the ventilatory strategy was changed back to the lung protective strategy, there was a decrease in most cytokines. IL, interleukin; TNF, tumor necrosis factor. (From Stüber F, Wrigge H, Schroeder S, et al: Kinetic and reversibility of mechanical ventilation-associated pulmonary and systemic inflammatory response in patients with acute lung injury. Intensive Care Med 2002;28:834–841.)

## REFERENCES

1. Acute Respiratory Distress Syndrome Network: Ventilation with lower tidal volumes as compared with traditional tidal volumes for acute lung injury and the acute respiratory distress syndrome. N Engl J Med 2000;342:1301–1308.

2. Bernard GR, Artigas A, Brigham KL, et al: Report of the American-European Consensus Conference on Acute Respiratory Distress Syndrome: Definitions, mechanisms, relevant outcomes, and clinical trial coordination. Consensus Committee. J Crit Care 1994;9:72–81.

3. International Consensus Conferences in Intensive Care Medicine: Ventilator-associated lung injury in ARDS. Am J Respir Crit Care Med 1999;160:2118–2124.

4. Ricard JD: Barotrauma during mechanical ventilation: Why aren't we seeing any more? Intensive Care Med 2004;30: 533–535.

5. Gattinoni L, Pesenti A: The concept of "baby lung." Intensive Care Med 2005;31:776–784.

6. Gattinoni L, Pesenti A, Avalli L, et al: Pressure-volume curve of total respiratory system in acute respiratory failure: Computed tomographic scan study. Am Rev Respir Dis 1987;136:730–736.

7. Slutsky AS: Lung injury caused by mechanical ventilation. Chest 116:S9–S15, 1999.

8. Mead J, Takishima T, Leith D: Stress distribution in lungs: A model of pulmonary elasticity. J Appl Physiol 1970;28: 596–608.

9. Steinberg JM, Schiller HJ, Halter JM, et al: Alveolar instability causes early ventilator-induced lung injury independent of neutrophils. Am J Respir Crit Care Med 2004;169:57–63.

10. Muscedere JG, Mullen JB, Gan K, et al: Tidal ventilation at low airway pressures can augment lung injury. Am J Respir Crit Care Med 1994;149:1327–1334.

11. Taskar V, John J, Evander E, et al: Surfactant dysfunction makes lungs vulnerable to repetitive collapse and reexpansion. Am J Respir Crit Care Med 1997;155:313–320.

12. Dreyfuss D, Saumon G: Ventilator-induced lung injury: Lessons from experimental studies. Am J Respir Crit Care Med 1998;157:294–323.

13. Verbrugge SJ, Bohm SH, Gommers D, et al: Surfactant impairment after mechanical ventilation with large alveolar surface area changes and effects of positive end-expiratory pressure. Br J Anaesth 1998;80:360–364.

14. Webb HH, Tierney DF: Experimental pulmonary edema due to intermittent positive pressure ventilation with high inflation pressures: Protection by positive end-expiratory pressure. Am Rev Respir Dis 1974;110:556–565.

15. Dreyfuss D, Soler P, Basset G, et al: High inflation pressure pulmonary edema: Respective effects of high airway pressure, high tidal volume, and positive end-expiratory pressure. Am Rev Respir Dis 1988;137:1159–1164.

16. Dreyfuss D, Saumon G: Barotrauma is volutrauma, but which volume is the one responsible? Intensive Care Med 1992;18: 139–141.

17. Hernandez LA, Peevy KJ, Moise AA, et al: Chest wall restriction limits high airway pressure-induced lung injury in young rabbits. J Appl Physiol 1989;66:2364–2368.

18. Coker PJ, Hernandez LA, Peevy KJ, et al: Increased sensitivity to mechanical ventilation after surfactant inactivation in young rabbit lungs. Crit Care Med 1992;20:635–640.

19. Dreyfuss D, Soler P, Saumon G: Mechanical ventilation-induced pulmonary edema: Interaction with previous lung alterations. Am J Respir Crit Care Med 1995;151:1568–1575.

20. Vlahakis NE, Hubmayr RD: Cellular stress failure in ventilator-injured lungs. Am J Respir Crit Care Med 2005;171: 1328–1342.

21. Tremblay LN, Slutsky AS: Ventilator-induced injury: From barotrauma to biotrauma. Proc Assoc Am Physicians 1998;110:482–488.

22. Tremblay L, Valenza F, Ribeiro SP, et al: Injurious ventilatory strategies increase cytokines and c-fos m-RNA expression in an isolated rat lung model. J Clin Invest 1997;99:944–952.

23. van Kaam AH, Dik WA, Haitsma JJ, et al: Application of the open-lung concept during positive-pressure ventilation reduces pulmonary inflammation in newborn piglets. Biol Neonate 2003;83:273–280.

24. Imai Y, Parodo J, Kajikawa O, et al: Injurious mechanical ventilation and end-organ epithelial cell apoptosis and organ dysfunction in an experimental model of acute respiratory distress syndrome. JAMA 2003;289:2104–2112.

25. Slutsky AS, Tremblay LN: Multiple system organ failure: Is mechanical ventilation a contributing factor? Am J Respir Crit Care Med 1998;157:1721–1725.

26. Dos Santos CC, Slutsky AS: The contribution of biophysical lung injury to the development of biotrauma. Annu Rev Physiol 2006;68:585–618.

27. Dos Santos CC, Slutsky AS: Mechanisms of ventilator-induced lung injury: A perspective. J Appl Physiol 2000;89: 1645–1655.

28. Uhlig S: Ventilation-induced lung injury and mechanotransduction: Stretching it too far? Am J Physiol 2002;282:L892–L896.

29. Haitsma JJ, Uhlig S, Goggel R, et al: Ventilator-induced lung injury leads to loss of alveolar and systemic compartmentalization of tumor necrosis factor-alpha. Intensive Care Med 2000;26: 1515–1522.

30. Dehoux MS, Boutten A, Ostinelli J, et al: Compartmentalized cytokine production within the human lung in unilateral pneumonia. Am J Respir Crit Care Med 1994;150:710–716.

31. Ranieri VM, Suter PM, Tortorella C, et al: Effect of mechanical ventilation on inflammatory mediators in patients with acute respiratory distress syndrome: A randomized controlled trial. JAMA 1999;282:54–61.

32. Ranieri VM, Giunta F, Suter PM, et al: Mechanical ventilation as a mediator of multisystem organ failure in acute respiratory distress syndrome. JAMA 2000;284:43–44.

33. Hickling KG, Henderson SJ, Jackson R: Low mortality associated with low volume pressure limited ventilation with permissive hypercapnia in severe adult respiratory distress syndrome. Intensive Care Med 1990;16:372–377.

34. Brochard L, Roudot-Thoraval F, Roupie E, et al: Tidal volume reduction for prevention of ventilator-induced lung injury in acute respiratory distress syndrome: The Multicenter Trial Group on Tidal Volume Reduction in ARDS. Am J Respir Crit Care Med 1998;158:1831–1838.

35. Brower RG, Shanholtz CB, Fessler HE, et al: Prospective, randomized, controlled clinical trial comparing traditional versus reduced tidal volume ventilation in acute respiratory distress syndrome patients. Crit Care Med 1999;27:1492–1498.

36. Stewart TE, Meade MO, Cook DJ, et al: Evaluation of a ventilation strategy to prevent barotrauma in patients at high risk for acute respiratory distress syndrome: Pressure- and Volume-Limited Ventilation Strategy Group. N Engl J Med 1998;338:355–361.

37. Brower RG, Matthay M, Schoenfeld D: Meta-analysis of acute lung injury and acute respiratory distress syndrome trials. Am J Respir Crit Care Med 2002;166:1515–1517.

38. Gajic O, Dara SI, Mendez JL, et al: Ventilator-associated lung injury in patients without acute lung injury at the onset of mechanical ventilation. Crit Care Med 2004;32:1817–1824.

39. Gajic O, Frutos-Vivar F, Esteban A, et al: Ventilator settings as a risk factor for acute respiratory distress syndrome in mechanically ventilated patients. Intensive Care Med 2005;31:922–926.

40. Amato MB, Barbas CS, Medeiros DM, et al: Effect of a protective-ventilation strategy on mortality in the acute respiratory distress syndrome. N Engl J Med 1998;338: 347–354.

41. De Durante G, Del Turco M, Rustichini L, et al: ARDSNet lower tidal volume ventilatory strategy may generate intrinsic positive end-expiratory pressure in patients with acute respiratory distress syndrome. Am J Respir Crit Care Med 2002;165: 1271–1274.

42. Lee CM, Neff MJ, Steinberg KP, et al: Effect of low tidal volume ventilation on intrinsic PEEP in patients with acute lung injury. Am J Respir Crit Care Med 2001;163:A765.

43. Brower RG, Lanken PN, MacIntyre N, et al: Higher versus lower positive end-expiratory pressures in patients with the acute respiratory distress syndrome. N Engl J Med 2004;351: 327–336.

44. Ferguson ND, Kacmarek RM, Chiche JD, et al: Screening of ARDS patients using standardized ventilator settings: Influence on enrollment in a clinical trial. Intensive Care Med 2004;30:1111–1116.

45. Esteban A, Anzueto A, Frutos F, et al: Characteristics and outcomes in adult patients receiving mechanical ventilation: A 28-day international study. JAMA 2002;287: 345–355.

46. Ferring M, Vincent JL: Is outcome from ARDS related to the severity of respiratory failure? Eur Respir J 1997;10: 1297–1300.

47. Parsons PE, Eisner MD, Thompson BT, et al: Lower tidal volume ventilation and plasma cytokine markers of inflammation in patients with acute lung injury. Crit Care Med 2005;33:1–6; discussion 230–232.

48. Headley AS, Tolley E, Meduri GU: Infections and the inflammatory response in acute respiratory distress syndrome. Chest 1997;111:1306–1321.

49. Roumen RM, Hendriks T, van der Ven-Jongekrijg J, et al: Cytokine patterns in patients after major vascular surgery, hemorrhagic shock, and severe blunt trauma: Relation with subsequent adult respiratory distress syndrome and multiple organ failure. Ann Surg 1993;218:769–776.

50. Stüber F, Wrigge H, Schroeder S, et al: Kinetic and reversibility of mechanical ventilation-associated pulmonary and systemic inflammatory response in patients with acute lung injury. Intensive Care Med 2002;28:834–841.

# CHAPTER 6

# Role of Changes in Body Temperature in Acute Lung Injury

Younsuck Koh and Chae-Man Lim

## CASE DISCUSSION

A 20-year-old woman was admitted to the medical intensive care unit at the Asan Medical Center, Seoul, with rapidly worsening dyspnea that had commenced the day before. A week earlier, she had developed dry cough, fever, and scanty whitish sputum with diffuse myalgia. Until this episode, she was a healthy adult, 160 cm tall and weighing 56 kg, with no history of medical illnesses such as tuberculosis, hepatitis, diabetes, or hypertension. At the initial physical examination, her vital signs were blood pressure 143/93 mm Hg, body temperature 36.5°C, heart rate 150 beats/min, respiration rate 36 breaths/min. She appeared alert but acutely ill, with severe dyspnea. Her lung sounds were decreased in both upper lung fields, without definite crackles or wheezes. Although rapid, her heart sounds were normal, and no murmur or gallop was heard. Her extremities were cold and deeply cyanotic. Physical examination of other parts of the patient's body revealed nothing remarkable.

Initial laboratory data included the following: complete blood count—white blood cells, 12,300/mm³; hemoglobin, 16.7 g/dL; platelets, 164 × 10³/mm³; hematocrit, 48.9%; chemistry—calcium, 8.0 mg/dL; glucose, 164 mg/dL; blood urea nitrogen, 10 mg/dL; creatinine, 1.0 mg/dL; protein, 5.9 g/dL; albumin, 2.8 g/dL; aspartate aminotransferase, 81 IU/L; alanine aminotransferase, 21 IU/L; alkaline phosphatase, 81 IU/L; total bilirubin, 0.7 mg/dL; cholesterol, 112 mg/dL; electrolytes—sodium/ potassium/chloride/total carbon dioxide ($CO_2$), 136/ 3.8/100/16.6 mEq/L; coagulation—prothrombin time, 75.2%; activated partial thromboplastin time, 44.6 seconds; urinalysis unremarkable; C-reactive protein, 54.7 mg/dL. Her initial arterial blood gas (ABG) analysis under room air revealed the following: pH, 7.329; arterial partial pressure of $CO_2$ ($PaCO_2$), 37.0 mm Hg; arterial partial pressure of oxygen ($PaO_2$), 13.7 mm Hg; base excess, −6.2 mEq/L; bicarbonate, 19.0 mEq/L; arterial oxygen saturation ($SaO_2$), 15.1%. Her initial chest radiograph is shown in Figure 6.1 *(left)*.

Our initial diagnosis was severe community-acquired pneumonia, on the basis of which antibiotics (ceftriaxone, high-dose ciprofloxacin, and clindamycin) were started immediately after procuring sputum, blood, and urine for microbiologic studies. On the evening of admission (day 1), however, the patient's temperature rose to 40.9°C, and ABG analysis under 10 cm $H_2O$ positive end-expiratory pressure, 100% oxygen, and 26 cm $H_2O$ pressure control level did not improve significantly: pH, 7.468; $PaCO_2$, 31.7 mm Hg; $PaO_2$, 39.9 mm Hg; base excess, −0.4 mEq/L; bicarbonate, 22.7 mEq/L; $SaO_2$, 77.7%. To correct the refractory hypoxia, we initiated inhalation of nitric oxide at 10 ppm, as well as prone positioning and an alveolar recruitment maneuver, but these had no effect. On day 2, her ABG analysis results were as follows: pH, 7.418; $PaCO_2$, 33.3 mm Hg; $PaO_2$, 42.8 mm Hg; base excess, −3.1 mEq/L; bicarbonate, 21.6 mEq/L; and $SaO_2$, 79.8%. Because of the moribund hypoxemia and worsening of pneumonic infiltrates, we initiated hypothermia at 35±1°C.

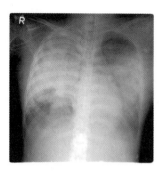
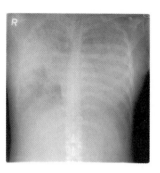
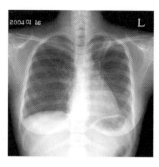

**Figure 6.1** A chest radiograph taken about 2 weeks after hospital discharge suggested active tuberculosis at the apex of the left lung, although this could not be demonstrated by culture.

Her ABG analysis on day 3, although acidotic, was slightly improved: pH, 7.294; $PaCO_2$, 53.2 mm Hg; $PaO_2$, 58.0 mm Hg; base excess, –0.8 mEq/L; bicarbonate, 25.9 mEq/L; and $SaO_2$, 86.0%. At this time, her antibiotic regimen was changed to cover all possible typical and atypical pneumonia pathogens, including *Mycobacterium tuberculosis*. Because there was no significant improvement in clinical signs and chest radiography (Fig. 6.1, *middle*), methylprednisolone was started at 1 mg/kg twice daily. By day 5, her $PaO_2$ rose to more than 60 mm Hg, and from day 6, the soft and hard pulmonary infiltrates began to recede, leading to a decrease in ventilatory support and oxygen requirement. On day 8, her ABG analysis under oxygen 60% was acceptable. Hypothermia was therefore halted, and she was passively rewarmed. On day 12, the patient was extubated, and on day 14 all antimicrobials, except antituberculous medication, were discontinued, and methylprednisolone was tapered. The patient was discharged neurologically intact on day 26, and she was breathing room air without dyspnea or any other significant organ insufficiency. A chest radiograph taken about 2 weeks after hospital discharge (Fig. 6.1, *right*) suggested active tuberculosis at the apex of the left lung, although this could not be demonstrated by culture. Figure 6.2 shows a summary of the patient's $PaO_2$, $SaO_2$, and rectal temperature (°C) during the first week after admission.

## GENERAL PRINCIPLES

Acute lung injury (ALI)/acute respiratory distress syndrome (ARDS) is one of the main causes of mechanical ventilation and mortality in the intensive care unit. ALI, which is associated with uncontrolled lung inflammation, manifests as increased capillary endothelial and alveolar epithelial permeability and results in refractory hypoxemia. Many inflammatory mediators, including proinflammatory cytokines, reactive oxygen species, and nitric oxide, are involved in the initiation and propagation of injury to endothelial and epithelial cells that delay the repair processes of these cells.

Despite intensive research over many decades, no effective therapy targeting the underlying pathophysiology has been introduced in large-scale human trials. The use of low tidal volume with titration of positive end-expiratory pressure is the only current approach to have an impact on mortality.[1] Most patients with ARDS die of multiorgan failure rather than of irreversible respiratory failure, a finding indicating that ALI is closely associated with other organs through neurologic, biochemical, metabolic, and inflammatory reactions. Moreover, the lungs may play an important role in the development of nonpulmonary organ failure in ALI. Therefore, new therapies attacking the underlying pathophysiology are needed to reduce the mortality of patients with ALI.

Since ancient times, therapeutic manipulation of body temperature has been tried in many disorders. Body temperature affects the immune system and tissue metabolism, as well as the intrinsic physical condition of the biomembrane by altering membrane fluidity.[2] Most patients with ALI have alterations in body temperature.

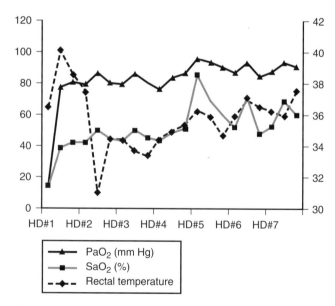

**Figure 6.2** A summary of the patient's arterial partial pressure of oxygen ($PaO_2$), arterial oxygen saturation ($SaO_2$), and rectal temperature (°C) during the first week after admission.

To preserve the function of vital organs, clinicians have attempted to reduce fever or to induce hypothermia, thus reducing tissue metabolism in severely hypoxemic patients such as those with ALI. The biologic importance of altered body temperature or induction of hypothermia in ALI, however, has not been well addressed. We therefore review the biologic roles of the heat shock response (HSR) and induced hypothermia, with a focus on ALI.

## ROLE OF THE HEAT SHOCK RESPONSE IN ACUTE LUNG INJURY

### Heat Shock Protein: A Molecular Chaperone

Heat shock proteins (HSPs) are a group of stress proteins that protect essential cell components from various types of harmful damage. These proteins have been remarkably conserved throughout evolution in almost every living cell. Their name derives from their production in *Drosophila* following elevations in temperature. HSPs are present in the cytosol, mitochondrion, endoplasmic reticulum, and nucleus. HSPs are a group of small polypeptides, and HSP families are classified by their molecular mass, which ranges from 8 to 110 kDa.[3] HSPs are expressed under normal conditions and after stress. Constitutively expressed HSPs, which are expressed under normal cellular conditions, serve vital functions in the maintenance and repair of intracellular proteins. Stress-inducible HSPs are expressed not only in response to elevations in temperature, but also in response to nonthermal insults. HSPs induced by moderate stress protect the organism from even more severe stress. The HSP70 family, which is found in organisms ranging from prokaryotes to mammals, is the most extensively studied. This family includes the constitutive HSP73 and

inducible HSP72 proteins. Lung has been shown to express HSP70 both constitutively and in response to stress.[3]

Although expression of HSPs induces stress tolerance, the prolonged expression of these proteins within cells is toxic. Therefore, expression of HSPs is tightly regulated within cells.[4] Under unstressed conditions, HSPs are bound to heat shock transcription factors (HSFs) in the cytosol of mammalian cells, but they dissociate in response to stress. Once dissociated, HSPs are free to bind denatured proteins. Separated HSFs are phosphorylated by protein kinase C or other serine/threonine kinases and then trimerize.[5] These trimerized HSFs enter the nucleus and bind to heat shock elements (HSEs) in the promoters of HSP genes, thereby leading to increased synthesis of HSPs. Under unstressed conditions, the ku protein, a constitutive HSE-binding factor, binds to HSE and prevents HSF binding.[6] The translated HSPs migrate to the cytosol. The HSFs also migrate into the cytosol and bind inactive HSPs, thus inhibiting further synthesis of HSPs (Fig. 6.3).

HSP70 seems to modulate cytokine production or the tolerance of individual cells to cytokines produced by endotoxin exposure resulting from participation in the control of cytokine gene expression and signal transduction.[7] The HSR can induce expression of the I-κB gene,[8] a natural inhibitor of NF-κB, which is critical in initiating the production of many inflammatory mediators. In respiratory cells, induced HSPs also stabilize I-κBα by preventing tumor necrosis factor-α (TNF-α)–induced-I-κB kinase activation and thus resulting in the inhibition of NF-κB activations.[9] HSP72 prevents the effector steps of stress-induced programmed cell death.[10] One antiapoptotic mechanism is the inhibition of c-Jun N-terminal kinase activation, which is critical for apoptosis.[11] HSP70 expression is impaired in septic rat lungs,[12] as well as in the peripheral blood lymphocytes of patients with severe sepsis.[13] Preemptive induction of HSP70

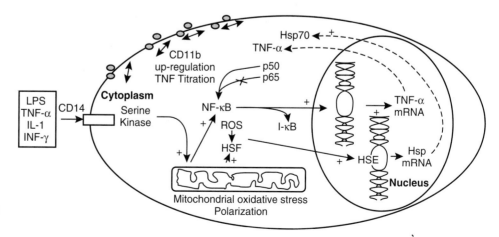

**Figure 6.3** Schematic representation of the interaction between heat shock protein and proinflammatory mediators (+, activation; –, inhibition).

expression reduces organ dysfunction and mortality in animal models of sepsis.[14] In rats, high level constitutive expression of human inducible HSP70 was shown to protect the myocardium from ischemia and reperfusion injury.[15] Moreover, gene transfer of HSP70 protected lung grafts from ischemia-reperfusion injury in an animal model.[16]

## Heat Shock Response in Experimental Models of Acute Lung Injury

The HSR is defined by the rapid expression of HSPs when cells, tissues, or organisms encounter various forms of environmental stress.[17] The response to brief heat shock has been reported to last for several minutes, resulting in biologic changes that make individual cells in the lung less susceptible to endotoxin. The HSR protects mice and rats against the lethal effects of endotoxin[18] and attenuates phospholipase $A_2$–induced ALI.[19] In a rat

model of intra-abdominal sepsis produced by cecal perforation, the HSR reduced both the mortality rate and histologic lung damage.[20] These effects of the HSR were also observed in rats following ALI induced by TNF-α or lipopolysaccharide (LPS).[21,22] In rats given LPS intravenously after heat pretreatment, alveolar spaces were relatively well preserved compared with rats given LPS alone.[23] In LPS-treated rats without heat pretreatment (Fig. 6.4$B_1$, electron microscopy [EM]; magnification × 4000), thickened interstitium, along with increases in interstitial cells and neutrophil infiltration, was observed. Lamellar body vacuoles were vacant in type II epithelial cells (*arrow* in Fig. 6.4$B_1$), and the alveolar space was obliterated with debris. In addition, an area was observed in which endothelial cell membranes were disrupted and fused with neutrophils (*arrow* in Fig. 6.4$B_2$, EM; magnification × 10,000). In heat- and LPS-treated rats (Fig. 6.4$C_1$, EM; magnification × 4000), however, these types of damage were less visible. The membrane

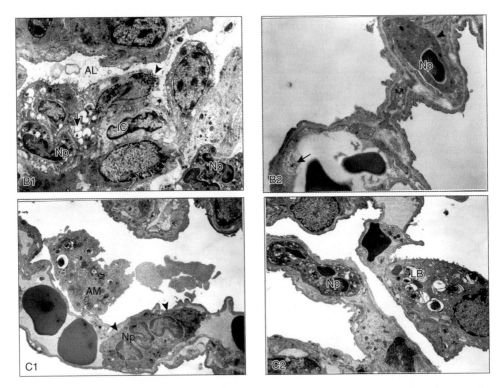

**Figure 6.4**   Histopathologic features of lung in a lipopolysaccharide (LPS)-treated rat without ($B_1$ and $B_2$) and with ($C_1$ and $C_2$) heat pretreatment, as determined by electron microscopy using an uranyl acetate, lead citrate stain.[23] In LPS-treated rats without heat pretreatment, the interstitium is thickened, with interstitial cell and neutrophil infiltration. Lamellar body vacuoles are vacant in type II epithelial cells, and the alveolar air space is obliterated. Also observed is an area in which the endothelial cell membranes are disrupted and fused with neutrophils (e.g., *arrow* in $B_2$). In LPS-treated rats with heat pretreatment, endothelial cells have a normal membrane structure, and neutrophils are not fused with endothelial cell membranes (*arrowhead* in $C_1$). The *asterisk* in $C_1$ indicates thickened interstitium. Alveolar macrophages in $C_1$ are filled with phagocytized debris. Lamellar body structure is well preserved in type II epithelial cells with intact basement membrane, and the alveolar space is relatively well preserved ($C_2$). $B_1$, LPS without heat pretreatment (magnification × 4000). $B_2$, LPS without heat pretreatment (magnification × 10,000). $C_1$ and $C_2$, LPS with heat-pretreatment (magnification × 4000). AL, alveolar space; AM, alveolar macrophage; En, endothelial cells; IC, interstitial cell; LB, lamellar body in type II cell; Np, neutrophil.

structure of these endothelial cells was normal, and neutrophils did not fuse with the membrane (see Fig. 6.4$C_1$ *and* $C_2$, EM; magnification × 4000). Lamellar body structures were well preserved in type II epithelial cells with intact basement membrane, and alveolar air space was relatively well preserved (see Fig. 6.4$C_2$, EM; magnification × 4000). In an ex vivo rat model, the HSR administered 18 hours before injurious mechanical ventilation attenuated ventilator-induced lung injury, as measured by lung compliance and the concentration of proinflammatory cytokines in lung lavage fluids.[24]

The amount of HSP72 protein has been shown to increase in the lung tissue of heat-pretreated rats, a finding suggesting that HSP72 is associated with improvements in ALI induced by various insults. In addition, the time course of formation and decay of HSP72 was shown to parallel the survival curve from endotoxin challenge,[25] and induction of HSP72 was found to prevent neutrophil-mediated human endothelial cell necrosis.[26] Heat pretreatment attenuates the recruitment into the lung of neutrophils, which play a central role in endotoxin-induced ALI.[27] Myeloperoxidase activity in the lung tissue of heat-pretreated, endotoxin-treated rats was decreased to the level observed in control rats.[22] Although HSP70 has been reported to participate in the control of cytokine gene expression and may alter their transcriptional pathways, the effects of brief heat shock on cytokine production is probably not universal. For example, in LPS-stimulated rats, heat stress decreased the peak plasma concentrations of TNF-$\alpha$[28] and interleukin (IL)-1$\beta$.[29] In studies of peritoneal macrophages and blood monocytes, HSP70 accumulation resulted in a decrease in TNF and IL-1 production, whereas IL-6 production was not changed.[30,31] We found, however, that heat pretreatment had no effect on the levels of TNF-$\alpha$, IL-1$\beta$, and interferon-$\gamma$ in plasma and bronchoalveolar lavage (BAL) fluid.[23]

Heating an animal for a brief period to ameliorate ALI can provoke a full systemic stress response. Depending on the heat shock period, hyperthermia significantly affects various cellular pathways, including protein synthesis. Adenoviral transfer of HSP70 into pulmonary epithelium ameliorated ALI in a rat model of cecal ligation and perforation, including decreased interstitial and alveolar edema, decreased neutrophil accumulation, and a twofold reduction in 48-hour mortality compared with the control group.[32]

In summary, these experimental results suggest that HSP70 can attenuate the pathophysiology of ALI. However, further investigation to determine which HSPs would be beneficial in an already injured lung is warranted.

## Clinical Aspects

Fever is frequently encountered in patients with ALI; however, its significance in host defense is not yet known.

It has been hypothesized that fever evolved as an adaptive host defense response to various stresses in vertebrates and invertebrates. Although prolonged high fever (>40°C) can injure the central nervous system and other body systems, low-grade fever (<39°C) need not be treated unless it makes the patient very uncomfortable. Biomedical research has revealed the potential benefits of the HSR, as described earlier. Moreover, some pathogenic microorganisms have decreased viability at high temperatures. Induction of HSP70 in peripheral blood mononuclear cells was lower in patients with severe sepsis than in healthy controls, a finding suggesting that the former had already been stimulated by endogenous mediators.[13] Therefore, understanding the biologic consequences of fever in septic patients may be important for their clinical management. In patients with ARDS, which is accompanied by serious hypoxemia, a reasonable approach may be to reduce fever or induce hypothermia to decrease systemic oxygen consumption. The decision to begin antipyretic therapy should be based on an evaluation of the relative risks and benefits of fever in each patient. Although there is little clinical evidence showing a relationship between HSPs and ALI, alveolar macrophages of patients with ARDS expressed high levels of HSP72 mRNA, and alveolar macrophages with high levels of HSP72 had low respiratory burst activity.[33] HSP70 inducibility in peripheral blood monocytes was decreased in patients with ARDS, and the degree was correlated with disease severity.[34]

## Methods to Induce Heat Shock Response

The HSR is induced by thermal or nonthermal stresses. In mammals, HSPs are induced by a fever temperature 3° to 5°C higher than normal.[35] Nonthermal inducers include sodium arsenite, herbimycin A, heavy metals such as cadmium and zinc, inflammation, circulatory shock, and ischemia and reperfusion injury.[17] There is as yet no optimal way to induce HSPs without harm or to transfer HSPs into patients with ALI. Induction of the HSR by heating or by sodium arsenite administration is not readily applicable to patients with ALI. Adenoviral transfer of HSPs would be a solution to this problem.[16]

## Future Directions

Many experimental results support the notion that the HSR may protect the lungs against ALI induced by various insults. To date, however, there is no strong evidence that induction of the HSR or delivery of HSPs after initiation of proinflammatory signal attenuates the pathophysiology of ALI. Preemptive induction of HSP70 expression would be a valuable therapeutic option in ALI. Gene therapy using adenoviruses to deliver HSPs directly into the lung might be a solution.

However, preemptive induction of HSP70 should address many related issues, including delivery methods, timing, frequency, and dose. Answering these questions may provide a better understanding for the pathogenesis of ALI.

## ROLE OF HYPOTHERMIA IN ACUTE LUNG INJURY

Induced hypothermia has long been employed in medicine to preserve tissue integrity in the context of compromised oxygenation, for example, during surgery under circulatory arrest, ischemic brain injury, and ex vivo organ preservation.[36–39] Besides its effect on metabolism, hypothermia has been shown to modulate the inflammatory response of the host.[40–42] In particular, the down-regulation of the number and activity of neutrophils during hypothermia[40,41] could be relevant to the treatment of septic ALI because the latter syndrome is characterized by intense neutrophil-mediated inflammation.[43]

### Effects of Hypothermia on Critical Organ Systems

#### Brain

During hypothermia in mammals, the global cerebral metabolic rate for glucose and oxygen is decreased, whereas glycolysis is enhanced through intracellular alkalinization.[44] Compared with normothermia, brain ischemic tolerance is thus longer during hypothermia, 11 to 19 minutes at 28°C and 39 to 65 minutes at 18°C in humans.[45] In this regard, many studies have shown that hypothermia is effective in attenuating brain injury associated with hypoxia and ischemia.[37,38,46–50] Cerebral protection resulting from profound hypothermia can be readily correlated with a decrease in the cerebral requirement for oxygen.[51] Unlike the mechanism of cerebral protection by profound hypothermia, however, cerebral protection by mild hypothermia is thought to be related to as yet unidentified mechanisms involving ion homeostasis, membrane stability, enzyme functions, neurotransmitter release or reuptake, and cellular structure.[52,53]

#### Cardiovascular System

Cardiac output has been shown to decrease in proportion to the degree of hypothermia.[54] Most of the decrease in cardiac output is attributable to the decrease in heart rate, because stroke volume is relatively preserved. The decrease in heart rate by hypothermia is associated with the suppression of both pacemaker activity and conduction velocity.[55] During hypothermia, left ventricular compliance decreases, and diastolic pressure of the left ventricle increases.[56] With alteration of the pressure-volume relationship, contractility of the left ventricle is decreased.

In the peripheral circulation, many changes occur during hypothermia. Blood becomes more viscous,[57] and systemic vascular resistance increases,[58] with the latter serving to preserve blood flow to the heart and brain.[58,59] Although oxygen consumption of the myocardium decreases during hypothermia,[60] blood and nutrient supply to the myocardium is relatively well preserved.[58] During moderate hypothermia, coronary arterial resistance increases, and thus coronary blood flow decreases.[46,61] With deeper than moderate hypothermia, however, coronary blood flow may increase as a result of direct cold-induced vasodilation.[62,63]

### Lung

In terms of ventilatory mechanics, hypothermia decreases lung compliance,[64] respiration rate, and tidal volume.[65] If moderate hypothermia is maintained over a longer period of time, ventilatory function will return to the level observed during normothermia, suggesting that the transient alteration in ventilatory function accompanying hypothermia is related to a change in central chemoreceptor sensitivity to $CO_2$.[65] During hypothermia, pulmonary vascular resistance increases, mostly because of an increase in pulmonary venous resistance.[66] Morphology of the lung parenchyma is minimal during surface cooling, whereas hypothermia associated with cardiopulmonary bypass is known to induce lung parenchymal damage, pulmonary edema, atelectasis, and interstitial/intra-alveolar hemorrhage.[67] Hypoxic pulmonary vasoconstriction, an innate protective mechanism against hypoxia associated with shunt, may be disrupted during hypothermia.[68]

### Immunologic-Inflammatory System

Considerable animal and human evidence indicates that mild core hypothermia directly impairs immune function. Various components of the immune system, such as natural killer cell activity[69] and cell-mediated antibody production,[70,71] are adversely affected by exposure to cold. Neutrophils are especially sensitive to hypothermia. Quantitatively, hypothermia has been shown to decrease the number of circulating neutrophils and to suppress the release of neutrophils from the bone marrow induced by endotoxin or other stimuli.[40] Qualitatively, hypothermia has been shown to decrease the in vivo migration of neutrophils,[41] which may occur at different levels of cell-tissue interaction through the suppression of endothelial expression of E-selectin[72] or the suppression of β-integrin expression by extravasated neutrophils themselves.[73] The production of oxygen radicals by neutrophils is also decreased during hypothermia.[74]

At the molecular level, hypothermia attenuates the release of various cytokines, such as IL-1β, IL-2, IL-6, and IL-8, compared with normothermia.[61,75,76]

The normal increase in IL-1β RNA observed in rats following traumatic brain injury was shown to be suppressed by hypothermia.[61] In a recent animal study, the level of IL-1β in BAL fluid induced by endotoxin administration was lower during hypothermia compared with normothermia, whereas the level of IL-10, a potent anti-inflammatory cytokine, in BAL fluid was higher during hypothermia than during normothermia.[76] In contrast, production of the proinflammatory cytokine TNF-α may be up-regulated by hypothermia.[76,77]

Relatively little is known about whether and how hypothermia influences macrophages in various organ systems, including alveolar macrophages in the lung. In a recent animal study, alveolar macrophage functions in the endotoxin-challenged lung were inhibited during hypothermia, as evidenced by the release of TNF-α, the earliest proinflammatory cytokine secreted in response to endotoxin.[78] In other studies, peritoneal macrophages exhibited lower phagocytic activity during hypothermia than during normothermia.[79,80] Furthermore, the proliferation and inflammatory response of microglia, the macrophages of the central nervous system, are reduced during hypothermia.[81,82]

## Clinical Aspects of Hypothermia

### Experiences in Acute Lung Injury

Because of its cerebroprotective effect in ischemia and suppression of neutrophil-mediated inflammation, hypothermia may be of therapeutic or preventive potential in ALI. There have been a few anecdotal reports on the use of hypothermia in moribund patients with ALI/ARDS.[69,83,84] Hypothermia was used to reduce cardiac output in five patients with acute respiratory failure who were undergoing extracorporeal membrane lung perfusion, and it led to the survival of four of these patients.[83] Hypothermia was also used in conjunction with high-frequency jet ventilation in a moribund patient with respiratory failure, who subsequently survived the refractory hypoxia.[49] There have been few controlled studies on the effect of hypothermia in the context of ALI/ARDS. In a study of induced hypothermia of 32° to 35° C in 19 patients with septic ARDS, oxygen extraction increased, shunt decreased, and mortality decreased, compared with control patients.[85] Several investigational studies support the usefulness of hypothermia in treating ARDS. Hypothermia either before or after treatment resulted in an attenuation of ALI.[76,86] This was associated with a decrease in endotoxin-induced neutrophil sequestration in the lung and decreased production of proinflammatory cytokines such as IL-1β. Oxidative burst of neutrophils, as assessed by phorbol myristate acetate, was also attenuated during hypothermia.[87] In another study, hypothermia appeared to attenuate hemorrhage, permeability edema, and

epithelial injury in lungs sustaining mechanical hyperinflation.[88] Through its low-flow state, hypothermia can be a paradigm of "lung rest" preventing the development of ventilator-induced lung injury, because this is partly aggravated by circulatory overload.[57]

### Complications of Hypothermia

Mild to moderate intraoperative hypothermia results in a significant increase in wound infections through decreased availability of subcutaneous oxygen from thermoregulatory vasoconstriction.[89,90] Hypothermia also directly impairs the immune function of the host, as discussed earlier.

**Cardiac Effects** Perioperative hypothermia may precipitate myocardial ischemia or ventricular arrhythmias through as yet unclear mechanisms.[91,92] In particular, fatal ventricular arrhythmias may occur at core temperatures lower than 28°C.[93] Apart from perioperative reports, however, the incidence of adverse cardiac events during the application and withdrawal of mild hypothermia has not been significant.[37,38,85]

**Pulmonary Effects** Hypothermia itself can increase pulmonary vascular resistance,[66] decrease lung compliance,[64] and induce minimal congestion and patchy atelectasis of the lung.[67] Monitoring of pulse oximetry may be difficult during hypothermia.[94]

**Coagulopathies** Hypothermia generally increases blood loss.[95] Although platelet count remains normal,[96] hypothermia has been shown to induce morphologic changes in platelet structure,[97,98] as well as the release of a circulating anticoagulant with heparin-like effects.[87] Hypothermia of 35°C or lower has been shown to prolong activated partial thromboplastin time by 10% compared with 37°C.[99] Fibrinolysis is largely unaffected by mild hypothermia.[100]

**Pharmacokinetics and Pharmacodynamics** The enzymes that moderate organ function and metabolize most drugs are highly temperature sensitive. The pharmacokinetic properties of drugs administered during hypothermia, however, have not been fully elucidated. In one study, the duration of action of vecuronium more than doubled in patients assigned to 2°C core hypothermia.[101]

### Methods for the Induction and Withdrawal of Therapeutic Hypothermia

There are several methods for inducing hypothermia, each with its own advantages and disadvantages. Surface cooling using cold gas or ice packs is a practical method for the induction of mild hypothermia.[37,38] In contrast, the pulmonary circulation can be adopted as a heat exchanger using a cold medium such as perfluorocarbon.[102–104] The optimal depth and duration of hypothermia have not yet been determined, let alone the method of rewarming. Because of the scarcity of clinical and experimental data, mild hypothermia (33° to 34°C) appears to be a prudent bedside application of this still experimental therapy.[37,38,52,85,105] Many recent clinical trials have chosen 12 to 24 hours for the duration of hypothermia, followed by passive rewarming over 12 to 24 hours.[37,38,105] The method and potential complications of rewarming from hypothermia remain largely unanswered.

## Future Directions

In view of the profound effects of hypothermia on inflammatory cellular activities and oxygen metabolism, the therapeutic use of hypothermia seems a plausible option in patients with ALI/ARDS. Detailed protocols for the bedside application of hypothermia have not yet been determined, however, especially in regard to the optimal depth and duration of hypothermia, the pharmacokinetics of drugs commonly used in these diseases, and the method of rewarming that best preserves the benefits while avoiding physiologic rebound associated with hypothermia.

## REFERENCES

1. Acute Respiratory Distress Syndrome Network: Ventilation with lower tidal volumes as compared with traditional tidal volumes for acute lung injury and the acute respiratory distress syndrome. N Engl J Med 2000;342:1301–1308.
2. Kozak W: Fever: A possible strategy for membrane homeostasis during infection. Perspect Biol Med 1993;37:14–34.
3. De Maio A: Heat shock proteins: Facts, thoughts, and dreams. Shock 1999;11:1–12.
4. Theodorakis NG, Drujan D, De Maio A: Thermotolerant cells show an attenuated expression of HSP70 after heat shock. J Biol Chem 1999;274:12081–12086.
5. Kiang JG, Tsokos GC: Heat shock protein 70 kDa: Molecular biology, biochemistry, and physiology. Pharmacol Ther 1998;80:183–201.
6. Li GC, Yang SH, Kim D, et al: Suppression of heat-induced HSP70 expression by the 70-kDa subunit of the human Ku autoantigen. Proc Natl Acad Sci U S A 1995;92: 4512–4516.
7. Moseley PL: Heat shock proteins and the inflammatory response. Ann N Y Acad Sci 1998;856:206–213.
8. Wong HR, Ryan M, Wispe JR: The heat shock response inhibits inducible nitric oxide synthase gene expression by blocking I kappa-B degradation and NF-kappa B nuclear translocation. Biochem Biophys Res Commun 1997;231:257–263.
9. Yoo CG, Lee S, Lee CT, et al: Anti-inflammatory effect of heat shock protein induction is related to stabilization of I kappa B alpha through preventing I kappa B kinase activation in respiratory epithelial cells. J Immunol 2000;164:5416–5423.
10. Mosser DD, Caron AW, Bourget L, et al: Role of the human heat shock protein HSP70 in protection against stress-induced apoptosis. Mol Cell Biol 1997;17:5317–5327.
11. Meriin AB, Yaglom JA, Gabai VL, et al: Protein-damaging stresses activate c-Jun N-terminal kinase via inhibition of its dephosphorylation: A novel pathway controlled by HSP72. Mol Cell Biol 1999;19:2547–2555.
12. Weiss YG, Bouwman A, Gehan B, et al: Cecal ligation and double puncture impairs heat shock protein 70 (HSP-70) expression in the lungs of rats. Shock 2000;13:19–23.
13. Schroeder S, Lindemann C, Hoeft A, et al: Impaired inducibility of heat shock protein 70 in peripheral blood lymphocytes of patients with severe sepsis. Crit Care Med 1999;27:1080–1084.
14. Bruemmer-Smith S, Stuber F, Schroeder S: Protective functions of intracellular heat-shock protein (HSP) 70-expression in patients with severe sepsis. Intensive Care Med 2001;27: 1835–1841.
15. Plumier JC, Ross BM, Currie RW, et al: Transgenic mice expressing the human heat shock protein 70 have improved post-ischemic myocardial recovery. J Clin Invest 1995;95:1854–1860.
16. Hiratsuka M, Mora BN, Yano M, et al: Gene transfer of heat shock protein 70 protects lung grafts from ischemia-reperfusion injury. Ann Thorac Surg 1999;67:1421–1427.
17. Malhotra V, Wong HR: Interactions between the heat shock response and the nuclear factor-kappa B signaling pathway. Crit Care Med 2002;30:S89–S95.
18. Ryan AJ, Flanagan SW, Moseley PL, et al: Acute heat stress protects rats against endotoxin shock. J Appl Physiol 1992;73: 1517–1522.
19. Villar J, Edelson JD, Post M, et al: Induction of heat stress proteins is associated with decreased mortality in an animal model of acute lung injury. Am Rev Respir Dis 1993;147: 177–181.
20. Villar J, Ribeiro SP, Mullen JB, et al: Induction of the heat shock response reduces mortality rate and organ damage in a sepsis-induced acute lung injury model. Crit Care Med 1994;22: 914–921.
21. Koh Y, Lim CM, Kim MJ, et al: The effect of heat shock response on the tumor necrosis factor-alpha–induced acute lung injury in rats. Tuberc Respir Dis 1997;44:1343–1352.
22. Koh Y, Lim CM, Kim MJ, et al: Heat shock response decreases endotoxin-induced acute lung injury in rats. Respirology 1999;4:325–330.
23. Koh Y, Lee YM, Lim CM, et al: Effects of heat pretreatment on histopathology, cytokine production, and surfactant in endotoxin-induced acute lung injury. Inflammation 2001;25:187–196.
24. Ribeiro SP, Rhee K, Tremblay L, et al: Heat stress attenuates ventilator-induced lung dysfunction in an ex vivo rat lung model. Am J Respir Crit Care Med 2001;163:1451–1456.
25. Hotchkiss R, Nunnally I, Lindquist S, et al: Hyperthermia protects mice against the lethal effects of endotoxin. Am J Physiol 1993;265:R1447–R1457.
26. Wang JH, Redmond HP, Watson RW, et al: Induction of heat shock protein 72 prevents neutrophil-mediated human endothelial cell necrosis. Arch Surg 1995;130:260–1265.
27. Smith ME, Gunther R, Gee M, et al: Leukocytes, platelets, and thromboxane A2 in endotoxin-induced lung injury. Surgery 1981;90:102–107.
28. Ribeiro SP, Villar J, Slutsky AS: Induction of the stress response to prevent organ injury. New Horiz 1995;3:301–311.
29. Hall TJ: Role of HSP70 in cytokine production. Experientia 1994;50:1048–1053.
30. Ensor JE, Wiener SM, McCrea KA, et al: Differential effects of hyperthermia on macrophage interleukin-6 and tumor necrosis factor-alpha expression. Am J Physiol 1994;266: C967–C974.

31. Snyder YM, Guthrie L, Evans GF, et al: Transcriptional inhibition of endotoxin-induced monokine synthesis following heat shock in murine peritoneal macrophages. J Leukoc Biol 1992;51:181–187.

32. Weiss YG, Maloyan A, Tazelaar J, et al: Adenoviral transfer of HSP-70 into pulmonary epithelium ameliorates experimental acute respiratory distress syndrome. J Clin Invest 2002;110:801–806.

33. Kindas-Mugge I, Pohl WR, Zavadova E, et al: Alveolar macrophages of patients with adult respiratory distress syndrome express high levels of heat shock protein 72 mRNA. Shock 1996;5:184–189.

34. Durand P, Bachelet M, Brunet F, et al: Inducibility of the 70 kD heat shock protein in peripheral blood monocytes is decreased in human acute respiratory distress syndrome and recovers over time. Am J Respir Crit Care Med 2000;161:286–292.

35. Lindquist S, Craig EA: The heat-shock proteins. Annu Rev Genet 1988;22:631–677.

36. Rittenhouse EA, Mori H, Dillard DH, et al: Deep hypothermia in cardiovascular surgery. Ann Thorac Surg 1974;17:63–98.

37. Hypothermia after Cardiac Arrest Study Group: Mild therapeutic hypothermia to improve the neurologic outcome after cardiac arrest. N Engl J Med 2002;346:549–556.

38. Bernard SA, Gray TW, Buist MD, et al: Treatment of comatose survivors of out-of-hospital cardiac arrest with induced hypothermia. N Engl J Med 2002;346:557–563.

39. Belzer FO, Southard JH: Principles of solid-organ preservation by cold storage. Transplantation 1988;45:673–676.

40. Biggar WD, Bohn D, Kent G: Neutrophil circulation and release from bone marrow during hypothermia. Infect Immun 1983;40:708–712.

41. Biggar WD, Bohn DJ, Kent G, et al: Neutrophil migration in vitro and in vivo during hypothermia. Infect Immun 1984;46:857–859.

42. Irazuzta JE, Pretzlaff R, Rowin M, et al: Hypothermia as an adjunctive treatment for severe bacterial meningitis. Brain Res 2000;881:88–97.

43. Weiland JE, Davis WB, Holter JF, et al: Lung neutrophils in the adult respiratory distress syndrome: Clinical and pathophysiologic significance. Am Rev Respir Dis 1986;133:218–225.

44. Erecinska M, Thoresen M. Silver IA: Effects of hypothermia on energy metabolism in mammalian central nervous system. J Cereb Blood Flow Metab 2003;23:513–530.

45. Greeley WJ, Kern FH, Ungerleider RM, et al: The effect of hypothermic cardiopulmonary bypass and total circulatory arrest on cerebral metabolism in neonates, infants, and children. J Thorac Cardiovasc Surg 1991;101:783–794.

46. Ginsberg MD, Sternau LL, Globus MY-T, et al: Therapeutic modulation of brain temperature: Relevance to ischemic brain injury. Cerebrovasc Brain Metab Rev 1992;4:189–225.

47. Maher J, Hachinski V: Hypothermia as a potential treatment for cerebral ischemia. Cerebrovasc Brain Metab Rev 1993;5:277–300.

48. Barone FC, Feuerstein GZ, White RF: Brain cooling during transient focal ischemia provides complete neuroprotection. Neurosci Biobehav Rev 1997;21:31–44.

49. Colbourne F, Sutherland G, Corbett D: Postischemic hypothermia: A critical appraisal with implications for clinical treatment. Mol Neurobiol 1997;14:171–201.

50. Wagner CL, Eicher DJ, Katikaneni LD, et al: The use of hypothermia: A role in the treatment of neonatal asphyxia? Pediatr Neurol 1999;21:429–443.

51. Michenfelder JD, Milde JH: The effect of profound levels of hypothermia (below 14 degrees C) on canine cerebral metabolism. J Cereb Blood Flow Metab 1992;12:877–880.

52. Soukup J, Zauner A, Doppenberg EM, et al: Relationship between brain temperature, brain chemistry and oxygen delivery after severe human head injury: The effect of mild hypothermia. Neurol Res 2002;24:161–168.

53. Lanier WL: Cerebral metabolic rate and hypothermia: Their relationship with ischemic neurologic injury. J Neurosurg Anesthesiol 1995;7:216–221.

54. Rittenhouse EA, Ito CS, Mohri H, et al: Circulatory dynamics during surface-induced deep hypothermia and after cardiac arrest for one hour. J Thorac Cardiovasc Surg 1971;61:359–369.

55. Mouritzen CV, Andersen MN: Mechanisms of ventricular fibrillation during hypothermia: Relative changes in myocardial refractory period and conduction velocity. J Thorac Cardiovasc Surg 1966;51:579–584.

56. Remensnyder JP, Austen WG.: Diastolic pressure-volume relationships of the left ventricle during hypothermia. J Thorac Cardiovasc Surg 1965;49:339–351.

57. Eckmann DM, Bowers S, Stecker M, et al: Hematocrit, volume expander, temperature, and shear rate effects on blood viscosity. Anesth Analg 2000;91:539–545.

58. Zarins CK, Skinner DB: Circulation in profound hypothermia. J Surg Res 1973;14:97–104.

59. Delin NA, Kjartansson KB, Pollock L, et al: Redistribution of regional blood flow in hypothermia. J Thorac Cardiovasc Surg 1965;49:511–516.

60. Russ C, Lee JC: Effect of hypothermia on myocardial metabolism. Am J Physiol 1965;208:1253–1258.

61. Goss JR, Styren SD, Miller PD, et al: Hypothermia attenuates the normal increase in interleukin 1 beta RNA and nerve growth factor following traumatic brain injury in the rat. J Neurotrauma 1995;12:159–167.

62. Berne RM: The effect of immersion hypothermia on coronary blood flow. Circ Res 1954;2:236–242.

63. Berne RM: Cardiodynamics and the coronary circulation in hypothermia. Ann N Y Acad Sci 1959;80:365–383.

64. Deal CW, Osborn JJ, Louis E, et al: Respiratory work in relation to cardiopulmonary bypass. Thorax 1967;22:139–141.

65. Blair E, Esmond WG, Attar S, et al: The effect of hypothermia on lung function. Ann Surg 1964;160:814–823.

66. Stern S, Braun K: Pulmonary arterial and venous response to cooling: Role of alpha-adrenergic receptors. Am J Physiol 1970;219:982–985.

67. Ashmore PG, Wakeford J, Harterre D: Pulmonary complications of profound hypothermia with circulatory arrest in experimental animal. Can J Surg 1964;41:93–96.

68. Benumof JL, Wahrenbrock EA: Dependency of hypoxic pulmonary vasoconstriction on temperature. J Appl Physiol 1977;42:56–58.

69. Hurst JM, deHaven CB, Branson R, et al: Combined use of high-frequency jet ventilation and induced hypothermia in the treatment of refractory respiratory failure. Crit Care Med 1985;13:771–772.

70. Cheng YS, Yin FH, Foundling S, et al: Stability and activity of human immunodeficiency virus protease: Comparison of the natural dimer with a homologous, single-chain tethered dimer. Proc Natl Acad Sci U S A 1990;87:9660–9664.

71. Beilin B, Shavit Y, Razumovsky J, et al: Effects of mild perioperative hypothermia on cellular immune responses. Anesthesiology 1998;89:1133–1140.

72. Johnson M, Haddix T, Pohlman T, et al: Hypothermia reversibly inhibits endothelial cell expression of E-selectin and tissue factor. J Card Surg 1995;10:428–435.

73. Rowin ME, Xue V, Irazuzta J: Hypothermia attenuates beta1 integrin expression on extravasated neutrophils in an animal model of meningitis. Inflammation 2001;25:137–144.

74. Wenisch C, Narzt E, Sessler DI, et al: Mild intraoperative hypothermia reduces production of reactive oxygen intermediates by polymorphonuclear leukocytes. Anesth Analg 1996;82:810–816.

75. Nandate K, Vuylsteke A, Crosbie AE, et al: Cerebrovascular cytokine responses during coronary artery bypass surgery: specific production of interleukin-8 and its attenuation by hypothermic cardiopulmonary bypass. Anesth Analg 1999;89:823–828.

76. Lim CM, Kim MS, Ahn JJ, et al: Hypothermia protects against endotoxin-induced acute lung injury in rats. Intensive Care Med 2003;29:453–459.

77. Wan S, Yim AP, Arifi AA, et al: Can cardioplegia management influence cytokine responses during clinical cardiopulmonary bypass? Ann Thorac Cardiovasc Surg 1999;5:81–85.

78. Lim CM, Kim EK, Koh Y, et al: Hypothermia inhibits cytokine release of alveolar macrophage and activation of nuclear factor kappa B in endotoxemic lung. Intensive Care Med 2004;30:1638–1644.

79. Salman H, Bergman M, Bessler H, et al: Hypothermia affects the phagocytic activity of rat peritoneal macrophages. Acta Physiol Scand 2000;168:431–436.

80. Houstek J, Holub M: Cold-induced changes in brown adipose tissue thermogenic capacity of immunocompetent and immunodeficient hairless mice. J Comp Physiol 1994;164:459–463.

81. Si QS, Nakamura Y, Kataoka K: Hypothermic suppression of microglial activation in culture: Inhibition of cell proliferation and production of nitric oxide and superoxide. Neuroscience 1997;81:223–229.

82. Inamasu J, Suga S, Sato S, et al: Post-ischemic hypothermia delayed neutrophil accumulation and microglial activation following transient focal ischemia in rats. J Neuroimmunol 2000;109:66–74.

83. Zapol WM, Qvist J, Pontoppidan H, et al: Extracorporeal perfusion for acute respiratory failure: Recent experience with the spiral coil membrane lung. J Thorac Cardiovasc Surg 1975;69:439–449.

84. Moonka R, Gentilello L: Hypothermia induced by continuous arteriovenous hemofiltration as a treatment for adult respiratory distress syndrome: A case report. J Trauma 1996;40:1026–1028.

85. Villar J, Slutsky AS: Effects of induced hypothermia in patients with septic adult respiratory distress syndrome. Resuscitation 1993;26:183–192.

86. Chin JY, Koh Y, Lim CM: Effect of mild hypothermia on endotoxin-induced acute lung injury in rats. J Jpn Respir Soc 2004;42:61.

87. Paul J, Cornillon B, Baguet J, et al: In vivo release of a heparin-like factor in dogs during profound hypothermia. J Thorac Cardiovasc Surg 1981;82:45–48.

88. Lim CM, Hong SB, Koh Y, et al: Hypothermia attenuates vascular manifestations of ventilator-induced lung injury in rats. Lung 2003;181:23–34.

89. Kurz A, Sessler DI, Lenhardt R: Perioperative normothermia to reduce the incidence of surgical-wound infection and shorten hospitalization: Study of Wound Infection and Temperature Group. N Engl J Med 1996;334:1209–1215.

90. Tayefeh F, Kurz A, Sessler DI, et al: Thermoregulatory vasodilation increases the venous partial pressure of oxygen. Anesth Analg 1997;85:657–662.

91. Frank SM, Fleisher LA, Breslow MJ, et al: Perioperative maintenance of normothermia reduces the incidence of morbid cardiac events: A randomized clinical trial. JAMA 1997;277:1127–1134.

92. Insler SR, O'Connor MS, Leventhal MJ, et al: Association between postoperative hypothermia and adverse outcome after coronary artery bypass surgery. Ann Thorac Surg 2000;70:175–181.

93. Janssens U, Schneider B, Hanrath P: Electrocardiographic changes in unintentional hypothermia: The J wave. Intensive Care Med 1998;24:1118–1119.

94. Kober A, Scheck T, Lieba F, et al: The influence of active warming on signal quality of pulse oximetry in prehospital trauma care. Anesth Analg 2002;95:961–966.

95. Schmied H, Kurz A, Sessler DI, et al: Mild hypothermia increases blood loss and transfusion requirements during total hip arthroplasty. Lancet 1996;347:289–292.

96. Kettner SC, Sitzwohl C, Zimpfer M, et al: The effect of graded hypothermia (36 degrees C–32 degrees C) on hemostasis in anesthetized patients without surgical trauma. Anesth Analg 2003;96:1772–1776.

97. Faraday N, Rosenfeld BA: In vitro hypothermia enhances platelet GPIIb-IIIa activation and P-selectin expression. Anesthesiology 1998;88:1579–1585.

98. Ferrell JE Jr, Martin GS: Platelet tyrosine-specific protein phosphorylation is regulated by thrombin. Mol Cell Biol 1988;8:3603–3610.

99. Felfernig M, Blaicher A, Kettner SC, et al: Effects of temperature on partial thromboplastin time in heparinized plasma in vitro. Eur J Anaesthesiol 2001;18:467–470.

100. Watts DD, Trask A, Soeken K, et al: Hypothermic coagulopathy in trauma: Effect of varying levels of hypothermia on enzyme speed, platelet function, and fibrinolytic activity. J Trauma 1998;44:846–854.

101. Heier T, Caldwell JE, Sessler DI, et al: Mild intraoperative hypothermia increases duration of action and spontaneous recovery of vecuronium blockade during nitrous oxide-isoflurane anesthesia in humans. Anesthesiology 1991;74:815–819.

102. Harrison MR, Hysing ES, Bo G: Control of body temperature: Use of respiratory tract as a heat exchanger. J Pediatr Surg 1977;12:821–828.

103. Forman DL, Bhutani VK, Tran N, et al: A new approach to induced hypothermia. J Surg Res 1986;40:36–42.

104. Hong SB, Koh Y, Shim TS, et al: Physiologic characteristics of cold perfluorocarbon-induced hypothermia during partial liquid ventilation in normal rabbits. Anesth Analg 2002;94:157–162.

105. Marion DW, Obrist WD, Carlier PM, et al: The use of moderate therapeutic hypothermia for patients with severe head injuries: A preliminary report. J Neurosurg 1993;79:354–362.

## SUGGESTED READINGS

Clardy CW, Edwards KM, Gay JC: Increased susceptibility to infection in hypothermic children: Possible role of acquired neutrophil dysfunction. Pediatr Infect Dis 1985;4:379–382.

Dreyfuss D, Saumon G: Ventilator-induced lung injury: Lessons from experimental studies. Am J Respir Crit Care Med 1998;157:294–323.

Hohn DC, MacKay RD, Halliday B, et al: Effect of oxygen tension on microbicidal function of leukocytes in wounds and in vitro. Surg Forum 1976;27:18–20.

Ning XH, Chen SH, Xu CS, et al: Hypothermia preserves myocardial function and mitochondrial protein gene expression during hypoxia. Am J Physiol 2003;285:H212–H219.

van Oss CJ, Absolom DR, Moore LL, et al: Effect of temperature on the chemotaxis, phagocytic engulfment, digestion and $O_2$ consumption of human polymorphonuclear leukocytes. J Reticuloendothel Soc 1980;27:561–565.

Wollenek G, Honarwar N, Golej J, et al: Cold water submersion and cardiac arrest in treatment of severe hypothermia with cardiopulmonary bypass. Resuscitation 2002;52:255–263.

# CHAPTER 7

# Severe Acute Respiratory Syndrome (SARS)

Gavin M. Joynt

Severe acute respiratory syndrome (SARS) is a viral pneumonia caused by a newly described coronavirus (SARS-CoV). During the SARS epidemic of November 2002 to July 2003, more than 8000 people in 26 countries on five continents were infected, of whom 774 lost their lives.[1] Sporadic, non–laboratory-associated cases of SARS have since been reported from southern China and highlight the possibility of repeated epidemics.

## PATHOPHYSIOLOGY

SARS is the consequence of human infection with the SARS-CoV. SARS-CoV has been repeatedly isolated from the nasopharynx, respiratory secretions, feces, and blood of patients with SARS, and seroconversion has been consistently demonstrated in survivors.[2–4] Individuals with potential exposure to SARS cases, but who do not develop the clinical syndrome, generally do not show evidence of seroconversion.[5] Direct evidence of causation is provided by the observation that experimental infection of cynomolgus macaques with SARS-CoV results in a similar clinical and histologic respiratory disease to that observed in humans.[6] The causative link between the SARS-CoV and SARS has therefore been well established; however, the pathophysiologic mechanisms by which this syndrome occurs are less clear.

Clinical observation and histologic studies confirm that the pathologic effects of infection are largely, but not exclusively, confined to the respiratory tract. Bronchial epithelial denudation, loss of cilia, and squamous metaplasia occur early.[7] In lung tissue, an early phase of hyaline membrane formation, edema, and pneumocyte proliferation is followed by diffuse alveolar damage characterized by an exudative and proliferative phase.[7,8] Although these features appear similar to findings in acute respiratory distress syndrome (ARDS), characteristics such as predominant macrophage proliferation in consolidated areas and the presence of multinucleate giant cells are more specific for SARS and may suggest an important role for proinflammatory cytokines in the pathogenesis of SARS.[7] Some data suggest that the viral load in the respiratory secretions of patients with SARS is characterized by a peak occurring around the 10th day of illness followed by a decrease in viral load, concomitant with the appearance of an antibody response to the virus.[9] However, in most patients, clinical deterioration occurs progressively during the second week of illness despite a stable or decreasing viral load. This time course supports the suggestion that part of the lung damage may be immunopathologic.[8,9] Serum cytokine levels in patients with SARS have been measured. Observational data suggest that proinflammatory cytokines such as tumor necrosis factor and interleukin (IL)-6, IL-8, and IL-16 are increased and peak during the 8th to 14th day following illness onset.[10]

Diarrhea is the most commonly reported sign of gastrointestinal involvement reported in patients with SARS.[11] Viral particles have been detected in splenic tissue and the gastrointestinal tract[12]; however, no cytolytic damage or inflammatory change has been histologically demonstrated in the small or large bowel. Although subclinical myocardial diastolic dysfunction in patients with SARS has been described, histologic examination of cardiac muscle did not reveal any evidence of endocarditis, interstitial lymphocytic infiltrate, or myocardial cell necrosis.[13] The cause of the dysfunction may be related to the effects of mechanical ventilation or circulating cytokines.

In summary, the pathophysiology of SARS remains obscure. The common presenting features (see later), many of which are similar to other viral infections, may be the consequence of viral replication, proinflammatory mediator production, or other as yet undiscovered mechanisms. The severe and largely isolated respiratory system manifestations typical of SARS are associated with evidence of both viral replication and proinflammatory mediator release, but exact pathophysiologic mechanisms are unknown. As has now been demonstrated in other infective conditions, it is also possible that genetic predisposition may play a role in determining the progression and ultimate severity of illness in individuals, but no published data as yet support this hypothesis.

## CLINICAL PRESENTATION

Patients usually present with fever, chills, rigors, myalgia, and headache. A nonproductive cough is present in only approximately 50% of patients on presentation. Sore throat and rhinorrhea are infrequent (Fig. 7.1).[8] Common laboratory features include an elevated serum lactate dehydrogenase concentration, lymphopenia, hypocalcemia,

and moderate thrombocytopenia.[8,14] The respiratory syndrome caused by SARS-CoV typically has an insidious onset. Although fever and other systemic symptoms may improve during the first week, particularly if anti-inflammatory therapy is used, the more important markers of clinical deterioration are progressive hypoxia and dyspnea, accompanied by the progression of pulmonary infiltrates on chest radiograph (Fig. 7.2).[8] Respiratory symptoms worsen slowly but steadily and reach a peak in the most severe cases during the first 10 to 15 days.[15] Published data consistently show that the time from symptom onset to intensive care unit (ICU) admission in these severe cases was approximately 8 to 10 days.[16–18] During the outbreak, approximately 20% to 30% of all patients with SARS required ICU admission.[8,9,14,16–19]

Admission to the ICU is almost always the consequence of progressive, severe respiratory failure. Current series reported an inability to maintain arterial oxygen saturation greater than 90% to 92% despite administration of supplemental oxygen at concentrations of more than 50% to 60% as criteria for admission to ICU

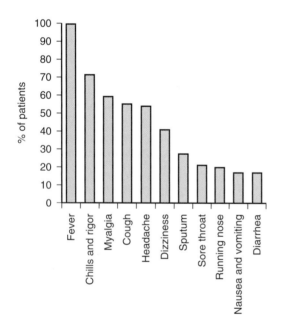

**Figure 7.1** Frequency of distribution of symptoms of patients presenting with severe acute respiratory syndrome (SARS). (Adapted from Lee N, Hui D, Wu A, et al: A major outbreak of severe acute respiratory syndrome in Hong Kong. N Engl J Med 2003;348:1986–1994.)

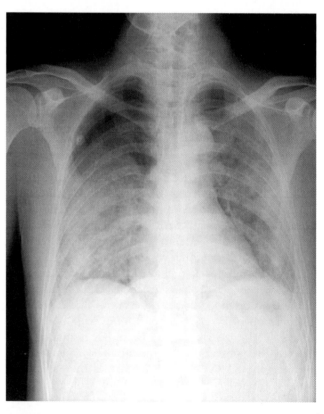

**Figure 7.2** Chest radiograph showing bilateral heterogeneous consolidation in both lungs in a 47-year-old male patient with severe acute respiratory syndrome (SARS). The patient has a small, spontaneous right pneumothorax. No pleural effusion or cardiomegaly is seen.

for monitoring. In the currently reported ICU series, more than 90% of patients met the clinical criteria of ARDS following admission (acute onset of bilateral diffuse pulmonary infiltrates on chest radiograph, a ratio of arterial oxygen tension to fractional inspired oxygen concentration ($PaO_2/FiO_2$) of less than 200 mm Hg, and the absence of left atrial hypertension[20]).[16–18] Median Acute Physiology and Chronic Health Evaluation (APACHE) II scores were reported to range between 11 and 19.5, and most patients had isolated respiratory failure on admission.[16–18]

## DIAGNOSIS

During the early outbreak, the World Health Organization (WHO) and the Centers for Disease Control and Prevention (CDC) criteria, comprising clinical, epidemiologic, and laboratory features for the diagnosis of SARS, were successfully used.[21] Briefly, these criteria were as follows. Patients demonstrating the clinical features of a temperature higher than 38°C and one or more clinical findings of respiratory illness (e.g., cough, shortness of breath, difficulty breathing, or hypoxia), as well as the epidemiologic features of travel within 10 days of onset of symptoms to an area with current suspected community transmission of SARS, or close contact within 10 days of onset of symptoms with a person known or suspected to have SARS, were considered suspect cases. Probable cases were defined as those having the foregoing features, as well as evidence of pneumonia on a chest radiograph or computed tomography scan. Because of the variable performance of laboratory testing for SARS at this time, case classification did not rely on laboratory criteria.

Currently, in the absence of an outbreak and endemic areas, epidemiologic criteria are of very limited use in assisting diagnosis. Only specific epidemiologic criteria, such as a history of laboratory exposure to the SARS virus, remain important. The current laboratory diagnostic criteria from the CDC are therefore important and stringent. They require the detection of antibody to SARS-CoV in a serum sample, or the detection of SARS-CoV RNA by reverse transcriptase–polymerase chain reaction (RT-PCR) in two samples, or the isolation of SARS-CoV with confirmation by a PCR assay or the isolation of SARS-CoV.[22] Findings must be verified in an appropriate WHO-certified laboratory. The use of RT-PCR is problematic, however, because interpretation requires some understanding of test parameters. Peiris and colleagues found that the sensitivity of RT-PCR assay is highly dependent on the type of specimen tested and the time of collection of specimens with respect to the day of onset of symptoms.[9] In particular, the viral load as detected by RT-PCR seems to follow a triphasic pattern with a peak on day 10. Sensitivity for respiratory specimens collected at presentation is low (32%), but it increases to approximately 70% during the second week. Yam and associates found that the sensitivities of RT-PCR performed on nasopharyngeal specimens and throat swabs collected between day 1 and day 5 after admission were 61% to 68% and 65% to 72%, respectively.[23] However, repeated testing on respiratory specimens increases sensitivity to 75% to 79%. The sensitivities on urine and fecal specimens collected between day 5 and day 10 after admission are lower (50% to 60%). The optimal strategy in using RT-PCR assay remains to be defined.

The risk of false-positive results from SARS-CoV testing remains high given the current low prevalence of the disease. The burden on the health care system for contact tracing and isolation of patients with false-positive results can be significant. The WHO currently recommends SARS-CoV testing in low-risk areas *only* when there is clustering of cases fulfilling the clinical case definition of SARS in an acute care facility within the same 10-day period of onset of illness or in cases epidemiologically linked to a laboratory where specimens of SARS-CoV are handled. Routine testing of SARS-CoV in cases of atypical pneumonia unexplained by another cause is reserved for areas of potential reemergence of the infection such as Guandong in southern China.

The absence of antibody to SARS-CoV in a convalescent-phase serum sample obtained more than 28 days after symptom onset is recommended for exclusion of probable and suspected cases of SARS. With serologic tests, there is also the possibility of cross-reactions among coronaviruses.[24] Although seroconversion may occur earlier, it is not useful for diagnosing or excluding acute disease; therefore, RT-PCR assay, albeit less than ideal, remains the best current method of detecting early clinical infection.

## VENTILATORY SUPPORT AND OUTCOME

Several studies have identified prognostic factors for ICU admission. These include older age (especially patients >60 years), the presence of comorbidities (particularly diabetes mellitus and hepatic or cardiac disease), and elevated lactate dehydrogenase levels on admission to the hospital.[13,14,25] The treatment of patients admitted to the ICU is mainly confined to routine organ support; beyond routine organ support protocols, the medical therapy of patients with SARS is controversial. Although antiviral agents were extensively used in reported series, clinical data supporting the efficacy of these agents are lacking.[26–28] Anti-inflammatory therapy and immuno-modulation with steroids, particularly high-dose methylprednisolone, have been used, and although observational data in SARS suggest that high-dose methylprednisolone may be helpful in modulating the lung injury,[18,29–32] no high-quality outcome data support their use. The use of steroids for the treatment of ARDS in general remains controversial.[33–35] High-dose methylpred-nisolone may also potentially cause serious side effects, notably osteonecrosis, which can have significant long-term debilitating effects.[15] Intravenous immunoglobulin, immunoglobulin M–enriched immunoglobulin, and plasma from patients in the convalescent phase have been used in critically ill patients with SARS; however, clinical efficacy is unproven.

Severe hypoxia or the development of respiratory exhaustion leads to mechanical ventilation in 50% to 85% of patients admitted to the ICU.[16–18] Based on the similar-ity of the clinical,[13,14, 16–18] radiologic,[36] and pathologic[7,13] features, the severe hypoxemic respiratory failure associated with SARS-CoV infection appears to resemble other forms of ARDS. It therefore appears prudent to use a currently accepted ventilation strategy for patients with ARDS.[37,38] Such a strategy to minimize ventilator-associated lung injury and to improve mortality includes ventilation with low tidal volumes, optimizing positive end-expiratory pressure (PEEP) to keep the lungs continuously recruited, minimizing the inspired oxygen concentration to decrease oxygen toxicity, and accepting moderately abnormal phys-iologic blood gas values when appropriate.[39,40] All reported ICU studies to date have documented attempts to limit tidal volume to 6 to 8 mL/kg estimated lean body weight, to limit the plateau or peak airway pressure to less than 30 to 35 cm $H_2O$, to titrate PEEP to minimize the inspired oxygen concentration, and to target moderate arterial oxygen saturation (88% to 95%) while allowing the arterial partial pressure of carbon dioxide ($PaCO_2$) to rise if necessary, provided the pH is greater than 7.15.

Prone position ventilation is a technique that often improves oxygenation in ARDS.[41] Although one large, randomized, controlled trial of prone ventilation showed no improvement in mortality or organ dysfunction overall, this approach may be of benefit in more severely ill patients.[42] Prone ventilation was utilized to a varying degree in mechanically ventilated patients with SARS; however, not enough data are available to draw any conclusions regarding efficacy.[16–18] In our unit, the expe-rience with prone ventilation was one of extreme inter-patient variability in response (determined by improved oxygenation in the prone position). The use of nitric oxide in ARDS has not been shown to improve out-come, and anecdotally, the experience in Toronto and Singapore also demonstrates little benefit from nitric oxide in patients with SARS.[16,17]

Few data on noninvasive positive pressure ventilation in SARS have yet been reported, but it is our opinion that this mode of ventilation be avoided because of the risk of infected aerosol generation from inevitable mask leakage and high gas-flow compensation.[18,43] An unex-pectedly high incidence of barotrauma-related air leak has been reported in patients with SARS. Pneumothorax, pneumomediastinum, and subcutaneous emphysema, alone or in combination, occurred in 20% and 30% of patients admitted to ICU.[16–18] This incidence is high compared with rates previously reported in ARDS.[39,44] The risk does not seem to be associated with the use of excessive tidal volume or airway pressure,[16,18] and it is not limited to patients receiving mechanical ventilation.[18] The exact mechanisms for this observation are unclear, but computed tomography studies in patients with SARS have shown that the diffuse alveolar damage observed in SARS progresses to fibrosis and the formation of cysts,[45] and rupture of these cysts during or after formation could contribute to extraparenchymal gas leaks.

Data from the ICU patients of one cohort showed an association between more negative average 24-hour fluid balance and good outcome.[18] This finding corresponds with those in ARDS of non-SARS origin in which some evidence indicates that restrictive fluid management is associated with better oxygenation, lower mortality, and fewer patient ventilator days.[46,47] Causation is not proved, but it may be prudent to restrict fluid intake while maintaining adequate mean arterial pressure and organ perfusion with the appropriate use of diuretics and vasopressors. Hypotension is not a common feature of SARS, and its presence should prompt an active search for possible nosocomial infections.

Nosocomial infections are an expected complication, and in the Singapore series, 12 of 46 patients (26%) developed positive blood cultures.[17] In our unit, we observed a high incidence of ventilator-associated pneu-monia (37 episodes per 1000 ventilator days) and a high incidence of methicillin-resistant *Staphylococcus aureus* acquisition within the ICU (about 25% of SARS admis-sions). Possible contributing factors included the use of steroids, an increase in the use of prophylactic and pre-emptive antibiotics, prolonged mechanical ventilation, and the routine use of gloves and gowns, which have been shown to be associated with poor hand hygiene compliance.

ICU admission carries a high mortality rate. For patients with SARS who were admitted to the ICU, the 28-day mortality was 34% in Toronto, 37% in Singapore, and 26% in Hong Kong (with a median APACHE II score of 19.5, 18, and 11, respectively).[16–18] Longer follow-up showed a slightly higher mortality.[17] Patients who died were more often older, had higher APACHE II scores, had greater comorbidities, and were more likely to have had bilateral radiologic infiltrates on hospital admission.[16,18] Long-term complications for ICU survivors include residual pulmonary abnormalities, muscle weakness, post-traumatic stress disorder and depression, and other long-term complications of corticosteroid treatment, such as osteonecrosis.[15]

In a six-month follow up study of a cohort of SARS patients, exercise capacity and health status of SARS survivors was considerably lower than that of a normal population at 6 months.[48] Most pulmonary function test parameters were minimally impaired, although significant impairment in surface area for gas exchange was noted in 15.5% of survivors. The functional disability appeared disproportionate to the degree of lung function impairment and may have been related to additional factors such as muscle deconditioning and steroid myopathy. Lung function tests at 6 months showed moderate, but significantly lower forced vital capacity (FVC), total lung capacity (TLC), and carbon monoxide transfer factor (TLCO) in survivors who had required ICU support than in those who were treated on general wards, although no significant differences were noted in 6MWD and respiratory muscle strength.[48]

A striking feature during the epidemic was its high rate of nosocomial transmission of SARS, particularly to health care workers.[1] In addition to the risk from direct patient exposure, many procedures in the ICU, such as intubation, bronchoscopy, or the use of nebulizers and Venturi-type oxygen masks, pose an additional risk of transmission of SARS-CoV to the health care worker. Because the disease has the ability to produce significant morbidity and to incapacitate staff for long periods, staff protection is critical to ensure the continued provision of adequate ICU services. The CDC issued guidelines and recommendations on infection control in health care facilities.[49] It is considered prudent by some clinicians to adopt contact and airborne infection isolation precautions, in addition to standard precautions.[50,51] Patient isolation in rooms with appropriate air-change performance,[52] as well as the appropriate and strictly enforced use of gloves and gowns, particulate, respirators and eye protection, is required.[49–51,53]

Ventilator circuits should be isolated from the environment by the use of filters, scavenging, and closed-suction systems, for example. Environmental cleansing with appropriate solutions such as chloride and hypochlorite is an important component of infection control. Staff members should be fully informed regarding relevant advances in knowledge of SARS and properly educated on infection control precautions.[53] Psychological support should be offered to the staff.

Critical care resources can be significantly strained during a SARS outbreak, as a result of an influx of patients with SARS, the closing of institutions for quarantine, and illness or quarantine of health care workers.[16]

One important lesson learned from SARS is that prospective local and regional contingency planning for major infectious disease outbreaks is critical if adequate ICU services are to be maintained.[50]

## REFERENCES

1. World Health Organization: Summary table of SARS cases by country, 1 November 2002–7 August 2003. Available at http://www.who.int/csr/sars/country/2003_08_15/en/index.html. Accessed 14 April 2007.
2. Kuiken T, Fouchier RA, Schutten M, et al: Newly discovered coronavirus as the primary cause of severe acute respiratory syndrome. Lancet 2003;362:263–270.
3. Drosten C, Gunther S, Preiser W, et al: Identification of a novel coronavirus in patients with severe acute respiratory syndrome. N Engl J Med 2003;348:1967–1976.
4. Ksiazek TG, Erdman D, Goldsmith CS, et al: A novel coronavirus associated with severe acute respiratory syndrome. N Engl J Med 2003;348:1953–1966.
5. Chan PKS, Ip M, Ng KC, et al: Seroprevalence of severe acute respiratory syndrome (SARS)–associated coronavirus among healthcare workers after a major outbreak of SARS in a regional hospital. Emerg Infect Dis 2003;9:1453–1454.
6. Fouchier RA, Kuiken T, Schutten M, et al: Aetiology: Koch's postulates fulfilled for SARS virus. Nature 2003;423:240.
7. Nicholls JM, Poon LL, Lee KC, et al: Lung pathology of fatal severe acute respiratory syndrome. Lancet 2003;361:1773–1778.
8. Lee N, Hui D, Wu A, et al: A major outbreak of severe acute respiratory syndrome in Hong Kong. N Engl J Med 2003;348:1986–1994.
9. Peiris JS, Chu CM, Cheng VC, et al: Clinical progression and viral load in a community outbreak of coronavirus-associated SARS pneumonia: A prospective study. Lancet 2003;361:1767–1772.
10. Beijing Group of National Research Project for SARS: Dynamic changes in blood cytokine levels as clinical indicators in severe acute respiratory syndrome. Chin Med J 2003;116:1283–1287.
11. Cheng VCC, Hung IFN, Tang BSF, et al: Viral replication in the nasopharynx is associated with diarrhea in patients with severe acute respiratory syndrome. Clin Infect Dis 2004;38:467–475.
12. Leung WK, To KF, Chan PK, et al: Enteric involvement of severe acute respiratory syndrome-associated coronavirus infection. Gastroenterology 2003;125:1011–1017.
13. Li SS, Cheng CW, Fu CL, et al: Left ventricular performance in patients with severe acute respiratory syndrome: A 30-day echocardiographic follow-up study. Circulation 2003;108:1798–1803.
14. Booth CM, Matukas LM, Tomlinson GA, et al: Clinical features and short-term outcomes of 144 patients with SARS in the greater Toronto area. JAMA 2003;289:2801–2809.
15. Peiris JS, Yuen KY, Osterhaus AD, Stohr K: The severe acute respiratory syndrome. N Engl J Med 2003;349:2431–2441.
16. Fowler RA, Lapinsky SE, Hallett D, et al: Critically ill patients with severe acute respiratory syndrome. JAMA 2003;290:367–373.
17. Lew TWK, Kwek T-K, Tai D, et al: Acute respiratory distress syndrome in critically ill patients with severe acute respiratory syndrome. JAMA 2003;290:374–380.
18. Gomersall CD, Joynt GM, Lam P, et al: Short term outcome of critically ill patients with severe acute respiratory syndrome. Intensive Care Med 2004;30:381–387.

19. Choi KW, Chau TN, Tsang O, et al: Outcomes and prognostic factors in 267 patients with severe acute respiratory syndrome in Hong Kong. Ann Intern Med 2003;139:715–723.

20. Bernard GR, Artigas A, Brigham KL, et al: The American-European Consensus Conference on ARDS: Definitions, mechanisms, relevant outcomes, and clinical trial coordination. Am J Respir Crit Care Med 1994;149:818–824.

21. Centers for Disease Control and Prevention: Updated interim US case definition for severe acute respiratory syndrome (SARS): Update, April 30, 2003. Available at http://www.cdc.gov/ncidod/sars/casedefinition.htm. Accessed 3 May 2003.

22. In the Absence of SARS-CoV Transmission Worldwide: Guidance for Surveillance, Clinical and Laboratory Evaluation, and Reporting Version 2. http://www.cdc.gov/ncidod/sars/absenceofsars.htm. Accessed 16 April 2007.

23. Yam WC, Chan KH, Poon LM, et al: Evaluation of reverse transcription-PCR assays for rapid diagnosis of severe acute respiratory syndrome associated with a novel coronavirus. J Clin Microbiol 2003;41:4521–4524.

24. World Health Organization (WHO) guidelines for the global surveillance of severe acute respiratory syndrome (SARS). Updated recommendations, October 2004. http://www.who.int/csr/resources/publications/WHO_CDS_CSR_ARO_2004_1/en/. Accessed 24 April 2007.

25. Tsui PT, Kwok ML, Yuen H, Lai ST: Severe acute respiratory syndrome: Clinical outcome and prognostic correlates. Emerg Infect Dis 2003;9:1064–1069.

26. Chu CM, Cheng VC, Hung IF, et al: The role of lopinavir/ritonavir in the treatment of SARS: Initial virological and clinical findings. Thorax 2004;59:252–256.

27. Hsu LY, Lee CC, Green JA, et al: Severe acute respiratory syndrome (SARS) in Singapore: Clinical features of index patient and initial contacts. Emerg Infect Dis 2003;9:713–717.

28. Chan KS, Lai ST, Chu CM: Treatment of severe acute respiratory syndrome with lopinavir/ritonavir: A multicentre retrospective matched cohort study. Hong Kong Med J 2003;9:399–406.

29. Zhao Z, Zhang F, Xu M, et al: Description and clinical treatment of an early outbreak of severe acute respiratory syndrome (SARS) in Guangzhou, PR China. J Med Microbiol 2003;52:715–720.

30. So LK, Lau AC, Yam LY, et al: Development of a standard treatment protocol for severe acute respiratory syndrome. Lancet 2003;361:1615–1617.

31. Ho JC, Ooi GC, Mok TY, et al: High dose pulse versus non-pulse corticosteroid regimens in severe acute respiratory syndrome. Am J Respir Crit Care Med 2003;168:1449–1456.

32. Sung JJ, Wu A, Joynt GM, et al: Severe acute respiratory syndrome: Report of treatment and outcome after a major outbreak. Thorax 2004;59:414–420.

33. Thompson BT: Glucocorticoids and acute lung injury. Crit Care Med 2003;31:S253–S257.

34. Meduri GU, Headley AS, Golden E, et al: Effect of prolonged methylprednisolone therapy in unresolving acute respiratory distress syndrome: A randomized controlled trial. JAMA 1998;280:159–165.

35. Brun-Buisson C, Brochard L: Corticosteroid therapy in acute respiratory distress syndrome: Better late than never? JAMA 1998;280:182–183.

36. Antonio GE, Wong KT, Chu WC, et al: Imaging in severe acute respiratory syndrome (SARS). Clin Radiol 2003;58:825–832.

37. Cordingley JJ, Keogh BF: The pulmonary physician in critical care: ventilatory management of ALI/ARDS. Thorax 2002;8:729–734.

38. Gattinoni L, Chiumello D, Russo R: Reduced tidal volumes and lung protective ventilatory strategies: Where do we go from here? Curr Opin Crit Care 2002;8:45–50.

39. Acute Respiratory Distress Syndrome Network: Ventilation with lower tidal volumes as compared with traditional tidal volumes for acute lung injury and the acute respiratory distress syndrome. N Engl J Med 2000;342:1301–1308.

40. Eichacker PQ, Gerstenberger EP, Banks SM, et al: Meta-analysis of acute lung injury and acute respiratory distress syndrome trials testing low tidal volumes. Am J Respir Crit Care Med 2002;166:1510–1514.

41. Ward NS: Effects of prone position ventilation in ARDS: An evidence-based review of the literature. Crit Care Clin 2002;18:35–44.

42. Gattinoni L, Tognoni G, Pesenti A, et al: Effect of prone positioning on the survival of patients with acute respiratory failure. N Engl J Med 2001;345:568–573.

43. Hui DS, Hall SD, Chan MT, et al. Noninvasive positive-pressure ventilation: An experimental model to assess air and particle dispersion. Chest 2006;130:730–740.

44. Anzueto A, Frutos-Vivar F, Esteban A, et al: Incidence, risk factors and outcome of barotrauma in mechanically ventilated patients. Intensive Care Med 2004;30:612–619.

45. Joynt GM, Antonio GE, Lam P, et al: Thin-section computed tomography abnormalities in patients with late adult respiratory distress syndrome (ARDS) caused by severe acute respiratory syndrome (SARS). Radiology 2004;230:339–346.

46. Humphrey H, Hall J, Sznajder I, et al: Improved survival in ARDS patients associated with a reduction in pulmonary capillary wedge pressure. Chest 1990;97:1176–1180.

47. Mitchell JP, Schuller D, Calandrino FS, et al: Improved outcome based on fluid management in critically ill patients requiring pulmonary catheter catheterization. Am Rev Respir Dis 1992;145:990–998.

48. Hui DS, Joynt GM, Wong KT, et al. Impact of severe acute respiratory syndrome (SARS) on pulmonary function, functional capacity and quality of life in a cohort of survivors. Thorax. 2005;60:401–409.

49. Severe Acute Respiratory Syndrome (SARS) III. Infection Control in Healthcare facilities May 3, 2005 http://www.cdc.gov/ncidod/sars/guidance/I/healthcare.htm#3d11. Accessed 14 April 2007.

50. Gomersall CD, Tai DY, Loo S, et al. Expanding ICU facilities in an epidemic: Recommendations based on experience from the SARS epidemic in Hong Kong and Singapore. Intensive Care Med. 2006;32:1004–1013.

51. Li TS, Buckley TA, Yap FH, Joynt GM: Severe acute respiratory syndrome (SARS): Infection control. Lancet 2003;361:1386.

52. Garner JS: Hospital Infection Control Practices Advisory Committee: Guideline for isolation precautions in hospitals. Infect Control Hosp Epidemiol 1996;17:53–80.

53. Gomersall CD, Joynt GM, Ho OM, et al. Transmission of SARS to healthcare workers. The experience of a Hong Kong ICU. Intensive Care Med 2006;32:564–569.

# SECTION 2

## PHYSIOLOGY AND PATHOPHYSIOLOGY OF VENTILATION

# CHAPTER 8

# Anatomy

Konrad Morgenroth and Michael Ebsen

## MORPHOLOGY OF THE UPPER AIRWAYS

The upper airways consist of the nose, the paranasal sinuses, the pharynx, and the larynx. The lower airways start in the area of the larynx below the glottis and continue inferiorly to the trachea. At the border from the upper to the middle third, the trachea enters the thorax. From this point on, the airways are part of the rhythmic respiration cycle, which leads to restriction during expiration and expansion during inspiration.

## TRACHEOBRONCHIAL TREE

The trachea begins with the cricoid cartilage of the larynx and reaches, at a dorsal angle of 30 degrees, 10 to 12 cm into the thorax. At the level of the fifth thoracic vertebra, the trachea divides into the left and right main bronchi. The trachea is framed by 15 to 20 horseshoe-shaped cartilagines. The open ends of these cartilaginous rings are sealed posteriorly by the membranous trachealis muscle, to form the paries membranaceus tracheae or posterior tracheal wall. With the relaxation of these muscles and of the connective tissue as a result of aging, this wall can lose elasticity.

The right main bronchus has a length of 2.5 cm, and the left main bronchus is 5 cm long. The lumen of the right main bronchus is larger than that of the left, and the bronchus itself shows a steeper orientation than its counterpart on the left. Two to 3 cm inferiorly, the superior lobe bronchus branches from the right main bronchus. From this point on, the bronchus is called the intermediate

bronchus, which is then divided into the right middle lobe and the right lower lobe bronchi. The left main bronchus is divided directly after passing the aortic arch into the left superior lobe and inferior lobe bronchi. In the superior lobe bronchus, the division into segmental bronchi takes place shortly after the division from the main bronchus. In the midsized bronchi, cartilage and peribronchial glands are scant. Stability of the bronchial wall in this region is only partly provided by the cartilaginous structures. The smaller bronchi have an increase in smooth muscle fibers and a dense network of capillaries (Fig. 8.1).

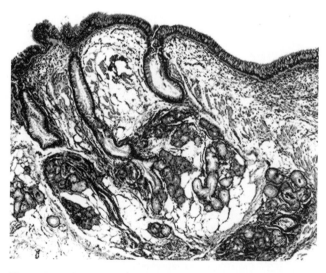

**Figure 8.1**  Structure of the bronchial mucosa. On the surface is ciliated stratified epithelium. In the subepithelial connective tissue are peribronchial glands with their ducts, which extend to the surface of the mucosa (hematoxylin and eosin; magnification × 240).

## BRONCHIAL EPITHELIUM

The trachea and bronchi are lined by stratified ciliated epithelium. The height of the epithelium decreases as the bronchial tree branches. Four different cell types can be found in the epithelium: basal cells, ciliated cells, goblet cells, and clear cells, which belong to the diffuse neuroendocrine system or amine precursor uptake and decarboxylation (APUD) system. The epithelium sits on a basement membrane, which has a thickness of 10 µm. The basement membrane serves as a foundation for the epithelium, but it also has important barrier functions for the submucosa. It therefore plays an important role in the processes of defense, growth, and repair of the mucosa (Fig. 8.2).

Basal cells are located in the lower parts of the epithelium directly above the basement membrane. These cells are usually configured like a pyramid, with the basement membrane on the bottom and the top pointing to the surface of the epithelium. Basal cells are connected over varying finger-shaped dentations and desmosomes to the adjacent epithelial cells. Hemidesmosomes are found at the base of the cells. The basal cell nucleus is large, mainly round to oval. Few mitochondria and little endoplasmic reticulum are found in the cytoplasm, which is crossed by tubular and filamentous components of the cytoskeleton. From these undifferentiated cells, ciliated cells and goblet cells originate after cell injury and loss.

Ciliated cells comprise the main cell group in the respiratory epithelium (Fig. 8.3). The ratio of goblet cells to ciliated cells is 1:4 in the upper and middle parts of bronchial system. Ciliated cells are located, with a small portion of cytoplasm, on the basement membrane and

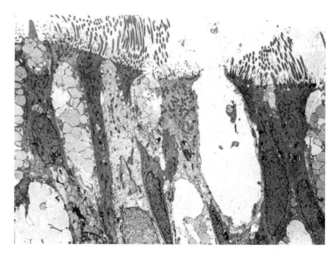

**Figure 8.3** Ultrastructure of the bronchial epithelium. In the goblet cells, different stages of mucus maturation and secretion are evident. Ciliated cells show regularly arranged cilia. In the cytoplasm in the apical areas is a dense arrangement of mitochondria (magnification × 480).

reach through the basal cells to the epithelial surface. The oval nucleus is present in the middle third of these cells. In the cytoplasm, which has a loose structure, scattered ribosomes are found, sometimes in groups. The endoplasmic reticulum is sparse. The Golgi apparatus is present near the nucleus. In the cytoplasm, numerous mitochondria are formed; these mitochondria are found in apical cell locations and have an elongated configuration. Mitochondria serve in the production of adenosine triphosphate, which is necessary for ciliary movement. Single lysosomes are also found in the cytoplasm, although their function remains unclear.

The surface of ciliated cells is covered with 200 to 300 cilia. Cilia, which comprise part of the cytoplasm, have an average length of 5 µm and a thickness of 0.2 to 0.3 µm (Fig. 8.4). Cilia are enveloped by an elementary membrane, which stays in direct continuity with the outer cell membrane, and are characterized by a typical inner structure. In the center are two microtubules, which extend to the top of the cilia. Under the outer elementary membrane, nine microtubules or so-called doublets are located in a ringlike pattern. Each doublet has a complete tubule (A subfiber) and an attached three-fourths circle of B subfiber. From the A subfiber, two rows of side arms, the outer and inner dynein arms, protrude toward the B subfiber of the adjacent doublet, and one radial spoke extends to the central pair.

The central tubules end freely in the narrow tip of the cilia, and the peripheral tubules fuse together in the tip. The basal bodies of the cilia are located directly under the cell membrane. The basal bodies or kinetosomes are cylindrical bodies 0.5 µm long. Their wall consists of nine groups of three tubules in a ringlike pattern.

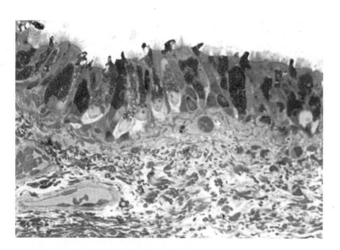

**Figure 8.2** Structure of the bronchial epithelium, with regularly arranged goblet cells showing different stages of mucus production. Among them are ciliated cells. Under the epithelial cells is the basement membrane. Beneath it are connective tissue and a capillary (basic fuchsin and methylene blue; magnification × 1200).

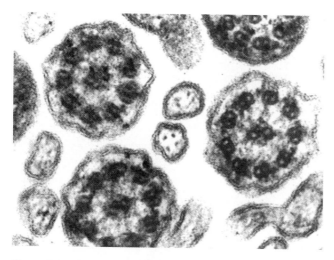

**Figure 8.4** Cross sections of cilia with typical tubules and dynein arms and radial spokes. On the surface is the doubled outer membrane. Among the cilia are microvilli (magnification × 5000).

Two of these tubules form the outer tubules of the cilia. Among the cilia, small protrusions of the cell membrane, the so-called microvilli, are formed. From the cytoplasm, filamentous structures of the cytoskeleton extend into the microvilli.

The mucus-producing cells of the respiratory epithelium are called goblet cells because of their shape. The central parts of these cells are formed by mucus. Like the ciliated cells, goblet cells sit on the basement membrane and reach through the basal cells to the surface of the epithelium (Fig. 8.5). The number of goblet cells decreases in the lower airways, and their number may vary in disease. Goblet cells show different stages of mucus formation and maturation. The components for mucus production are delivered from the capillaries and by diffusion through the basement membrane. Synthesis starts in the endoplasmic reticulum. The formed parts of the mucus are stored in the Golgi apparatus. In the Golgi apparatus, the maturation and the configuration of the viscoelastic properties of the mucus take place. The mucus precursor droplets have a flocky appearance which is changing to the apical cell component as the fluid content increases. With increasing maturation, the membranes of the vesicles become thinner and finally disrupt. Several confluent mucus droplets form a mucus plug. The other components of cytoplasm are pushed to the periphery of the cell. The intracytoplasmic mucus complex protrudes into the bronchial lumen (Fig. 8.6). The cell membrane opens, and the mucus is released (Fig. 8.7). The released mucus comes into contact with the gel phase of the mucus layer and is transported with the mucus stream. After the release of the mucus, formation of new mucus starts again in the goblet cell.

The cytoplasm of the goblet cells is dense at the beginning of the mucus formation cycle, and it contains mitochondria and membranes of the endoplasmic reticulum covered with ribosomes. The goblet cell nucleus is characterized by a dense chromatin structure and is located in the basal areas of the cell. Adjacent to the nucleus is a prominent Golgi apparatus, which is formed by small saccules and a rim of vesicles.

The cell membrane forms toward the bronchial lumen microvilli, which are reaching in the sol phase of the mucus stream. It is thought that this serves to increase the cell surface and that it has a function in the resorption of substances from the sol phase.

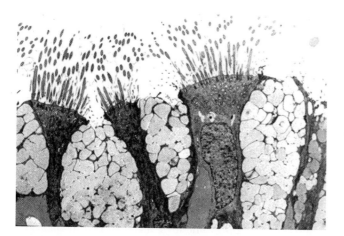

**Figure 8.5** Mucus formation in the goblet cells. In the cytoplasm, dense formations of mucus complexes show confluence in the apical areas. In the outer parts of the cell, few organelles are present (magnification × 2500).

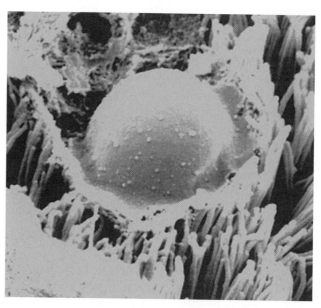

**Figure 8.6** Surface structure of the bronchial epithelium. In advanced stages of mucus formation, the mucus complex protrudes into the bronchial lumen (REM; magnification × 5000).

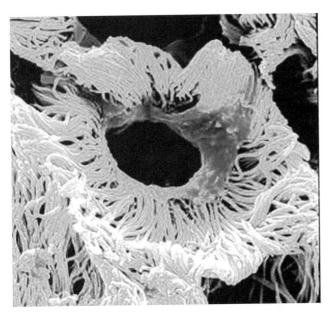

**Figure 8.7** Release of the mucus. After mucus maturation is complete, the cell membrane is disrupted, and the mucus is released. The mucus itself is transported by the adjacent cilia (REM; magnification × 3000).

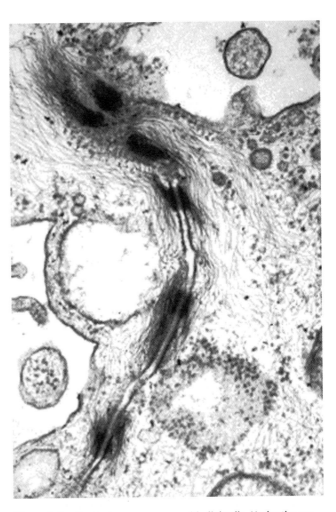

**Figure 8.8** Contact zones among epithelial cells. Under the surface membranes are tight-junctions. Beneath them are the zonulae adherentes and desmosomes. Filamentous and tubulous parts of cytoplasm extend into these contact zones (magnification × 25000).

Among the epithelial cells is a complex network of connections. Directly under the cell surface, membranes fuse to form tight junctions (Fig. 8.8). The tight junctions are built up in the whole circumference of the cell and have a gridlike appearance. Under this area is the zonula adhaerens, in which the cells are divided by a gap of 150 to 200 Å. The cell membrane is thickened circumferentially by short filaments. The adjacent desmosomes form these discontinuous zonula adherentes between the cell membranes. They form identical halves surrounding a glycoprotein-rich substance of fine, crosswise filaments. Into these filaments are integrated other filaments arising from the cytoskeleton. In the lower parts of the epithelium, the desmosomes are loosely arranged. Additionally in this area so called gap junctions are found.

Clear cells of the bronchial epithelium are called Kultschinsky cells, after their first describer. These cells belong to the diffuse neuroendocrine system, the APUD system. Catecholamines can be stored and degraded in these cells. Similar cells are found in the pancreas, the urogenital system, the endocrine system, and the mucosa of the gastrointestinal tract. The biologic relevance of this system is still in question. Neuroendocrine tumors can arise from these cells (Fig. 8.9).

These round cells are distributed irregularly in the epithelium. They have a clear cytoplasmic matrix, with loosely arranged neurosecretory granules. At the cell surface, single direct contacts to nerve fibers are formed. The neuroendocrine substances can be elucidated by immunohistochemical analysis.

## PERIBRONCHIAL GLANDS

Most mucus is produced by the peribronchial submucosal glands. These glands are tubuloacinar mixed glands with serous and mucous acini and a common duct system (Fig. 8.10). The glands' ducts are diagonally oriented, with a funnel-shaped part directly before their opening. The ducts are lined by ciliated epithelium. The glands lie in loose connective tissue between bundles of smooth muscles and cartilage. The number of glands decreases at the periphery of the tracheobronchial tree. The configurations of the glands vary from trees consisting of several branched glands to two-gland tubes. These glands are most prominent (1 gland/mm²) in midsized bronchi. The serous and mucous glands cells are distributed in distinct areas of the gland.

The gland acini contain groups of epithelial cells that form 0.5-μm mucus granules in their cytoplasm and are

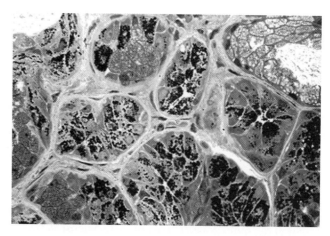

**Figure 8.10** Acini of a peribronchial gland. Serous epithelial cells contain densely arranged granules apically and in the cytoplasm. Adjacent mucous cells with light granules are visible. Their nucleus is found at the base of the cells (magnification × 380).

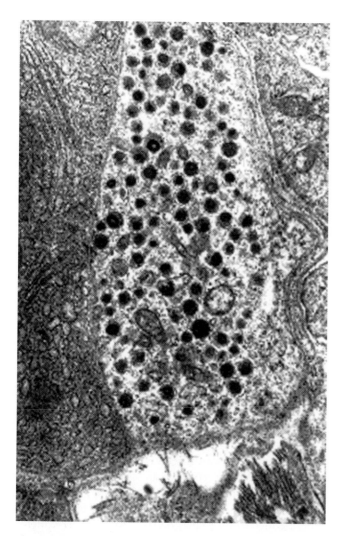

**Figure 8.9** Neuroendocrine cells. In the basal layer of the epithelium are cells with densely arranged neuroendocrine granules. They are located directly on the basement membrane (magnification × 12000).

called serous cells. The nucleus is found in the middle third of these cells, and the granules form in the apical regions of the cytoplasm. The second group of gland cells is known as mucous cells. They resemble the goblet cells of the respiratory epithelium. Mucous cells have densely packed granules, and their nucleus is located in the basal cytoplasm. The acinar cells are surrounded by spindle-shaped myoepithelial cells. The differentiation of serous and mucous gland cells is probably an expression of varying stages of mucus maturation in the cells.

The synthesis of mucus in mucous cells begins with the formation of electron-dense vacuoles from the Golgi saccules. These granules of mucus migrate to the apical cell areas. With loosening and swelling, the maturation of the mucus takes place. The secretion granules enlarge and confluence (Fig. 8.11). The cytoplasm diminishes, and larger complexes of mucus form. The apical cell membrane disrupts, and the mucus extends to the acinar lumen.

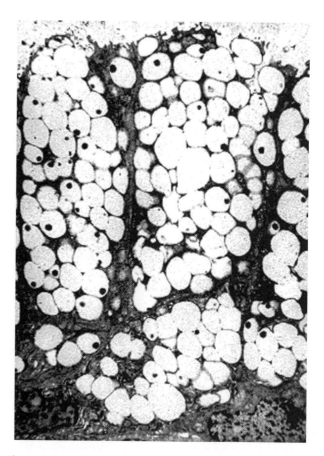

**Figure 8.11** Mucus maturation in mucous epithelial cells of a peribronchial gland. In the cytoplasm, mucus complexes are surrounded by a membrane. They show confluence in the apical cell areas. The nuclei lie at the base of the cells (magnification × 4100).

Depending on the stage of mucus maturation, peroxisomes are found in cytoplasm. Peroxisomes contain oxidative and antioxidative enzymes and are located close to the preliminary secretion vacuoles. It is very probable that substances produced by the peroxisomes are released together with the mucus (Fig. 8.12).

The formation of mucus in serous cells is characterized by the formation of electron-dense granules originating in the membrane of the Golgi apparatus. The granules migrate to the apical cell area. After a circumscript opening of the cell membrane the mucus component is released into the acinar lumen.

The acinar spindle-shaped myoepithelial cells are found in the outer zone. These cells have a dense network of filaments in their cytoplasm. It is believed that the contraction of these cells is related to secretion mechanisms.

## MORPHOLOGY OF THE SMALL AIRWAYS

After the 20th branching of the bronchial system, the airways are called bronchioles. They have a diameter of 0.5 to 0.15 mm. The bronchioli respiratorii form the transformation zone between the airways and the gas exchanging system of the respiratory tract. The bronchioles are supplied by the pulmonary artery and function in gas exchange. After the third branching, they become the ductuli alveolares (see Fig. 8.10), and then the alveoli. These terminal parts of the respiratory system, including the alveolar ducts and the alveoli, form the terminal respiratory unit.

The walls of the peripheral branches of the bronchial system have a similar morphologic structure. However, some distinct differences contribute to the functional properties of these airway structures. The lumen of the nonrespiratory bronchioles measures 2 mm, and these bronchial segments have no cartilage. The outer wall is composed of loose connective tissue and loosely arranged, gridlike smooth muscle fibers.

Mucus in this area is produced by the mucosa itself, which contains several goblet cells. The number of cilia on the surface of the ciliated cell is less than in central parts of the airways. The cilia themselves are shorter, whereas the goblet cells are plumper and have a broad part of their cytoplasm attached to the basement membrane (Fig. 8.13).

After the 20th branching, the airways show changes in their morphology and their mechanisms of mucus production. In the epithelium of the respiratory bronchioles, ciliated and nonciliated cells, or the Clara cells, also known as bronchiolar exocrine cells, are arranged next to each other (Fig. 8.14). The number of ciliated cells decreases in the periphery, whereas the number of Clara cells increases. The terminal bronchioles widen in inspiration and collapse at end expiration. Stable conditions of the wall structures are essential for ventilation of the alveoli (Fig. 8.15).

In the respiratory bronchioles, serous secretions are formed, consisting of proteins, polysaccharides, cholesterol, and surfactant from the alveolar system. Secretion is influenced by β-adrenergic agonists and probably also by prostaglandins. Clara cell secretion is regulated by apocrine mechanisms (Fig. 8.16). Clara cells have direct contact with the basement membrane. A dense network of rough endoplasmic reticulum in the cytoplasm indicates high metabolic activity. Around the nucleus are two

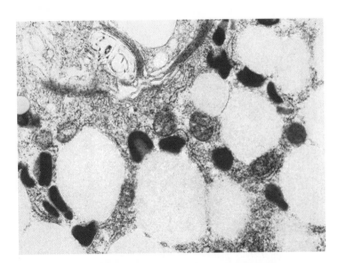

**Figure 8.12** Mucus maturation in a peribronchial gland. The components of the mucus are synthesized in the endoplasmic reticulum. After passage through the Golgi apparatus, vacuoles with a loose structure develop. Among them are peroxisomes (magnification × 8200).

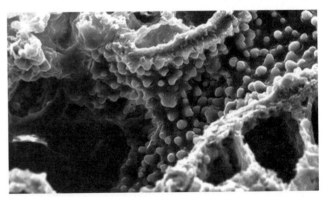

**Figure 8.13** Cross section of a bronchiole. Inside, cylindrical epithelium with few goblet cells and irregularly dispersed ciliated cells are visible. Beneath is loose connective tissue with elastic fibers. In the outer areas are smooth muscles and connective tissue (magnification × 700).

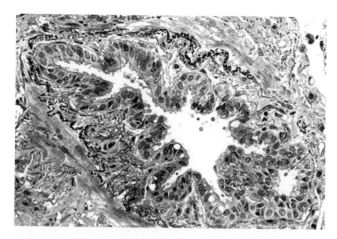

**Figure 8.14** Terminal bronchiole at the border to the alveolar duct. On the surface of the mucosa, mucus protrusions of the Clara cells are noted (REM; magnification × 240).

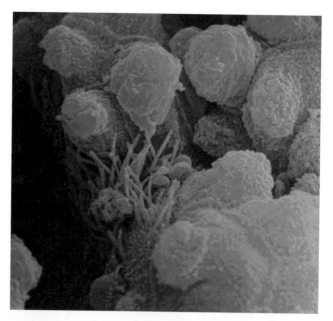

**Figure 8.16** Structure of Clara cells. On the cell surface are protrusions. Between the Clara cells are ciliated cells (REM; magnification × 5000).

Golgi apparatus. The mitochondria are evenly distributed in the cytoplasm.

As mucus forms, the cells grow and develop a flat, rounded, hilltop-like protrusion into the bronchial lumen (Fig. 8.17). The cell surface has irregularly distributed microvilli. The predominant parts of the endoplasmic reticulum and the nucleus are translocated from the middle areas to the apical areas of the cell. At the same time, granules with a dense matrix form and are surrounded by a single membrane. The cell surface protrudes, with a clear, granular matrix toward the lumen. At the periphery and at the height of the original cell membrane, a vesicular structure develops and forms a new cell membrane (Fig. 8.18). These new membranous

structures can become confluent, and the apical vesicular protrusions can be removed from the cell surface in a manner resembling a zip fastener. The cell compartments are seen as dense membranous structures above the cilia.

## Bronchial Muscles

The width of the bronchial lumen is determined by the tone of the smooth muscles of the bronchial wall. Smooth muscle tone is regulated by the nervous system. The arrangement of the muscular system depends on the diameter of the various airway regions. In the main bronchi, there is a band of muscles between the U-shaped cartilagines. In the smaller bronchi, the muscles connect the tips of the cartilagines. The midsized and small bronchi possess a spiral muscle layer with fibers in longitudinal and circular orientation.

In the larger airways, muscle contraction can narrow the bronchial lumen, whereas relaxation can widen it. Through the arrangement of the fibers, bronchial constriction also shortens the airway. The muscle bundles have a spindle-shaped configuration. In the center of the cells is a rodlike dentate nucleus; regularly dispersed myofilaments are found in the cytoplasm (Fig. 8.19). Mitochondria and rough and smooth endoplasmic reticulum are arranged on both sides of the nucleus. Additionally, glycogen granules and a Golgi apparatus are present. The muscle cells are surrounded by a basement membrane. Among these cells, small amounts of collagen and elastic fibers are detectable. Beneath the cell

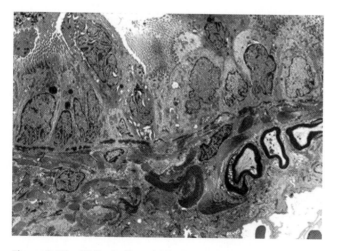

**Figure 8.15** Wall of a bronchiole. In the epithelium among the ciliated cells are Clara cells with apical protrusions. The cells are broadly based on the basement membrane. In the adjacent connective tissue, elastic fibers are found. Beneath are smooth muscles and a nerve fiber (magnification × 2500).

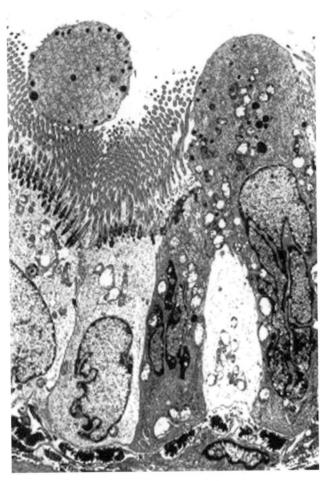

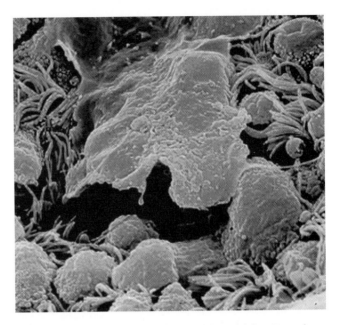

**Figure 8.18** Secretion in the terminal bronchioles. From the Clara cells, mucus complexes are released and form mucus plaques above the epithelium and the cilia. They are situated directly on the watery sol phase and can be transported by the ciliary movement (REM; magnification × 5000).

**Figure 8.17** Apocrine mucus formation in Clara cells. On the cell surface are protrusions with granular and tubular architecture in the cytoplasm. Adjacent granules with a dense structure are surrounded by a membrane. The nucleus is indented, with perinuclear endoplasmic reticulum and mitochondria. Adjacent ciliated cells are noted (magnification × 8000).

The viscoelastic properties of the gel phase determine its fluidity. These properties are responsible for the attachment of inhaled particles at the mucosal layer and for the transport of these particles to the environment. The adhesiveness of the mucus is an important component of the clearance mechanisms, although it can also lead to adherence of the mucus on the bronchial mucosa.

surface ribosomes, smooth endoplasmic reticulum and some pinocytotic vesicles are found.

## Mucus Layer

Under normal circumstances, the bronchial mucosa shows a smoothly functioning system of mucus formation and transport. The mucus is formed by two distinct layers located directly above the epithelium (Fig. 8.20). There is a continuous watery phase (sol phase), which covers the surface of the epithelium from the periphery to the central parts of the bronchial tree (Fig. 8.21). The sol phase is in direct contact with the hypophase of the surfactant layer of the alveolar system. The watery mucous components surround the microvilli and the cilia. A discontinuous, gelid, viscous layer is situated above the watery phase, probably suspended over it.

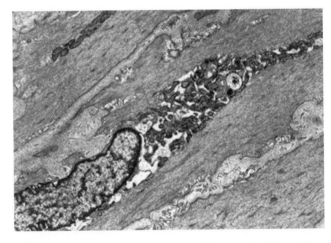

**Figure 8.19** Bronchial muscle system. The muscle cells contain long, indented nuclei, with perinuclear endoplasmic reticulum and mitochondria. In the cytoplasm, filamentous contractile structures are visible. In the vicinity of the cells, a broad basement membrane and some collagen bundles are found (magnification × 6000).

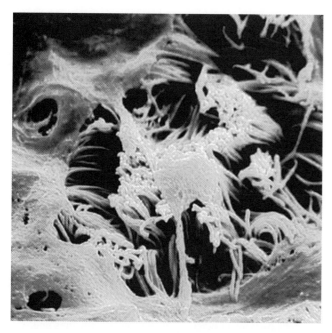

**Figure 8.20** Mucus layer over the bronchial epithelium. Mucus plaques of changing size are noted. The gelid mucus layer is found over the sol phase and the cilia (REM; magnification × 1800).

Surfactant material is probably transported to the bronchi during expiration (Fig. 8.22). It decreases the adhesive power between the sol phase and the hypophase and regulates the water content of the sol phase. This process allows regular transport of the mucus. The effectiveness of ciliary function depends on the configuration and the height of the sol phase of the mucus.

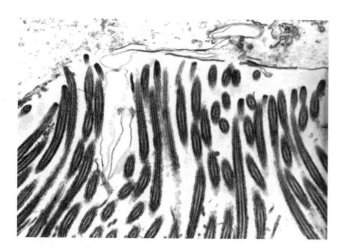

**Figure 8.21** Mucus layer over the bronchial epithelium. The gelid sol phase is arranged over the tips of the cilia. Between the cilia and the mucus complexes are formations of thin, contrast-rich lamellae. In the vicinity are cilia in the watery sol phase (magnification × 8000).

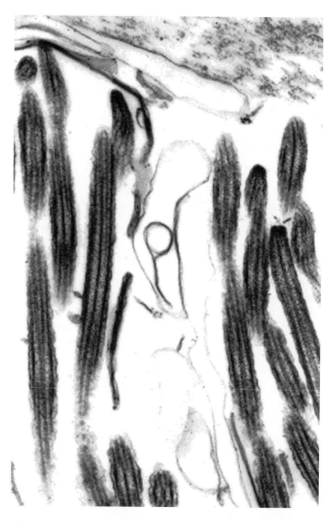

**Figure 8.22** Mucus layer over the bronchial epithelium. Between the gelid mucus phase and the watery sol phase, formations of surfactant are found. Surfactant decreases adhesiveness at the border of the two phases so the cilia can move in the mucus phase. Among the cilia are vesicular components of surfactant in the sol phase (magnification × 15000).

## Innervation

The functions of the bronchial clearance mechanisms are based on strict coordination of mucus production, ciliary activity, and bronchial muscular tone. The integration of these functions is regulated by an autonomous regulation mechanism and by differentiated innervation.

Airway functions are maintained even after interruption of the nerve supply, for example, after organ transplantation; therefore, an autonomous mechanism of regulation has been postulated. Experimental investigations propose that information can be received by cellular structure, for example, by the microvilli, and can be transported horizontally from cell to cell using components of the cytoskeleton (Fig. 8.23). In the transport of information, the cell-cell contact zones play a very important role. Under normal circumstances, the highly

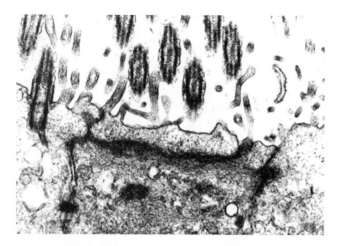

**Figure 8.23** Autonomic regulation at the bronchial epithelium. Components of the cytoskeleton participate in the transmittal of information among the cells. Filamentous and tubulous parts of this system are found in the apical regions of the bronchial epithelial cells. The filamentous structures are part of the tight junctions. They are arranged directly under the cell membrane and adjacent to the basal bodies of the cilia (magnification × 10000).

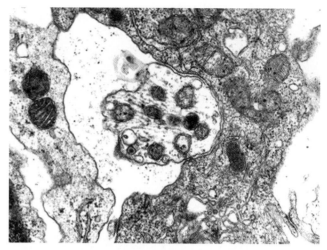

**Figure 8.24** Innervation of the bronchial mucosa. Distal branches of nerve fibers extend through the basement membrane into the epithelium. They follow the intracellular gaps and have broad contact zones with the epithelial cells. On cross sections of these fibers, typical microtubules and small mitochondria are noted (magnification × 9500).

differentiated innervation moderates autonomous regulation, so fast and effective adaptation to changing environmental conditions is guaranteed.

The human lung has strong cholinergic parasympathetic innervation, whereas the adrenergic sympathetic component is less developed. Comparison of functional and morphologic investigations demonstrates that the human lung is mainly innervated by parasympathetic nerve fibers arising from the vagus nerve. A combination of myelinated and nonmyelinated nerve fibers and ganglion cells forms the plexus bronchialis, which is located in the hilar lung area. This plexus is divided into the plexus bronchiales. The plexus peribronchialis has several multipolar ganglion cells, which have axons mixed with fibers of the vagus nerve and the sympathetic nerve fibers. The ratio of myelinated to nonmyelinated nerve fibers 1:50 in the hilar region and 1:100 at the periphery.

The axons are enveloped by Schwann cells. Several myelinated and nonmyelinated axons are found in the cytoplasm of a single Schwann cell. From the nerve complexes of the peribronchial plexus, fine fibers migrate to single structures of the bronchial mucosa. They extend to the epithelium, the bronchial muscular system, and the peribronchial glands.

In the bronchial epithelium, efferent and afferent fibers are detectable. The afferent sensory fibers show circumscribed nodules directly beneath the epithelium. They are arranged as sensory organs in the upper layers of the epithelium.

The efferent fibers branch from the subepithelial nerve fibers, extend to the epithelium through the basement membrane, and thus leave the Schwann sheath. These fibers are located in the intracellular gaps in the apical region (Fig. 8.24). On cross and longitudinal sections, neurotubules can be detected. The fibers contain regularly arranged small mitochondria, as well as granules in the periphery that are separated by a single membrane. These fibers contain dense granular material and have a light matrix. The differentiation between adrenergic and cholinergic fibers is morphologically not possible.

The nerve endings are located in the upper epithelial layers in cell membrane invaginations. Between the nerve fiber and the cell membrane is a gap of 120 nm (Fig. 8.25). The functional nervous system regulation of the peribronchial glands is determined by parasympathetic cholinergic fibers. Secretion can be stimulated by cholinergic substances. In the connective tissue, the nerve fibers are adjacent to the acinar gland structures and are in nearly direct contact with the acini. On cross sections of the axons, vesicles of varying diameters that carry catecholaminergic transmitter substances can be seen. After losing the Schwann sheath, the axons migrate directly into the acini after they have passed the basement membrane. The nerve endings have direct contact with secretory cells by means of synapses (Fig. 8.26). The peripheral nerve nodules simultaneously are in contact with myoepithelial cells.

Terminal branches of the plexus peribronchialis supply the smooth muscle of the bronchial wall. In these areas, a dense network of fine fibers is developed. Single branches of the peribronchial plexus extend to single muscle fibers and are related in the form of large nerve complexes to the single muscle bundles. From this complex, fine fibers are located among single muscle cells. These branches have synaptic contacts with muscle cells (Fig. 8.27).

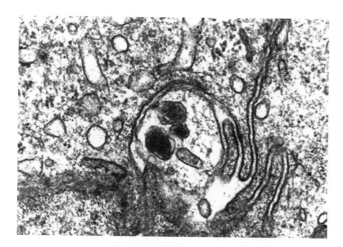

**Figure 8.25** Innervation of the bronchial mucosa: cross section of an intraepithelial nerve fiber directly under the surface of the epithelium. The fiber is located to, and is close to, the cell membrane of the epithelial cell. In this section, a small mitochondrion and neuroendocrine granules are visible (magnification × 12000).

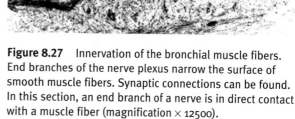

**Figure 8.27** Innervation of the bronchial muscle fibers. End branches of the nerve plexus narrow the surface of smooth muscle fibers. Synaptic connections can be found. In this section, an end branch of a nerve is in direct contact with a muscle fiber (magnification × 12500).

The nerve endings are located in loose connective tissue and are covered by basement membrane. Neurosecretory granules are regularly found in these fibers.

## Submucosa

The submucosa of the bronchial mucosa consists of loose connective tissue, in which capillaries, lymphatic vessels, and nerves can be found. It contains the peribronchial glands and the central parts of the bronchial system cartilage. In this zone, mobile cells are found in the submucosa and serve as a reagible cell population in local immunologic defense.

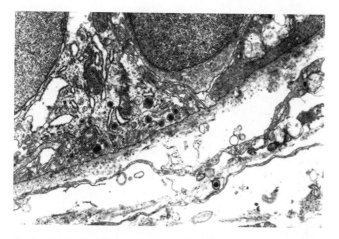

**Figure 8.26** End branches of a peribronchial plexus contacting the outer zones of the acini of peribronchial glands after passing the basement membrane. Synapses between mucus-producing cells and myoepithelial cells are noted (magnification × 16000).

The lamina propria is larger centrally than peripherally. Capillaries are present in a network of collagen and elastic bundles and extend nearly to the basement membrane of the surface epithelium (Fig. 8.28). The blood supply of the trachea is from branches of the thyroid artery and anastomoses of the bronchial arteries. The blood supply of the lower parts of the trachea and the bronchi is guaranteed by bronchial wall arteries from the descending aorta, the intercostal artery, and the internal mammary artery. The venous blood flow from the trachea follows the venous plexus of the thyroid blood vessels, and the intrapulmonary airways are drained by the pulmonary veins.

In the zone of the different fibers, mast cells are irregularly distributed. These cells are mainly arranged in the vicinity of the vessels, the muscle fibers, and the peribronchial glands. They are characterized by typical intracytoplasmic granules and have thin microvilli on the surface (Fig. 8.29). These active cells can traverse the surface epithelium to enter the bronchial lumen.

In the tunica propria, lymphocytes and plasma cells can be found loosely dispersed. They are mainly detected in the vicinity of the peribronchial glands. Plasma cells produce immunoglobulin A, which is bound to a secretory component in the epithelial gland cells and is secreted in the bronchial lumen.

Only single macrophages in the lumina and in the bronchial wall can be observed. They may contain organic and inorganic particles from breathed air.

Lymphatic tissue is found in all areas of the tracheobronchial wall. The distribution of this tissue shows great individual and age-dependent variability. It consists of intrapulmonary lymph nodes, bronchus-associated

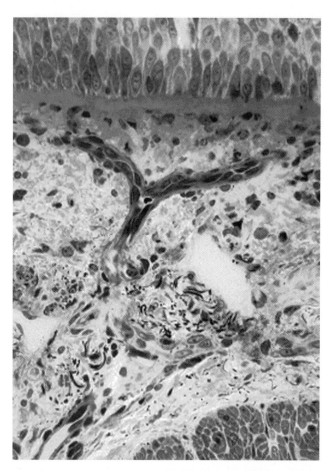

**Figure 8.28** Submucosa. Beneath the bronchial epithelium and among the bronchial muscle fibers is loose connective tissue with a dense network of capillaries. The capillaries are found directly under the basement membrane of the bronchial epithelium. In the connective tissue, single lymphocytes and plasma cells are noted (basic fuchsin and methylene blue; magnification × 420).

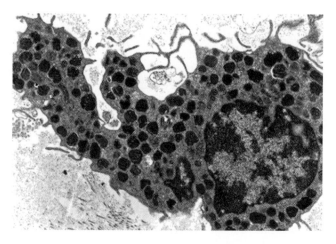

**Figure 8.29** Mast cell in the submucosa of the bronchial mucosa. On the cell surface are small microvilli. In the cytoplasm are densely arranged granules with a lamellar structure. Also visible is an eccentrically located indented nucleus. In the vicinity are filamentous components of the connective tissue (magnification × 8000).

## Type I Pneumocytes

Type I pneumocytes cover approximately 95% of the alveolar surface. Their diameter is 50 µm, and their overall extension is 2300 µm. These cells have few organelles. They are characterized by a flat appearance and are 0.1 to 0.2 µm thick. The flat cytoplasmic protrusions overlap and touch during inspiration and expiration. Between the adjacent cells, tight junctions are present

lymphoid tissue (BALT), which can be compared with the Peyer plaques from the gut, and lymphoreticular aggregates. This area is important for the transport of interstitial fluid in the lymph nodes.

## ALVEOLAR SYSTEM

The gas-exchanging surface structures of the lung are organized in form of bleblike alveoli, of which 30 million are formed. They have diameters up to 250 µm and are able to respond to the different demands of inspiration and expiration. Alveoli are connected by one to seven cores (pores of Kohn), which are 2 to 13 µm in diameter. The inside of the alveolus is covered by a flat epithelial layer, in which two cell types, type I and type II pneumocytes, can be differentiated (Fig. 8.30).

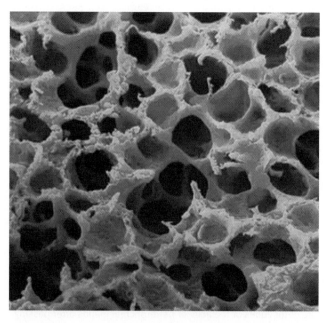

**Figure 8.30** Alveolar system. Divided by the thin interstitium are several alveoli with a smooth surface (REM; magnification × 200).

and surround the pneumocytes like a collar. Type I pneumocytes have a continuous basement membrane that is fused with the basement membrane of the endothelial cells of the alveolar capillaries (Fig. 8.31). These capillaries are located directly beneath the alveolar lining cells. The epithelial cells, the basement membrane, and the endothelial cells of the capillaries form the barrier of gas exchange in the alveolar wall. The thickness of this barrier measures 0.5 to 0.7 μm (Fig. 8.32).

## Type II Pneumocytes

Type II pneumocytes have a cubic shape and a diameter of 9 μm. They lie isolated among the type I pneumocytes. Rarely, small groups of two or three type II pneumocytes can be observed. On their surface, they characteristically contain many microvilli (Fig. 8.33). The cytoplasm is rich in organelles. Rough endoplasmic reticulum, free ribosomes, mitochondria, lysosomes, multivesicular bodies, and a prominent Golgi apparatus can be found. The nucleus is located centrally and has a well-formed nucleolus. The most impressive and characteristic morphologic features are lamellar bodies, which measure 0.2 to 2 μm in diameter (Fig. 8.34). They comprise 25% of the cytoplasm of type II pneumocytes. These lamellar bodies are meant to be the substrate of the synthetic activity of the pneumocytes. These structures are equated with the surface active substances (surfactant) that are formed in the cytoplasm of these cells.

## Interstitium

The small area of tissue among the alveoli is mainly formed by the alveolar capillaries. The capillaries are

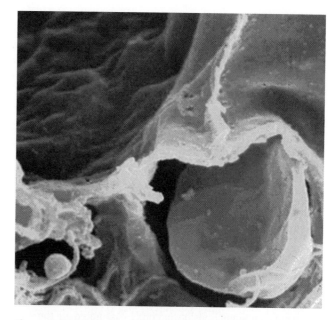

**Figure 8.32**   Alveolar wall. Regularly arranged type I pneumocytes are seen, as well as a thin alveolar membrane. In this section, one capillary with one erythrocyte are visible (REM; magnification × 7500).

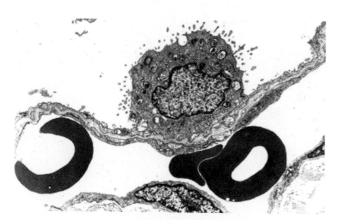

**Figure 8.31**   Alveolar wall. The alveolus is lined by flat alveolar epithelial cells (type I pneumocytes). In the center is a cubic type II pneumocyte. The alveolar membrane is formed by the fused basement membrane of the alveolar epithelium and the capillary endothelium. In the lumen of the capillary are erythrocytes. In the interstitium are loosely arranged collagen bundles (magnification × 3500).

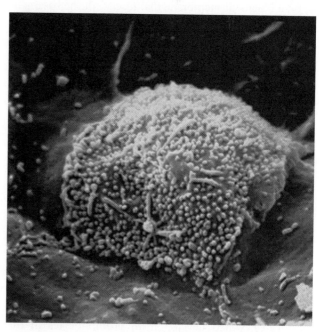

**Figure 8.33**   Surface structure of a type II pneumocyte. On the surface are several microvilli in the alveolus. The adjacent alveolar epithelial cells overlap. On the surface of a type I pneumocyte are few microvilli (REM; magnification × 5000).

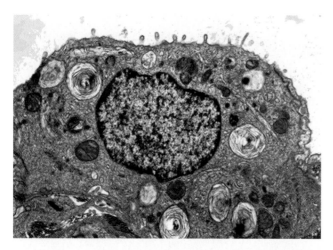

**Figure 8.34** Structure of a type II pneumocyte. On the surface are several microvilli. A centrally located nucleus is visible, as well as perinuclear endoplasmic reticulum and Golgi apparatus. Irregularly located osmiophilic lamellar bodies are seen. The basement membrane is visible inferiorly. Also noted are the adjacent portions of a type I pneumocyte (magnification × 4500).

arranged in a network around the alveoli. The flat endothelial cells have small protrusions against the capillary wall and a nucleus containing a few organelles. The capillary wall is covered with thin cytoplasmic branches. These branches overlap and form contact zones, which are characterized by fine filamentous cytoplasmic condensations. In the cytoplasm of the endothelial cells, many pinocytotic vesicles can be detected. The endothelial cells lie on a basement membrane that fuses with the basement membrane of the alveolar epithelium in areas of direct contact. Between the capillaries are single fibrocytes, which form a loose network and stabilize the alveolar structure (see Fig. 8.26). In the interstitium, single lymphocytes and monocytes can be observed. They serve as a reagible cell pool for local immunologic reactions. Additionally, single nerve fibers can be seen in the interstitium.

### Alveolar Macrophages

Even under normal circumstances, macrophages are loosely dispersed in the alveoli. They are able to phagocytose and destroy inhaled particles, such as infectious or inorganic particles, dead cells, and irregularly formed surfactant. Although many particles are taken up during inhalation, the alveolar space is normally sterile. The number and degree of macrophage activity increase during infection and after inhalation of certain environmental particles. Macrophages originate from blood monocytes, which develop from promonocytes in the bone marrow. Macrophages reach the capillary bed of the alveolar wall through the vascular system. They are located in the interstitium initially, and through gaps in the alveolar epithelium, they can enter the alveolar space.

Macrophage size increases in the alveoli (Fig. 8.35). These structures have a diameter of 10 to 15 μm and a nucleus located mostly in the cell's periphery. In the cytoplasm, endoplasmic reticulum, some small mitochondria, and a few lysosomes are found. One or two Golgi apparatus can be observed adjacent to the nucleus (Fig. 8.36).

Depending on functional status, phagolysosomes can be detected, with varying inclusions. Macrophages have a large surface area, which can change depending on the state of activation. On the surface, microplicae are found in several patterns. Furthermore, large cytoplasmic protrusions can be present and used for transport along the alveolar epithelium (Fig. 8.37). Macrophages use these protrusions to make contact with particles that should be phagocytosed.

The functional cytochemical and morphologic characteristics of alveolar macrophages differ from those of macrophages in other regions of the body. It is thought that these functional characteristics, especially their activity, result from the initial phagocytosis of the surfactant in the alveolar lumen.

## ACINUS

Lung tissue is organized in acini, which comprise the functional unit for gas exchange distal to the terminal (lobular) bronchioles. The acini are formed by the

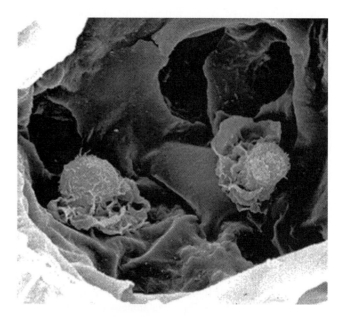

**Figure 8.35** Structure of the alveolar macrophages. These cells migrate through the gaps between the alveolar epithelial cells arising from the interstitium. They move on the surface of the epithelium (REM; magnification × 2400).

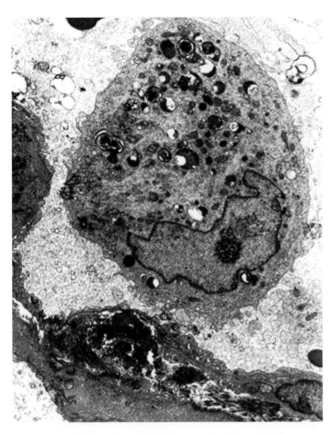

**Figure 8.36** Alveolar macrophage, with an eccentrically located indented nucleus and a prominent nucleolus. In the cytoplasm are several Golgi apparatus. Lysosomes and phagolysosomes are also seen, some with a lamellar architecture. The cell migrates with the help of the microvilli along the surface of the epithelium. In the vicinity are complexes of surfactant (magnification × 12000).

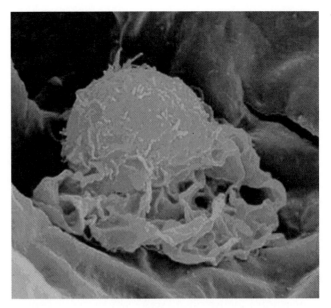

**Figure 8.37** Surface structure of a macrophage. On the surface are irregularly dispersed microvilli and microplicae. The cell is in direct contact with the alveolar epithelium (REM; magnification × 6500).

bronchioli respiratorii, the ductuli alveolares, the alveoli, and the local pulmonary vessels. An acinus has a diameter of 7.5 to 8.5 mm and contains 3000 to 4000 alveoli. The whole lung consists of 15,000 to 20,000 acini. Under certain circumstances, the acinus can be demonstrated radiographically. The acinus has a wedgelike appearance. With the conducting terminal bronchiole and the conducting pulmonal artery at the top and the capillaries and the pulmonal vein at the outer edge, the acinus forms the smallest morphologically detectable unit of the lung.

## PULMONARY CIRCULATION

### Pulmonary Arteries

The truncus pulmonalis begins at the pulmonic valve and is divided into the right and left pulmonary artery. The right pulmonary artery follows the aortic arch horizontally. In the mediastinum, the arteries of the upper lobe branch from the main vessel. The interlobular artery lies in front of the lower lobe bifurcation, inferior to the main bronchi. The shorter left artery runs cranial and dorsally. It is divided into the upper and lower lobe vessels. In the lung parenchyma, the division into the different vascular branches takes place.

The vascular architecture derives from the elasticity of the arteries. The wall is thinner than that of the aorta. The smaller arteries, beginning with a diameter of 1 mm, lose their elasticity and develop circular muscle fibers. In the precapillary areas, these muscle fibers are no longer detectable.

### Pulmonary Veins

The pulmonary veins do not follow the bronchial tree. Instead, they have a horizontal course. The four pulmonary veins lead to the left atrium. Histologically, the pulmonal veins have an irregular muscular layer and a thick adventitia. The venules have the same architecture as the arterioles.

The pulmonary arteries provide the lung with functional and nutritional circulation. The bronchial arteries supply the bronchial system up to the terminal bronchioles and are responsible for the blood supply of the visceral pleura, the lymphatic system of the lung, and the walls of the intrapulmonary vessels. Arteriovenous and bronchopulmonary artery anastomoses form various connections in the pulmonary circulation system. At the periphery, they have a common capillary network. A portion of this network, especially in the proximal bronchial tree, leads to the small bronchial veins, which themselves lead to the azygos and hemiazygos veins. The right bronchial artery derives from the aorta, and the left bronchial artery derives from the third or fourth intercostal artery or the subclavian artery.

## LYMPHATIC VESSEL SYSTEM

Lymphatic drainage is performed by a superficial and deep peribronchial network of vessels. In the alveolar septa, no lymphatic vessels are found. They lie in the loose connective tissue of the bronchioli respiratorii and continue into the perilobular, intralobular, perivenous, and subpleural connective tissue. Several anastomoses are established in the hilar region to connect the vessel systems of adjacent organ systems, including the thorax and the parietal pleura. Through transdiaphragmatic connections, the lymphatic vessel system makes contact with the abdominal region. A larger part of the left lung is drained by the right tracheobronchial lymph nodes. The right bronchomediastinal trunk and the right lymphatic trunk lead to the right vein angle.

## SURFACTANT SYSTEM

Surfactant is a mixture of substances produced by the alveolar epithelium to decrease surface tension of the lung. These substances are produced and released by type II pneumocytes. The effect of surface tension on the mechanical characteristics of the lung and on ventilation was first described by Neergard in 1929. A comparison of pressure-volume graphs of air-filled and fluid-filled lungs showed that surface tension was the decisive retraction power in the alveolar system. The lung's elasticity has an influence of only 25% to 35%. Therefore, it was concluded that there had to be a detergent in the lung that functioned as an "antiatelectasis factor" for surface tension during ventilation.

This mixture of substances consists of 90% lipids and 10% proteins. The main fraction of the phospholipids consists of phosphatidylcholine, and the lipids are predominantly cholesterine. The alveolar surface is covered by two layers or phases: the upper phase of phospholipids and the lower watery alveolar phase. In the protein fraction, four surfactant-associated proteins (SPs) have been detected: SPA, B, C, and D. They have a special importance for intracellular transport, exocytosis, surface active properties, and endocytosis of surfactant components.

The secretion is carried out in the alveolar system by cubic alveolar epithelial cells. The substances necessary

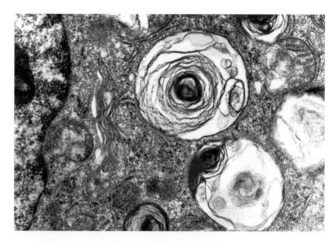

**Figure 8.38** Surfactant system. After passage through the Golgi apparatus, the components of the surfactant are stored in form of lamellar bodies in the cytoplasm. Among the lamellar bodies are single mitochondria (magnification $\times$ 16500).

for surfactant synthesis are delivered by blood vessels (Fig. 8.38). By diffusion, these substances reach the cytoplasm of type II pneumocytes. The proteins are synthesized in the endoplasmic reticulum and are transported to the Golgi apparatus and to the multivesicular bodies. Finally, these proteins reach the lamellar bodies, in which intracellular transport takes place. The contents of the osmiophilic bodies are secreted on the cell surface by merocrine mechanisms.

Surfactant covers a 70-Å thick osmiophilic layer, the invisible and alternating high hypophase over the alveolar epithelium (Fig. 8.39). By its surface active properties, this layer guarantees the focal collapse of the alveoli

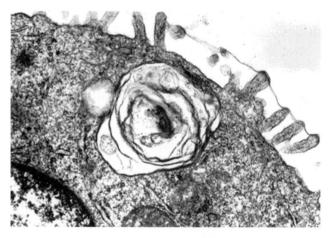

**Figure 8.39** Arrangement of the surfactant over the surface epithelium. At the surface of the epithelial cells over the hypophase is a broad layer of an osmiophilic, contrast-rich lamella. This layer extends to the microvilli. In the cytoplasm of the pneumocyte directly under the cell membrane is an osmiophilic lamellar body (magnification $\times$ 17000).

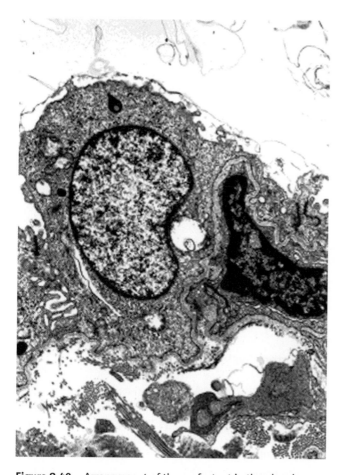

**Figure 8.40**  Arrangement of the surfactant in the alveolar duct. Over the cubic epithelial cell of the alveolar duct is a regularly arranged surfactant layer over the hypophase. Microvilli extend to this formation. Under the epithelial cell is a basement membrane. In the adjacent connective tissue are smooth muscle fibers (magnification × 5200).

during expiration and the unfolding and extension during inspiration. Surfactant evenly covers the cell membranes of the alveolar epithelium, so infectious agents that are taken up with the inhaled air cannot reach these membranes.

The epithelium of the alveolar duct is also covered with surfactant (Fig. 8.40). Surfactant particles can be detected in the sol phase of the mucus in the bronchioles and in bronchial epithelium. Probably, some surfactant shifts from the alveolar space over the alveolar duct into the bronchial system. This portion of surfactant improves the gliding properties of the gelid, sticky bronchial mucus. The height of the thin sol phase over the bronchial epithelium, in which the cilia are moving, is likely regulated by these surfactant particles.

## SUGGESTED READINGS

Clara M. (1937) Zur Histologie des Bronchialepthels. Z. mikr.-anat. Forsch.41, 321.

Morgenroth K. (1986) Das Surfactantsystem der Lunge. W. De Gruyter Berlin New York.

Morgenroth K., Bolz J. (1985)  Morphological feature of the interaction between mucus and surfactant on the bronchial mucosa. Respiration 47, 225–231.

Morgenroth K., Hörstebrock U. (1978) Transmissions- und rasterelektronenmikroskopische Untersuchungen zur Struktur der Clarazellen des Bronchialsystems. Arzeneim.-Forsch. Drug. Res. 28, 911–917.

Von Neergard K. Wirz K. (1929) Neue Auffassung über einen Begriff der Atemmechanik. Z. Ges. Exp. Med. 66, 373–381.

Weibel, E. R., Gil (1968) Electron microscopic demonstration of an extracellular duplex lining of alvioli. Resp. Physiol. 4, 42–57.

Shimura S., Takishima T. (1994) Airway submucosal secretion. In Takishima T., Shimura S. Airway secretion. Marcel Dekker New York Basel Hong Kong 325–386.

# CHAPTER 9

# Lung Mechanics in Health

Edgardo D'Angelo

## STATICS

The statics of the respiratory system and its component parts is studied by determining and analyzing the corresponding volume-pressure (V-P) relationships. These relationships are usually represented as single lines, implying that (a) static pressures depend on volume alone and (b) pressure across any respiratory structure can be dealt with as a single value. Static pressures differ, however, depending on the volume and time history of the respiratory system, and curves obtained as volume is changed in progressive steps from minimal to maximal lung volume and back again are loops, called *hysteresis loops*. In the respiratory system, hysteresis is attributed to both viscoelasticity (i.e., a rate-dependent phenomenon) and plasticity (i.e., a rate-independent phenomenon). Indeed, only plasticity should be held responsible for static hysteresis, which in mechanical analogues is produced by Prandtl bodies. There is no information concerning pressure related to tissue plasticity in humans; however, it has been suggested that this pressure component should be very small in the tidal volume range.[1] Moreover, the static pressure across the lung and chest wall varies at different sites because of the effects of gravity and different shapes of these two structures.[2] It is therefore important to keep in mind that the balance between the lung and the chest wall under physiologic conditions results from a wide distribution of pressures. In addition, the static pressure across the respiratory system may become nonuniform under conditions involving airway closure. Nevertheless, for analytic purposes, the static V-P relationship is hereafter considered as a single function.

## Respiratory System

The net pressure developed by the respiratory system under static conditions (Pst,rs) results from the forces exerted by its elastic elements and equals the difference between alveolar pressure (PA) and body surface pressure (Pbs). Conversely, Pst,rs indicates the pressure that the respiratory muscles must exert to maintain that lung volume with open airways, provided shape of the respiratory system is kept fixed. For a given volume, the elastic energy and hence the elastic pressure are minimal for the configuration occurring during paralysis, and they are increased whenever that configuration is changed.

In anesthetized paralyzed subjects, the V-P curve of the respiratory system has been assessed using various methods, thus leading to different evaluations of the elastic properties. Because of the very low ratio of carbon dioxide output to oxygen consumption ($V_{CO_2}/V_{O_2}$), lung volumes can be markedly overestimated when these curves are obtained in steps through subsequent inflations and deflations, the more so the greater number of steps and the longer the periods between successive volume changes.[3] This situation causes overestimation of both compliance and hysteresis. An additional source of variability could be the anesthetic agents, because they have been shown to affect the P-V curve of excised dog lungs differently.[4] Moreover, V-P curves have been obtained only for volumes greater than the functional residual capacity (FRC), which is the resting volume of the respiratory system in paralyzed subjects, and have been rarely extended to Pst,rs of 30 cm $H_2O$ or greater.

Figure 9.1 shows the inflation V-P curve of the respiratory system and its component parts obtained during

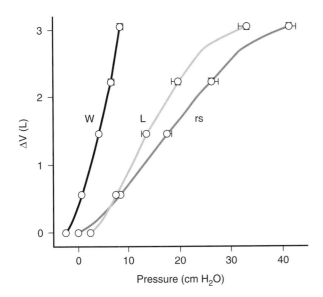

**Figure 9.1** Relationship between lung volume above functional residual capacity (FRC) and quasistatic pressure across the respiratory system (rs), lung (L) and chest wall (w) in 13 paralyzed anesthetized normal subjects. Bars: SE.
(Adapted from D'Angelo E, Tavola M, Milic-Emili J: Volume and time dependence of respiratory system mechanics in normal anaesthetized paralysed humans. Eur Respir J 2000;16:665–672).

anesthesia and paralysis in recumbent normal subjects ventilated on zero end-expiratory pressure. The V-P curve is slightly sigmoidal, and the compliance of the respiratory system ($Crs = \Delta V / \Delta P$) therefore changes with the inflation volume. The initial inflection ("knee") in the inflation V-P curve occurs at Pst,rs of 2 to 3 cm $H_2O$, but in certain subjects it occurs at Pst,rs as high as

5 cm $H_2O$, whereas in others it is essentially absent.[5,6] The presence of the knee, together with its variable position in the inflation V-P curve, makes Crs assessed as the ratio of volume to pressure changes at a given pressure questionable. In a substantial volume range above the initial knee, the inflation V-P curve of the respiratory system, as well as that of its component parts, is almost linear, and the slope of the V-P curve in this volume range probably gives a true measure of Crs that can be used for comparison among subjects and conditions.

Table 9.1 summarizes the reported average values of Crs, besides CL and CW. As pointed out earlier, the largest percentage of the variability among studies is likely caused by the different methods and anesthetics employed, but a substantial fraction could be the result of the various ways and volume ranges in which Crs was computed. Conversely, it has been shown that Crs does not change progressively with time during anesthesia, with repeated inflations to high distending pressures, with increasing the depth of anesthesia, or with muscle paralysis.[6–10]

## Lung and Chest Wall

Because the chest wall (W) and lung (L) are placed pneumatically in series, the volume changes of the chest wall ($\Delta Vw$) and the lung ($\Delta VL$) should be the same, except for blood shifts, and should be equal to those of the respiratory system ($\Delta Vrs$), whereas the algebraic sum of the pressure exerted by the lungs (PL) and the chest wall (Pw) equals the pressure of the respiratory system. It follows that the reciprocal of Crs equals the sum of the reciprocals of lung (CL) and chest wall compliance (CW). The pressure exerted by the lung is the difference between

**Table 9-1** Quasistatic Compliance of Respiratory System, Lung, and Chest Wall in Anesthetized Paralyzed Normal Subjects Lying Supine*

| Number of Subjects | Age (yr) | Crs (cm $H_2O$/L) | CL (cm $H_2O$/L) | Cw (cm $H_2O$/L) | Reference |
|---|---|---|---|---|---|
| 15 | 40 (18–63) | 0.064±0.004 | 0.097±0.007 | 0.204±0.023 | 6 |
| 10 | 38 (21–49) | 0.090±0.010 | 0.171±0.016 | 0.221±0.047 | 32 |
| 22 | 47 (29–68) | 0.113±0.005 | 0.204±0.018 | 0.305±0.024 | 33 |
| 5 | 27 (24–29) | 0.099±0.011 | 0.140±0.016 | 0.430±0.118 | 10 |
| 5 | 26 (23–28) | 0.087±0.005 | 0.168±0.012 | 0.212±0.048 | 9 |
| 18 | 31 (17–42) | 0.071±0.006 | 0.112±0.008 | 0.161±0.010 | 49 |
| 17 | 43 | 0.081±0.004 | 0.150±0.013 | 0.203±0.018 | 82 |
| 15 | 20 (14–28) | 0.083±0.007 | 0.141±0.012 | 0.210±0.021 | 5 |

*Values are mean ±SE.
CL, lung compliance; Crs, respiratory system compliance; CW, chest wall compliance.

PA and pleural surface pressure (Ppl); that exerted by the chest wall is the difference between Ppl and Pbs. Thus, the resting volume of the respiratory system is reached when the inward recoil of the lung is balanced by the outward recoil of the chest wall (i.e., PL + Pw = 0). In paralyzed subjects, Pw is equal to Ppl, the latter obtained from esophageal pressure (Pes) measurements; the interpretation of Ppl requires caution, however.[11,12]

The V-P relationships of the chest wall and lungs above FRC are curvilinear: the former decreases its curvature with increasing lung volume, and the opposite is true for the latter, except in the initial part, which is usually convex toward the pressure axis (see Fig. 9.1). There is, however, a substantial range of volumes slightly above FRC in which the V-P curves of both the lung and chest wall are nearly linear: in this volume range, CW has been usually found to be larger than CL (see Table 9.1).

Although the fall in Crs at high lung volumes is entirely the result of the decrease of CL, the low Crs at low inflation pressures is also caused by the chest wall, although to a lesser extent than the lungs (see Fig. 9.1). However, the intersubject variability of the position of the initial knee in the inflation V-P curve of the respiratory system should reflect that of the lung V-P curve only.[5] Moreover, the initial knee is abolished when a positive end-expiratory pressure (PEEP) of 5 cm $H_2O$ is applied.[6,13] These observations suggest that the progressive increase in CL and Crs with increasing the lung volume to more than FRC results from reopening of small airways and recruitment of dependent lung units. Owing to the low values of FRC in recumbent, anesthetized normal subjects and the presence of a vertical gradient of Ppl, it seems likely that small airways in the dependent part of the lung are exposed to zero or positive pressure, and thus they collapse. As a consequence, an inverse relationship should exist between normalized FRC and the position of the initial knee along the pressure axis. Unfortunately, no pertinent data are available.

Lung volume changes occur because of the displacement of the rib cage facing the lung (rc,L) and of the diaphragm-abdomen (di-ab). From this viewpoint, these two structures may be considered to operate in parallel: hence Pw = Prc,L = Pdi-ab, ΔVw = ΔVrc,L + ΔVdi-ab, and Cw = Crc,L + Cdi-ab. This model was used by Wade[14] and Agostoni and colleagues[15] to construct the V-P curve of the pulmonary part of the rib cage and diaphragm-abdomen in normal subjects during voluntary relaxation. Partitioning of ΔVw has also been made between two parallel pathways represented by the entire rib cage (rc) and the diaphragm-abdominal wall (di-ab,w), respectively: hence ΔVw = ΔVrc + ΔVdi-ab,w, Pw = Prc = Pdi-ab,w, and Cw = Crc + Cdi-ab,w.[8,16] The latter model has been used to assess the V-P curves of the chest wall and its component parts of supine anesthetized paralyzed normal subjects.[17] In the volume range FRC

to FRC+1.13 L, Crc was approximately 2.5 times greater than Cdi-ab,W, thus contributing 70% to 75% of CW and hence of ΔV. Lower values of Crc/Cdi-ab,w likely applied to the subjects studied by Jones and associates[18] and Vellody and colleagues,[19] because the contribution of rib cage displacement to ΔV was only 48% and 27%, respectively. In the mechanically ventilated subject, the Crc/Cdi-ab,w ratio should be relevant in determining the alveolar ventilation-perfusion (VA/Q) distribution and the efficiency of gas exchange.

## Effects of Anesthesia and Paralysis

The most frequently reported effect of general anesthesia in normal supine subjects is a reduction of FRC; according to Rehder and Marsh,[20] this decrease is given by ΔFRC = 10.18 − 0.23 age − 46.7 weight/height, where age, weight, and height are in years, kilograms, and centimeters, respectively, and ΔFRC is expressed as the percentage of FRC while awake. Such a decrease occurs also in the prone posture, but not in the sitting position or probably the lateral decubitus position.[21,22] Several mechanisms have been invoked to explain the reduction of FRC in recumbent, anesthetized subjects; the marked intersubject variability of this reduction (Fig. 9.2) suggests that

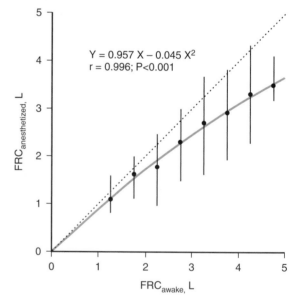

$$Y = 0.957\,X - 0.045\,X^2$$
$$r = 0.996;\ P < 0.001$$

**Figure 9.2** Relationship between functional residual capacity (FRC) in the awake and anesthetized states assessed in 128 subjects. The *symbols* are mean of values falling within each subsequent 0.5-L interval beginning with 1-L FRC awake. The *continuous line* is the best fit through mean values. Bars: range. (Data from Rehder K, Marsh M: Respiratory mechanics during anesthesia and mechanical ventilation. In Macklem PT, Mead J [eds]: Handbook of Physiology: The Respiratory System, Mechanics of Breathing, sect 3, vol 3. Bethesda, MD: American Physiological Society, 1986, pp 737–752.)

this decrease depends on several factors, none of which consistently prevails.

Tonic activity of both inspiratory rib cage muscles and the diaphragm has been suggested to augment the chest wall recoil in awake subjects.[8,23,24] However, this tone is minimal in the supine position, when ΔFRC is large, and it is greater in the erect posture, when ΔFRC is absent.[8,23] Perhaps tonic activity affects only the shape of the diaphragm, because these morphologic changes are not followed by any net cephalad displacement of the diaphragm with induction of anesthesia and paralysis.[8,16,25] The shape of the chest wall also changes with anesthesia: the anteroposterior diameters of both the rib cage and the abdomen decrease, whereas the transverse diameters increase.[19] Conversely, it is unclear whether the volume of the thoracic cavity is effectively reduced because of these dimensional changes.[7,8,26] Finally, expiratory activity that appears in abdominal muscles with anesthesia[27] does not seem a main factor in lowering FRC, because FRC does not change with muscular paralysis.[10]

Increases in intrathoracic blood volume up to 0.3 L have been reported to occur with anesthesia and paralysis.[7,8] Although these changes could be large enough to account for the reported reductions in FRC, the lack of an established intrasubject relationship with the fall of FRC prevents any firm conclusion concerning the role of blood shifts.

As for FRC changes, those in the elastic recoil of the respiratory system also show great intersubject variability, a finding suggesting that the same factors could be responsible for both effects. In this connection, the entity of the resting volume with anesthesia may be critical: indeed, no change in Crs occurs in sitting subjects both during anesthesia, when FRC does not fall, and with submaximal muscular paralysis, when FRC decreases because of blood shift, but Crs remains greater than in awake, supine subjects.[22,28]

The fall of FRC with general anesthesia in recumbent normal subjects reflects the fact that, under these conditions, the balance between the outward recoil of the chest wall and the inward recoil of the lungs occurs at lower lung volume. The majority of evidence suggests that the decrease in Crs is mainly the result of changes in lung mechanical properties, under both quasistatic[6,9,10] and dynamic conditions,[29–31] although some authors found no change.[32,33] Several mechanisms can lower $C_L$, such as increased smooth muscle tone or stimulation of other contractile elements in the airways or lung parenchyma, atelectasis, small airway closure, and changes in surfactant function. Lung V-P curves on inflation from FRC are often S shaped (see Fig. 9.1), a finding that could indicate small airway opening and alveolar recruitment, as mentioned earlier. In supine anesthetized paralyzed normal subjects, atelectasis that eventually develops during ventilation on zero end-expiratory pressure is eliminated with inflations to $P_A$ of 30 cm $H_2O$ or greater.[34] Such alveolar recruitment can quantitatively account for both the increase in $C_L$ and the leftward shift of the static V-P curve of the lung observed with PEEP ventilation in some anesthetized paralyzed normal subjects.[13] However, similar changes in lung mechanics have also been observed in normal, seated subjects after maintained hyperinflation and have been attributed to changes in either pulmonary blood volume or airway muscle tone.[35–37] Finally, Westbrook and colleagues[10] suggested that changes in $C_L$ are secondary to a rightward shift of V-P curve of the chest wall leading to volume reduction, because ventilation at low lung volumes in awake, normal subjects is eventually associated with increased lung recoil, probably as a result of higher surface tension.[38] This sequence of events contrasts with the observation that, in supine anesthetized paralyzed subjects, $C_L$, although increased with PEEP, remains substantially lower[13] than that reported by Agostoni and Hyatt[39] for awake supine subjects at comparable lung volumes.

The V-P curve of the chest wall seems to undergo only relatively minor changes with anesthesia and paralysis in the supine posture, in spite of substantial changes in configuration (see earlier). Quasistatic $C_W$ is similar to that reported for awake supine subjects during relaxation (see Table 9.1),[39] but the outward recoil could be reduced at low lung volumes.[10] Indeed, the increase in $C_W$ with PEEP in anesthetized paralyzed subjects is only one fourth of that occurring over the same range of lung volume during relaxation in awake supine subjects.[13]

Changes in the elastic properties of lung and chest wall with anesthesia and paralysis, together with the dependent alterations in chest wall configuration, should likely influence the distribution of inspired gas during mechanical ventilation. Only part of the differences in the distribution of ventilation observed in most postures between awake spontaneously breathing and anesthetized paralyzed subjects can be attributed to differences in the distribution of forces applied by the respiratory muscles and ventilator.[40] Indeed, the direction of changes in regional ventilation with anesthesia and paralysis in different postures is not always consistent with the known pattern of respiratory muscle activation in awake subjects, in which more or less pronounced changes in the distribution of inspired gas occur in all but the prone posture.[40] Although several mechanisms, such as mechanical interdependence of lung parenchyma, collateral ventilation, and lobar sliding, may limit the modification of regional ventilation, the changes in chest wall shape occurring with anesthesia should therefore influence regional lung expansion and hence the distribution of regional $C_L$. Moreover, although these changes imply relatively minor modifications in the overall compliance, they may reflect important changes in regional $C_W$ and thus may further influence the distribution of ventilation.

## DYNAMICS

The pressure that opposes the driving pressure arises from the following: (a) elastic forces within the lung and chest wall, including those required to compress or decompress the intrathoracic gases and to distort the respiratory system from the relaxed configuration; (b) viscous forces related to flow of gas along the airways and of lung and chest wall tissues; (c) viscoelastic forces resulting from stress adaptation units within the tissues of lung and chest wall; (d) plastoelastic forces, as reflected by differences in elastic recoil pressure of the lung or chest wall at isovolume between inflation and deflation under true static conditions; and (e) inertial forces of tissues and gas in the airways. Among these factors, items a to c provide the relevant pressures that under normal conditions oppose the driving pressure developed by the respiratory muscles or the ventilator in spontaneously breathing or mechanically ventilated, anesthetized subjects. Dynamic forces that more commonly develop in opposition to the driving pressures are discussed first; static forces are described earlier. Next, the dynamic performance of the respiratory system and of its component parts, the lung and chest wall, is considered.

### Viscous Forces

The pressure that causes the flow of gases along the airways is the difference between $P_A$ and airway opening pressure, but the direct measure of $P_A$ is clearly impossible in humans. On the basis of postmortem measurements of airway dimensions, Rohrer[41,42] proposed the following relationships between gas flow ($\dot{V}$) and the pressure dissipated within the airways (Pres) or airway resistance (Raw)

$$Pres = K_1 \cdot \dot{V} + K_2 \cdot \dot{V}^2 \qquad (1)$$

$$Raw = K_1 + K_2 \cdot \dot{V} \qquad (2)$$

where K1 and K2 are constants. Moreover, Raw has been shown also to depend on lung volume, according to[43]

$$Gaw = 1/Raw = a + b \cdot V \qquad (3)$$

where $a$ and $b$ are constants. Although the physical meaning originally assigned to K1 and K2 is no longer accepted, Rohrer's equations are still widely used, because they provide a close description of experimental data.[44] Conversely, the values of K1 and K2 reported in the literature vary substantially, mainly because of differences in the techniques used to obtain the relevant measures, besides experimental conditions. The average values of the constants in Equations 1 to 3 for the interrupter resistance of the respiratory system obtained in anesthetized paralyzed normal subjects lying supine are given in Table 9.2. In mechanically ventilated subjects, evaluation of K1 and, especially, K2 is made difficult by the presence of the endotracheal tube (ETT): because the ETT resistance in situ may differ from that in vitro,[45] the use of the subtraction technique to correct for the ETT resistance could become inadequate (see Table 9.2). During general anesthesia, a further source of variability is represented by the anesthetics agents, which may affect the bronchomotor tone differently.[20,46] Of the two methods currently used to estimate airflow resistance, the body plethysmographic and the interrupter method, only the latter can be applied in anesthetized subjects. This method allows the computation of viscous resistance as the ratio of the sudden pressure change that occurs with rapid airway occlusion to the flow existing immediately before the occlusion (Fig. 9.3). Depending on whether airway opening, esophageal, or transpulmonary pressure is being measured, this ratio gives the interrupter resistance of the respiratory system (Rint,rs), chest wall (Rint,w), and lung (Rint,l), respectively. In anesthetized paralyzed subjects, airway opening pressure is usually measured at the proximal end of the ETT; therefore, Rint includes the ETT resistance, which is strongly flow dependent. Because corrections of EET

| Table 9-2 | Constants K1 and K2 in Equation 2 and constants a and b in Equation 3 for the Interrupter Resistance of the Respiratory System in Anesthetized Paralyzed Normal Subjects Lying Supine* | | | | |
|---|---|---|---|---|---|
| K1 (cm $H_2O$/sec/L) | K2 (cm $H_2O$/sec²/L) | a (L/sec/cm $H_2O$) | b (sec/cm $H_2O$) | Number of Subjects | Reference |
| 1.47±0.08 | 0.058±0.028 | 0.64±0.05 | 0.13±0.02 | 28 | 5 |
| 1.87±0.10 | 0.367±0.027 | | | 26 | 13, 49 |

*Values are mean ±SE. K1 and K2 were computed from measurements performed at volumes 0.41–0.76 L greater than functional residual capacity and flows from 0.22 to 1.31 L/sec, with[13,49] or without the need of correction for the endotracheal tube resistance (see text). Constants a and b were computed from measurements performed at volumes from 0.5 to 3.2 L greater than functional residual capacity and flows of 0.82–0.97 L/sec.

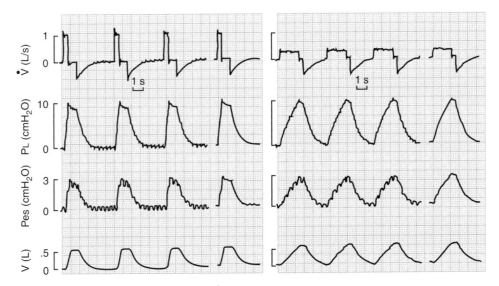

**Figure 9.3** Records of flow ($\dot{V}$), changes in transpulmonary ($P_L$) and esophageal pressure (Pes) and in lung volume (V) of three consecutive breaths and after ensemble average of 33 to 35 consecutive breaths pertaining to the same condition, obtained in a paralyzed anesthetized normal subject during ventilation with high-inflation (*left*) and low-inflation flow (*right*). (Adapted from D'Angelo E, Prandi E, Tavola M, et al: Chest wall interrupter resistance in anesthetized paralyzed humans. J Appl Physiol 1994;77:883–887.)

resistance are often problematic, especially when the ETT has been kept in place for some time, assessment of Rint,rs and Rint,L is best performed by measuring airway opening pressure in the trachea, a few centimeters away from the distal end of the ETT. Table 9.3 shows the mean values of Rint,rs, Rint,L, and Rint,w thus obtained in supine anesthetized paralyzed normal subjects, whereas Figure 9.4 illustrates the dependence of Rint,rs on flow and volume greater than FRC.

Assessment of Rint,w in humans is problematic because rapid airway occlusions are rarely associated with evident sudden changes in Pes both in spontaneously breathing[47] and mechanically ventilated anesthetized paralyzed subjects.[13,48,49] However, with the use of a rapid airway shutter and ensemble averaging of 30 to 40 tests breaths to allow for cardiac artifacts (see Fig. 9.3), Rint,w has been assessed in mechanically ventilated anesthetized paralyzed normal subjects. In the range 0.24 to 1.12 L/second, Rint,w was independent of flow, and it amounted to approximately 0.25% Rint,rs.[50] Because the measurements of Rint,rs in intubated subjects were based on tracheal pressure changes, upper airway resistance was obviously not included; therefore, in anesthetized subjects ventilated through a mask, Rint,w should represent a substantially lower fraction of Rint,rs. This explains the results obtained by Liistro and associates,[51] who found Rint,rs close to Raw measured with the body plethysmographic method in awake, normal subjects.

**Table 9-3** Interrupter Resistance and Quasistatic Elastance of the Respiratory System, Lung, and Chest Wall in Anesthetized Paralyzed Normal Subjects Lying Supine*

| Rint,rs (cm H$_2$O/sec/L) | Rint,L (cm H$_2$O/sec/L) | Rint,w (cm H$_2$O/L) | Est,rs (cm H$_2$O/L) | Est,L (cm H$_2$O/L) | Est,w H$_2$O/sec/L) | Number of Subjects | Reference |
|---|---|---|---|---|---|---|---|
| 1.54±0.13 | 1.13±0.11 | 0.41±0.03 | | | | 12 | 50 |
| 1.48±0.07 (1.12–1.65) | | | 15.0±0.7 (10.1–19.3) | 9.3±0.5 | 5.8±0.4 | 28 | 5 |

*Values are mean ±SE; range in parentheses. Values refer to measurements performed in the volume and flow range 0.41–0.76 L greater than functional residual capacity and 0.22–1.31 L/sec, respectively.

Est, quasistatic elastance; L, lung; Rint, interrupter resistance; rs, respiratory system; w, chest wall.

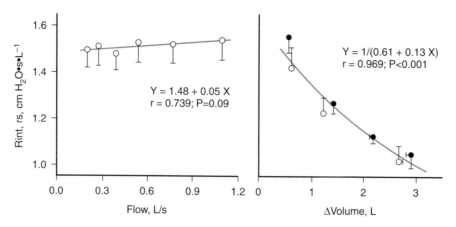

**Figure 9.4** *Left*: Relationship between inflation flow and interrupter resistance of the respiratory system (Rint,rs) obtained in 30 paralyzed anesthetized normal subjects. Bars: SE. *Right*: Relationship between volume above functional residual capacity (FRC) and Rint,rs in 13 (*closed symbols*) and 15 paralyzed anesthetized normal subjects (*open symbols*) ventilated on zero end-expiratory pressure with different tidal volumes and with fixed tidal volume (0.61±0.05 L) on zero and positive end-expiratory pressure of 9 and 23 cm $H_2O$, respectively. Bars: SE. (*Left*, Data from D'Angelo E, Tavola M, Milic-Emili J: Volume and time dependence of respiratory system mechanics in normal anaesthetized paralysed humans. Eur Respir J 2000;16:665–672; and D'Angelo E, Calderini E, Tavola M, et al: Effect of PEEP on respiratory mechanics in anesthetized paralyzed humans. J Appl Physiol 1992;73:1736–1742; *right*, data from D'Angelo E, Tavola M, Milic-Emili J: Volume and time dependence of respiratory system mechanics in normal anaesthetized paralysed humans. Eur Respir J 2000;16:665–672.)

Moreover, Rint,w should become a negligible fraction of Rint,rs in patients with increased Raw. Indeed, in patients with adult respiratory distress syndrome, Rint,w was normal (0.3±0.1 cm $H_2O$ L/second), and it amounted to only approximately 6% of Rint,rs.[52]

Whereas Rint,w reflects the viscous resistance of chest wall tissues, Rint,L should correspond to the sum of Raw and the viscous resistance of lung tissues. However, using the alveolar capsule technique in open-chest dogs[53] and rats,[54] investigators showed that the pulmonary tissues do not contribute appreciably to Rint,L, whereby Rint,L is approximately equal to Raw. In the normal tidal volume range, Rint,L should represent a constant fraction (~0.75) of Rint,rs, because both Rint,L and Rint,w are essentially independent of $\dot{V}$.[13] In contrast, any dependence of Rint,rs on $\dot{V}$ and $\Delta V$ should reflect that of Rint,L, because Rint,w is independent of both $\dot{V}$ and $\Delta V$.

The directly measured (no need of correction for ETT resistance) Rint,rs is flow independent,[5,50] at least in the range of 0.2 to 1.3 L/second, in line with the observations of Jonson and colleagues,[1] which were also based on tracheal pressure measurements. In mechanically ventilated subjects, the effective resistance of the respiratory system becomes markedly flow dependent, however, because of the presence of the ETT and, during expiration, the expiratory valve of the ventilator. This has the consequence that, for a given tidal volume and breath timing, both mean resistive pressure and viscous work depend on the shape of the flow wave, the more so the greater the value of the constant K2 and the mean flow.[55]

## Viscoelastic Forces

The pressure developed by viscoelastic elements cannot be measured directly, but it can be assessed by the slow change of pressure that takes place when airflow is suddenly stopped and the volume is kept fixed until pressure becomes constant or nearly so. This phenomenon, usually referred to as *stress relaxation*, provides the basis of the rapid airway occlusion method that has been used in anesthetized paralyzed humans and animals for determining the viscoelastic properties of lung and chest wall, besides the viscous resistance and quasistatic elastance. Figure 9.5 illustrates the rapid airway occlusion method as applied during constant flow inflation in an anesthetized paralyzed normal subject: (a) the immediate drop in PL (Pmax − P1) with airway occlusion divided by the flow preceding the occlusion ($\dot{V}$) gives Rint,L; (b) the slow decay in PL and Pes to a nearly constant value achieved in 3 to 4 seconds represents the viscoelastic pressure dissipation (Pvisc = P1 − Pst), which, divided by $\dot{V}$ or $\Delta V$, gives the additional resistance ($\Delta R = Pvisc/\dot{V}$) or elastance ($\Delta E = Pvisc/\Delta V$) resulting from the viscoelastic behavior of the lung and chest wall tissues, respectively; and (c) the apparent plateau of PL and Pes (Pst) represents the quasistatic recoil pressure that, divided by the volume change, gives the quasistatic elastance (Est = Pst/$\Delta V$) of the lung and chest wall, respectively. Figure 9.6 depicts the simplest model, originally proposed by Mount,[56] that satisfactorily reproduces the time course of Pes and PL in experiments like those presented in Figure 9.5: both the lung and chest wall

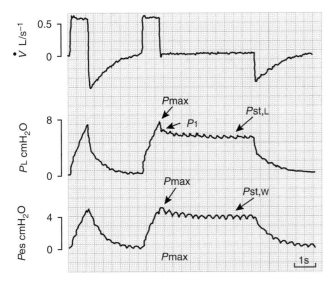

**Figure 9.5** Records of flow ($\dot{V}$) and changes in transpulmonary pressure (PL) and esophageal pressure (Pes) in a paralyzed anesthetized normal subject in whom, during constant-flow inflation of 0.55 L/second, the airway was rapidly occluded at a lung volume of 0.6 L greater than functional residual capacity (FRC).

submodels comprise a dashpot, Rint,L (~Raw) and Rint,W, respectively, arranged in parallel with a Kelvin body, which consists of a spring representing the quasi-static elastance (Est,L and Est,W) in parallel with Maxwell body. The latter is made by a spring (Evisc,L and Evisc,W) and dashpot (Rvisc,L and Rvisc,W) arranged serially, which, together with the corresponding time constant ($\tau$visc,L = Rvisc,L/Evisc,L and $\tau$visc,W = Rvisc,W/Evisc,W), accounts for the viscoelastic behavior. Because with constant flow inflation

$$\Delta R = Rvisc \ (1 - e^{-TI/\tau visc}) \qquad (4)$$

the viscoelastic parameters Rvisc, $\tau$visc, and Evisc can be computed from $\Delta R$ values of test breaths with different durations of inflation (TI) and fixed $\Delta V$.

The lungs and chest wall comprise a large number of elements that very likely possess different mechanical properties. The model in Figure 9.6 is clearly too simple to be a comprehensive representation of the respiratory system. On the basis of stress relaxation data obtained in excised cat lungs, Hildebrandt[57] proposed a plastoelastic linear viscoelastic model in which the viscoelastic compartment is made by elements with a continuous spectrum of time constants and the mechanical analogue is represented by a number of Maxwell bodies arranged in parallel. Other models suggested so far[58-60] basically represent developments of Hildebrandt's model. In contrast, Mount's model is useful because it mimics adequately the most common and fundamental aspects of respiratory dynamics in a more direct way. Moreover, it has been shown[5] that the performance of the Mount and Hildebrandt models in fitting impedance data obtained in normal subjects with the forced oscillation technique over an extended frequency range are essentially the same (see later).

Viscoelastic constants assessed in normal anesthetized paralyzed human subjects with the technique of rapid airway occlusion at end inflation are independent of flow and volume up to 1.3 L/second and FRC+3 L, respectively.[5,13,48,49] Their average values are given in Table 9.4, together with those of Est obtained in the normal tidal volume range. Conversely, Sharp and associates[61] found that stress adaptation in the respiratory system, lung, and chest wall of anesthetized paralyzed normal subjects became somewhat larger at high lung volumes.

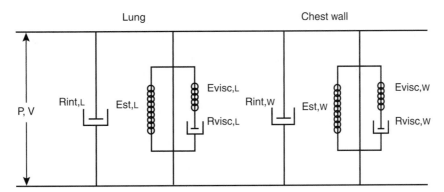

**Figure 9.6** A mechanical viscoelastic model for interpretation of respiratory mechanics. The respiratory system consists of two parallel units, that is, lung (L) and chest wall (W), each made by a dashpot (interrupter resistance: Rint,L ≈ airway resistance and Rint,W, respectively) in parallel with a Kelvin body, which, in turn, consists of a spring (static elastance: Est,L and Est,W, respectively) in parallel with a Maxwell body. The latter, with its spring Evisc (viscoelastic elastance) and dashpot Rvisc (viscoelastic resistance) arranged serially, represents the viscoelastic (*stress adaptation*) unit. The distance between the horizontal bars is analogous to lung volume (V), and force applied to the bars is analogous to pressure applied to the respiratory system (P).

| Table 9-4 | Viscoelastic Resistance, Elastance, and Time Constant of the Respiratory System, Lung, and Chest Wall in Anesthetized Paralyzed Normal Subjects Lying Supine* | |
| --- | --- |
| Rvisc,rs (cm $H_2O$/sec/L) | 6.14±0.81 (3.78–7.74) |
| Rvisc,L (cm $H_2O$/sec/L) | 3.79±0.62 (1.58–6.06) |
| Rvisc,w (cm $H_2O$/sec/L) | 2.41±0.36 (1.47–3.19) |
| Evisc,rs (cm $H_2O$/L) | 4.93±0.43 (2.96–6.71) |
| Evisc,L (cm $H_2O$/L) | 3.04±0.59 (1.35–5.49) |
| Evisc,w (cm $H_2O$/L) | 1.92±0.26 (1.13–2.44) |
| τvisc,rs (sec) | 1.28±0.15 (0.84–1.86) |
| τvisc,L (sec) | 1.27±0.22 (0.30–2.68) |
| τvisc,w (sec) | 1.27±0.17 (0.53–2.06) |

*Values are mean ±SE; range in parentheses. Values are from measurements performed in 51 subjects,[5,13,49] with flows and volumes up to 1.3 L/sec and 3 L greater than functional residual capacity, respectively.
Evisc, viscoelastic elastance; L, lung; rs, respiratory system; Rvisc, viscoelastic resistance; τvisc, viscoelastic time constant; w, chest wall.

Although this observation may indicate increased Rvisc and Evisc, because τvisc computed from the pressure decay during the end-inspiratory phase hold did not change with lung volume, it is more likely explained by the limitations of the adopted procedure.[5] Hence, lungs and chest wall behave as an essentially linear viscoelastic system. Conversely, evaluation of viscoelastic properties from single ΔR measures could be misleading: because of their time dependence (see Equation 4), comparison of ΔR values requires that the duration of inflation be kept the same.

## Dynamic Performance

Respiratory system mechanics under dynamic conditions in mechanically ventilated patients are often investigated by using a multiple linear regression to fit the equation

$$Ptr = E \cdot \Delta V + R \cdot \dot{V} \qquad (5)$$

to measures of tracheal pressure (Ptr), volume changes from the end-expiratory lung volume (ΔV), and flow ($\dot{V}$), obtained throughout the breathing cycle. Because of viscoelastic properties and marked flow dependence of the expiratory valve of the ventilators, this analysis yields higher correlation coefficients if it is limited to the inflation phase. To account for continuously applied end-expiratory pressures, a constant is often added to the right hand of Equation 5. This approach is widely used because it is not time consuming and is easily implemented with commonly available facilities. Generally, E and R in the foregoing equation are referred to as respiratory system elastance and resistance, respectively. Substitution of Ptr with PL or Pes would yield lung and chest wall E and R, respectively. Provided the breathing pattern is kept fixed, this approach may be useful for studies such as the changes of gross mechanical features over extended periods of time, the dose-response characteristics of bronchomotor agents,[62] and, with adequate refinements, the rapid mechanical changes during drug uptake and clearance.[63] In contrast, it assumes that E and R are constant throughout the data being analyzed, independent of ΔV, $\dot{V}$, and breath timing. Therefore, the single-compartment, linear resistance-elastance model in Equation 5 is unable fully to describe the actual behavior of the respiratory system and its component parts, particularly when breathing frequency is lower than 0.5 Hz (see later).

The viscoelastic elements within the lung and chest wall confer time dependence of elastance and resistance. With reference to the model in Figure 9.6, at high respiratory frequencies ($f$), there will be insufficient time for the energy stored in springs Evisc to dissipate through dashpots Rvisc, whereas at low $f$, most of applied energy will dissipate through dashpots Rvisc, and little will be stored in springs Evisc. This implies that dynamic lung and chest wall elastance (Edyn) should increase with increasing $f$, and the opposite is true for dynamic resistance, usually referred to as effective resistance (Reff). Hence, Edyn should approach the corresponding values of Est + Evisc at high $f$, whereas Reff should tend to Rint + Rvisc at low $f$. During sinusoidal breathing, Edyn and Reff should change with frequency according to the following functions[49]

$$Edyn = Est + \Delta E$$
$$= Est + Evisc \cdot \omega^2 \cdot \tau visc^2/(1 + \omega^2 \cdot \tau visc^2) \quad (6)$$

and

$$Reff = Rint + \Delta R = Rint + Rvisc/(1 + \omega^2 \cdot \tau visc^2) \quad (7)$$

where $\omega$ is angular frequency ($2\pi f$). Figure 9.7 shows the relationship of lung and chest wall Evisc and $\Delta R$ to frequency computed for $\Delta V$ in the normal tidal volume range according to Equations 6 and 7, using the average values of the constants reported in Tables 9.3 and 9.4. Both Edyn,L and Edyn,W increase with $f$ and approach plateau values at $f$ of approximately 0.5 Hz, when Edyn,L and Edyn,W become about 38% and 26% higher than Est,L and Est,W, respectively. In contrast, $\Delta R$ decreases with increasing $f$, and the contribution of viscoelastic resistance to both Reff,L and Reff,W becomes negligible at $f$ greater than or equal to 0.5 Hz. No allowance of

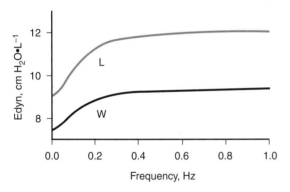

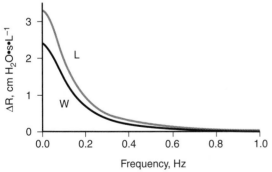

**Figure 9.7** Relationships between frequency and dynamic elastance (Edyn) or additional resistance of the respiratory system ($\Delta R$) during sinusoidal ventilation computed according to Equations 6 and 7, respectively, using average values of respiratory system static elastance (Est), viscoelastic elastance (Evisc), and viscoelastic resistance (Rvisc) in Tables 9.3 and 9.4.

possible contributions related to plastoelastic properties has been made in the foregoing computations, but such contributions should be trivial with $\Delta V$ in the normal tidal volume range.[1,64] Hence, at $f$ greater than or equal to 0.5 Hz, the respiratory system behaves effectively as a single compartment consisting of an essentially fixed elastance (Ers = Est,rs + Evisc,rs) served by a resistance Rint,rs = Raw + Rint,W. Because Raw is approximately equal to Rint,L, and neglecting the volume dependence of Raw (see Equation 3), which is trivial in the tidal volume range, the driving pressure during inflation should change according to

$$P_{(t)} = Ers \cdot \Delta V_{(t)} + (Rint,W + Rint,L + K_1) \cdot \dot{V}_{(t)}$$
$$+ K_2 \cdot \dot{V}_{(t)}^2 \quad (8)$$

where $K_1$ and $K_2$ account for the ETT resistance.

Time dependency of respiratory elastance and resistance has been also described by numerous investigators using the forced oscillation technique in studies in animals and humans. When impedance data obtained with this method are interpreted according to Hildebrandt's model, the following relationships hold for dynamic elastance[5]:

$$Edyn = A + B \cdot (0.25 + \log \omega) \quad (9)$$

and effective resistance

$$Reff = Rv + Rtis = Rv + 0.683B/\omega \quad (10)$$

respectively, where A and B are constants, Rv represents all viscous resistances, like Rint in Mount's model (see Fig. 9.6), and Rtis is tissue viscance. Both Hildebrandt and Mount models have been shown to describe equally well the respiratory impedance of anesthetized paralyzed dogs,[65] awake normal subjects relaxing in the seated posture,[5,66,67] and anesthetized paralyzed normal subjects[68,69] and patients,[70] except possibly at very low frequencies. Under this condition, the contribution of plastoelasticity may eventually become appreciable because of the small $\Delta V$ used with the forced-oscillation method, whereas plastoelastic pressure dissipation cannot be detected with the rapid end-inspiratory occlusion method. However, in anesthetized paralyzed humans, the latter method, although probably more time consuming, is technically easier to implement than the forced oscillation technique, which has major methodologic problems.

Time dependency of pulmonary and, hence, respiratory system Edyn and Reff can also be caused by time-constant inequality within the lung.[71] Although there is no certain means to distinguish between the contribution of viscoelastic properties and time-constant inequality to $\Delta R$ and $\Delta E$, it seems likely that the latter contributes substantially to the increased time dependency of $\Delta R$ observed in mechanically ventilated patients,[52,72,73] whereas in normal subjects such contribution is probably negligible. Hence, the substantial time dependency of Edyn and Reff observed in paralyzed anesthetized normal subjects should reflect primarily the viscoelastic properties of both lung and chest wall.

Viscoelasticity also influences the pattern of lung emptying, especially during passive expiration. The classical model of the respiratory system described by Equation 5 is characterized by a single time constant ($\tau rs = Rrs/Ers$): accordingly, the time course of passive volume emptying should be described by a monoexponential function

$$V(t) = V_O \cdot e^{-t/\tau rs} \qquad (11)$$

where $t$ is time from the onset of expiration and $V_O$ is the inflation volume. This equation is the kernel of various methods of measurement of respiratory mechanics, such as that based on the addition of known expiratory resistances[74] and the single breath method.[75] In contrast, Bates and colleagues[76] observed, in paralyzed dogs, that the expiratory volume-time profile was better described by a biexponential function

$$V(t) = A_1 \cdot e^{-t/\tau 1} + A_2 \cdot e^{-t/\tau 2} \qquad (12)$$

where $t$ is time from the onset of expiration, and $A_1$, $A_2$, $\tau 1$, and $\tau 2$ are constants that depend on Rvisc, Evisc, Rint, and Est, besides elastic recoil pressure at the onset of expiration.[77] $\tau 1$ and $\tau 2$ are complex parameters that do not correspond to $\tau visc$ and $\tau rs$ in Equations 4 and 11, respectively. A biexponential decay of lung volume during expiration has also been observed in normal anesthetized paralyzed normal subjects and has been related to the viscoelastic properties of the respiratory system.[78] Using a different approach, Jonson and associates[1] also concluded that in paralyzed normal humans, the time course of the decay from end-inspiratory volumes in the normal range can be adequately explained by the viscoelastic model in Figure 9.6. The effective time course of volume decay during expiration in paralyzed normal subjects is, however, more complex than that of Equation 12, because airflow occurs through the ETT and the expiratory valve of the ventilator, which exhibit marked flow dependence of resistance. A more accurate description of volume and pressure time course during passive expiration in mechanically ventilated subjects can be found elsewhere.[55]

Viscoelasticity also affects the driving pressure and airway resistance during expiration. Because part of the energy spent to inflate the respiratory system is used to elongate the springs of the viscoelastic elements (see Fig. 9.6), the stored elastic pressure can be recovered during expiration to overcome Raw. According to Equation 4,

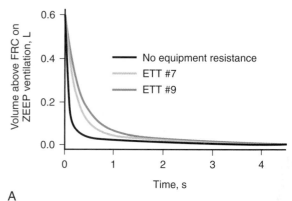

A

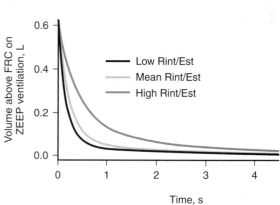

B

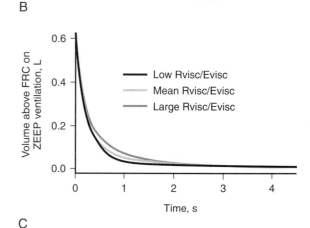

C

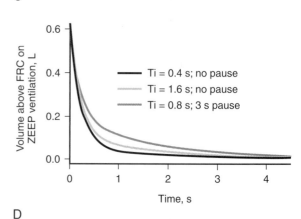

D

**Figure 9.8** The effects on the volume time course of passive expiration resulting from the following: *(a)* equipment resistance; *(b)* various combinations of interrupter resistance (Rint) and quasistatic elastance (Est) *(c)* viscoelastic resistance (Rvisc) and elastance (Evisc) of the respiratory system; and *(d)* pattern of the preceding constant-flow inflation. The volume-time profile was computed according to Equation 11A in reference 55. The duration of inspiration was 0.8 seconds from *(a)* to *(c)*, whereas in all instances, expiration started from 0.6 L greater than functional residual capacity (FRC). Constants K1 and K2 of endotracheal tubes (ETT) and expiratory port of the ventilator were taken from reference 55. The values of respiratory system Rint, Est, Rvisc, and Evisc used for computations in *(a)* and *(d)*, and in "mean" of *(b)* and *(c)* were the corresponding average values in Tables 9.3 and 9.4, whereas the values in parentheses provided the largest and lowest possible Rint/Est and Rvisc/Evisc ratios used for "high" and "low" in *(b)* and *(c)*, respectively.

◄─────────────────

this additional recoil pressure (see PL-Pst in Figure 9.5) is given by $\dot{V} \cdot Rvisc \cdot (1 - e^{-TI/\tau visc})$; therefore, it should be larger the higher $\dot{V}$ and/or $f$ and should progressively decrease and eventually vanish during end-inspiratory occlusion. Indeed, passive lung deflation is faster following rapid inflation, whereas flow is reduced if expiration is preceded by a breath-hold (see Fig. 9.5; Fig. 9.8D). Further contribution to faster expiration by viscoelastic mechanisms results from decreased Raw. Owing to the recoil pressure developed by the viscoelastic elements, the effective pull exerted by the parenchyma on intrathoracic airways becomes larger than that related to lung expansion alone, airway dilation ensues, and Raw and hence Rint,L are reduced. The presence of these viscoelastic effects has been shown to have an important effect on the interpretation of common tests of respiratory function.[79-81]

Passive expiration is hindered by the resistance of the equipment, essentially the ETT and the expiratory valve of the ventilator, a combination of high Rint and low Est values, as well as large τvisc. Indeed, once the elastic energy stored in springs, Evisc at the end of inspiration is dissipated in the dashpot Rvisc (see Fig. 9.6), the viscoelastic elements are eventually compressed, and hence brake expiration. This situation also occurs with prolonged inspiratory duration at fixed inflation volume or insertion of an end-inspiratory occlusion, because the elastic energy stored in springs Evisc at end inspiration is reduced or eventually abolished under these conditions. Figure 9.8 summarizes the effects that the equipment resistance, Rint and Est combinations, τvisc, and pattern of inspiration exert on the computed time course of expired volume during mechanical ventilation of normal subjects on zero end-expiratory pressure. With the average values of Rint, Est, and τvisc reported in Tables 9.3 and 9.4, an expiratory duration of 2 seconds ensures a

practically complete volume decay to FRC, provided an ETT no. 7 or larger is used. Indeed, with the commonly used ventilator settings (inspiratory duration, 0.8 to 1 second; expiratory duration, ≥2 seconds; tidal volume 8 to 12 mL/kg), no intrinsic PEEP (PEEPi) and dynamic hyperinflation were found in paralyzed anesthetized normal subjects.[79-81] Dynamic hyperinflation and PEEPi readily develops when the expiratory duration is 1 second or less or the equipment resistance is too large relative to Est. However, even with an expiratory duration of 2 seconds, significant PEEPi values (~1 cm $H_2O$) could also occur in normal subjects provided they exhibit the combination of the largest and lowest observed value of Rint and Est, respectively (see Fig. 9.8B), or provided ventilator settings include an end-inspiratory pause or a long inspiratory duration (see Fig. 9.8D).

## REFERENCES

1. Jonson B, Beydon L, Brauer K, et al: Mechanics of respiratory system in healthy anesthetized humans with emphasis on viscoelastic properties. J Appl Physiol 1993;75:132–140.
2. Agostoni E: Mechanics of the pleural space. Physiol Rev 1972;52:57–128.
3. Gattinoni L, Mascheroni D, Basilico E, et al: Volume/pressure curve of total respiratory system in paralysed patients: Artefacts and correction factors. Intensive Care Med 1987;13:19–23.
4. Woo SW, Berlin D, Hedly-Whyte J: Surfactant function and anesthetic agents. J Appl Physiol 1969;26:571–577.
5. D'Angelo E, Tavola M, Milic-Emili J: Volume and time dependence of respiratory system mechanics in normal anaesthetized paralysed humans. Eur Respir J 2000;16:665–672.
6. Howell JBL, Peckett BW: Studies of the elastic properties of the thorax of supine anaesthetized paralysed human subjects. J Physiol (Lond) 1957;136:1–19.
7. Hedenstierna G, Löfström B, Lundh R: Thoracic gas volume and chest-abdomen dimensions during anesthesia and muscle paralysis. Anesthesiology 1981;55:499–506.
8. Krayer S, Rehder K, Beck KC, et al: Quantification of thoracic volumes by three-dimensional imaging. J Appl Physiol 1987;62:591–598.
9. Rehder K, Mallow JE, Fibuch EE, et al: Effects of isoflurane anesthesia and muscle paralysis on respiratory mechanics in normal man. Anesthesiology 1974;41:477–485.
10. Westbrook PR, Stubbs SE, Sessler AD, et al: Effects of anesthesia and muscle paralysis on respiratory mechanics in normal man. J Appl Physiol 1973;34:81–86.
11. D'Angelo E: Techniques for studying the mechanics of the pleural space. In Otis AB (ed): Techniques in Life Science, part 2, vol P415. Amsterdam: Elsevier, 1984, pp 1–32.
12. Milic-Emili J: Measurements of pressures in respiratory physiology. In Otis AB (ed): Techniques in Life Science, part 2, vol P412. Amsterdam: Elsevier, 1984, pp 1–22.
13. D'Angelo E, Calderini E, Tavola M, et al: Effect of PEEP on respiratory mechanics in anesthetized paralyzed humans. J Appl Physiol 1992;73:1736–1742.
14. Wade OL: Movements of the thoracic cage and diaphragm in respiration. J Physiol (Lond) 1954;124:193–212.
15. Agostoni E, Mognoni P, Torri G, Saracino F: Relation between changes of rib cage circumference and lung volume. J Appl Physiol 1965;20:1179–1186.

16. Krayer S, Rehder K, Vettermann J, et al: Position and motion of the human diaphragm during anesthesia-paralysis. Anesthesiology 1989;70:891–898.

17. Grimby G, Hedenstierna G, Löfström B: Chest wall mechanics during artificial ventilation. J Appl Physiol 1975;38:576–580.

18. Jones JG, Faithfull D, Jordan C, Minty B: Rib cage movement during halothane anaesthesia in man. Br J Anaesth 1979;51:399–407.

19. Vellody VP, Nassery M, Dius WS, Sharp JT: Effects of body position change on thoracoabdominal motion. J Appl Physiol 1978;45:581–589.

20. Rehder K, Marsh M: Respiratory mechanics during anesthesia and mechanical ventilation. In Macklem PT, Mead J (eds): Handbook of Physiology: The Respiratory System, Mechanics of Breathing, sect 3, vol 3. Bethesda, MD: American Physiological Society, 1986, pp 737–752.

21. Hedenstierna C, Bindslev L, Santesson J, Norlander DP: Airway closure in each lung of anesthetized human subjects. J Appl Physiol 1981;50:55–64.

22. Rehder K, Sittipong R, Sessler AD: The effects of thiopental-meperidine anesthesia with succinylcholine paralysis on functional residual capacity and dynamic lung compliance in normal sitting man. Anesthesiology 1972;37:395–398.

23. Druz WS, Sharp JT: Activity of respiratory muscles in upright and recumbent humans. J Appl Physiol 1981;51:1552–1561.

24. Muller N, Volgyesi G, Becker L, et al: Diaphragmatic muscle tone. J Appl Physiol 1979;47:279–284.

25. Drummond GB, Allan PL, Logan MR: Changes in diaphragmatic position in association with the induction of anaesthesia. Br J Anaesth 1986;58:1246–1251.

26. Hedenstierna G, Strandberg A, Brismar B, et al: Functional residual capacity, thoracoabdominal dimensions, and central blood volume during general anesthesia with muscle paralysis and mechanical ventilation. Anesthesiology 1985;62:247–254.

27. Freund F, Roos A, Dodd RB: Expiratory activity of the abdominal muscles in man during general anesthesia. J Appl Physiol 1964;19:693–697.

28. Kimball WR, Loring SH, Basta SJ, et al: Effects of paralysis with pancuronium on chest wall statics in awake humans. J Appl Physiol 1985;58:l638–1645.

29. Gold ML, Helrich M: Pulmonary compliance during anesthesia. Anesthesiology 1965;26:281–288.

30. Hedenstierna G, McCarthy G: Mechanics of breathing, gas distribution and functional residual capacity at different frequencies of respiration during spontaneous and artificial ventilation. Br J Anaesth 1975;47:706–712.

31. Wu N, Miller WF, Luhn NR: Studies of breathing in anesthesia. Anesthesiology 1956;17:696–707.

32. Foster CA, Heaf PJD, Semple SJG: Compliance of the lung in anesthetized paralyzed subjects. J Appl Physiol 1957;11:383–384.

33. Van Lith P, Johnson FN, Sharp JT: Respiratory elastances in relaxed and paralyzed states in normal and abnormal men. J Appl Physiol 1967;23:475–486.

34. Brismar B, Hedenstierna G, Lundquist H, et al: Pulmonary densities during anesthesia with muscular relaxation: A proposal of atelectasis. Anesthesiology 1985;62:422–428.

35. Duggan CJ, Castle WD, Berend N: Effects of continuous positive airway pressure breathing on lung volume and distensibility. J Appl Physiol 1990;68:1121–1126.

36. Goldberg HS, Mitzner W, Adams K, et al: Effect of intrathoracic pressure on pressure-volume characteristics of the lung in man. J Appl Physiol 1975;38:411–417.

37. Hillman DR, Finucane KE: The effect of hyperinflation on lung elasticity in healthy subjects. Respir Physiol 1983;54:295–305.

38. Young SL, Tierney DF, Clements JA: Mechanism of compliance change in excised rat lungs at low transpulmonary pressure. J Appl Physiol 1970;29:780–785.

39. Agostoni E, Hyatt R: Static behavior of the respiratory system. In Macklem PT, Mead J (eds): Handbook of Physiology: The Respiratory System, Mechanics of Breathing, sect 3, vol 3. Bethesda, MD: American Physiological Society, 1986, pp 113–130.

40. Rehder K, Knopp TJ, Sessler AD: Regional intrapulmonary gas distribution in awake and anesthetized-paralyzed prone man. J Appl Physiol 1978;45:528–535.

41. Rohrer F: Physiologie der Atembewegung. In Bethe ATJ, von Bergmann G, Embden G, Ellinger A (eds): Handbuch der Normalen und Pathologischen Physiologie, vol 2. Berlin: Springer-Verlag, 1925, pp 70–127.

42. Rohrer F: Der Stromungswiderstand in den menschlichen Atemwegen und der Einfluss der unregelmassigen Verzweigung des Bronchialsystems auf den Atmungsverlaud verschiedenen Lungenbezirken. Arch Gesamte Physiol Mens Tiere 1915;162:225–299.

43. Briscoe WA, DuBois AB: The relationship between airway resistance, airway conductance and lung volume in subjects of different age and body size. J Clin Invest 19587:1279–1285.

44. Mead J, Agostoni E: Dynamics of breathing. In Fenn OW, Rahn H (eds): Handbook of Physiology: Respiration, vol 1. Washington, DC: American Physiological Society, 1964, pp 411–427.

45. Wright PE, Marini JJ, Bernard GR: In vitro versus in vivo comparison of endotracheal tube airflow resistance. Am Rev Respir Dis 1989;140:10–16.

46. D'Angelo E, Salvo Calderini I, Tavola M: The effects of $CO_2$ on respiratory mechanics in normal anesthetized paralyzed humans. Anesthesiology 2001;94:604–610.

47. Mead J, Whittenberger JL: Evaluation of airway interruption technique as a method for measuring pulmonary air-flow resistance. J Appl Physiol 1954;6:408–416.

48. D'Angelo E, Calderini E, Torri G, et al: Respiratory mechanics in anesthetized-paralyzed humans: Effects of flow, volume and time. J Appl Physiol 1989;67:2556–2564.

49. D'Angelo E, Robatto F, Calderini E, et al: Pulmonary and chest wall mechanics in anesthetized paralyzed humans. J Appl Physiol 1991;70:2602–2610.

50. D'Angelo E, Prandi E, Tavola M, et al: Chest wall interrupter resistance in anesthetized paralyzed humans. J Appl Physiol 1994;77:883–887.

51. Liistro GD, Stanescu D, Rodenstein D, Veriter C: Reassessment of the interruption technique for measuring flow resistance in humans. J Appl Physiol 1989;67:933–937.

52. D'Angelo E, Calderini E, Robatto FM, et al: Lung and chest wall mechanics in patients with acquired immunodeficiency syndrome and severe *Pneumocystis carinii* pneumonia. Eur Respir J 1997;10:2343–2350.

53. Bates JHT, Ludwig MS, Sly PD, et al: Interrupter resistance elucidated by alveolar pressure measurement in open-chest normal dogs. J Appl Physiol 1988;65:408–414.

54. Saldiva PHN, Zin WA, Santos RLB, et al: Alveolar pressure measurement in open-chest rats. J Appl Physiol 1992;72:302–306.

55. D'Angelo E, Rocca E, Milic-Emili J: A model analysis of the effects of different inspiratory flow patterns on inspiratory work during mechanical ventilation. Eur Respir Mon 1999;4:279–295.

56. Mount LE: The ventilation flow-resistance and compliance of rat lungs. J Physiol (Lond) 1955;127:157–167.

57. Hildebrandt J: Pressure-volume data of cat lung interpreted by a plastoelastic linear viscoelastic model. J Appl Physiol 1970;28:365–372.

58. Fredberg JJ, Stamenovic D: On the imperfect elasticity of lung tissue. J Appl Physiol 1989;67:2408–2419.

59. Hoppin FG, Stothert JC, Greaves IA, et al: Lung recoil: Elastic and rheological properties. In Mead J, Macklem PT (eds): Handbook of Physiology: The Respiratory System, Mechanics of Breathing, sect 3, vol 3. Bethesda MD, American Physiological Society, 1986, pp 195–216.

60. Stamenovic D, Glass GM, Barnas GM, Fredberg JJ: Viscoplasticity of respiratory tissues. J Appl Physiol 1990;69:973–988.

61. Sharp JT, Johnson FN, Goldberg NB, Van Lith P: Hysteresis and stress adaptation in the human respiratory system. J Appl Physiol 1967;23:487–497.

62. Ludwig MS, Romero PV, Bates JHT: A comparison of the dose-response behavior of canine airways and parenchyma. J Appl Physiol 1989;67:1200–1225.

63. Lauzon AM, Bates JHT: Estimation of time-varying respiratory mechanical parameters by recursive least squares. J Appl Physiol 1991;71:1159–1165.

64. Shardonofsky FR, Sato J, Bates JHT: Quasi-static pressure-volume hysteresis in the canine respiratory system in vivo. J Appl Physiol 1990;68:2230–2236.

65. Hantos Z, Daróczy B, Suki B, et al: Forced oscillation impedance of the respiratory system at low frequencies. J Appl Physiol 1986;60:123–132.

66. Lutchen KR, Jackson AC: Effects of tidal volume and methacholine on low frequency total respiratory impedance in dogs. J Appl Physiol 1990;68:2128–2138.

67. Suki B, Peslin R, Duvivier C, Farré R: Lung impedance of respiratory system in healthy humans measured by forced oscillations from 0.01 to 0.1 Hz. J Appl Physiol 1989;67: 1623–1629.

68. Navajas D, Farrè R, Carnet J, et al: Respiratory input impedance in anesthetized paralyzed patients. J Appl Physiol 1990;69: 1372–1379.

69. Peslin R, Da Silva FJ, Duvivier C, Chabot F: Respiratory mechanics studied by forced oscillations during artificial ventilation. Eur Respir J 1993;6:772–784.

70. Beydon L, Malassiné P, Lorino AM, et al: Respiratory resistance by end-inspiratory occlusion and forced oscillations in intubated patients. J Appl Physiol 1996;80:1105–1111.

71. Otis AB, McKerrow CB, Bartlett RA, et al: Mechanical factors in distribution of pulmonary ventilation. J Appl Physiol 1956;8: 427–443.

72. Eissa NT, Ranieri VM, Corbeil C, et al: Analysis of behavior of the respiratory system in ARDS patients: Effects of flow, volume, and time. J Appl Physiol 1991;70:2719–2729.

73. Guèrin C, Coussa M-L, Eissa NT, et al: Lung and chest wall mechanics in mechanically ventilated COPD patients. J Appl Physiol 1993;74:1570–1580.

74. McIlroy MB, Tierney DF, Nadel JA: A new method of measurement of compliance and resistance of lungs and thorax. J Appl Physiol 1963;18:424–427.

75. Zin WA, Pengelly LD, Milic-Emili J: Single-breath method for measurement of respiratory system mechanics in anesthetized animals. J Appl Physiol 1982;52:1266–1271.

76. Bates JHT, Decramer M, Chartrand D, et al: Volume-time profile during relaxed expiration in the normal dog. J Appl Physiol 1985;59:732–737.

77. Bates JHT, Decramer W, Zin WA, et al: Respiratory resistance with histamine challenge by single-breath and forced oscillation methods. J Appl Physiol 1986;61:873–880.

78. Chelucci GL, Brunet F, Dall'Ava-Santucci, J et al: A single-compartment model cannot describe passive expiration in intubated, paralysed humans. Eur Respir J 1991;4:458–464.

79. D'Angelo E, Prandi E, Marazzini L, Milic-Emili J: Dependence of maximal flow-volume curves on time course of preceding inspiration in patients with chronic obstructive pulmonary disease. Am J Respir Crit Care Med 1994;150:1581–1586.

80. D'Angelo E, Prandi E, Milic-Emili J: Dependence of maximal flow-volume curves on time-course of preceding inspiration. J Appl Physiol 1993;75:1155–1159.

81. Santus P, Pecchiari M, Carlucci P, et al: Bronchodilation test in COPD: Effect of inspiratory manoeuvre preceding forced expiration. Eur Respir J 2003;21:82–85.

## SUGGESTED READINGS

Konno K, Mead J: Measurement of the separate volume changes of rib cage and abdomen during breathing. J Appl Physiol 1967;22: 407–422.

Konno K, Mead J: Static volume-pressure characteristics of the rib cage and abdomen. J Appl Physiol 1968;24:544–548.

# CHAPTER 10

# Lung Mechanics in Disease

Claude Guérin, Antonia Koutsoukou, Joseph Milic-Emili, and Edgardo D'Angelo

Patients with chronic respiratory disease often require mechanical ventilation because of respiratory failure. The incidence of acute respiratory failure requiring mechanical ventilation is particularly high for patients with chronic obstructive pulmonary disease (COPD). Hence it is not surprising that many investigators have studied lung mechanics in this disease. In contrast, our knowledge of lung mechanics in other respiratory diseases is limited: pertinent studies in spontaneously breathing and, particularly, mechanically ventilated patients are in fact very few. Additionally, obesity is a rapidly growing problem in most developed countries, and obese subjects are becoming common in the intensive care unit (ICU). A section on respiratory mechanics in obesity is thus provided.

## CHRONIC OBSTRUCTIVE PULMONARY DISEASE

Since the early 1990s, several investigations performed in intubated patients have led to better understanding of the abnormalities of respiratory mechanics in patients with COPD and acute ventilatory failure (AVF). Remarkably, in these patients, the present choice of ventilator settings stems mostly from physiologic studies and not from recommendations based on randomized controlled studies. Moreover, the physiologic studies have provided the background information for respiratory monitoring during mechanical ventilation.

The AVF of COPD is a true respiratory *decompensation* because the compensatory mechanisms evolved over the prolonged chronic state suddenly become insufficient. The respiratory muscles are no longer able to sustain the rapidly increasing mechanical loads, and the result is a breakdown of the subtle equilibrium between muscle adaptation and increasing loading. By increasing respiratory loading, dynamic hyperinflation (DH) plays a crucial role in the genesis of AVF.

### Pulmonary Hyperinflation

In healthy individuals at rest, the end-expiratory lung volume (i.e., the functional residual capacity [FRC]) corresponds to the relaxation volume of the respiratory system (Vr) (i.e., the lung volume at which the static recoil pressure of the relaxed respiratory system is nil). Pulmonary hyperinflation, which is defined as an increase in FRC higher than the predicted normal range, may be caused by increased Vr as a result of loss of lung recoil (e.g., emphysema) or dynamic pulmonary hyperinflation. The latter occurs whenever the expiratory flow is impeded (e.g., increased airway resistance) or the duration of expiration is insufficient to allow the lungs to deflate to the Vr before the next inspiration (e.g., increased breathing frequency). Expiratory flow may also be reduced by other mechanisms, such as persistent contraction of the inspiratory muscles during expiration and expiratory narrowing of the glottic aperture. In patients with COPD, DH is mainly caused by tidal expiratory flow limitation (EFL). Healthy subjects do not exhibit EFL even during maximal exercise. In contrast, in patients with COPD, tidal EFL with concurrent DH may be present even at rest and may play a central role in causing dyspnea, exercise intolerance, and AVF.

### Expiratory Flow Limitation

The term EFL should be used only to describe a condition in which expiratory flow at a given lung volume cannot be augmented in spite of further increases of the transpulmonary and alveolar pressure. Thus, EFL reflects effort independence of maximal expiratory flow ($\dot{V}$max) at that volume. Two main mechanisms promote the occurrence of tidal EFL, namely, reduction of $\dot{V}$max and increase in ventilatory requirements. In normal individuals at rest, the expiratory flow reserve (i.e., the difference between $\dot{V}$max and actual expiratory flows) is very high (Fig. 10.1, *left*), whereas patients with severe COPD may not have any flow reserve left (Fig. 10.1, *right*). In the latter condition, ventilation can be augmented only by increasing the operational lung volume, thus causing DH, with a concurrent increase in $\dot{V}$max, or by decreasing the duration of inspiration with a concurrent increase in time available for expiration. The expiratory flow reserve can be reduced by (a) airway obstruction and lowered $\dot{V}$max (see Fig. 10.1, *right*) and (b) reduced FRC resulting from recumbency or disease (obesity, congestive heart failure). A fall in the expiratory flow reserve also occurs with aging, because $\dot{V}$max decreases. Patients with COPD and AVF are usually old, often obese, and axiomatically recumbent in the ICU. In addition, their impaired pulmonary gas exchange implies increased ventilatory requirement, further promoting tidal EFL. Accordingly, tidal EFL is almost invariably present in patients with COPD and AVF.

In mechanically ventilated patients, tidal EFL can be measured using the negative expiratory pressure (NEP) method.[1] Although a prototype of a ventilator equipped with a NEP device has been built and provides easy and accurate assessment of EFL,[2] it is not commercially available.

## Intrinsic Positive End-Expiratory Pressure

Under normal conditions, the end-expiratory elastic recoil pressure of the respiratory system (Pst,rs) is zero.

In this case, the alveolar pressure becomes subatmospheric, and gas flows into the lungs as soon as the inspiratory muscles contract. When breathing takes place at lung volumes greater than Vr (i.e., when DH is present), the Pst,rs and hence the alveolar pressure are positive. This pressure has been termed intrinsic end-expiratory positive pressure (PEEPi). When PEEPi is present, onset of inspiratory muscle activity and inspiratory flow are not synchronous: inspiratory flow starts only when the pressure developed by the inspiratory muscles exceeds PEEPi.[3] In this respect, PEEPi acts as an inspiratory threshold load, increasing the inspiratory work of breathing. This places a further burden on the inspiratory muscles, which, in addition, operate under disadvantageous force-length and geometric conditions.[4]

DH occurs not only during spontaneous breathing, but also possibly in passively ventilated patients if the expiratory time is less than the time required to reach Vr. In mechanically ventilated patients with COPD, the factors promoting PEEPi and DH are related to the patient (EFL, bronchoconstriction, secretions), the ventilator (large tidal volume [VT], short expiratory time), or the equipment (high-resistance endotracheal tube, ventilator tubing, expiratory valve).

During mechanical ventilation of relaxed subjects, PEEPi can be suspected by inspection of the flow-time tracings that are displayed on the screen of most modern ICU ventilators. With DH, the flow does not reach zero at the end of expiration (Fig. 10.2), and in fact, DH can be quantified by prolonging expiration until flow becomes nil and Vr is eventually reached.[5] Monitoring the time course of flow is therefore required to minimize unwarranted hyperinflation by adjusting the ventilator settings.

During mechanical ventilation, PEEPi cannot be directly assessed by inspecting the pressure at airway opening.

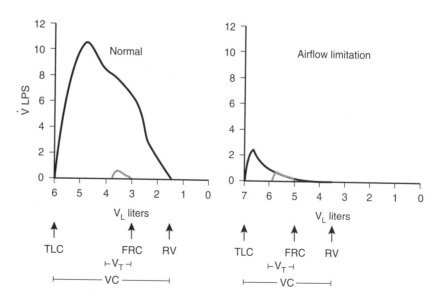

**Figure 10.1**  Flow-volume curves during quiet and forced expiration in a normal subject *(left)* and a patient with severe chronic obstructive pulmonary disease (COPD) *(right)*. Although in the normal subject there is a considerable expiratory flow reserve in the resting tidal volume (VT) range, in the patient, the tidal expiratory flow is maximal (i.e., expiratory flow limitation is present). The latter promotes an increase in functional residual capacity (FRC) with concomitant reduction of inspiratory capacity (total lung capacity [TLC] − FRC). RV, residual volume; VC, vital capacity.

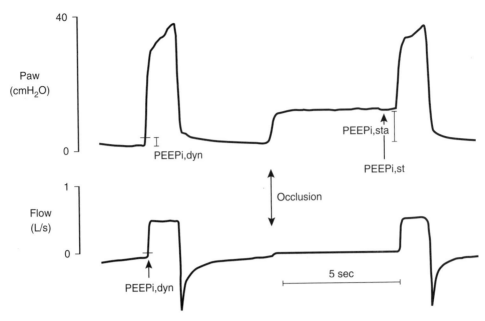

**Figure 10.2** Time course of pressure at airway opening (Pao) and flow during mechanical ventilation with constant-flow inflation. At end expiration of the regular cycle, flow is not zero *(first arrow)*, a finding reflecting hyperinflation and intrinsic positive end-expiratory pressure (PEEPi). Static PEEPi (PEEPi,st) *(third arrow)* is obtained from the end-expiratory occlusion. Dynamic PEEPi (PEEPi,dyn) is change in Pao required to initiate mechanical inflation. (From Maltais F, Reissmann H, Navalesi P, et al: Comparison of static and dynamic measurements of intrinsic PEEP in mechanically ventilated patients. Am J Respir Crit Care Med 1994;150:1318–1324.)

To measure PEEPi, the expiratory port must be occluded by pressing a specific knob that is available in all modern ICU ventilators. Such an end-expiratory occlusion provides static PEEPi (PEEPi,st) (see Fig. 10.2), which reflects the average value of the end-expiratory Pst,rs from lung regions with markedly different time constants. The pressure that the ventilator generates before the start of inflation is dynamic PEEPi (PEEPi,dyn) (see Fig. 10.2). Because PEEPi,dyn is always lower than PEEPi,st, PEEPi,dyn/PEEPi,st is less than 1. In patients with COPD and AVF, activity of abdominal muscles is frequent.[6] This abdominal contraction generates increased end-expiratory alveolar pressure. Thus, accurate measurement of PEEPi during spontaneous breathing or assisted ventilation requires absence of abdominal muscle contraction or assessment of its contribution.[7,8]

## Closing Volume

Assessment of the closing volume (CV) was originally performed by inhaling a bolus of xenon-133 at the onset of an inspiratory vital capacity maneuver: during the subsequent expiration, the concentration of the tracer suddenly increased, reflecting the onset of airway closure at the bottom of the lungs.[9] The volume at which this occurs is termed CV. Small airway closure is a common phenomenon in stable patients with COPD.[10] Behind closed airways there is gas trapping, so that, with the progression of peripheral airway disease, CV becomes larger than FRC,[10] with consequent maldistribution of ventilation and impaired gas exchange.

In relaxed, mechanically ventilated patients with AVF, the CV has been indirectly assessed by constructing the quasistatic inflation volume-pressure (V-P) curve of the respiratory system (Fig. 10.3): this curve exhibits an inflection point at low lung volumes that reflects the critical opening pressure (Po) and volume (Vo), which are the pressure and volume, respectively, at which previously closed small airways reopen.[11] In seven patients with COPD, Vo was greater than the end-expiratory lung volume on ZEEP, a finding indicating that some peripheral airways were probably closed throughout the breathing cycle, whereas others cyclically opened and closed. In contrast, in three patients with COPD, Vo was lower than the end-expiratory lung volume on ZEEP, a finding indicating an absence of peripheral airway closure during baseline ventilation. Other implications of these findings are discussed later.

## Elastance

Only a few studies have assessed the quasistatic inflation V-P curve of anesthetized paralyzed patients with COPD.[12–14]

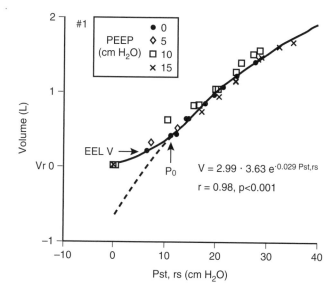

**Figure 10.3** Relationship of inflation volume to static pressures of respiratory system (Pst,rs) in a representative patient with chronic obstructive pulmonary disease (COPD) and in acute ventilatory failure, ventilated with four levels of positive end-expiratory pressure (PEEP). Volumes are referred to relaxation volume (Vr) measured at all levels of applied PEEP. The volume-pressure curve exhibits an inflection point (Po) above which the experimental points are fitted to the following function: $V = Vmax - b\ e^{-kPst,rs}$, where Vmax is the extrapolated volume at infinite Pst,rs, $b$ is the difference between Vmax and the predicted lung volume at zero Pst,rs, and k is a constant. (From Guérin C, LeMasson S, de Varax R, et al: Small airway closure and positive end-expiratory pressure in mechanically ventilated patients with chronic obstructive pulmonary disease. Am J Respir Crit Care Med 1997;155:1949–1956.)

In the $V_T$ range, the quasistatic elastance of the respiratory system (Est,rs) is similar in these patients and in normal anesthetized paralyzed subjects, provided measurements obtained with the same procedure are compared. This also applies to quasistatic lung elastance (Est,L).[12,13] This similarity may be surprising, but in patients with COPD and AVF, factors with decreasing (e.g., pulmonary emphysema) and increasing (e.g., DH, small airway closure, atelectasis) effects on Est are simultaneously operating, likely with a different impact. Indeed, much higher values of Est,rs have been found during the first day of mechanical ventilation in patients with COPD who exhibited more marked DH, besides pulmonary edema.[15]

In normal anesthetized and paralyzed, mechanically ventilated subjects, dynamic elastance ([Edyn]; i.e., tidal pressure swing divided by inflation volume [$\Delta V$]) is always larger than Est at any given $\Delta V$; the difference between Edyn and Est ($\Delta E$) reflects the additional elastic pressure stored in the tissue viscoelastic units and contributions of time-constant inhomogeneities.[16,17]

Moreover, Edyn is time (frequency) dependent, because it increases with increasing the inflation flow ($\dot{V}$) at constant $\Delta V$ and decreases with increasing $\Delta V$ at constant $\dot{V}$, whereas Est is independent of breath frequency (Fig. 10.4). The same observations have been made in anesthetized paralyzed patients with COPD and AFV.[13] In these patients, however, both the magnitude of $\Delta Ers$ and its dependence on $\dot{V}$ and $\Delta V$ were markedly enhanced with respect to those occurring in normal anesthetized and paralyzed, mechanically ventilated subjects, a finding implying increased viscoelastic work (see later). Both increased $\Delta Ers$ and enhanced frequency dependence were the result of lung mechanical behavior, and the mechanical properties of the chest wall were essentially the same in normal subjects and in patients with COPD (Fig. 10.4).[13,17] Therefore, it seems likely that changes in $\Delta Ers$ are mainly the result of pulmonary time-constant inhomogeneities, which should be substantial in patients with COPD.

## Resistance

Respiratory system resistance (Rrs) can be partitioned into interrupter resistance (Rint,rs), which mainly reflects airway flow resistance, and additional resistance ($\Delta Rrs$), which reflects pressure dissipation caused by tissue viscoelastic properties or time-constant inequality. In relaxed, mechanically ventilated subjects, both resistances

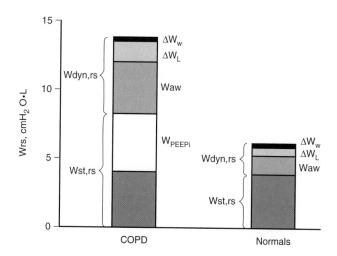

**Figure 10.4** Average relationships of static (st; *circles*) and dynamic (dyn; *triangles*) elastance of lung (EL) and chest wall (Ew) to inflation flow at fixed inflation volume of 0.73 L in 10 patients with chronic obstructive pulmonary disease (closed symbols) and 18 normal subjects (open symbols). *Bars* are SE. (Data from D'Angelo E, Robatto FM, Calderini E, et al: Pulmonary and chest wall mechanics in anesthetized paralyzed humans. J Appl Physiol 1991;70:2602–2610; and Guérin C, Coussa ML, Eissa NT, et al: Lung and chest wall mechanics in mechanically ventilated COPD patients. J Appl Physiol 1993;74:1570–1580.)

are greater in patients with COPD than in normal subjects.[13,14,16] Moreover, Rint,rs and ΔRrs exhibit greater flow and time dependence, respectively, in patients with COPD than in normal subjects, because, with fixed inflation volume, the former increases linearly, whereas the latter decreases progressively with increasing inflation flow.[13,16] Hence Rrs depends on the respective contributions of Rint,rs and ΔRrs. In patients with COPD and AVF, Rrs is maximal at low inflation flow and decreases with increasing flow to a minimal value that occurs at inflation flows of approximately 1 L/second.[14] The latter is commonly selected during mechanical ventilation.

## Work of Breathing

The components of the inspiratory work of breathing (WI,rs) were described for similar VT and inflation flow in 10 patients with COPD and AVF[18] and in 18 normal subjects.[16] WI,rs was twice as high in patients with COPD as in normal subjects (Fig. 10.5). The increase was mainly the result of work done to overcome PEEPi (WPEEPi) and increased airway resistance (Waw). The WPEEPi, which was absent in normal subjects, accounted for 57% of the overall increase of WI,rs, whereas that of Waw accounted for 34%. The remaining 9% of ΔWI,rs was the result of work to overcome viscoelastic forces or energy dissipated because of time-constant inequality (ΔWL). The increase in ΔWL is associated with flow and time dependence of dynamic pulmonary elastance, which is markedly greater in patients with COPD than in normal subjects. In normal lungs, the small changes of lung elastance with flow reflect viscoelastic behavior, whereas in patients with COPD, the large changes probably also reflect increased time-constant inequality within the lungs.

## Implications for Management

Application of PEEP during controlled mechanical ventilation is still controversial in COPD. PEEP may be used to avoid cyclic opening and closing of the peripheral airways and hence may prevent lung parenchyma from further inflammation and damage.[19] The level of PEEP must be selected (Fig. 10.3).[11] If PEEP is less than Po, some of the previously closed peripheral airways will remain open throughout the breathing cycle, thus improving the distribution of ventilation. The changes in lung volume and alveolar pressure as PEEP approaches Po are probably too small to worsen pulmonary hemodynamics. If PEEP is greater than Po, most airways should be open, end-expiratory lung volume should increase along the static V-P curve, but hemodynamic worsening is likely.[11,20]

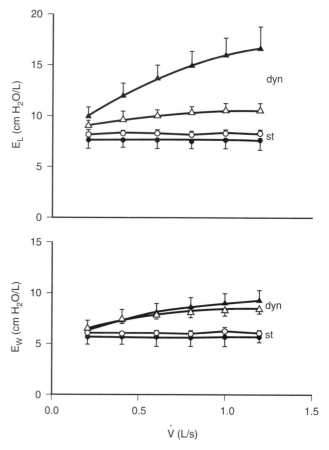

**Figure 10.5** Mean values of the components of inspiratory work of breathing (WI,rs) in 10 patients with chronic obstructive pulmonary disease (COPD) and 18 anesthetized and paralyzed normal subjects ventilated with similar inflation flow (0.8 L/s) and volume (0.73 L). Wst,rs, total static work; WPEEPi, total static work due to PEEPi; Wdyn,rs, total dynamic work; Waw, dynamic work due to airway resistance; ΔWL, additional dynamic work done on the lung due to viscoelastic properties of the tissues and time constant inequality; ΔWw, additional dynamic work done on the chest wall due to viscoelastic properties of the tissues and time constant inequality.

During weaning from mechanical ventilation, continuous positive applied pressure up to 15 cm $H_2O$ reduces the work of breathing and the breathlessness.[21] Selected to counterbalance PEEPi,dyn, low levels of PEEP combined with pressure support or proportional assisted ventilation can also reduce the respiratory drive and risk of fatigue by further unloading the respiratory muscles.[7,22]

Bronchodilating agents, particularly $\beta_2$-agonists, are widely used in patients with COPD and AVF.[23] Investigators showed that salbutamol increases V̇max in the majority of stable patients with COPD, who, although still flow limited, can therefore breathe at lower lung volumes, thus reducing DH.[24,25] During mechanical ventilation, the inhalation route is preferred, provided the recommendations for improving delivery are followed.[26] Small-volume nebulizers or metered dose inhalers with inhalation chamber have a similar effect.[27,28]

## CYSTIC FIBROSIS

No study investigated respiratory mechanics of patients with cystic fibrosis during AVF. In stable patients, average values ($\pm$SD) for PEEPi,dyn, dynamic lung compliance, and resistance during quiet breathing were found to be 1$\pm$1 cm $H_2O$, 0.12$\pm$0.06 L/cm $H_2O$, and 7.3$\pm$5.6 cm $H_2O$/L/second, respectively.[29] These patients also exhibit marked DH, independent of age and EFL.[29–31] Conflicting results exist regarding the prevalence of EFL and the appropriate method to assess EFL. With the NEP method, tidal EFL was found in 3 out of 22 young and adult patients[30] and in 4 out of 17 young patients,[31] whereas using the traditional spirometric approach, flow-limited patients increased to 10 and 7, respectively.

## RESTRICTIVE LUNG DISEASE

In stable, spontaneously breathing patients with neuromuscular diseases, Est,rs was 1.5 to 2 times higher than in controls, whereas Rrs averaged 17 cm $H_2O$/L/second.[32] Under the same conditions, Rrs averaged 16 cm $H_2O$/L/second in patients with sarcoidosis.[33] In mechanically ventilated patients with end-stage interstitial lung fibrosis[34] and severe kyphoscoliosis,[35] both Est,rs and Rrs are markedly increased compared with COPD (Table 10.1). This may explain why, once intubated, these patients become ventilator dependent, a situation that raises ethical considerations.[36] EFL seems to be rare in stable, spontaneously breathing patients with restrictive respiratory disorders: it was found in only 1 of 19 patients with severe kyphoscoliosis.[37]

## OBESITY

Obesity is a metabolic disease characterized by excessive accumulation of adipose tissue. It has become a major health concern because 35% of the population in North

---

**Table 10-1** Respiratory Mechanics in Patients with Acute or Chronic Ventilatory Failure and in Normal Subjects, Anesthetized and Paralyzed, Intubated, and Mechanically Ventilated on Zero End-Expiratory Pressure

|  | COPD[13] | Kyphoscoliosis[80] | Interstitial Lung Fibrosis[34] | Normal Subjects[16] |
|---|---|---|---|---|
| Number of patients | 10 | 7 | 7 | 18 |
| EFL | Common[81] | Not evaluated | Not evaluated | Not evaluated |
| $\Delta$FRC (L) | 0.34 | Not evaluated | Not evaluated | 0 |
| PEEPi (cm $H_2O$) | 5.7 | 1.8 | Negligible | 0 |
| Rrs (cm $H_2O$/L/sec) | 12.8 | 20.0 | 16.7 | 5.0 |
| Rint,rs (cm $H_2O$/L/sec) | 7.2 | 6.2 | 13.7 | 2.23 |
| $\Delta$Rrs (cm $H_2O$/L/sec) | 5.6 | 14.0 | 4.0 | 2.73 |
| Est,rs (cm $H_2O$/L) | 12.6 | 28 | 51.9 | 14.5 |
| Inflation flow (L/sec) | 0.80 | 0.28 | 0.60 | 0.56 |
| Inflation volume (L) | 0.73 | 0.47 | 8 mL/kg | 0.47 |

COPD, chronic obstructive pulmonary disease; EFL, expiratory flow limitation; Est,rs, static elastance of the respiratory system; $\Delta$FRC, end-expiratory lung volume above relaxation volume; PEEPi, intrinsic positive end-expiratory pressure; Rrs, Rint,rs, $\Delta$Rrs, total, interrupter, and additional resistances of the respiratory system.

America and 15% to 20% in Europe is obese.[38] In healthy people, fat constitutes approximately 15% to 30% of body mass, whereas it amounts to 40% to 60% in obesity. The severity of obesity is assessed in terms of the extent by which body weight exceeds ideal weight, as predicted by age, height, and gender. Obesity is considered mild or severe when body weight lies between 120% and 150% or exceeds 150% of ideal weight, respectively. However, the most common index of obesity is the body mass index (BMI), which is the quotient of body weight and height squared. The upper limit of normal BMI is 25 kg/m$^2$: values greater than 30 kg/m$^2$ correspond to obesity, and values in excess of 40 kg/m$^2$ correspond to morbid obesity.

Obesity, even without concomitant diseases, is associated with altered respiratory function during spontaneous breathing as well as during anesthesia and mechanical ventilation. It is important to identify pulmonary function abnormalities in obese patients, because they are at greater risk of developing further respiratory impairment when they are exposed to other factors associated with increased respiratory morbidity, such as cigarette smoking, respiratory infections, and thoracic or abdominal surgery.

## Respiratory Function during Spontaneous Breathing

In simple obesity, the expiratory reserve volume (ERV) and FRC are increased, whereas residual volume (RV), vital capacity (VC), and total lung capacity (TLC) are essentially normal.[39] Moreover, the FRC may fall below the CV.[40,41] These volume changes are mainly the result of those in the static properties of the chest wall that, in turn, are usually attributed to mass loading.[42,43] A slight reduction in lung compliance has also been reported and related to increased intrapulmonary blood volume and airway closure in the dependent lung zones.[39,44] Relative to normal values, the total respiratory system compliance decreases more in the supine than in the sitting position, because of the greater degree of chest wall compression and cranial displacement of the diaphragm in the former posture.[45]

Morbidly obese subjects exhibit increased airway and Rrs, the latter significantly correlated with BMI.[46,47] Because there is a close correlation between airway conductance and lung volume, it was concluded that the major reason for increased Rrs in obesity is the reduction of FRC. However, measurements with the forced oscillation technique have shown that Rrs is increased in excess of that accountable for by the reduction in FRC.[48]

## Gas Exchange

Severely obese subjects at rest are often hypoxemic, with a widened alveolar-arterial oxygen tension gradient.[49–51]

Direct evidence of ventilation-perfusion mismatch resulting from peripheral airway closure in sitting obese subjects was provided by Holley and colleagues,[51] who found that during quiet breathing, the distribution of the inspired gas was preferential to the upper lobes in subjects with ERV lower than 0.3 L, whereas it was more uniform in subjects with ERV greater than 0.4 L. Similarly, Hedenstierna and colleagues[40] found that the degree of hypoxemia was correlated with the magnitude of airway closure, which was greater in obese subjects with small lung volumes and in the supine position.[52] Even though obesity requires higher ventilation to maintain normal partial arterial carbon dioxide pressure, most subjects are eucapnic. To meet the increased ventilatory demand, obese subjects increase their minute ventilation mainly by increasing the respiratory rate, which may be up to 50% higher than in normal subjects, whereas the V$_T$ is either normal or increased.[53,54]

In obesity, the work of breathing is 60% higher than normal, and the energy cost of breathing can increase by as much as fourfold.[39,55] Accordingly, the maximum voluntary ventilation (MVV) is abnormally low,[39,56] especially in subjects who at rest exhibit small V$_T$s, small inspiratory and expiratory flow rates, and more air trapping.[57] Although low MVV has been attributed to changes in chest wall mechanics,[58] air trapping could also play a role by placing the inspiratory muscles at a mechanical disadvantage and reducing their strength.[57]

## Peripheral Airway Closure

Tidal breathing at low lung volume promotes peripheral airway closure in the dependent lung zones.[35,59,60] Although in young, normal adults, FRC is considerably larger than CV, in young obese subjects CV is substantially increased in both the sitting and the supine positions,[40,49] so peripheral airway closure can occur during tidal breathing.[52] This should cause impairment of gas exchange and risk of injury to peripheral airways resulting from mechanical stresses related to their cyclic opening and closing (see later). Moreover, peripheral airway closure should reduce $\dot{V}$ max, because the lung units served by these airways cease to contribute to the expiratory flow.

## Expiratory Flow Limitation

EFL is commonly seen during spontaneous breathing in morbidly obese subjects, particularly in the supine position.[50,61] This is the result of reduced $\dot{V}$max in the V$_T$ range, lowered FRC, and higher ventilatory requirements consequent to increased metabolic demands. Because the FRC is lower in the supine than in the sitting position,[62] tidal EFL is more common in the former position. Tidal EFL entails cyclic airway dynamic compression and reexpansion of peripheral airways. This, together with cyclic opening and closing of peripheral airways, may result in increased risk of peripheral airway injury.[63]

In the presence of predisposing conditions such as shortening of expiratory time resulting from rapid breathing, augmented minute ventilation caused by high ventilatory demand, and increased airway resistance caused by reduced lung volumes, EFL can produce DH and PEEPi by preventing the respiratory system from reaching its Vr during expiration. In fact, the presence of PEEPi has been documented in supine morbidly obese subjects.[61] As mentioned earlier, PEEPi represents an a threshold load that must be overcome by the inspiratory muscles during tidal breathing. This is an important mechanism leading to dyspnea in morbidly obese subjects.[64]

## Respiratory Function during Anesthesia and Mechanical Ventilation

General anesthesia impairs pulmonary function even in normal individuals, and it results in decreased oxygenation.[65] It also causes a reduction in FRC of up to 50% of the preanesthesia value.[66,67] Computed tomography has shown that pulmonary atelectasis is a common finding in anesthetized subjects, because it occurs in 85% to 90% of healthy adults. Atelectasis develops within minutes after the induction of anesthesia, and in normal subjects, up to 15% of the entire lung may be atelectic, particularly the basal regions; the result is a 5% to 10% shunting of cardiac output.[53] In morbidly obese subjects, general anesthesia causes much more atelectasis than in subjects of normal weight.[53] The formation of atelectasis during anesthesia and mechanical ventilation has been ascribed to a decreased ventilation-perfusion ratio ($\dot{V}A/\dot{Q}$) in dependent lung units and gas absorption during the apnea following hyperventilation with pure oxygen before intubation.[67,68]

The increased abdominal mass and pressure of morbidly obese subjects cause cephalad displacement of the diaphragm and reduction in the passive movements of its dependent part; the results are lowered end-expiratory volume, decreased respiratory system compliance, and increased respiratory resistance.[69,70] In contrast, the viscoelastic properties are little affected by the increased body mass.[69] Moreover, as FRC becomes less than CV, airway closure will be present during tidal breathing; together with alveolar collapse, this leads to abnormal $\dot{V}A/\dot{Q}$ distribution. Indeed, a substantial impairment of oxygenation has been reported in anesthetized, morbidly obese subjects, both preoperatively and postoperatively.[40,68,70,71]

Because of the decrease of FRC with anesthesia and paralysis, a high prevalence of EFL and PEEPi should be predictable in obese subjects. Indeed, morbidly obese, postoperative mechanically ventilated subjects commonly exhibit EFL (Fig. 10.6, *left*) with concomitant PEEPi.[70] PEEPi was significantly correlated to the extent of EFL percentage of VT but not to inspiratory Rrs or its

components, because in the presence of EFL, the rate of lung emptying is independent of inspiratory resistance.[72,73] Nonsignificant differences in respiratory mechanics and blood gases were found between EFL and non-EFL subjects. The finding that postoperative blood gases do not differ between EFL and non-EFL individuals indicates that tidal EFL does not play a primary role in pulmonary gas exchange, as in spontaneously breathing subjects.[50]

## Effect of Positive End-Expiratory Pressure

The effect of PEEP on respiratory mechanics and blood gases in morbidly obese, mechanically ventilated subjects was studied by Pelosi and colleagues,[74] who applied PEEP of 10 cm $H_2O$ to nine such patients after abdominal surgery. These investigators found a significant reduction in Est,rs that was attributed to recruitment of atelectatic alveoli or opening of closed airways and a small but significant improvement in arterial oxygenation correlated with the amount of recruited volume. In a similar group of subjects, Koutsoukou and associates applied PEEP large enough (4 to 16 cm $H_2O$) to abolish EFL (Fig. 10.6, *right*) and found a significant reduction in PEEPi, Est,rs, and Rrs, but no effect on gas exchange.[70] However, in both studies, oxygenation remained markedly abnormal after application of PEEP, probably reflecting atelectasis. In this connection, in healthy anesthetized subjects, quasistatic inflation pressures of at least 30 cm $H_2O$ are required to reduce atelectasis substantially.[68]

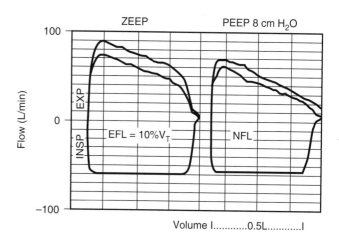

**Figure 10.6** Flow-volume loops of negative expiratory pressure (NEP) test breath *(thin line)* and preceding control breath *(heavy line)* in a morbidly obese subject on zero end-expiratory pressure (ZEEP) and after application of 8 cm $H_2O$ of positive end-expiratory pressure (PEEP). On ZEEP, expiratory flow limitation amounted to 10% tidal volume (VT), whereas it was absent on PEEP. On-line record from an Evita 2 screen (Draeger, Lubeck, Germany). (From Koutsoukou A, Koulouris N, Bekos B, et al: Expiratory flow limitation in morbidly obese postoperative mechanically ventilated patients. Acta Anaesthesiol Scand 2004;48:1080–1088.)

## Clinical Considerations

Peripheral airway closure and EFL, which are common in morbidly obese subjects,[50,51,61] may lead to mechanical injury of the peripheral airways[75,76] and alteration of the contractile properties of airway smooth muscle.[77] In fact, it has been shown that in normal open-chest rabbits, low-volume ventilation with physiologic $V_T$, which entails cyclic opening and closing of peripheral airways, leads within 3 to 4 hours to a persistent increase in airway resistance and damage of respiratory and membranous bronchioles, characterized by epithelial necrosis and sloughing.[75] This could explain why Rrs is abnormally high in supine, spontaneously breathing, morbidly obese subjects.[48] In addition, model analyses suggest that (a) heterogeneous peripheral airway constriction amplifies airflow-related shear stress within the peripheral airways with risk of injury even in the absence of airway closure,[76] and (b) breathing at low lung volume increases the rate of stress generation in airway smooth muscle leading to bronchial hyperresponsiveness.[77] Although these effects may occur during long-standing spontaneous breathing at low lung volumes, the risk of injury should be greater during mechanical ventilation. With constant flow inflations, there is a rapid initial increase in airway pressure that, by snapping open the closed or compressed airways and generating high shear stresses, enhances peripheral airway injury, as shown in open-chest rabbits ventilated with different inflation flows.[78] Indeed, by lowering the surface tension and reducing the shear stress that occur with cyclic opening and closing of the peripheral airways, intratracheal instillation of exogenous surfactant in anesthetized and paralyzed, open chest rabbits largely prevented the histological and functional alterations of prolonged mechanical ventilation at low lung volume.[79] Accordingly, to abolish the risk of peripheral airway injury, PEEP should be applied to increase the end-expiratory lung volume to more than the CV as well as the EFL volume, thus requiring the assessment of EFL. Furthermore, avoidance of rapid increase in airway pressure at the onset of lung inflation by using lower constant flows or sinusoidal and not decelerating flows seems important.

In summary, morbidly obese subjects manifest important changes in respiratory function both during spontaneous breathing and mechanical ventilation. The presence of peripheral airway closure and tidal EFL promotes peripheral airway injury and may accelerate the abnormalities of lung function. The risk of injury is expected to be higher during mechanical ventilation, particularly if it involves high-pressure transients. This implies that external PEEP should be applied to these subjects to reduce and eventually abolish peripheral airway closure and EFL.

## REFERENCES

1. Valta P, Corbeil C, Lavoie A, et al: Detection of expiratory flow limitation during mechanical ventilation. Am J Respir Crit Care Med 1994;150:1311–1317.
2. Armaganidis A, Stavrakaki-Kallergi K, Koutsoukou A, et al: Intrinsic positive end-expiratory pressure in mechanically ventilated patients with and without tidal expiratory flow limitation. Crit Care Med 2000;28:3837–3842.
3. Maltais F, Reissmann H, Navalesi P, et al: Comparison of static and dynamic measurements of intrinsic PEEP in mechanically ventilated patients. Am J Respir Crit Care Med 1994;150:1318–1324.
4. Decramer M, Derom E, Gosselink R: Respiratory muscle mechanics in chronic obstructive pulmonary disease and acute respiratory failure. In Lenfant C (ed): Acute Respiratory Failure in Chronic Obstructive Pulmonary Disease. Bethesda, MD: Marcel Dekker, 1996, pp 47–64.
5. Tuxen DV: Detrimental effects of positive end-expiratory pressure during controlled mechanical ventilation of patients with severe airflow obstruction. Am Rev Respir Dis 1989;140:5–9.
6. Ninane V, Rypens F, Yernault JC, De Troyer A: Abdominal muscle use during breathing in patients with chronic airflow obstruction. Am Rev Respir Dis 1992;146:16–21.
7. Appendini L, Patessio A, Zanaboni S, et al: Physiologic effects of positive end-expiratory pressure and mask pressure support during exacerbations of chronic obstructive pulmonary disease. Am J Respir Crit Care Med 1994;149:1069–1076.
8. Lessard MR, Lofaso F, Brochard L: Expiratory muscle activity increases intrinsic positive end-expiratory pressure independently of dynamic hyperinflation in mechanically ventilated patients. Am J Respir Crit Care Med 1995;151:562–569.
9. Dollfuss R, Milic-Emili J, Bates DV: Regional ventilation of the lung studied with boluses of $^{133}$Xenon. Respir Physiol 1967;2:234–246.
10. McCarthy DS, Spencer R, Greene R, Milic-Emili J: Measurement of "closing volume" as a simple and sensitive test for early detection of small airway disease. Am J Med 1972;52:747–753.
11. Guérin C, LeMasson S, de Varax R, et al: Small airway closure and positive end-expiratory pressure in mechanically ventilated patients with chronic obstructive pulmonary disease. Am J Respir Crit Care Med 1997;155:1949–1956.
12. Van Lith P, Johnson FJ, Sharp JT: Respiratory elastances in relaxed and paralyzed states in normal and abnormal men. J Appl Physiol 1967;23:475–486.
13. Guérin C, Coussa ML, Eissa NT, et al: Lung and chest wall mechanics in mechanically ventilated COPD patients. J Appl Physiol 1993;74:1570–1580.
14. Tantucci C, Corbeil C, Chassé M, et al: Flow resistance in patients with chronic obstructive pulmonary disease in acute respiratory failure: Effects of flow and volume. Am Rev Respir Dis 1991;144:384–389.
15. Broseghini C, Brandolese R, Poggi G, et al: Respiratory mechanics during the first day of mechanical ventilation in patients with pulmonary edema and chronic airway obstruction. Am Rev Respir Dis 1988;138:355–361.
16. D'Angelo E, Calderini E, Torri G, et al: Respiratory mechanics in anesthetized paralyzed humans: effects of flow, volume and time. J Appl Physiol 1989;67:2556–2564.
17. D'Angelo E, Robatto FM, Calderini E, et al: Pulmonary and chest wall mechanics in anesthetized paralyzed humans. J Appl Physiol 1991;70:2602–2610.

18. Coussa ML, Guérin C, Eissa NT, et al: Partitioning of work of breathing in mechanically ventilated COPD patients. J Appl Physiol 1993;75:1711–1719.

19. Milic-Emili J: Does mechanical injury of the peripheral airways play a role in the genesis of COPD in smokers? COPD 2004;1:141–149.

20. Ranieri VM, Giuliani R, Cinnella G, et al: Physiologic effects of positive end-expiratory pressure in patients with chronic obstructive pulmonary disease during acute ventilatory failure and controlled mechanical ventilation. Am Rev Respir Dis 1993;147:5–13.

21. Petrof BJ, Calderini E, Gottfried SB: Effect of CPAP on respiratory effort and dyspnea during exercise in severe COPD. J Appl Physiol 1990;69:179–188.

22. Appendini L, Purro A, Gudjonsdottir M, et al: Physiologic response of ventilator-dependent patients with chronic obstructive pulmonary disease to proportional assist ventilation and continuous positive airway pressure. Am J Respir Crit Care Med 1999;159:1510–1517.

23. Schumaker GL, Epstein SK: Managing acute respiratory failure during exacerbation of chronic obstructive pulmonary disease. Respir Care 2004;49:766–782.

24. Pecchiari M, Pelucchi A, D'Angelo E, et al: Effect of heliox breathing on dynamic hyperinflation in COPD patients. Chest 2004;125:2075–2082.

25. Tantucci C, Duguet A, Similowski T, et al: Effect of salbutamol on dynamic hyperinflation in chronic obstructive pulmonary disease patients. Eur Respir J 1998;12:799–804.

26. Dhand R, Tobin MJ: Inhaled bronchodilator therapy in mechanically ventilated patients. Am J Respir Crit Care Med 1997;156:3–10.

27. Duarte AG, Momii K, Bidani A: Bronchodilator therapy with metered-dose inhaler and spacer versus nebulizer in mechanically ventilated patients: Comparison of magnitude and duration of response. Respir Care 2000;45:817–823.

28. Guérin C, Chevre A, Dessirier P, et al: Inhaled fenoterol-ipratropium bromide in mechanically ventilated patients with chronic obstructive pulmonary disease. Am J Respir Crit Care Med 1999;159:1036–1042.

29. Pradal U, Polese G, Braggion C, et al: Determinants of maximal transdiaphragmatic pressure in adults with cystic fibrosis. Am J Respir Crit Care Med 1994;150:167–173.

30. Goetghebeur D, Sarni D, Grossi Y, et al: Tidal expiratory flow limitation and chronic dyspnoea in patients with cystic fibrosis. Eur Respir J 2002;19:492–498.

31. Tauber E, Fazekas T, Eichler I, et al: Negative expiratory pressure: A new tool for evaluating lung function in children? Pediatr Pulmonol 2003;35:162–168.

32. Baydur A: Respiratory muscle strength and control of ventilation in patients with neuromuscular disease. Chest 1991;99:330–338.

33. Baydur A, Carlson M: Respiratory mechanics by the passive relaxation technique in conscious healthy adults and patients with restrictive respiratory disorders. Chest 1994;105:1171–1178.

34. Nava S, Rubini F: Lung and chest wall mechanics in ventilated patients with end stage idiopathic pulmonary fibrosis. Thorax 1999;54:390–395.

35. Caro CG, Butler J, DuBois AB: Some effects of restriction of chest cage expansion on pulmonary function in man: An experimental study. J Clin Invest 1960;39:573–583.

36. Blivet S, Philit F, Sab JM, et al: Outcome of patients with idiopathic pulmonary fibrosis admitted to the ICU for respiratory failure. Chest 2001;120:209–212.

37. Baydur A, Milic-Emili J: Expiratory flow limitation during spontaneous breathing: Comparison of patients with restrictive and obstructive respiratory disorders. Chest 1997;112:1017–1023.

38. Jack DB: Fighting obesity the Franco-British way. Lancet 1996;347:1756.

39. Rochester DF: Obesity and abdominal distention. In Roussos C (ed): The Thorax. Part C: Disease. New York: Marcel Dekker, 1995, pp 1951–1973.

40. Hedenstierna G, Santesson J, Norlander O: Airway closure and distribution of inspired gas in the extreme obese, breathing spontaneously and during anesthesia with intermittent positive pressure ventilation. Acta Anaesthesiol Scand 1976;20:334–342.

41. Vaughan RW, Cork RC, Hollander D: The effect of massive weight loss on arterial oxygenation and pulmonary function tests. Anesthesiology 1981;54:325–328.

42. Barrera F, Reitenberg MM, Winters WL: Pulmonary function in the obese patient. Am J Med Sci 1967;254:785–796.

43. Naimark A, Cherniack RM: Compliance of the respiratory system and its component in health and obesity. J Appl Physiol 1960;15:377–382.

44. Rochester DF, Enson Y: Current concepts in the pathogenesis of the obesity-hypoventilation syndrome. Am J Med 1974;57:402–420.

45. Bae J, Ting EY, Giuffrida JG: The effect of changes in the body position of obese patients on pulmonary volume and ventilatory function. Bull N Y Acad Med 1976;52:830–837.

46. Sharp JT, Henry JP, Sweany SK, et al: The total work of breathing in normal and obese men. J Clin Invest 1964;43:728–739.

47. Zerah F, Harf A, Perlemuter L, et al: Effects of obesity on respiratory resistance. Chest 1993;103:1470–1476.

48. Yap JCH, Gilbey HS, Pride NB: Effects of posture on respiratory mechanics in obesity. J Appl Physiol 1995;79:1199–1205.

49. Farebrother MJB, McHardy GJR, Munro JF: Relation between pulmonary gas exchange and volume before and after substantial weight loss in obese subjects. BMJ 1974;3:391–393.

50. Ferretti A, Giampiccollo P, Cavalli A, et al: Expiratory flow limitation and orthopnea in massively obese subjects. Chest 2001;119:1401–1408.

51. Holley H, Milic-Emili J, Becklake M, Bates D: Regional distribution of pulmonary ventilation and perfusion in obesity. J Clin Invest 1967;46:475–481.

52. Douglas FG, Chong PY: Influence of obesity on peripheral airway patency. J Appl Physiol 1972;33:559–563.

53. Eichenberger AS, Proietti S, Wicky S, et al: Morbid obesity and postoperative pulmonary atelectasis: An underestimated problem. Anesth Analg 2002;95:1788–1792.

54. Sampson MG, Grassino AE: Load compensation in obese patients during tidal breathing. J Appl Physiol 1983;55:1269–1276.

55. Kress JP, Pohlman AS, Alverdy J, Hall JB: The impact of morbid obesity on oxygen cost of breathing at rest. Am J Respir Crit Care Med 1999;160:883–886.

56. Biring MS, Lewis MI, Liu JT, Mohsenifar Z: Pulmonary physiologic changes of morbid obesity. Am J Med Sci 1999;318:293–297.

57. Sahebjami H, Gartside PS: Pulmonary function in obese subjects with a normal $FEV_1/FVC$ ratio. Chest 1996;110:1425–1429.

58. Ray CS, Sue DY, Bray G, et al: Effects of obesity on respiratory function. Am Rev Respir Dis 1983;128:501–506.

59. Burger EJ, Macklem PT: Airway closure: Demonstration by breathing 100% $O_2$ at low lung volumes and by N2 washout. J Appl Physiol 1968;25:139–148.

60. Hughes JM, Rosenzweig DY, Kivitz PB: Site of airway closure in excised dog lungs: Histologic demonstration. J Appl Physiol 1970;29:340–344.

61. Pankow W, Podszus T, Gutheil T, et al: Expiratory flow limitation and intrinsic positive end-expiratory pressure in obesity. J Appl Physiol 1998;85:1236–1243.

62. Agostoni E, Hyatt RE: Static behavior of the respiratory system. In Macklem PT, Mead J (eds): Handbook of Physiology: The Respiratory System, Mechanics of Breathing, sect 3, vol 3. Bethesda, MD: American Physiological Society, 1986, pp 113–130.

63. Koutsoukou A, Bekos B, Sotiropoulou C, et al: Effects of positive end-expiratory pressure on gas exchange and expiratory flow limitation in adult respiratory distress syndrome. Crit Care Med 2002;30:1941–1949.

64. Sahebjami H: Dyspnea in obese healthy men. Chest 1998;114:1373–1377.

65. Moller JT, Johannessen NW, Berg H, et al: Hypoxemia during anesthesia: An observer study. Br J Anaesth 1991;66:437–444.

66. Don HF, Wahba WM, Craig DB: Airway closure, gas trapping and the functional residual capacity during anesthesia. Anesthesiology 1972;36:533–539.

67. Hedenstierna G, Stranberg A, Brismar B, et al: Functional residual capacity, thoracoabdominal dimensions, and central blood volume during general anesthesia with muscle paralysis and mechanical ventilation. Anesthesiology 1985;62:247–254.

68. Rothen HU, Sporre B, Englberg G, et al: Re-expansion of atelectasis during anesthesia: A computed tomography study. Br J Anaesth 1993;71:788–795.

69. Pelosi P, Croci M, Ravagnan I, et al: Total respiratory system, lung and chest wall mechanics in sedated-paralyzed postoperative morbidly obese patients. Chest 1996;109:144–151.

70. Koutsoukou A, Koulouris N, Bekos B, et al: Expiratory flow limitation in morbidly obese postoperative mechanically ventilated patients. Acta Anaesthesiol Scand 2004;48:1080–1088.

71. Pelosi P, Croci M, Ravagnan I, et al: The effect of body mass on lung volumes, respiratory mechanics, and gas exchange during general anesthesia. Anesth Analg 1998;87:654–660.

72. Dawson SV, Elliot EA: Wave-speed limitation on expiratory flow: A unifying concept. J Appl Physiol 1977;43:498–515.

73. Macklem P, Mead J: Resistance of central and peripheral airways measured by a retrograde catheter. J Appl Physiol 1967;22:395–401.

74. Pelosi P, Ravagnan I, Giurati G, et al: Positive end-expiratory pressure improves respiratory function in obese but not in normal subjects during anesthesia and paralysis. Anesthesiology 1999;91:1221–1231.

75. D'Angelo E, Pecchiari M, Baraggia P, et al: Low-volume ventilation induces peripheral airways injury and increased airway resistance in normal open-chest rabbits. J Appl Physiol 2002;92:949–956.

76. Nucci G, Suki B, Lutchen K: Modeling air-flow related shear stress during heterogeneous constriction and mechanical ventilation. J Appl Physiol 2003;95:348–356.

77. McClean MA, Matheson MJ, McKay K, et al: Low lung volume alters contractile properties of airway smooth muscle in sheep. Eur Respir J 2003;22:50–56.

78. D'Angelo E, Pecchiari M, Saetta M, et al: Dependence of lung injury on inflation rate during low volume ventilation in normal open-chest rabbits. J Appl Physiol 2004;97:260–268.

79. D'Angelo E, Pecchiari M, Gentile G: Dependence of lung injury on surface tension during low volume ventilation in normal open-chest rabbits. J Appl Physiol 2007;102:174–182.

80. Conti G, Rocco M, Antonelli M, et al: Respiratory system mechanics in the early phase of acute respiratory failure due to severe kyphoscoliosis. Intensive Care Med 1997;23:539–544.

81. Alvisi V, Romanello A, Badet M, et al: Time course of expiratory flow limitation in COPD patients during acute respiratory failure requiring mechanical ventilation. Chest 2003;123:1625–1632.

## SUGGESTED READINGS

Rodarte JR, Hyatt RE, Cortese DA: Influence of expiratory flow on expiratory capacity at low expiratory flow rates. J Appl Physiol 1975;39:60–65.

Rossi A, Santos C, Roca J: Effects of PEEP on V/Q mismatching in ventilated patients with chronic airflow obstruction. Am J Respir Crit Care Med 1994;149:1077–1084.

Thomas PS, Cowen ERT, Hulands G, et al: Respiratory function in the morbidly obese before and after weight loss. Thorax 1989;44:382–386.

# CHAPTER 11

# Muscle Function

Theodoros Vassilakopoulos, Ioanna Sigala, and Charis Roussos

The respiratory muscles are the only muscles, along with the heart, that have to work continuously, although intermittently, to sustain life. They have to move repetitively a complex elastic structure, the thorax, to achieve the entry of air into the lung and thence gas exchange. The great number of these muscles mandates that they should interact properly to perform their task despite their different anatomic locations, geometric orientations, and motor innervation. They should also be able to adapt to a variety of working conditions and respond to many different chemical and neural stimuli.

Describing the function of the respiratory muscles in a single chapter is extremely difficult. We therefore present certain aspects of respiratory muscle function that are relevant to an understanding of the role of these muscles in breathing. Accordingly, we first discuss the functional anatomy of the respiratory muscles. Next we describe the elastic properties of the thorax that the muscles must move to achieve ventilation in the section on the statics of breathing. The ability to take a breath depends on the balance between the inspiratory load and neuromuscular competence. However, the respiratory muscles must contract continuously to sustain life, and the ability to do this depends on the balance between energy supplies and demands. Consequently, we deal with the parameters of these balances and the way in which they interact in the section on the ability to breathe. The factors that could impair the force-generating capacity of the respiratory muscles are then discussed. The respiratory muscles are plastic structures that adapt to changes in level of the load they are facing. The impact of increased load and inactivity on the respiratory muscles is the topic of the last two sections of this chapter.

## FUNCTIONAL ANATOMY

### Intercostal Muscles

The intercostal muscles are two thin layers of muscle fibers occupying each of the intercostal spaces. They are termed external and internal because of their surface relations, the external being superficial to the internal. The muscle fibers of the two layers run approximately at right angles to each other, and both layers are thicker behind than in front.[1]

The external intercostals extend from the tubercles of the ribs dorsally to the costochondral junctions ventrally, and their fibers are oriented obliquely, downward and forward, from the rib above to the rib below. Near the costochondral junctions, the external intercostals are replaced by a fibrous aponeurosis, the anterior intercostal membrane that extends to the anterior end of the intercostal space.

The internal intercostals begin posteriorly as the posterior intercostal membrane on the inner aspect of the external intercostal muscles. From approximately the angle of the rib, the internal intercostal muscles run obliquely, upward and forward from the superior border of the rib and costal cartilage below, to the floor of the subcostal groove of the rib and the edge of the costal cartilage above, ending at the sternocostal junctions.

Although the intercostal spaces have two layers of intercostal muscle fibers in their lateral portion, they contain a single muscle layer in their ventral and dorsal portion. Ventrally, between the sternum and the costochondral junctions, the only fibers are those of the internal intercostal muscles; these are particularly thick in this region of the rib cage, where they are conventionally called the parasternal intercostals. Dorsally, from the angles of the ribs to the vertebrae, the only fibers come from the external intercostal muscles. These latter, however, are duplicated by a spindle-shaped muscle that runs in each interspace from the tip of the transverse process of the vertebra to the angle of the rib below; this muscle is the levator costae. All the intercostal muscles are innervated by the intercostal nerves.

The respiratory action of the intercostal muscles has been a matter of controversy throughout medical history. The most influential theory proposed to explain this action was that of Hamberger (1749), who based it on geometric considerations (Fig. 11.1): when an intercostal muscle contracts in one interspace, it pulls the upper rib downward and the lower rib upward. The actual movement of the ribs depends on the relative amount of torque around the center of rotation (the vertebral articulations) acting on the two points of attachment of the muscle to the respective ribs: the external intercostals run obliquely downward and forward, so their insertion to the lower rib is more distant from the center of rotation than their insertion to the upper rib. Hence when these muscles contract, the

torque acting on the lower rib is greater than that acting on the upper rib, and its net effect is to raise the ribs. The reverse is true for the internal intercostals, which run upward and forward, so their action is to lower the ribs to which they are attached. The parasternal intercostals are part of the internal intercostal layer, but their action is referred to the sternum, rather than to the vertebral column (i.e., the center of rotation is the sternocostal junctions); therefore, by similar arguments, their contraction should raise the ribs.[2]

The Hamburger theory is incomplete, however, and cannot entirely explain the actions of the intercostal muscles on the ribs for two reasons.[3,4] First, the Hamburger model is planar, whereas in reality the ribs are curved. As a result, the changes in length of the intercostal muscles during a given rotation of the ribs (hence their mechanical advantage and action on the ribs) vary as a function of the position of the muscle fibers along the rib. Thus, during cranial rotation of the ribs, their curvature causes changes in muscle length that are greater in the dorsal region, decrease progressively as one moves around the rib cage, and are reversed as one approaches the sternum. This finding is in contrast to the Hamberger model, which predicts equal shortening of all external intercostals and equal lengthening of all internal intercostals during cranial rotation of two adjacent ribs. Second, the Hamburger model states that all the ribs rotate by equal amounts around parallel axes so the distance between adjacent ribs remains constant. In fact, the radii of curvature of different ribs are different, increasing from the top downward, so their rotations are similarly different. Consequently, there is a change in intercostal muscle length owing to the changes in the distance between the ribs from the top downward.

Despite the inaccuracies included in the Hamberger model, its predictions seem valid because experimental data suggest that the external intercostals, the parasternal intercostals, and the levatores costarum have an inspiratory action on the rib cage, whereas the internal intercostals are expiratory. During breathing at rest, normal humans have inspiratory activity in the parasternal intercostals.[5,6] This finding suggests that in humans the contribution of the parasternal intercostals to resting breathing is greater than that of the external intercostals. During loaded breathing, the activation of the external intercostals and levatores costarum increases, although the mechanical effectiveness of this reserve "load-compensating" system is relatively small.[7]

A clearly illustrative clinical example of the "isolated" inspiratory action of the intercostals is offered by patients who suffer from bilateral diaphragmatic paralysis. In these patients, inspiration is accomplished solely by the rib cage muscles. As a result, the rib cage expands during inspiration, and the pleural pressure falls. Because the diaphragm is flaccid and no transdiaphragmatic pressure can be

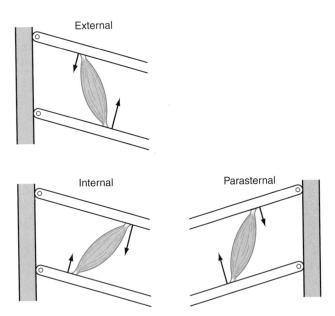

**Figure 11.1** Diagram illustrating Hamberger's theory. In each panel, the *hatched area* represents the center of rotation (the spine for internal and external intercostal muscles and the sternum for parasternal muscles), and the *two bars oriented obliquely* represent two adjacent ribs. The intercostal muscles are depicted as single bundles, and the torques acting on the ribs during contraction of these muscles are represented by *arrows.* (From DeTroyer A, Loring SH: Actions of the respiratory muscles. In Roussos C [ed]: The Thorax. New York: Marcel Dekker, 1995.)

developed, the fall in pleural pressure is transmitted to the abdomen, thus causing an equal fall in abdominal pressure. Hence the abdomen moves paradoxically inward during inspiration, thus opposing the inflation of the lung. In fact, this paradoxic motion is the cardinal sign of diaphragmatic paralysis on clinical examination and is invariably present in the supine posture, during which the abdominal muscles usually remain relaxed during the whole respiratory cycle. On the contrary, this sign may be absent in the erect posture, in which some patients partially compensate for diaphragmatic paralysis by contracting the abdominal muscles during expiration, thus displacing the abdomen inward and the diaphragm cranially into the thorax. Relaxation of the abdominal muscles at the onset of inspiration may then cause outward motion of the abdominal wall and (passive) descent of the diaphragm that removes the characteristic paradoxic inspiratory inward abdominal motion.

## Diaphragm

The floor of the thoracic cavity is closed by a thin musculotendinous sheet of complex structure and development, the diaphragm, which is anatomically unique among the skeletal muscles in that its fibers radiate from a central tendinous structure (the central tendon) to insert peripherally into skeletal structures. The central tendon of the diaphragm is thin, strong, and roughly trilobed. It has the shape of a boomerang, with its two ends pointing posterolaterally.[8] The central part is fused above with the fibrous pericardial sac, and both structures at this point are derived from the embryonic septum transversum.

The muscle of the diaphragm, all of which inserts into the central tendon, falls into two main components, according to its point of origin: the crural (vertebral) part and the costal (sternocostal) part. The crural (vertebral) part of the diaphragm arises from the crura and the three aponeurotic arcuate ligaments. The crura are strong, tapering tendons attached vertically to the anterolateral aspects of the bodies and intervertebral disks of the first three lumbar vertebrae on the right and two on the left. An ill-defined, fibrous thickening arch between the two crura forms the median arcuate ligament. A tendinous medial arcuate ligament passes from the crus on each side across the psoas major muscle to the tip of the transverse process of the first lumbar vertebra. From this point, a lateral arcuate ligament then runs to the 12th rib crossing the quadratus lumborum muscle. The medial and lateral arcuate ligaments are firmly adherent to the posterior body wall fused to the sheath and fascia of psoas and quadratus lumborum muscles, respectively. Muscle fibers arising from the crura and the arcuate ligaments pass upward to insert into the posterior border of the central tendon, overlapping to some extent and passing behind the fibers ascending from the 12th rib.

The costal (sternocostal) part of the diaphragm arises from the xiphoid process and the lower end of the sternum and the costal cartilages of the lower six ribs. From the back of the xiphoid process and the lower end of the sternum, muscle fibers pass almost horizontally backward into the anterior border of the central tendon. Separated from the sternal portion by a small gap, the sternocostal triangle, muscle fibers arise from the inner aspects of each costal cartilage from the 7th rib to the tip of the 12th rib. These costal fibers run cranially so they are directly apposed to the inner aspect of lower rib cage, thus creating a zone of apposition. Only at higher levels does an angle open up between them and the chest wall, and finally they converge horizontally onto the anterior, lateral, and, to some extent, posterior borders of the central tendon and increase progressively in length around the chest and from front to back. Frequently, a triangular gap remains between the fibers from the 12th rib and the most lateral fibers from the lateral arcuate ligament, thereby leaving a muscular deficiency, the vertebrocostal trigone.

The shape of the relaxed diaphragm at functional residual capacity (FRC) is that of two domes joined by a saddle that runs from the sternum to the anterior surface of the spinal column.[9,10] The free surface curves to join the inside of the rib cage and then continues downward so the diaphragm becomes cylindric in the zone of apposition. The height of this zone in the standing human at rest is about 6 to 7 cm in the midaxillary line and occupies 25% to 30% of the total internal surface area of the rib cage. The motor innervation of the diaphragm is from the phrenic nerves, which also provide a proprioceptive supply to the muscle. When tension develops within the diaphragmatic muscle fibers, a caudally oriented force is applied on the central tendon, and the dome of the diaphragm descends. This descent has two effects. First, it expands the thoracic cavity along its craniocaudal axis, and consequently the pleural pressure falls. Depending on whether the airways are open or closed, lung volume increases or alveolar pressure falls. Second, it produces caudal displacement of the abdominal visceral contents and an increase in the abdominal pressure that, in turn, results in an outward motion of the ventral abdominal wall. Furthermore, diaphragmatic contraction acts to displace the bony rib cage both directly through the insertions of the costal diaphragmatic fibers onto the ribs and indirectly through the effect of changing the pleural and abdominal pressures. Thus, when the diaphragm contracts, a cranially oriented force is applied by the costal diaphragmatic fibers to the upper margins of the lower six ribs that has the effect of lifting and rotating them outward (insertional force). The actions mediated by the changes in pleural and abdominal pressures are more complex: if one assumes that the diaphragm is the only muscle acting on the rib cage, it appears that it has two opposing effects when it contracts. On the upper rib cage, it causes a decrease in the anteroposterior (AP) diameter, and this expiratory action is primarily the result of the fall in pleural pressure.[11] On the lower rib cage, it causes an expansion that is more pronounced along its transverse diameter than along its AP diameter. In fact, this is the pattern of chest wall motion observed in tetraplegic patients with transection injury at the C5 segment or below who have complete paralysis of the inspiratory muscles except for the diaphragm. This inspiratory action on the lower rib cage is caused by the concomitant action of two different forces, the "insertional" force already described and the "appositional" force. The zone of apposition makes the lower rib cage, in effect, part of the abdominal container, and measurements in dogs have established that, during breathing, the changes in pressure in the pleural recess between the apposed diaphragm and the rib cage are almost equal to the changes in abdominal pressure.[12] Pressure in this pleural recess rises rather than falls during inspiration, a finding indicating that the rise in abdominal pressure is truly transmitted through the apposed diaphragm to expand the lower rib cage. This mechanism of diaphragmatic action has been termed the *appositional force*, and its magnitude depends directly on the size of the zone of apposition and on the rise in abdominal pressure and indirectly on the resistance provided by the abdominal contents to diaphragmatic descent. Clearly, for a given diaphragmatic contraction, the appositional force is greater when the rise in abdominal pressure and the zone of apposition are larger and when the resistance to diaphragmatic descent is higher because in this case the dome of the diaphragm descends less, the zone of apposition remains significant throughout inspiration, and the rise in abdominal pressure is larger. An illustrative clinical example of this latter effect is provided by tetraplegic patients: when the compliance of their abdomen decreases either by having them in the seated position or by means of a pneumatic cuff or an elastic binder around the abdomen, the expansion of the lower rib cage during inspiration is accentuated.[13] The greater area of apposed diaphragm at the sides of the rib cage, compared with that at the front, presumably accounts for the finding that the human diaphragm has a greater expanding action on the transverse than on the AP diameter of the lower rib cage.[11]

The balance between pleural pressure and the insertional and appositional forces of the diaphragm is also markedly affected by changes in lung volume. As lung volume decreases to less than FRC, the zone of apposition increases in size,[14] and the fraction of the rib cage exposed to pleural pressure decreases. As a result, the appositional force increases, whereas the effect of pleural pressure diminishes, so the inspiratory action of the diaphragm on the rib cage is enhanced. Conversely, as lung volume increases, the zone of apposition decreases in size, and a larger fraction of the rib cage becomes exposed to pleural pressure. Hence the diaphragm's inspiratory action on the rib cage diminishes.[2,14–16] When lung volume approaches total lung capacity (TLC), the zone of apposition all but disappears,[14] and the diaphragmatic muscle fibers become oriented internally as well as cranially. As in the eviscerated animal, the insertional force of the diaphragm is then expiratory, rather than inspiratory, in direction. These two effects of increasing lung volume account for the inspiratory decrease in the transverse diameter of the lower rib cage in subjects with emphysema and severe hyperinflation (Hoover's sign).

The relationship between the lung volume and the mechanical effectiveness/advantage of the diaphragm is more pronounced whenever the lung volume changes acutely. When the lung volume increases chronically, some form of adaptation takes place to compensate partially for the mechanical disadvantage created for the diaphragm. In fact, it has been shown that in emphysematous hamsters the diaphragm drops out sarcomeres, resulting in a leftward shift of the whole length-tension curve so the muscle adapts to the shorter operating length.[17] The extent to which this adaption occurs in humans remains unclear as yet.

Although diaphragmatic contraction alone causes distortion of the rib cage at all lung volumes, normal humans breathing at rest expand the rib cage without distortion. Thus, during inspiration, the AP and transverse diameters of the lower rib cage increase proportionately and synchronously, and the AP diameter of the upper rib cage increases as well. This finding implies that, even during resting breathing, normal humans contract other muscles that expand the upper rib cage and increase the AP diameter of the lower rib cage.

## Neck Muscles

### Sternocleidomastoids

The sternocleidomastoids arise from the mastoid process and descend to the ventral surface of the manubrium sterni and the medial third of the clavicle. Their neural supply is from the accessory nerve. The action of the sternocleidomastoids is to displace the sternum cranially during inspiration, to expand the upper rib cage more in its AP diameter than in its transverse one, and to decrease the transverse diameter of the lower rib cage. This is inferred from the measurements of chest wall motion in subjects with transection of the upper cervical spinal cord,[18] in which the sternocleidomastoids are the only muscles spared. In essence, their isolated action counteracts the isolated action of the diaphragm on the upper rib cage.

In normal subjects breathing at rest, however, the sternocleidomastoids are inactive, recruited only when the inspiratory muscle pump is abnormally loaded or when ventilation increases substantially.[19,20] Therefore, they should be considered accessory muscles of inspiration.

## Scalenes

The scalenes comprise three muscle bundles that run from the transverse processes of the lower five cervical vertebrae to the upper surface of the first two ribs. They receive their neural supply mainly from the lower five cervical segments. Their action is to increase (slightly) the AP diameter of the upper rib cage.[21] Although earlier studies[22] had suggested that the scalenes function as accessory muscles of inspiration, more recent data[23] provide convincing evidence that these muscles are invariably active during inspiration. In fact, seated normal subjects cannot breathe without contracting the scalenes even when they reduce the required inspiratory effort by reducing tidal volume considerably.[23] Therefore, the scalenes in humans are primary muscles of inspiration, and their contraction is an important determinant of the expansion of the upper rib cage during breathing.

## STATICS OF BREATHING

The respiratory system is an elastic structure; that is, if a force is applied to it, it changes volume, and when the force is released, it returns to its resting configuration. Rohrer[23] proposed in 1916 that movement of the respiratory system is caused by pressure differences across the system to overcome the elastic resistance to volume change (elastic load), the frictional resistance to flow (resistive load), and the inertial resistance to mass acceleration (inertial load). The main function of the respiratory muscles is to provide the required pressure across the respiratory system to achieve its movement and thus the entry of air into the thorax. Although the act of breathing incorporates all the components initially described by Rohrer, it is really didactic to isolate each one and determine the pressure required to overcome each of the elastic, resistive, and inertial loads.

The term *statics of breathing* refers to the pressure-volume relationship of the respiratory system. As the origin of the word static implies (static is a Greek word meaning "with no movement"), this relationship has to be determined with no movement of air (no resistive pressure losses) and no acceleration of tissues (no inertial pressure losses) to reflect the elastic behavior of the respiratory system (elastic load).

One of the first experimental descriptions of the static properties of the respiratory system was that of Rahn and colleagues in 1946.[24] Normal subjects were asked to inspire a volume of air from a spirometer and then to relax against an occluded airway with an open glottis for a few seconds. This was repeated at various lung volumes. The pressure at the mouth was measured together with the lung volume and was recorded on an X-Y plot. Because under these conditions there is no flow of air within the airways, the pressure at the mouth equals the pressure in the airways and that of the alveoli. Consequently, the difference between the pressure in the mouth and the atmospheric pressure (i.e., body surface pressure) represents the distending pressure of the respiratory system. The volume at zero pressure is the resting volume of the respiratory system where mouth pressure equals zero and is the FRC. The horizontal distance from the solid line to the zero-pressure ordinate indicates total respiratory system distending (elastic) pressure (Pel,rs) and is negative (subatmospheric) below FRC and positive above FRC. Although Rahn and associates[24] reasoned that total pressure at the mouth is the sum of the pressures exerted by the elastic recoil properties of the chest wall (Pel,W) and the lung (Pel,L) (i.e., Pel,rs = Pel,L + Pel,W), these investigators were unable to measure these parameters directly. The best they could do was to use published values of the lung's in vitro pressure-volume relationship and to plot them on the pressure-volume diagram; then by subtracting Pel,L from Pel,rs at any volume, they calculated Pel,W (Fig. 11.2). This diagram illustrates that lung recoil is positive at all lung volumes above residual volume (RV). On the contrary, the chest wall exhibits more complex behavior: from RV to approximately 60% of vital capacity (VC), the chest wall exerts outward elastic pressure (i.e., tends to expand). At FRC, which is approximately 40% of VC, there is an equilibrium between the inward pressure of the lungs and the outward pressure exerted by the rib cage; hence alveolar and mouth pressures are zero. From 60% of VC to TLC, the chest wall recoil is inward and is additive to that of the lungs.

The next major advance in the study of the statics of breathing came with the introduction of the esophageal balloon technique,[25] which allowed the measurement of esophageal pressure as an estimate of pleural pressure (PPL) and consequently the partitioning of the respiratory system into its two components: lungs and chest wall. Because both share the same volume change, pressure partitioning is all that is necessary. Accordingly, Heaf and Prime[26] and Campbell[27] modified the Rahn diagram by plotting lung volume against PPL under two conditions (Fig. 11.3): during breath-holding with the glottis open (which is achieved by the coordinated action of the inspiratory muscles) and during relaxation of the respiratory muscles with the airway occluded. Under the first condition, because there is no movement of air and the airway (glottis) remains open, the pressure in the

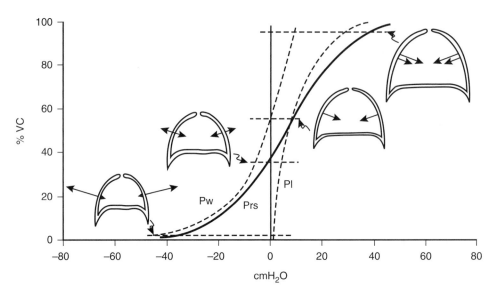

**Figure 11.2** Static volume-pressure curves of the lung (Pl), chest wall (Pw), and total respiratory system (Prs) during relaxation in the sitting posture. The static forces of the lung and the chest wall are pictured by *arrows* in the side drawings. The dimensions of the arrows are not to scale; the volume corresponding to each drawing is indicated by *horizontal broken lines*. (From Rahn H, Otis AB, Chadwick LE, Fenn WO: The pressure-volume diagram of the thorax and lung. Am J Physiol 1946;146:161–178, as modified by Agostoni E, Mead J: Statics of the respiratory system. In Fenn WO [ed]: Handbook of Physiology. Section 3: Respiration, vol 1. Washington, DC: American Physiological Society, 1964.)

mouth (i.e., the same with the atmospheric pressure) equals the pressure in the alveoli (i.e., Pm = Patm = PaLV). The difference between this pressure and the PPL (i.e., PaLV − PPL) represents the distending pressure of the lung (Pel,L). Because pressures are measured relative to Patm (i.e., Patm is considered to be zero), under this condition Pel,L = −$P_{PL}$ ⇒ $P_{PL}$ = −Pel,L. Accordingly, if lung volume were plotted against PPL, the pressure-volume relationship of the lung would be obtained (*left curve* on Fig. 11.3). Under the second condition, the respiratory muscles are relaxed, and so the difference between PPL and body surface pressure (i.e., Patm) represents the distending pressure of the chest wall: Pel,W = PPL − Patm. Because Patm = 0, Pel,W = PPL, and if lung volume were plotted against PPL, the pressure-volume relationship of the chest wall would be obtained (*right curve* on Fig. 11.3). This is identical to the chest wall pressure-volume curve in the Rahn diagram. The two curves intersect at approximately −5 cm H₂O, the PPL value at resting FRC. The horizontal distance between the two curves gives the elastic pressure that must be developed (by either the respiratory muscles or the ventilator) to displace the system above or below its equilibrium volume (where the two curves intersect) and thus corresponds to the pressure-volume relationship of the entire respiratory system.

Neglecting dynamic considerations, the left-hand curve shows the pleural pressure-volume relationship during spontaneous breathing when airway pressure is near zero. The right-hand curve shows the pleural pressure-volume relationships during mechanical ventilation (when the respiratory muscles are relaxed), and the distance between the curves approximates alveolar pressure during mechanical ventilation.[28]

Note that this analysis considers the chest wall as a single compartment model (i.e., as having a single degree of freedom). This means that it is possible to measure the change in a single dimension of the chest wall and solve for changes in all other dimensions. Of course, the contribution of the abdomen, diaphragm, or rib cage to the volume displacements cannot be differentiated. Before this volume partitioning could be attempted, one had to know the pressures acting on these different compartments. This became possible after the work of Agostoni and Rahn,[29] who developed the method of measuring transdiaphragmatic pressure as the difference between gastric and esophageal pressure. By measuring gastric pressure as an index of abdominal pressure (Pab) and esophageal pressure as an index of pleural pressure, these investigators accomplished the pressure partitioning necessary to determine the pressures displacing the abdomen (Pab), as well as those acting on the inner surface of the rib cage (PPL). This set the stage for partitioning of the chest wall elastic properties into those of the abdomen and the rib cage. Although several techniques and models for this

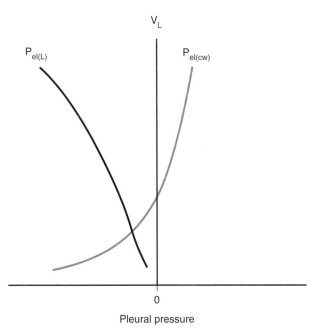

**Figure 11.3** Pressure-volume curves of lung and chest wall. Esophageal pressure as estimate of pleural pressure (PPL) on the horizontal axis is plotted against volume on the vertical axis. Data were obtained from normal young men under two conditions. *Left curve*, Pel(L) is the pressure-volume relationship when the lung is held inflated by the respiratory muscles with the glottis open and thus negative of transpulmonary pressure (alveolar minus pleural pressure). *Right curve*, Pel(cw) is the pressure-volume curve during muscular relaxation against an occluded airway. The curve defines the transthoracic pressure (pleural minus atmospheric pressure)–volume relationship. (From Rodarte JH: Lung and chest wall mechanics: Basic concepts. In Scharf SM [ed]: Heart-Lung Interactions in Health and Disease. New York: Marcel Dekker, 1989.)

partitioning have been proposed,[30–33] the one introduced by Konno and Mead[34] has gained wide acceptance and will be further analyzed. These investigators measured the surface motion displacements of the rib cage and abdomen and used them to represent the corresponding volume changes in both sitting and supine normal subjects keeping a fixed body position. These investigators hypothesized that the chest wall has two degrees of freedom (i.e., can accommodate lung volume by displacing the rib cage or diaphragm and abdomen independently, as parallel pathways). The sum of both displacements was monotonically related to changes in lung volume. AP displacements of the rib cage and abdominal wall were initially measured on many different chest wall surface points by means of linear differential transducers. Displacement of loci on the middle sternum and above the umbilicus were found to be those that best represent the volume displacement relationship of the rib cage and abdomen, respectively. The investigators recognized that in the boundary between the rib cage and the abdomen,

there were more degrees of freedom. Even more degrees of freedom emerged by considering the cranial movement of rib cage[35] and by allowing flexion of the spine. Konno and Mead[34] expressed chest wall configuration by plotting rib cage versus abdominal AP wall dimensions (Fig. 11.4).[36] Each point in the diagram (i.e., each pair of AP dimensions) would represent a unique configuration of the chest wall at volumes from TLC to RV. The *dashed line* encircling the data points in Figure 11.4 represents the limits of possible configurations. The *continuous line* from RV to TLC represents the chest wall configurations (i.e., pairs of AP dimensions) obtained when the corresponding lung volumes were held by relaxing against a closed airway. This relaxation curve represents the minimum energy configuration at each lung volume, and distortion away from this configuration requires energy. If at any point along the relaxation line the subject closes the airway and shifts volume between the abdominal and rib cage compartments while lung volume remains constant (isovolume maneuver), the AP diameters of the rib cage and the abdomen will follow a line with a negative slope (i.e., the AP diameter of the

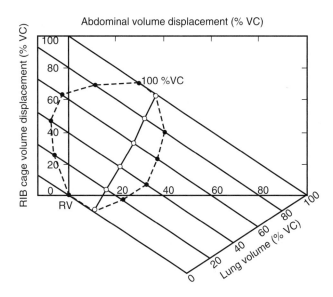

**Figure 11.4** The Konno-Mead diagram. The rib cage anteroposterior dimensions are plotted against the abdominal anteroposterior dimensions. The displacements are expressed as a percentage of total over the vital capacity (VC) relative to values at active residual volume (RV). The *solid line with open points* indicates the configurations in relaxed states from total lung capacity (TLC) (100%) isovolume obtained by shifting volume from abdomen to chest and vice versa and by keeping a closed glottis (isovolume maneuvers). The area enclosed by the *dashed line* illustrates a range of possible configurations produced by submaximal contraction of rib cage and abdominal muscles. (From Smith J, Loring S: Passive mechanical properties of the chest wall. In Handbook of Physiology. Section 3: The Respiratory System, vol 3, part 2. Washington, DC: American Physiological Society, 1986.)

abdomen becomes smaller when the AP diameter of the rib cage becomes bigger and vice versa). In reality, these isovolume isopleths are flat loops showing hysteresis rather than lines. The AP diameter can be derived not only by linear pressure transducers, as originally described, but also with the use of magnetometers or Respitrace (respiratory inductive plethysmography bands), which, in fact, measures a cross-sectional area that is less susceptible to local distortion than with magnetometers.[37] Calibration of chest wall dimensions can be achieved by doing isovolume maneuvers at different lung volumes (e.g., at 20% intervals of the VC, as indicated in Fig. 11.4), thus providing a quantitative link between configuration and lung volume. The measurement of chest wall displacements has become a useful method to monitor ventilation noninvasively, and it has a precision to within approximately 10% of spirometric measurements.

By combining the pressure partitioning of Agostoni and Rahn with the volume partitioning already presented, one can measure the elastic properties of the rib cage and abdomen separately.[38] In the upright, standing position, the abdomen is considerably less compliant than the rib cage because the action of gravity causes the abdominal contents to stretch the anterior abdominal wall; in the supine position, however, abdominal compliance increases markedly.[39] As a result, abdominal motion during breathing is more prominent in the supine position than in the upright position.[40]

The Konno-Mead method does not measure displacement of the diaphragm. The actual lung volume displaced by the diaphragm is included in both rib cage expansion and abdominal displacement, and the exact contribution of the diaphragm to the two compartments remains a matter of controversy despite thorough investigation and ingenious theoretical analysis. This stems from the complex actions of the diaphragm and the finding that the rib cage and the diaphragm-abdomen complex, rather than being two independent pathways, seem to be mechanically coupled in ways that are not well understood. Detailed presentation of this challenging area of controversy is beyond the scope of this chapter, however, and the interested reader should consult several excellent reviews.[39-41]

## ABILITY TO BREATHE: LOAD/CAPACITY BALANCE

For a human to take a spontaneous breath, the inspiratory muscles must generate sufficient force to overcome the elastance of the lungs and chest wall (lung and chest wall elastic loads) as well as the airway and tissue resistance (resistive load). This requires an adequate output of

the centers controlling the muscles, anatomic and functional nerve integrity, unimpaired neuromuscular transmission, an intact chest wall, and adequate muscle strength. This can be schematically represented by considering the ability to take a breath as a balance between inspiratory load and neuromuscular competence (Fig. 11.5). Under normal conditions, this system is polarized in favor of neuromuscular competence (i.e., there are reserves that permit considerable increases in load). However, for humans to breathe spontaneously, the inspiratory muscles should be able to sustain the previously mentioned load over time and also adjust the minute ventilation in such a way that there is adequate gas exchange. The ability of the respiratory muscles to sustain this load without the appearance of fatigue is called *endurance* and is determined by the balance between energy supplies and energy demands (Fig. 11.6).

Energy supplies depend on the inspiratory muscle blood flow, the blood substrate (fuel) concentration and arterial oxygen content, the muscle's ability to extract and utilize energy sources, and the muscle's energy stores.[42,43] Under normal circumstances, energy supplies are adequate to meet the demands, and a large recruitable reserve exists (see Fig. 11.6).

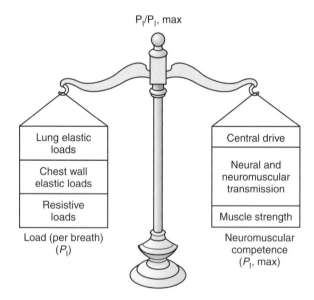

**Figure 11.5** The ability to take a spontaneous breath is determined by the balance between the load imposed on the respiratory system (PI) and the neuromuscular competence of the ventilatory pump (PImax). Normally this balance weighs in favor of competence, thus permitting significant increases in load. However, if the competence is, for whatever reason, reduced to less than a critical point (e.g., drug overdose, myasthenia gravis), the balance may then weigh in favor of load, thus rendering the ventilatory pump insufficient to inflate the lungs and chest wall. (From Vassilakopoulos T, Zakynthinos S, Roussos C: Respiratory muscles and weaning failure. Eur Respir J 1996;9:2383–2400.)

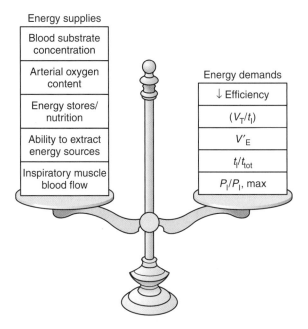

Energy supplies

- Blood substrate concentration
- Arterial oxygen content
- Energy stores/ nutrition
- Ability to extract energy sources
- Inspiratory muscle blood flow

Energy demands

- ↓ Efficiency
- $(V_T/t_I)$
- $V'_E$
- $t_I/t_{tot}$
- $P_I/P_I$, max

**Figure 11.6** Respiratory muscle endurance is determined by the balance between energy supplies and demands. Normally, the supplies meet the demands, and a large reserve does exist. Whenever this balance weighs in favor of demands, the respiratory muscles ultimately become fatigued, leading to inability to sustain spontaneous breathing. (From Vassilakopoulos T, Zakynthinos S, Roussos C: Respiratory muscles and weaning failure. Eur Respir J 1996;9:2383–2400.)

Energy demands increase proportionally with the mean tidal pressure developed by the inspiratory muscles (PI) expressed as a fraction of maximum (PI/PImax), the minute ventilation (VE), the inspiratory duty cycle (TI/TTOT), and the mean inspiratory flow rate (VT/TI) and are inversely related to the efficiency of the muscles.[42,43] Fatigue develops when the mean rate of energy demands exceeds the mean rate of energy supply[44] (i.e., when the balance is polarized in favor of demands)

$$Ud > Us \; \frac{W}{E} > Us \qquad (1)$$

where W is the mean muscle power, E is efficiency, Ud is energy demand, and Us is energy supply.

Bellemare and Grassino[45] suggested that the product of TI/TTOT and the mean transdiaphragmatic pressure expressed as a fraction of maximal (Pdi/Pdimax) defines a useful tension-time index (TTIdi) that is related to the endurance time (i.e., the time that the diaphragm can sustain the load imposed on it). Whenever TTIdi is smaller than the critical value of 0.15, the load can be sustained indefinitely, but when TTIdi exceeds the critical zone of 0.15 to 0.18, the load can be sustained

only for a limited time period (i.e., the endurance time). This was found to be inversely related to TTIdi. By analogy, a TTI was calculated for the rib cage muscles:

$$TTIrc = \text{mean value } P_{PL}/P_{PLmax} \; TI/TT \qquad (2)$$

where $P_{PL}$ is the pleural pressure, and the critical value was found to be 0.30.[46] The TTI concept is assumed to be applicable not only to the diaphragm, but also to the respiratory muscles as a whole:[47]

$$TTI = \frac{PI}{PI_{max}} \bullet \frac{T_I}{T_{TOT}} \qquad (3)$$

where PI = mean inspiratory pressure per breath and PImax = maximal inspiratory pressure. Because we have stated that endurance is determined by the balance between energy supply and demand, TTI of the inspiratory muscles has to be in accordance with the energy balance view. In fact, as Figure 11.6 demonstrates, PI/PImax and TI/TTOT, which constitute the TTI, are among the determinants of energy demands; an increase in either that will increase the TTI value will also increase the demands. The energy balance may then weigh in favor of demands leading to fatigue. Furthermore, Roussos and colleagues[48] directly related PI/PImax to the endurance time. The critical value of PI/PImax that could be generated indefinitely at FRC was approximately 0.60. Greater values of PI/PImax ratio were inversely related to the endurance time in a curvilinear fashion. When lung volume was increased from FRC to FRC + 1/2 inspiratory capacity, the critical values of PI/PImax and the endurance time were diminished greatly (20% to 25% of PImax).

What determines the PI/PImax ratio, however? The nominator, the mean inspiratory pressure, is determined by the elastic and resistive loads imposed on the inspiratory muscles. The denominator, the maximum inspiratory pressure, is determined by the neuromuscular competence (i.e., the maximum inspiratory muscle activation that can be achieved). It follows, then, that the value of PI/PImax is determined by the balance between load and competence (see Fig. 11.5). However, PI/PImax is also one of the determinants of energy demands (see Fig. 11.6); therefore, the two balances (i.e., between load and competence and energy supply and demand) are in essence linked, creating a system. Schematically, when the central hinge of the system moves upward, or is at least horizontal, spontaneous ventilation can be sustained indefinitely (Fig. 11.7). One can easily see that the ability of a subject to breathe spontaneously depends on the fine interplay of many different factors. Normally, this interplay moves the central hinge far upward and creates a great ventilatory reserve for the healthy individual.

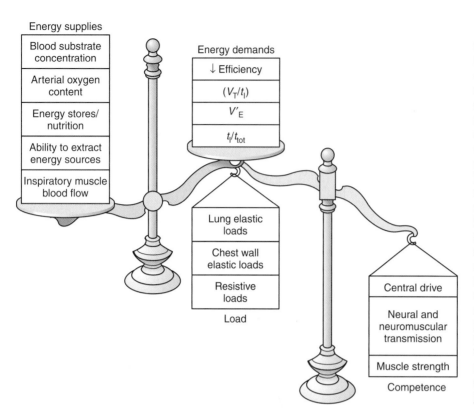

**Figure 11.7** The system of two balances incorporating the various determinants of load, competence, energy supplies, and demands is represented schematically. The PI/PImax that was one of the determinants of energy demands (see Fig. 11.6) is replaced by its equivalent: the balance between load and neuromuscular competence (see Fig. 11.5). In fact, this is the reason that the two balances are linked. When the central hinge of the system moves upward or is at least at a horizontal level, an appropriate relationship between ventilatory needs and neurorespiratory capacity exists, and spontaneous ventilation can be sustained. In healthy persons, the hinge moves far upward to create a large reserve. (From Vassilakopoulos T, Zakynthinos S, Roussos C: Respiratory muscles and weaning failure. Eur Respir J 1996;9:2383–2400.)

When the central hinge of the system, for whatever reason, moves downward, spontaneous ventilation cannot be sustained, and ventilatory failure ensues, ultimately necessitating mechanical ventilation.

## FACTORS IMPAIRING MUSCLES' FORCE-GENERATING CAPACITY

### Decreased Neuromuscular Competence

Proper function of the respiratory muscles requires an adequate output of the centers controlling them, anatomic and functional integrity of the nerves supplying them, unimpaired neuromuscular transmission, and adequate muscle strength. A defect at any of these levels would obviously decrease neuromuscular competence and thus the muscles' force-generating capacity.

### Decreased Respiratory Drive

Central nervous system (CNS) depression caused by neurologic damage, toxic-metabolic encephalopathy, or drug overdose (sedatives, narcotics) is commonly the cause of decreased drive to the respiratory muscles. Metabolic alkalosis is another potential factor. Furthermore, occult hypothyroidism, sleep deprivation, and starvation are recognized as potential causes of

decreased respiratory drive.[49] Dysfunction of the respiratory center may be caused by bulbar poliomyelitis, myotonic dystrophy, or acid maltase deficiency.[50] Alterations in central respiratory control may also develop in patients with neuromuscular disorders that do not produce specific dysfunction of the respiratory center. These alterations may be related to sleep-induced hypoventilation.[51]

### Decreased Neural and Neuromuscular Transmission

Neural transmission to the respiratory muscles may be interrupted in phrenic nerve or spinal cord transection. Transmission may also be impaired in phrenic nerve injury (thermal, hypoxic, or traction injury during cardiac surgery[52]), demyelinating diseases, immunologic conditions (e.g., Guillain-Barré syndrome,[50,53] multiple sclerosis) or toxin-induced disorders (e.g., diphtheria), or in diseases affecting the lower motoneurons, whether infectious (e.g., poliomyelitis) or degenerative (e.g., amyotrophic lateral sclerosis). Various other neuropathies could also be included, but are rare enough not to merit special mention in this context.

Neuromuscular transmission, in turn, may be impaired by toxins (e.g., botulism that inhibits presynaptic acetylcholine release), an episode of myasthenia gravis, and drugs (organophosphate poisoning, aminoglycosides, and, especially, neuromuscular blockers).[50,54] Critical illness polyneuropathy is a syndrome of prolonged muscle weakness or paralysis typically manifesting as failure to wean from mechanical ventilation.[50,55] The cause is unknown, although sepsis, multiple organ failure, shock, hypoxia, medications, and prolonged use of neuromuscular blocking agents have been implicated.[56] Electrophysiologic studies reveal abnormalities primarily characterized by axonal degeneration.[50,56,57] Although critical illness polyneuropathy is usually improved in parallel with the underlying disease, weaning is difficult, and the mortality rate is high in these patients.[50,56]

## Muscle Weakness

Muscle weakness, a condition in which the capacity of a rested muscle to generate force is impaired, can be caused by a variety of reasons: (1) inflammatory, alcohol, and thyroid myopathies; (2) muscular dystrophies; (3) myopathies induced by drugs, especially cortico-steroids,[58,59] antibiotics (aminoglycosides), and relaxants; (4) malnutrition[60–62] and muscle atrophy (especially important in the critically ill patient); (5) obesity[63]; (6) electrolyte imbalances, including hypocalcemia,[64] hypokalemia,[65] hypophosphatemia,[66,67] and both hypomagnesemia[68] and hypermagnesemia[65]; (7) hypercapnia (acute)[69] and acidosis,[70,71] which are important factors in the development of muscular weakness because most patients who increase their carbon dioxide tension ($P_{CO_2}$) enter a vicious cycle in which the increased $P_{CO_2}$ reduces muscle strength,[69] ventilatory failure is thus worsened, and $P_{CO_2}$ is further increased; (8) mechanical disadvantage; (9) sepsis and endotoxic shock; and (10) disuse atrophy.

With regard to mechanical disadvantage, hyperinflation is a factor. Respiratory muscles, like other skeletal muscles, obey the length-tension relationship. At any given level of activation, changes in muscle fiber length alter active and passive tension and thus modify actin-myosin interaction. At a concrete fiber length (Lo), active tension is maximal, whereas below or above this, it declines. Respiratory muscle length depends largely on lung volume and, to a lesser extent, on thoracoabdominal configuration.[35,72,73] The exact in vivo relationships have not been defined in detail. However, it is believed, based on animal experiments,[74,75] that Lo for inspiratory muscles (diaphragm and intercostals) is near RV. In addition, a relationship between lung volume and diaphragmatic fiber length in humans has been confirmed[76] that could entirely explain the decreases in pressure with increasing lung volume by corresponding decreases in contractility. Hyperinflation, then, causes a decrease in the respiratory muscles' length and a change in their geometry that clearly decreases PImax. However, an important distinction should be made between the chronic, slowly developing static hyperinflation resulting from loss of lung elastic recoil and the acute, rapidly developing dynamic hyperinflation caused by bronchoconstriction, respiratory tract infection, or abnormally increased frequency of

breathing (see the earlier discussion of the diaphragm). In fact, it has been shown that changes in inspiratory muscle characteristics can compensate for the decrease in the operating length caused by hyperinflation. In emphysematous hamsters, the diaphragm drops out sarcomeres, thus resulting in a leftward shift of the whole length-tension curve so the muscle adapts to the shorter operating length.[17] These alterations in muscle fiber length-tension characteristics may help to restore the mechanical advantage of the diaphragm in chronically hyperinflated states, although the extent to which this adaptation occurs in humans remains unclear.

Indirect evidence for the existence of such an adaptation in humans comes from the work of Similowski and co-workers,[77] who studied the contractile properties of the human diaphragm of well-nourished, stable, chronically hyperinflated patients with chronic obstructive pulmonary disease (COPD). These investigators showed that, at comparable lung volumes, the twitch transdiaphragmatic pressure (i.e., the Pdi developed in response to supramaximal bilateral phrenic nerve stimulation) was higher in the patients than in the normal controls, whereas the reverse was true when Pdi twitch was measured at the corresponding FRCs. Thus, in chronically hyperinflated patients with COPD, some form of adaptation (length adaptation being the most probable) must have accounted for the better contractile performance of the diaphragm at the same lung volumes compared with physiologically normal persons. This adaptation may partially counterbalance the deleterious effects of hyperinflation on the contractility and inspiratory action of the diaphragm in patients with COPD. Furthermore, changes in thoracoabdominal configuration also alter the fiber length and the pressure generated independently of changes in lung volume. In fact, Grassino and colleagues[35] found that Pdi at the same lung (isolung) volume and a given level of excitation depended on thoracoabdominal configuration. Pdi decreased when rib cage volume decreased. Thus, it can be assumed that, at any given lung volume, an inward paradoxic rib cage movement would decrease PImax because it would lower rib cage volume. This is observed in patients with neuromyopathies (e.g., tetraplegia) or COPD (Hoover's sign). Changes in thoracoabdominal configuration can also explain the decrease in PImax observed in patients with kyphoscoliosis.[78]

As noted earlier and as convincingly evident from animal models, sepsis and endotoxic shock pose a potentially great threat to respiratory muscle contractility.[79–84] This is especially important for mechanically ventilated patients because mechanical ventilation, per se, greatly increases the risk of infection and sepsis, thus potentially initiating a vicious cycle.

Another factor mentioned earlier is disuse atrophy. Artificial ventilation may be followed by respiratory muscle weakness resulting from atrophy (secondary to disuse). This is likely because muscles that are used most often, such as the inspiratory muscles (particularly the diaphragm), atrophy the fastest,[85] as discussed at the end of this chapter.

## ADAPTATION OF THE RESPIRATORY MUSCLES TO INCREASED LOAD

### Immune Response to Loaded Breathing

The respiratory muscles are plastic organs that respond to either acute or chronic increases of their activity with structural and functional changes—adaptation. Strenuous resistive breathing, that accompanies many disease states as COPD and asthma, represents a form of "exercise" for the respiratory muscles that initiates an inflammatory response consisting of elevation of plasma cytokines and recruitment and activation of lymphocyte subpopulations.[86] These cytokines do not originate from monocytes, but are instead produced within the diaphragm secondary to the increased muscle activation. More specifically, levels of interleukin-6 (IL-6) and, to a lesser extent, IL-1β, tumor necrosis factor-α (TNF-α), IL-10, IL-4, and interferon-γ (IFN-γ) increase in the diaphragm of rats undergoing inspiratory resistive loading in a time-dependent manner (Fig. 11.8).[87] Oxidative stress is a major stimulus for the cytokine induction secondary to loaded breathing. The administration of antioxidants and reactive oxygen species scavengers in healthy subjects undergoing resisting breathing reverses the observed increase of IL-1β and TNF-α in plasma, whereas it greatly limits the increase of IL-6.[88] In addition, in vitro experiments have proven that reactive oxygen species can stimulate the induction of IL-6 from myoskeletal cells in a manner that involves the transcriptional activation of the IL-6 gene through a NF-κB–dependent pathway.[89] Consequently, the diaphragm is the only proven source of cytokine induction secondary to loaded breathing, and oxidative stress is the only proven stimulus. More studies are needed to elucidate other potential sources and stimuli.

Loaded breathing–induced cytokine up-regulation may have many implications in respiratory muscle function that could be both adaptive and maladaptive. The production of cytokines within the diaphragm may be mediating the diaphragm muscle fiber injury that occurs with strenuous contractions or may contribute to the expected repair process. These cytokines may also compromise diaphragmatic contractility or contribute to the development of muscle cachexia.

### Muscle Injury

Strenuous resistive breathing results in diaphragmatic injury in both animals and humans.[90–92] The mechanisms

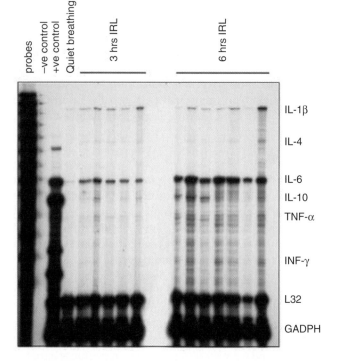

**Figure 11.8** Resistive loading and intradiaphragmatic cytokine expression. Representative autoradiograph of ribonuclease protection assay performed on diaphragm muscle samples obtained after 3 hours *(lanes 5 to 9)* and 6 hours *(lanes 10 to 16)* of inspiratory resistive loading (IRL). *Lanes 1 to 3*, Probe, negative (–ve) control and positive (+ve) control, respectively. *Lane 4*, Diaphragm of a quietly breathing rat. A total of 10 μg RNA was used in each lane. (From Vassilakopoulos T, Divangahi M, Rallis G, et al: Differential cytokine gene expression in the diaphragm in response to strenuous resistive breathing. Am J Respir Crit Care Med 2004;170:154–161.)

involved are not definitely established, and it is tempting to speculate that intradiaphragmatic cytokine induction could be involved in mediating the injurious process,[87] by recruiting initially neutrophils and later monocytes within the muscle, and augmenting oxidative stress in a paracrine fashion,[93] which could contribute to muscle injury.[90] Cytokines and cytokine receptors are up-regulated in the muscles in various forms of muscle injury,[94] as well as in muscle diseases such as critical illness polyneuropathy and myopathy.[95] However, the cytokine response is not only maladaptive. In fact, not only are proinflammatory cytokines such as IL-1β, TNF-α, and IFN-γ induced, but also anti-inflammatory cytokines such as IL-4, IL-10, and IL-6 (which has some proinflammatory but mainly anti-inflammatory properties[96]) are up-regulated,[87] a finding suggesting that some of these cytokines may serve to control local inflammation.[96]

### Muscle Regeneration

Cytokines are also essential in orchestrating muscle recovery after injury. Cytokines such as TNF-α, IL-6,

LIF (leukemia inhibitory factor), and IL-1β and their cognate receptors are up-regulated in skeletal muscle after injury.[94,97-100] These cytokines enhance proteolytic removal of damaged proteins and damaged cells (through recruitment and activation of phagocytes) and activate satellite cells.[101,102] Satellite cells are quiescent cells of embryonic origin that reside in the muscle and are transformed into myocytes either during the normal muscle remodeling or when the muscle becomes injured, to replace damaged myocytes.[103]

## Muscle Contractility

Cytokines may affect contractility of the diaphragm. TNF-α impairs contractility of the diaphragm.[104,105] The intradiaphragmatic expression of cytokines and especially TNF-α with the attendant contractility-depressing effect may contribute to the development of peripheral muscle fatigue (i.e., decreased force production on constant electrical stimulation of the muscle) observed after resistive loading.[106] The intradiaphragmatic expression of cytokines and especially TNF-α may also explain the observation that force decline after resistive loading is proportionally greater than the observed muscle injury.[107] Whereas force declines by as much as 30%, the degree of injury is only 9%, a finding suggesting that other factors in addition to injury depress the contractility of the diaphragm.[107]

## Respiratory Muscle Fatigue

In daily life, the word *fatigue* is usually used to express tiredness or weakness. A National Heart, Lung and Blood Institute workshop defined fatigue as the loss of capacity to develop force and/or velocity in response to a load that is reversible by rest.[108] According to this definition, fatigue may be present before the point at which a muscle is unable to continue to perform a particular task (task failure). In applying this concept to the inspiratory muscles, one could conclude that they may be fatigued before there is hypercapnia because of their inability to continue to generate sufficient pressure to maintain alveolar ventilation.[109] Fatigue should be distinguished from weakness in which reduced force generation is fixed and not reversed by rest, although the presence of weakness may itself predispose a muscle to fatigue.

The site and mechanism of fatigue remain controversial. Theoretically, the site of fatigue may be located at any link in the long chain of events involved in voluntary muscle contraction leading from the brain to the contractile machinery. It is not certain whether failure to generate force results from reduced central motor output (central fatigue) or from failure at the neuromuscular junction and/or within the muscle machinery (peripheral fatigue). For the respiratory system, the following question arises: Do the respiratory controllers become too tired to drive the muscles to maintain adequate ventilation when the respiratory system is presented with a fatiguing load, or do the muscles become unable to generate the required force despite an adequate neural drive? Although no definite answer can be given, at least for the diaphragm when fatigue is induced by an intermittent contraction breathing protocol, approximately 50% of the force decline can be attributed to reduced central motor drive, and the remainder can be attributed to peripheral muscle contractile failure.[108] However, it is not yet clear whether such a CNS depression is the result of primary central failure or of an adaptation of the CNS to the changes in the contracting muscles that reflects a protective mechanism to prevent an undue reduction of intrinsic muscle fiber strength.

## Central Fatigue

Central fatigue is considered present when a maximal voluntary contraction generates less force than does maximal electrical stimulation.[110,111] If maximal electrical stimulation superimposed on a maximal voluntary contraction can potentiate the force generated by a muscle, a component of central fatigue is said to exist. This procedure applied to the diaphragm consists of the twitch occlusion test, which may separate central from peripheral fatigue.[112,113] This test examines the transdiaphragmatic pressure (Pdi) response to bilateral phrenic nerve stimulation superimposed on graded voluntary contractions of the diaphragm. Normally, the amplitude of Pdi twitches in response to phrenic nerve stimulation decreases as the voluntary Pdi increases.[112] During maximal voluntary contractions of the diaphragm (Pdimax), no superimposed twitches can be detected. When diaphragmatic fatigue was induced either by resistive loads or by expulsive contractions against a bounded abdominal wall,[113] superimposed twitches could be demonstrated at the limits of diaphragmatic endurance, but not at the start of the experiment. At these limits, voluntary Pdimax had decreased by 50%, whereas the Pdimax estimated from the twitch occlusion had decreased by only 25%. Consequently, at the limits of diaphragmatic endurance, although peripheral fatigue was present, a significant portion of the reduction in the force was the result of failure of the CNS to activate the diaphragm completely. Similar results were also reported by McKenzie and associates in 1992 for fatigue induced by diaphragmatic expulsive maneuvers.[114]

Central fatigue may be caused by a reduction in the number of motor units that can be recruited by the motor drive or by a decrease in motor unit discharge rates, or both. However, central fatigue should not be confused with the progressive decrease in firing rate during maximum contraction because, in this case, as opposed to fatigue, superimposed supramaximal electric tetanic stimulation does not increase muscle force.[115]

The observed decreased central firing rate during fatigue[116] may, in fact, be a beneficial adaptive response: fatigue is characterized by slowing of the muscle contractile speed. In addition, for any muscle or motor unit, the minimum excitation frequency required to generate force and tetanic fusion (i.e., maximum force) is proportional to its contractile speed. Thus, if during fatigue the degree of contractile slowing matches the decline in motoneuron firing rate, the latter does not result in any additional reduction in muscle force. On the contrary, it would avoid the failure of impulse propagation associated with high-frequency fatigue as well as the complete depletion of vital chemicals within the muscle cell that could otherwise occur if high-frequency excitation were maintained. This brings up the question of how such an adaptation is initiated. It seems likely that activation of muscle afferents by some fatigue-induced change within the muscle inhibits motoneuron activity by reducing its firing rate. Although unequivocal proof is lacking, it has been shown that afferent information through large (type I and II) and especially small (type III and IV) fibers affects the central respiratory controller's discharge in terms of firing rate, firing time, and frequency of breathing[117]; the latter is observed in states of diaphragmatic fatigue in both animals and humans.[118] These sensory fibers are activated primarily by extracellular metabolic changes (e.g., low pH, ischemia, increased osmolarity) and some substances.[81] It is therefore tempting to hypothesize that, as the contractile properties and the diaphragmatic chemistry change during fatigue, respiratory muscle afferents through the phrenic nerve may affect the output of respiratory centers in terms of firing rate or timing.

This hypothesis is further supported by animal experiments in which endogenous opioid pathways are activated in response to acute, intense flow-resistive loading, thus reducing overall ventilatory output[119–121] (Fig. 11.9); this reduction, secondary to increased endorphin activity, is signaled by small fiber afferents stimulated by lactate accumulation and pH fall in the respiratory muscles.[119] Thus, it is possible that afferents, through the small fibers during loaded breathing in various clinical states, modulate endogenous opioids[122,123] as an adaptive response, thereby minimizing breathlessness and avoiding or delaying the onset of respiratory muscle fatigue.

In summary, as fatigue ensues, central discharge rate decreases, either as primary central failure (central fatigue) or as an adaptive response preventing the muscle's self-destruction by excessive activation. The importance of central fatigue in clinical ventilatory failure remains uncertain.

## Peripheral Fatigue

This type of fatigue may occur because of failure of impulse propagation across the neuromuscular junction and/or over the muscle surface membrane (transmission fatigue) or because of failure of the contractile apparatus of the muscle fibers (impaired excitation-contraction coupling). During artificial stimulation of a motoneuron, especially at high frequencies, muscle force declines

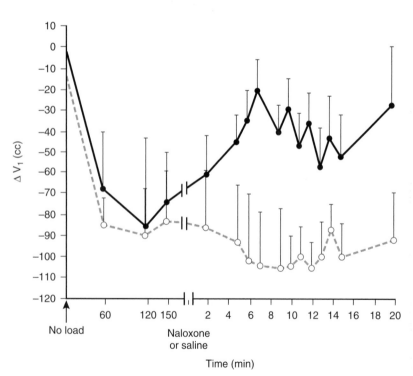

**Figure 11.9** Tidal volume response of unanesthetized goats to 2.5 hours of high-inspiratory, flow-resistive loading before and following the administration of naloxone (*filled circles*) or saline (*open circles*). Tidal volume, which fell considerably during loading, increased significantly but transiently after naloxone administration, whereas saline had no effect. (Note the change in time scale on the X-axis.) The data indicate that an increase in airway resistance can activate the endogenous opioid system. Furthermore, the increase in tidal volume immediately following naloxone suggests that these potentially fatiguing loads reduce tidal volume before the onset of overt muscle fatigue by a mechanism that, in addition to the direct mechanical effect of the load, involves the endogenous opioid system. Data are presented as mean±SEM. (From Scardella AT, Parisi RA, Phair DK, et al: The role of endogenous opioids in the ventilatory response to acute flow-resistive loads. Am Rev Respir Dis 1986;133:26–31.)

rapidly in association with the decline in action potential amplitude. This response, known as high-frequency fatigue (Fig. 11.10), is attributed to transmission fatigue. The site of this type of fatigue may be located postsynaptically (from a decrease in end-plate excitability) or presynaptically (probably in fine terminal filaments of the motor nerve or less frequently from depletion of synaptic transmitter substance).[124]

The development of this type of failure during voluntary contraction is questionable because each motor unit is excited at a rate matched to its particular contractive properties. In fact, evoked muscle compound action potential (M-wave) amplitudes are generally found to remain unimpaired, and, in addition, no unique relationship between muscle force and activity on electromyography (EMG) has been observed.[108] Evidence that neuromuscular transmission and cell membrane excitation are adequate during fatigue produced by voluntary contractions was found in experiments in dogs in cardiogenic and septic shock.[83,125] As the diaphragm became fatigued, the relationship of integrated phrenic nerve activity (Ephr) and diaphragmatic EMG increased proportionally so their relationship remained unaltered. However, these experiments may not be specific in testing this question; for example, changes in the wave form of action potential through the run may have compensated for discrepancies between Ephr and EMG. Teleologically, transmission block could be beneficial in some instances. As suggested by some authors,[126] if failure

occurs at the neuromuscular junction or in the excitation of the cell membrane, it may protect the muscle against excessive depletion of its adenosine triphosphate (ATP) stores, which would lead to rigor mortis. If high-frequency fatigue is the result of failure of the neuromuscular junction, it may be speculated that such a failure can exist in the human diaphragm. In fact, it has been clearly shown that normal subjects breathing against inspiratory loads develop high-frequency fatigue,[127] which may reflect neuromuscular junction failure.

All processes that link the electrical activation of the muscle fiber and the various metabolic and enzymatic processes providing energy to the contractile machinery are called *excitation-contraction coupling processes*. Impaired excitation contraction coupling is thought to be responsible when the loss of force is not accompanied by a parallel decline in the electrical activity.[128] This type of fatigue is characterized by a selective loss of force at low frequencies of stimulation (low-frequency fatigue) (see Fig. 11.10), despite maintenance of the force generated at high frequencies of stimulation, a finding indicating that the contractile proteins continue to generate force. This type of fatigue is not related to depletion of ATP or phosphocreatine (PCr) and is characteristically long lasting, taking several hours to recover. The mechanism of this type of fatigue is not well known. It may occur because of a reduced supply of calcium ($Ca^{2+}$) or a change in the affinity of the troponin binding site for $Ca^{2+}$. These defects would reduce the twitch and hence would reduce the force developed at low stimulation. In contrast, at higher stimulation frequencies, a relatively normal force can be generated when the interior of the fiber is saturated with $Ca^{2+}$.[129] Other possibilities include structural damage[129] or an alteration in the compliance of the series elastic component of the muscle.[130]

Low-frequency fatigue occurs during high-force contractions and is less likely to develop when the forces generated are smaller, even if these are maintained for longer periods, thereby achieving the same total work. It thus appears likely that muscle ischemia and reliance on anaerobic metabolism are important factors in the generation of low-frequency fatigue.

In this regard, impaired excitation-contraction coupling occurred in the diaphragm of the dog during cardiogenic or septic shock[83,125]; despite a threefold increase of the integrated EMG, Pdi decreased (Fig. 11.11). Low-frequency fatigue and, by inference, impaired excitation-contraction coupling has also been found in the diaphragm and sternomastoid of normal subjects after they breathed against very high inspiratory resistance.[127,131]

Because low-frequency fatigue impairs force generation at physiologic firing frequencies, ventilation may be reduced. To compensate for low-frequency fatigue, motoneuron firing frequency must be increased, or

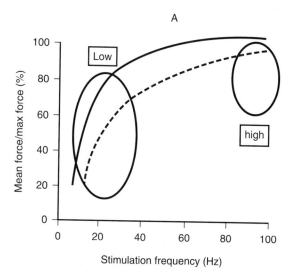

**Figure 11.10** Frequency-force curve of skeletal muscles illustrating the curve for fresh muscle *(solid line)* and a shift to the right with fatigue *(dashed line)*. (From Moxham J, Edwards RH, Aubier M, et al: Changes in EMG power spectrum (high-to-low ratio) with force fatigue in humans. J Appl Physiol 1982;53: 1094–1099.)

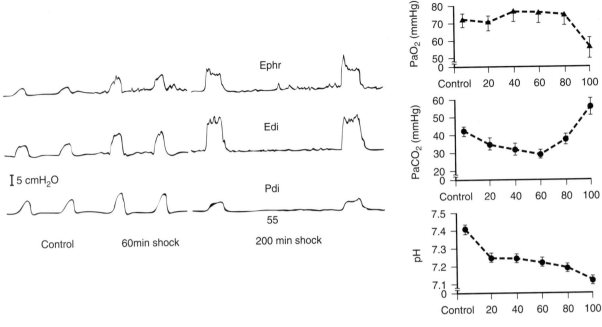

**Figure 11.11** *Left,* Representative tracing of one dog during endotoxic shock showing changes in integrated phrenic neurogram (Ephr) *(top),* integrated diaphragmatic electromyogram (Edi) *(middle),* and transdiaphragmatic pressure (Pdi) *(bottom). Left,* During control; *middle,* 60 minutes after the onset of endotoxic shock; *right,* 200 minutes after the onset of endotoxic shock and before the death of the animal. *Right,* Time course of mean arterial oxygen tension (Pao$_2$) *(top),* carbon dioxide tension (Paco$_2$) *(middle),* and mean arterial pH *(bottom)* for 10 dogs breathing spontaneously. *Points,* means; *bars,* ±SE. Note the significant fall of Pao$_2$ and the rise of Paco$_2$ before the death of these animals. (From Hussain SN, Simkus G, Roussos C: Respiratory muscle fatigue: A cause of ventilatory failure in septic shock. J Appl Physiol 1985;58:2033–2040.)

additional contractile units must be recruited, by an increase in central respiratory drive. This can be demonstrated by recording the smoothed and rectified EMG (SREMG) from the sternomastoid during the production of standard forces when the muscle has low-frequency fatigue compared with the response obtained for fresh muscle.[131] Depression of respiratory drive by hypoxia or drugs could therefore impair compensatory responses, and ventilation would then become inadequate.

### Metabolic Considerations in Muscle Fatigue

Most studies conclude that the major factors underlying neuromuscular fatigue occur within the muscle fibers and mainly result from depletion of muscle energy stores or pH changes from lactate accumulation.[108] The substances directly involved in the transformation of chemical energy into mechanical work in skeletal muscles are ATP, adenosine diphosphate (ADP), inorganic phosphate (Pi), hydrogen ions (H$^+$), magnesium ions (Mg$^{2+}$), and PCr. ATP leaves the mitochondria and diffuses in the contractile machinery of the cell, where

ATPase enzymes hydrolyze one of the pyrophosphate bonds and liberate large quantities of energy in the process:

$$MgATP + H_2O \xrightarrow{ATPases} MgADP + Pi + H^+ + Energy \quad (4)$$

PCr is used to regenerate ATP:

$$MgADP + PCr \rightleftharpoons MgATP + Cr \quad (5)$$

Metabolic changes may cause fatigue either through a reduction of high-energy compounds (e.g., PCr and ATP) or through an accumulation of breakdown products (e.g., Pi, H$^+$, lactate).

ATP is the immediate energy source for energy-requiring processes such as cross-bridge cycling and ion pumping, and a significant reduction of the myoplasmic ATP concentration would affect cell function. Generally reported reductions of ATP in fatigue are small (from approximately 6 to 5 mM) and would, if representative, be unlikely to affect cell function. However, several studies have found considerably larger reductions (up to approximately 50%).[132] Furthermore, local concentrations at sites where ATP turnover is particularly high may well be lower than the cell average (e.g., in the narrow space between the t-tubules and the terminal cisternae of the sarcoplasmic reticulation, called the triad).[133] Historically, lactic acid accumulation has received great attention as the cause of fatigue in the skeletal muscles. Similarly, blood lactate elevation has been found in subjects breathing through high inspiratory loads to exhaustion,[134] but there is no direct evidence that the lactic acid produced by the respiratory muscles is the culprit in fatigue. However, animals in cardiogenic shock develop substantially less lactic acidosis if they are mechanically ventilated than if they are breathing spontaneously,[135] a finding indicating that the respiratory muscles produce great amounts of lactic acid if they are working under fatiguing conditions.

The effects of lactic acid on force generation are believed to be mediated by lowering the pH. $H^+$ and Pi are among the breakdown products of energy metabolism that have the greatest effect on the contractile apparatus.[136] An increased concentration of these ions results in both reduced maximum tension production (i.e., tension at saturating $Ca^{2+}$ concentration) and reduced myofibrillar $Ca^{2+}$ sensitivity.[137] In addition, $H^+$ exerts a direct negative effect on the contractile process itself, which is not related to pH.[137]

The increase in energy demands in the working skeletal muscles, including the respiratory muscles, is provided mainly by the combustion of fat, blood glucose, and glycogen of the muscle. During submaximal prolonged heavy exercise, exhaustion coincides with the depletion of muscle glycogen, whereas exercise capacity is enhanced when the storage of muscle glycogen is increased.[138] Similar observations have been made in the diaphragm of dogs with low cardiac output.[135] However, why glycogen depletion coincides with fatigue is not clear. During prolonged intermittent heavy exercise that depends on aerobic metabolism, the rate of utilization of fatty acids and glucose is high; although these substances circulate in large amounts in the bloodstream, they cannot provide sufficient energy to the muscle to meet the demands. Hence muscle glycogen must be used to supplement the bloodborne fuels, and fatigue will occur when it is depleted.

Oxygen-derived free radicals have been implicated as mediators of respiratory muscle dysfunction,[139] particularly diaphragm fatigue, because pretreatment with free radical scavengers (e.g., N-acetylcysteine,[140] dimethylsulfoxide, lazaroid agents) resulted in a reduction in the rate at which diaphragm fatigue developed in response to oxidative stress. However, the precise source of free radicals, the particular physiologic conditions under which they can be generated, and the protective mechanism of different free radical scavengers in the respiratory muscles remain unclear.[139]

To summarize, glycogen depletion, lactic acid accumulation, acidosis of every kind, inability to utilize bloodborne substances, decrease in the rate of ATP hydrolysis, and increased oxygen-derived free radical production affect loss of force. However, the exact interplay of all these factors is not yet identified in either the diaphragm or the other skeletal muscles.

## Integrated View of Respiratory Muscle Fatigue

Fatigue is likely to be the result of a dynamic process in which compensatory mechanisms are overwhelmed in a closed-loop system consisting of central motor drive, peripheral impulse propagation, excitation-contraction coupling, depletion of energy substrates, or metabolite accumulation and feedback-modulating reflexes.[108] The site of fatigue may be placed at any level from the CNS to the contractile machinery depending on the experimental setting. For an individual muscle, a close relationship exists between excitation and energy metabolism. It has been shown that a protective mechanism may exist at the site of the action potential or beyond, so when fuel is depleted, failure of the activation system occurs and in extreme fatigue prevents the muscle from destroying itself, which would happen if the ATP level fell to zero. A decrease in excitation may result from failure of the neuromuscular junction,[126] or it may stem from a reduced rate of firing by the CNS,[115] or both. In the respiratory system, in addition to the reduction in firing frequency, the CNS may respond by altering the frequency and the duty cycle. Although it has not yet been proved, such an alteration in the responses of central controllers could be brought about by afferents from the fatiguing inspiratory muscles and the chest wall. These small (types III and IV) fibers possibly reduce central respiratory output by modulating endorphins as an adaptive response to avoid or delay respiratory muscle fatigue.

An alternate, not mutually exclusive mechanism reducing central respiratory output (see earlier) is the production of cytokines by the strenuously contracting diaphragm secondary to resistive loading. Cytokines, especially IL-1β and IL-6, are very strong stimulants of the hypothalamic-pituitary-adrenal (HPA) axis,[141–143] and they exhibit significant synergism.[144] Both these cytokines stimulate concomitant adrenocorticotropic hormone (ACTH) and β-endorphin release by the pituitary gland. Strenuous inspiratory resistive breathing that induces plasma cytokines stimulates the HPA axis and results in increased levels of circulating β-endorphin and ACTH[86] (Fig. 11.12).

It is tempting to speculate that HPA axis stimulation may occur secondary to the increased levels in circulating proinflammatory cytokines induced by strenuous resistive breathing. This notion is supported by the different time courses of cytokine and hormonal elevations (cytokine elevation appearing first, followed by the

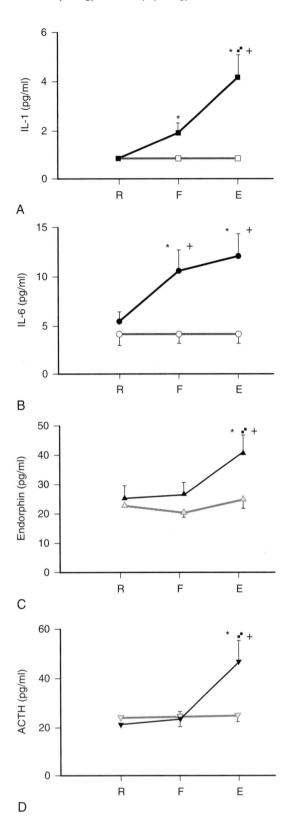

**A**

**B**

**C**

**D**

**Figure 11.12** The plasma cytokine and hypothalamic pituitary responses to resistive breathing. Mean plasma level of interleukin (IL)-1β *(A)*, IL-6 *(B)*, β-endorphin *(C)*, and adrenocorticotropic hormone (ACTH; *D*) at rest (R), at the point where the subjects could not generate the target maximum inspiratory pressure (75% of maximum, 45 minutes after the beginning of resistive breathing; *F*), and at the end of resistive breathing (15 minutes later, at 60 minutes from the beginning; *E*). From *F* to *E*, subjects were put through an alinear resistance to the maximum they could achieve. Data are presented as mean ±SEM. *Filled squares*, high-load run; *open squares*, moderate-load run; *number sign*, statistically significant difference (*P* <.05) from R; *paragraph sign*, statistically significant difference (*P* <.05) from F; *plus sign*, statistically significant difference (*P* <.01) from the moderate-load run. (From Vassilakopoulos T, Zakynthinos S, Roussos C: Strenuous resistive breathing induces proinflammatory cytokines and stimulates the HPA axis in humans. Am J Physiol 1999;277:R1013–R1019.)

increase in β-endorphin and ACTH level) (see Fig. 11.12). Furthermore, the increase in IL-6 was strongly correlated with the increase in both β-endorphin and ACTH, thus implying a causative role of the IL-6 for the HPA axis stimulation secondary to resistive breathing. The ACTH response may represent an attempt of the organism to reduce the injury occurring in the respiratory muscles through the production of glucocorticoids by the adrenals, which suppress induction of inflammatory genes, and induction of the acute-phase response proteins from the liver, which serve as antiproteases.[141]

The elaboration of β-endorphins decreases the activation of the respiratory muscles and changes the pattern of breathing, which becomes rapid and shallow. This is probably an attempt by the respiratory controller to reduce the strenuous respiratory muscle contractions (and thus the accompanying muscle injury), through the decline in tidal volume at the expense of increased respiratory frequency. In animals, adequate evidence supports this concept.[119,120,145,146] It was demonstrated that resistive loading resulted in a progressive reduction in tidal volume, which was partially reversed by administration of the opioid antagonist naloxone[146,147] (see Fig. 11.9). An increase in β-endorphin in the cisternal cerebrospinal fluid was also detected.[146] In humans, an increase in the β-endorphin plasma level was measured secondary to resistive breathing.[86,148] It was also demonstrated that naloxone could restore the load compensatory reflex in patients with COPD in whom it was initially absent.[123] Such a strategy, representing an adaptive response much in the way that β-endorphins are generated in response to chronic pain, certainly minimizes dyspnea and may avoid or delay the onset of

**Figure 11.13** Integrated view of the origin and functional consequences of resistive breathing–induced cytokines. Resistive breathing results in the generation of oxidative stress and the induction of cytokines within the diaphragm, secondary to the increased muscle activation. Oxidative stress is a major stimulus for this cytokine induction. Cytokines stimulate the hypothalamic-pituitary-adrenal axis either hematogenously or by stimulation of small afferent nerve fibers, leading to production of adrenocorticotropic hormone (ACTH) and β-endorphins. The ACTH response may represent an attempt of the organism to reduce the injury occurring in the respiratory muscles through the production of glucocorti-coids by the adrenals and the induction of acute-phase response proteins. The β-endorphin response would decrease the activation of the respiratory muscles and change the pattern of breathing, which becomes more rapid and shallow, possibly in an attempt to reduce or prevent further injury to the respiratory muscles. POMC, pro-opiomel-aninocortin; ROS, reactive oxygen species. (From Vassilakopoulos T, Roussos C, Zakynthinos S: The immune response to resistive breathing. Eur Respir J 2004;24:1033–1043.)

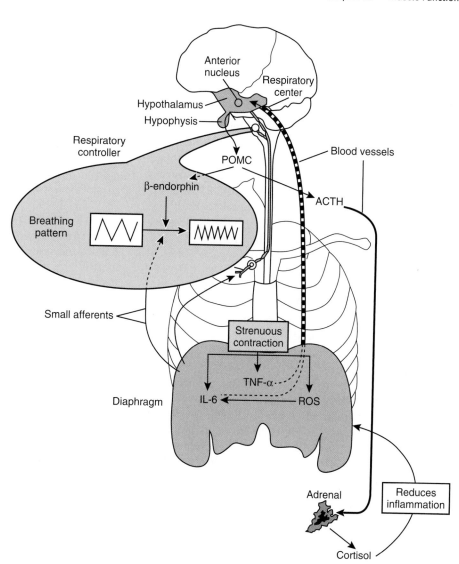

respiratory muscle peripheral fatigue, thus protecting the ventilatory pump from exhaustion. However, it may result in hypoventilation and the development of hypercapnia (Fig. 11.13).

## What Is the Role of Fatigue in the Patient Who Fails to Wean?

Consideration of the imbalance between energy supply and energy demand of the respiratory muscles suggests that inspiratory muscle fatigue is frequently a final common pathway leading to inability to sustain spontaneous breathing and thus to weaning failure.[149] In a very influential study, Cohen and associates[150] studied 12 patients with various disorders leading to hypercapnic respiratory failure after discontinuing mechanical ventilation. The power spectrum of diaphragmatic surface EMG activity was analyzed. A sustained reduction of the H/L ratio of the EMG power spectrum to less than 80% of the initial value was taken as indicative that diaphrag-matic fatigue would ensue. Seven patients showed evidence on EMG of inspiratory muscle fatigue. Electrical fatigue was followed by respiratory alternans and/or paradoxic inward movement of the abdominal wall during inspiration (abdominal paradox). However, it is possible that these changes may not reflect inspira-tory muscle fatigue per se, but rather alternations in central drive resulting from excessive loading response.[151] Nevertheless, such high inspiratory loads observed during weaning failure eventually lead the ventilatory pump to exhaustion and overt fatigue, which is, undoubtedly, a terminal event.

Respiratory muscle maximum relaxation rate (MRR) has been measured during the weaning process and has been demonstrated to slow in those patients failing to wean; it has also remained unchanged in patients who were weaned successfully.[152] This finding suggests that during failed weaning trials, a fatigue process is initiated peripherally into the respiratory muscles; associated with the slowing of MRR, it is likely that the central drive is modulated.[153]

Furthermore, using electrical criteria similar to those used by Cohen and associates,[150] Brochard and co-workers[154] found that seven out of eight patients who met the usual criteria for weaning but who failed to wean exhibited a sustained reduction of the H/L ratio of the EMG power spectrum of the diaphragm during spontaneous breathing, followed by decreased tidal volume, an increased respiratory rate, and the development of hypercapnia. All these patients had increased energy demands, as evidenced by the oxygen consumption of the respiratory muscles and the work of breathing per unit of time, W, that was always higher than 8 to 10 L/minute. When pressure support was applied, thus reducing the work performed by the muscles, the reduced H/L ratio was prevented. Impaired diaphragmatic function during weaning was also implicated by Pourriat and co-workers,[155] who studied diaphragmatic function and the pattern of breathing in patients with COPD who were being weaned from mechanical ventilation after acute respiratory failure. These investigators noted that when Pdi was expressed as a fraction of the maximal Pdi (Pdimax), this value reached a mean of 46% in the group failing to wean. According to Roussos and Macklem,[106] a Pdi/Pdimax ratio greater than 40% cannot be tolerated for long periods without fatigue of the diaphragm. It has also been possible in these patients to measure the load imposed on the respiratory muscles and their capacity. When the ratio of load to capacity (i.e., PI/PImax ratio) is high, weaning fails.[156] In fact, PI/PImax had an excessively high mean value amounting to $0.42 \pm 0.11$ in patients failing at discontinuation of mechanical ventilation.[156] Additionally, dynamic hyperinflation amounting to $0.25 \pm 0.19$ l was present in almost all patients. When the PI/PImax ratio was plotted against the dynamic increase in FRC to account for the effect of hyperinflation, 13 out of 31 patients (42%) were placed above a hypothetic critical line representing the critical inspiratory pressure above which fatigue may occur. In addition, all patients were gathered around the critical line (Fig. 11.14).[156]

Following these observations, patients who had initially failed to wean from mechanical ventilation but who were successfully weaned on a later occasion were prospectively studied.[157] Compared with success, during failure, patients had greater intrinsic positive end-expiratory pressure, dynamic hyperinflation, total resistance, ratio of mean to maximum inspiratory pressure, TTI and power, less maximum inspiratory pressure, and a breathing pattern that was more rapid and shallow (ratio of frequency to tidal volume, f/VT). To clarify on pathophysiologic

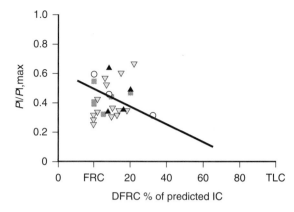

**Figure 11.14** Pressure-volume diagram similar to that of Roussos and associates[48] plotting the PI/PImax ratio against a dynamic increase in FRC (DFRC) expressed as a percentage of predicted inspiratory capacity (IC). The PI/PImax ratio is the mean inspiratory pressure per breath expressed as a fraction of the maximum. Each *closed symbol* refers to a patient. The *solid line* was constructed from data in normal subjects and represents the critical inspiratory pressures above which fatigue may occur. At normal FRC, the critical inspiratory pressure per breath above which fatigue may occur in normal subjects is about 50% of PImax, whereas at FRC + 1/2 IC, this critical pressure is 25% to 30% of the maximum. All patients had excessively high values of the PI/PImax ratio, clustering around the critical line, rather than remaining away from it, as happens in normal subjects. *Closed circles,* exacerbated chronic obstructive pulmonary disease (COPD); *closed squares,* adult respiratory distress syndrome (ARDS); *closed downward triangles,* other pulmonary diseases; *closed upward triangles,* acute respiratory failure of extrapulmonary origin. (From Zakynthinos SG, Vassilakopoulos T, Roussos C: The load of inspiratory muscles in patients needing mechanical ventilation. Am J Respir Crit Care Med 1995;152:1248–1255.)

grounds what determines an inability to wean from mechanical ventilation, multiple logistic regression analyses with the weaning outcome as the dependent variable were performed. The TTI and the f/VT ratio were the only significant variables in the model. Thus, the TTI and the f/VT were the major pathophysiologic determinants of the weaning outcome. The increased TTI, which was higher than the critical threshold of 0.15 during failure, was again suggestive of the presence of fatigue (Fig. 11.15). However, the diagnosis of diaphragmatic fatigue requires the demonstration of reduced force generation by the diaphragm on constant levels of stimulation.[108]

Evidence does not support the existence of low-frequency fatigue (the type of fatigue that is long lasting, taking more than 24 hours to recover) in patients who fail to wean despite the excessive respiratory muscle load.[158] The twitch transdiaphragmatic pressure elicited by magnetic stimulation of the phrenic nerve was not

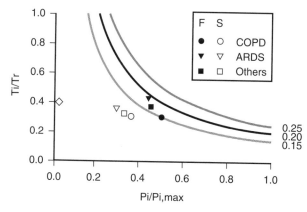

**Figure 11.15** Diagram similar to the isodiaphragmatic tension-time index (iso-TTdi) plot of Bellemare and Grassino[45] constructed from the data of our patients. *Ordinate,* Inspiratory to total cycle duration ratio (TI/Ttot) at the end of the spontaneous breathing trial. *Abscissa,* Mean inspiratory pressure, expressed as a fraction of maximum (PI/PImax). The product of each combination of the two variables is the TTI of global inspiratory muscles. Three iso-TTI isopleths are drawn for reference. Each *closed symbol* refers to the mean value of each group during weaning failure. Each *open symbol* refers to the mean value of each group during weaning success. The *open diamond* represents the average TTI of 10 normal subjects breathing with a minute volume similar to the mean minute volume of our patients. ARDS, adult respiratory distress syndrome; COPD, exacerbated chronic obstructive pulmonary disease; F, weaning failure; S, weaning success. (From Vassilakopoulos T, Zakynthinos S, Roussos C: The tension-time index and the frequency/tidal volume ratio are the major pathophysiologic determinants of weaning failure and success. Am J Respir Crit Care Med 1998;158:378–385.)

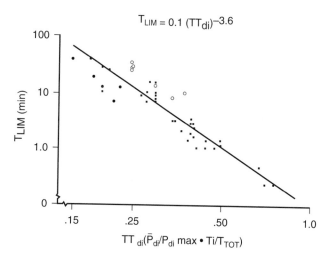

**Figure 11.17** Relationship between time limit (TLIM) and tension-time index of the diaphragm (TTdi). The two scales are logarithmic. TLIM, the time elapsed from the onset of the contraction to the time at which a target tension can no longer be sustained. (From Bellemare F, Grassino A: Effect of pressure and timing of contraction on human diaphragm fatigue. J Appl Physiol 1982;53:1190–1195.)

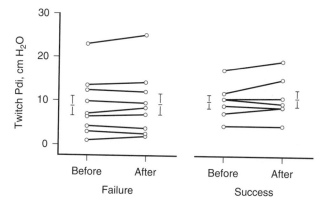

**Figure 11.16** Transdiaphragmatic twitch pressure (twitch Pdi), recorded before and 30 minutes after a weaning trial in nine patients who failed weaning *(closed symbols, left panel)* and seven weaning success patients *(open symbols, right panel)*. Twitch Pdi did not differ between the groups before the trial, and it did not decrease after the trial in either group. *Bars* represent group mean ± SE. (From Laghi F, Cattapan SE, Jubran A, et al: Is weaning failure caused by low-frequency fatigue of the diaphragm? Am J Respir Crit Care Med 2003;167:120–127.)

altered before and after the failing weaning trials (Fig. 11.16).[158] The TTI of the diaphragm was 0.17 to 0.22 during failing weaning trials.[158] Bellemare and Grassino[45] reported that the relationship between the TTI of the diaphragm (TTdi) and time to task failure in healthy subjects follows an inverse power function: time to task failure = 0.1 (TTdi)$^{-3.6}$ (Fig. 11.17). Based on this formula, the expected times to task failure would be 59 to 13 minutes. The average value of the TTI of the diaphragm during the last minute of the trial was 0.26, and the patients with weaning failure would be predicted to sustain this effort for another 13 minutes before developing diaphragmatic fatigue.[158] Thus, the reason for the lack of low-frequency respiratory muscle fatigue development despite the excessive load is that physicians have adopted criteria for the definition of spontaneous breathing trial failure and thus termination of unassisted breathing that lead them to put patients back on the ventilator before the development of low-frequency respiratory muscle fatigue.

The lack of fatigue, however, does not mean that the loaded breathing associated with weaning failure is not injurious for the respiratory muscles. Both animal models and human data have shown that breathing against such loads (TTIdi, 0.17 to 0.22) can injure respiratory muscles.[90] Nevertheless, this injury peaks at about 3 days after the excessive loading, a time that coincides with the documented decline in the force-generating capacity of the diaphragm at this later point.[90] Thus, although weaning failure is not associated with low-frequency fatigue of the diaphragm at the time of termination of spontaneous breathing trials, it may lead to the onset of an injurious process in the respiratory muscles that is expected to peak later.

## ADAPTATION OF THE RESPIRATORY MUSCLES TO INACTIVITY

Respiratory muscles adapt not only when they function against increased load but also when they become inactive, as happens when a mechanical ventilator undertakes their role as force generator to create the driving pressure permitting airflow into the lungs. Evidence supports the finding that the inactivity and unloading of the diaphragm caused by mechanical ventilation are harmful, resulting in decreased diaphragmatic force-generating capacity, diaphragmatic atrophy, and diaphragmatic injury, conditions described by the term *ventilator-induced diaphragmatic dysfunction* (VIDD).[159]

In the intact diaphragm of various animal species (including primates) studied in vivo after a period of controlled mechanical ventilation (CMV), transdiaphragmatic pressure generation caused by phrenic nerve stimulation declines at both submaximal and maximal stimulation frequencies (20 to 100 Hz) in a time-dependent manner.[160–162] The decline is evident early and worsens as mechanical ventilation is prolonged. Within a few days (3 days in rabbits,[162] 5 days in piglets,[161] 11 days in baboons[160]), the pressure-generating capacity of the diaphragm declines by 40% to 50%. The endurance of the diaphragm is also significantly compromised, as suggested by the reduced ability of animals to sustain an inspiratory resistive load.[160]

The decreased force-generating capacity is not secondary to changes in lung volume because transpulmonary pressure and dynamic lung compliance do not change. Moreover, it is not caused by changes in abdominal compliance, given the nearly stable abdominal pressure over the observation period and the similar results obtained with abdominal wrapping, which prevents changes in abdominal compliance.[160,161]

Neural or neuromuscular transmission remains intact, as reflected by the lack of changes in phrenic nerve conduction (latency) and the stable response to repetitive stimulation of the phrenic nerve.[161] In contrast, the decrease in the compound muscle action potential suggests that excitation-contraction coupling or membrane depolarization may be involved in the dysfunction.[161] Thus, the mechanical ventilation–induced impairment in force-generating capacity appears to reside within the myofibers.[159]

In vitro results of isometric (both twitch and tetanic) tension development in isolated diaphragmatic strips confirm the in vivo findings,[85,163–166] and they suggest that the decline in contractility is an early (12 hours)[165] and progressive phenomenon.[165,167] Isometric force development declines by 30% to 50% after 1 to 3 days of CMV in rats and rabbits, although this time course may be prolonged in piglets,[161] a finding that could suggest that the bigger the species, the longer it takes for VIDD to develop.

The mechanisms of VIDD are not fully elucidated. Muscle atrophy, oxidative stress, structural injury, and muscle fiber remodeling have been documented after CMV.[159] The precise contribution of each in the development of VIDD has to be defined.

Muscle atrophy results from a combination of decreased protein synthesis and increased proteolysis,[168] and both mechanisms have been documented in VIDD.[169,170] From the three intracellular proteolytic systems of mammalian cells (lysosomal proteases, calpains, and proteasome), both calpains and the proteasome are activated to induce atrophy secondary to CMV.[170] The proteasome is a multiple-subunit multicatalytic complex that exists in two major forms: the core 20S proteasome can be free or bound to a pair of 19S regulators to form the 26S proteasome (Fig. 11.18). The 26S proteasome is activated in ventilator-induced cachexia.[167,171] Shanely and colleagues showed that CMV resulted in a fivefold increase in 20S proteasome activity,[170] which is specialized in degrading proteins oxidized by reactive oxygen species.[172] Oxidative damage of a protein results in its partial unfolding, exposing hidden hydrophobic residues; therefore, an oxidized protein does not need to be further modified by ubiquitin conjugation to confer a hydrophobic patch, nor does it require energy from ATP hydrolysis to unfold (Fig. 11.19).[173]

This result is in concert with evidence of oxidative stress–induced modification of proteins obtained from the diaphragms of animals subjected to CMV.[170,174] Oxidative stress is augmented in the diaphragm after CMV, as indicated by increased protein oxidation and lipid peroxidation byproducts.[170,174] The onset of oxidative modifications is rapid, occurring within the first 6 hours of the institution of CMV.[174] Oxidative stress can modify many critical proteins involved in energetics, excitation-contraction coupling, and force generation. Accordingly, CMV-induced diaphragmatic protein oxidation was evident in insoluble (but not soluble) proteins with molecular masses of approximately 200, 128, 85, and 40 kDa.[174] These findings raise the possibility that actin (40 kDa) and myosin (200 kDa) undergo oxidative modification during CMV.[174] This intriguing possibility awaits confirmation by more specific identification of the modified proteins.

Structural abnormalities of different subcellular components of diaphragmatic fibers have been found after CMV.[162,175,176] The changes consist of disrupted myofibrils, increased numbers of lipid vacuoles in the sarcoplasm,

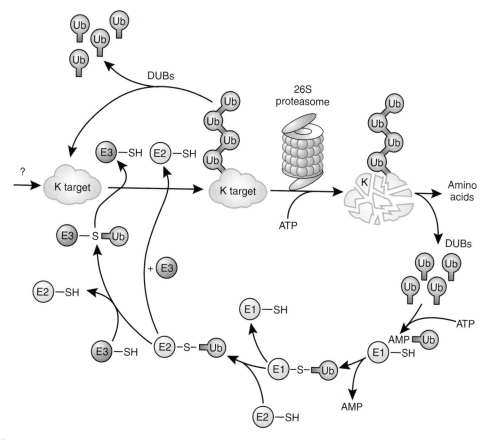

**Figure 11.18** The ubiquitin-proteasome pathway of proteolysis. Proteins degraded by the ubiquitin-proteasome pathway are first conjugated to ubiquitin (Ub in *A*). The process of linking ubiquitin to lysine residues in proteins destined for degradation involves the activation of ubiquitin by the E1 enzyme in a reaction dependent on adenosine triphosphate (ATP). Activated ubiquitin is transferred to an E2 carrier protein and then to the substrate protein, a reaction catalyzed by an E3 enzyme. This process is repeated as multiple ubiquitin molecules are added to form a ubiquitin chain. In ATP-dependent reactions, ubiquitin-conjugated proteins are recognized and bound by the 19S complex, which releases the ubiquitin chain and catalyzes the entry of the protein into the 20S core proteasome (*B*). Degradation occurs in the 26S core proteasome, which contains multiple proteolytic sites within its two central rings. Peptides produced by the proteasome are released and are rapidly degraded to amino acids by peptidases in the cytoplasm or are transported to the endoplasmic reticulum and used in the presentation of class I antigens. The ubiquitin is not degraded but is released and reused. ADP, adenosine diphosphate; PP1 pyrophosphate; SH, sulfhydryl.

and abnormally small mitochondria containing focal membrane disruptions. Similar alterations were observed in the external intercostals muscles of ventilated animals, but not in the hind limb muscle.[175] The structural alternations in the myofibrils have detrimental effects on diaphragmatic force-generating capacity; the number of abnormal myofibrils is inversely related to the force output of the diaphragm.[162] However, further studies are needed to elucidate the amount of activity that the respiratory muscles should have to prevent VIDD and whether periods of intermittent activity (i.e., "exercise" of the respiratory muscles) can prevent or attenuate VIDD.

## Clinical Relevance of Ventilator-Induced Diaphragmatic Dysfunction

Do we have evidence of VIDD in patients? Although conclusive data do not exist, several intriguing observations suggest that VIDD may occur clinically. The twitch transdiaphragmatic pressure elicited by magnetic stimulation of the phrenic nerves is reduced in ventilated patients compared with physiologically normal subjects[177] and in patients ready to undergo weaning trials.[158] Diaphragmatic atrophy was documented (by ultrasound) in a tetraplegic patient after prolonged CMV;[178] the time course of atrophy, however, was not

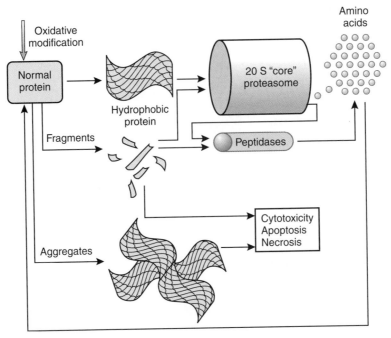

**Figure 11.19** Proposed scheme for oxidation-induced protein degradation by the 20S proteasome or fragmentation and aggregation. Mild oxidative stress modifies cellular proteins, thus generating hydrophobic protein patches that bind to the 20S proteasome and ensure rapid degradation. Because most oxidatively modified proteins are efficiently degraded, there is little chance for further oxidation reactions to cause protein fragmentation or aggregation. Under conditions of severe oxidative stress, however, or if proteasome activity declines during aging or disease, the production of protein fragments and of cross-linked and oxidized protein aggregates increases. Some of the fragments are still degraded by the 20S proteasome (alone or in cooperation with cellular peptidases), but some may have cytotoxic biomimetic effects. Cross-linked and oxidized protein aggregates still tend to bind to the proteasome, which they then irreversibly inhibit. This process can cause a progressively worsening cycle of protein oxidation and increasing accumulation that is ultimately cytotoxic.

established. Furthermore, denervation atrophy removes substances originating from the nerve that are trophic for the muscle, and this is not the case for VIDD, because neural and neuromuscular functions remain intact. The presence of confounding factors, such as disease states (e.g., sepsis) and drug therapy (e.g., corticosteroids, neuromuscular blocking agents), makes documentation of VIDD difficult in a clinical setting.[159] Nevertheless, retrospective analysis of postmortem data from neonates who received ventilator assistance for 12 days or more immediately before death revealed diffuse diaphragmatic myofiber atrophy (small myofibers with rounded outlines) that was not present in extradiaphragmatic muscles.[179]

The typical clinical scenario in which to suspect VIDD is a patient who fails to wean from CMV because of respiratory muscle dysfunction.[159] Other known causes of respiratory muscle weakness such as shock, ongoing sepsis, major malnutrition, electrolyte disturbances, and neuromuscular disorders, are excluded. For example, prolonged neuromuscular blockade can be ruled out by

the lack of an abnormal response to train-of-four stimulation; critical illness polyneuropathy can be excluded by the absence of neuropathic changes on electrophysiologic testing; and acute quadriplegic myopathy can be excluded by the lack of corticosteroid exposure history (or by muscle biopsy in indeterminate cases).[180]

## REFERENCES

1. Osmond DG: Functional anatomy of the chest wall. In Roussos C (ed): The Thorax. New York: Marcel Dekker, 1995.
2. DeTroyer A, Loring SH: Actions of the respiratory muscles. In Roussos C (ed): The Thorax. New York: Marcel Dekker, 1995.
3. Saumarez RC: An analysis of action of intercostal muscles in human upper rib cage. J Appl Physiol 1986;60:690–701.
4. Wilson TA, De Troyer A: Respiratory effect of the intercostal muscles in the dog. J Appl Physiol 1993;75:2636–2645.
5. De Troyer A, Sampson MG: Activation of the parasternal intercostals during breathing efforts in human subjects. J Appl Physiol 1982;52:524–529.
6. Whitelaw WA, Feroah T: Patterns of intercostal muscle activity in humans. J Appl Physiol 1989;67:2087–2094.

7. De Troyer A: The electro-mechanical response of canine inspiratory intercostal muscles to increased resistance: The cranial rib-cage. J Physiol (Lond) 1992;451:445–461.

8. Braun NM, Arora NS, Rochester DF: Force-length relationship of the normal human diaphragm. J Appl Physiol 1982;53:405–412.

9. Paiva M, Verbanck S, Estenne M, et al: Mechanical implications of in vivo human diaphragm shape. J Appl Physiol 1992;72:1407–1412.

10. Whitelaw WA: Shape and size of the human diaphragm in vivo. J Appl Physiol 1987;62:180–186.

11. Estenne M, De Troyer A: Relationship between respiratory muscle electromyogram and rib cage motion in tetraplegia. Am Rev Respir Dis 1985;132:53–59.

12. Urmey WF, De Troyer A, Kelly KB, Loring SH: Pleural pressure increases during inspiration in the zone of apposition of diaphragm to rib cage. J Appl Physiol 1988;65:2207–2212.

13. Mead J, Banzett RB, Lehr J, et al: Effect of posture on upper and lower rib cage motion and tidal volume during diaphragm pacing. Am Rev Respir Dis 1984;130:320–321.

14. Mead J, Loring SH: Analysis of volume displacement and length changes of the diaphragm during breathing. J Appl Physiol 1982;53:750–755.

15. D'Angelo E, Sant'Ambrogio G: Direct action of contracting diaphragm on the rib cage in rabbits and dogs. J Appl Physiol 1974;36:715–719.

16. De Troyer A, Sampson M, Sigrist S, Macklem PT: Action of costal and crural parts of the diaphragm on the rib cage in dog. J Appl Physiol 1982;53:30–39.

17. Farkas GA, Roussos C: Adaptability of the hamster diaphragm to exercise and/or emphysema. J Appl Physiol 1982;53:1263–1272.

18. De Troyer A, Estenne M, Vincken W: Rib cage motion and muscle use in high tetraplegics. Am Rev Respir Dis 1986;133:1115–1119.

19. Campbell EJ: The role of the scalene and sternomastoid muscles in breathing in normal subjects: An electromyographic study. J Anat 1955;89:378–386.

20. Raper AJ, Thompson WT Jr, Shapiro W, Patterson JL Jr: Scalene and sternomastoid muscle function. J Appl Physiol 1966;21:497–502.

21. Estenne M, De Troyer A: Relationship between respiratory muscle electromyogram and rib cage motion in tetraplegia. Am Rev Respir Dis 1985;132:53–59.

22. Campbell EJ: The role of the scalene and sternomastoid muscles in breathing in normal subjects: An electromyographic study. J Anat 1955;89:378–386.

23. De Troyer A, Estenne M: Coordination between rib cage muscles and diaphragm during quiet breathing in humans. J Appl Physiol 1984;57:899–906.

24. Rahn H, Otis AB, Chadwich LE, Fenn WO: The pressure-volume diagram of the thorax and lung. Am J Physiol 1946;146:161–178.

25. Agostoni E, Mead J: Statics of the respiratory system. In Fenn WO (ed): Handbook of Physiology. Section 3: Respiration, vol 1. Washington, DC: American Physiological Society, 1964.

26. Heaf PJ, Prime FJ: The mechanical aspects of artificial pneumothorax. Lancet 1954;267:468–470.

27. Campbell EJM: The Respiratory Muscles and the Mechanics of Breathing. Chicago: Year Book, 1958.

28. Rodarte JH: Lung and chest wall mechanics: Basic concepts. In Scharf SM (ed): Heart-Lung Interactions in Health and Disease. New York: Marcel Dekker, 1989.

29. Agostoni E, Rahn H: Abdominal and thoracic pressures at different lung volumes. J Appl Physiol 1960;15:1087–1092.

30. Bergofsky EH: Relative contributions of the rib cage and the diaphragm to ventilation in man. J Appl Physiol 1964;19:698–706.

31. Krnjevic K, Miledi R: Presynaptic failure of neuromuscular propagation in rats. J Physiol (Lond) 1959;149:1–22.

32. Wade OL: Movements of the thoracic cage and diaphragm in respiration. J Physiol (Lond) 1954;124:193–212.

33. Agostoni EP: Relation between changes on rib cage circumference and lung volume. J Appl Physiol 1965;20:1179–1186.

34. Konno K, Mead J: Measurement of the separate volume changes of rib cage and abdomen during breathing. J Appl Physiol 1967;22:407–422.

35. Grassino A, Goldman MD, Mead J, Sears TA: Mechanics of the human diaphragm during voluntary contraction: Statics. J Appl Physiol 1978;44:829–839.

36. Smith J, Loring S: Passive mechanical properties of the chest wall. In Handbook of Physiology. Section 3: The Respiratory System, vol 3, part 2. Washington, DC: American Physiological Society, 1986.

37. Sackner JD, Nixon AJ, Davis B, et al: Non-invasive measurement of ventilation during exercise using a respiratory inductive plethysmograph. I. Am Rev Respir Dis 1980;122:867–871.

38. Konno K, Mead J: Static volume-pressure characteristics of the rib cage and abdomen. J Appl Physiol 1968;24:544–548.

39. D'Angelo E, Agostoni E: Statics of the chest wall. In Roussos C (ed): The Thorax. New York: Marcel Dekker, 1995.

40. Grassino AE, Roussos C, Macklem PT: Static properties of the chest wall. In Crystal RG, Wea J (eds): The Lung: Scientific Foundations. New York: Raven Press, 1991.

41. Mead J, Loring SH, Smith JC: Volume displacements of the chest wall and their mechanical significance. In Roussos C (ed): The Thorax. New York: Marcel Dekker, 1995.

42. Macklem PT: Respiratory muscle dysfunction. Hosp Pract (Off Ed) 1986;21:83–86.

43. Roussos C, Macklem PT: The respiratory muscles. N Engl J Med 1982;307:786–797.

44. Monod H, Scherrer J: The work capacity of a synergistic muscular group. Ergonomics 1965;8:329–337.

45. Bellemare F, Grassino A: Effect of pressure and timing of contraction on human diaphragm fatigue. J Appl Physiol 1982;53:1190–1195.

46. Zocchi L, Fitting JW, Majani U, et al: Effect of pressure and timing of contraction on human rib cage muscle fatigue. Am Rev Respir Dis 1993;147:857–864.

47. Milic-Emili J: Is weaning an art or a science? Am Rev Respir Dis 1986;134:1107–1108.

48. Roussos C, Fixley M, Gross D, Macklem PT: Fatigue of inspiratory muscles and their synergic behavior. J Appl Physiol 1979;46:897–904.

49. Marini JJ: The physiologic determinants of ventilator dependence. Respir Care 1986;31:271–282.

50. Maher J, Rutledge F, Remtulla H, et al: Neuromuscular disorders associated with failure to wean from the ventilator. Intensive Care Med 1995;21:737–743.

51. Smith PE, Calverley PM, Edwards RH: Hypoxemia during sleep in Duchenne muscular dystrophy. Am Rev Respir Dis 1988;137:884–888.

52. Abd AG, Braun NM, Baskin MI, et al: Diaphragmatic dysfunction after open heart surgery: Treatment with a rocking bed. Ann Intern Med 1989;111:881–886.

53. Chevrolet JC, Deleamont P: Repeated vital capacity measurements as predictive parameters for mechanical ventilation need and weaning success in the Guillain-Barré syndrome. Am Rev Respir Dis 1991;144:814–818.

54. Segredo V, Caldwell JE, Matthay MA, et al: Persistent paralysis in critically ill patients after long-term administration of vecuronium. N Engl J Med 1992;327:524–528.

55. Bolton CF: Neuromuscular complications of sepsis. Intensive Care Med 1993;19(Suppl 2):S58–S63.

56. Witt NJ, Zochodne DW, Bolton CF, et al: Peripheral nerve function in sepsis and multiple organ failure. Chest 1991;99:176–184.

57. Spitzer AR, Giancarlo T, Maher L, et al: Neuromuscular causes of prolonged ventilator dependency. Muscle Nerve 1992;15:682–686.

58. Decramer M, Stas KJ: Corticosteroid-induced myopathy involving respiratory muscles in patients with chronic obstructive pulmonary disease or asthma. Am Rev Respir Dis 1992;146:800–802.

59. Douglass JA, Tuxen DV, Horne M, et al: Myopathy in severe asthma. Am Rev Respir Dis 1992;146:517–519.

60. Driver AG, LeBrun M: Iatrogenic malnutrition in patients receiving ventilatory support. JAMA 1980;244:2195–2196.

61. Driver AG, McAlevy MT, Smith JL: Nutritional assessment of patients with chronic obstructive pulmonary disease and acute respiratory failure. Chest 1982;82:568–571.

62. Kelly SM, Rosa A, Field S, et al: Inspiratory muscle strength and body composition in patients receiving total parenteral nutrition therapy. Am Rev Respir Dis 1984;130:33–37.

63. Wilson DO, Rogers RM, Wright EC, Anthonisen NR: Body weight in chronic obstructive pulmonary disease: The National Institutes of Health Intermittent Positive-Pressure Breathing Trial. Am Rev Respir Dis 1989;139:1435–1438.

64. Aubier M, Viires N, Piquet J, et al: Effects of hypocalcemia on diaphragmatic strength generation. J Appl Physiol 1985;58:2054–2061.

65. Knochel JP: Neuromuscular manifestations of electrolyte disorders. Am J Med 1982;72:521–535.

66. Aubier M, Murciano D, Lecocguic Y, et al: Effect of hypophosphatemia on diaphragmatic contractility in patients with acute respiratory failure. N Engl J Med 1985;313:420–424.

67. Fisher J, Magid N, Kallman C, et al: Respiratory illness and hypophosphatemia. Chest 1983;83:504–508.

68. Dhingra S, Solven F, Wilson A, McCarthy DS: Hypomagnesemia and respiratory muscle power. Am Rev Respir Dis 1984;129:497–498.

69. Juan G, Calverley P, Talamo C, et al: Effect of carbon dioxide on diaphragmatic function in human beings. N Engl J Med 1984;310:874–879.

70. Howell S, Fitzgerald RS, Roussos C: Effects of uncompensated and compensated metabolic acidosis on canine diaphragm. J Appl Physiol 1985;59:1376–1382.

71. Yanos J, Wood LD, Davis K, Keamy M III: The effect of respiratory and lactic acidosis on diaphragm function. Am Rev Respir Dis 1993;147:616–619.

72. Loring SH, Mead J, Griscom NT: Dependence of diaphragmatic length on lung volume and thoracoabdominal configuration. J Appl Physiol 1985;59:1961–1970.

73. Smith J, Bellemare F: Effect of lung volume on in vivo contraction characteristics of human diaphragm. J Appl Physiol 1987;62:1893–1900.

74. Farkas GA, Decramer M, Rochester DF, De Troyer A: Contractile properties of intercostal muscles and their functional significance. J Appl Physiol 1985;59:528–535.

75. Farkas GA, Rochester DF: Functional characteristics of canine costal and crural diaphragm. J Appl Physiol 1988;65:2253–2260.

76. Gauthier AP, Verbanck S, Estenne M, et al: Three-dimensional reconstruction of the in vivo human diaphragm shape at different lung volumes. J Appl Physiol 1994;76:495–506.

77. Similowski T, Yan S, Gauthier AP, et al: Contractile properties of the human diaphragm during chronic hyperinflation. N Engl J Med 1991;325:917–923.

78. Caro CG, Dubois AB: Pulmonary function in kyphoscoliosis. Thorax 1961;16:282–290.

79. Boczkowski J, Dureuil B, Branger C, et al: Effects of sepsis on diaphragmatic function in rats. Am Rev Respir Dis 1988;138:260–265.

80. Hussain SN, Graham R, Rutledge F, Roussos C: Respiratory muscle energetics during endotoxic shock in dogs. J Appl Physiol 1986;60:486–493.

81. Hussain SN, Magder S, Chatillon A, Roussos C: Chemical activation of thin-fiber phrenic afferents: Respiratory responses. J Appl Physiol 1990;69:1002–1011.

82. Hussain SN, Roussos C: Distribution of respiratory muscle and organ blood flow during endotoxic shock in dogs. J Appl Physiol 1985;59:1802–1808.

83. Hussain SN, Simkus G, Roussos C: Respiratory muscle fatigue: A cause of ventilatory failure in septic shock. J Appl Physiol 1985;58:2033–2040.

84. Rochester DF, Esau SA: Critical illness, infection, and the respiratory muscles. Am Rev Respir Dis 1988;138:258–259.

85. Le Bourdelles G, Viires N, Boczkowski J, et al: Effects of mechanical ventilation on diaphragmatic contractile properties in rats. Am J Respir Crit Care Med 1994;149:1539–1544.

86. Vassilakopoulos T, Zakynthinos S, Roussos C: Strenuous resistive breathing induces proinflammatory cytokines and stimulates the HPA axis in humans. Am J Physiol 1999;277:R1013–R1019.

87. Vassilakopoulos T, Divangahi M, Rallis G, et al: Differential cytokine gene expression in the diaphragm in response to strenuous resistive breathing. Am J Respir Crit Care Med 2004;170:154–161.

88. Vassilakopoulos T, Katsaounou P, Karatza MH, et al: Strenuous resistive breathing induces plasma cytokines: Role of antioxidants and monocytes. Am J Respir Crit Care Med 2002;166:1572–1578.

89. Kosmidou I, Vassilakopoulos T, Xagorari A, et al: Production of interleukin-6 by skeletal myotubes: Role of reactive oxygen species. Am J Respir Cell Mol Biol 2002;26:587–593.

90. Jiang TX, Reid WD, Road JD: Free radical scavengers and diaphragm injury following inspiratory resistive loading. Am J Respir Crit Care Med 2001;164:1288–1294.

91. Orozco-Levi M, Lloreta J, Minguella J, et al: Injury of the human diaphragm associated with exertion and chronic obstructive pulmonary disease. Am J Respir Crit Care Med 2001;164:1734–1739.

92. Reid WD, Belcastro AN: Time course of diaphragm injury and calpain activity during resistive loading. Am J Respir Crit Care Med 2000;162:1801–1806.

93. Reid MB, Li YP: Cytokines and oxidative signalling in skeletal muscle. Acta Physiol Scand 2001;171:225–232.

94. Warren GL, Hulderman T, Jensen N, et al: Physiological role of tumor necrosis factor alpha in traumatic muscle injury. FASEB J 2002;16:1630–1632.

95. De Letter MA, van Doorn PA, Savelkoul HF, et al: Critical illness polyneuropathy and myopathy (CIPNM): Evidence for local immune activation by cytokine-expression in the muscle tissue. J Neuroimmunol 2000;106:206–213.

96. Xing Z, Gauldie J, Cox G, et al: IL-6 is an antiinflammatory cytokine required for controlling local or systemic acute inflammatory responses. J Clin Invest 1998;101:311–320.

97. Cannon JG, Fielding RA, Fiatarone MA, et al: Increased interleukin 1 beta in human skeletal muscle after exercise. Am J Physiol 1989;257:R451–R455.

98. Kami K, Morikawa Y, Sekimoto M, Senba E: Gene expression of receptors for IL-6, LIF, and CNTF in regenerating skeletal muscles. J Histochem Cytochem 2000;48:1203–1213.

99. Kami K, Senba E: Localization of leukemia inhibitory factor and interleukin-6 messenger ribonucleic acids in

regenerating rat skeletal muscle. Muscle Nerve 1998;21: 819–822.

100. Kurek JB, Nouri S, Kannourakis G, et al: Leukemia inhibitory factor and interleukin-6 are produced by diseased and regenerating skeletal muscle. Muscle Nerve 1996;19:1291–1301.

101. Llovera M, Carbo N, Lopez-Soriano J, et al: Different cytokines modulate ubiquitin gene expression in rat skeletal muscle. Cancer Lett 1998;133:83–87.

102. Tsujinaka T, Kishibuchi M, Yano M, et al: Involvement of interleukin-6 in activation of lysosomal cathepsin and atrophy of muscle fibers induced by intramuscular injection of turpentine oil in mice. J Biochem (Tokyo) 1997;122:595–600.

103. Hawke TJ, Garry DJ: Myogenic satellite cells: Physiology to molecular biology. J Appl Physiol 2001;91:534–551.

104. Wilcox P, Milliken C, Bressler B: High-dose tumor necrosis factor alpha produces an impairment of hamster diaphragm contractility: Attenuation with a prostaglandin inhibitor. Am J Respir Crit Care Med 1996;153:1611–1615.

105. Wilcox PG, Wakai Y, Walley KR, et al: Tumor necrosis factor alpha decreases in vivo diaphragm contractility in dogs. Am J Respir Crit Care Med 1994;150:1368–1373.

106. Roussos CS, Macklem PT: Diaphragmatic fatigue in man. J Appl Physiol 1977;43:189–197.

107. Jiang TX, Reid WD, Road JD: Delayed diaphragm injury and diaphragm force production. Am J Respir Crit Care Med 1998;157:736–742.

108. National Heart, Lung and Blood Institute Workshop Summary: Respiratory muscle fatigue: Report of the Respiratory Muscle Fatigue Workshop Group. Am Rev Respir Dis 1990;142: 474–480.

109. Macklem PT: The importance of defining respiratory muscle fatigue. Am Rev Respir Dis 1990;142:274.

110. Bigland-Ritchie B, Jones DA, Hosking GP, Edwards RH: Central and peripheral fatigue in sustained maximum voluntary contractions of human quadriceps muscle. Clin Sci Mol Med 1978;54:609–614.

111. Merton PA: Voluntary strength and fatigue. J Physiol (Lond) 1954;123:553–564.

112. Bellemare F, Bigland-Ritchie B: Assessment of human diaphragm strength and activation using phrenic nerve stimulation. Respir Physiol 1984;58:263–277.

113. Bellemare F, Bigland-Ritchie B: Central components of diaphragmatic fatigue assessed by phrenic nerve stimulation. J Appl Physiol 1987;62:1307–1316.

114. McKenzie DK, Bigland-Ritchie B, Gorman RB, Gandevia SC: Central and peripheral fatigue of human diaphragm and limb muscles assessed by twitch interpolation. J Physiol (Lond) 1992;454:643–656.

115. Grimby L, Hannerz J, Hedman B: The fatigue and voluntary discharge properties of single motor units in man. J Physiol (Lond) 1981;316:545–554.

116. Bigland-Ritchie B, Johansson R, Lippold OC, Woods JJ: Contractile speed and EMG changes during fatigue of sustained maximal voluntary contractions. J Neurophysiol 1983;50:313–324.

117. Jammes Y, Buchler B, Delpierre S, et al: Phrenic afferents and their role in inspiratory control. J Appl Physiol 1986;60:854–860.

118. Cohen CA, Zagelbaum G, Gross D, et al: Clinical manifestations of inspiratory muscle fatigue. Am J Med 1982;73:308–316.

119. Petrozzino JJ, Scardella AT, Santiago TV, Edelman NH: Dichloroacetate blocks endogenous opioid effects during inspiratory flow-resistive loading. J Appl Physiol 1992;72:590–596.

120. Scardella AT, Parisi RA, Phair DK, et al: The role of endogenous opioids in the ventilatory response to acute flow-resistive loads. Am Rev Respir Dis 1986;133:26–31.

121. Scardella AT, Petrozzino JJ, Mandel M, et al: Endogenous opioid effects on abdominal muscle activity during inspiratory loading. J Appl Physiol 1990;69:1104–1109.

122. Bellofiore S, Di Maria GU, Privitera S, et al: Endogenous opioids modulate the increase in ventilatory output and dyspnea during severe acute bronchoconstriction. Am Rev Respir Dis 1990;142:812–816.

123. Santiago TV, Remolina C, Scoles V III, Edelman NH: Endorphins and the control of breathing: Ability of naloxone to restore flow-resistive load compensation in chronic obstructive pulmonary disease. N Engl J Med 1981;304: 1190–1195.

124. Krnjevic K, Miledi R: Presynaptic failure of neuromuscular propagation in rats. J Physiol (Lond) 1959;149:1–22.

125. Aubier M, Trippenbach T, Roussos C: Respiratory muscle fatigue during cardiogenic shock. J Appl Physiol 1981;51:499–508.

126. Kugelberg E, Lindegren B: Transmission and contraction fatigue of rat motor units in relation to succinate dehydrogenase activity of motor unit fibres. J Physiol (Lond) 1979;288:285–300.

127. Aubier M, Farkas G, De Troyer A, et al: Detection of diaphragmatic fatigue in man by phrenic stimulation. J Appl Physiol 1981;50:538–544.

128. Merton PA: Voluntary strength and fatigue. J Physiol (Lond) 1954;123:553–564.

129. Edwards RHT, Mills KR, Newham DJ: Greater low frequency fatigue produced by eccentric rather than concentric muscle contraction. J Physiol (Lond) 1981;317:17–24.

130. Vigreux B, Cnockaert JC, Pertuzon E: Effects of fatigue on the series elastic component of human muscle. Eur J Appl Physiol Occup Physiol 1980;45:11–17.

131. Moxham J, Wiles CM, Newham D, Edwards RH: Sternomastoid muscle function and fatigue in man. Clin Sci (Lond) 1980;59:463–468.

132. Nagesser AS, van der Laarse WJ, Elzinga G: Metabolic changes with fatigue in different types of single muscle fibres of *Xenopus laevis*. J Physiol (Lond) 1992;448:511–523.

133. Han JW, Thieleczek R, Varsanyi M, Heilmeyer LM Jr: Compartmentalized ATP synthesis in skeletal muscle triads. Biochemistry 1992;31:377–384.

134. Jardim J, Farkas G, Prefaut C, et al: The failing inspiratory muscles under normoxic and hypoxic conditions. Am Rev Respir Dis 1981;124:274–279.

135. Aubier M, Viires N, Syllie G, et al: Respiratory muscle contribution to lactic acidosis in low cardiac output. Am Rev Respir Dis 1982;126:648–652.

136. Westerblad H, Lannergren J: The relation between force and intracellular pH in fatigued, single *Xenopus* muscle fibres. Acta Physiol Scand 1988;133:83–89.

137. Westerblad H, Allen DG: Changes of myoplasmic calcium concentration during fatigue in single mouse muscle fibers. J Gen Physiol 1991;98:615–635.

138. Bergstrom J, Hermansen L, Hultman E, Saltin B: Diet, muscle glycogen and physical performance. Acta Physiol Scand 1967;71:140–150.

139. Anzueto A, Supinski GS, Levine SM, Jenkinson SG: Mechanisms of disease: Are oxygen-derived free radicals involved in diaphragmatic dysfunction? Am J Respir Crit Care Med 1994;149:1048–1052.

140. Shindoh C, DiMarco A, Thomas A, et al: Effect of N-acetylcysteine on diaphragm fatigue. J Appl Physiol 1990;68:2107–2113.

141. Chrousos GP: The hypothalamic-pituitary-adrenal axis and immune-mediated inflammation. N Engl J Med 1995;332:1351–1362.

142. Mastorakos G, Chrousos GP, Weber JS: Recombinant interleukin-6 activates the hypothalamic-pituitary-adrenal axis in humans. J Clin Endocrinol Metab 1993;77:1690–1694.

143. Watanabe T, Morimoto A, Tan N, et al: ACTH response induced in capsaicin-desensitized rats by intravenous injection of interleukin-1 or prostaglandin E. J Physiol (Lond) 1994;475:139–145.

144. Turnbull AV, Rivier CL: Regulation of the hypothalamic-pituitary-adrenal axis by cytokines: Actions and mechanisms of action. Physiol Rev 1999;79:1–71.

145. Petrozzino JJ, Scardella AT, Edelman NH, Santiago TV: Respiratory muscle acidosis stimulates endogenous opioids during inspiratory loading. Am Rev Respir Dis 1993;147:607–615.

146. Scardella AT, Santiago TV, Edelman NH: Naloxone alters the early response to an inspiratory flow-resistive load. J Appl Physiol 1989;67:1747–1753.

147. Scardella AT, Edelman NH: Central fatigue in respiratory control. In Roussos C (ed): The Thorax. New York: Marcel Dekker, 1995.

148. Wanke T, Lahrmann H, Auinger M, et al: Endogenous opioid system during inspiratory loading in patients with type I diabetes. Am Rev Respir Dis 1993;148:1335–1340.

149. Vassilakopoulos T, Zakynthinos S, Roussos C: Respiratory muscles and weaning failure. Eur Respir J 1996;9:2383–2400.

150. Cohen CA, Zagelbaum G, Gross D, et al: Clinical manifestations of inspiratory muscle fatigue. Am J Med 1982;73:308–316.

151. Tobin MJ, Perez W, Guenther SM, et al: Does rib cage-abdominal paradox signify respiratory muscle fatigue? J Appl Physiol 1987;63:851–860.

152. Goldstone JC, Green M, Moxham J: Maximum relaxation rate of the diaphragm during weaning from mechanical ventilation. Thorax 1994;49:54–60.

153. Bigland-Ritchie B, Donovan EF, Roussos CS: Conduction velocity and EMG power spectrum changes in fatigue of sustained maximal efforts. J Appl Physiol 1981;51:1300–1305.

154. Brochard L, Harf A, Lorino H, Lemaire F: Inspiratory pressure support prevents diaphragmatic fatigue during weaning from mechanical ventilation. Am Rev Respir Dis 1989;139:513–521.

155. Pourriat JL, Lamberto C, Hoang PH, et al: Diaphragmatic fatigue and breathing pattern during weaning from mechanical ventilation in COPD patients. Chest 1986;90:703–707.

156. Zakynthinos SG, Vassilakopoulos T, Roussos C: The load of inspiratory muscles in patients needing mechanical ventilation. Am J Respir Crit Care Med 1995;152:1248–1255.

157. Vassilakopoulos T, Zakynthinos S, Roussos C: The tension-time index and the frequency/tidal volume ratio are the major pathophysiologic determinants of weaning failure and success. Am J Respir Crit Care Med 1998;158:378–385.

158. Laghi F, Cattapan SE, Jubran A, et al: Is weaning failure caused by low-frequency fatigue of the diaphragm? Am J Respir Crit Care Med 2003;167:120–127.

159. Vassilakopoulos T, Petrof BJ: Ventilator-induced diaphragmatic dysfunction. Am J Respir Crit Care Med 2004;169:336–341.

160. Anzueto A, Peters JI, Tobin MJ, et al: Effects of prolonged controlled mechanical ventilation on diaphragmatic function in healthy adult baboons. Crit Care Med 1997;25:1187–1190.

161. Radell PJ, Remahl S, Nichols DG, Eriksson LI: Effects of prolonged mechanical ventilation and inactivity on piglet diaphragm function. Intensive Care Med 2002;28:358–364.

162. Sassoon CS, Caiozzo VJ, Manka A, Sieck GC: Altered diaphragm contractile properties with controlled mechanical ventilation. J Appl Physiol 2002;92:2585–2595.

163. Capdevila X, Lopez S, Bernard N, et al: Effects of controlled mechanical ventilation on respiratory muscle contractile properties in rabbits. Intensive Care Med 2003;29:103–110.

164. Gayan-Ramirez G, de Paepe K, Cadot P, Decramer M: Detrimental effects of short-term mechanical ventilation on diaphragm function and IGF-I mRNA in rats. Intensive Care Med 2003;29:825–833.

165. Powers SK, Shanely RA, Coombes JS, et al: Mechanical ventilation results in progressive contractile dysfunction in the diaphragm. J Appl Physiol 2002;92:1851–1858.

166. Yang L, Luo J, Bourdon J, et al: Controlled mechanical ventilation leads to remodeling of the rat diaphragm. Am J Respir Crit Care Med 2002;166:1135–1140.

167. Zhu E, Sassoon CS, Nelson R, et al: Early effects of mechanical ventilation on isotonic contractile properties and MAF-box gene expression in the diaphragm. J Appl Physiol 2005;99:747–756.

168. Hussain SN, Vassilakopoulos T: Ventilator-induced cachexia. Am J Respir Crit Care Med 2002;166:1307–1308.

169. Shanely RA, Van Gammeren D, Deruisseau KC, et al: Mechanical ventilation depresses protein synthesis in the rat diaphragm. Am J Respir Crit Care Med 2004;170:994–999.

170. Shanely RA, Zergeroglu MA, Lennon SL, et al: Mechanical ventilation-induced diaphragmatic atrophy is associated with oxidative injury and increased proteolytic activity. Am J Respir Crit Care Med 2002;166:1369–1374.

171. DeRuisseau KC, Kavazis AN, Deering MA, et al: Mechanical ventilation induces alterations of the ubiquitin-proteasome pathway in the diaphragm. J Appl Physiol 2005;98:1314–1321.

172. Davies KJ: Degradation of oxidized proteins by the 20S proteasome. Biochimie 2001;83:301–310.

173. Shringarpure R, Grune T, Mehlhase J, Davies KJ: Ubiquitin conjugation is not required for the degradation of oxidized proteins by proteasome. J Biol Chem 2003;278:311–318.

174. Zergeroglu MA, McKenzie MJ, Shanely RA, et al: Mechanical ventilation-induced oxidative stress in the diaphragm. J Appl Physiol 2003;95:1116–1124.

175. Bernard N, Matecki S, Py G, et al: Effects of prolonged mechanical ventilation on respiratory muscle ultrastructure and mitochondrial respiration in rabbits. Intensive Care Med 2003;29:111–118.

176. Radell P, Edstrom L, Stibler H, et al: Changes in diaphragm structure following prolonged mechanical ventilation in piglets. Acta Anaesthesiol Scand 2004;48:430–437.

177. Watson AC, Hughes PD, Louise HM, et al: Measurement of twitch transdiaphragmatic, esophageal, and endotracheal tube pressure with bilateral anterolateral magnetic phrenic nerve stimulation in patients in the intensive care unit. Crit Care Med 2001;29:1325–1331.

178. Ayas NT, McCool FD, Gore R, et al: Prevention of human diaphragm atrophy with short periods of electrical stimulation. Am J Respir Crit Care Med 1999;159:2018–2020.

179. Knisely AS, Leal SM, Singer DB: Abnormalities of diaphragmatic muscle in neonates with ventilated lungs. J Pediatr 1988;113:1074–1077.

180. Deem S, Lee CM, Curtis JR: Acquired neuromuscular disorders in the intensive care unit. Am J Respir Crit Care Med 2003;168:735–739.

# CHAPTER 12

# Surfactant Therapy

Diederik Gommers and Burkhard Lachmann

Historically, Kurt von Neergaard[1] was the first to suggest that surface tension plays an important role in lung elasticity. In 1929, he showed that the pressure necessary to fill the lung with liquid was less than half the pressure necessary to fill the lung with air, and he concluded that two thirds to three fourths of the elasticity of the lung was derived from interfacial forces.[1] The problem with his discovery was that this article was published in German, and, for 25 years, no scientists in the evolving field really took note of this publication. In 1954, Macklin[2] described the presence of a thin aqueous mucoid microfilm, formed from secretion of the granular pneumocytes, on the pulmonary alveolar walls and in constant slow movement toward the phagocytic pneumocytes and bronchioles. One year later, Pattle[3] noticed the remarkable stability of foam and bubbles from lung edema and healthy lung. He assumed that the walls of these bubbles consisted of surface-active material that would have to lower the surface tension to nearly zero. In 1957, Clements[4] was the first to prove the direct evidence of surface-active material in the lungs. He measured the surface tension of a surface film derived from the lung by using a Wilhelmy balance and demonstrated that the surface tension was not a constant value; when the surface was stretched, the tension was relatively high (40 dynes/cm), but when the surface area was decreased, the tension fell to 10 dynes/cm. Clements pointed out that such a reduction in surface tension during deflation in the lung would tend to stabilize the air spaces by permitting them to remain open at low lung volumes. Two years later, Avery and Mead[5] demonstrated that lung extracts of very small premature infants and of infants dying of hyaline membrane disease had much higher surface tension than normal lung extracts,

as a result of a deficiency in surface-active material. This was the first step toward extensive research on the surfactant system, and Fujiwara and colleagues, in 1980,[6] were the first to treat premature babies suffering from respiratory insufficiency with exogenous surfactant.

Since 1980, premature infants suffering from respiratory distress syndrome (RDS) resulting from surfactant deficiency have been successfully treated with exogenous surfactant, almost without any side effects.[7,8] Biochemical and biophysical abnormalities of the pulmonary surfactant system are also seen in other diseases such as acute lung injury (ALI) or acute RDS (ARDS)[9–11] and infectious lung disease,[12] as well as after cardiopulmonary bypass surgery.[13] Furthermore, investigators have demonstrated that nonoptimal ventilation may lead to disturbance of alveolar surfactant.[14] Results are available of limited clinical studies in which patients other than neonates with RDS were treated with exogenous surfactant.[15]

In this chapter, we describe the rationale for exogenous surfactant therapy in ARDS by reviewing experimental and clinical findings. Further, various factors that may influence a host's response to this therapy are discussed, and finally we speculate about future developments.

## OVERVIEW OF SURFACTANT

The main function of surfactant is to lower the surface tension at the air-liquid interface and thereby to allow normal breathing with the least possible effort. In addition, as alveolar size decreases during deflation of the lung, pulmonary surfactant ensures that surface tension falls approximately to zero and prevents alveolar collapse.[16] Thus, at small alveolar volumes, surface tension becomes a negligible force and tends to promote alveolar stability.[16] Other physiologic functions of the pulmonary surfactant system include mechanical stabilization of small airways, protection against lung edema, and defense against lung infections.[17]

Pulmonary surfactant has two major fractions: lipids and surfactant-specific proteins.[18] Although surfactant is mainly composed of lipids, proteins make up 10% of pulmonary surfactant. These proteins can be divided into two groups: the hydrophilic surfactant proteins SP-A and SP-D and the hydrophobic proteins SP-B and SP-C.[18]

Surfactant proteins play an important role in surfactant metabolism and function. Both SP-B and SP-C have been demonstrated to enhance lipid insertion into the monolayer at the air-liquid interface.[18] In this way, these proteins maintain a low surface tension and thereby protect the surface film from contamination by plasma proteins that can cause inactivation or degradation of the surfactant film. SP-A and SP-D are believed to be molecules of the innate immune system through their ability to recognize a broad spectrum of pathogens.[17] Several studies have shown that SP-A and SP-D interact with numerous viruses, bacteria, and fungi, as well as with inhaled glycoconjugate allergens, such as pollen grains and mite allergens. Furthermore, SP-A and SP-D have been shown to bind to alveolar macrophages, which carry receptors for SP-A and SP-D on their surface. In general, the interaction of SP-A with pathogens and phagocytes leads to an increased uptake of pathogens.[17]

Both natural and synthetic surfactant preparations have been successfully used in clinical trials in neonates suffering from RDS, but differences in efficacy have been noted.[8] The natural surfactants, which are obtained by organic solvent extraction of bovine or calf lung lavage (Alveofact, BLES, and Infasurf), minced bovine lungs (Surfacten and Survanta), or minced pig lungs (HL-10, Curosurf), contain 1% to 2% of SP-B and SP-C, whereas the available synthetic surfactants (Alec and Exosurf) are protein free.[19] From experimental studies, it is known that in contrast to the synthetic surfactants, the natural surfactants are characterized by rapid adsorption to the air-liquid interface, less sensitivity to inactivation by serum proteins, and almost immediate improvement of gas exchange.[19] It is assumed that the presence of the surfactant proteins in the natural surfactant preparations accounts for these differences.

Surfactant proteins, especially SP-A, SP-B, and SP-C, are almost exclusively secreted in the lung and are compartmentalized in the alveoli by apical secretion in the healthy lung. This exclusive characteristic could make surfactant proteins a highly specific biologic marker of lung injury or disease. In a study of patients with acute cardiogenic pulmonary edema, plasma levels of SP-A and SP-B were elevated at the time of diagnosis and continued to rise for 3 days before falling.[20] This temporal pattern is consistent with prolonged and initial worsening of cardiogenic pulmonary edema during the first 3 days,[20] a finding indicating the possible usefulness of plasma surfactant proteins as clinical markers of lung injury.

Surfactant can be impaired at different levels. An important cause can be degradation of lipids through phospholipases during inflammatory lung injury. Lytic enzymes of this kind can degrade and inactivate not only endogenous surfactant, but also exogenous lung surfactants used in treating clinical ALI and ARDS.[21] All current exogenous surfactant drugs contain substantial amounts of phospholipids including dipalmitoylphosphatidylcholine (DPPC), the most prevalent component of endogenous lung surfactant. Phospholipase-induced degradation of glycerophospholipids not only reduces the concentration of active surfactant, but also generates byproducts such as lysophosphatidylcholine and fluid free fatty acids that can further decrease surface activity through biophysical interactions.[21] Wang and co-workers demonstrated that a synthetic lipid (DPPC analogue) resistant to degradation by phospholipases in vitro had equal or lower dynamic surface tension compared with normal DPPC, and the addition of SP-B/SP-C further enhanced the in vitro characteristics.[21] Besides phospholipids, cholesterol is the major nonphospholipid component of surfactant (10 to 20 mol %), and cholesterol can lower surface tension.[22] This effect is dependent on cholesterol concentration and was more pronounced in the presence of SP-B.[22] This finding provides additional evidence that natural surfactant, containing SP-B and SP-C, is superior to surfactants lacking one of these components.[22]

## SURFACTANT AND ACUTE RESPIRATORY DISTRESS SYNDROME

In 1967, Ashbaugh and co-workers[23] described 12 adult patients with acute respiratory failure who did not respond to usual therapy. The clinical and pathologic features were very similar to those seen in neonates with RDS, so the name *adult* (later changed to *acute*) *respiratory distress syndrome* was introduced. ARDS has become a well-recognized condition that can result from numerous different causes, such as sepsis, polytrauma, aspiration, multiple organ failure, burns, pneumonia, near drowning, and acute pancreatitis, among others.[24] Despite diverse causes of ARDS, the common pathologic characteristic is increased alveolocapillary permeability associated with damage to the alveolar epithelium.

The mechanisms responsible for the injury to the alveolocapillary membrane are complex and are still under discussion. Active roles have been attributed to neutrophils, basophils, macrophages, platelets, arachidonic acid metabolites, oxygen-derived free radicals, complement, proteases, interleukins, serotonin, platelet-activating factor, tumor necrosis factor, surfactant-inhibiting plasma proteins, drugs, and many other substances. However, all these individual factors, which can lead to pulmonary edema, do not necessarily lead to ARDS. Therefore, another system must be involved to explain the functional changes as seen in ARDS. It is established that the capillary leakage combined with damage to the alveolar epithelium leads to an immediate, or moderately slow, loss of active surfactant by inactivation or depletion from the alveoli and small airways that is compensated by a release of stored surfactant from type II cells.[25] Thus, disease progression depends on the balance between new production and release of surfactant into the alveoli and its inactivation or loss from the alveoli and airways. If the synthesis is reduced (e.g., by influenza virus, hypoxia, or hyperoxia), an imbalance between new synthesis and demand will result. This will finally lead to a total loss of functional active surfactant, with resulting failure of the lung as a gas exchange organ.[26] Thus, in ARDS, the surfactant deficiency is a complication of lung injury rather than a primary etiologic factor, as in neonatal RDS.

Analyses of lung surfactant recovered in bronchoalveolar lavage (BAL) fluid from patients with ARDS, or from animal models of acute respiratory failure, demonstrate disturbances of the lung surfactant system.[27] Reduction of surfactant activity is associated with increased minimal surface tension of lung extracts or lung homogenates and with compositional changes of surfactant or decreased surfactant content of the lungs.[28] Ashbaugh and colleagues[23] were the first to demonstrate decreased lung compliance and increased minimal surface tension in lung extracts from two patients with ARDS. Since then, several studies have demonstrated qualitative and quantitative changes of surfactant in BAL fluid from patients with ARDS.[29–32] Gregory and colleagues[32] demonstrated that several of these alterations already occur in patients at risk of developing ARDS, a finding suggesting that these abnormalities of surfactant occur early in the disease process.

## SURFACTANT AND MECHANICAL VENTILATION

Several studies have shown that ventilator modes with large tidal volumes and high peak inspiratory pressures during mechanical ventilation affect the pulmonary surfactant system.[33] The exact mechanism by which the surfactant system is affected by mechanical ventilation is not yet entirely clear. One factor is that the surfactant in the alveolar lining is actively removed from the alveolus toward the larger airways; this can lead to a shortage of surfactant at the alveolar level that can cause the changes in surface tension characteristics in the lung seen during or after prolonged periods of mechanical ventilation.[34]

During end-expiration, the surfactant molecules covering the alveolar epithelium are compressed on the small alveolar area (leading to low surface tension or high surface pressure), thus preventing the alveoli from collapse. When the surface of the alveolus is smaller than the surface occupied by the surfactant molecules, the molecules are squeezed out of the surface of the alveolus and are forced toward the airways. These surfactant molecules are then unavailable to the alveoli and are eventually cleared from these alveoli. During the following inflation of the alveoli, the surface is replenished with surfactant molecules from the underlying hypophase, in which surfactant molecules in micelles are stored for later use. During the next expiration, the mechanism repeats itself, and again surfactant molecules are forced out of the alveolus and are subsequently replenished from the hypophase, in a continuing cycle.[35]

The amount of surfactant that must be produced and subsequently secreted by the alveolar type II cells is proportional to the loss of surface active molecules during the breathing cycle. When production and secretion of new surfactant molecules keep pace with consumption, no surfactant deficiency can occur, as in a normal, healthy lung.

Thus, mechanical ventilation should take place at a lung volume equal to or higher than the functional residual capacity level with the smallest possible volume and pressure changes. Another factor that may be important is that mechanical ventilation, especially in nonhomogeneous lungs, creates severe shear forces between open and closed airways and possible overstretch of the epithelium during the breathing cycle, thereby resulting in necrosis and desquamation of bronchiolar and alveolar epithelium.[36] The overstretch of the intercellular junctions of the epithelium leads to increased permeability, with resulting surfactant inhibition.

Gross and Narine[37] were the first to show that conversion of active into nonactive surfactant subfractions depends on cyclic changes in surface area in vitro. To maintain an adequate pool of functional surfactant subfraction in the air spaces in vivo, it is necessary to maintain a balance among secretion, uptake, and clearance of the active and nonactive surfactant subfractions.[38] In vivo studies by Veldhuizen and colleagues[39,40] in rabbits attributed the surfactant conversion to a change in alveolar surface area associated with mechanical ventilation. These investigators found that changing the respiratory rate did not affect the rate of conversion, but conversion of surfactant subfractions depended on tidal volume and time.[40]

## CLINICAL INVESTIGATIONS OF EXOGENOUS SURFACTANT IN ACUTE RESPIRATORY DISTRESS SYNDROME

For treatment of ARDS, a high concentration of surfactant is required to overcome the inhibitory effect of plasma components. This was first postulated by Lachmann[26] after treating the first adult patient, and it was later confirmed by the results of Gregory and associates[41] from a randomized pilot study in 59 patients with ARDS of different causes. In the latter study, four different dosing strategies were tested, and the results showed that maximum improvement in oxygenation, minimum ventilatory requirements, and the lowest mortality rate were obtained by using four doses of 100 mg/kg of a natural surfactant (total amount, 400 mg/kg). Walmrath and colleagues[42] reported an impressive acute improvement of arterial oxygenation in response to bronchoscopic application of a large quantity of natural surfactant (300 mg/kg) in 10 adult patients with severe ARDS and sepsis. In half of their patients, a second dose (200 mg/kg) was required within 24 hours to achieve a prolonged effect on gas exchange.

In contrast to these results, Anzueto and associates[43] demonstrated that administration of aerosolized artificial surfactant had no effect on mortality and lung function in a multicenter, randomized placebo-controlled trial in 725 patients with sepsis-induced ARDS. The authors speculated that one of the reasons for the lack of response could be that less than 25 mg surfactant/kg body weight was actually delivered into the lungs as a result of the method of administration, which is only one 16th of the dosage used by Gregory and colleagues.[43]

Kesecioglu and colleagues[44] determined the efficacy and safety of intratracheal instillation of a natural porcine surfactant (HL 10) in patients with ALI or ARDS in a prospective, randomized, multicenter, open-label, phase II study in Europe. Patients were randomized to receive standard therapy in addition to surfactant (n = 22) or standard therapy alone (n = 14). Dosage was from 200 mg phospholipids/kg ideal body weight (up to four doses in case of relapse). Efficacy variables were changes in the ratio of arterial oxygen tension to inspired fraction of oxygen ($PaO_2/FiO_2$), length of hospital stay, and 28-day mortality. Measures of oxygenation, duration of ventilation, and length of stay in the intensive care unit did not differ significantly between the two groups. However, 28-day mortality in the surfactant-treated group was 2 out of 22 (9%) versus 6 out of 14 (43%) in the control group ($P = .036$). Based on these promising results, these investigators concluded that surfactant therapy improved survival significantly, and a phase III trial has started.

Spragg and co-workers[45] published the results of a phase I/II trial in North America of a recombinant SP-C–based surfactant (Venticute) as treatment for ARDS. Patients were prospectively randomized to receive either standard therapy or standard therapy in addition to one or two doses of exogenous surfactant given four times over 24 hours. Surfactant administration was well tolerated. No significant benefit was associated with surfactant treatment. BAL fluid of treated patients at 48 hours reflected the presence of exogenous surfactant components but did not show evidence of improved surface tension–lowering function. However, interleukin-6 concentrations were significantly lower than control group values, consistent with an anti-inflammatory treatment effect. The presence of exogenous surfactant was not detected in BAL fluid obtained at 120 hours.[45] Future studies could rationally employ larger surfactant doses and a more prolonged dosing schedule. Data from this latter study have been used in the design of two phase III studies.

Preliminary reports available from the North American (n = 224) and European-South African (n = 224) studies, using a dose of 200 mg/kg phospholipids, showed significant improvements in oxygenation in both surfactant-treated groups compared with controls.[46] However, there were no differences in ventilator-free days or survival rates between the treatment groups and controls for either study. Nonetheless, post hoc analyses of the overall database did reveal that patients with ARDS secondary to direct insults such as pneumonia or aspiration (n = 154) had a lower mortality rate than their respective control groups (38.5% versus 25.9% in the North American study and 39.0% versus 25.5% in the European-South African study; not significant).[46] Taken together, this experience suggests that future studies could rationally be designed to employ higher doses of surfactant or a longer treatment period in specific patient populations.

Moller and colleagues[47] published data from a multicenter trial of surfactant with standardized treatment (n = 20) versus standard care (n = 15) in children with severe ARDS.[19] The primary end point was $PaO_2/FiO_2$ at 48 hours, and secondary end points were as follows: $PaO_2/FiO_2$ at 2, 4, 12, and 24 hours; survival; survival without rescue; and days on ventilator. Children received 100 mg/kg of natural bovine surfactant (Alveofact), and a second similar dose was given in case of relapse. A higher $PaO_2/FiO_2$ ratio was observed in the surfactant-treated group 2 hours after the first dose; at 48 hours, there was a trend toward a higher $PaO_2/FiO_2$ ratio.[47] The rate of rescue therapy was significantly lower in the surfactant-treated group. A significant difference in

$PaO_2/FiO_2$ in favor of surfactant at 48 hours was found in the subgroup with an initial $PaO_2/FiO_2$ ratio higher than 65 and in patients without pneumonia. These investigators concluded that surfactant therapy in severe ARDS improves oxygenation immediately after administration. This improvement is sustained only in the subgroup of patients without pneumonia and in those with an initial $PaO_2/FiO_2$ ratio higher than 65.

Gregory and colleagues[48] showed additional information on bronchopulmonary segmental lavage in 22 patients with ARDS who were treated with Surfaxin (synthetic surfactant) following up on the results of Wisell and associates.[49] Increasing concentrations of Surfaxin were administered: 22.8 g (n = 5), 34.2 g (n = 6), 57 g (n = 6), and 61 g (n = 5) of phospholipids. The primary end points were safety and tolerability. Mortality, ventilator-free days, and number of patients alive and free of mechanical ventilation were secondary outcome parameters. Patients receiving the higher doses of phospholipids had zero mortality. In total, 67% of the patients receiving the high-phospholipid dose of 57 g were alive and free of mechanical ventilation at day 28, and 100% of the patients receiving 61 g of phospholipids were alive and free of mechanical ventilation at day 28. The safety review committee determined that the procedure was generally safe and tolerable and that it was appropriate to proceed to the second part of the study, to evaluate the safety and preliminary efficacy of Surfaxin versus standard of care. The primary end point is the number of patients alive and free of mechanical ventilation at the end of day 28.[48]

The positive results of two preliminary pilot studies led to a multicenter trial of Calfactant (a natural surfactant containing high levels of SP-B) compared with placebo in 153 infants, children, and adolescents with respiratory failure from ALI.[50] Calfactant administration early in the course of pediatric acute respiratory failure resulted in acute improvement in oxygenation and was associated with significant lower mortality. The primary outcome variable, ventilator-free days, was not significantly different among the groups. There was no difference in long-term complications.

## POTENTIAL FACTORS AFFECTING SURFACTANT RESPONSIVENESS

An important aspect of surfactant response is the time at which surfactant is given. In a model of acid aspiration, we[51] showed that respiratory failure could be prevented when exogenous surfactant was given before deterioration of lung function (i.e., within 10 minutes after acid aspiration), whereas after development of respiratory failure, exogenous surfactant served only to prevent further deterioration of lung function but did not restore gas exchange. In the model of repeated saline BAL, Ito and associates,[52] and later our group,[53] demonstrated that exogenous surfactant at an early stage of lung injury resulted in sustained improvement of lung function, whereas lung function deteriorated when surfactant was given at a relatively late time point in lung injury, as a result of an increased amount of protein.

Rasaiah and co-workers[54] investigated the effect of early treatment with surfactant in mice with abdominal sepsis by cecal ligation. Administering exogenous surfactant at the time of surgery did not affect lung mechanics or interleukin-6 levels in either the cecal ligation–treated or sham groups at 18 hours. However, the animals that underwent cecal ligation and that received surfactant had a lower mortality than their non–surfactant-treated counterparts.[54] Mechanical ventilation in the nontreated animals induced severe lung impairment, whereas treatment with surfactant prevented this condition.[54] Therefore, it is expected that early treatment of patients with ARDS may require smaller amounts of exogenous surfactant, and the outcome results will probably be better.

The optimal method to deliver exogenous surfactant in adults is not yet known. Possibilities include aerosol delivery, continuous infusion, BAL, or bolus administration. The last method has been used in most animal studies, clinical case reports, and neonates with RDS.[8,9] The advantage of this method of instillation is that it is rapid and can deliver the large quantities of surfactant that are necessary, especially in ARDS, to overcome the inhibitory effects of the serum proteins present in the alveoli. Van der Bleek and colleagues[55] also demonstrated that the distribution of endotracheal instilled surfactant is more homogeneous after a large bolus than after a smaller one. This finding was confirmed by Segerer and colleagues,[56] who demonstrated homogeneous pulmonary surfactant distribution after bolus instillation, whereas distribution after slow tracheal infusion of exogenous surfactant was extremely uneven. In the latter study, the distribution of surfactant was closely related to its effect on pulmonary gas exchange.[56] Results from studies in premature animals showed that administration of surfactant directly after birth gives a more homogeneous distribution than in animals ventilated before treatment.[57] Instillation of surfactant into lungs filled with intrapulmonary fluid could be compared with instillation of a very large bolus of surfactant into sick lungs. Therefore, one may speculate that one has to fill up at least the total dead space of the lungs with surfactant suspension for a more even distribution. The disadvantage of the bolus instillation technique is the relatively large amount of fluid that has to be instilled. However, Gilliard and associates[58] demonstrated that the volume of fluid in which surfactant is administered is rapidly absorbed; 30 minutes after surfactant instillation, there was no significant difference between the lung weights of animals with lung injury that received 5 mL and those of animals receiving 50 mL of surfactant suspension. Thus, results of studies in which exogenous bolus instillation shows heterogeneous distribution may be explained by too small an amount of fluid in each single bolus.[58–60]

In addition, exogenous surfactant delivered as an aerosol has been investigated.[59,60] The rationale is that, with this method of instillation, a smaller volume of liquid will be instilled into the lungs at one time and distribution will be more homogeneous. In two different animal models, Lewis and colleagues[59,60] demonstrated that the distribution pattern was more homogeneous after aerosolized surfactant administration. However, these investigators found that tracheally instilled surfactant was superior to aerosolized surfactant in improving blood gases, whereas there was no difference in improvement of lung mechanics. These researchers suggested that "the low quantities of aerosolized surfactant deposited in the lungs limited the physiologic responses." In this study, only $6.1\pm2.2\%$ of the total aerosolized surfactant was recovered in the peripheral lung tissue, whereas after bolus instillation, $51\pm2\%$ of the instilled surfactant was recovered.[60] These investigators concluded the following: "a disadvantage of aerosolized surfactant administration is the relatively long time period required to administer significant quantities of exogenous surfactant due to the inefficiencies of aerosol deposition." Moreover, aerosolized surfactant could not be considered cost effective because large quantities of surfactant are required. The same group of investigators also showed that it was impossible to improve gas exchange after aerosolized surfactant in a nonuniform pattern of lung injury.[61] In this study, the less injured areas of the lung received relatively more surfactant than the severely injured areas. These researchers concluded that "one should be cautious in administering aerosolized surfactant to patients with ARDS who have nonuniform infiltrates on chest radiograph," but this a contradiction because ARDS-affected lungs are always injured in a nonuniform way.[62]

An alternative approach to administer surfactant is by BAL. We[63] showed that BAL with a diluted surfactant suspension (3.3 mg/mL, 30 mL/kg) was as effective as high-bolus administration (200 mg/kg) to improve gas exchange in a model of acid aspiration. In BAL-treated rabbits, Balaraman and associates[64] demonstrated that the effectiveness of a synthetic surfactant, which has not been shown to be highly effective in various animal models,[65,66] was enhanced by administering the surfactant by means of a lavage procedure compared with normal bolus administration. Further, Enhorning[67] suggested that saline lavage could also be used to reduce the protein content intra-alveolarly, which would be beneficial in the treatment of ARDS. This idea was investigated by Kobayashi and associates,[68] who demonstrated that a relatively low dose of exogenous surfactant (75 mg/kg) could improve gas exchange only after intra-alveolar edema was removed by BAL with saline in rabbits with severe respiratory failure resulting from acid aspiration. However, BAL with saline also removes the endogenous surfactant and leads to further deterioration of pulmonary function.[69] Therefore, we[53] performed BAL with a diluted surfactant suspension before surfactant therapy and showed that this combination was the optimal treatment regimen compared with the alternatives in a model of severe respiratory failure.

Various surfactant preparations are already available on the market and have been used successfully in worldwide clinical trials in neonates with RDS.[9] In BAL-treated rats, we[19] compared eight clinically used surfactants under standardized conditions. We confirmed the previous results of several animal studies,[65,66] as well as studies in neonates with RDS,[70,71] that the natural surfactant preparations, which contain the hydrophobic peptides SP-B and SP-C, are more effective in improving lung function immediately after instillation than the artificial surfactant preparations without surfactant proteins. In the same study,[19] we showed that the effect of surfactants on oxygenation was, in general, dose dependent, and we found marked differences in response pattern among the natural surfactants, especially when positive end-expiratory pressure was reduced at the end of the study protocol.

Several experimental studies have shown that the ventilator pattern strongly influences exogenous surfactant efficacy.[72–77] Froese and associates[74] demonstrated that, in BAL-treated rabbits, the effect of exogenous surfactant on arterial oxygenation remained stable only in combination with high-frequency oscillatory ventilation (HFOV) at high lung volume and not with HFOV at low lung volume or with conventional mechanical ventilation (CMV) at high or low lung volume. High lung volume means that lungs are actively opened (reexpanded) and are then kept expanded by using relative high mean airway pressures.[76] These results are in contrast to our findings,[77] in which surfactant therapy in combination with HFOV was not superior to CMV in increasing lung function or in reducing lung injury in BAL-treated rabbits. Further, it has been shown that HFOV also has a beneficial effect on exogenous surfactant composition by reducing the conversion of exogenously administered surfactant into small aggregate (nonactive) forms.[74] This finding has been attributed to the small alveolar volume changes with HFOV. However, we have shown that this can also be obtained with CMV by using small pressure amplitudes and high end-expiratory pressures.[78]

## FUTURE DEVELOPMENTS

Currently, exogenous surfactant therapy in adults with ARDS has failed to demonstrate any beneficial effect on outcome of either mortality or ventilator-free days. In neonates with RDS, surfactant therapy has proven to be efficacious, and in pediatric patients with ARDS, exogenous surfactant has reduced morbidity and mortality. Why are the results so different between adult and pediatric patients with ARDS? It has become clear that several factors may influence the surfactant response, such as timing of administration, composition or dose of surfactant, technique of instillation, and applied ventilation strategies. Future research should focus on these factors before one can conclude that exogenous surfactant has no place in the treatment of ALI/ARDS.

With further evidence that surfactant may play a role in host defense, therapeutic strategies aimed at preventing progressive lung dysfunction in various lung diseases can be developed. Finally, the expansive properties of pulmonary surfactant suggest that exogenous surfactant could be exploited as a carrier for drugs to the alveolar compartment of the lung.[79] Although each agent with its mode of action in the alveolar space and the lung interstitium could be considered for this route of administration, antimicrobial agents are the focus of interest.

## REFERENCES

1. Von Neergaard K: Neue Auffassungen über einen Grund-begriff der Atemmechanik. Z Ges Exp Med 1929;66:373–394.
2. Macklin CC: The pulmonary alveolar mucoid film and the pneumocytes. Lancet 1954;2:1099–1104.
3. Pattle RE: Properties, function, and origin of the alveolar lining layer. Nature 1955;175:1125–1126.
4. Clements JA: Surface tension of lung extracts. Proc Soc Exp Biol Med 1957;95:170–172.
5. Avery ME, Mead J: Surface properties in relation to atelectasis and hyaline membrane disease. Am J Dis Child 1959;97:517–523.
6. Fujiwara T, Maeta H, Chida S, et al: Artificial surfactant therapy in hyaline-membrane disease. Lancet 1980;1:55–59.
7. Segerer H, Obladen M: Surfactant substitution treatment of neonatal respiratory distress syndrome. Pediatr Rev 1990;5:67–82.
8. Jobe AH: Pulmonary surfactant therapy. N Engl J Med 1993;328:861–868.
9. Lewis JF, Jobe AH: Surfactant and the adult respiratory distress syndrome. Am Rev Respir Dis 1993;147:218–233.
10. Holm BA, Matalon S: Role of pulmonary surfactant in the development and treatment of adult respiratory distress syndrome. Anesth Analg 1989;69:805–818.
11. Lachmann B, Danzmann E: Acute respiratory distress syndrome. In Robertson B, van Golde LMG, Batenburg JJ (eds): Pulmonary Surfactant. Amsterdam: Elsevier, 1984, pp 505–548.
12. Brogden KA: Changes in pulmonary surfactant during bacterial pneumonia. Antonie van Leeuwenhoek 1991;59:215–223.
13. Johansson J, Curstedt T, Robertson B: The proteins of the surfactant system. Eur Respir J 1994;7:372–391.
14. Verbrugge SJ, Lachmann B: Mechanisms of ventilation-induced lung injury: Physiological rationale to prevent it. Monaldi Arch Chest Dis 1999;54:22–37.
15. Lewis JF, Veldhuizen R: The role of exogenous surfactant in the treatment of acute lung injury. Annu Rev Physiol 2003;65:613–642.
16. Lachmann B, Winsel K, Reutgen H: Der Anti-Atelektase-Faktor der Lunge I. Z Erkr Atm 1972;137:267–287.
17. Rozendaal BAWM van, Golde LMG van, Haagsman HP: Localization and functions of SP-A and SP-D at mucosal surfaces. Pediatr Pathol Mol Med 2001;20:319–339.
18. Notter R: Lung surfactants: Basic science and clinical applications. In Lenfant C (ed): Lung Biology in Health and Disease. New York: Marcel Dekker, 2000, pp 305–308.
19. Gommers D, Van't Veen A, Verbrugge SJC, Lachmann B: Comparison of eight surfactant preparations on improvement of blood gases in lung-lavaged rats. Appl Cardiopulm Pathophysiol 1998;7:95–102.
20. De Pasquale CG, Arnolda LF, Doyle IR, et al: Prolonged alveolocapillary barrier damage after acute cardiogenic pulmonary edema. Crit Care Med 2003;31:1060–1067.
21. Wang Z, Schwan AL, Lairson LL, et al: Surface activity of a synthetic lung surfactant containing a phospholipase-resistant phosphonolipid analog of dipalmitoyl phosphatidylcholine. Am J Physiol 2003;285:L550–L559.
22. Diemel RV, Snel MM, Golde LM van, et al: Effects of cholesterol on surface activity and surface topography of spread surfactant films. Biochemistry 2002;41:15007–15016.
23. Ashbaugh DG, Bigelow DB, Petty TL, Levine BE: Acute respiratory distress in adults. Lancet 1967;2:319–323.
24. Bernard GR, Artigas A, Brigham KL, et al: The consensus committee: Report of the American-European consensus conference on ARDS: Definitions, mechanisms, relevant outcomes and clinical trial coordination. Intensive Care Med 1994;20:225–232.
25. Seeger W, Günther A, Walmrath HD, et al: Alveolar surfactant and adult respiratory distress syndrome. Clin Invest 1993;71:177–190.
26. Lachmann B: The role of pulmonary surfactant in the pathogenesis and therapy of ARDS. In Vincent JL (ed): Update in Intensive Care and Emergency Medicine. Berlin: Springer-Verlag, 1987, pp 123–134.
27. Spragg RG, Gilliard N, Richman P, et al: The adult respiratory distress syndrome: Clinical aspects relevant to surfactant supplementation. In Robertson B, Golde LMG van, Batenburg JJ (eds): Pulmonary Surfactant. Amsterdam: Elsevier, 1992, pp 685–703.
28. Veldhuizen RAW, McCaig LA, Akino T, Lewis JF: Pulmonary surfactant subfractions in patients with the acute respiratory distress syndrome. Am J Respir Crit Care Med 1995;152:1867–1871.
29. Hallman M, Spragg R, Harrell JH, et al: Evidence of lung function abnormality in respiratory failure: Study of bronchoalveolar lavage phospholipids, surface activity phospholipase activity, and plasma myoinositol. J Clin Invest 1982;70:673–683.
30. Pison U, Seeger W, Buchorn R, et al: Surfactant abnormalities in patients with respiratory failure after multiple trauma. Am Rev Respir Dis 1989;140:1033–1039.
31. Veldhuizen RAW, McCaig LA, Akino T, Lewis JF: Pulmonary surfactant subfractions in patients with the acute respiratory

distress syndrome. Am J Respir Crit Care Med 1995;152: 1867–1871.

32. Gregory TJ, Longmore WJ, Moxley MA, et al: Surfactant chemical composition and biophysical activity in acute respiratory distress syndrome. J Clin Invest 1991;88:1976–1981.

33. Verbrugge SJC, Böhm SH, Gommers D, et al: Surfactant impairment after mechanical ventilation with large alveolar surface area changes and effects of positive end-expiratory pressure. Br J Anaesth 1998;80:360–364.

34. Greenfield LJ, Ebert PA, Benson DW: Effect of positive pressure ventilation on surface tension properties of lung extracts. Anaesthesia 1964;25:312–316.

35. Bos JAH, Lachmann B: Effects of artificial ventilation on surfactant function. In Rügheimer E (ed): New Aspects of Respiratory Failure. Berlin: Springer-Verlag, 1992, pp 194–208.

36. Nilsson R, Grossmann G, Robertson B: Lung surfactant and the pathogenesis of neonatal bronchiolar lesions induced by artificial ventilation. Pediatr Res 1978;12:249–255.

37. Gross NJ, Narine KR: Surfactant subtypes of mice: Metabolic relationship and conversion in vitro. J Appl Physiol 1989;66:414–421.

38. Magoon MW, Wright JR, Baritussio A, et al: Subfractions of lung surfactant: Implications for metabolism and surface activity. Biochim Biophys Acta 1983;750:18–31.

39. Ito Y, Veldhuizen RAW, Yao LJ, et al: Ventilation strategies affect surfactant aggregate conversion in acute lung injury. Am J Respir Crit Care Med 1997;155:493–499.

40. Veldhuizen RAW, Marcou J, Yao LJ, et al: Alveolar surfactant aggregate conversion in ventilated normal and injured rabbits. Am J Physiol 1996;270:L152–L158.

41. Gregory TJ, Steinberg KP, Spragg R, et al: Bovine surfactant therapy for patients with acute respiratory distress syndrome. Am J Respir Crit Care Med 1997;155;1309–1315.

42. Walmrath D, Gunther A, Ghofrani HA, et al: Bronchoscopic surfactant administration in patients with severe adult respiratory distress syndrome and sepsis. Am J Respir Crit Care Med 1996;154:57–62.

43. Anzueto A, Baughmann RP, Guntupalli KK, et al: Aerosolized surfactant in adults with sepsis-induced acute respiratory distress syndrome N Engl J Med 1996;334:1417–1421.

44. Kesecioglu J, Schultz MJ, Lundberg D, et al: Treatment of acute lung injury (ALI/ARDS) with surfactant. Am J Respir Crit Care Med 2001;163:A819.

45. Spragg RG, Lewis JF, Wurst W, et al: Treatment of acute respiratory distress syndrome with recombinant surfactant protein C surfactant. Am J Respir Crit Care Med 2003;167:1562–1566.

46. Lewis JF, Brackenbury A: Role of exogenous surfactant in acute lung injury. Crit Care Med 2003;31:S324–S328.

47. Moller JC, Schaible T, Roll C, et al: Surfactant ARDS Study Group. Treatment with bovine surfactant in severe acute respiratory distress syndrome in children: A randomized multicenter study. Intensive Care Med 2003;29:437–446.

48. Gregory TJ, Hite RD, Hicklin G, et al: Dose escalation study of Surfaxin delivered via bronchopulmonary segmental lavage (BPSL) in patients with ARDS. Am J Respir Crit Care Med 2003;167:A178.

49. Wiswell TE, Smith RM, Katz LB, et al: Bronchopulmonary segmental lavage with Surfaxin (KL[4]-surfactant) for acute respiratory distress syndrome. Am J Respir Crit Care Med 1999;160:1188–1195.

50. Wilson DF, Thomas NJ, Markovitz BP, et al: Effect of exogenous surfactant (Calfactant) in pediatric acute lung injury. JAMA 2005;293:470–476.

51. Eijking EP, Gommers D, So KL, et al: Prevention of respiratory failure after hydrochloric acid aspiration by intratracheal surfactant instillation in rats. Anesth Analg 1993;76:472–477.

52. Ito Y, Goffin J, Veldhuizen R, et al: Timing of exogenous surfactant administration in a rabbit model of acute lung injury. J Appl Physiol 1996;80:1357–1364.

53. Gommers D, Eijking EP, So KL, et al: Bronchoalveolar lavage with a diluted surfactant suspension prior to surfactant instillation improves the effectiveness of surfactant therapy in experimental acute respiratory distress syndrome (ARDS). Intensive Care Med 1998;24:494–500.

54. Rasaiah VP, Malloy JL, Lewis JF, Veldhuizen RA: Early surfactant administration protects against lung dysfunction in a mouse model of ARDS. Am J Physiol 2003;284: L783–L790.

55. van der Bleek J, Plötz FB, van Overbeek M, et al: Distribution of exogenous surfactant in rabbits with severe respiratory failure: The effect of volume. Pediatr Res 1993;34:154–158.

56. Segerer H, van Gelder W, Angenent FWM, et al: Pulmonary distribution and efficacy of exogenous surfactant in lung-lavaged rabbits. Pediatr Res 1993;34:490–494.

57. Jobe A, Ikegami M, Jacobs H, Jones S: Surfactant and pulmonary blood flow distributions following treatment of premature lambs with natural surfactant. J Clin Invest 1984;73:848–856.

58. Gilliard N, Richman PM, Merritt A, Spragg RG: Effect of volume and dose on the pulmonary distribution of exogenous surfactant administered to normal rabbits or to rabbits with oleic acid lung injury. Am Rev Respir Dis 1990;141:743–747.

59. Lewis JF, Ikegami M, Higuchi R, et al: Nebulized vs. instilled exogenous surfactant in an adult lung injury model. J Appl Physiol 1991;71:1270–1276.

60. Lewis JF, Tabor B, Ikegami M, et al: Lung function and surfactant distribution in saline-lavaged sheep given instilled vs. nebulized surfactant. J Appl Physiol 1993;74:1256–1264.

61. Lewis JF, Ikegami M, Jobe AH, Absolom D: Physiologic responses and distribution of aerosolized surfactant (Survanta) in a nonuniform pattern of lung injury. Am Rev Respir Dis 1993;147:1364–1370.

62. Gattinoni L, D'Andrea L, Pelosi P, et al: Regional effects and mechanism of positive end-expiratory pressure in early adult respiratory distress syndrome. JAMA 1993;269:2122–2127.

63. Eijking EP, Gommers D, So KL, et al: Surfactant treatment of respiratory failure induced by hydrochloric acid aspiration in rats. Anesthesiology 1993;78:1145–1151.

64. Balaraman V, Sood SL, Finn KC, et al: Physiologic response and lung distribution of lavage versus bolus Exosurf in piglets with acute lung injury. Am J Respir Crit Care Med 1996;153: 1838–1843.

65. Cummings JJ, Holm BA, Hudak ML, et al: A controlled clinical comparison of four different surfactant preparations in surfactant-deficient preterm lambs. Am Rev Respir Dis 1992;145:999–1004.

66. Häfner D, Beume R, Kilian U, et al: Dose-response comparisons of five lung surfactant factor (LSF) preparations in an animal model of adult respiratory distress syndrome (ARDS). Br J Pharmacol 1995;115:451–458.

67. Enhorning G: Surfactant replacement therapy in adult respiratory distress syndrome. Am Rev Respir Dis 1989;140:281–283.

68. Kobayashi T, Ganzuka M, Tanigushi J, et al: Lung lavage and surfactant replacement for hydrochloric acid aspiration in rabbits. Acta Anaesthesiol Scand 1990;34:216–221.

69. Lachmann B, Robertson B, Vogel J: In vivo lung lavage as an experimental model of the respiratory distress syndrome. Acta Anaesthesiol Scand 1980;24:231–236.

70. Soll RF, Vermont-Oxford Neonatal Network: A multicenter, randomized trial comparing synthetic surfactant with modified bovine surfactant extract in the treatment of neonatal respiratory distress syndrome. Pediatrics 1996;97:1–6.

71. Hudak ML, Farrell EE, Rosenberg AA, et al: A multicenter randomized, masked comparison trial of natural versus synthetic surfactant for the treatment of respiratory distress syndrome. J Pediatr 1996;128:396–406.

72. Kobayashi T, Kataoka H, Ueda T, et al: Effects of surfactant supplement and end-expiratory pressure in lung-lavaged rabbits. J Appl Physiol 1984;57:995–1001.

73. Rider ED, Jobe AH, Ikegami M, Sun B: Different ventilation strategies alter surfactant responses in preterm rabbits. J Appl Physiol 1992;73:2089–2096.

74. Froese AB, McCulloch PR, Sugiura M, et al: Optimizing alveolar expansion prolongs the effectiveness of exogenous surfactant therapy in the adult rabbit. Am Rev Respir Dis 1993;148:569–577.

75. Ito Y, Manwell SEE, Kerr CL, et al: Effects of ventilation strategies on the efficacy of exogenous surfactant therapy in a rabbit model of acute lung injury. Am J Respir Crit Care Med 1998;157:149–155.

76. McCulloch PR, Forkert PG, Froese AB: Lung volume maintenance prevents lung injury during high frequency oscillatory ventilation in surfactant-deficient rabbits. Am Rev Respir Dis 1988;137:1185–1192.

77. Gommers D, Hartog A, Schnabel R, et al: Surfactant therapy in combination with high frequency oscillatory ventilation is not superior to conventional mechanical ventilation in reducing lung injury in lung-lavaged rabbits. Eur Respir J 1999;14:738–744.

78. Verbrugge SJC, Gommers D, Lachmann B: Conventional ventilation modes with small pressure amplitudes and high positive end-expiratory pressure levels optimize surfactant therapy. Crit Care Med 1999;27:2724–2728.

79. Gommers D, Van't Veen A, Lachmann B: Usefulness of a combination of exogenous surfactant with inhaled nitric oxide or antibiotics to improve lung function in acute respiratory failure. J Jpn Med Soc Biol Interface 1996; 27:5–9.

# CHAPTER 13

# Diffusion and Mechanical Ventilation

Hervé Guénard

Pulmonary function tests are usually performed in patients with chronic respiratory diseases, with the objective of providing individualized therapy. The Acute Respiratory Distress Syndrome (ARDS) Network trial demonstrated the major influence of mechanical ventilation on ARDS prognosis and further highlighted the importance of the mechanical properties of the respiratory system in acute disease. Some mechanical ventilators now allow the measurement of the quasistatic compliance of the respiratory system and thus provide a unique opportunity to individualize mechanical ventilation in the intensive care unit according to specific patients' needs. At present, pulmonary function testing in mechanically ventilated patients is restricted to oxygenation determination. Inasmuch as both an ongoing process (e.g., acute injury) and mechanical ventilation may affect the components of diffusion and resulting oxygenation in complex ways, bedside diffusion testing constitutes an optimal way to tailor mechanical ventilation to each patient's requirements.

This chapter details the physical processes involved in lung diffusion and emphasizes the physiologic components that may be affected by both respiratory diseases and mechanical ventilation. Diffusion measurement is the only available test that may directly assess impairment of the vascular bed, which is an independent prognostic factor in ARDS.[1]

Gases in the lung move according to two physical processes. In the first process, the pressure applied to fluid pushes all the gases in one direction (i.e., the force moving the gas mixture is outside it); this is bulk flow or convective flow. In the second process, the gases move inside a fluid, liquid or gaseous, according to their gradients of partial pressures (i.e., the driving forces are in the gas mixture); this flow is diffusive. Both types of flow can combine to enhance or reduce the transport of a given gas.

Flow of respiratory gases (i.e., oxygen [$O_2$] and carbon dioxide [$CO_2$]) in the body is either convective or diffusive. Both types of flow may occur at the transition between the two processes, such as within the lung in the distal airways. In the deep lung, the speed of convective flow slows sufficiently to become negligible compared with diffusive flow. Therefore, $O_2$ reaches the membrane by diffusion, the same process by which $CO_2$ leaves the alveoli. The transport of gases through the membrane is mostly diffusive because the membrane is in the form of a gel; the liquid in the interstitium is thought to have negligible convection.

In capillary blood, close to the endothelium, plasma is variably stirred. An unstirred layer with thickness dependent on blood flow can be present, and the same applies to red blood cells. Thus, $O_2$ has to diffuse through these layers and through the red cell membrane before reacting rapidly with hemoglobin (Hb). $CO_2$, which is less reactive with Hb but is stored in bicarbonate form mainly in the red blood cells, follows a reverse path.

The systemic circulation brings both these gases to the periphery by convection. $O_2$ crosses the capillary walls in tissues by diffusion attracted by the lower $O_2$ partial pressure. A cascade of morphologic structures is traversed: interstitial liquid, cellular membrane, protoplasm, and mitochondrial membrane. $CO_2$ production in the peripheral cells maintains a high partial pressure that drives a diffusive process toward the capillary. It is then mostly transformed into bicarbonate and is transported by convection to the heart and lung.

Diseases may alter each step in the transfer of $O_2$ and $CO_2$ from the atmosphere to the cells or back.

This chapter focuses on lung diffusion alterations while acknowledging that the transfers of both gases are serial processes; therefore, these transport processes may be limited at every step in the chain. Separating diffusion from convection processes is often simplistic in complex disorders.

Several factors must be considered when following the step-by-step transport of $O_2$ in the lung, as described earlier: (1) diffusion alterations in the gas phase and the possibility to enhance or reduce the diffusivity of gases by changing either the inspired mixture or the pattern of ventilation; (2) alterations in the membrane structure, which are common in many diseases; and (3) lung microcirculation alterations either in specific vascular diseases such as pulmonary emboli or associated with many other pulmonary diseases.

Although tests of diffusivity of gases within the lung are used routinely in conscious patients, such is not the case in patients who are receiving mechanical ventilation. Fast, reliable, and simple tests are needed to provide information on gas lung transfer. As new advances are made in this field, progress will be expected.

## DIFFUSION IN THE GAS PHASE OF THE LUNG

The total area of the airways greatly increases with the generation of bronchi. Morphologically, this increase is usually compared to a trumpet or, more accurately, to a pinhole because the section surface of the alveoli is approximately 300,000-fold that of the trachea. The flow velocity (v) in a given generation is the ratio of total flow ($\dot{V}$) to the section surface (S): $\dot{V}/S$. At rest, mean flow is on the order of $10^{-4}$ m³/second, S in the trachea is approximately $3 \cdot 10^{-4}$/m², and v in meters per second is $10^{-4}/3 \cdot 10^{-4}$ (i.e., 0.3 m/second). Reaching the alveoli, this velocity would be 300,000-fold less (i.e., 1 μm/second). Therefore, diffusivity becomes increasingly predominant from one generation to another of greater order. The section surface increases with lung volume, that is, an increase in lung volume decreases flow velocity. Flow in the upper airways and in the first generations of bronchi follows a convective turbulent pattern. Even the trachea and the bronchi, which are tubular, do not allow the establishment of true laminar flow as these tubes are too small in diameter length.

At each generation, dichotomies create eddies supplying the turbulent pattern. The flow is more laminar in peripheral airways, owing to the decrease in flow speed with the increasing total cross section near the alveoli. These physical processes are schematically shown in Figure 13.1.

One model, developed by Paiva,[2] focuses on the transition between molecular diffusion and convective flow, whereas other models have focused on intra-airway transport.[3] The efficiency of gas transport in the lung is a function of the position of both the diffusion front (Fig. 13.1A) and the turbulent/laminar front (Fig. 13.1B). A shift of these fronts toward the alveoli enhances gas exchange, as intended by the different techniques used in mechanical ventilation without the help of high driving pressure. High instantaneous flow would indeed move both fronts toward the alveoli; however, this approach would require more driving pressure to push gas into the lung. Because mechanical distension of the lung increases the accumulated cross section of the bronchial tree, the high level of positive end-expiratory pressure (PEEP) often used to keep open some lung regions would have the drawback of reducing flow velocity in the deep lung and of moving the diffusive front toward the mouth. For instance, in dogs ventilated at high frequency, $CO_2$ elimination was greater when lung volume was reduced by compression of the thorax with slight external positive pressure.[4] Inversely, constant flow ventilation, in which a catheter delivers a constant flow of gas into the trachea with no thoracic motion, moves the diffusion front toward the mouth (see Fig. 13.1A) and induces hypercapnia, with arterial oxygenation dependent on the fraction of $O_2$ in inspired gas ($FIO_2$).[5] Owing to the high flow, the other front should move deeper into the lung (see Fig. 13.1B, on the *left*); however, this movement is extremely sensitive to the position

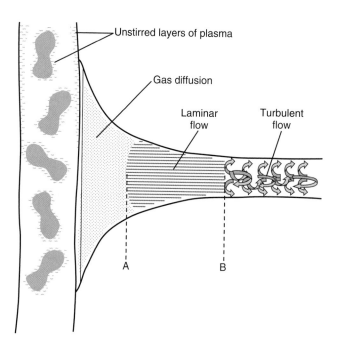

**Figure 13.1** These schematic drawings show that the efficiency of gas transport in the lung is a function of the position of both the diffusion front *(A)* and the turbulent/laminar front *(B)*.

of the catheter in the airway and thus leads to great heterogeneity in the distribution of convective flow.[6,7]

Heart motion may add convective flow (cardiogenic mixing) to gas diffusion in the lungs. Apart from constant flow ventilation, the effectiveness of cardiogenic mixing in enhancing the diffusive transport of the gases at the periphery of the lung in patients is unknown. Pericarditis, which dampens the transmission of these movements, is known to decrease the partial arterial pressure of $O_2$ ($PaO_2$) in some experimental conditions.[8] Cardiogenic mixing may increase $O_2$ transport only during hypoventilation.[9] Another experimental study suggested that long-term conventional ventilation reduces the efficiency of cardiac mixing, likely through a decrease in lung compliance.[10]

The ease with which a gas (e.g., $O_2$) is transported by molecular diffusion is quantified by its conductance, which is a function of the gradient of $O_2$ along its pathway from the distal airways to the alveoli and the binary coefficient of diffusion of $O_2$ in the other gases, mainly nitrogen ($N_2$). One application of this theoretic approach is the use of helium (He) instead of $N_2$, for two reasons: (1) the binary diffusion coefficient of $O_2$ in He is 2.5-fold that in $N_2$[11] (thus affecting diffusion); (2) the specific weight of He is seven times less than that of $N_2$, and its kinematic viscosity is seven times that of $N_2$ (thus affecting the work of breathing).

$He/O_2$ (heliox) breathing has been used successfully to ventilate infants with respiratory distress syndrome of prematurity.[12] Compared with nitrox (air with added $O_2$), heliox improved ventilation efficiency, increased the $PaO_2/FiO_2$ ratio, and decreased the duration of intubation. However, the mechanism of the improvement did not rely on improved diffusivity of $O_2$ in He, but rather on the decrease in the inspiratory pressure needed to ventilate the infants. In healthy adults, heliox breathing has been shown to reduce carbon monoxide (CO) transfer by 20% to 30%[13] and to induce slight hypoxemia.[14] Indeed, the positive effect of the increase in diffusivity of $O_2$ in heliox is reduced by the shift of the transition front between convective and diffusive flows within the airways toward the mouth (see the right shift in Fig. 13.1$A$). This shift increases the path length for diffusion in the gas phase and induces slight hypoxemia in healthy persons. As a result of its molecular weight and its viscosity, heliox favors the development of laminar flow, which needs less of a pressure drop for a given flow than does turbulent flow (see the right shift in Fig. 13.1$B$). For a given ventilation regimen, heliox needs less driving pressure than nitrox, and for a given pressure, more ventilation is delivered with heliox. In patients with chronic obstructive pulmonary disease (COPD), heliox breathing did not change the distributions of ventilation and perfusion, as assessed by the inert gas method (parallel heterogeneity), but it did induce a diffusion defect for $O_2$, likely by increasing the pathway for this process.[15]

In adult patients, heliox may have a role in the treatment of acute asthma or COPD, although this indication is debated.[16–18] High-frequency jet ventilation (HFJV) with heliox allows better ventilation in models of experimental stenosis.[19] In patients undergoing laryngoscopy, HFJV with heliox provided a greater ventilatory flow rate than did nitrox, with other variables kept constant.[20] Heliox has been used successfully with high percussive ventilation in the management of severe respiratory failure.[21] Heliox is less efficient than a mixture of sulfur hexafluoride ($SF_6$) and $O_2$ mixture in eliminating $CO_2$ during constant flow ventilation. The likely reason is the shift of the diffusion and convection fronts toward the mouth with heliox because the $SF_6/O_2$ mixture, owing to its high density, moves the convection front toward the alveoli.[22]

Diffusion in the gas phase may also play a role in impaired gas exchange in patients with severe lung distension. In patients with COPD, the alveoli and distal bronchi are enlarged by the disease and are distended by trapping; patients with severe acute asthma may also have severe lung distension. Investigators have shown that patients with lung distension increase their single-breath CO transfer with the duration of apnea, whereas the expired fraction of the inert gas, usually He, used to measure the lung volume, decreases with time.[23,24] These findings suggest that the pathway for diffusion in the gas phase is increased in these patients. The implications of reduced diffusion in the gas phase in patients receiving mechanical ventilation have not been studied. Increasing lung volume by increasing end-expiratory pressure allows recruitment of a previously poorly ventilated area and reduction of the heterogeneities of ventilation and ventilation-perfusion ratios. In one study, weaning from mechanical ventilation in patients with COPD had deleterious effects on these ratios, and pressure support ventilation restored better distributions.[25] However, the induced distension impeded the diffusion of $O_2$ in the gas phase, an effect hidden by the improvement in ventilation distribution.

Diffusion hypoxia is a transient effect observed when a patient ventilated with a relatively soluble anesthetic gas such as nitrous oxide ($N_2O$) is switched to air breathing. This transient hypoxia results from the difference in the kinetics of the transfer of $N_2O$ and $N_2$.[26,27] This effect can be avoided by using less soluble anaesthetic gas such as xenon.[28,29] The occurrence of diffusion hypoxia in patients is debated.[30]

## ALVEOLOCAPILLARY MEMBRANE TRANSFER

### Alveolar Membrane

This membrane is irregular in thickness, sometimes a fraction of a micrometer, but nearly 10 μm in other places and covered by pneumocytes. The membrane is frequently appended to a capillary when it is not simply separating two alveoli. Therefore, the membrane is an effective site for gas exchange either with blood or between alveoli. The membrane is made of three thin sheets: the epithelial sheet derived from type 1 epithelial cells, the fused basement membrane, and the endothelial cells. It ranges in thickness between 0.1 and 0.2 μm at the thinnest part to less than 1 μm at the thickest part.[31] The transfer of gases through the membrane (Dm) depends on its surface (S) and is inversely related to its mean thickness (μm):

$$Dm = d \times S/\mu m$$

where d is the diffusivity of the gas, dependent on its solubility in plasma and its molecular weight. Increasing lung volume would change neither the surface nor the thickness if the alveoli act like bellows, and the transfer of gases would be unaffected. If alveoli behave like elastic balloons or bubbles, an increase in lung volume would increase the surface of the membrane and would reduce its thickness, with a resulting increase in gas transfer. The folding of the membrane modulates its thickness and thus prevents its thickening during expiration.[32]

All experimental studies agree that the transfer of test gases (nitric oxide [NO] and CO) increases with lung volume; however, the correlation between theoretic and measured transfer is not always strong. The model of the bubble suggests an increase in surface and a decrease in thickness that can easily be calculated, leading to a power (4/3) relationship between the transfer (TL) and lung volume (V), as follows: $TL = kV^{4/3}$.[33] The experimental relationships give power coefficients that are widely scattered around 1 among subjects and studies,[34] findings likely suggesting that the thickness of the membrane does not decrease during inflation. These relationships were obtained in healthy subjects who voluntarily altered their lung volumes. It is unlikely that the same would hold true in patients intubated and ventilated with positive pressure, because a large increase in lung volume would require high positive pressure, which could induce collapse of some lung capillaries and reduce the effective surface of exchange. This point is discussed later.

Diseases may reduce lung surface or increase membrane thickness. Reduction in the exchanging lung surface can result from pulmonary resection, alveolar destruction in COPD or chronic restrictive lung diseases, and alveolar flooding or filling by secretions, cells, and proteins. Increased membrane lung thickness can be caused by an increase in capillary pressure, an increase in permeability of the membrane, and any inflammatory process. The increase in pulmonary capillary pressure is common in heart failure and leads to membrane thickening.

In acute conditions, the thickening is reversible as a result of interstitial edema, whereas in chronic conditions, thickening is caused by remodeling of the membrane.[35] Ultrafiltration, which reduces lung fluid overload, does not increase the membrane component of CO transfer.[36] An increase in capillary pressure is also common in ARDS,[37] in addition to the increase in membrane permeability. Alterations in both surface and thickness can be present, as in ARDS. Conventional mechanical ventilation with PEEP should, by increasing lung volume, increase the surface and reduce the thickness of the membrane. Dm measurement in mechanically ventilated patients is of interest in ascertaining optimal ventilatory settings and therapies. NO transfer measurement would be sufficient for this purpose, as described later.

## Capillaries

Diffusion of gases from the gas phase within the capillaries is important and complex. Blood within the capillary is a heterogeneous fluid in which gases are partly transported in plasma by convection; however, two unstirred layers of plasma adhering to the endothelium and the red blood cells thicken the diffusive path for $O_2$, which also includes the red blood cell membrane. The effects of these layers on diffusion have been analyzed theoretically.[38] However, there is no way at present to determine the impact of these concepts in patients.

The volume of blood in capillaries (Vc) is a key point in the diffusion process because it is a determinant, with cardiac blood flow (Q̇c), of the transit time (τT) of the blood in the lung: τT = Vc/Q̇c. Because Vc is approximately 80 mL and Q̇c is 80 mL/second at rest, τT is approximately 1 second in healthy young adults; however, it decreases with age as Vc decreases. Some elderly persons have Vc as low as 10 mL, and with normal cardiac blood flow of 80 mL/second, τT would be 120 milliseconds, a threshold value for the $O_2$ equilibration between alveolar and blood. In this condition, any slight decrease in Vc or increase in Q̇c would induce hypoxemia. Alterations in Vc or Q̇c resulting from diseases or therapies would have the same effect.

Another key point in the diffusion process within the capillary is the capacitance (β) of the gas in the blood; this is also called the effective solubility of the gas in blood. β is proportional to the slope of the concentration versus gas partial pressure curve. The flow of gas that is transferred through the membrane is a function of $\beta \times \dot{Q}$, where Q̇ is the blood flow.[39] If the gas has a high capacitance, the membrane should have a conductance for that gas (Dm) that is high enough to allow the transfer; if not, the transfer will be limited. Conversely, if the gas has low solubility, its transfer will depend greatly on blood flow. A gas with a high $Dm/(\beta \times \dot{Q})$ ratio has a limited perfusion transfer, whereas a gas with a low ratio has a membrane-limited transfer. Therefore, gases with very high capacitance, such as NO, have transfers limited by the membrane.

$O_2$ has either a low capacitance at normal arterial partial pressure or a high capacitance at low partial pressure; in the latter case, the membrane can limit the $O_2$ transfer. This limitation is modulated by blood flow. In healthy persons, the membrane limitation appears only in conditions of deep hypoxia with increased cardiac blood flow, such as while climbing to the summit of Mount Everest. In patients, this phenomenon can be present even at rest. Patients with interstitial pulmonary fibrosis have a low $Dm/\dot{Q}$ ratio,[40] which, associated with hypoxemia, is a condition of membrane limitation for $O_2$ transfer.

### Determinants of Blood Capillary Volume

Three main factors determine Vc: the number of lung capillaries, the mean transmural capillary pressure (mtPcap), and the distensibility or recruitment of the capillaries.

### Capillary Number

Vc increases during childhood and reaches a maximum in young adulthood, a finding suggesting an increase in the density of capillaries during growth associated with an increase in lung volume.[41] However, nothing seems to be known about their change in length. In elderly persons, this density decreases slowly to the 60s and then more markedly thereafter. Because Vc is dependent on lung volume, use of the ratio of Vc to alveolar volume (Vc/Va) is more appropriate. The heterogeneity of human Vc/Va is large; for a given age, the ratio of one standard deviation to the mean (variation coefficient) is approximately 20% in an unselected healthy population of 315 adults (personal data). Among factors explaining this heterogeneity is the physical activity status of the individual. Training exercise is known to increase both Dm and Vc in patients with chronic heart failure.[42] Hypoxemia is known to induce angiogenesis in the lung either experimentally in rats[43] or in persons living at high altitude.[44] The deleterious effect of 100% $O_2$ breathing is well known,[45] whereas the effect of prolonged exposure to hyperoxic mixture on Vc is not. A morphologic study of lung in rats that had undergone lobe resection and had received 70% $O_2$ for 14 days suggested few alterations in postresectional lung growth but an increase in density of type 2 cells, fibroblasts, and neutrophils, along with interstitial edema.[46]

### Mean Transmural Capillary Pressure

mtPcap is the difference between mean capillary pressure (mPcap) and mean alveolar pressure (mPa). Positive continuous breathing pressure reduces the transmural pressure, and the reverse is true for negative pressure breathing. Human mPcap can be estimated using a simple bicompartmental model of the lung.[47] The model includes an arterial component serially feeding capillary-venous component. The fall in pressure at the tip of a catheter at the onset of occlusion of a small pulmonary artery allows one to calculate mPcap. This parameter depends on several hemodynamic factors: pressure and resistance up to the capillaries (i.e., mean pulmonary artery pressure [mPAP] and arterial resistance) and pressure and resistance down to the capillaries (i.e., wedge pressure and venous resistance). Unfortunately, mPcap is seldom measured because the procedure necessitates right-sided heart catheterization and repeated arterial occlusion maneuvers. mPcap is measured in the middle part of the lung. This pressure is different from one zone to another, and it increases from zone 1 to zone 3. The elevation in mPcap is a main determinant of an increase in Vc by recruitment or distension of capillaries. This increase is also a determinant of the filtration of fluid in the interstitium at the origin of pulmonary edema. An increase in mPAP elevates Vc when the mPAP rise is not the result of augmented pulmonary arterial resistance. In fact, patients with primary pulmonary hypertension have a low Vc, a finding suggesting that the increase in arterial resistance is relatively greater than that in mPAP.[48,49] An increase in cardiac blood flow in patients with normal arterial resistance elevates mPAP, mPcap, and Vc. All studies agree that physical activity induces an increase in mPAP and Vc, by means of elevated $\dot{Q}c$.

Recruitment and distensibility of capillaries are not easily distinguished. The opening of a previously closed capillary is a physiologic adaptation of muscle likely resulting from alterations in tissue oxygenation. Such alterations are unlikely within an alveolus filled with alveolar gas. Nevertheless, the videomicroscopic observations made by Baumgartner and colleagues[50] confirmed wide heterogeneity of perfusion of capillary segments within alveoli. Following a given increase in the perfusion pressure, recruitment appears different from one trial to another.

Lung capillaries are more distensible than capillaries in other parts of the body.[51] Distension, as recruitment, is an adaptation to the increase in capillary pressure. By increasing diameter and volume, resistance of the capillary is reduced, and tT is prolonged, thus giving more time for $O_2$ pressure in the blood to equilibrate with Pa. Distensibility of capillaries in patients is not yet measurable but can be estimated when changing either the inside capillary pressure (mPcap) or the Pa during breathing with positive or negative pressure. An easy way to increase mPcap is to change body position. Switching from the standing to the lying position removes the blood from the lower part of the body and increases all thoracic blood volumes including Vc. Breathing briefly under negative continuous pressure increases Vc by elevating transmural capillary pressure. When a person is standing, the blood moves downward, and Vc decreases. Positive pressure breathing reduces transmural capillary pressure and thus reduces Vc. This finding was shown in nine healthy subjects undergoing intermittent positive pressure ventilation. A 10-hPa PEEP regimen reduced Vc from a mean of 82 to 56 mL (i.e., 68%).[52] Similar PEEP in dogs reduced the elimination of CO.[53] The effect of positive or negative pressure breathing was related to the value of the applied pressure. The distensibility and compressibility of capillaries appeared scattered among individuals. Unfortunately, no measurement of mtPcap seems to have been made under these conditions. The effect of negative or positive pressure breathing on transcapillary pulmonary pressure is therefore unclear. If the changes in PA do not modify mPcap, then mtPcap would change by the same amount. Continuous positive pressure of 10 hPa would reduce mtPcap by 10 hPa, and, conversely, continuous negative pressure of 10 hPa would increase mtPcap by 10 hPa. This seems unlikely, at least for 10-hPa positive pressure, because the normal mPcap value is close to 10 hPa (26), and most capillaries would collapse (50% if the distribution of the capillary pressure in the lung was symmetric). As already mentioned, the Vc decrease with 10-hPa positive pressure is 32% in healthy persons. In patients with ARDS, mPcap is increased, and its value is independent under PEEP of 5 to 16 hPa.[37] Although distensibility and recruitment of capillaries cannot be measured accurately, the previously described techniques have demonstrated that some diseases are associated with low capillary distensibility (diabetes,[54] primary pulmonary artery hypertension[55]). Furthermore, the pressure-induced effects of mechanical ventilation on capillaries should be kept in mind.

### Physiopathology of Lung Capillaries

Capillaries may be reduced in number. In healthy persons, Vc decreases with age, mainly after the 60s.[56] When compared with young adults, healthy persons in their 50s have a slight reduction of capillary density, as estimated by morphometry.[57] This reduction can be accentuated by diseases such as emphysema, in which alveolar and capillary surfaces are decreased,[58] or interstitial lung disease, in which microvascular lesions are common.[59]

Pulmonary resection induces an acute reduction in Vc that can be compensated for by the increase of distensibility and the recruitment; if not, a rise in capillary pressure and pulmonary edema may result. In the long term, postresectional growth can compensate, at least in part, for the loss of Vc (and Dm).

Capillaries can be collapsed by the occlusion of arteries, as in pulmonary emboli, although the back pressure from the left atria can be sufficient to keep open capillaries in the dependent region of the lung. The consensus in the literature is that Dm is more greatly reduced than Vc, as a secondary consequence of occlusion on the alveolar membrane.[49] The interpretation of the alteration in Dm and Vc in these patients is not easy because, after thromboendarterectomy, there is a discrepancy between the improvement in hemodynamic parameters and the lack of increase in Dm and Vc.[60] Another cause of capillary collapse is the fall in blood pressure, as happens physiologically in the less dependent part of the lung during diastole. In disease, a fall in mPAP decreases pressure in all capillaries. Experimental massive hemorrhage reduced Vc to 43% in rats.[61]

Obstruction of capillaries by thrombosis is common in patients with COPD,[62] and it reduces both Dm and Vc. Platelets aggregate in the microcirculation of the lung in patients with COPD,[63] as well as in patients with asthma.[64]

## MEASUREMENTS OF CARBON MONOXIDE AND NITRIC OXIDE TRANSFERS

The lung transfer of a gas x (or lung conductivity or conductance) is defined by the ratio of its flow through the lung ($\dot{V}x$) to the difference between the PA and the mPcap of this gas ($PAx - mPcapx$):

$$TLx = \dot{V}x / (PAx - mPcapx)$$

mPcap of $O_2$ or $CO_2$ is not easy to calculate because both pressures are present in the venous blood, and the instantaneous values of these pressures vary along the capillary. For CO, which is nearly absent from blood (HbCO is usually <1% in nonsmokers), or for NO, which has an even lower endogenous pressure, the assumption that their mPcap is nil when these gases are breathed shortly at low fraction can be made because of their high affinities for Hb. For these gases, except for CO in smokers, $TLx = \dot{V}x / PAx$. In smokers or patients intoxicated by CO, the back pressure of CO in the venous blood has to be taken into account.

The fixation of CO or NO to Hb is characterized by specific conductivity ($\theta x$, flow of the gas fixed by 1 g of Hb by a unit of partial pressure); the greater the conductivity is, the greater the volume of gas will be transferred. In vitro, the values of conductivity are as follows, in decreasing order: $NO > CO_2 > O_2 > CO$.[38] In vivo, owing to the convective transport of red blood cells, the values are greater; NO conductivity can be assumed to be infinite, whereas CO has limited conductivity inversely dependent on $PO_2$.[65] When CO and NO are inspired, their fractions in the alveolar space decrease according to their uptake by the blood through the membrane. Because the conductivity of NO for the blood is infinite, the only limitation for the transfer of this gas is the membrane conductivity for NO (DmNO). The transfer of NO is therefore equal to DmNO.[66] The interpretation of a fall in TLNO in a patient is straightforward: reduction in Dm (i.e., reduction in surface of the membrane or increase in membrane thickness). The transfer of CO is more complex because CO has finite conductivity in the blood. The flow of CO combined with Hb for a unit of partial pressure depends on the Hb mass within the capillaries, which, in turn, depends on the concentration of Hb and on Vc ([Hb] × Vc × θCO). Patients with anemia have less transfer than patients with polycythemia, other variables being equal. CO passes through the lung following two conductivities (or conductances): that of the membrane DmCO and that of the blood: [Hb] × Vc × θCO. Because conductivities are in series, the total conductivity or transfer mainly depends on the smaller of the two. The relationship with total conductivity or TL is as follows:

$$1/TLCO = 1/Dm + 1/([Hb] \times Vc \times \theta CO).$$

In this equation, θCO depends on mPcapO$_2$, which has to be taken in account in patients (see later).

Calculations of Dm and Vc can be made by one of two methods. The first is to measure the transfer twice, once using a relatively low fraction of O$_2$ and then using a higher fraction, which should give a lower value of transfer. This method is not applicable to patients receiving a high fraction of O$_2$ to maintain normal blood oxygenation. By knowing mPmcapO$_2$ in both situations, the respective values of θCO can be deduced. A set of two equations is obtained to allow calculations of Dm and Vc. The second method, which is more recent,[66] comprises one step, in which both CO and NO transfers are measured simultaneously. DmNO and DmCO are related by a coefficient that is close to 2: DmCO = DmNO/2.[13] Introducing this DmCO value in the TLCO equation allows one to calculate the Vc.

mPcapO$_2$ can be calculated using either TLCO or TLNO. Whatever the method used, calculations of O$_2$ consumption (V̇O$_2$) and of the PA of O$_2$ (PAO$_2$) are necessary:

$$PaO_2 - mPcapO_2 = \dot{V}O_2 / K \times TL$$

where K is a coefficient (1.23 for CO and 0.64 for NO[67]).

## Methods of Measurement

The transfer of CO can be measured using several methods: single breath, rebreathing, and steady state. Measurements can be made under normal circumstances with a given fraction of O$_2$ and with a hyperoxygenated mixture allowing the calculation of Dm and Vc.[65] The drawback of this technique is the need to repeat the transfer measurements with two different mixtures; this

process is time consuming and reduces the accuracy of the results.[24] The NO transfer measurement, which depends only on Dm,[66] can be combined with the CO transfer measurement to allow the calculation of Vc and Dm in one step.[24,68] All these methods can putatively be adapted to a mechanically ventilated patient if the ventilator can accommodate the required maneuvers.

### Single-Breath Method

The single-breath method[65] is well adapted to patients who are ventilating spontaneously even with support. A deep exhalation is first requested, then a rapid inspiration, followed by apnea that should be, according to the recommendations, 8 seconds long, and finally a rapid expiration, during which a sample of gas is taken. The main problem for the patient is to hold his or her breath for 8 seconds. Because the transfer of gases is time dependent only in patients with distension, 8 seconds of apnea are useless in patients without distension, and 4 seconds would be sufficient. In patients with distension, even 8 seconds of apnea are not sufficient to obtain a stable value of the transfer. Therefore, in the current practice of managing patients with severe or acute diseases, a 4-second duration for apnea can be chosen, as long as one keeps in mind that the results may incorporate a possible limitation of the transfer in the gas phase. Any reduction in lung distension increases the transfer.

Single-breath measurement in an intubated, mechanically ventilated patient requires a forced inflation of the test mixture with positive pressure, apnea maintained at positive pressure (~20 hPa), and then a free expiration during which the alveolar gas is sampled. The positive pressure alters the transfer of CO by reducing Vc and then Dm.[69] This technique is therefore not adapted to intubated patients. However, it is useful in patients who are ventilated with extrathoracic negative pressure because intrathoracic pressure is normal in this condition.[70]

### Rebreathing Method

The rebreathing method[65] is easier to perform in patients who are mechanically ventilated. The basic principle is to allow the patient to rebreathe in a bag with a volume of gases of approximately 80% of the patient's vital capacity. The bag is in a box that can be ventilated by the ventilator. The patient can be ventilated either directly or through the box with the mixture contained in the bag. The mixture is composed of an inert gas (usually 10% He) to calculate lung volume, a tracer gas for the transfer (usually 0.3% CO), and O$_2$ at a fraction equivalent to that given to the patient. During 30 to 45 seconds, the patient rebreathes in this bag. The decrease in the CO fraction at each breath is measured. The calculation takes into account the fractions of CO at two times, t1 and t2, of the rebreathing period, the alveolar volume and the time difference. This method was adapted by Clark and associates[71] and MacNaughton and colleagues[52] to patients in intensive care. In these patients, the volume of the bag is reduced to 1 L, and the rebreathing duration is decreased to six cycles. The setting of the ventilator, including PEEP value, is kept constant during the rebreathing period. In patients with ARDS, the measurements of TLCO with two different fractions of $O_2$, allowing calculation of Vc and Dm, gave a true improvement in the understanding of the physiopathologic features of each patient. There was a straightforward relationship between Vc and the pulmonary vascular resistance as well as between oxygenation and functional residual capacity. Furthermore, the improvement in TLCO from day to day was a good prognostic sign.

## Steady-State Method

The steady-state method is not used in mechanically ventilated patients. The principle is to add the test gases to the inspired gas and to sample the alveolar gas at each expiration to measure the He and CO (or NO) fractions. Once the He fraction is stabilized, the steady state is reached, and the transfer can be calculated. The drawbacks of this method are its duration ($\geq 2$ minutes) and the fact that if repeated measurements are needed, the percentage of HbCO will rise and the back pressure of CO will need to be taken into account. The rebreathing method therefore seems to be the best method to use in intubated patients.

The three methods described previously for the measurement of CO transfer can be used simultaneously for NO transfer determinations. The transfer of NO is much faster than that of CO because the membrane conductance is twice that of CO and the blood conductance is infinite. The inspired concentration of NO is about 40 ppm, a thousand times that of endogenous NO. It could be less with the steady-state method and more with the rebreathing method, to keep a measurable concentration in the expired gas. The single-breath method with NO is increasingly used routinely even in severely ill patients, and it does not need fast-responding analyzers. Use of the other methods is limited by the necessity to analyze NO with a chemoluminescent fast analyzer, which is expensive. However, the steady-state method[72,73] and the rebreathing method[74] have been tested and validated with NO. Measuring the transfer of NO without CO transfer gives straightforward information on the state of the lung membrane, information that can be helpful to patients in critical care. This measurement can be performed repetitively because NO does not accumulate in the blood.

## CONCLUSION

Measuring NO or CO transfer provides helpful physiopathologic information on the membrane and lung capillaries. It may also contribute to the adjustment of ventilator settings and can, in some diseases, indicate prognosis.

The development of this field will thus be of interest to intensive care physicians.

## ACKNOWLEDGMENT

I want to thank C. Delclaux for his helpful comments and for revising the manuscript.

## REFERENCES

1. Brower RG, Lanken PN, MacIntyre N, et al: Higher versus lower positive end-expiratory pressures in patients with the acute respiratory distress syndrome. N Engl J Med 2004;22;351:327–336.
2. Paiva M: Theoretical studies of gas mixing in the lung. In Engel LA, Paiva M (eds): Gas Mixing and Distribution in the Lung. New York: Marcel Dekker, 1985, pp 221–285.
3. Slutsky ASZ, Kamm RD, Drazen JM: Alveolar ventilation at high frequencies using tidal volume smaller than the anatomical dead space. In Engel LA, Paiva M (eds): Gas Mixing and Distribution in the Lung. New York: Marcel Dekker, 1985, pp 137–176.
4. Baum M, Mutz N, Benzer H: Influence of end-expiratory lung volume on carbon dioxide elimination during high frequency ventilation in dogs. Br J Anaesth 1989;63(Suppl 1):53S–58S.
5. Breen PH, Sznajder JI, Morrison P, et al: Constant flow ventilation in anesthetized patients: Efficacy and safety. Anesth Analg 1986;65:1161–1169.
6. Venegas JG, Yamada Y, Hales CA: Contributions of diffusion jet flow and cardiac activity to regional ventilation in CFV. J Appl Physiol 1991;71:1540–1553.
7. Ingenito E, Kamm RD, Watson JW, Slutsky AS: A model of constant-flow ventilation in a dog lung. J Appl Physiol 1988;64:2150–2159.
8. Kelly SM, Brancatisano AP, Engel LA: Effect of cardiogenic gas mixing on arterial $O_2$ and $CO_2$ tensions during breath holding. J Appl Physiol 1987;62:1453–1459.
9. Slutsky AS, Khoo MC, Brown R: Simulation of gas transport due to cardiogenic oscillations. J Appl Physiol 1985;58:1331–1339.
10. Lichtwarck-Aschoff M, Suki B, Hedlund A, et al: Decreasing size of cardiogenic oscillations reflects decreasing compliance of the respiratory system during long-term ventilation. J Appl Physiol 2004;96:879–884.
11. Chang HK, Farhi LE: Ternary diffusion and effective diffusion coefficients in alveolar spaces. Respir Physiol 1980;40:269–279.
12. Elleau C, Galperine RI, Guenard H, Demarquez JL: Helium-oxygen mixture in respiratory distress syndrome: A double-blind study. J Pediatr 1993;122:132–136.
13. Guénard H, Chaussain M, Lebeau C: Respiratory gas exchange under normobaric helium-oxygen breathing at rest and during muscular exercise. Bull Eur Physiopathol Respir 1978;14:417–429.
14. Thiriet M, Douguet D, Bonnet JC, et al: The effect on gas mixing of a He-$O_2$ mixture in chronic obstructive lung diseases. Bull Eur Physiopathol Respir 1979,15:1053–1068.
15. Manier G, Guenard H, Castaing Y, Varene N: Inert gas study of heliox gas exchange in patients with COPD. Bull Eur Physiopathol Respir 1983;19:401–406.
16. Chevrolet JC: Helium mixtures in the intensive care unit. Crit Care 2001;5:179–181.

17. Burns SM: Ventilating patients with acute severe asthma: What do we really know? AACN Adv Crit Care 2006;17:186–193.

18. Tassaux D, Gainnier M, Battisti A, Jolliet P: Helium-oxygen decreases inspiratory effort and work of breathing during pressure support in intubated patients with chronic obstructive pulmonary disease. Intensive Care Med 2005;31:1501–1507.

19. Buczkowski PW, Fombon FN, Russell WC, Thompson JP: Effects of helium on high frequency jet ventilation in model of airway stenosis. Br J Anaesth 2005;95:701–705.

20. Cros AM, Guenard H, Boudey C: High-frequency jet ventilation with helium and oxygen (heliox) versus nitrogen and oxygen (nitrox). Anesthesiology 1988;69:417–419.

21. Stucki P, Scalfaro P, de Halleux Q, et al: Successful management of severe respiratory failure combining heliox with noninvasive high-frequency percussive ventilation. Crit Care Med 2002;30:692–694.

22. Luijendijk SC, van der Grinten CP: The ratio of the alveolar ventilations of $SF_6$ and He in patients with lung emphysema and in healthy subjects. Respir Physiol Neurobiol 2002;130:69–77.

23. Graham BL, Mink JT, Cotton DJ: Effect of breath-hold time on DLCO(SB) in patients with airway obstruction. J Appl Physiol 1985;58:1319–1325.

24. Moinard J, Guenard H: Determination of lung capillary blood volume and membrane diffusing capacity in patients with COLD using the NO-CO method. Eur Respir J 1990;3:318–322.

25. Ferrer M, Iglesia R, Roca J, et al: Pulmonary gas exchange response to weaning with pressure-support ventilation in exacerbated chronic obstructive pulmonary disease patients. Intensive Care Med 2002;28:1595–1599.

26. Einarsson S, Stenqvist O, Bengtsson A, et al: Nitrous oxide elimination and diffusion hypoxia during normo- and hypoventilation. Br J Anaesth 1993;71:189–193.

27. Einarsson S, Cerne A, Bengtsson A, et al: Should nitrous oxide be discontinued before desflurane after anaesthesia with desflurane/$N_2O$? Acta Anaesthesiol Scand 1997;41:1285–1291.

28. Calzia E, Stahl W, Handschuh T, et al: Continuous arterial $P(O_2)$ and $P(CO_2)$ measurements in swine during nitrous oxide and xenon elimination: Prevention of diffusion hypoxia. Anesthesiology 1999;90:829–834.

29. Hecker K, Baumert JH, Horn N, Rossaint R: Xenon, a modern anaesthesia gas. Minerva Anestesiol 2004;70:255–260.

30. Jeske AH, Whitmire CW, Freels C, Fuentes M: Noninvasive assessment of diffusion hypoxia following administration of nitrous oxide-oxygen. Anesth Prog 2004;51:10–13.

31. Weibel ER, Federspiel WJ, Fryder-Doffey F, et al: Morphometric model for pulmonary diffusing capacity. I. Membrane diffusing capacity. Respir Physiol 1993;93:125–149.

32. Lebecque P, Mwepu A, Veriter C, et al: Hysteresis of the alveolar capillary membrane in normal subjects. J Appl Physiol 1986;60:1442–1445.

33. Tsoukias NM, Wilson AF, George SC: Effect of alveolar volume and sequential filling on the diffusing capacity of the lungs. I. Theory. Respir Physiol 2000;20:231–249.

34. Stam H, Kreuzer FJ, Versprille A: Effect of lung volume and positional changes on pulmonary diffusing capacity and its components. J Appl Physiol 1991;71:1477–1488.

35. Guazzi M: Alveolar-capillary membrane dysfunction in heart failure: Evidence of a pathophysiologic role. Chest 2003;124:1090–1102.

36. Agostoni PG, Guazzi M, Bussotti M, et al: Lack of improvement of lung diffusing capacity following fluid withdrawal by ultrafiltration in chronic heart failure. J Am Coll Cardiol 2000;36:1600–1604.

37. Nunes S, Ruokonen E, Takala J: Pulmonary capillary pressures during the acute respiratory distress syndrome. Intensive Care Med 2003;29:2174–2179.

38. Chakraborty S, Balakotaiah V, Bidani A: Diffusing capacity reexamined: Relative roles of diffusion and chemical reaction in red cell uptake of $O_2$, CO, $CO_2$, and NO. J Appl Physiol 2004;97:2284–2302.

39. Kobayashi H, Pelster B, Piiper J, Scheid P: Diffusion and perfusion limitation in alveolar $O_2$ exchange: Shape of the blood $O_2$ equilibrium curve. Respir Physiol 1991;83:23–34.

40. Yamaguchi K, Mori M, Kawai A, et al: Inhomogeneities of ventilation and the diffusing capacity to perfusion in various chronic lung diseases. Am J Respir Crit Care Med 1997;156:86–93.

41. Rouatbi S, Ouahchi YF, Ben Salah C, et al: Facteurs physiologiques influençant le volume capillaire pulmonaire et la diffusion membranaire. Rev Mal Respir 2006;23:211–218.

42. Guazzi M, Reina G, Tumminello G, Guazzi MD: Improvement of alveolar-capillary membrane diffusing capacity with exercise training in chronic heart failure. J Appl Physiol 2004;97:1866–1873.

43. Howell K, Preston RJ, McLoughlin P: Chronic hypoxia causes angiogenesis in addition to remodelling in the adult rat pulmonary circulation. J Physiol (Lond) 2003;547:133–145.

44. De Bisschop C, Ajata A, Huez S, et al: Increase in lung capillary blood volume in native highlanders: Angiogenesis? Eur Respir J Suppl 50 2006;28:407s.

45. Harris JB, Chang LY, Crapo JD: Rat lung alveolar type I epithelial cell injury and response to hyperoxia. Am J Respir Cell Mol Biol 1991;4:115–125.

46. Cui DJ, Jafri A, Thet LA: Effect of 70% oxygen on postresectional lung growth in rats. J Toxicol Environ Health 1988;25:71–86.

47. Baconnier PF, Eberhard A, Grimbert FA: Theoretical analysis of occlusion techniques for measuring pulmonary capillary pressure. J Appl Physiol 1992;73:1351–1359.

48. Borland C, Cox Y, Higenbottam T: Reduction of pulmonary capillary blood volume in patients with severe unexplained pulmonary hypertension. Thorax 1996;51:855–856.

49. Steenhuis LH, Groen HJ, Koeter GH, van der Mark TW: Diffusion capacity and haemodynamics in primary and chronic thromboembolic pulmonary hypertension. Eur Respir J 2000;16:276–281.

50. Baumgartner WA Jr, Jaryszak EM, Peterson AJ, et al: Heterogeneous capillary recruitment among adjoining alveoli. J Appl Physiol 2003;5:469–476.

51. Glazier JB, Hughes JM, Maloney JE, West JB: Measurements of capillary dimensions and blood volume in rapidly frozen lungs. J Appl Physiol 1969;1:65–76.

52. MacNaughton PD, Morgan CJ, Denison DM, Evans TW: Measurement of carbon monoxide transfer and lung volume in ventilated subjects. Eur Respir J 1993;6:231–236.

53. Breen PH, Mazumdar B: How does positive end-expiratory pressure decrease $CO_2$ elimination from the lung? Respir Physiol 1996;103:233–242.

54. Fuso L, Cotroneo P, Basso S, et al: Postural variations of pulmonary diffusing capacity in insulin-dependent diabetes mellitus. Chest 1996;110:1009–1013.

55. Horn M, Hooper W, Brach B, et al: Postural changes in pulmonary blood flow in pulmonary hypertension: A noninvasive technique using ventilation-perfusion scans. Circulation 1982;66:621–626.

56. Georges R, Saumon G, Loiseau A: The relationship of age to pulmonary membrane conductance and capillary blood volume. Am Rev Respir Dis 1978;117:1069–1078.

57. Verbeken EK, Cauberghs M, Mertens I, et al: The senile lung: Comparison with normal and emphysematous lungs. I. Structural aspects. Chest 1992;101:793–799.

58. Vlahovic G, Russell ML, Mercer RR, Crapo JD: Cellular and connective tissue changes in alveolar septal walls in emphysema. Am J Respir Crit Care Med 1999;160:2086–2092.

59. Magro CM, Allen J, Pope-Harman A, et al: The role of microvascular injury in the evolution of idiopathic pulmonary fibrosis. Am J Clin Pathol 2003;119:556–567.

60. Bernstein RJ, Ford RL, Clausen JL, Moser KM: Membrane diffusion and capillary blood volume in chronic thromboembolic pulmonary hypertension. Chest 1996;110:1430–1436.

61. Vock R, Weibel ER: Massive hemorrhage causes changes in morphometric parameters of lung capillaries and concentration of leukocytes in microvasculature. Exp Lung Res 1993;19:559–577.

62. Voelkel NF, Cool CD: Pulmonary vascular involvement in chronic obstructive pulmonary disease. Eur Respir J Suppl 2003;46:28S–32S.

63. Ferroni P, Basili S, Martini F, et al: Soluble P-selectin as a marker of platelet hyperactivity in patients with chronic obstructive pulmonary disease. J Invest Med 2000;48:21–27.

64. Taytard A, Guenard H, Vuillemin L, et al: Platelet kinetics in stable atopic asthmatic patients. Am Rev Respir Dis 1986;134:983–985.

65. Hughes JM, Bates DV: Historical review: The carbon monoxide diffusing capacity (DLCO) and its membrane (DM) and red cell (Theta.Vc) components. Respir Physiol Neurobiol 2003;138:115–142.

66. Guénard H, Varene N, Vaida P: Determination of lung capillary blood volume and membrane diffusing capacity in man by the measurements of NO and CO transfer. Respir Physiol 1987;70:113–120.

67. Heller H, Schuster KD: Model analysis on alveolar-capillary $O_2$ equilibration during exercise. Nitric Oxide 2006;16:131–134.

68. Borland CD, Higenbottam TW: A simultaneous single breath measurement of pulmonary diffusing capacity with nitric oxide and carbon monoxide. Eur Respir J 1989;2:56–63.

69. Nijenhuis FC, Jansen JR, Versprille A: Components of carbon monoxide transfer at different alveolar volumes during mechanical ventilation in pigs. Clin Physiol 1997;17:225–236.

70. Asada M, Nakayama K, Kaneko K, et al: CO diffusing capacity during continuous negative extra-thoracic pressure [Japanese]. Masui 1991;40:1492–1494.

71. Clark EH, Jones HA, Hughes JM: Bedside rebreathing technique for measuring carbon-monoxide uptake by the lung. Lancet 1978;1:791–793.

72. Glénet SN, de Bisschop CM, Dridi R, Guénard HJ: Membrane conductance in trained and untrained subjects using either steady state or single breath measurements of NO transfer. Nitric Oxide 2006;25:199–208.

73. Borland C, Mist B, Zammit M, Vuylsteke A: Steady-state measurement of NO and CO lung diffusing capacity on moderate exercise in men. J Appl Physiol 2001;90:538–544.

74. Phansalkar AR, Hanson CM, Shakir AR, et al: Nitric oxide diffusing capacity and alveolar microvascular recruitment in sarcoidosis. Am J Respir Crit Care Med 2004;169:1034–1040.

# CHAPTER 14

# Acid-Base Balance and Kidney-Lung Interaction

Rinaldo Bellomo and John A. Kellum

When considering all the issues related to mechanical ventilation and its physiologic effects and the role of mechanical ventilation in patient management, the critical care physician is faced with several important pathophysiologic considerations that relate to acid-base control: How does mechanical ventilation affect acid-base balance? What is the role of mechanical ventilation in the control of acid-base balance? How does the effect of mechanical ventilation relate to that of the other major acid-base controlling organ, the kidney? How does function of the kidney (native or artificial), in turn, affect the requirements and specifications of mechanical ventilation?

Most clinicians are familiar with the paradigm that there is essentially *only* one way in which the lung affects acid-base balance: through its effect on the tension of carbon dioxide ($CO_2$) in plasma. By eliminating $CO_2$ through the act of ventilation, the lung controls the volatile component of the Henderson-Hasselbalch acid-base equation and thereby affects acid-base balance and pH. Accordingly, by choosing the settings of the ventilator, the clinician may influence acid-base balance either by allowing the patient to set its own ventilation (and arterial $CO_2$ tension [$PaCO_2$]) or by taking full control of it and thereby completely determining the patient's $PaCO_2$.

Similarly, most clinicians believe they have a reasonable understanding of how the kidney responds to changes in $PaCO_2$ generated by changes in mechanical or spontaneous ventilation. They believe in the paradigm that changes in the renal handling of bicarbonate ($HCO_3^-$) allow the kidney to either retain or lose $HCO_3^-$ in a way that is directed toward the reestablishment of acid-base balance and pH homeostasis. According to this paradigm, the accumulation of $CO_2$ (increased $PaCO_2$) in blood generates "renal $HCO_3^-$ retention" by the kidney that, in turn, acts as a counterweight to the acidifying effect of $CO_2$ and maintains pH within a narrow physiologic band. Similarly, the sufficiently prolonged maintenance of a low $PaCO_2$ increases the excretion of $HCO_3^-$ through the kidneys and induces a degree of counterbalancing acidosis, which also restores the pH to normal values. Within these paradigms, the lung and ventilation are known to be rapid in their responses and effects (seconds to minutes), and the renal adjustments are known to take place more slowly (hours to days).

Fewer critical care clinicians, however, are familiar with primary disorders of renal acid-base control and how such disorders can affect the need for adjustments in mechanical ventilation. Even fewer are familiar with the profound and variable acid-base effects that renal replacement therapy (RRT) techniques can induce in patients in intensive care units (ICUs) who are receiving mechanical ventilation. Furthermore, fewer still are familiar with the concept that the paradigms currently used to understand all the foregoing effects and interactions are being questioned by the emergence of a different paradigm, which represents a particularly powerful challenge to the conventional understanding of the regulation of serum $HCO_3^-$ concentration and to the mechanisms responsible for changes in the nonvolatile component of acid-base balance.

Given the foregoing considerations, in this chapter we explore the effects of mechanical ventilation on acid-base balance from the point of view of the kidney (native or artificial), the effect of kidney function (or dysfunction) on the nonvolatile component of acid-base balance, and the effect of the artificial kidney on acid-base physiology, as well as ways in which both native and artificial kidneys may affect ventilation. More important, however, we begin by reviewing some fundamental aspects of acid-base regulation. We present the conventional paradigm of acid-base balance control and compare such ideology to that proposed by a newer paradigm (the so-called Stewart approach). We then discuss many of the important implications of these two different approaches for our understanding of the pathophysiology of acid-base disorders during mechanical ventilation and renal disease and how they may assist us in understanding the mechanisms underlying kidney-lung interaction in the control of acid-base balance.

## HISTORY OF THE CONVENTIONAL ACID-BASE PARADIGM

To understand the two major paradigms currently offered to explain how acid-base balance is controlled by lung and kidney, clinicians need to understand some of the history of acid-base ideology. In the late 1800s, Arrhenius, a Swedish physicist, developed two chemical concepts important to acid-base physiology. The first was a new approach to the dissociation of chemical salts into electrolytes; for this work, Arrhenius almost failed his doctorate but was later awarded the Nobel Prize. The second concept was a new definition of an acid as a substance that, when added to a solution, increases the hydrogen ion (H$^+$) concentration. The next important development was the work of a Boston physician, Henderson, in the early 1900s. From in vitro work, Henderson rewrote the law of mass action equation for acid-base physiology to describe the role of weak acids in maintaining "neutrality regulation in the animal organism." The Henderson equation applies particularly to HCO$_3^-$ and carbonic acid (H$_2$CO$_3$), where k is a constant:

$$[H^+] = k \times [H_2CO_3]/[HCO_3^-]$$

Over the next 20 years, a new definition of acid was then developed by Bronstead, who stated that an acid is a substance that donates H$^+$ in solution. Bronstead noted that an Englishman, Lowry, had developed a similar definition. This became the Bronstead-Lowry definition, still the dominant definition of an acid. The operative and scientific superiority in the biologic field of this later definition of acid compared with that of Arrhenius remains unknown.

Sorensen, a chemist, made two further contributions. First, he developed the concept of taking the negative log to the base ten of the H$^+$ concentration, which he called pH. Second, he called chemicals that reduced pH changes in solutions "buffers," after the springs on the end of railway carriages. Hasselbalch, a physician-farmer, combined Sorensen's work with Henderson's to produce the Henderson-Hasselbalch equation:

$$pH = pKa + \log_{10} [HCO_3^-]/[H_2CO_3]$$

where pKa is the negative log of the dissociation constant.

Whether concepts such as buffers and the continued use of a logarithmic scale for changes in H$^+$ activity are useful or necessary in modern medicine remains doubtful.

Over the next 50 years, acid-base physiology centered on the Henderson-Hasselbalch equation, not because it provided an explanation for what happens in the body (it does not), but rather because it simplified a complex system and offered the ability to predict the value for one variable when the other two are known. Later, the P$CO_2$ was substituted for carbonic acid (the former became easier to measure). The nonvolatile, or metabolic, component was interpreted, although not proven, as being the result of the body's controlling plasma HCO$_3^-$ concentration. Acid-base physiology became simple: the lung controls CO$_2$, and the kidney regulates HCO$_3^-$. The two together rule pH. One difficulty in the clinical application of this paradigm was that changes in HCO$_3^-$ had to be interpreted while allowing for simultaneous changes in P$CO_2$. To deal with this problem, Schwartz and Relman, Boston physicians, produced "rules of thumb." The rules of thumb were equations to determine whether the simultaneous changes in HCO$_3^-$ and CO$_2$ were a single process, such as in metabolic acidosis with compensation, or mixed processes.

In the 1960s, Siggard-Anderson, a Danish physician, introduced base excess (BE) as a measure of metabolic acid-base status. The use of BE did not require calculating the rules of thumb. BE assumes a P$CO_2$ of 40 mm Hg and includes the plasma HCO$_3^-$ concentration in the calculation. The subsequent controversy between Boston and Copenhagen over the merits of the "rules of thumb" versus BE was known as "the great trans-Atlantic debate," and it continues to this day.

This conventional paradigm is extraordinarily simple: acid-base control is regulated by the two organs that control PaCO$_2$ and HCO$_3^-$. The lung controls PaCO$_2$, and the kidney controls HCO$_3^-$. If one organ malfunctions, the other compensates by acting to preserve a normal or near normal pH.

The seductiveness of such a system is great and lies in its simplicity. The naivete of believing that the human body, which controls all aspects of homeostasis through multiple complex systems, should make an exception in the case of acid-base physiology is intellectually almost unforgivable.

## NEW PARADIGM

In the late 1970s and early 1980s, in two articles and a book, Peter Stewart, a Canadian-American physiologist working at Brown University in Providence, Rhode Island, introduced a new approach to acid-base physiology and disorders.[1] While using $P_{CO_2}$, Stewart used two other variables, the strong-ion difference (SID) and the total concentration of weak acid ($A_{TOT}$), instead of $HCO_3^-$. Stewart based his work on several chemical principles, particularly electroneutrality, conservation of mass, and dissociation of electrolytes and water. Unfortunately for the ongoing debate, Stewart died in 1993.

The main principles of Stewart's approach are that three important independent factors control the acid-base status of a physiologic solution: $P_{CO_2}$, SID, and the $A_{TOT}$. The role of $CO_2$ controlled by the lungs is similar to that described by the Henderson-Hasselbalch approach. Strong ions are those ions that are completely dissociated in solution. The most important strong ions are sodium ($Na^+$) and chloride ($Cl^-$). The important factor in determining pH is the difference between the strong ions, rather than the absolute concentrations of the ions. As the SID falls, the dissociation of plasma water increases and the $H^+$ concentration increases. This approach is summarized in Figure 14.1. Lactate is treated as a strong ion because, with a pKa of 3.9, it is almost completely dissociated at pH 7.40. The major participating ions in the regulation of the SID are therefore several: NaCl, potassium, magnesium, calcium, lactate, sulfate, pyruvate, urate, and all other fully dissociated acids found in plasma in millimolar concentration. The pH control system is affected by multiple variables, not just two.

The most important weak acids in plasma are albumin, as shown by Figge and associates[2] using magnetic resonance technology, and, to a lesser extent, phosphate.

Stewart emphasized that the foregoing three independent factors must be considered simultaneously. These independent factors control dependent factors, which include $HCO_3^-$, hydroxyl ions, and $H^+$.

The source of $H^+$ in the Stewart approach is the dissociation of water molecules. Important underlying factors are the temperature-dependent dissociation constants of weak acids, including carbonic acid, and the dissociation constant of water. We consider this novel approach to be more useful clinically.

## DIFFERENCE BETWEEN THE TWO PARADIGMS

For several reasons, Stewart's work has provoked, and continues to provoke, strong adverse reaction from those committed to the Henderson-Hasselbalch approach. First, Stewart rejected $HCO_3^-$ as a vital controlling factor. Second, he emphasized the essential role of strong ions; he saw hydrochloric acid as acidifying not because it brings $H^+$ into a solution but because it brings a strong anion, $Cl^-$, without strong cations. The addition of $Cl^-$ decreases the SID, releases $H^+$ from water, and induces a decrease in pH. Stewart saw $NaHCO_3$ as alkalinizing, not because it provides $HCO_3^-$ (a buffer in conventional parlance) but because it increases the serum $Na^+$ concentration and thereby the SID, with the opposite effect of adding $Cl^-$. Third, Stewart rejected the notion of buffers and instead talked of weak acids. Fourth, he rejected pH in favor of a return to $H^+$ concentration. Last, he returned to the Arrhenius definition of an acid: a substance that, when added to a solution, increases the $H^+$ concentration. This definition accommodates both $CO_2$ and strong anions.

Not surprisingly, Stewart's ideology is anathema to those who believe in the conventional view. Nonetheless, many groups have continued Stewart's work in clinical applications, particularly in critical care, in exercise physiology, and in veterinary applications.

## APPLICATION OF THE TWO PARADIGMS TO LUNG AND KIDNEY FUNCTION

The conventional paradigm explains the function of the lung in terms of acid-base control as simply related to its ability to control $P_{aCO_2}$, the volatile component of the acid-base equation. If $P_{aCO_2}$ increases as a result of relative hypoventilation, then respiratory (*ventilatory* is a more appropriate term) acidosis will occur. If $P_{aCO_2}$ decreases consequent to relative hyperventilation, then respiratory (ventilatory) alkalosis will occur. In response

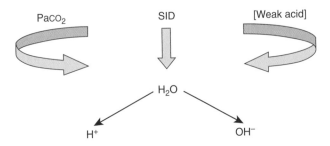

**Figure 14.1** Schematic representation of Stewart's regulation of acid-base balance. The source of hydrogen ions is plasma water dissociation. Its dissociation is dependent on three factors: carbon dioxide ($CO_2$), the total weak-acid concentration ($A_{TOT}$), and the strong-ion difference.

to these changes, which can be quite rapid and may or may not be sustained, the kidney reacts by either retaining or eliminating more $HCO_3^-$. This $HCO_3^-$ retention buffers the effect of $CO_2$ and restores pH toward normal. Although we have a reasonable understanding of how the respiratory center regulates ventilation and $CO_2$ removal or retention in response to changes in cerebrospinal fluid pH, we do not know how the kidney senses the need to alter its handling of acid-base control. A passive mechanism dependent on the tension of $CO_2$ in plasma is postulated but not proven. According to the conventional paradigm, all tubular cells secrete $H^+$ into the lumen. This secretion occurs as $CO_2$ is transformed into carbonic acid and is then dissociated into $HCO_3^-$ and $H^+$, which are then exchanged for $Na^+$ through a countertransport mechanism ($Na^+$ moves into the cell and $H^+$ into the lumen).

According to the Stewart approach, however, there is no countertransport mechanism. $Na^+$ is simply reabsorbed by energy-requiring mechanisms. As $Na^+$ shifts from the lumen (urine), the SID of urine falls, the dissociation of urine water increases, and $H^+$ is released, as measured for decades by micropipetting technology. Both paradigms acknowledge an $H^+$ concentration increase in urine and the movement of $Na^+$ from lumen to cell. However, they offer different mechanistic explanations. Neither approach can currently be proven right or wrong. As $Na^+$ is reabsorbed, it contributes to an increased SID in the body (alkalinizing effect). According to the conventional paradigm, as $H^+$ ions are excreted, $HCO_3^-$ ions are retained through a $CO_2$ shuttle, with the $CO_2$ generated in the lumen by the reaction of $HCO_3^-$ with $H^+$ and then leading to more $HCO_3^-$ generation inside the cell.

According to the Stewart approach, $HCO_3^-$ concentration changes as a dependent factor simply because the SID has changed: the shift in SID alters pH, which changes the state of the carbonic acid–$HCO_3^-$ system and decreases the amount of dissociated weak acid ($HCO_3^-$). As seen earlier, the conventional approach invokes an extraordinary series of steps. The new paradigm invokes only one: $Na^+$ movement from lumen to blood.

## QUANTIFICATION OF ACID-BASE DISORDERS

Although the understanding of the pathogenesis of an acid-base disorder is now quite different, not only does the traditional approach to quantifying an acid-base disorder still "work," but also it is entirely complementary to this physical chemical analysis. In fact, the standard BE (SBE) that can be used to quantify the amount of change in

SID has occurred from baseline with $CO_2$ and $A_{TOT}$ constant. The SBE can be thought of as the amount of change in the SID that is required in order to restore the pH to 7.40, given a $P_{CO_2}$ of 40 mm Hg (a negative SBE refers to the amount the SID must increase) and a normal $A_{TOT}$. This is because the SID is essentially equal to the buffer base described by Singer and Hastings, and BE quantifies the change in buffer base. SBE is theoretically superior to BE because the former has been "standardized" to account for the difference between $CO_2$ equilibration in vitro compared with in vivo. Although SBE is not strictly comparable to the change in SID because it deals with whole blood as opposed to plasma, the two are generally close enough for most clinical circumstances. Thus, SBE provides an estimate of the amount of strong anion that needs to be removed or strong cation that needs to be added to normalize the pH. For example, to change the SBE from −20 to −10 mEq/L by adding $NaHCO_3$, the serum $Na^+$ concentration would need to be increased by 10 mEq/L.

Schlichtig and co-workers described the changes in SBE that occur with acute and chronic disorders of $Pa_{CO_2}$. The SBE does not change with acute changes in $Pa_{CO_2}$. During chronic respiratory acidosis or alkalosis, the change in the SBE is equal to $0.4 \times (Pa_{CO_2} - 40)$. Similarly, the expected change $Pa_{CO_2}$ for a given abnormality in SBE is as follows: for acidosis, the decrease in $Pa_{CO_2}$ is equal to the change in SBE; for alkalosis, the increase in $Pa_{CO_2}$ is equal to $0.6 \times SBE$.

## ANION GAP

When the SID decreases, metabolic acidosis ensues. When this occurs as a result of increased $Cl^-$, the anion gap (AG), which is a measure of missing charge, does not change (so-called hyperchloremic acidosis). However, when other anions are present, the AG increases. Unfortunately, the accuracy of the AG is questionable in certain clinical situations, particularly in critically ill patients, who are frequently hypoalbuminemic and acidotic. In contrast, the strong-ion gap (SIG) is calculated from the SID, $A_{TOT}$, and $Pa_{CO_2}$, and it is thus sensitive to changes in albumin and phosphate. The SIG is positive when unmeasured anions outnumber unmeasured cations and negative when unmeasured cations outnumber unmeasured anions. Unexplained anions, and in some cases cations, have been found in the circulation of patients with a variety of diseases and in animals under experimental conditions. Normally, the SIG is zero, whereas the AG is 8 to 12 mEq/L. The AG is an estimate of the sum of SIG plus the dissociated form of $A_{TOT}$ ($A^-$). Thus, subtracting $A^-$ from the AG approximates the SIG. A convenient and reasonably accurate way to estimate A⁻ is to use the following formula:

$$\text{"Normal" AG} = 2 \text{ (albumin g/dL)} + 0.5 \text{ (phosphate mg/dL)}$$

Or, for international units:

$$\text{"Normal" AG} = 0.2 \text{ (albumin g/L)} + 1.5 \text{ (phosphate mmol/L)}$$

Figge and colleagues[3] showed that, in most critically ill patients, the "normal" AG can be estimated by using 2.5 times the albumin concentration in grams per deciliter (or 0.25 for albumin in grams per deciliter). However, if the serum phosphate concentration is significantly abnormal, this estimate will be inaccurate. Thus, *the AG must always be adjusted for the effect of hypoalbuminemia.* In a critically ill patient with an albumin concentration of 1.5 g/dL, a normal unadjusted AG gap can coexist with a lactate concentration of 6 mmol/L.

The origin of anions other than Cl⁻ varies depending on the population studied. Ketones, organic acids accumulating in renal failure, and toxins are important causes in appropriate patient groups. In critically ill patients, lactate is a particularly important cause. Lactate is a strong ion because at pH within the physiologic range, it is almost completely dissociated (i.e., the pK of lactate is 3.9; at a pH of 7.4, 3162 lactate ions are dissociated for every one that is not). Because the body can produce and dispose of lactate rapidly, lactate functions as one of the most dynamic components of the SID. Lactate therefore can produce significant acidemia. However, critically ill patients often have hyperlactatemia that is much greater than the amount of acidosis seen. Physical chemistry also allows us to understand how hyperlactatemia may exist without metabolic acidosis. First, acid is not "generated" apart from lactate through "unreversed adenosine triphosphate hydrolysis," as some investigators have suggested. Phosphate is a weak acid and does not contribute substantially to metabolic acidosis even under extreme circumstances. Furthermore, the H⁺ concentration is not determined by how much H⁺ is produced or removed from the plasma but rather by changes in one of the three independent variables (SID, $P_{CO_2}$, or $A_{TOT}$). Virtually anywhere in the body, pH is greater than 6.0, and lactate behaves as a strong ion. Its generation then decreases the SID and results in increased water dissociation and thus increased H⁺ concentration.

How then can the plasma lactate concentration be increased and the H⁺ concentration not? There are two possible answers. First, if lactate is added to the plasma, not as lactic acid but rather as the salt of a strong acid (i.e., Na⁺ lactate), there will be little change in the SID.

This is because a strong cation (Na⁺) is being added along with a strong anion. In fact, as lactate is then removed by metabolism and is transformed into $CO_2$ which is then exhaled, the remaining Na⁺ will increase the SID, and metabolic alkalosis will result. Hence it would be possible to give enough lactate to increase the plasma lactate concentration slightly without any major change in H⁺ concentration. However, the amount of exogenous lactate required would be very large. This is because normal metabolism results in the turnover of approximately 1500 to 4500 mmol/day of lactic acid. Thus, only very large amounts of lactate infused rapidly will result in appreciable increases in the plasma lactate concentration, or such changes may result from failure of lactate-metabolizing organs. The kidney is thought responsible for approximately 30% of the metabolism of lactate. In the setting of rapid lactate infusion (lactated Ringer's solution) or hemofiltration, mild acidosis may occur until the lactate is metabolized (usually within several minutes) (Fig. 14.2). A more important mechanism whereby hyperlactatemia exists without acidemia (or with less acidemia than expected) is when the SID is corrected by the elimination of another strong anion from the plasma, as demonstrated by Madias and colleagues.[4] In the setting of sustained lactic acidosis induced by lactic acid infusion, these investigators found that Cl⁻ moves out of the plasma space to normalize pH. Under these conditions, hyperlactatemia may persist, but BE may be normalized by compensatory mechanisms to restore the SID. Armed with these fundamental insights into the possible mechanisms for the regulation of

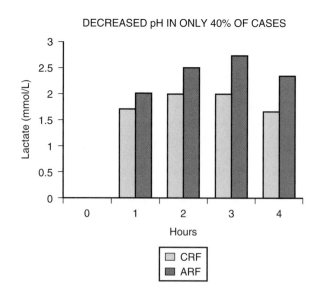

**Figure 14.2** Changes in lactate levels during hemofiltration with lactate-buffered fluid in patients with chronic renal failure (CRF) and acute renal failure (ARF). Although lactate levels rose in all patients, only some patients experienced a change in pH.

acid-base balance, we can now consider pathophysiologic states and the possible interactions between lung and kidney.

## ACUTE RENAL FAILURE

Acute renal failure (ARF) in critically ill patients is still associated with a poor prognosis. Metabolic acid-base disorders, especially acidosis, are particularly common in these patients. The pathogenesis of such acidosis remains poorly understood because its main cause in ARF is not fully understood.

Classically, metabolic acidosis in renal failure is described as high-AG metabolic acidosis. However, in the clinical setting, the AG is not always elevated. This finding can lead clinicians to diagnostic and therapeutic confusion. In these situations, quantitative analysis using the Stewart approach can, again, be helpful. In this regard, Rocktaeschel and associates[5] examined the acid-base status of patients with ARF by means of the strong-ion method and demonstrated several features. First, critically ill patients with ARF are typically acidemic compared with control patients. Second, this acidemia is secondary to metabolic acidosis with a mean BE of approximately −7 mEq/L, which is consequent to the accumulation of lactate, phosphate, and unmeasured anions (possible candidates for these unmeasured anions include sulfate, urate, hydroxypropionate, oxalate, and furanpropionate). Third, in these patients, there is also a marked failure to alter the apparent SID (SIDa) to achieve a degree of metabolic compensation. Despite this finding, one half of the patients with ARF had an AG within the normal range. The reason for the normal AG, as explained earlier, is that these acidifying disorders are attenuated by concomitant metabolic alkalosis, which is essentially secondary to hypoalbuminemia. Hypoalbuminemia lowers the AG and masks the presence of acidifying anions to those clinicians using conventional acid-base analysis.

An interesting feature is that most of the patients analyzed in the study by Rocktaeschel and colleagues were mechanically ventilated. Thus, in spontaneous mode, these patients were unable to compensate, or, more likely, in conventional mode, no adjustment was made to ensure ventilatory compensation. This may appear surprising to some clinicians because persistent acidosis has been demonstrated to be an indicator of poor prognosis. Furthermore, there is a rationale for the need to correct severe acidosis that lies in the potential adverse cellular effects of such metabolic disturbance on myocardial function, arrhythmia risk, and pulmonary vascular tone. Conversely, very few studies have established that clinically significant benefits may arise from the full correction of such acidosis. It was a matter of debate for many that the Acute Respiratory Distress Syndrome Network (ARDS Network) protocol for the ventilation of ARDS patients pursued normal or near-normal pH at the cost of respiratory rates close to 40 breaths/minute, instead of accepting a degree of hypercapnia.

Nonetheless, when the syndrome of severe ARF develops and acidemia occurs, ventilatory compensation is only a short-term option. The correct approach to management relies on the initiation of RRT. In fact, RRT techniques such as intermittent hemodialysis (IHD), continuous venovenous hemofiltration (CVVH), continuous venovenous hemodialysis (CVVHD), and continuous venovenous hemodiafiltration (CVVHDF) have been successfully applied to the treatment of critically ill patients with ARF to improve fluid overload, uremia, and acid-base disorders for decades.

The use of RRT and adjustments in the replacement solutions administered to acidotic, critically ill patients with ARF can have a substantial effect on acid-base homeostasis. Furthermore, so-called high-volume hemofiltration (HVHF) may have an even stronger effect on acid-base disorders. Therefore, improving our understanding of the impact of RRT on acid-base disorders and gaining insight into the nature of such disorders and the mechanisms of action of RRT are important.

### Effect of Renal Replacement Therapy on Acid-Base Balance

There are two major modalities of RRT. One is intermittent and the other continuous. Few studies have been done to determine which modality is better in terms of acid-base control. Uchino and colleagues[6] compared the effect on acid-base balance of IHD and CVVHDF. Before treatment, metabolic acidosis was common in both groups (63.2% for IHD and 54.3% for CVVHDF). Both IHD and CVVHDF corrected metabolic acidosis. However, the rate and degree of correction differed significantly. CVVHDF normalized metabolic acidosis more rapidly and more effectively in the first 24 hours than IHD ($P < .01$). IHD was also associated with a higher incidence of metabolic acidosis than CVVHDF during the subsequent 2-week treatment period ($P < .005$). Accordingly, CVVHDF can be considered physiologically superior to IHD in the correction of metabolic acidosis.

The overwhelming superiority of continuous RRT (CRRT) in terms of control of acidosis was also established in comparison with peritoneal dialysis (PD); all patients randomized to CVVH achieved correction of acidosis by 50 hours of treatment compared with only 15% of those treated by PD ($P < .001$). Clearly, CRRT is a powerful tool for the control of acid-base balance in the absence of adequate or sufficient renal function.

How does CRRT correct acidosis? To seek to understand the mechanisms by which CRRT corrects metabolic acidosis in ARF, Rocktaschel and colleagues[7] studied the effect of CVVH on acid-base balance using the strong-ion method. Before commencing CVVH, patients had acidemia secondary to metabolic acidosis. This acidosis was the result of increased unmeasured anions (SIG, 12.3 mEq/L), hyperphosphatemia, and hyperlactatemia. It was attenuated by the alkalizing effect of hypoalbuminemia. Once CVVH was commenced, acidemia was corrected within 24 hours. This change was associated with a decreased SIG, phosphate, and $Cl^-$ concentration. This correction was so powerful and dominant that, after 3 days of CVVH, patients went on to develop alkalemia secondary to metabolic alkalosis ($HCO_3^-$, 29.8 mmol/L; BE, 6.7 mmol/L). This alkalemia appeared to result from a further decrease in SIG and a further decrease in serum phosphate concentration in the setting of persistent hypoalbuminemia. Hence CVVH appears to correct metabolic acidosis in ARF through its effect on unmeasured anions, phosphate, and $Cl^-$. Once hemofiltration is established, it becomes the dominant force in controlling metabolic (nonvolatile) acid-base status and often leads to alkalosis. In spontaneously but mechanically supported ventilating patients (pressure support ventilation) and in the absence of other factors, a change in pH from 7.4. to 7.5 may require a decrease in ventilation by 10% to 20% to restore normal pH.

## Effect of Replacement Fluid Composition (Lactate, Acetate, Bicarbonate, and Citrate)

The exchange of approximately 30 L/day of plasma water by CRRT is necessary to achieve adequate control of uremia and acid-base disorders in ARF. During CRRT, according to conventional acid-base thinking, there is a substantial loss of endogenous $HCO_3^-$ that has to be substituted by the addition of buffer substances (Stewart approach and explanation: there is loss of a fluid with an SID of between 30 and 40 mEq/L that must be replaced by a fluid with a similar SID).

Lactate, acetate, and $HCO_3^-$ have typically been used as buffers (or SID generators, according to Stewart) during RRT. Citrate has been used as both a buffer and an anticoagulant. Because these buffers affect acid-base balance, we must understand their physiologic characteristics.

$HCO_3^-$ has the major advantage of being the most physiologic anion equivalent. However, the production of a commercially available $HCO_3^-$–based solution is not easy because of the formation of calcium and magnesium salts during long-term storage. Furthermore, the cost of this solution is approximately three times higher than that of other buffer solutions. Accordingly, acetate and lactate have been used widely for RRT. Under normal conditions, acetate is rapidly converted on a 1:1 basis to $CO_2$ by both liver and skeletal muscle. Lactate is also rapidly converted in the liver on a 1:1 basis.

Studies of acetate-based solutions show that such solutions appear to exert a negative influence on mean arterial blood pressure and cardiac function in critically ill patients. Morgera and associates[8] compared acid-base balance between acetate-buffered and lactate-buffered replacement fluids and reported that the acetate-buffered solution was associated with a significant lower pH and $HCO_3^-$ levels than the lactate-buffered solution. However, the acetate-buffered solution had 9.5 mmol/L less buffer than the lactate-buffered solution. Therefore, the difference is likely simply a matter of dose rather than of choice of buffer. From the Stewart point of view, the acetate-buffered solution contained 8 mmol/L of $Cl^-$ more than the lactate-buffered solution to achieve electrical equilibrium. This composition reduces the SID of the replacement fluid and acidifies blood more.

Thomas and associates[9] studied the effects of lactate-buffered versus $HCO_3^-$–buffered fluids. Hemofiltration fluids contained either 44.5 mmol/L $Na^+$ lactate or 40.0 mmol/L $NaHCO_3$ with 3 mmol/L of lactate (43 mmol/L). Lactate-buffered fluids contained 142 mmol/L of $Na^+$ and 103 mmol/L of $Cl^-$ (SID = 39), and $HCO_3^-$–buffered fluids contained 155 mmol/L of $Na^+$ and 120 mmol/L of $Cl^-$ (SID = 35). Lactate rose from approximately 2 to 4 mmol/L when lactate-based fluids were given but not with $HCO_3^-$. Both therapies resulted in a similar improvement in metabolic acidosis. Potentially, the lactate-buffered fluid could have had a more alkalinizing effect. However, the accumulation of lactate in blood may have offset this effect and attenuated the trend toward a higher BE with the lactate-buffered fluids.

Tan and colleagues[10] studied the acid-base effect of CVVH with lactate-buffered or $HCO_3^-$ buffered solution. The lactate-buffered solution had an SID of 46 mEq/L versus 35 mEq/L for the $HCO_3^-$ fluid. From the Stewart point of view, the lactate-buffered solution should have led to a greater amount of alkalosis. However, this study showed a significant increase in plasma lactate levels (Fig. 14.3) and a decrease in BE with the lactate-buffered solution (Fig. 14.4). Lactate, if not metabolized and still present in blood, acts as a strong anion, which would have the same acidifying effect as $Cl^-$. Accordingly, iatrogenic hyperlactatemia can cause metabolic acidosis with a lowered serum $HCO_3^-$ (Fig. 14.5). The controversy can, of course, also be explained by the failure to convert exogenous lactate into $HCO_3^-$ (conventional paradigm).

Most commercially available replacement fluids are buffered with approximately 40 to 46 mmol/L of lactate. In most patients, the administration of such replacement fluid maintains a normal serum $HCO_3^-$ level

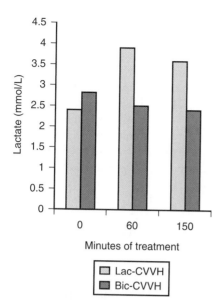

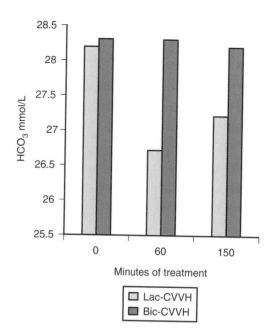

**Figure 14.3** Changes in lactate levels with continuous venovenous hemofiltration (CVVH) using either bicarbonate-based replacement fluids (Bic-CVVH) or lactate-buffered replacement fluids (Lac-CVVH). The latter fluids induced a significant increase in lactate levels.

**Figure 14.5** Changes in bicarbonate levels with continuous venovenous hemofiltration (CVVH) using either bicarbonate-based replacement fluids (Bic-CVVH) or lactate-buffered replacement fluids (Lac-CVVH). The latter fluids induce an initial significant decrease in bicarbonate levels that is slowly and spontaneously corrected.

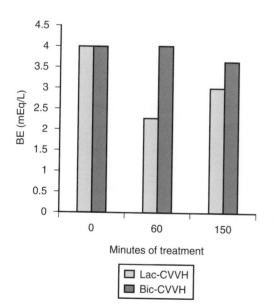

**Figure 14.4** Changes in base excess (BE) with continuous venovenous hemofiltration (CVVH) using either bicarbonate-based replacement fluids (Bic-CVVH) or lactate-buffered replacement fluids (Lac-CVVH). The latter fluids induce an initial significant decrease in BE that is slowly and spontaneously corrected.

without any significant increase in blood lactate concentration. Because the ability of the liver to metabolize lactate is in the range of approximately 100 mmol/hour, even CVVH at 2 L/hour exchange would still deliver less than the normal liver can handle.

However, if lactate-based dialysates or replacement fluids are used, in some patients with liver dysfunction or shock, the administration of lactate-buffered fluids can induce significant hyperlactatemia and acidosis because the metabolic rate is insufficient to meet the additional lactate load. Although lactate normally acts as a buffer by being removed from the circulation and thereby lowering the SID, if lactate is only partly metabolized and accumulates in plasma water, it acts like a strong anion. Thus, hyperlactatemia decreases the SIDa, which results in increased dissociation of plasma water and thereby lowers the pH.

Citrate has been used for regional anticoagulation. During this procedure, citrate is administered to the circuit before the filter and chelates calcium, thus impeding coagulation. Once citrate enters the circulation, it is metabolized to $CO_2$ and then $HCO_3^-$ on a 1:3 basis; thus, 1 mmol of citrate yields 3 mmol of $CO_2$ and then $HCO_3^-$.

Under these circumstances, citrate acts as the buffer as well as the anticoagulant. If the method described by Mehta and colleagues[11] is applied, approximately 48 mmol/hour of $HCO_3^-$ equivalent are given as citrate. This rate of alkali administration may result in metabolic alkalosis (≤25% of cases). Attention must be paid to patients with liver disease who may not be able to metabolize citrate. In these patients, citrate may accumulate and may result in severe ionized hypocalcemia and metabolic acidosis because the citrate anion ($C_6H_5O_7^{3-}$) acts as an unmeasured anion and increases the SIG, which has acidifying effects.

According to conventional thinking, when oxidizable anions are used in the replacement fluids, the anion (acetate, lactate, and citrate) must be completely oxidized to $CO_2$ and water to generate $HCO_3^-$. If the metabolic conversion of non-$HCO_3^-$ anions proceeds without accumulation, their buffering capacity will be equal to that of $HCO_3^-$. Thus, the effect on acid-base status depends on the buffer concentration and transformation, rather than on the kind of buffer used. If transformation is not adequate, an $HCO_3^-$ deficit will develop. According to the Stewart paradigm, when the metabolic conversion is impaired, the increased blood concentration of the anion in question simply leads to an increased concentration of lactate (if lactate is the anion) or an increased concentration of unmeasured anions (if acetate and citrate are the anions). All anions in blood lower the SID and acidify blood. The nature and extent of these acid-base changes are governed by the intensity of plasma water exchange or dialysis, by the buffer content of the replacement fluid or dialysate, and by the metabolic rate of these anions. If $HCO_3^-$ fluid is used, according to the Stewart approach, the SID will be modified as $HCO_3^-$ becomes $CO_2$, which is removed by the lung, and $Na^+$ remains in blood to increase the SID and thereby alkalinize blood. The SID of the replacement fluid determines pH.

## Effect of High-Volume Hemofiltration on Acid-Base Balance

HVHF has been applied to the treatment of patients with septic shock, with favorable hemodynamic results. However, if commercial lactate-buffered replacement fluid is used during HVHF, patients may receive more than 270 mmol/hour of exogenous lactate. This lactate load could overcome endogenous lactate metabolism even in healthy subjects and could result in progressive hyperlactatemia. This risk is even greater in sick patients with impaired lactate metabolism. Hyperlactatemia has been reported during lactate-buffered fluid administration in critically ill patients with ARF treated with intermittent hemofiltration and a lactate load of 190 to 210 mmol/hour. Such hyperlactatemia may induce metabolic acidosis. Cole and associates[12,13] studied the effect of HVHF on acid-base balance. HVHF with lactate-buffered replacement fluids (6 L/hour of lactate-buffered fluids) induced iatrogenic hyperlactatemia. Plasma lactate levels increased from a median 2.51 mmol/L

to a median of 7.3 mmol/hour at 2 hours. This change was accompanied by a significant decrease in $HCO_3^-$ and BE (Fig. 14.6). However, such hyperlactatemia had only a mild and transient acidifying effect. A decrease in $Cl^-$ and $A_{TOT}$ and the removal of unmeasured anions (decrease in SIG) all rapidly compensated for this effect (Fig. 14.7). Thus, the final effect was that HVHF induced only a minor change in pH from 7.42 to 7.39 at 2 hours. In the period from 2 to 8 hours, the blood lactate concentration remained stable at approximately 7 to 8 mmol/L, whereas compensatory effects continued and restored $HCO_3^-$ levels to 27.2 mmol/L and pH to 7.44 by 8 hours of treatment.

Although the $Cl^-$ concentration in the replacement fluid was high compared with the serum $Cl^-$ level, a progressive decrease in $Cl^-$ was observed. This could have resulted from $Cl^-$ losses in excess of gains. To confirm this possibility, Uchino and colleagues[14] examined the sieving coefficient (the ratio between a solute in the effluent and the same solute in plasma water) for $Cl^-$ during HVHF and showed a sieving coefficient for $Cl^-$ greater than 1. Another possible explanation for hypochloremia is the intracellular movement of $Cl^-$ in response to metabolic acidosis ($Cl^-$ shift), a physiologic phenomenon already known to occur in venous blood. A decrease in $A_{TOT}$ was explained by the aggregate minor changes in albumin and phosphate. The changes in SIG appeared most likely to result from simple filtration of unmeasured anion.

Consequently, HVHF with lactate-buffered fluids induced marked hyperlactatemia but did not induce progressive acidosis. However, caution should be exerted in

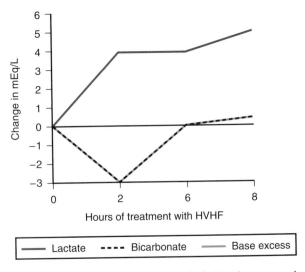

**Figure 14.6** Changes in base excess (BE), bicarbonate, and lactate levels with high-volume hemofiltration using lactate-buffered replacement fluids. The dramatic lactate level increase induces an initial fall in bicarbonate and BE that is slowly and spontaneously corrected.

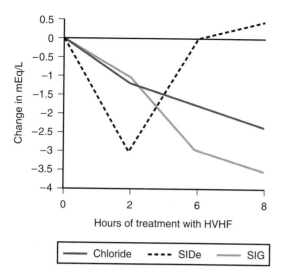

**Figure 14.7** Changes in strong-ion gap (SIG), strong-ion difference effective (SIDe), and chloride levels with high-volume hemofiltration (HVHF) using lactate-buffered replacement fluids. HVHF decreases the SIG and chloride levels and thus compensates for the changes in lactate levels that lead to a relatively rapid correction of SIDe.

particular patients who have marked pretreatment hyperlactatemia (>5 mmol/L) or liver dysfunction or in whom the intensity of HVHF exceeds 6 L/hour of plasma water exchange. $HCO_3^-$ use is warranted in such patients. These observations should remind clinicians that the liver, to name an obvious component of acid-base physiology, is a powerful regulator of lactate levels. Accordingly, to consider kidney-lung interactions as the sole controlling system for acid-base balance is wrong, and the liver needs to be taken into account in any description of nonvolatile acid-base control.

## LIVER IN ACID-BASE CONTROL

Not all anions appearing in the blood of critically ill patients can be identified by routine biochemical measures. The SID method, however, can be used to detect unexplained anions because the SIDa calculated from the routinely measurable ions should be equal to the effective (SIDe) derived from the remaining charges attributable to $CO_2$ and ATOT. If a difference exists between the SIDa and SIDe, then unmeasured anions must be present because of the law of isoelectricity. This difference has been termed the SIG to distinguish it from the AG.

Unlike the AG, the normal SIG has not been defined. However, only very few anions are not measured by routine laboratory methods, are found in millimolar or substantial micromolar concentrations, and are not used for the SID equation. Such anions include urate, pyruvate,

sulfate, ascorbate, citrate, glutamate, aspartate, pyroglutamate, and few other metabolites. From knowledge obtained from measurements in normal humans, these anions should not account for more than 2 to 3 mEq/L. However, this gap does not need to be filled by strong ions. Some weak acids may also play a role.

Unmeasured anions (detected using SIG calculations but not formally identified) have been reported in the blood of patients with sepsis and liver disease. These anions may be the source of much or some of the unexplained acidosis seen in patients with critical illness. The presence of unexplained anions in the blood of patients with sepsis and liver disease was investigated further in an animal model of sepsis using endotoxemia. In this study, investigators found that during control conditions, the liver cleared unmeasured anions from the circulation (mean flux, −0.34 mEq/minute). With early endotoxemia, however, the liver switched to release of unmeasured anions (0.12 mEq/minute, $P < .005$). These data suggest that the liver has a role in systemic acid-base balance by way of regulating anion fluxes apart from metabolism of lactate. The liver also regulates acid-base balance through its effect on proteins.

## Effects of Plasma Proteins on Acid-Base Balance

Considerable controversy has developed regarding classification of acid-base derangements occurring as a result of abnormalities in weak acids (ATOT). A sudden decrease in ATOT produces alkalosis, whereas an increase is acidifying. Some investigators have advocated a third classification for this effect, perhaps termed *proteinaceous acidosis or alkalosis*, to be added to metabolic (SID) and respiratory ($PCO_2$) acidosis or alkalosis. Others have strenuously objected. The debate may actually prove moot in light of more recent evidence. First, when the SID of critically ill patients was compared with SBE, the intercept for SBE = 0 was found to be 30 to 35 mEq/L, rather than 40 to 42 mEq/L, as in healthy individuals. Thus, in these critically ill patients, many of whom had a decreased ATOT secondary to hypoalbuminemia, the SID was reduced even when there was no apparent acid-base disorder. The reason for this is obvious from a physical chemical perspective. As a patient's albumin decreases, so does ATOT and thus A−. This decrease in weak acid has a slightly alkalinizing effect. Thus, decreased albumin synthesis by the liver induces metabolic alkalosis. The body could adapt to this change by retaining $CO_2$, but it appears to reserve this adaptation for changes in SID. Instead, the body adapts to a decreased ATOT by decreasing the SID.

Although one may be tempted to classify this adaptation as a mixed acid-base disorder, as hypoalbuminemic alkalosis with compensatory metabolic acidosis, a patient in whom SID fails to reduce the SID in response to a decrease in ATOT should be considered to have metabolic alkalosis as a consequence of failed renal homeostatic mechanisms (e.g., secondary to hypovolemia), not pro- teinaceous alkalosis secondary to hypoalbuminemia. The findings of Wilkes in critically ill patients and of Wooten in mathematical simulations appear to support this assertion. Both authors demonstrated that the set point for the SID to achieve a normal pH given a normal PCO2 changes with changes in ATOT. Furthermore, although the loss of weak acid from the plasma space is an alkalinizing process, there is no evidence that the body regulates ATOT to maintain acid-base balance. Nonetheless, the regulation of albumin synthesis by the liver is another important way in which this organ participates in setting the acid-base balance from the point of view of its nonvolatile component.

## SPECIFIC DISORDERS OF RENAL ACID-BASE CONTROL

A group of disorders of kidney function is characterized by a reduction of acid excretion that is out of proportion to reductions in glomerular filtration rate. This group of disorders is referred to as *renal tubular acidoses*. Their major characteristic from the point of view of conventional acid-base physiology is that they all have so-called hyperchloremic nonanion gap acidosis. The conventional explanation for such acidoses differs according to the type but includes failure to excrete $H^+$ or $H^+$ back diffusion or deficient $HCO_3^-$ reabsorption in the proximal tubule with $HCO_3^-$ wasting or alterations in ammonium ion excretion. The Stewart explanation is simple: failure to excrete $Cl^-$ normally.

The mechanisms at work in these disorders are becoming more relevant to the critical care physician because these conditions, particularly type 4 renal tubular acidosis, occur in the setting of diabetic nephropathy, nephrosclerosis related to hypertension, and chronic tubulointerstitial nephropathy resulting from immunosuppressive agents such as cyclosporine and FK-506. These patients increasingly populate ICUs, and their acid-base disorders require greater awareness. Despite the increased presence of so-called hyperchloremic acidosis secondary to renal dysfunction, by far the most common cause of hyperchloremic acidosis is iatrogenic and derives from the administration of $Cl^-$-rich intravenous fluids. The effect of these fluids on acid-base balance is particularly pronounced when there is concomitant renal dysfunction and the kidney is unable to dispose of the additional $Cl^-$ load rapidly. The clinical significance of such iatrogenic hyperchloremic (low SID) acidosis is unknown. It is typically seen with the rapid administration of large amounts of saline, as occurs during the resuscitation of trauma patients, the initiation of cardiopulmonary bypass with a saline pump prime, or the administration of $Cl^-$-rich colloid solutions in the ICU.

It is very important for the critical care physician to be aware of this iatrogenic syndrome so that diagnostic errors are avoided. In particular, if lactate measurements are not readily available, the lower $HCO_3^-$ levels and greater base deficit that develop as a consequence of the administration of such $Cl^-$-rich fluids (fluids with an SID of zero) may induce to clinicians to believe that either resuscitation has been inadequate or that other organic causes of such acidosis exist. These erroneous beliefs may then lead to unnecessary fluid overload, investigations, or even exploratory surgery. Irrespective of the source of any acidosis, however, much controversy surrounds the issue of whether acidosis should be treated per se.

## TREATMENT OF ACIDOSIS AND ACIDEMIA

Whether induced by the accumulation of the lactate anion or by the accumulation of other anions ($Cl^-$, ketones, exogenous acids, acids associated with renal failure), severe acidosis may be associated with inadequate physiologic compensation and may lead to acidemia. Although clinicians agree that treatment of such acidemia and acidosis should first and foremost involve correction of its cause, it is controversial whether some or all of these patients should also receive alkalinizing solutions such as $NaHCO_3$.

The biologic rationale for administering $NaHCO_3$ rests on three major considerations: (1) low pH is harmful to the organism (e.g., impairs myocardial contractility and induces pulmonary vasoconstriction), (2) intravenous $NaHCO_3$ can increase pH, and (3) any adverse effects of $NaHCO_3$ are outweighed by its benefits. However, concerning the first point, evidence that low pH decreases myocardial contractility is mostly based on data from isolated animal heart muscle preparations. In whole-animal preparations, the effects of acidosis on contractility are much more difficult to document. In humans, data from patients with permissive hypercapnia or with diabetic ketoacidosis support the view that there is marked tolerance to low pH without major adverse effects. Furthermore, data suggest that acidosis may protect cells from anoxia, chemical hypoxia, and reperfusion injury. With regard to the effect of pH on pulmonary vascular tone, the increase induced by a change in pH from 7.4 to 7.2 is likely small and is not clinically relevant in patients who do not already have a degree of pulmonary hypertension or right ventricular dysfunction.

Of course, the effects of acidosis, particularly metabolic acidosis, are diverse. Acidosis can affect blood pressure as well as hepatic and renal blood flow, although the underlying mechanisms of these effects are uncertain. An increase of inducible nitric oxide synthase, which can lead to vasodilatation, has been shown in both in vitro models and animal studies. Furthermore, it has been demonstrated that hyperchloremic acidosis increases lung and intestinal injury and decreases gut barrier function. Acidosis has also many untoward effects on metabolism. Glucose metabolism is impaired by the induction of insulin resistance and the inhibition of anaerobic glycolysis. Furthermore, there is induction of protein breakdown and decreased muscle protein synthesis. Hyperchloremic acidosis has proinflammatory effects documented in vitro and in animal models. Hydrochloric acid infusion increases the release of nitric oxide and increases the ration of interleukin-6 to interleukin-10. In addition, hydrochloric acid increased NF-κB DNA binding in lipopolysaccharide-stimulated pulmonary macrophage-like cells. Thus, it seems plausible that hyperchloremic acidosis may influence sepsis-induced inflammation and, potentially, lung injury.

With regard to the concern that intravenous $NaHCO_3$ can increase pH, clinical studies show that the effect of up to 2 mmol/kg of $NaHCO_3$ on human pH is small, with increments in the range of 0.05 to 0.15. In addition, $NaHCO_3$ fails to increase intracellular pH predictably and often appears to induce a decrease instead. Changes in blood pH may also decrease oxygen delivery to tissues by changing the dissociation curve of hemoglobin. Thus, the efficacy of $NaHCO_3$ in increasing pH where it matters is unclear. The hemodynamic effects of intravenous $NaHCO_3$ have been studied in humans with mild to moderate acidosis. These effects were indistinguishable from those of an equivalent amount of $Na^+$ delivered as saline. In uncontrolled studies of patients with diabetic ketoacidosis, no benefits could be seen, and delayed clearance of ketones and lactate was documented. $HCO_3^-$ also lowers ionized calcium concentrations and $Pao_2$ in animals and in nonacidemic patients with congestive cardiac failure. Thus, the safety of intravenous $HCO_3^-$ remains untested. Other alkalinizing preparations exist:

1. Carbicarb (equimolar mixture of $Na^+$ carbonate and $NaHCO_3$).
2. Dichloroacetate (an agent that stimulates pyruvate dehydrogenase and lowers lactate levels).
3. *Tris*-hydroxymethyl aminomethane (THAM).

Carbicarb has also undergone limited studies in humans, and its role is unclear. Dichloroacetate was tested in a large, randomized controlled trial in patients with lactic acidosis. In this trial, dichloroacetate was found efficacious in lowering lactate levels and in increasing $HCO_3^-$ concentration and pH. However, it did not achieve any changes in hemodynamics or clinical outcomes.

THAM appears to improve contractility in isolated rabbit ear preparations. However, no controlled studies are available to support its use in humans with acidemia.

Given the foregoing considerations, the administration of intravenous $NaHCO_3$ in patients with acidemia remains one of the most controversial areas of anesthetic and critical care practice. As in other similar areas of controversy, the intensity of opinion is inversely proportional to the quality and amount of evidence available. Data are insufficient to support the use of intravenous $NaHCO_3$ in patients with acidemia. There are also insufficient data to ban the use of $NaHCO_3$ in these patients. If a decision is made to administer intravenous $NaHCO_3$, we recommend that it should occur with close hemodynamic and biochemical monitoring and that the agent be administered in the presence of a physician and by continuous infusion to achieve specified biochemical and physiologic targets.

The general principles described earlier apply to general populations and offer an understanding of how fluid administration, kidney function, liver function, and physician intervention may alter acid-base balance from the point of view of its nonvolatile component. Understanding of these effects and knowledge of the homeostatic response of the lung to changes in metabolic acid-base status are fundamental in guiding ICU clinicians in their appreciation of how these events can affect the patient's ventilatory behavior in the setting where mechanical ventilation is supportive (spontaneously set but assisted, as is the case for all noninvasive modalities and pressure support ventilation). These issues are also fundamental in informing physicians' choices where mechanical ventilation is controlled (set by the physician, as is the case during any form of fully controlled and or mandatory ventilation). Nonetheless, specific clinical situations exist in which the interactions between kidney (native or artificial) and lung (including issues of mechanical ventilation) require specific comments.

## Permissive Hypercapnia

In some centers, the technique of permissive hypercapnia is practiced. Typically, this approach is applied to mechanically ventilated patients with ARDS or marked airflow limitation (exacerbation of chronic obstructive pulmonary disease [COPD] or asthma). The rationale for permissive hypercapnia is that it allows either low tidal volumes (avoidance of volutrauma in ARDS) or reduction in excessive air trapping with risk of barotrauma (asthma or COPD). A physiologic consequence of hypercapnia is the development of respiratory (ventilatory) acidosis. The clinical consequences of such acidosis are not well understood. Some clinicians believe them to be important and to require treatment.

This view may particularly apply to patients who display signs of clinically important right ventricular dysfunction.

In ARDS, one approach may be simply to increase the respiratory rate and readjust the ventilation to minimize the degree of $CO_2$ accumulation. This approach, however, would likely be dangerous in COPD and asthma. Another approach would be to infuse $NaHCO_3$ (a fluid with a large SID in Stewart parlance) continuously to induce metabolic alkalosis (i.e., increase the SID) and rapidly readjust pH toward normal. This approach may be feasible and reasonably safe in selected patients, but it can result in clinically important fluid overload or hypernatremia in others, particularly in the setting of renal dysfunction. Such fluid overload could then aggravate the severity of ARDS or complicate the course of COPD or asthma in patients with the onset of pulmonary congestion.

In other patients with concurrent metabolic lactic acidosis, the amounts of $NaHCO_3$ necessary to control acid-base status may be extraordinary (200 mL/hour) and very likely to induce volume overload. In these difficult patients, we believe that continuous hemofiltration offers a solution that combines the avoidance of volume problems, the full correction of acidosis (if so desired), and the control of uremia if the patient has concurrent renal dysfunction. In a patient with a serum $HCO_3^-$ concentration of 20 mmol/L, CVVH in postdilution, using an $HCO_3^-$-buffered fluid at a concentration of 35 mmol/L and a fluid exchange rate of 4 L/hour, will provide the equivalent of a continuous infusion of approximately 50 to 60 mmol/hour. If this is still deemed an insufficient dose, either the exchange rate can be increased or, more cheaply, an $HCO_3^-$ infusion can be started at whatever dose the clinician believes appropriate. The additional volume can be removed during CVVH, so that fluid overload is completely prevented while acid-base status is altered. In short, the availability of CVVH makes the regulation of acid-base balance possible under even the most extreme circumstances. However, whether such regulation changes clinical outcome remains unknown.

## Effect of Metabolic Acidosis on Ventilation

In occasional patients undergoing weaning from mechanical ventilation, even small increases in ventilatory requirements make the difference between success or failure in liberating patients from mechanical ventilation. In some of these patients, an additional ventilatory burden may be imposed by the presence of persistent metabolic acidosis (iatrogenic or secondary to renal dysfunction). In these patients, the kidney may be unable to achieve independent control of acid-base status, for several reasons. In this situation, there is typically a mixed acid-base picture that includes hyperchloremia and the accumulation of renal unexcreted anions. An initial approach is directed at the correction of hyperchloremia (low-SID state). This can be achieved by the judicious mixing of loop diuretic–induced $Cl^-$ loss and the administration of $Cl^-$-poor (normal or near-normal SID) fluid such as lactated Ringer's solution. If renal dysfunction is significant, CRRT or slow extended daily dialysis (SLEDD) for a period of 1 to 2 days may be sufficient to achieve the desired goal.

In other patients, admission to ICU is characterized by profound metabolic acidosis. For example, a patient with septic shock who has received massive fluid resuscitation and who presented with prolonged hypotension leading to ischemic hepatitis may have combined lactic acidosis and hyperchloremic (low-SID) iatrogenic acidosis with a BE of −20 mEq/L and perhaps even evidence of myocardial dysfunction on echocardiography. Such a patient may have a pH of 6.9. In this setting, most clinicians would consider that the correction of acidemia would be beneficial and would consider strategies to achieve it. One way to improve pH rapidly is to implement a hyperventilation strategy. However, even lowering the $PaCO_2$ to 10 to 15 mm Hg represents only a short-term response and cannot successfully correct this disorder alone. In such patients, the administration of intravenous $HCO_3^-$ is also a useful initial strategy, but the dose required to correct the acidosis even partially is in the range of 150 to 200 mmol/hour. In this setting, the kidney cannot make the necessary adjustments because their magnitude is beyond its ability to do so even under normal circumstances and because ARF typically develops in this setting. The only way to sustain correction of acid-base disorders of this magnitude is through the application of RRT techniques. In this setting, CRRT therapies are necessary because the disorder will not resolve within hours, but if the patient survives, the condition will slowly resolve within days, and maintenance of homeostasis will be required 24 hours a day.

## Effect of Metabolic Alkalosis on Spontaneous Ventilation

Rarely, patients develop profound metabolic alkalosis (pH > 7.6), typically in the setting of high gastrointestinal obstruction with large gastric aspirates ($Cl^-$ loss leading to an increase in SID) and hypoalbuminemia. In some of these patients, $PaCO_2$ may rise to more than 60 mm Hg and may independently induce somnolence and further hypoventilation with $CO_2$ narcosis, which may require endotracheal intubation for airway protection. Such patients are rare but provide an interesting challenge, particularly if they have renal dysfunction or end-stage renal failure as the background to their inability to make the necessary adjustments in terms of renal $Cl^-$ retention.

In this setting, patients typically require repletion of the intravascular and extravascular compartment with a $Cl^-$-rich fluid (SID = 0). This can be typically achieved with saline and, as is often necessary, with the addition of potassium Cl and magnesium Cl. If a patient also has congestive cardiac failure and no intravascular volume deficit but simply developed alkalosis because of an ill-advised aspirate replacement strategy that included relatively $Cl^-$-poor fluids (Ringer's solution), then saline administration may be deleterious unless it is delivered within the setting of simultaneous RRT. The $HCO_3^-$ and $Na^+$ content of such RRT can be adjusted to facilitate restoration of acid-base homeostasis.

## Effect of Mechanical Ventilation of Renal Acid-Base Handling

The effect of mechanical ventilation per se on renal function is poorly understood. The effect beyond the possible changes in $PaCO_2$ is even less clearly understood. This limited understanding derives from the finding that mechanical ventilation in humans occurs in the setting of surgery or disease. Nonetheless, the available evidence indicates that mechanical ventilation is responsible for increased reabsorption of water and $Na^+$ through an effect on vasopressin release and the angiotensin-aldosterone system. The effect of such changes on acid-base balance can be expected to induce a degree of metabolic alkalosis independent of the renal response to changes in $PaCO_2$. Work by Imai and colleagues[15] highlighted that the way in which ventilation is applied can induce distal organ injury involving the kidney. In an elegant study in animals ventilated with high tidal volumes, these investigators demonstrated the induction of tubular apoptosis, which was prevented by low–tidal volume ventilation. Furthermore, plasma from patients who had received high–tidal volume ventilation was able to induce renal cell apoptosis in vitro.

These novel observations indicate that humoral factors can participate in cross-organ talk and that mechanical ventilation may well affect the way the kidney works beyond its straightforward effect on $PaCO_2$. Equally, acute uremia may affect lung function in ways we do not yet fully understand and that go beyond the simple induction of metabolic acidosis or fluid overload.

## CONCLUSIONS

The mechanisms responsible for human acid-base balance are a matter of controversy. Conventional paradigms are being challenged by modern ideology.

Irrespective of the mechanisms at play, derangements in the control of the nonvolatile component of acid-base balance have major repercussions on the need for and settings of mechanical ventilation. Similarly, some strategies of mechanical ventilation and pulmonary disease profoundly affect the way in which the kidney has to adjust its function. Other factors such as liver function and fluid therapy are also important. In some cases, the kidney is unable to achieve the desired adjustments, and artificial renal support becomes necessary. In the ICU, CRRTs offer the ability to control fully the nonvolatile component of acid-base balance 24 hours a day. Critical care physicians need to understand the therapeutic options available and the limitations of these options, to offer their patients thoughtful and successful interventions.

## REFERENCES

1. Stewart PA: Modern quantitative acid-base chemistry. Can J Physiol Pharmacol 1983;61:1444–1461.
2. Figge J, Mydosh T, Fencl V: Serum proteins and acid-base equilibria: A follow-up. J Lab Clin Med 1992;120:713–719.
3. Figge J, Jabor A, Kazda A, Fencl V: Anion gap and hypoalbuminemia. Crit Care Med 1998;26:1807–1810.
4. Madias NE, Homer SM, Johns CA, Cohen JJ: Hypochloremia as a consequence of anion gap metabolic acidosis. J Lab Clin Med 1984;104:15–23.
5. Rocktaeschel J, Morimatsu H, Uchino S, et al: Acid-base status of critically ill patients with acute renal failure: Analysis based on Stewart-Figge methodology. Crit Care 2003;7:60–66.
6. Uchino S, Bellomo R, Ronco C: Intermittent versus continuous renal replacement therapy in the ICU: Impact on electrolyte and acid-base balance. Intensive Care Med 2001;27:1037–1043.
7. Rocktaschel J, Morimatsu H, Uchino S, et al: Impact of continuous veno-venous hemofiltration on acid-base balance. Int J Artif Organs 2003;26:19–25.
8. Morgera S, Heering P, Szentandrasi T, et al: Comparison of a lactate- versus acetate-based hemofiltration replacement fluid in patients with acute renal failure. Renal Fail 1997;19:155–164.
9. Thomas AN, Guy JM, Kishen R, et al: Comparison of lactate and bicarbonate buffered hemofiltration fluids: Use in critically ill patients. Nephrol Dial Transplant 1997;12:1212–1217.
10. Tan HK, Uchino S, Bellomo R: The acid-base effects of continuous hemofiltration with lactate or bicarbonate buffered replacement fluids. Int J Artif Organs 2003;26:477–483.
11. Mehta RL, McDonald B, Aguilar M, Ward DM: Regional citrate anticoagulation for continuous arteriovenous hemodialysis in critically ill patients. Kidney Int 1990;38:976–981.
12. Cole L, Bellomo R, Journois D, et al: High volume hemofiltration in human septic shock. Intensive Care Med 2001;27:978–986.
13. Cole L, Bellomo R, Baldwin I, et al: The impact of lactate-buffered high volume hemofiltration on acid-base balance. Intensive Care Med 2003;29:1113–1120.
14. Uchino S, Cole L, Morimatsu H, et al: Solute mass balance during isovolaemic high volume hemofiltration. Intensive Care Med 2003;29:1541–1546.
15. Imai Y, Parodo J, Kajikawa O, et al: Injurious mechanical ventilation and end-organ epithelial cell apoptosis and organ dysfunction in an experimental model of acute respiratory distress syndrome. JAMA 2003;289:2104–2112.

## SUGGESTED READINGS

Brivet F, Kleinknecht D, Loirat P: Acute renal failure in intensive care units—Causes, outcome, and prognostic factors: A prospective, multicenter study. Crit Care Med 1996;24:192–198.

Burchardi H, Kaczmarczyk G: Effects of mechanical ventilation on the kidney. Curr Opin Crit Care 1998;4:341–346.

Cohen RD, Iles RA: Lactic acidosis. Clin Endocrinol Metab 1980;9:513–527.

Davenport A, Will E, Davison AM: The effect of lactate-buffered solutions on the acid-base status of patients with renal failure. Nephrol Dial Transplant 1989;4:800–804.

Heering P, Ivens K, Thumer O, et al: Acid-base balance and substitution fluid during continuous hemofiltration. Kidney Int 1999;56:S37–S40.

Hoste EA, Kellum JA: Acute renal failure in the critically ill: Impact on morbidity and mortality. Contrib Nephrol 2004;144:1–11.

Kellum JA: Determinants of blood pH in health and disease. Critical Care 2000;4:6–14.

Kellum JA, Bellomo R, Kramer DJ, Pinsky MR: Hepatic anion flux during acute endotoxemia. J Appl Physiol 1995;78:2212–2217.

Kellum JA, Bellomo R, Kramer DJ, Pinsky MR: Splanchnic buffering of metabolic acid during early endotoxemia. J Crit Care 1997;12:7–12.

Kellum JA, Bellomo R, Kramer DJ, Pinsky MR: Etiology of metabolic acidosis during saline resuscitation in endotoxemia. Shock 1998;9:364–368.

Kellum JA, Kramer DJ, Pinsky MR: Strong ion gap: A methodology for exploring unexplained anions. J Crit Care 1995;10: 51–55.

Kellum JA, Song M, Li J: Lactic and hydrochloric acids induce different patterns of inflammatory response in LPS-stimulated RAW 264.7 cells. Am J Physiol 2004;286:R686–R692.

Kellum JA, Song M, Venkataraman R: Effects of hyperchloremic acidosis on arterial pressure and circulating inflammatory molecules in experimental sepsis. Chest 2004;125:243–248.

Kierdorf H, Sieberth HG: Continuous treatment modalities in acute renal failure. Nephrol Dial Transplant 1995;10:2001–2008.

Kirshbaum B: Effect of hemodialysis on the hypersalphatemia of chronic renal failure. ASAIO J 1998;44:314–318.

Leblanc M, Kellum JA: Biochemical and biophysical principles of hydrogen ion regulation. In Ronco C, Bellomo R (eds): Critical Care Nephrology. Dordrecht, Netherlands: Kluwer Academic Publishers, 1998, pp 261–277.

Levraut J, Ciebiera JP, Jambou P, et al: Effect of continuous venovenous hemofiltration with dialysis on lactate clearance in critically ill patients. Crit Care Med 1997;25:58–62.

Magder S: Pathophysiology of metabolic acid-base disturbances in patients with critical illness. In Ronco C, Bellomo R (eds): Critical Care Nephrology. Dordrecht, Netherlands: Kluwer Academic Publishers, 1998, pp 279–296.

Mansell MA, Morgan SH, Moore L, et al: Cardiovascular and acid-base effects of acetate and bicarbonate haemodialysis. Nephrol Dial Transplant 1987;1:229–232.

Prough DS, Bidani A: Hyperchloremic metabolic acidosis is a predictable consequence of intraoperative infusion of 0.9% saline. Anesthesiology 1999;90:1247–1249.

Phu MH, Hien TT, Hoang NT, et al: Hemofiltration and peritoneal dialysis in infection-associated acute renal failure. N Engl J Med 2002;347:895–902.

Salem MM, Mujais SK: Gaps in the anion gap. Arch Intern Med 1992;152:1625–1629.

Saman S, Opie LH: Mechanism of reduction of action potential duration of ventricular myocardium by exogenous lactate. J Mol Cell Cardiol 1984;10:659–662.

Spiegel DM, Ullian ME, Zerbe GO, Berl T: Determinant of survival and recovery in acute renal failure patients dialysed in the intensive care unit. Am J Nephrol 1991;11:44–47.

Scheingraber S, Rehm M, Sehmisch C, Finsterer U: Rapid saline infusion produces hyperchloremic acidosis in patients undergoing gynecologic surgery. Anesthesiology 1999;90:1265–1270.

Wendon J, Smithies M, Sheppard M, et al: Continuous high volume venovenous hemofiltration in acute renal failure. Intensive Care Med 1989;15:358–363.

# CHAPTER 15

# Heart-Lung Interactions

Indra Singh and Michael R. Pinsky

The most basic function of the cardiovascular and pulmonary systems is to provide an adequate supply of oxygen ($O_2$) to tissues and organ systems to meet the metabolic demands of the body. Under normal physiologic conditions, the lungs maintain the arterial $O_2$ content ($CaO_2$) within normal limits. A responsive heart and circulatory autonomic control ensures adequate $O_2$ delivery ($DO_2$). Under conditions of increased metabolic demands, whether physiologic (e.g., exercise, pregnancy) or pathologic (e.g., trauma, infections), $DO_2$ may not be sufficient, and artificial pulmonary or cardiac support may be required. Preexisting disease states of either or both systems confound this adaptive process. Various pulmonary diseases, artificial ventilation, and ventilatory maneuvers can have profound effects not only on gas exchange but also on cardiac output. Similarly, cardiac diseases can affect pulmonary function. Therefore, it is necessary to understand the interactions between the cardiovascular and pulmonary systems during spontaneous and artificial ventilation, for better application and withdrawal of various ventilatory therapies and for improved patient outcomes.

The hemodynamic effects of ventilation can be examined in various ways. All forms of ventilation alter lung volume to achieve a given minute ventilation necessary for gas exchange. Spontaneous ventilation increases lung volume by muscular contraction, whereas positive pressure ventilation increases lung volume by increasing airway pressure (Paw). Thus, both forms of ventilation increase lung volume, but the changes in intrathoracic pressure (ITP) are direct opposites. Accordingly, the hemodynamic differences between spontaneous and positive pressure ventilation are related to the directionally different changes in ITP and the energy needed to create these changes. Thus, one useful approach to describing the hemodynamic effects of ventilation is first to describe the metabolic demands placed on the cardiovascular system by spontaneous ventilatory efforts, then the effects of changes in lung volume, and finally the effects of both increases and decreases in ITP. These separations of hemodynamic interactions are arbitrary, but they do allow one to comprehend the complex processes that result in the observed heart-lung interactions commonly seen in critically ill patients. We use this approach to describe the specific effects of ventilation on the circulation and then group these effects by specific disease process.

## VENTILATION AS EXERCISE

Breathing is a dynamic process that requires muscular contraction and thus blood flow, energy, and $O_2$ and produces $CO_2$. Under normal conditions, the work cost of breathing is very low and is almost not measurable except by the most sensitive of metabolic techniques; breathing requires less than 5% of total $O_2$ consumption. However, in the setting of lung disease, the work cost of breathing can increase markedly and often becomes the primary limiting factor in performing tasks. Ventilatory work arises from the generation of transpulmonary pressure and can be quantified by the pressure-time product of inspiration and transpulmonary pressure. Although a discussion of the work of breathing is beyond the scope of this chapter, both elastic work and resistive work represent the dynamic components. Hyperinflation, upper airway obstruction, and decreased gas exchange efficiency reflect more dynamic qualities of ventilatory work. In some critically ill patients with limited cardiac reserve (as a result of ischemia or congestive heart failure [CHF]), the work of breathing induces a marked increase in respiratory muscle $O_2$ demand that may increase the global $O_2$ demands beyond the capability of these patients' already decompensated cardiovascular reserve. In various lung diseases (e.g., pulmonary edema, airway obstruction, acute respiratory distress syndrome [ARDS]), the increased work of breathing requires in excess of 25% of total $O_2$ consumption. In a low cardiac output state, blood flow to respiratory muscles is inadequate, resulting in hypoxia and lactic acidosis. Respiratory muscles fail despite high respiratory drive; the results are alveolar hypoventilation, respiratory acidosis, and, ultimately, respiratory death despite the presence of potentially normal lungs. Intubation and mechanical ventilation, when adjusted to metabolic demands, must reduce the work of breathing and reduce cardiovascular stress.

Like all exercise, increased work of breathing elevates both cardiac output and $O_2$ extraction, thus decreasing mixed venous $O_2$ saturation ($SvO_2$) for a given cardiac output and $CaO_2$. If initiation of mechanical ventilation reduces $O_2$ consumption, then $SvO_2$ will increase. Assuming that the intrapulmonary shunt remains constant, the arterial partial pressure of $O_2$ ($PaO_2$) will also increase, despite no actual improvement in gas exchange efficiency. Furthermore, if cardiac output is limited, the reduced metabolic demand from the respiratory muscles will allow blood originally delivered to these muscles to be diverted elsewhere. If the patient is already in circulatory shock, the increased blood flow to other hypoperfused tissues may also result in a decrease in blood lactate levels without any change in cardiac output or $DO_2$.

## EFFECT OF CHANGES IN LUNG VOLUME

### Autonomic Tone

The lung is richly innervated with autonomic nerves that sense lung volume and vascular pressure changes as well as causing bronchomotor and vasomotor shifts and alterations in cardiac inotropy and chronotropy. Small increases in lung volume (<10 mL/kg) elevate heart rate by vagal withdrawal. This phenomenon is referred to as *respiratory sinus arrhythmia*. Respiratory sinus arrhythmia reflects the existence of a normal autonomic state and a responsive cardiovascular system. This arrhythmia disappears in dysautonomic states, such as diabetes mellitus. Some degree of respiration-related change in heart rate is intrinsic to the heart itself because it is seen in cardiac transplant recipients whose hearts are denervated.

This respiratory sinus arrhythmia probably functions directly through right atrial mechanoreceptors. Lung inflation to larger tidal volumes (>15 mL/kg) also causes sympathetic withdrawal that rapidly becomes the dominant force. This condition manifests itself as bradycardia, vasodilatation, and decreased cardiac contractility.

Although commonly seen only in neonates and with high-frequency ventilation, potentially selected lung hyperinflation, as may occur when ventilating patients with ARDS who have otherwise normal tidal volumes that overdistend their noncollapsed alveoli, can induce the same sympathetic withdrawal effect, although this has not been studied. Mild hypoxemia and hypercarbia stimulate sympathetic tone and thereby increase cardiac output and blood pressure. Presumably, these effects overshadow the hyperinflation-induced sympathetic withdrawal effects in this setting. However, profound hypoxemia ($PaO_2$ <35 mm Hg) and severe acidemia (pH <7.25) blunt the vascular response to sympathetic stimulation and cause cardiovascular collapse despite increased circulating levels of catecholamines.

### Pulmonary Vascular Resistance

Ventilation affects pulmonary vascular resistance (PVR) by two different mechanisms. It can have direct mechanical effects on pulmonary vascular bed, and it can influence factors causing hypoxic vasoconstriction.

The pulmonary circulation can be divided into two anatomically distinct vascular regions, based on pressures that surround them: alveolar vessels and extra-alveolar vessels. Alveolar vessels consist of arterioles, venules, and capillaries that sense alveolar pressure (Palv) as their surrounding pressure. Extra-alveolar vessels are large pulmonary arteries and veins, the intrathoracic component of the large systemic vessels, and the heart, which sense ITP as their surrounding pressure. As lung volume increases, transpulmonary pressure increases, with the absolute increase in lung volume defined by the respiratory system compliance. However, transpulmonary pressure is Palv minus ITP. Thus, increasing lung volume induces a parallel increase in the extravascular pressure gradient. As the alveoli expand from residual volume, resistance of alveolar capillaries gradually increases to maximum at total lung capacity as a result of their compression from this increasing transpulmonary pressure. Whereas resistance of extra-alveolar vessels gradually decreases as the lung expands, as the radial forces resisting lung expansion increase the diameter of both the large airways (thus decreasing airway resistance) and the extra-alveolar vessels. The opposite occurs with decreasing lung volumes.

Hypoxic pulmonary vasoconstriction develops when regional alveolar $PO_2$ ($PaO_2$) decreases to less than 60 mm Hg. Hypoxic pulmonary vasoconstriction is mediated, in part, by variation in synthesis and release of nitric oxide by pulmonary vascular endothelium. As the lung volume decreases to less than functional residual capacity (FRC), the terminal airways collapse because the radial forces distending them are lost. The obstructed terminal airways rapidly have their $O_2$ absorbed by the perfused blood and become hypoxemic. Thus, as a result of hypoxic pulmonary vasoconstriction, pulmonary vasomotor tone and therefore PVR increase.

Critically ill patients with various pulmonary disorders have marked regional variation in PVR. Diseased areas of lung may experience region-specific hypoxia and consequently may display local vasoconstriction and elevated vascular resistance, thus minimizing the intrapulmonary shunt that would otherwise occur if no vasoconstriction were present. PVR is a dynamic measurement with regional variations. PVR measured by pulmonary artery catheter gives only a mean PVR value that may not reflect pulmonary resistance in different regions of the lung. If alveolar hypoxia is generalized, however, or if systemic acidosis develops, then global pulmonary vasomotor tone will increase, thus increasing PVR and placing a marked afterload on the right ventricle. This may result in reduced right ventricular (RV) output with systemic venous congestion, without any associated left ventricular (LV) failure. The net effect is that PVR is lowest at FRC and increases as the lung volume either increases or decreases from it (Fig. 15.1).

Based on this discussion, it should be clear that positive end-expiratory pressure (PEEP), by increasing transpulmonary pressure at end-expiration, may either increase or decrease PVR, depending on the final end-expiratory lung volume created. The initiation of positive pressure ventilation and the application of PEEP increase both Palv and ITP. However, the degree of elevation of the two differs and is not parallel, depending on various factors such as airway resistance and lung and chest wall compliance (see later). If the lungs were already expanded, then the elevated Palv and ITP would

increase lung volume further, thereby increasing PVR. If, however, regions of the lung were collapsed, and PEEP recruited collapsed alveoli by refreshing them with $O_2$ and reversing hypoxic pulmonary vasoconstriction, then PVR would decrease. Therefore, positive pressure ventilation and PEEP can increase or decrease PVR, depending on underlying lung condition and changes in lung volumes.

## Ventricular Interdependence

The right and left ventricles interact in two ways. First, blood flow to one ventricle eventually flows to the other because they are connected in series. Thus, decreases in RV output during positive pressure ventilation, for example, result in a subsequent decrease in LV output in a few beats. Similarly, reduced LV output leads to elevated PVR over time and to reduced RV output. This series interaction is of primary importance in most circumstances.

Changes in biventricular performance also have a more direct interaction owing to their intimate relationship wherein they share a common interventricular septum and common pericardium and are housed in a common cardiac fossa within the thorax. The two ventricles are separated from each other by an interventricular septum and are surrounded by a restrictive pericardium, which resists acute distention, although it can distend gradually over time. This is called pericardial constraint and it can result in significant hemodynamic consequences as seen in cardiac tamponade. Pericardial volume limitation is the primary factor governing diastolic ventricular interdependence.

Ventricular output depends on diastolic filling. During diastole, the interventricular septum is flaccid, and its position is determined by pressure difference on either side (i.e., LV end-diastolic pressure [LVEDP] minus RV end-diastolic pressure [RVEDP]). It is also called the *transseptal pressure gradient*. As the volume of two ventricles increases acutely (volume overload or CHF), because of the effect of pericardial constraint, the volume of one ventricle increases at the expense of the other, with a corresponding shift in the transseptal gradient. This process is called *direct ventricular interaction*. Its relevance came to light in the 1980s with the application of echocardiography, and it has significant clinical importance. In a state of acute pulmonary hypertension resulting from either acute LV dysfunction or primary pulmonary disease (acute pulmonary embolism), RVEDP increases greatly as compared with LVEDP. This situation leads to changes in the transseptal gradient, shifts the septum to the left, and thus reduces LV diastolic compliance. As a result, LV end-diastolic volume (LVEDV) and cardiac output are decreased. Treating this condition with a fluid challenge makes

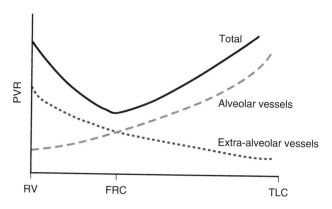

**Figure 15.1** Effects of changes in lung volumes on pulmonary vascular resistance. See text for details.

matters worse and increases RVEDP further. Thus, patients with a low cardiac output state caused by RV failure should not be treated with intravenous fluids except when the low cardiac output state is the result of RV infarction, in which case there is no pulmonary hypertension. The same principle applies in chronic lung diseases associated with chronic pulmonary hypertension, although the effect is seen at higher filling pressures (Fig. 15.2).

## EFFECTS OF CHANGES IN INTRATHORACIC PRESSURE

### Relationships among Right Atrial, Right Ventricular, and Pericardial Pressures

The right atrium is a thin-walled chamber with very low transmural pressure. Therefore, in normal circumstances, right atrial intracavitary pressure corresponds to pericardial pressure. Changes in right atrial pressure closely reflect pericardial pressure changes. The right ventricle has high diastolic compliance and discharges into a very compliant pulmonary circulation. Transmural RVEDP does not change even if right atrial pressure becomes elevated with excess volume loading, which, in fact, represents elevated pericardial pressure. RV volume increases as a result of conformational changes rather than of myocardial stretch. Transmural RVEDP increases

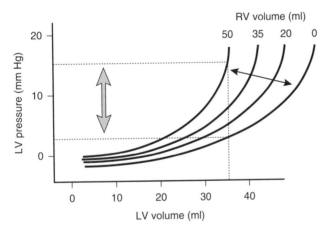

**Figure 15.2** Schematic diagram of the effect of increasing right ventricular (RV) volumes on the left ventricular (LV) diastolic pressure-volume (filling) relationship. Note that increasing RV volumes decrease LV diastolic compliance, such that a higher filling pressure is required to generate a constant end-diastolic volume. (Adapted from Taylor RR, Covell JW, Sonnenblick EH, Ross J Jr: Dependence of ventricular distensibility on filling the opposite ventricle. Am J Physiol 1967;213:711–718.)

in the presence of ischemia, hypertrophy, or increased pericardial compliance.

### Venous Return

Venous return to the right atrium is the most important factor determining cardiac output, provided both ventricles and the pulmonary circulation are normal. Venous return to the right atrium from the systemic venous reservoir occurs along the venous pressure gradient. It is the difference between the mean systemic filling pressure and the right atrial pressure. During spontaneous inspiratory effort, ITP and pericardial pressures fall to less than atmospheric pressure, thus reflecting a decrease in right atrial pressure. This increases the pressure gradient and venous return. Under normal conditions, the right ventricle and pulmonary circulation are highly compliant. Thus, this increase in venous return during inspiration does not result in any significant RVEDP or pulmonary artery pressure change. During loaded inspiratory effort, as occurs in airway obstruction, large negative swings in ITP occur. This results in higher pressure gradients for venous return. If this situation is allowed to continue, it will result in an abnormally high volume of venous return, acute dilatation of the right ventricle, and heart failure. The right ventricle is protected against this acute distention by a phenomenon called *flow limitation*. During these loaded inspiratory efforts, intra-abdominal pressure also becomes negative, thus leading to collapse of large veins and limiting the quantity of venous return (Fig. 15.3).

Positive pressure ventilation with reasonable tidal volumes (<10 mL/kg) and Paw reduces venous return during inspiration as a result of the decreased venous pressure gradient. It also reduces afterload. The net result in a patient with a healthy heart is decreased stroke volume and pulse pressure, because vasomotor tone does not change from beat to beat. This effect is further accentuated in cases of low intravascular volume. This finding forms the basis for diagnosing preload responsiveness in critically sick patients who are receiving mechanical ventilation. In patients with LV dysfunction and with high preload, the effect of positive pressure ventilation is the opposite, leading to increased stroke volume with a decline in afterload. Moreover, cardiac efficiency increases with decreased preload (Figs. 15.4 and 15.5). In all these evaluations, we presume that the patient has no outflow obstruction or valvular dysfunction.

During mechanical ventilation, positive pressure inspiration increases ITP and right atrial pressure, with resulting decreased venous pressure gradient and thus reduced RV filling and RV stroke volume. This situation has been clearly validated in human patients during Doppler flow studies showing inferior vena cava flow variation with ventilatory cycles. The decrease in venous

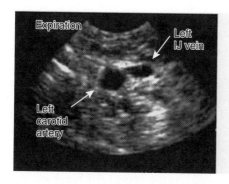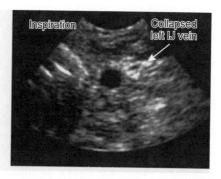

**Figure 15.3** Effects of respiration on venous diameter. Transverse view of the left carotid and internal jugular vein in a spontaneously breathing patient sitting in bed at 30 degrees. The patient was febrile and dehydrated. A near-total collapse of the vein (which is of small caliber) can be appreciated on inspiration (*right*) compared with expiration (*left*). (Courtesy of Dr. Yanick Beaulieu.)

return during positive pressure inspiration is usually lower than would be expected by the degree of increase in right atrial pressure. Various animal studies and subsequent studies in humans showed that, during positive pressure inspiration, the descent of the diaphragm increases intra-abdominal pressure. This elevation of intra-abdominal pressure increases mean systemic filling pressure and minimizes the change in the venous pressure gradient. If the abdominal cavity is open, as in laparotomy, venous return will decrease remarkably with positive pressure inspiration, an effect that can be minimized with volume resuscitation (Fig. 15.6). The application of PEEP also increases hepatic venous resistance to portal flow by elevating right atrial pressure and thus

decreasing portal venous flow, increased pooling of blood in the splanchnic compartment, and reduced venous return to the right atrium. Therefore, the effect of positive pressure ventilation and PEEP on venous return to the right atrium in an individual patient can be positive, negative, or absent, depending on the various factors outlined earlier (Fig. 15.7).

## Preload

Clinicians frequently make the error of assuming that pulmonary artery occlusion pressure (PAOP) is a

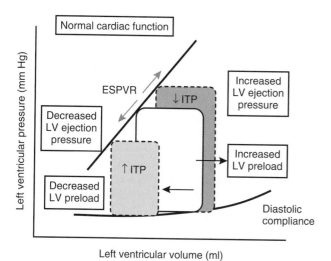

**Figure 15.4** The effect of increasing (gray shade) and decreasing (green shade) intrathoracic pressure on the pressure-volume loop of the cardiac cycle. The slope of the left ventricular (LV) end-systolic pressure-volume relationship (ESPVR) is proportional to contractility. The slope of the diastolic LV pressure-volume relationship defines diastolic compliance.

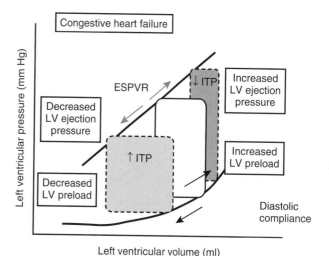

**Figure 15.5** The effect of increasing (*gray shade*) and decreasing (*green shade*) intrathoracic pressure on the left ventricular (LV) pressure-volume loop of the cardiac cycle in congestive heart failure when LV contractility is reduced and intravascular volume is expanded. The slope of the LV end-systolic pressure-volume relationship (ESPVR) is proportional to contractility. The slope of the diastolic LV pressure-volume relationship defines diastolic compliance.

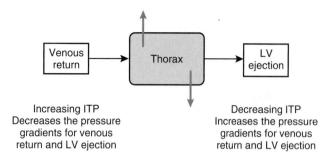

**Figure 15.6** Hemodynamic effects of changes in intrathoracic pressure. Schematic diagram of the effect of increasing or decreasing intrathoracic pressure on the left ventricular (LV) filling (venous return) and ejection pressure.

measure of LV preload. PAOP is a measure of intracavitary LVEDP. Under normal conditions, when there is no diastolic dysfunction and pericardial pressures are low, PAOP correlates well with LV preload. However, in truth, this is transmural LVEDP, which correlates with LVEDV and is correctly the measure of LV preload (transmural LVEDP equals intracavitary LVEDP minus pericardial pressure). Under normal conditions (with low pericardial pressures), intravascular volume expansion increases both intracavitary LVEDP and transmural LVEDP, and thus both correlate with LVEDV. However, in the presence of external constraint, either

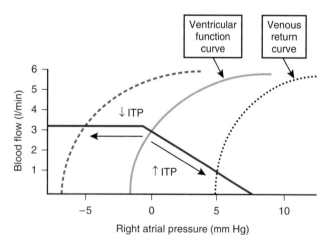

**Figure 15.7** Changes in intrathoracic pressure alter the relationships among cardiac output, venous return, and right atrial pressure. Schematic representation of the effects of increasing or decreasing intrathoracic pressure (ITP) on steady-state venous return. Note that decreases in ITP that decrease right atrial pressure to less than zero relative to atmospheric pressure increase venous return only by a limited amount, whereas increases in ITP progressively decrease venous return to a complete circulatory standstill.

pericardial constraint or the application of positive pressure ventilation and PEEP, a disparity occurs between the changes in intracavitary LVEDP and those in transmural LVEDP (and therefore LVEDV). Similarly, during acute or chronic RV volume expansion, intracavitary LVEDP increases, whereas transmural LVEDP and LVEDV may actually decrease. This effect results from ventricular interdependence (see earlier). Thus, when a patient receives positive pressure ventilation with PEEP, PAOP increases and cardiac output decreases (reduced cardiac work). In the past, this situation was presumed to result from the negative effect of PEEP on LV contractility. However, it is actually caused by decreased transmural LVEDP and LVEDV and can be easily reversed with volume expansion to bring preload to pre-PEEP levels.

## Afterload

LV afterload is a measure of maximal systolic wall tension, which, according to the Laplace equation, is as follows:

$$\text{LV afterload} \propto \text{Transmural LV pressure} \times \text{Radius of curvature of LV (LV volume)}$$

$$\text{Transmural LV pressure (LV ejection pressure)} = \text{Intracavitary LV pressure} - \text{Pericardial pressure}$$

Maximal LV systolic wall tension occurs at the end of isometric contraction when the radius of the curvature is maximal and the transmural pressure is the difference between intracavitary LV pressure (diastolic aortic pressure) and pericardial pressure. During LV ejection, afterload decreases despite a slight increase in ejection pressure resulting from the decline in radius of the curvature as LV volume decreases. During a loaded spontaneous inspiratory effort, as seen with airway obstruction, a negative swing in ITP increases transmural LV pressure for a given LV volume and aortic pressure and results in increased afterload and thus increased myocardial $O_2$ consumption. This is a cardiac stress test, and in patients with low cardiac reserve, it can precipitate myocardial ischemia and heart failure. The application of positive pressure ventilation increases ITP and thus reduces LV ejection pressure besides decreasing LVEDV by direct compression and reduced venous return. The net results are reduced afterload and myocardial $O_2$ consumption. In addition, the work of breathing is reduced, and global $O_2$ demand is thus decreased. This situation offloads an ischemic and failing left ventricle. Weaning from mechanical ventilation acts as a stress test, and patients with poor LV function may fail a weaning trial despite good lung mechanics if this factor is not taken into consideration.

## Interactions among Airway Pressure, Lung Volume, and Intrathoracic Pressure

An oversimplification of cardiopulmonary physiology in patients receiving positive pressure ventilation that relates hemodynamic changes to Paw has resulted in confusion in the literature and in the minds of physicians caring for these patients. This situation has occurred because Paw can easily be measured in patients receiving mechanical ventilation, and changes in Paw are frequently associated with some changes in lung volumes and pleural pressure. Bedside clinical decisions based on changes in Paw associated with certain changes in hemodynamic parameters may frequently result in the institution of therapies that are wrong. Numerous studies have shown that the major determinants of the hemodynamic effects of ventilation result from changes in ITP, lung volumes, and pericardial pressure. A change in Paw does not necessarily result in a change in ITP of the same magnitude. The fraction of change in Paw that is transmitted to ITP depends on lung compliance, chest wall compliance, frequency and type of ventilation, and airway resistance. In spontaneously breathing individuals, negative swings in ITP generate tidal volumes the magnitude of which depends on airway resistance and lung compliance. Thus, if an increase in airway resistance or lung compliance exists, a greater negative swing in ITP will be required to generate the same tidal volume. Increasing the work of breathing by placing a greater demand on a limited cardiovascular system will have serious hemodynamic consequences.

During mechanical ventilation, Paw measured at the endotracheal tube is a sum of the pressure required to overcome airway resistance and Palv. Provided airway resistance is normal, Paw correlates well with Palv. A fraction of Palv is utilized to expand the lung (lung volume change) and is called *transpulmonary pressure*, and the rest is used for chest wall expansion (ITP change). In healthy individuals, compliance of the lung and the chest wall is equal. Thus, 50% of Palv change is a change in transpulmonary pressure, and the remainder is a shift in ITP that influences hemodynamics. Thus:

$$\Delta Paw \propto \Delta\ Palv = \Delta\ Transpulmonary\ pressure + \Delta\ ITP$$

As the transpulmonary pressure increases, it expands lungs by a volume that depends on compliance. As the lungs expand, they press on the surrounding structures, distort these structures, and cause their surface pressures to rise. Various studies have shown that, in diseased or healthy lungs, the ITP rise will be similar to the volume increase, although the change in Paw will be dissimilar (Fig. 15.8). The pressure is higher in diseased lungs because the transpulmonary pressure is high.

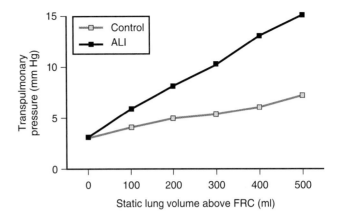

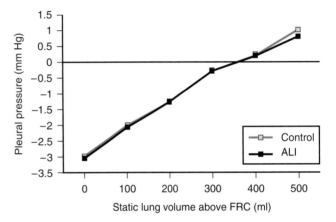

**Figure 15.8** Relation between airway pressure (Paw) and tidal volume (Vᴛ) and between pleural pressure (Ppl) and Vᴛ in control and oleic acid–induced acute lung injury (ALI) conditions in a canine model. Note that despite greater increases in Paw for the same Vᴛ during ALI as compared with control conditions, Ppl and Ppc increase similarly during both control and ALI conditions for the same increase in Vᴛ. (From Romand JA, Shi W, Pinsky MR: Cardiopulmonary effects of positive pressure ventilation during acute lung injury. Chest 1995;108:1041–1048.)

Because the change in ITP is similar, so are the hemodynamic effects. Clinically, patients with primary lung disease (primary ARDS) who have decreased lung compliance have a greater fraction of increase in Paw utilized for transpulmonary pressure change and a minimal change in ITP and thus hardly any effect on hemodynamic parameters. In contrast, in patients with low chest wall compliance (secondary ARDS, intra-abdominal pressure increase), a greater fraction of Paw increase is spent in overcoming chest wall compliance, thus resulting in a higher increase in ITP and greater hemodynamic consequences.

It is also clinically relevant to understand that the chest wall consists of structures with different compliance. The anterior chest wall and the lateral chest wall have higher compliance than the posterior chest wall and the cardiac fossa (Fig. 15.9). The diaphragm also displays high compliance. During delivery of a positive pressure

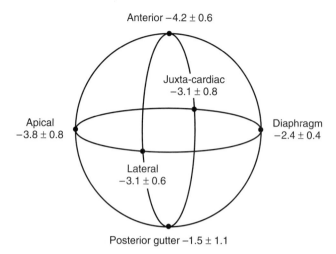

**Figure 15.9** Apneic pleural pressure (Ppl) (mean ± SE) in mm Hg for six pleural regions of the right hemothorax of an intact supine canine model. ANT, anterior; AP, apical; DI, diaphragmatic; JC, juxtacardiac; LAT, lateral; PG, posterior gutter; *ellipses,* regional measurements defining three orthogonal planes. (From Novak R, Matuschak GM, Pinsky MR. J Appl Physiol 1995;65:1314–1323.)

tidal breath, the juxtacardiac pleural pressure increases most and the diaphragmatic pleural pressure least. However, increase in intra-abdominal pressure resulting from gut wall swelling or distention can significantly lower compliance, with a significant rise in ITP and hemodynamic effects. Thus, a clinician may wrongly assume, in a patient with abdominal distention, that the lung is injured and less compliant. Increasing Paw further to overcome this stiffness will increase ITP further; greater hemodynamic consequences will result, without improving gas exchange. Normally, pericardial pressure is low, and an increase in juxtacardiac pleural pressure is linearly transmitted to the pericardium. An increase in pericardial pressure reduces LV diastolic compliance and also decreases transmural LV pressure and thus afterload. Diastolic compliance is further reduced by the effects of ventricular interdependence. Reduced venous return results in low LVEDV. Low cardiac output in patients who are receiving positive pressure ventilation is the result of reduced preload and not of decreased contractility, as could be erroneously deduced. The initial increase in ITP increases only juxtacardiac pleural pressure without affecting pericardial pressure and thus has no hemodynamic effects. Once juxtacardiac pleural pressure rises above pericardial pressure, a further increase in ITP linearly raises both pressures.

## ENDOCRINE EFFECTS OF HEART-LUNG INTERACTION

During acute respiratory failure, clinically significant disturbances occur in the hormonal systems involved in salt and water homeostasis. These systems are further influenced by the application of positive pressure ventilation and PEEP. Atrial natriuretic peptide (ANP) is released from secretory granules in the atrial myocytes in response to stretch. ANP acts on the kidneys directly and causes natriuresis and diuresis. It also acts on the hypothalamus, where it suppresses the release of antidiuretic hormone and inhibits the renin-angiotensin-aldosterone system. High levels of ANP are seen in patients with pulmonary disorders associated with cor pulmonale and right atrial stretch. In vitro studies have shown that vasopressin, epinephrine, and phenylephrine may increase ANP secretion. Mechanical ventilation and PEEP increase ITP, a change that decreases intrathoracic blood volume and offloads the right atrium. This situation reduces plasma levels of ANP and causes antidiuresis. In addition, levels of vasopressin, renin, aldosterone, and angiotensin II are elevated. The net result is salt and water retention. The clinical significance lies in the finding that when such patients are weaned from mechanical ventilation and are extubated, fluid shift may impair gas exchange, and extubation may fail. Studies have shown beneficial effects of infusion of ANP on gas exchange by inducing diuresis in patients with ARDS who are receiving mechanical ventilation.

## CLINICAL APPLICATIONS OF HEART-LUNG INTERACTION

We have seen that positive pressure ventilation and PEEP can have variable effects on hemodynamics depending on underlying pulmonary and extrapulmonary disease, intravascular volume status, lung volumes, lung compliance, chest wall compliance, airway resistance, RV function, and LV function. In general, positive pressure ventilation reduces venous return by decreasing venous pressure gradient and reduces afterload by reducing transmural LV pressure and LVEDV. Ventilation also affects PVR, which increases as lung volume increases from FRC. PEEP opens up collapsed alveoli, improves ventilation-perfusion (V/Q) mismatch, and may reduce PVR by removing hypoxic pulmonary vasoconstriction. However, this is not so simple. Acute lung injury and ARDS affect lungs in a nonhomogeneous fashion. Some areas of lung are normal, whereas other areas have collapsed alveoli with low compliance. PEEP may overdistend normal alveoli. This hyperinflation compresses alveolar vessels and increases PVR. Collapsed alveoli are opened up with PEEP; alveolar vessels of these alveoli then open up, and their resistance falls.

### Acute Lung Injury/Acute Respiratory Distress Syndrome

Since its description more than 25 years ago, ARDS has received considerable attention in critical care medicine.

Whenever the lungs are exposed to an insult, a host response is mounted in the form of close interactions between the cellular and humoral immune systems. The net result is damage to the epithelial and endothelial regions of lung, although injury to one or the other may predominate. Insult to the lungs may be direct or indirect as a result of responses to systemic inflammatory processes. The prevalent damage following a direct insult is intra-alveolar, with alveolar filling by edema, fibrin, collagen, neutrophil aggregates, or blood. It is often described as *pulmonary consolidation*. When lungs are involved in systemic inflammation (an indirect insult), the initial injury is to the vascular endothelium, and it results in microvascular congestion and interstitial edema, whereas alveolar spaces are relatively spared. Frequently, both processes overlap to varying degrees. Formerly, based on chest radiographs, ARDS was presumed to be a homogeneous alteration of the lung parenchyma. Computed tomographic imaging completely changed this assumption. ARDS involves nonhomogeneous pulmonary infiltrates, primarily distributed in dependent regions, with relative sparing of nondependent regions. Accordingly, the lung in ARDS can be modeled as comprising three zones: normally inflated lungs (the baby lung, nondependent), recruitable (collapsed lung that could be opened with adequate inflation pressure), and consolidated lung (lung with alveolar filling that cannot be opened by increasing Palv).

Baby lung is not an anatomic reality, but rather a functional concept. Early in the course of ARDS caused by an indirect insult, the lungs are characterized by diffuse edema, with the superimposed pressure causing atelectasis and collapse of dependent lung zones. The maneuver of prone positioning does not help by redistributing edema fluid because the interstitial edema, being rich in proteins, is not free to move. Instead, prone positioning helps by relieving compression from superimposed pressure.

## Recruitment and Oxygenation

Opening pressures, required to inflate the collapsed airways and alveoli, are much greater than pressures required to keep the lungs open (PEEP). Recruitment helps to provide a more homogeneous distribution of tidal volumes and consequently results in reduced V/Q mismatch and improved oxygenation. In nondependent lung regions, increasing PEEP causes overdistention of alveoli and decreased regional compliance. In dependent lung regions, PEEP maintains recruitment of collapsing alveoli and increases compliance. Opening of alveoli in dependent lung regions reduces the shunt fraction and thereby improves oxygenation. Excessive PEEP overstretches the alveoli in nondependent lung regions, thus reducing ventilation and causing hypercarbia, sometimes seen with excessive PEEP. There is no ideal PEEP, and it is always a compromise between inflation of collapsed alveoli and overstretching of others.

## Respiratory Elastance

*Elastance*, the reciprocal of compliance, is the pressure required to inflate the lungs. One half of this pressure is spent to inflate the lungs, and the other half is used to inflate the chest wall in normal lungs. Normally, the elastance of the lungs and chest wall is similar. In ARDS from direct injury (primary ARDS), the elastance of the chest wall remains normal. The net effect is that transpulmonary pressure is increased, whereas pleural pressure remains the same. In ARDS resulting from direct injury, increasing Paw applied to improve the V/Q mismatch has little effect on cardiac dimensions and cardiopulmonary hemodynamics. The reverse is true in patients with ARDS from an indirect insult (secondary ARDS). In these patients, chest wall elastance is increased much more than lung elastance, thus resulting in increased pleural pressure as Paw increases. In addition, in secondary ARDS, intra-abdominal pressures are elevated, because most of the causes of secondary ARDS lie in the abdomen. This situation adversely affects the extrapulmonary elastance. Therefore, the cardiac dimensions are diminished, and cardiopulmonary hemodynamics are adversely affected. In ARDS of any cause, pulmonary artery pressure and PVR are elevated as a result of multiple factors, such as compression of vessels (from superimposed pressure), endothelial swelling, medial hypertrophy, and vasoconstriction. The net effect of all this is an increased work cost of breathing, which a patient cannot sustain alone.

## Ventilation Strategy

No single ventilatory strategy is most beneficial in all patients. An individualized approach has to be adopted, depending on a patient's baseline cardiopulmonary status and the cause of ARDS. Various studies have shown deleterious effects of high tidal volumes (>10 mL/kg), in the form of elevated levels of inflammatory mediators. Clinically relevant beneficial effects of low tidal (6 mL/kg) volumes, even allowing permissive hypercapnia, were clearly shown by an ARDS Network trial, although considerable controversy was generated by the study design. Other studies failed to show any benefits of a low–tidal volume strategy. Effort should be made to keep plateau pressure lower than 30 cm $H_2O$. Higher ITP has a more profoundly negative effect on cardiac output in secondary ARDS than in primary ARDS (see earlier). This situation is made worse by low intravascular volumes. Higher tidal volumes and not Paw negatively affect RV afterload. Whichever ventilatory strategy is adopted, the following three principles should be followed: (1) avoid large swings in ITP, (2) minimize the work cost of breathing, and (3) return end-expiratory lung volume to FRC. Pressure support ventilation is possibly the best weaning method because it is associated with the least swings in ITP and therefore is less stressful.

## Asthma

During quiet breathing in physiologically normal persons, air flow changes from turbulent to laminar as the air passes from the trachea to around the second-generation bronchi. In patients with exacerbations of asthma, turbulent flow occurs more frequently, thereby increasing the work of breathing. To overcome increased airway resistance, more negative ITP is generated by the inspiratory muscles. This exaggerated negative swing in ITP augments venous return and leads to increased RVEDV, higher lung blood volume, and higher lung volume at end-inspiration. Because of ventricular interdependence, LV diastolic compliance is decreased, and LV afterload is increased (the effect of more negative ITP). The net hemodynamic effect is decreased stroke volume during spontaneous inspiratory effort against bronchospasm. With further worsening of asthma, PVR is increased, thus reducing RV output. An increase in venous return occurs only to a certain extent and is restricted by flow limitation resulting from venous collapse. A further decrease in ITP increases LV afterload without increasing venous return. Removing these markedly negative swings in ITP should disproportionately reduce LV afterload more than decrease venous return (preload). Assisted ventilation with endotracheal intubation and positive pressure ventilation not only reduces the work of breathing but also removes these negative swings in ITP. High levels of positive pressure during assisted ventilation may markedly reduce venous return, thereby jeopardizing cardiac output and possibly leading to circulatory collapse. This situation can be worsened by coexisting hypovolemia and the development of auto-PEEP and is further compounded by withdrawal of sympathetic activity as the patient is sedated and intubated. Therefore, patients with severe asthma characterized by hypoxemia and hypercarbia may need not only positive pressure ventilation and bronchodilation but also fluid replacement.

## Chronic Obstructive Pulmonary Disease

Chronic obstructive pulmonary disease (COPD) has two different underlying pathophysiologic conditions, and they affect hemodynamics differently. Chronic bronchitis is characterized by airway obstruction as the primary component, with hemodynamic effects resembling those of asthma. Conversely, emphysema is characterized by air space destruction, airway obstruction, and damage to alveolar capillaries. Usually, both conditions coexist, although one disorder may predominate in any given patient. Patients with predominant emphysema have a higher residual volume and total lung capacity. Vital capacity is diminished, and compliance is high. Alveolar ventilation and gas exchange are affected, leading to hypercarbia and hypoxemia. Hypoxemia causes pulmonary vasoconstriction and therefore elevated PVR and chronic cor pulmonale. To generate adequate tidal volume, the inspiratory muscles have to generate higher negative pressures that increase the work of breathing. Noninvasive positive pressure ventilation has been shown to improve outcomes in patients with COPD exacerbation. In addition, positive pressure ventilation has mortality benefits in stable patients with COPD who have hypoxemia when they breathe room air. By relieving hypoxia, alveolar vasoconstriction is reversed, and RV afterload is reduced.

During positive pressure ventilation, patients with airway obstruction can develop intrinsic PEEP and dynamic hyperinflation of lungs that lead to elevated Paw. Because lung elastance is low, a higher fraction of Paw is transmitted to the pleura. High ITP adversely affects venous return and RV afterload. This situation may lead to circulatory collapse when patients with an exacerbation of COPD receive mechanical ventilation. Intrinsic (auto) PEEP also increases the work of breathing. The adverse effects of intrinsic PEEP can be minimized by several approaches. First, one can treat the underlying bronchospasm and airway inflammation. Second, by prolonging the expiratory time (shorten the I:E ratio), more time is allowed for exhalation. This can be achieved either by shortening the inspiratory time (increasing flow rate or decreasing tidal volume) or by decreasing the respiratory rate. Third, one can apply increasing levels of extrinsic PEEP to minimize the work cost of spontaneous efforts. Extrinsic PEEP helps to eliminate auto-PEEP by a "waterfall effect." Finally, one can increase intravascular volume by fluid resuscitation.

## Congestive Heart Failure

Heart failure can have two underlying pathophysiologic processes. It can result from either systolic or diastolic dysfunction. Both types of disorder can coexist in a single patient, and treatments for both types differ. Patients with systolic dysfunction are usually volume overloaded (higher preload), whereas those with diastolic dysfunction need higher than usual preload. Echocardiography helps in differentiating the two conditions. Diastolic dysfunction is characterized by reversal of E/A ratio during LV diastolic filling. Long-standing diastolic dysfunction ultimately leads to systolic dysfunction. Patients with chronic stable CHF are usually asymptomatic in the resting state. In a state of decompensation or during development of acute CHF (e.g., myocardial ischemia, arrhythmia) there is elevation of left atrial pressure. Lung compliance decreases. Resulting pulmonary edema leads to hypoxemia from

V/Q mismatch. Patients need to develop more negative pressures to ventilate, thus leading to a higher $O_2$ demand that their already stressed cardiovascular system is unable to meet. Their hearts are already near the plateau of the Frank-Starling curve. Treatment in such conditions involves reducing preload (diuresis, venodilatation), reducing afterload (arterial vasodilatation), and improving contractility (inotropes). Positive pressure ventilation (endotracheally or noninvasively) helps in acute CHF exacerbation in multiple ways. By increasing ITP, it reduces venous return and decreases preload. It also results in decreased RV dimension, thereby leading to increased LV diastolic compliance and increased LVEDV (ventricular interdependence; see earlier). Similarly, diuresis helps. Increased ITP reduces afterload ($\propto$ aortic pressure – ITP). Assisted ventilation also offloads respiratory muscles and reduces $O_2$ requirements. As in ARDS, application of increasing levels of extrinsic PEEP helps in oxygenation by bringing FRC toward normal and thus improving V/Q mismatch. Positive pressure ventilation helps to buy time to address the underlying cause of CHF exacerbation.

Weaning from mechanical ventilation requires special attention to cardiovascular status. If cardiac insufficiency persists, weaning will fail. The process of weaning, by removing the beneficial effects of positive pressure ventilation, places an extra metabolic burden on the cardiovascular system. Needless to say, cardiovascular and pulmonary insufficiency must be resolved if weaning is to succeed.

## Hemodynamic Monitoring: Pulse Pressure Variation, Systolic Pressure Variation, and Preload Responsiveness

Respiration-induced changes in pulse volume have long been known in the form of pulsus paradoxus. Interest has renewed in the value of variation in systolic arterial pressure and pulse pressure with ventilation and in their role in assessing preload responsiveness. Measurements of preload such as left atrial pressure, right atrial pressure, and RVEDV do not help in the estimation of preload responsiveness because preload is not preload responsiveness. In a sedated patient receiving mechanical ventilation with low tidal volume (<10 mL/kg), systolic pressure and arterial pulse pressure depend on vasomotor tone and stroke volume. Because vasomotor tone does not normally change from beat to beat, any variation in systolic arterial pressure ($\Delta$SP) and pulse pressure ($\Delta$PP) with positive pressure inspiration will result from a change in stroke volume. As previously discussed, positive pressure inspiration reduces venous return, which is further accentuated in hypovolemic patients. This results in reduced stroke volume manifesting as a decline in pulse pressure and systolic pressure. The greater the degree of variation in systolic and pulse pressure, the greater will be the increase in stroke volume in response to fluid challenge. This finding was validated in a study of patients in septic shock (Figs. 15.10 and 15.11).

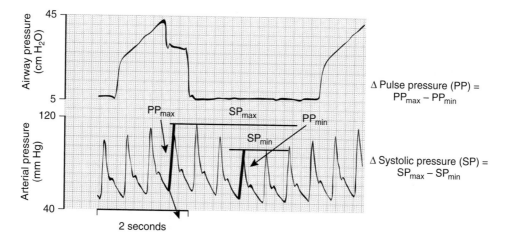

$\Delta$ Pulse pressure (PP) = $PP_{max} - PP_{min}$

$\Delta$ Systolic pressure (SP) = $SP_{max} - SP_{min}$

**Figure 15.10** Simultaneous recording of systemic arterial and airway pressure curves in one illustrative patient with large systolic and pulse pressure variations. Systolic and diastolic pressures were measured on a beat-to-beat basis, and pulse pressure was calculated as the difference between systolic and diastolic pressures. Maximum and minimum values for systolic and pulse pressures ($PP_{max}$ and $PP_{min}$, respectively) were determined over a single respiratory cycle. The respiratory changes in pulse pressure ($\Delta$PP) were calculated as the difference between $PP_{max}$ and $PP_{min}$ divided by the mean of the two values and were expressed as a percentage. The respiratory changes in systolic pressure ($\Delta$SP) were evaluated using a similar formula. (From Michard F, Boussat S, Chemla D, et al: Relation between respiratory changes in arterial pulse pressure and fluid responsiveness in septic patients with acute circulatory failure. Am J Respir Crit Care Med 2000;162:134–138.)

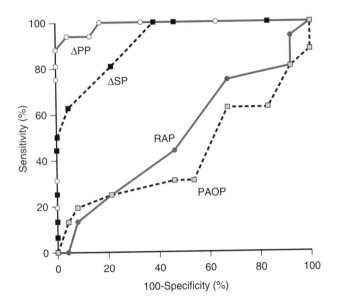

**Figure 15.11** Receiver operating characteristic (ROC) curves. The ability of the respiratory changes in pulse pressure (ΔPP), the respiratory changes in systolic pressure (ΔSP), the right atrial pressure (RAP), and the pulmonary artery occlusion pressure (PAOP) to discriminate between responders (cardiac index increase = 15%) and nonresponders to volume expansion is compared. The area under the ROC curve for ΔPP was greater than those for ΔSP, RAP, and PAOP ($P < .01$). (From Michard F, Boussat S, Chemla D, et al: Relation between respiratory changes in arterial pulse pressure and fluid responsiveness in septic patients with acute circulatory failure. Am J Respir Crit Care Med 2000;162:134–138.)

## CONCLUSION

In critically ill patients, lung compliance and chest wall compliance are frequently altered. The result is an increase in the work of breathing that a patient with cardiovascular insufficiency may not be able to tolerate and that may lead to the initiation of mechanical ventilation. Positive pressure ventilation has significant effects on hemodynamic status resulting from alterations in preload and afterload. These effects are accentuated in patients with hypovolemia and cardiovascular insufficiency. In addition, positive pressure ventilation helps by removing negative swings in ITP and associated adverse effects on hemodynamics. PEEP opens up collapsed alveoli thus improving V/Q mismatch and gas exchange. PEEP also lowers PVR by removing hypoxic alveolar vasoconstriction in diseased alveoli, but it may adversely affect normal alveoli. Thus, the overall effects on PVR may be variable. Weaning from mechanical ventilation once the underlying lung disorder is resolved is a process of transition from positive pressure ventilation to spontaneous breathing. At that time, consideration should also be given to the patient's cardiovascular status because occult cardiac failure may be unmasked, resulting in failed extubation.

## ACKNOWLEDGMENT

This work was supported in part by the federal government (GM61992–03, NHLBI K–24 HL67181–01A2, and NRSA 2–T32 HL07820–06).

## SUGGESTED READINGS

Andrivet P, Adnot S, Sanker S, et al: Hormonal interactions and renal function during mechanical ventilation and ANF infusion in humans. J Appl Physiol 1991;70:287–292.

Belenkie I, Smith ER, Tyberg JV: Ventricular interaction: From bench to bedside. Ann Med 2001;33:236–241.

Chihara E, Hasimoto S, Kinoshita T, et al: Elevated mean systemic filling pressure due to intermittent positive-pressure ventilation. Am J Physiol 1992;262:H1116–H1121.

Denault AY, Gorscan J III, Pinsky MR: Dynamic effects of positive-pressure ventilation on canine left ventricular pressure-volume relations. J Appl Physiol 2001;91:298–308.

Gattinoni L, Marini JJ: Ventilatory management of acute respiratory distress syndrome: A consensus of two. Crit Care Med 2004;32:250–255.

Michard F, Boussat S, Chemla D, et al: Relation between respiratory changes in arterial pulse pressure and fluid responsiveness in septic patients with acute circulatory failure. Am J Respir Crit Care Med 2000;162:134–138.

Pelosi P, D'onofrio D, Chiumello D, et al: Pulmonary and extrapulmonary acute respiratory distress syndrome are different. Eur Respir J 2003;42(Suppl):48S–56S.

Pinsky MR: Breathing as exercise: The cardiovascular response to weaning from mechanical ventilation. Intensive Care Med 2000;26:1164–1166.

Pinsky MR, Guimond JG: The effects of positive end-expiratory pressure on heart-lung interactions. J Crit Care 1991;6:1–11.

Stock MC, David DW, Manning JW, Ryan ML: Lung mechanics and oxygen consumption during spontaneous ventilation and severe heart failure. Chest 1992;102:279–283.

# CHAPTER 16

# Gastrointestinal-Lung Interactions

Enrico Calzia and Peter Radermacher

Mechanical ventilation (MV) interferes with visceral organ function, in part as a result of well-known heart-lung interactions. In fact, because of the increase in intrathoracic pressure (ITP), MV markedly affects hemodynamics, especially when positive end-expiratory pressure (PEEP) is applied.[1-3] These interactions, which mainly lead to a reduction in cardiac output, are crucially important to understanding the impact of MV with PEEP on critically ill patients, and the reader with a special interest in these fundamental topics should refer to Chapter 15.

Under normal circumstances, a substantial portion of the cardiac output crosses the splanchnic and non-splanchnic abdominal regions before entering the thorax and returning to the right side of the heart. Impedance of abdominal venous return may thus be a further mechanism by which MV impairs whole hemodynamics independent of organ interactions at the thoracic level. Indeed, as we discuss in this chapter, experimental evidence indicates that MV and PEEP may also directly affect the regional circulation, not only by heart-lung interactions but also by increasing resistance to flow at the abdominal level.[4,5] In particular, limitations in blood flow to the hepatosplanchnic organs under such circumstances[4,6-9] may be of crucial importance in critically ill patients.

This chapter first summarizes our present knowledge on the effects of MV on the perfusion and function of the hepatosplanchnic organs. Much of this knowledge is based on experimental data from animal studies that provide a fundamental understanding of the basic physiologic mechanisms involved in these interactions. The main focus of this chapter, however, is on data obtained from human studies from the past several decades that give us a fairly clear picture of the clinical effects of PEEP ventilation on hepatosplanchnic perfusion and function. Furthermore, our discussion focuses on the potential impact on hepatosplanchnic function and circulation of therapeutic approaches widely used in intensive care units (ICUs) to support lung function in patients with acute respiratory failure (e.g., prone position, partial spontaneous breathing, and permissive hypercapnia).

## POSITIVE END-EXPIRATORY PRESSURE INDUCES MECHANICAL EFFECTS ON HEPATOSPLANCHNIC VASCULATURE

Unimpeded abdominal venous return is of crucial importance to hemodynamics, not only because of the large amount of blood that returns to the heart across this vascular region but also because of the large capacitance of the hepatosplanchnic vasculature, which is involved in the regulation of circulating blood volume. The basic mechanisms acting to regulate blood flow across the abdominal organs and thus influencing cardio-circulatory homeostasis have been studied extensively, albeit mainly in animals.[5,10] Further experiments performed by the same group focused more closely on the effects of MV with PEEP on liver blood flow.[11,12] The physical bases of the interactions between MV and hepatosplanchnic perfusion and between MV and abdominal venous return, respectively, are the increase in intra-abdominal pressure and the caudal displacement of the diaphragm. The first effect was shown theoretically and experimentally to affect venous return in dogs with closed and open abdomens, an effect that was highly dependent on the actual intravascular blood volume.[5,10] By analyzing the abdominal compartment in terms of vascular zones (analogous to the well-known models of pulmonary circulation), Takata and colleagues were able to show that abdominal venous return increased once the inferior vena cava (IVC) pressure exceeded the sum of abdominal pressure and venous closure pressure, a situation consistent with a sufficient intravascular volume loading. In contrast, once IVC pressure falls to less than the sum of abdominal and venous closure pressures, as may occur with low intravascular fluid volume, a pressure gradient across the diaphragm develops along the IVC, consistent with a vascular waterfall.[10] Furthermore, the caudal displacement of the diaphragm may directly increase intrahepatic resistance to flow by liver compression, which apparently occurs even with an open abdomen and thus is not necessarily related to intra-abdominal pressure.[5]

This latter interaction had been suggested earlier by Alexander,[13] as well as by Johnson and Hedley-Whyte, who found that continuous positive pressure ventilation increased resistance to flow through the choledochoduodenal junction.[14] More recently, however, an MV-induced increase in intrahepatic resistance failed to be confirmed either by Matuschak and colleagues[15] or by Bredenberg and associates.[16] A possible explanation for these conflicting results may be derived from data presented by Brienza and associates,[4] who suggested that increased intrahepatic vascular resistance may be counteracted by increased intravascular volume, according to the well-known distensible properties of the hepatic vascular resistance.[17]

With respect to liver perfusion, the experiments by Brienza and colleagues are fundamental to understand how PEEP ventilation interferes with the regulation of blood flow across the hepatosplanchnic region. The results may be summarized as follows: (1) the presence of a vascular waterfall[18,19] keeps portal blood flow and hence splanchnic venous return stable up to the point when hepatic outflow pressure exceeds portal closure pressure, (2) the distensibility of the portal vascular bed allows flow resistance to be decreased once outflow pressure exceeds portal closure pressure,[17] and (3) hepatic artery flow is not characterized by a classic waterfall inasmuch as closure pressure rises with the outflow pressure.[11,12] As shown experimentally, the first two mechanisms, which under physiologic conditions act to maintain constant splanchnic venous return regardless of changes in central venous pressure, may be affected by PEEP ventilation. In this animal study,[4] the PEEP-related increase in right atrial pressure was shown to be transmitted to the portal vein, in contrast to the expected dilatation of the portal vasculature.[17] However, flow resistance across this vascular section did not decrease, but rather increased, probably owing to direct compression of the

intrahepatic vessels.[4] These observations are consistent with human data, in which PEEP ventilation was shown to shift blood volume toward the intestine and the liver as the largest capacitance region while partially depleting the intrathoracic vascular bed.[20] In this study by Peters and colleagues, PEEP-induced changes in liver blood volume were relatively small when compared with changes in the intestine, thus indicating that PEEP may indeed act to compress the liver even in human subjects.

Similar to the effects on portal circulation, in the animal experiment by Brienza and colleagues, hepatic arterial resistance was found to be increased under PEEP ventilation. Probably, this effect is due to the elevated tissue pressure which results from the diaphragm displacement. The so-called hepatic artery buffer response (HABR) was proven to be intact at all PEEP levels; that is, the effects of this physiologic mechanism on liver hemodynamics were apparently counterbalanced by direct mechanical compression. According to these experimental data, the HABR was found to work properly even in anesthetized human subjects under PEEP ventilation (Fig. 16.1).[21] The HABR is an important mechanism, mainly responsible for compensating fluctuations in portal vein flow (normally ~75% of total hepatic blood flow), thus maintaining a constant total liver blood flow. Furthermore, the HABR permits separate regulation of hepatic and intestinal blood flow and thus controls the physiologic functions linked to hepatic blood flow and volume independent of the intestinal blood supply.[22] In summary, this fundamental mechanism, which has been shown to be affected by some

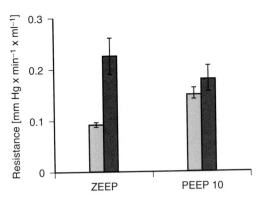

**Figure 16.1** The diagram demonstrates the effects of the hepatic artery buffer response in humans during mechanical ventilation with positive end-expiratory pressure (PEEP). Mesenteric vascular resistance (*dark bars*) increases under PEEP of 10 cm $H_2O$ and is accompanied by a simultaneous decrease in hepatic arterial vascular resistance (*white bars*). (Data [mean ± SEM] from Aneman A, Eisenhofer G, Fändriks L, et al: Splanchnic circulation and regional sympathetic outflow during perioperative PEEP ventilation in humans. Br J Anaesth 1999;82:838–842.)

pathologic conditions,[23] was found to be basically unaltered by PEEP ventilation in animals[4] and humans.[21]

All the available data have been obtained in animals or humans during PEEP ventilation but without specific pathologic conditions. Because conditions such as endotoxic shock have been shown to alter splanchnic hemodynamics, it is conceivable that PEEP ventilation may have a far more impressive impact on liver and gut perfusion under such circumstances. Thus, a detailed analysis of the role of PEEP ventilation on hepatosplanchnic circulation and function under such critical circumstances will require further research.

## HEPATOSPLANCHNIC PERFUSION IS REDUCED DURING MECHANICAL VENTILATION WITH POSITIVE END-EXPIRATORY PRESSURE IN HUMANS

Even when stable systemic arterial pressure is maintained, the application of positive airway pressure results in a marked decrease in human cardiac output.[21,24,25] In dogs, analogous changes in cardiac output under PEEP ventilation up to 20 mm Hg were found to be affiliated with a redistribution of blood flow that favored brain, heart, and adrenals at the expense of blood flow to stomach, pancreas, and thyroid gland.[8] Neither hepatic nor intestinal perfusion seemed to be the subject of redistribution in that study, because flow decreased proportionally to cardiac output. These data on mesenteric blood flow are particularly noteworthy because they are in contrast to later results[7] (see later).

A second, simultaneously published study in eight critically ill patients demonstrated that the ratio between hepatic plasma flow and cardiac output remained constant, at a value of approximately 0.15 when PEEP was increased up to 20 cm $H_2O$.[9] Interpreting data on total hepatic blood or plasma flow is not easy, however, because of the HABR, which, as just explained, compensates for the portal vein flow decrease to keep the total hepatic perfusion stable. The key question—whether the fall in *both* hepatic artery and portal blood flow is simply proportional to the decrease in cardiac output or is further modulated by neural or humoral mechanisms related to the redistribution of blood flow among different organs—remained open and was raised again a few years later by Winsö and co-workers.[7] Their study confirmed that portal blood flow falls with cardiac output during MV with PEEP of 5 and 10 cm $H_2O$ in anesthetized patients undergoing cholecystectomy or hepatic tumor resection (Fig. 16.2). Even in that study, the ratio of both variables did not change, except from a statistically significant increase once PEEP was set back to zero at the end of the experiment. In contrast, a small but

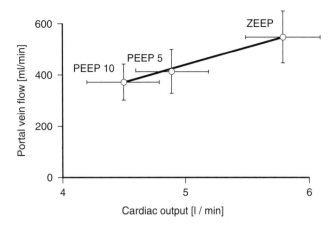

**Figure 16.2** Portal blood flow falls linearly with cardiac output in mechanically ventilated humans once positive end-expiratory pressure (PEEP) of 5 and 10 cm $H_2O$ is used. (Data [mean ± SD] from Winsö O, Biber B, Gustavsson B, et al: Portal blood flow in man during graded positive end-expiratory pressure ventilation. Intensive Care Med 1986;12:80–85.)

statistically significant increase in preportal vascular resistance was observed under MV with PEEP. The authors of this study suspected the presence of long-standing bloodborne mechanisms as a possible cause of this finding.

Some animal and human studies have revealed increments in vasopressin or renin-angiotensin activity as potential mechanisms in the regulation of hemodynamics during PEEP ventilation.[6,24,25] Similarly, experimental data have suggested an increase in sympathetic activity under PEEP ventilation in awake humans[26] and animals,[27,28] activity that may potentially interfere with regional resistance to blood flow in terms of redistribution mechanisms. However, a PEEP-related increase in sympathetic activity failed to be confirmed in human patients during general anesthesia.[29] An investigation by Aneman and colleagues seemed to exclude a role for sympathetic nerve activity in the observed down-regulation of mesenteric and portal venous blood flow during PEEP ventilation.[21] Unfortunately, other possible mediators, such as vasopressin or angiotensin II, were not measured in this study. This study by Aneman and colleagues clearly demonstrated the effects of the buffer response between hepatic arterial and portal venous blood supply. This mechanism is apparently intact, and, despite the altered distribution of perfusion between the two vessels, maintains a constant ratio of total hepatic blood flow to cardiac output in healthy humans during MV with PEEP. This study basically confirmed the previous observations made by Beyer and colleagues[8] in animals and by Bonnet and associates[9] in ventilated human subjects.

A more recent investigation, performed by Kiefer and colleagues on six ventilated patients who were suffering from acute lung injury, failed to confirm any effect of small PEEP increments on cardiac output and hepatosplanchnic perfusion.[30] In this study, PEEP and MV were adjusted to keep airway pressures within the linear part of the pressure-volume curve. The fairly moderate PEEP levels applied in this study, titrated according to the lower inflection point determined on the pressure-volume curve of the respiratory system, may be one explanation for the apparent absence of any interaction between MV and hemodynamics. Furthermore, the intravascular fluid volume of these patients had been accurately replaced in this study before PEEP was increased. As also stated by the authors, this approach may also have prevented major changes in hemodynamics, thus emphasizing the role of adequate intravascular volume replacement during MV with PEEP (discussed in the next section). Conversely, these data clearly suggest that the potentially deleterious effect of PEEP may disappear when increments in airway pressure are titrated according to the thoracopulmonary pressure-volume curve, as when the PEEP maneuver restores functional residual capacity and thereby optimizes the relationship between pulmonary vascular resistance and lung volume, such as in patients with acute respiratory distress syndrome (ARDS), in contrast to patients with exacerbated chronic obstructive pulmonary disease (COPD).[31]

In conclusion, in healthy humans, total hepatic blood or plasma flow seems to decrease in linear relation to cardiac output during PEEP ventilation. This relatively stable perfusion does not necessarily mean that hepatic artery flow and portal vein flow both decrease to the same degree as cardiac output, but rather, the HABR permits increased hepatic artery blood flow and thus

compensates for elevated preportal (mesenteric) resistance. The exact mechanism by which these changes in preportal resistance are mediated remains controversial.

## ADEQUATE INTRAVASCULAR FLUID VOLUME REPLACEMENT COMPENSATES FOR HEMODYNAMIC CHANGES AND PRESERVES DECREASES IN HEPATOSPLANCHNIC PERFUSION

Volume expansion is a common therapeutic tool used to counteract the hemodynamic effects of MV with PEEP. At the cardiac level, MV- and PEEP-related increases in ITP result in raised right atrial pressure. Thus, the pressure gradient for venous return, which corresponds to the difference between mean filling pressure and right atrial pressure, is reduced, and a decrease in cardiac output is the obvious result. Consequently, expanding intravascular volume increases mean filling pressure and restores pressure gradient and cardiac output, as demonstrated experimentally. As extensively reviewed elsewhere,[2] the effects of volume expansion on cardiac output are widely dependent on the actual myocardial state and seem to be far less impressive or are even reversed with a failing myocardium.[31-33]

Restoring cardiac output by volume expansion should also restore hepatosplanchnic perfusion during PEEP ventilation. Indeed, this effect was clearly demonstrated in animals by Brienza and associates[4] during MV with PEEP of 15 cm $H_2O$, as well as by Matuschak and colleagues[15] during MV with PEEP of 10 cm $H_2O$ (Fig. 16.3). In both studies, changes in hepatic perfusion

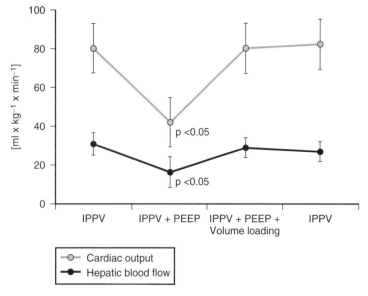

**Figure 16.3** Cardiac output and steady state mean hepatic outflow proportionately fall once positive end-expiratory pressure (PEEP) of 10 cm $H_2O$ is applied during intermittent positive pressure ventilation (IPPV). Replacement of intravascular fluid volume restores initial values for cardiac output and for mean hepatic outflow. (Data [mean ± SD] from Matuschak GM, Pinsky MR, Rogers RM: Effects of positive end-expiratory pressure on hepatic blood flow and performance. J Appl Physiol 1987;62:1377–1383.)

were completely reversed once cardiac output was restored by intravascular fluid volume replacement.

As explained earlier, restoration of hepatosplanchnic perfusion by intravascular volume replacement is expected to result from increased ventricular preload, but this effect may be in part achieved by preventing impeded venous return at the abdominal level. According to Takata and colleagues,[5,10] maintaining sufficient intravascular fluid volume prevents the IVC from collapsing as a result of PEEP-related increments in abdominal pressure. Furthermore, these authors suggested that, with adequate intravascular filling volume, the pressure exerted on the liver as a result of diaphragmatic descent expressed blood stored in the hepatic vasculature into the IVC, thus augmenting venous return. In contrast, in hypovolemia, the IVC collapsed, and blood recruitment from liver storage was not sufficient to maintain stable venous return and thus cardiac output.

All the available data clearly demonstrate the crucial role of adequate volume treatment to prevent decreases in hepatosplanchnic perfusion during MV with PEEP. According to these data, the results presented by Kiefer and associates[30] may be in part explained by the adequate intravascular volume state achieved in their patients before PEEP was increased. The animal models presented by Takata and colleagues[5,10] are particularly interesting, although they are not based on human data, because they clearly explain how the actual intravascular fluid volume of MV-treated subjects may indeed interfere with hemodynamics at the hepatosplanchnic organ level.

## HEPATIC METABOLISM AND OXYGENATION DURING POSITIVE END-EXPIRATORY PRESSURE VENTILATION

Examining the effects of MV and PEEP on hepatic perfusion, as we have mainly so far, tells only part of the story. After all, could it be reasonable to think that the intrinsic metabolic activity of the liver would be disturbed in these circumstances? Indeed, hepatic clearance function has been suggested to be largely related to total hepatic blood flow,[34,35] thus emphasizing the fundamental role of an intact HABR for maintaining not only perfusion but also the normal metabolic functions of the liver.[22] These interpretations may underscore the crucial importance of the finding that the HABR was found to be unaltered by PEEP ventilation in humans,[21] even though in dogs the HABR-related decrease in hepatic artery resistance was partially counterbalanced by the pressure exerted on the liver during PEEP ventilation.[4]

In a few investigations, hepatic performance was studied directly, mainly by measuring indocyanine green (ICG)

clearance during PEEP ventilation.[15,30,36] One of these studies,[15] performed in MV-treated dogs, revealed some alterations in hepatic clearance function, even though the clinical significance of these changes remains unclear. However, ICG clearance increased during MV with PEEP of 10 cm $H_2O$, once intravascular fluid volume had been adequately replaced to restore cardiac output to control conditions. The authors interpreted their data as the result of augmentation of transsinusoidal plasma movement by PEEP-induced increases in hepatic back pressure. The result was an increase in transsinusoidal ICG passage into the hepatic extracellular space that led to enhanced uptake. In contrast, two more recent investigations, by Krenn and associates[36] and Kiefer and colleagues,[30] did not reveal any particular effect of PEEP ventilation on hepatic metabolic performance quantified in terms of ICG clearance. In both studies, cardiac output also remained stable with PEEP. In contrast to the experimental study by Matuschak and associates,[15] in which intravascular fluid volume was given during the experiment to demonstrate the effects of adequate volume filling on cardiac output and hepatic perfusion as well as on performance, in the two latter studies no comparison between low and high intravascular volume states was intended. Instead, the authors emphasized that intravascular volume was adequate just before PEEP was increased, a situation that may well explain the stability not only hemodynamically, but also in terms of hepatic perfusion and metabolic performance. In conclusion, no available evidence indicates that hepatic metabolic function may be seriously impaired by MV or PEEP alone, once intravascular fluid volume and cardiac output are kept at adequate levels.

A large body of evidence suggests that the mesenteric organs and the liver may compensate for a decreased oxygen supply resulting from decreased perfusion by adequately increasing uptake. In fact, oxygen delivery to the liver normally widely exceeds demand, thus permitting a wide range for regulation through increased uptake without deleterious effects.[34,37,38] This phenomenon was observed not only when reduced oxygen delivery was induced by experimental hemodilution,[38] but also when oxygen uptake was increased by dinitrophenol[34] or lactic acidosis.[39] In experimentally induced endotoxic shock, hepatic oxygen extraction capability was found to be increased even by normovolemic hemodilution.[40]

Actually, there is no evidence that oxygenation of the hepatosplanchnic region may be compromised in humans by MV or PEEP alone. In fact, the investigation by Aneman and colleagues[21] revealed decreased mesenteric oxygen delivery but stable mesenteric oxygen consumption during PEEP ventilation, achieved by increasing the extraction rate. In contrast, in these patients, hepatic oxygen delivery was not affected by MV with PEEP. This result is fully consistent with an intact

HABR, even though the maintenance of hepatic perfusion rather than oxygenation is considered the target of the HABR.[35] In accordance with these data, the previously mentioned investigation by Winsö and colleagues also revealed increased preportal oxygen extraction and stable oxygen consumption, although oxygen delivery was reduced during PEEP ventilation.[7]

Although these data suggest that mesenteric and hepatic oxygenation is not likely to be seriously impaired by MV, the data were obtained in subjects without severely compromised physiologic conditions. Actually, however, there are no sufficient data to evaluate the extent to which, in pathologic conditions commonly encountered in MV-treated ICU patients, MV- and PEEP-induced suppression of hepatosplanchnic circulation may contribute to compromise of oxygenation in this region, especially if arterial oxygenation is decreased.

## WEANING IS EXERCISE: MAY IT COMPROMISE GASTROINTESTINAL AND HEPATIC PERFUSION AND FUNCTION?

The occurrence of gastrointestinal symptoms related to some kinds of physical exercise is well known to physiologists.[41] Since the middle of the last century, reduced splanchnic blood flow has been regarded as a probable cause of these disturbances,[42,43] but even now the discussion of the underlying mechanisms remains open.[41] These observations are relevant to our discussion inasmuch as spontaneous breathing performed by mechanically supported patients has to be considered a form of physical exercise.[44] Potentially, there are different goals of spontaneous breathing during MV. The first one is weaning, which is obviously a mandatory phase of any ventilator therapy but is known to increase oxygen consumption of the whole organism and to burden the cardiovascular system.[45,46] The second one is the knowledge we have gained in the last few years, that preserved spontaneous breathing during MV may beneficially influence the physiologic functions of different organs, although the clinical relevance of these effects is not yet known.[47]

In the last few years, many investigators have contributed to define a clear picture of the complex physiologic effects related to weaning and have shown that the success or failure of weaning may be associated with certain cardiovascular responses. Accordingly, while investigating a series of 19 patients, Jubran and associates[48] found that weaning failure was related to a decrease in convective oxygen transport and an increase in peripheral oxygen extraction, which was reflected by a concomitant decrease in mixed venous oxygen saturation. With regard to the gastrointestinal system, a prospective study performed by Bouquillon and colleagues[49] confirmed these

findings in 27 patients with COPD who were undergoing 2-hour weaning trials with pressure supported spontaneous breathing. In fact, during this pressure support period, 16 patients, who were successfully extubated after the trial, revealed a mean statistically significant increase in gastric mucosal blood flow as determined by laser Doppler flowmetry. In contrast, in the 11 patients in whom the weaning trial failed, gastric mucosal blood flow decreased as a potential indicator of an inadequate cardiovascular response. According to more recent investigations,[50] the data presented by Bouquillon and colleagues[49] seem to reflect, at least qualitatively, a normal physiologic response to physical stress. In fact, Rokyta and co-workers[50] found that during submaximal exercise in normal, healthy volunteers, increases in the gastric mucosal–arterial partial pressure of carbon dioxide ($PaCO_2$) difference paralleled alterations in systemic energy status. These results indicate a limitation in energy supply to the gastric mucosa under these conditions, a finding consistent with the decrease in blood flow to this region observed by Bouquillon and associates in patients with COPD during weaning from MV.

However, as shown in a prospective study by De Backer and co-workers,[51] in patients undergoing cardiac or vascular surgery, when interpreting the type of cardiovascular response observed during weaning, one should consider that this reaction may be limited by the actual cardiovascular condition. These authors were able to demonstrate that, in patients after abdominal aortic surgery, postoperative weaning induced an increase in cardiac index. In contrast, after cardiac surgery, especially after cardiac transplantation, the cardiac index showed only minor changes, and the weaning-related increase oxygen consumption was achieved by increasing the oxygen extraction rate. Even these patients were successfully weaned, despite hemodynamic responses to weaning resembling those that indicated weaning failure in previous studies.[48,49]

The data of Putensen and colleagues[47,52] on the effects of MV combined with preserved spontaneous breathing apparently indicate that, despite exercise, spontaneous breathing may also have beneficial effects on pulmonary gas exchange and may support systemic as well as regional perfusion. These authors mainly investigated the physiologic effects of airway pressure release ventilation, a ventilator mode corresponding to continuous positive airway pressure switching at predefined time intervals between two different pressure levels. The results of these animal and human studies revealed that simultaneous active and passive breathing slightly but clearly improves not only the ventilation-perfusion ratio at the alveolar level but also systemic blood flow.[47,52] In patients with acute lung injury, an improvement of renal perfusion was confirmed under these conditions when compared with controlled MV.[53] With regard to intestinal blood flow, only experimental data from an animal study are available to date.[54] However, these data apparently confirm a beneficial effect of spontaneous breathing even for perfusion of this organ region.

Currently, there are no data to evaluate the clinical significance of these effects with regard to patient outcomes. However, the available data do give us an idea why and to which extent spontaneous breathing may not be simply a burden on the cardiovascular system and on other organ systems in MV-treated patients but may at least partially contribute to maintain normal organ functions.

## HYPOCAPNIA, HYPERCAPNIA, AND HEPATOSPLANCHNIC PERFUSION

For decades, attention has focused on the effects of changes in $PaCO_2$ on hepatosplanchnic perfusion and oxygenation. This interest was mainly derived from the observations that hypercapnia and hypocapnia induce major hemodynamic effects systemically as well as on regional blood flow.[55-57] More recently, however, interest in the role of hypoventilation- and hyperventilation-induced variations of $CO_2$ tension ($PCO_2$) has increased because these variations are among the therapeutic goals of ventilator therapy. In fact, since the article published in 1990 by Hickling and colleagues,[58] permissive hypercapnia has become a common tool for lung-protective ventilation.[59,60] The exact role of hypercapnia itself, which mainly derives from the intention to protect lung tissue from stretching forces by limiting tidal volumes, remains a matter of debate.[61] Nevertheless, the use of hypercapnia is presumably a widespread and accepted practice during MV, especially in patients with ARDS.

Only a few investigations have dealt with the effects of hypercapnia on hepatosplanchnic perfusion or function, and some of the data are controversial.[62-65] A major problem with such studies is that significant changes in ventilatory pattern, which may be necessary to induce corresponding changes in $PCO_2$, may also influence whole and regional hemodynamics simply by affecting the ITP. An interesting approach to this problem was presented by Kiefer and colleagues.[66] These authors induced an increase in $PCO_2$ by inserting an additional dead space into the ventilatory circuit in six sedated and paralyzed patients with ARDS who were receiving controlled MV. After a period of 60 minutes, these investigators measured splanchnic blood flow by a primed continuous infusion of ICG and energy balance of the hepatosplanchnic region by determining the gastric mucosal–$PaCO_2$ difference and splanchnic lactate-pyruvate exchange. Comparing these data with those obtained under baseline conditions before and after induction of moderate hypercapnia, these investigators did not observe any change induced by their intervention. This finding suggests that acute, moderate $PCO_2$ changes are not likely to affect splanchnic perfusion and metabolism seriously. Obviously, these results have important limitations because they were obtained in a small group of patients, and the $PCO_2$ changes induced by the additional dead space were minimal when compared with those observed when protective ventilation and permissive hypercapnia were applied in clinical practice. Nevertheless, they are the only existing data on this topic obtained in MV-treated human subjects.

Interest in the effects of hyperventilation-induced hypocapnia on organ blood flow or oxygen consumption arose from past recommendations of this therapeutic option for patients with head trauma, even though the debate about the usefulness of this approach is ongoing.[67,68] One investigation,[69] in 11 MV-treated patients with isolated head trauma and stable hemodynamic status, revealed that moderate hypocapnia induced for 24 hours by increasing tidal volumes and respiratory rate to achieve $PaCO_2$ values not less than 25 mm Hg did not alter hepatic hemodynamics or hepatosplanchnic oxygenation. In this study, cardiovascular performance was not impaired by hyperventilation, despite a small increase in mean airway pressure under these conditions that may have contributed to the observed stability of hepatosplanchnic perfusion and function. In summary, currently available scientific data appear to indicate that moderate changes in $PaCO_2$ have no major impact on hepatosplanchnic perfusion and function.

## PRONE POSITION IS APPARENTLY SAFE IN MECHANICALLY VENTILATED PATIENTS WITH STABLE HEMODYNAMICS

Turning the patient from the supine to the prone position has become one of the most widespread measures to support gas exchange in MV-treated patients suffering from acute lung injury or ARDS.[70,71] However, because the gastrointestinal system is usually considered a potential factor in multiple organ failure in critically ill patients,[72] the safety of this intervention has been questioned by different investigators.[73-75] Kiefer and associates[75] investigated the effects of prone positioning on intragastric pressure and the gastric mucosal–$PaCO_2$ difference over a median period of 6.5 hours in 25 MV-treated surgical patients. These investigators found that turning patients to the prone position did not affect the $PCO_2$ gradient; however, in 9 of 11 patients, in whom intragastric pressure increased in the prone position, the gastric mucosal–$PaCO_2$ gradient also increased. Furthermore, in this study, systemic hemodynamics did not differ between the supine and the prone position.

Further investigations by Matejovic and associates[73] and Hering and colleagues[74,76] did not reveal major changes when the patients were turned from the supine to the prone position. The first study enrolled 11 patients with acute lung injury who required MV. The effects of supine and prone positioning were evaluated in terms of intra-abdominal pressure, hepatosplanchnic blood flow measured by the steady-state ICG technique,[77] and gastric mucosal–PaCO$_2$ gap. All parameters tested remained unchanged in both positions, a finding suggesting that prone positioning did not compromise hepatosplanchnic perfusion or gastric mucosal energy balance in this group of patients. Similarly, the study by Hering and associates in 12 MV-treated patients with acute lung injury did not reveal any negative effect of prone positioning on hepatic ICG kinetics and gastric intramucosal energy balance. In this study, only a minor increase in intra-abdominal pressure was found to occur when the patients were turned from the supine to the prone position.

In summary, based on these data, it does not seem likely that prone positioning should seriously impair hepatosplanchnic perfusion or function in MV-treated, critically ill patients. However, two limitations may be of particular relevance in ICU patients. First, because all patients enrolled in these studies had stable hemodynamics, we cannot ascertain the effects of prone positioning in patients with compromised cardiovascular conditions. Second, for the same reason, it cannot be excluded that under particular conditions intra-abdominal pressure may increase up to critical values and may thus compromise hepatosplanchnic perfusion or function.

## REFERENCES

1. Miro AM, Pinsky MR: Heart-lung interactions. In Tobin MJ (ed): Principles and Practice of Mechanical Ventilation. New York: McGraw-Hill, 1994, pp 647–671.
2. Pinsky MR: Heart-lung interactions. In Pinsky MR, Dhainaut JF (eds): Pathophysiologic Foundations of Critical Care. Baltimore: Williams & Wilkins, 1993, pp 472–490.
3. Pinsky MR: The hemodynamic consequences of mechanical ventilation: An evolving story. Intensive Care Med 1997;23:493–503.
4. Brienza N, Revelly JP, Ayuse T, et al: Effects of PEEP on liver arterial and venous blood flows. Am J Respir Crit Care Med 1995;152:504–510.
5. Takata M, Robotham JL: Effects of inspiratory diaphragmatic descent on inferior vena caval venous return. J Appl Physiol 1992;72:597–607.
6. Aneman A, Ponten J, Fandriks L, et al: Hemodynamic, sympathetic and angiotensin II responses to PEEP ventilation before and during administration of isoflurane. Acta Anaesthesiol Scand 1997;41:41–48.
7. Winsö O, Biber B, Gustavsson B, et al: Portal blood flow in man during graded positive end-expiratory pressure ventilation. Intensive Care Med 1986;12:80–85.
8. Beyer J, Beckenlechner P, Messmer K: The influence of PEEP ventilation on organ blood flow and peripheral oxygen delivery. Intensive Care Med 1982;8:75–80.
9. Bonnet F, Richard C, Glaser P, et al: Changes in hepatic flow induced by continuous positive pressure ventilation in critically ill patients. Crit Care Med 1982;10:703–705.
10. Takata M, Wise RA, Robotham JL: Effects of abdominal pressure on venous return: Abdominal vascular zone conditions. J Appl Physiol 1990;69:1961–1972.
11. Beloucif S, Brienza N, Andreoni K, et al: Distinct behavior of portal venous and arterial vascular waterfalls in porcine liver. J Crit Care 1995;10:104–114.
12. Brienza N, Ayuse T, O'Donnell CP, et al: Regional control of venous return: Liver blood flow. Am J Respir Crit Care Dis 1995;152:511–518.
13. Alexander RS: Influence of the diaphragm upon portal blood flow and venous return. Am J Physiol 1951;167:738–748.
14. Johnson EE, Hedley-Whyte J: Continuous positive-pressure ventilation and choledochoduodenal flow resistance. J Appl Physiol 1975;39:937–942.
15. Matuschak GM, Pinsky MR, Rogers RM: Effects of positive end-expiratory pressure on hepatic blood flow and performance J Appl Physiol 1987;62:1377–1383.
16. Bredenberg CE, Paskanik A, Fromm D: Portal hemodynamics in dogs during mechanical ventilation with positive end-expiratory pressure. Surgery 1981;90:817–822.
17. Lautt WW, Legare D: Passive autoregulation of portal venous pressure: Distensible hepatic resistance. Am J Physiol 1992;263:G702–G708.
18. Mitzner W: Hepatic outflow resistance, sinusoid pressure, and the vascular waterfall. Am J Physiol 1974;227:513–519.
19. Permutt S, Riley RL: Hemodynamics of collapsible vessels with tone: The vascular waterfall. J Appl Physiol 1963;18:924–932.
20. Peters J, Hecker B, Neuser D, et al: Regional blood volume distribution during positive and negative airway pressure breathing in supine humans. J Appl Physiol 1993;75:1740–1747.
21. Aneman A, Eisenhofer G, Fändriks L, et al: Splanchnic circulation and regional sympathetic outflow during perioperative PEEP ventilation in humans. Br J Anaesth 1999;82:838–842.
22. Lautt WW: Mechanism and role of intrinsic regulation of hepatic arterial blood flow: Distensible hepatic resistance. Am J Physiol 1990;249:G549–G556.
23. Ayuse T, Brienza N, Revelly JP, et al: Alterations in liver hemodynamics in an intact porcine model of endotoxic shock. Am J Physiol 1995;268:H1106–H1114.
24. Annat G, Viale JP, Bui Xuan B, et al: Effect of PEEP ventilation on renal function, plasma renin, aldosterone, neurophysins and urinary ADH, and prostaglandins. Anesthesiology 1983;58:136–141.
25. Khambatta HJ, Baratz RA: IPPB, plasma ADH, and urine flow in conscious man. J Appl Physiol 1972;33:362–364.
26. Tanaka S, Sagawa S, Miki K, et al: Changes in muscle sympathetic nerve activity and renal function during positive-pressure breathing in humans. Am J Physiol 1994;266:R1220–R1228.
27. Sellden H, Sjövall H, Ricksten SE: Sympathetic nerve activity and central hemodynamics during mechanical ventilation with positive end-expiratory pressure in rats. Acta Physiol Scand 1986;127:51–60.
28. Chernow B, Soldano S, Cook D, et al: Positive end-expiratory pressure increases plasma catecholamine levels in non–volume loaded dogs. Anaesth Intensive Care 1986;14:421–425.
29. Sellgren J, Ponten J, Wallin BG: Characteristics of muscle nerve sympathetic activity during general anaesthesia in humans. Acta Anaesthesiol Scand 1992;36:336–345.

30. Kiefer P, Nunes S, Kosonen P, et al: Effect of positive end expiratory pressure on splanchnic perfusion in acute lung injury Intensive Care Med 2000;26:376–383.

31. Pinsky MR: Heart-lung interactions during positive-pressure ventilation. New Horiz 1994;4:443–456.

32. Räsänen J, Nikki P, Heikkila J: Acute myocardial infarction complicated by respiratory failure: The effects of mechanical ventilation. Chest 1984;85:21–28.

33. Räsänen J, Vaisanen IT, Heikkila J, et al: Acute myocardial infarction complicated by left ventricular dysfunction and respiratory failure: The effects of continuous positive airway pressure. Chest 1985;87:158–162.

34. Lautt WW: Control of hepatic arterial blood flow: Independence from liver metabolic activity. Am J Physiol 1980;239:H559–H564.

35. Lautt WW: Mechanism and role of intrinsic regulation of hepatic arterial blood flow: Hepatic arterial buffer response. Am J Physiol 1985;249:G549–G556.

36. Krenn CG, Krafft P, Schaefer B, et al: Effects of positive end-expiratory pressure on hemodynamics and indocyanine green kinetics in patients after orthotopic liver transplantation. Crit Care Med 2000;28:1760–1765.

37. Bredfeldt JE, Riley EM, Groszmann RJ: Compensatory mechanisms in response to an elevated hepatic oxygen consumption in chronically ethanol-fed rats. Am J Physiol 1985;248:G507–G512.

38. Lautt WW: Control of hepatic and intestinal blood flow: Effect of isovolemic haemodilution on blood flow and oxygen uptake in the intact liver and intestines. J Physiol (Lond) 1977;265:313–326.

39. Hughes RL, Mathie RT, Fitch W, et al: Liver blood flow and oxygen consumption during metabolic acidosis and alkalosis in the greyhound. Clin Sci 1980;60:355–361.

40. Creteur J, Sun Q, Abid O, et al: Normovolemic hemodilution improves oxygen extraction capabilities in endotoxic shock. J Appl Physiol 2001;91:1701–1707.

41. Gil SM, Yazaki E, Evans DF: Aetiology of running-related gastrointestinal dysfunction: How far is the finishing line? Sports Med 1998;26:365–378.

42. Bradley SE: Variations in hepatic blood flow in man during health and disease. N Engl J Med 1949;240:456.

43. Wade OL, Combes B, Childs AW, et al: The effects of exercise on the splanchnic blood flow and splanchnic blood volume in normal men. Clin Sci 1956;13:457–463.

44. Pinsky MR: Breathing as exercise: The cardiovascular response to weaning from mechanical ventilation. Intensive Care Med 2000;26:1164–1166.

45. Kemper M, Weissman C, Askanasi J, et al: Metabolic and respiratory changes during weaning from mechanical ventilation. Chest 1987;92:979–983.

46. Pinsky MR: Cardiovascular effects of ventilatory support and withdrawal. Anaesth Analg 1994;79:567–576.

47. Putensen C, Räsänen J, Lopez F, et al: Effect of interfacing between spontaneous breathing and mechanical cycles on the ventilation-perfusion distributions in canine lung injury. Anesthesiology 1994;81:921–930.

48. Jubran A, Mathru M, Dries D, et al: Continuous recordings of mixed venous oxygen saturation during weaning from mechanical ventilation and the ramifications thereof. Am J Respir Crit Care Med 1998;158:1763–1769.

49. Bocquillon N, Mathieu D, Neviere R, et al: Gastric mucosal pH and blood flow during weaning from mechanical ventilation in patients with chronic obstructive pulmonary disease. Am J Respir Crit Care Med 1999;160:1555–1561.

50. Rokyta R, Matejovic M, Novak I, et al: Submaximal exercise in healthy volunteers: The relationship between gastric mucosal and systemic energy status. Pflugers Arch 2002;443:852–857.

51. De Backer D, El Haddad P, Preiser JC, et al: Hemodynamic responses to successful weaning from mechanical ventilation after cardiovascular surgery. Intensive Care Med 2000;26:1201–1206.

52. Putensen C, Mutz NJ, Putensen-Himmer G, et al: Spontaneous breathing during ventilatory support improves ventilation-perfusion distributions in patients with acute respiratory distress syndrome. Am J Respir Crit Care Med 1999;159:1241–1248.

53. Hering R, Peters D, Zinserling J, et al: Effects of spontaneous breathing during airway pressure release ventilation on renal perfusion and function in patients with acute lung injury. Intensive Care Med 2002;28:1426–1433.

54. Hering R, Viehöfer A, Zinserling J, et al: Effects of spontaneous breathing during airway pressure release ventilation on intestinal blood flow in experimental lung injury. Anesthesiology 2003;99:1137–1144.

55. Cullen D, Eger E: Cardiovascular effects of carbon dioxide in man. Anesthesiology 1974;41:345–349.

56. Price H: Effects of carbon dioxide on the cardiovascular system. Anesthesiology 1960;6:652–663.

57. Noble MIM, Trenchard D, Guz A: Effect of changes in $PaCO_2$ and $PaO_2$ on cardiac performance in conscious dogs. J Appl Physiol 1967;22:147–152.

58. Hickling KG, Henderson SJ, Jackson R: Low mortality associated with low volume pressure limited ventilation with permissive hypercapnia in severe adult respiratory distress syndrome. Intensive Care Med 1990;16:372–377.

59. Amato MB, Barbas CS, Medeiros DM, et al: Effect of a protective-ventilation strategy on mortality in the acute respiratory distress syndrome. N Engl J Med 1998;338:347–354.

60. Acute Respiratory Distress Syndrome Network: Ventilation with lower tidal volumes as compared with traditional tidal volumes for acute lung injury and the acute respiratory distress syndrome. N Engl J Med 2000;342:1301–1308.

61. Laffey JG, O'Croinin D, McLoughlin P, et al: Permissive hypercapnia: Role in protective lung ventilatory strategies. Intensive Care Med 2004;30:347–356.

62. Fujita Y, Sakai T, Ohsumi A, et al: Effects of hypocapnia and hypercapnia on splanchnic circulation and hepatic function in the beagle. Anesth Analg 1989;69:152–157.

63. Hughes RL, Mathie RT, Campbell D, et al: Effect of hypercarbia on hepatic blood flow and oxygen consumption in the greyhound. Br J Anaesth 1979;51:289–296.

64. Juhl B, Einer-Jensen N: The effect on the splanchnic blood flow and cardiac output of various carbon dioxide concentration during fluroxene anaesthesia. Acta Anaesthesiol Scand 1977;21:449.

65. Epstein RM, Wheeler HO, Frumin MJ, et al: The effect of hypercapnia on estimated hepatic blood flow, circulating splanchnic blood volume, and hepatic sulphobromophthalein clearance during general anaesthesia in man. J Clin Invest 1961;40:592–598.

66. Kiefer P, Nunes S, Kosonen P, et al: Effect of an acute increase in $PCO_2$ on splanchnic perfusion and metabolism. Intensive Care Med 2001;27:775–778.

67. Coles JP, Minhas PS, Fryer TD, et al: Effect of hyperventilation on cerebral blood flow in traumatic head injury: Clinical relevance and monitoring correlates. Crit Care Med 2002;30:1950–1959.

68. Brain Trauma Foundation: The American Association of Neurological Surgeons: The Joint Section on Neurotrauma and Critical Care. Hyperventilation. J Neurotrauma 2000;17:513–520.

69. Ichai C, Levraut J, Baruch I, et al: Hypocapnia does not alter hepatic blood flow or oxygen consumption in patients with head injury. Crit Care Med 1998;26:1725–1730.

70. Gattinoni L, Tognoni G, Pesenti A, et al: Effect of prone positioning on the survival of patients with acute respiratory failure. N Engl J Med 2001;345:568–573.

71. Pelosi P, Tubiolo D, Mascheroni D, et al: Effects of the prone position on respiratory mechanics and gas exchange during acute lung injury. Am J Respir Crit Care Med 1998;157:387–393.

72. Brinkmann A, Calzia E, Träger K, et al: Monitoring the hepatosplanchnic region in the critically ill patient. Intensive Care Med 1998;24:542–556.

73. Matejovic M, Rokyta R Jr, Radermacher P, et al: Effect of prone position on hepato-splanchnic hemodynamics in acute lung injury. Intensive Care Med 2002;28:1750–1755.

74. Hering R, Vorwerk R, Wrigge H, et al: Prone positioning, systemic hemodynamics, hepatic indocyanine green kinetics, and gastric intramucosal energy balance in patients with acute lung injury. Intensive Care Med 2002;28:53–58.

75. Kiefer P, Morin A, Putzke C, et al: Influence of prone position on gastric mucosal–arterial $P_{CO_2}$ gradients. Intensive Care Med 2001;27:1227–1230.

76. Hering R, Wrigge H, Vorwerk R, et al: The effects of prone positioning on intraabdominal pressure and cardiovascular and renal function in patients with acute lung injury. Anesth Analg 2001;92:1226–1231.

77. Uusaro A, Ruokonen E, Takala J: Estimation of splanchnic blood flow by the Fick principle in man and problems in the use of indocyanine green. Cardiovasc Res 1995;30:106–112.

# CHAPTER 17

# Kidney-Lung Interactions

Sean M. Bagshaw and Rinaldo Bellomo

Kidney function and lung function are closely interconnected, and dysfunction in either or both of these organ systems is highly prevalent in critically ill patients. The practice of critical care demands an intimate knowledge of the link between both normal and abnormal kidney and lung function. Lung injury impairs gas exchange and elicits systemic inflammation that can have direct consequences on kidney function. Likewise, the extracellular fluid expansion and metabolic disarray resulting from acute renal failure (ARF) can impose several physiologic challenges to normal lung function. Artificial organ support, in the form of mechanical ventilation (MV) or renal replacement therapy (RRT), is regularly introduced in the routine care of critically ill patients. MV can elicit important declines in kidney function. RRT, administered as either hemodialysis or continuous hemofiltration, can impair or improve lung function, depending on the clinical circumstances. This chapter focuses on the physiology of kidney-lung interaction and how it pertains to the care of critically ill patients.

## PHYSIOLOGIC EFFECT OF MECHANICAL VENTILATION ON KIDNEY FUNCTION

Most critically ill patients require MV during admission to intensive care, whether for disease-specific indications such as acute respiratory distress syndrome (ARDS) or simply for routine postoperative care. The application of positive pressure MV in these patients, particularly with positive end-expiratory pressure (PEEP), can have important physiologic effects on kidney function. Although the precise effects are not completely understood,

many experimental and clinical studies have clearly established an association between MV (and PEEP) and alterations in kidney function (Box 17.1).

The positive pressure applied during MV acts to increase intrathoracic, intrapleural, and intra-abdominal pressures both during inspiration and for the duration of the respiratory cycle, and even more so with the use of PEEP. This increase in intrathoracic pressure, monitored clinically by changes in mean airway pressure, can stimulate an array of hemodynamic, neural, and hormonal

---

**BOX 17-1**

**Summary of the Potential Physiologic Mechanisms of Altered Kidney Function with Mechanical Ventilation and Positive End-Expiratory Pressure**

Altered cardiovascular function
  Reduced cardiac output
  Reduced renal blood flow
  Altered distribution of intrarenal blood flow
  Raised inferior vena cava and renal vein pressure
Alterations in neurohormonal activation
  Sympathetic nervous system stimulation
  Renin-angiotensin-aldosterone system stimulation
  Reduced atrial natriuretic peptide secretion
  Increased vasopressin secretion
Possible causes of exaggerated mechanical
  ventilation effects
  Intravascular volume depletion
  Poor baseline cardiac performance
  Alterations in pulmonary compliance
  Prior chronic kidney disease
  Prior chronic pulmonary disease

responses that collectively act on the kidney to reduce renal perfusion, reduce the glomerular filtration rate (GFR), and inhibit excretory function. Kidney function per se may not be impaired with MV, but rather, the kidney is appropriately responding to these stimuli by reducing osmolar, sodium, and water clearance. At the bedside, this condition may manifest as an increase in surrogate markers of kidney function (i.e., creatinine, urea), oliguria, and a positive fluid balance with edema formation.

These hemodynamic, neural, and hormonal effects on kidney function may be further exacerbated by additional factors such as baseline cardiac performance, intravascular volume status, and dynamic changes in pulmonary compliance. Similarly, the presence of preexisting comorbid illness (i.e., chronic kidney disease, chronic obstructive pulmonary disease [COPD]) has the potential to exaggerate the influence of MV on kidney function.

## Alterations in Cardiovascular Function

The rise in intrathoracic pressure with MV (and PEEP) can act to reduce intrathoracic blood volume, decrease transmural pressure, reduce right ventricular preload, increase right ventricular afterload, exert alterations to pulmonary vascular resistance and volume, and contribute to changes in left ventricular filling and geometry. Together, these effects can cause a significant decrease in cardiac output.

Several clinical studies have found that MV (especially with increasing levels of PEEP) exerts immediate effects on kidney function characterized by reduced renal blood flow (RBF).[1] The effect on renal perfusion is likely more pronounced in the setting of intravascular volume depletion and preserved pulmonary compliance. Normal lung compliance permits a greater relative proportion of positive pressure to be transmitted to the pleural space and great vessels and acts to reduce transmural pressures and cardiac output. Mirro and colleagues[2] found that even modest increases in mean airway pressure contributed to considerable declines in cardiac output and renal perfusion. These physiologic responses appeared to occur before any noticeable evidence of change in mean arterial pressure.[2] However, reductions in RBF have not been confirmed in other experimental studies despite similar undesirable reductions in kidney excretory function and fluid retention.[3]

The amount of PEEP applied can further exacerbate the renal response to MV. Annat and associates[1] found that 10 cm $H_2O$ of PEEP was associated with early decreases in RBF, GFR, and urine output in a small cohort of critically ill patients. These authors further suggested that these physiologic effects could generally be reversed after the removal of PEEP. Another small study

of critically ill trauma patients reported that levels of PEEP greater than 6 cm $H_2O$ were independently associated with the development of ARF.[4] In this study, ARF developed in 73% of patients who were receiving levels of PEEP greater than 6 cm $H_2O$, but in only 36% of those receiving levels of PEEP lower than 6 cm $H_2O$.

Kidney function may also be sensitive to the strategy of MV used in addition to the level of PEEP applied. This was shown by Gattinoni and colleagues[5] in a sheep model in which low-frequency ventilation (PEEP at 5 cm $H_2O$) with extracorporeal carbon dioxide ($CO_2$) removal attenuated the decline in cardiac output and kidney function with improved creatinine clearance and urine output when compared with controlled MV (PEEP at 5 cm $H_2O$). Selecting an MV strategy that incorporates spontaneous breathing has also been suggested to attenuate the decline in kidney function with MV.[6] Spontaneous MV modes may aid to counter the impact of raised intrathoracic pressure with MV and may restore pulmonary and systemic hemodynamics towards normal. Spontaneous MV allows for an increase in diaphragmatic activity. Further, spontaneous MV is often associated with reductions in mean airway pressure, intrapleural pressure, and pressure exerted on the inferior vena cava. These effects, representing restoration of more normal physiology, can lead to augmented venous return and cardiac output that translate into benefits for the renal circulation and kidney function. The benefits of spontaneous MV were shown in a clinical study in which the use of a fully controlled mode of MV appeared to worsen kidney function when compared with an intermittent strategy of mandatory MV.[7] However, these findings were not confirmed in another, more recent study.[8] Spontaneous strategies are appealing, to reduce sedation and to wean patients from MV; however, the role of increased sympathetic activity from pain, discomfort, or patient-ventilator dyssynchrony that may occur and may potentially further worsen the kidney-lung interaction is unknown.

The intrarenal distribution of blood flow may also be affected by MV and may contribute to impaired kidney function.[9-11] Experimental data show that MV could potentially shunt intrarenal flow from the cortical to the medullary circulation, and such redistribution was associated with declines in creatinine clearance and urine output. However, additional studies failed to corroborate these findings reliably.[3,9,11,12] Thus, whether MV can have an important effect on the distribution of intrarenal blood flow remains uncertain.

The increase in intrathoracic pressure with MV can transmit across the diaphragm to raise intra-abdominal pressure. This has been postulated as another mechanism whereby MV can adversely affect kidney function. The result is compression of the inferior vena cava and renal veins.[13-15] This effect has been shown in experimental studies in which impaired renal venous outflow, by reducing effective renal perfusion pressure, was associated with reductions in RBF and kidney function.[13,15]

## Alterations in Neurohormonal Activation

Several neurohormonal mechanisms, in addition to the aforementioned hemodynamic effects, have been found to contribute to alterations in kidney function during MV. Raised intrathoracic pressure, by altering transmural pressures, reducing cardiac output, and unloading intrathoracic baroreceptors, can initiate a cascade of compensatory neurohormonal events that culminate in altered renal perfusion and kidney excretory function. However, the alterations induced by MV (and PEEP) on these neurohormonal systems and their effects on kidney function are poorly understood. Nonetheless, the principal mechanisms hypothesized to contribute include increased systemic and renal sympathetic nervous activity, increased activation of the renin-angiotensin-aldosterone system, increased secretion of vasopressin, and inhibited release of atrial natriuretic peptide (ANP).

Clinical studies have shown increased sympathetic outflow in response to MV (and PEEP).[16] An increase in sympathetic activity can result in renal vasoconstriction and increased renal tubular reabsorption, and it can act to stimulate the renin-angiotensin-aldosterone axis directly. Farge and associates[16] observed that the reduction in kidney excretory function with MV (and PEEP) was associated with increased plasma renin activity and serum norepinephrine and epinephrine levels. This finding suggested an important role for sympathetic activation and stimulation of the renin-angiotensin-aldosterone axis. Boemke and colleagues[17] found evidence of increased plasma renin activity and aldosterone levels despite complete renal denervation in conscious dogs ventilated with PEEP, a finding suggesting that activation of the renin-angiotensin-aldosterone axis occurred independent of renal sympathetic tone. Annat and colleagues[1] found that short exposure to MV with PEEP significantly increased plasma renin activity and aldosterone levels. However, these authors found that the effects on kidney function were reversed when PEEP was withdrawn, and they also suggested that the immediate effects of PEEP were hemodynamic, and the neurohormonal responses were more likely to contribute to reduced kidney excretory function and fluid retention during prolonged ventilation with PEEP. In addition, the raised intrathoracic pressure seen during MV has also been speculated to act on pulmonary endothelial angiotensin-converting enzyme and to promote an increase in circulating angiotensin II.

ANP, which is released by the atria in response to an increase in atrial stretch or transmural pressure, has potent diuretic and natriuretic properties. In addition, ANP may act to reduce renal sympathetic activity, plasma renin activity, and aldosterone secretion. Evidence of a decrease in circulating ANP levels has been shown to occur in response to ventilation with PEEP, a decrease that is approximately proportional to the change in mean airway pressure.[18] Further, Christensen and associates[19] found that PEEP ventilation in conscious dogs resulted in a drop in plasma ANP levels that correlated with significant fluid retention. This causal relationship was further supported after the addition of an infusion of ANP induced an increase in sodium excretion and urine output. Similar findings were reported by Andrivet and colleagues, who found that PEEP ventilation reduced plasma ANP levels, but diuresis and natriuresis increased in response to an infusion of ANP.[20,21] Although these studies provide evidence that ANP may have a central role in reducing kidney excretory function associated with MV, these findings have not been shown in other experimental studies.[22]

Vasopressin is released from the posterior pituitary gland in response to changes in intravascular volume status or osmolarity. The stimulus for secretion originates, in part, from reflexes in intrathoracic baroreceptors in the aorta and carotid arteries and from stretch receptors in the atria. An increase in intrathoracic pressure brought about by MV (and PEEP) and the resulting reduction in transmural filling pressures and cardiac output act to stimulate an increase in secretion of vasopressin independent of serum osmolality. Numerous experimental and clinical studies found an increase in serum vasopressin after initiation of PEEP ventilation.[1,17,22,23] However, another small study in critically ill patients failed to corroborate these findings.[16] Vasopressin can exert a variety of antidiuretic and antinatriuretic effects on kidney function by altering intrarenal hemodynamics, reducing GFR, increasing sodium reabsorption in the thick ascending loop of Henle, and increasing the permeability of collecting tubules to increase reabsorption of water. The net effect of vasopressin is a decrease in kidney excretory function with sodium and fluid retention.

Intravascular volume expansion can mitigate the negative hemodynamic and neurohormonal consequences of MV on kidney function.[24] Experimental studies have shown that MV with volume expansion has little measurable effect on renal sympathetic tone, plasma renin activity, or vasopressin secretion.[22,25] Although this may be a logical strategy to minimize the potential negative influence of MV on kidney function, intravascular volume expansion may be undesirable in many patients, in particular those with poor underlying cardiac performance or ARDS. The risks and benefits of fluid therapy under these circumstances must be carefully considered.

Additional studies have explored the biologic effects of other vasoactive substances including nitric oxide, bradykinins, prostaglandins, and endothelin, which may play a role in modulating the renal response to MV.

However, although there maybe biologic rationale for each of these compounds, the specific impact of these substances on kidney function during MV has yet to be well characterized.

## Injurious Mechanical Ventilation

Particular strategies of MV are now recognized to contribute to or to provoke ventilator-induced lung injury (VILI) (Table 17.1). Evidence suggests that the pathophysiology of VILI is multifactorial and results from the combined effects of volutrauma (excessive tidal or end-expiratory volumes), barotrauma (excessive end-inspiratory peak and plateau pressures), atelect-trauma (cyclic opening and closing of alveolar units), and biotrauma (local release of inflammatory mediators from injured lung). Injurious MV can initiate a cascade of events that result in an increase in systemic inflammation and adversely affect kidney function. These events are discussed further in the next section.

## PHYSIOLOGIC EFFECT OF LUNG FAILURE ON KIDNEY FUNCTION

Injury to the lungs, such as in ARDS, can contribute to downstream kidney dysfunction through impairment in gas exchange and an increase in systemic inflammation. Few clinical studies have specifically described the clinical outcome and prognosis of patients presenting with acute lung injury or ARDS who then develop ARF. However, a small retrospective study by Valta and colleagues[26] found a high incidence of combined organ failure in critically ill patients with ARDS. Another study, by Fowler and associates,[27] found an elevated serum urea in 25% patients with ARDS. Of course, kidney function may be worsened by measures to optimize lung function, such as lung-protective MV strategies and fluid restriction or diuresis.

## Alterations in Gas Exchange

Abnormalities in gas exchange are commonplace in critically ill patients with lung injury. The initiation of MV is often needed in these patients, with the aim of restoring normal gas exchange. However, in many instances, such as in ARDS or diseases with marked air-flow limitations (i.e., asthma or COPD), achieving normal gas exchange may not be possible. The end result is that such patients may undergo MV with variable degrees of hypoxemia or hypercapnia.

The exact mechanisms by which hypoxemia leads to impaired kidney function are not completely understood; however, they are likely multifactorial and relate to various changes in cardiovascular function, sympathetic nervous and renin-angiotensin aldosterone system activation, and modulation of additional vasoactive mediators (Box 17.2). There are conflicting experimental studies describing the acute kidney effects of hypoxemia.[28-30] Bruns and colleagues[28] described significant reductions in RBF in response to hypoxia in dogs. The reduced perfusion in this study was associated with a decrease in GFR and excretory function. However, additional studies did not corroborate the finding that moderate to severe hypoxemia impairs oxygen delivery, renal perfusion, or kidney function, and these other studies suggested that kidney function is more sensitive to altered cardiovascular performance than to hypoxemia per se.[31-33] Evidence from clinical studies has generally focused on hypoxemic patients with COPD. In one small study, reversal of hypoxemia was associated with significant increases in RBF.[34] However, Reihman and associates[35] suggested that exposure to hypoxemia in stable patients with COPD impaired GFR and excretory function independent of RBF. These authors speculated that hypoxemia could impair local autoregulation of the GFR and could contribute to sodium and fluid retention.

| Table 17-1 | Mechanisms of Ventilator-Induced Lung Injury |
|---|---|
| Volutrauma | Ventilation with excessive tidal or end-expiratory volumes |
| Barotrauma | Ventilation with excessive end-inspiratory or plateau pressures |
| Atelect-trauma | Ventilation below lower inflection point on pressure-volume curve with cyclic opening and closing of alveoli |
| Biotrauma | Local and systemic release of inflammatory mediators |

---

BOX 17-2

**Proposed Mechanisms of Hypoxemia during Hemodialysis**

Ventilation-perfusion mismatch
    Pulmonary leukocyte sequestration
    Thromboemboli
    Silicone microemboli
Alveolar hypoventilation
    Carbon dioxide diffusion into dialysate
    Correction of metabolic acidosis

Hypercapnia can also exert adverse effects on kidney function. In patients with ARDS or marked airflow obstruction, hypercapnia is common and may worsen with lung-protective MV strategies and so-called permissive hypercapnia. The rationale for permissive hypercapnia is that it allows either low tidal volume ventilation (avoidance of volutrauma) or reduction in excessive air trapping (reduced risk of barotrauma). Hypercapnia has been correlated with reductions in RBF and altered kidney function.[36,37] The mechanisms of reduced RBF with hypercapnia are again likely multifactorial and result from enhanced sympathetic tone and altered cardiovascular function. Zillig and colleagues[33] found reductions in RBF in hypercapnic rats, although the effects on kidney function were variable. Similarly, clinical studies in healthy, normal volunteers and kidney transplant recipients (renal denervation) showed that hypercapnia leads to acute increases in renovascular resistance, and these changes can be independent of concomitant hypoxemia.[38] Acute hypercapnia can also result in respiratory (ventilatory) acidosis. Whether this acidosis can directly affect RBF and kidney function remains uncertain. However, Rose and associates[39] found no significant effect on kidney function in dogs with acute hypercapnic acidosis. Experimental and clinical data have further suggested that combined hypoxemia and hypercapnia may act synergistically to impair kidney function.[40] Sharkey and colleagues[38] found greater increases in renovascular resistance in healthy volunteers who were exposed to both hypoxemia and hypercapnia compared with exposure to either alone.

## Alterations in Systemic Inflammatory Mediators

Lung injury may result from underlying lung disease or the injurious application of MV. VILI is a well-recognized complication of MV and is primarily attributable to the use of excessive tidal or end-inspiratory volumes. However, the added effects of barotrauma, atelect-trauma, and biotrauma are probably important contributors. The mechanical disruption of the alveolar-capillary barrier, commonly referred to as *stress failure*, can induce release of local inflammatory mediators that can spill into the systemic circulation.[41] Numerous inflammatory mediators have been detected in the systemic circulation of lung injury patients, including interleukin-1 (IL-1), IL-6, IL-8, IL-10, and tumor necrosis factor-α (TNF-α).[42] Evidence has confirmed that systemic mediators can contribute to downstream extrapulmonary organ dysfunction.[43] In a murine model of lung injury, the application of injurious MV was associated with increased expression of IL-6 in kidney tissue.[44] Imai and associates[45] found increased rates of renal tubular apoptosis after exposure of rabbits to injurious MV that was further associated with impaired kidney function.

Clinical studies supported these findings and showed that VILI can worsen lung function, contribute to extrapulmonary organ dysfunction, and increase mortality in critically ill patients. Ranieri and colleagues[42] found that conventional MV in patients with ARDS was associated with sustained elevations in both bronchoalveolar and serum inflammatory cytokines. These authors further found that serum concentrations of IL-6 correlated with clinically evident reductions in kidney function.[46] Persistent elevations in inflammatory cytokines, in particular IL-6, were found in clinical studies to predict mortality in critically ill patients with ARF.[47] The kidneys appear to be particularly susceptible to the systemic inflammatory response from injurious MV. These inflammatory mediators may induce kidney dysfunction through alterations in systemic and renal hemodynamics, by induction of renal tubular cell apoptosis, or by exerting direct toxic effects in the kidney.

## PHYSIOLOGIC EFFECT OF ACUTE RENAL FAILURE ON LUNG FUNCTION

The loss of excretory function characterized by ARF is associated with the accumulation of metabolic waste products, nonvolatile acids, and extracellular volume expansion. Such a loss in kidney function can have clinically important and negative physiologic consequences on the normal function of other organ systems, in particular the lung (Fig. 17.1). However, there have been few experimental or clinical investigations into the mechanisms whereby ARF may alter lung function.

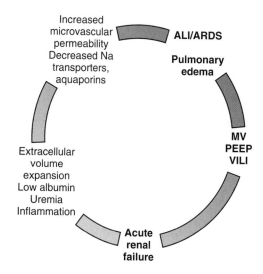

**Figure 17.1** Summary of the mechanism by which acute renal failure can impair lung function.

## Uremic Pneumonitis

Uremia (serum urea >20 mmol/L) has been associated with lung inflammation and injury, commonly referred to as *uremic pneumonitis*.[48] Although uremic pneumonitis may contribute to lung injury, this complication of ARF is now generally less common as a result of earlier initiation and the more efficient application of RRT. Abnormalities in serum phosphorus and calcium and metabolic acidosis from ARF have all been proposed to contribute to respiratory muscle weakness and dysfunction.[49] Various abnormalities in lung function have been described in patients with ARF, including obstructive and restrictive defects and impairment of diffusion capacity.[50] Uremia, hypervolemia, and hypoalbuminemia commonly seen in ARF can lead to pleural effusions and ascites. Large pleural effusions can worsen lung mechanics by causing significant restriction. Ascites can also impair mechanics by reducing functional residual capacity and causing diaphragmatic dysfunction. Although uncommon, the development of urinothorax from small defects in the diaphragm with leakage of ascitic fluid into the chest has been described. Uremic encephalopathy can cause an altered level of consciousness and alveolar hypoventilation and can predispose a patient to aspiration or poor clearance of secretions. Of course, consideration must be given to preexisting lung disease (i.e., pulmonary fibrosis, lung transplantation, drug toxicity) or other acute processes (i.e., pneumonia, sepsis) that may worsen in the setting of concomitant with ARF.

## Pulmonary Edema

Probably the most common pulmonary complication of ARF encountered in clinical practice is alveolar edema. The increased extracellular volume, altered pulmonary microvascular permeability, and reduced serum oncotic pressure described in patients with ARF can lead to an increase in extravascular lung water. This change can act to reduce pulmonary compliance, worsen lung function, and potentially lead to life-threatening alveolar flooding. Experimental studies found that extravascular lung water accumulates at a lower threshold in ARF.[51] This finding was attributed in part to the down-regulation of epithelial sodium transporters, sodium-potassium adenosine triphosphatases, and aquaporins at the alveolar-capillary barrier that result in a diminished capacity for clearance of alveolar fluid.[52,53] Extravascular lung water accumulation also occurs in response to altered microvascular permeability and reduced serum oncotic pressure seen in ARF, thus diminishing the gradient for fluid reabsorption.[51] In experimental studies, ARF was associated with up-regulation of pulmonary leukocyte adhesion molecules in a murine model. Further, ARF was associated with histologic evidence of interstitial edema and alveolar hemorrhage.

Finally, aberrance in these factors (hypervolemia, alveolar fluid removal, microvascular permeability, oncotic pressure) can be exaggerated in the critically ill patient, in particular in sepsis or trauma, in which profound systemic inflammation and aggressive fluid resuscitation can further contribute to both lung injury and ARF. The outcome of combined lung failure in the setting of ARF is generally poor. Chertow and associates[54–56] found that lung failure prompting MV in critically ill patients with ARF was independently associated with an increase in mortality.

## PHYSIOLOGIC EFFECT OF HEMODIALYSIS AND HEMOFILTRATION ON THE LUNG

Hemodialysis or continuous hemofiltration can have several important physiologic effects on lung function in patients with ARF.

### Alterations in Gas Exchange

Several clinical studies have shown evidence of gas exchange abnormalities during or immediately following hemodialysis. Hypoxemia is commonly observed during hemodialysis, although the exact mechanisms are poorly understood. Hypoxemia may occur in response to ventilation-perfusion mismatch or alveolar hypoventilation.[57] Hemodialysis with bioincompatible membranes (cellulose based) can elicit intense inflammation through activation of complement and leukocyte sequestration that can lead to lung injury. Similarly, thromboemboli, leukostasis, silicone microemboli from the blood pump tubing, and alterations in pulmonary perfusion have all been proposed as causes of ventilation-perfusion abnormalities. Alveolar hypoventilation may result from correction of metabolic acidosis or from the diffusion of $CO_2$ into the dialysate, can suppress the respiratory drive, and can cause clinically evident hypoxemia.[58]

### Beneficial Effects of Hemofiltration on Lung Function

Hemodialysis can also have beneficial effects on lung function in ARF.[59] Huang and colleagues[60] found reductions in respiratory drive and improved pulmonary mechanics after hemodialysis in a small cohort of MV-treated patients with ARF. These improvements were likely attributable to removal of excess extravascular lung water. Further, no significant episodes of hypoxemia or alveolar hypoventilation were reported.

Hemofiltration, depending on the flux of the hemofilter and volume of ultrafiltrate, can remove large-molecular-weight inflammatory mediators such as IL-1, IL-6, IL-8, and TNF-α. This effect has been shown in experimental and small clinical studies to improve right ventricular function and systemic hemodynamics, in particular in sepsis.[61-71] Whether these RRT modalities can translate into improved lung function in patients with lung injury remains uncertain; however, the early initiation of hemofiltration in ARF characterized by hypervolemia was found to have early and significant improvements in oxygenation.

Cardiac surgery with cardiopulmonary bypass (CPB) has been shown to elicit systemic inflammation that can contribute to both acute lung injury and kidney injury. Continuous hemofiltration can attenuate the systemic inflammatory response and reduce circulating inflammatory mediators after CPB. Huang and colleagues[72] found that hemofiltration during CPB reduced inflammatory mediators and was associated with improved pulmonary mechanics and oxygenation. Another study found that hemofiltration resulted in a shorter time to extubation following cardiac surgery with CPB.[73]

Patients with liver failure who are undergoing orthotopic liver transplantation commonly have perioperative impairment of lung function. Experimental data suggested that lung dysfunction is likely multifactorial and may result from preexisting lung disease (i.e., hepatopulmonary syndrome), massive blood loss and replacement, accumulation of excess extravascular lung water, splanchnic ischemia or reperfusion injury, and impaired kidney excretory function. Small clinical studies reported that continuous hemofiltration during and following orthotopic liver transplantation is associated with improved lung compliance and oxygenation while reducing extravascular lung water and fluid sequestration.[74,75]

## EFFECT OF FLUID THERAPY ON LUNG AND KIDNEY FUNCTION

Fluid therapy is considered a cornerstone of resuscitation of the critically ill patient. Similarly, fluid resuscitation is a primary strategy for preservation of kidney function in the patient with progressive increases in serum creatinine and urea or the development of oliguria. However, evidence suggests that there may be negative consequences to fluid therapy for both lung function and kidney function. Both the type of fluid and the quantity of fluid administered (or cumulative fluid balance) appear to have important implications for normal lung and kidney physiology in critical illness.

### Type of Fluid Therapy

Synthetic colloid therapies (i.e., hydroxyethyl starches) have been associated with declines in kidney function after cadaveric kidney transplantation. Patients administered

starches have been found to have higher postoperative serum creatinine values, greater need for RRT, and evidence of osmotic-nephrosis-like lesions on histologic evaluation.[76,77] Similar findings have been shown in critically ill patients after resuscitation for severe sepsis in whom the use of starches was associated with higher rates of ARF compared with other colloids or crystalloids.[78,79] The exact mechanism remains uncertain, although the hydroxyethyl starches may influence intrarenal hemodynamics or the GFR through alterations in vascular oncotic pressure.

In a small observational study of septic critically ill patients, Van Biesen and associates[80] compared the fluid intake of patients developing and not developing ARF. These authors found that patients with ARF had, on average, received a significantly higher volume of colloid resuscitation (2000 mL for ARF versus 1100 mL for no ARF) in the first 72 hours, even though both groups were administered similar volumes of crystalloid. Further, patients with ARF had evidence of higher filling pressures and a lower urine output despite diuretic therapy in the majority. Additional fluid loading in these patients, in spite of apparently optimal hemodynamics and intravascular volume status, failed to improve kidney function, although it contributed to a notable deterioration in oxygenation. It remains unclear from this study whether the differences are attributable to the type of fluid (i.e., colloid) or to the extra volume of fluid administered.

### Amount of Fluid Therapy

An increasing body of evidence suggests that a positive cumulative fluid balance can worsen the outcome in critically ill patients with lung injury.[81-83] The ARDS Clinical Trials Network completed the largest randomized trial assessing fluid therapy in patients with lung injury.[84] This trial compared restrictive and liberal strategies for fluid management in 1000 critically ill patients, mostly with pneumonia or sepsis, and evidence of acute lung injury. At 72 hours, patients receiving a restrictive fluid strategy had a nearly neutral fluid balance, whereas those in the liberal strategy were positive (>5 L). Although the study failed to show a difference in mortality between the strategies, a restrictive strategy improved lung function, increased in ventilator-free days, reduced length of stay in the intensive care unit (ICU), and, most important, was associated with no difference in nonpulmonary organ failure, specifically ARF. In fact, although the restrictive group had nonsignificant increases in serum creatinine and urea, there was a trend toward a reduced need for RRT. The indications for initiation of RRT were not provided, yet pulmonary complications likely contributed to the greater need for RRT in patients receiving a liberal fluid strategy (Box 17.3).

---

**BOX 17-3**

**Current Controversy: Fluid Management Strategy in Critically Ill Patients May Have Important Effects on Both Lung and Kidney Function**

- A large double-blind trial found that a restrictive fluid strategy that aimed for a neutral daily fluid balance, when compared with a liberal fluid strategy, although not improving mortality, was associated with significant improvements in markers of morbidity.
- The restrictive strategy improved lung function, reduced days on the ventilator, and shortened the intensive care unit stay.
- The restrictive strategy showed no increase in the rate of nonpulmonary organ failure, including acute renal failure.
- The restrictive strategy was associated with a reduced need for renal replacement therapy.

---

A restrictive fluid strategy, such as described earlier, requires not only judicious use of fluids, but also an aggressive method for fluid removal. Short of hemofiltration, patients are commonly given diuretics to promote natriuresis and diuresis that can translate into a reduction in extravascular lung water and improved lung function. The most common diuretic used is furosemide, a loop diuretic. Furosemide can also exert additional effects independent of its action on the kidney. In experimental studies, furosemide was shown to induce pulmonary vasodilation and to act as a weak bronchodilator, both of which can improve ventilation-perfusion matching.[85–87] A reduction in total serum protein, and hence colloid oncotic pressure, was shown to be predictive of a positive fluid balance and a worse outcome for patients with ARDS.[88] Experimental studies suggested that furosemide may also act to reduce extravascular lung water by causing an increase colloid oncotic pressure.[89] In a small, randomized trial, Martin and colleagues[90] found that furosemide combined with albumin administration in hypoproteinemic patients with lung injury resulted in greater improvements in oxygenation, net negative fluid balance, and hemodynamic stability compared with patients receiving furosemide alone.

## PULMONARY-RENAL SYNDROMES

The clinical presentation characterized by evidence of both diffuse alveolar hemorrhage (DAH) and acute glomerulonephritis typically defines the small spectrum of pulmonary renal syndromes.

### Diffuse Alveolar Hemorrhage

DAH is generally the result of immunologic, inflammatory, or mechanical injury with loss of integrity and disruption of the alveolar-capillary basement membrane.[91] The injury to pulmonary arterioles, venules, capillaries, and the alveolar septa results in bleeding into the alveolar space.[92] Clinically, DAH is manifest by variable degrees of hemoptysis, gas exchange abnormalities, specifically hypoxemia, and widespread pulmonary infiltrates. A deterioration in gas exchange that prompts MV is common. Bronchoscopy may be used to exclude airway obstruction secondary to blood clots. Acute glomerulonephritis represents inflammatory or immunologic injury to the renal glomeruli in the context of acute reductions in kidney function. Glomerular injury is manifest by evidence of active urinary sediment with variable amounts of hematuria (specifically if dysmorphic red blood cells are present), red blood cell casts, lipiduria, and proteinuria (Box 17.4).

### Wegener's Granulomatosis

Wegener's granulomatosis is a systemic form of vasculitis of small to medium-sized vessels that classically involves the upper and lower respiratory tracts and the kidneys. However, musculoskeletal, cutaneous, ocular, and nervous system involvement can also occur. Patients can present with nonspecific constitutional symptoms such as fever, weight loss, and fatigue. Upper airway symptoms include purulent or bloody rhinorrhea, nasal ulcerations, hoarseness, and stridor. Lower respiratory tract symptoms include cough, dyspnea, hemoptysis, and pleuritis. Hemoptysis may result from alveolar capillaritis or tracheobronchial disease. Pulmonary physiology and imaging are frequently abnormal. Although both obstructive and restrictive physiologic patterns have been described, airflow obstruction is most common. Chest radiographs have a variable appearance and may include cavitating nodules, patchy alveolar opacities, or pleural opacities. Kidney involvement is heralded by rapidly progressive glomerulonephritis (elevations in serum creatinine and urea) and the presence of active urinary sediment. The diagnosis is further supported by the

---

**BOX 17-4**

**Differential Diagnosis of Pulmonary Hemorrhage and Acute Renal Failure**

Wegener's granulomatosis
Goodpasture's syndrome
Systemic lupus erythematosus
Poststreptococcal glomerulonephritis
Henoch-Schönlein purpura
Pulmonary veno-occlusive disease
Drug toxicity (i.e., cocaine, sirolimus)
Severe pulmonary sepsis

---

presence of circulating antineutrophil cytoplasmic antibodies (ANCAs). The cytoplasmic subtype (c-ANCA) targeting the proteinase-3 (PR3) antigen is most consistent with generalized Wegener's granulomatosis, whereas the perinuclear subtype (p-ANCA) specific for the myeloperoxidase (MPO) antigen suggests a diagnosis of microscopic polyangiitis or Churg-Strauss syndrome. The diagnosis is further confirmed by tissue biopsy at a site of active disease, usually the upper airway, skin, or kidney. Treatment consists of high-dose corticosteroids, immunosuppressive therapy, and plasmapheresis.

## Goodpasture's Syndrome

Goodpasture's syndrome is caused by circulating anti–glomerular basement membrane (anti-GBM) antibodies directed against antigens with nearly identical epitopes present on both the glomerular and the alveolar-capillary basement membranes. The result is a clinical syndrome characterized by variable degrees of rapidly progressive glomerulonephritis and DAH. The clinical presentation is characterized by cough, dyspnea, and hemoptysis. Variable hypoxemia and gas exchange abnormalities with diffuse pulmonary infiltrates on chest radiograph are typically seen. Renal manifestations include active urinary sediment and evidence of acute rises in serum creatinine and urea. Systemic constitutional symptoms are typically absent. The diagnosis is strongly suspected by the clinical presentation and by the presence of circulating anti-GBM antibodies. Concomitant studies for ANCA antibodies should be performed because of overlap with Wegener's granulomatosis. However, the diagnosis is confirmed by evidence on renal biopsy of linear basement membrane staining of anti-GBM antibodies. The optimal treatment for Goodpasture's syndrome is early initiation of plasmapheresis combined with various regimens of systemic corticosteroids and immunosuppression with cyclophosphamide.

## Other Diseases

Several additional conditions warrant consideration for the patient with a suspected pulmonary-renal syndrome, including other immune-mediated diseases such as systemic lupus erythematosus, poststreptococcal glomerulonephritis, and additional causes of systemic vasculitis (i.e., Henoch-Schönlein purpura). Similarly, other conditions may mimic classic pulmonary-renal syndrome such as severe mitral stenosis or pulmonary veno-occlusive disease with pulmonary edema and a low cardiac output state, drug toxicity (i.e., cocaine, sirolimus), primary pulmonary infection or severe sepsis, and any cause of ARF with uremic-induced increases in pulmonary capillary permeability.

---

**BOX 17-5**

**Clinical Caveat: Effect of Fluid Therapy on Lung and Kidney Function**

- Synthetic colloid fluids, such as hydroxyethyl starch, may contribute to or worsen kidney function.
- The mechanism is not well understood, but it may involve alterations in glomerular oncotic pressure or renal hemodynamics.

---

## CONCLUSION

In conclusion, the normal physiologic functions of the kidneys and lungs are strongly linked. Dysfunction in both organs' systems is commonplace in critically ill patients, and the interaction can present unique challenges for the critical care clinician. MV, with or without PEEP, has a multitude of effects on kidney function by altering cardiovascular function and neurohormonal activation and by contributing to systemic inflammation. Hypoxemia, hypercapnia, and an increase in systemic inflammation can exert negative effects on renal perfusion and kidney function. ARF, in addition to leading to extracellular volume expansion, can impair gas exchange, weaken respiratory muscles, and down-regulate alveolar proficiency for fluid clearance. Although RRT can provoke gas exchange abnormalities, the timely commencement of RRT may improve lung function directly by reducing lung water and indirectly by various effects on cardiovascular function and systemic inflammation. Several issues of fluid therapy remain controversial in patients with multiorgan failure; however, more recent evidence supports restrictive strategies and a more judicious use of fluids. Pulmonary-renal syndromes are uncommon but represent important systemic diseases to identify because the prognosis is greatly improved by well-timed and aggressive therapy (Box 17.5).

## CASE STUDY

The patient is a 58-year-old woman with long-standing diabetes mellitus treated with insulin therapy, hypertension, and mild chronic kidney disease (baseline serum creatinine, 120 µmol/L) who presented to the hospital with a history of fever, cough, dyspnea, and diarrhea. Initial clinical examination found mild confusion (Glasgow Coma Scale, 13), a temperature of 38.9°C, a heart rate of 115 beats/minute, blood pressure of 84/48 mm Hg, a respiratory rate of 28 breaths/minute, and a pulse oximetry saturation of 90% on 8 L oxygen by mask. The chest radiograph showed extensive bilateral interstitial infiltrates with no evidence of pleural effusions. Laboratory values showed leukocytosis with left shift, mild thrombocytopenia, and the following: serum glucose, 15 mmol/L; serum sodium, 132 mEq/L; serum potassium, 4.8 mEq/L; and serum creatinine, 350 μmol/L. Arterial blood gas analysis showed the following: pH, 7.32; $PaCO_2$, 33 cm $H_2O$; $PaO_2$, 64 cm $H_2O$; and lactate, 3.4 mmol/L.

## What is your differential diagnosis for this patient's presentation?

## What would be your approach to management?

The patient was admitted to the ICU with a presumptive diagnosis of severe community-acquired pneumonia, sepsis syndrome, and multiorgan dysfunction. She was aggressively resuscitated with broad-spectrum antibiotics including macrolides, fluid therapy (5 L crystalloid), and vasopressors. An infusion of insulin was started to correct hyperglycemia. Her lung function quickly deteriorated, thus prompting intubation and MV with an inspired oxygen fraction ($FiO_2$) greater than 0.8 and PEEP at 12 cm $H_2O$. Her urine output remained less than 20 mL/hour. The laboratory results showed a positive urinary antigen test for *Legionella pneumophila*.

## What are the potential contributing factors to her oliguric ARF?

## What are the potential contributing factors to her lung function deterioration?

## What would be your approach to management at this time?

The patient was ventilated with a lung-protective strategy using low tidal volumes, PEEP, and limited end-inspiratory plateau pressures. This resulted in mild permissive hypercapnia and respiratory acidosis. These metabolic effects and those resulting from ARF were offset by initiation of continuous hemofiltration prescribed at a dose of 35 mL/kg/hour, using bicarbonate-based replacement fluid, and targeting a net negative fluid balance. Over the next 48 hours, the patient's lung function improved significantly and allowed for weaning to pressure support ventilation, PEEP of 5 cm $H_2O$, and an $FiO_2$ of 0.40. The metabolic acidosis, uremia, and excess extravascular fluid had improved, and the patient was now spontaneously producing urine at more than 40 mL/hour. Over the next 48 hours, she was weaned from the ventilator and from continuous hemofiltration and was discharged to the hospital ward.

# REFERENCES

1. Annat G, Viale JP, Bui Xuan B, et al: Effect of PEEP ventilation on renal function, plasma renin, aldosterone, neurophysins and urinary ADH, and prostaglandins. Anesthesiology 1983;58:136–141.
2. Mirro R, Busija D, Green R, Leffler C: Relationship between mean airway pressure, cardiac output, and organ blood flow with normal and decreased respiratory compliance. J Pediatr 1987;111:101–106.
3. Berry AJ, Geer RT, Marshall C, et al: The effect of long-term controlled mechanical ventilation with positive end-expiratory pressure on renal function in dogs. Anesthesiology 1984;61:406–415.
4. Vivino G, Antonelli M, Moro ML, et al: Risk factors for acute renal failure in trauma patients. Intensive Care Med 1998;24:808–814.
5. Gattinoni L, Agostoni A, Damia G, et al: Hemodynamics and renal function during low frequency positive pressure ventilation with extracorporeal $CO_2$ removal: A comparison with continuous positive pressure ventilation. Intensive Care Med 1980;6:155–161.
6. Hering R, Peters D, Zinserling J, et al: Effects of spontaneous breathing during airway pressure release ventilation on renal perfusion and function in patients with acute lung injury. Intensive Care Med 2002;28:1426–1433.
7. Steinhoff H, Falke K, Schwarzhoff W: Enhanced renal function associated with intermittent mandatory ventilation in acute respiratory failure. Intensive Care Med 1982;8:69–74.
8. Botha J, Mudholkar P, Le Blanc V: The effect of changing from pressure support ventilation to volume control ventilation on renal function. Crit Care Resusc 2005;7:303–309.
9. Hall SV, Johnson EE, Hedley-Whyte J: Renal hemodynamics and function with continuous positive-pressure ventilation in dogs. Anesthesiology 1974;41:452–461.
10. Priebe HJ, Hedley-Whyte J: Positive end-expiratory pressure (PEEP) and renal function. Anesthesiology 1982;57:144–145.
11. Moore ES, Galvez MB, Paton JB, et al: Effects of positive pressure ventilation on intrarenal blood flow in infant primates. Pediatr Res 1974;8:792–796.
12. Priebe HJ, Heimann JC, Hedley-Whyte J: Mechanisms of renal dysfunction during positive end-expiratory pressure ventilation. J Appl Physiol 1981;50:643–649.
13. Mullins RJ, Dawe EJ, Lucas CE, et al: Mechanisms of impaired renal function with PEEP. J Surg Res 1984;37:189–196.
14. Rossaint R, Krebs M, Forther J, et al: Inferior vena caval pressure increase contributes to sodium and water retention during PEEP in awake dogs. J Appl Physiol 1993;75:2484–2492.
15. Shinozaki M, Muteki T, Kaku N, Tsuda H: Hemodynamic relationship between renal venous pressure and blood flow regulation during positive end-expiratory pressure. Crit Care Med 1988;16:144–147.
16. Farge D, De la Coussaye JE, Beloucif S, et al: Interactions between hemodynamic and hormonal modifications during PEEP-induced antidiuresis and antinatriuresis. Chest 1995;107:1095–1100.
17. Boemke W, Krebs MO, Djalali K, et al: Renal nerves are not involved in sodium and water retention during mechanical ventilation in awake dogs. Anesthesiology 1998;89:942–953.
18. Kharasch ED, Yeo KT, Kenny MA, Buffington CW: Atrial natriuretic factor may mediate the renal effects of PEEP ventilation. Anesthesiology 1988;69:862–869.
19. Christensen G, Bugge JF, Ostensen J, Kiil F: Atrial natriuretic factor and renal sodium excretion during ventilation with PEEP in hypervolemic dogs. J Appl Physiol 1992;72:993–997.

20. Andrivet P, Adnot S, Brun-Buisson C, et al: Involvement of ANF in the acute antidiuresis during PEEP ventilation. J Appl Physiol 1988;65:1967–1974.

21. Andrivet P, Adnot S, Sanker S, et al: Hormonal interactions and renal function during mechanical ventilation and ANF infusion in humans. J Appl Physiol 1991;70:287–292.

22. Kaczmarczyk G, Jorres D, Rossaint R, et al: Extracellular volume expansion inhibits antidiuretic hormone increase during positive end-expiratory pressure in conscious dogs. Clin Sci (Lond) 1993;85:643–649.

23. Hemmer M, Viquerat CE, Suter PM, Vallotton MB: Urinary antidiuretic hormone excretion during mechanical ventilation and weaning in man. Anesthesiology 1980;52:395–400.

24. Venus B, Mathru M, Smith RA, et al: Renal function during application of positive end-expiratory pressure in swine: Effects of hydration. Anesthesiology 1985;62:765–769.

25. Rossaint R, Jorres D, Nienhaus M, et al: Positive end-expiratory pressure reduces renal excretion without hormonal activation after volume expansion in dogs. Anesthesiology 1992;77:700–708.

26. Valta P, Uusaro A, Nunes S, et al: Acute respiratory distress syndrome: Frequency, clinical course, and costs of care. Crit Care Med 1999;27:2367–2374.

27. Fowler AA, Hamman RF, Zerbe GO, et al: Adult respiratory distress syndrome: Prognosis after onset. Am Rev Respir Dis 1985;132:472–478.

28. Bruns FJ: Decrease in renal perfusion, glomerular filtration and sodium excretion by hypoxia in the dog. Proc Soc Exp Biol Med 1978;159:468–472.

29. Franklin KJ, McGee LE, Ullmann EA: Effects of severe asphyxia on the kidney and urine flow. J Physiol 1951;112:43–53.

30. Kilburn KH, Dowell AR: Renal function in respiratory failure: Effects of hypoxia, hyperoxia, and hypercapnia. Arch Intern Med 1971;127:754–762.

31. Gotshall RW, Miles DS, Sexson WR: Renal oxygen delivery and consumption during progressive hypoxemia in the anesthetized dog. Proc Soc Exp Biol Med 1983;174:363–367.

32. Gotshall RW, Miles DS, Sexson WR: The combined effects of hypoxemia and mechanical ventilation on renal function. Aviat Space Environ Med 1986;57:782–786.

33. Zillig B, Schuler G, Truniger B: Renal function and intrarenal hemodynamics in acutely hypoxic and hypercapnic rats. Kidney Int 1978;14:58–67.

34. Howes TQ, Deane CR, Levin GE, et al: The effects of oxygen and dopamine on renal and aortic blood flow in chronic obstructive pulmonary disease with hypoxemia and hypercapnia. Am J Respir Crit Care Med 1995;151:378–383.

35. Reihman DH, Farber MO, Weinberger MH, et al: Effect of hypoxemia on sodium and water excretion in chronic obstructive lung disease. Am J Med 1985;78:87–94.

36. Anderson RJ, Rose CE Jr, Berns AS, et al: Mechanism of effect of hypercapnic acidosis on renin secretion in the dog. Am J Physiol 1980;238:F119–F125.

37. Bersentes TJ, Simmons DH: Effects of acute acidosis on renal hemodynamics. Am J Physiol 1967;212:633–640.

38. Sharkey RA, Mulloy EM, O'Neill SJ: Acute effects of hypoxaemia, hyperoxaemia and hypercapnia on renal blood flow in normal and renal transplant subjects. Eur Respir J 1998;12:653–657.

39. Rose CE Jr, Walker BR, Erickson A, et al: Renal and cardiovascular responses to acute hypercapnic acidosis in conscious dogs: Role of renin-angiotensin. J Cardiovasc Pharmacol 1982;4:676–687.

40. Rose CE Jr, Kimmel DP, Godine RL Jr, et al: Synergistic effects of acute hypoxemia and hypercapnic acidosis in conscious dogs: Renal dysfunction and activation of the renin-angiotensin system. Circ Res 1983;53:202–213.

41. Chiumello D, Pristine G, Slutsky AS: Mechanical ventilation affects local and systemic cytokines in an animal model of acute respiratory distress syndrome. Am J Respir Crit Care Med 1999;160:109–116.

42. Ranieri VM, Suter PM, Tortorella C, et al: Effect of mechanical ventilation on inflammatory mediators in patients with acute respiratory distress syndrome: A randomized controlled trial. JAMA 1999;282:54–61.

43. Meduri GU, Headley S, Kohler G, et al: Persistent elevation of inflammatory cytokines predicts a poor outcome in ARDS: Plasma IL-1 beta and IL-6 levels are consistent and efficient predictors of outcome over time. Chest 1995;107:1062–1073.

44. Gurkan OU, O'Donnell C, Brower R, et al: Differential effects of mechanical ventilatory strategy on lung injury and systemic organ inflammation in mice. Am J Physiol 2003;285:L710–L718.

45. Imai Y, Parodo J, Kajikawa O, et al: Injurious mechanical ventilation and end-organ epithelial cell apoptosis and organ dysfunction in an experimental model of acute respiratory distress syndrome. JAMA 2003;289:2104–2112.

46. Ranieri VM, Giunta F, Suter PM, Slutsky AS: Mechanical ventilation as a mediator of multisystem organ failure in acute respiratory distress syndrome. JAMA 2000;284:43–44.

47. Simmons EM, Himmelfarb J, Sezer MT, et al: Plasma cytokine levels predict mortality in patients with acute renal failure. Kidney Int 2004;65:1357–1365.

48. Hopps HC, Wissler RW: Uremic pneumonitis. Am J Pathol 1955;31:261–273.

49. Bush A, Gabriel R: The lungs in uraemia: A review. J R Soc Med 1985;78:849–855.

50. Lee HY, Stretton TB, Barnes AM: The lungs in renal failure. Thorax 1975;30:46–53.

51. Slutsky RA, Day R, Murray M: Effect of prolonged renal dysfunction on intravascular and extravascular pulmonary fluid volumes during left atrial hypertension. Proc Soc Exp Biol Med 1985;179:25–31.

52. Rabb H, Chamoun F, Hotchkiss J: Molecular mechanisms underlying combined kidney-lung dysfunction during acute renal failure. Contrib Nephrol 2001;132:41–52.

53. Rabb H, Wang Z, Nemoto T, et al: Acute renal failure leads to dysregulation of lung salt and water channels. Kidney Int 2003;63:600–606.

54. Chertow GM, Lazarus JM, Paganini EP, et al: Predictors of mortality and the provision of dialysis in patients with acute tubular necrosis: The Auriculin Anaritide Acute Renal Failure Study Group. J Am Soc Nephrol 1998;9:692–698.

55. Chertow GM, Levy EM, Hammermeister KE, et al: Independent association between acute renal failure and mortality following cardiac surgery. Am J Med 1998;104:343–348.

56. Metnitz PG, Krenn CG, Steltzer H, et al: Effect of acute renal failure requiring renal replacement therapy on outcome in critically ill patients. Crit Care Med 2002;30:2051–2058.

57. Milner LS, Rothberg AD, Thomson PD, Stothart M: Sustained ventilation: Perfusion imbalance during hemodialysis. Int J Pediatr Nephrol 1983;4:89–92.

58. Pierson DJ: Respiratory considerations in the patient with renal failure. Respir Care 2006;51:413–422.

59. Zidulka A, Despas PJ, Milic-Emili J, Anthonisen NR: Pulmonary function with acute loss of excess lung water by hemodialysis in patients with chronic uremia. Am J Med 1973;55:134–141.

60. Huang CC, Tsai YH, Lin MC, et al: Respiratory drive and pulmonary mechanics during haemodialysis with ultrafiltration in ventilated patients. Anaesth Intensive Care 1997;25:464–470.

61. Grootendorst AF, van Bommel EF, van der Hoven B, et al: High volume hemofiltration improves right ventricular function in endotoxin-induced shock in the pig. Intensive Care Med 1992;18:235–240.

62. Grootendorst AF, van Bommel EF, van Leengoed LA, et al: High volume hemofiltration improves hemodynamics and survival of pigs exposed to gut ischemia and reperfusion. Shock 1994;2:72–78.

63. Bellomo R: Continuous hemofiltration as blood purification in sepsis. New Horiz 1995;3:732–737.

64. Bellomo R, Kellum JA, Gandhi CR, et al: The effect of intensive plasma water exchange by hemofiltration on hemodynamics and soluble mediators in canine endotoxemia. Am J Respir Crit Care Med 2000;161:1429–1436.

65. Bellomo R, Tipping P, Boyce N: Continuous veno-venous hemofiltration with dialysis removes cytokines from the circulation of septic patients. Crit Care Med 1993;21:522–526.

66. Bellomo R, Tipping P, Boyce N: Interleukin-6 and interleukin-8 extraction during continuous venovenous hemodiafiltration in septic acute renal failure. Ren Fail 1995;17:457–466.

67. Cole L, Bellomo R, Davenport P, et al: Cytokine removal during continuous renal replacement therapy: An ex vivo comparison of convection and diffusion. Int J Artif Organs 2004;27:388–397.

68. Cole L, Bellomo R, Hart G, et al: A phase II randomized, controlled trial of continuous hemofiltration in sepsis. Crit Care Med 2002;30:100–106.

69. Cole L, Bellomo R, Journois D, et al: High-volume haemofiltration in human septic shock. Intensive Care Med 2001;27:978–986.

70. Uchino S, Bellomo R, Goldsmith D, et al: Cytokine removal with a large pore cellulose triacetate filter: An ex vivo study. Int J Artif Organs 2002;25:27–32.

71. Uchino S, Bellomo R, Goldsmith D, et al: Super high flux hemofiltration: A new technique for cytokine removal. Intensive Care Med 2002;28:651–655.

72. Huang H, Yao T, Wang W, et al: Combination of balanced ultrafiltration with modified ultrafiltration attenuates pulmonary injury in patients undergoing open heart surgery. Chin Med J (Engl) 2003;116:1504–1507.

73. Oliver WC Jr, Nuttall GA, Orszulak TA, et al: Hemofiltration but not steroids results in earlier tracheal extubation following cardiopulmonary bypass: A prospective, randomized double-blind trial. Anesthesiology 2004;101:327–339.

74. Tuman KJ, Spiess BD, McCarthy RJ, et al: Effects of continuous arteriovenous hemofiltration on cardiopulmonary abnormalities during anesthesia for orthotopic liver transplantation. Anesth Analg 1988;67:363–369.

75. Sankary HN, Foster P, Tuman K, et al: Intraoperative continuous arterio-venous hemofiltration (CAVH): A method to diminish fluid sequestration during liver transplant operations. Transplant Proc 1989;21:2326–2327.

76. Legendre C, Thervet E, Page B, et al: Hydroxyethylstarch and osmotic-nephrosis–like lesions in kidney transplantation. Lancet 1993;342:248–249.

77. Cittanova ML, Leblanc I, Legendre C, et al: Effect of hydroxyethylstarch in brain-dead kidney donors on renal function in kidney-transplant recipients. Lancet 1996;348:1620–1622.

78. Schortgen F, Brochard L, Burnham E, Martin GS: Pro/con clinical debate: Hydroxyethylstarches should be avoided in septic patients. Crit Care 2003;7:279–281.

79. Schortgen F, Lacherade JC, Bruneel F, et al: Effects of hydroxyethylstarch and gelatin on renal function in severe sepsis: A multicentre randomised study. Lancet 2001;357:911–916.

80. Van Biesen W, Yegenaga I, Vanholder R, et al: Relationship between fluid status and its management on acute renal failure (ARF) in intensive care unit (ICU) patients with sepsis: A prospective analysis. J Nephrol 2005;18:54–60.

81. Sakr Y, Vincent JL, Reinhart K, et al: High tidal volume and positive fluid balance are associated with worse outcome in acute lung injury. Chest 2005;128:3098–3108.

82. Simmons RS, Berdine GG, Seidenfeld JJ, et al: Fluid balance and the adult respiratory distress syndrome. Am Rev Respir Dis 1987;135:924–929.

83. Humphrey H, Hall J, Sznajder I, et al: Improved survival in ARDS patients associated with a reduction in pulmonary capillary wedge pressure. Chest 1990;97:1176–1180.

84. Wiedemann HP, Wheeler AP, Bernard GR, et al: Comparison of two fluid-management strategies in acute lung injury. N Engl J Med 2006;354:2564–2575.

85. Ali J, Unruh H, Skoog C, Goldberg HS: The effect of lung edema on pulmonary vasoactivity of furosemide. J Surg Res 1983;35:383–390.

86. Ali J, Wood LD: Pulmonary vascular effects of furosemide on gas exchange in pulmonary edema. J Appl Physiol 1984;57:160–167.

87. Stevens EL, Uyehara CF, Southgate WM, Nakamura KT: Furosemide differentially relaxes airway and vascular smooth muscle in fetal, newborn, and adult guinea pigs. Am Rev Respir Dis 1992;146:1192–1197.

88. Martin GS: Fluid balance and colloid osmotic pressure in acute respiratory failure: Emerging clinical evidence. Crit Care 2000;4(Suppl 2):S21–S25.

89. Ali J, Duke K: Colloid osmotic pressure in pulmonary edema clearance with furosemide. Chest 1987;92:540–546.

90. Martin GS, Moss M, Wheeler AP, et al: A randomized, controlled trial of furosemide with or without albumin in hypoproteinemic patients with acute lung injury. Crit Care Med 2005;33:1681–1687.

91. Franks TJ, Koss MN: Pulmonary capillaritis. Curr Opin Pulm Med 2000;6:430–435.

92. Collard HR, Schwarz MI: Diffuse alveolar hemorrhage. Clin Chest Med 2004;25:583–592, vii.

# CHAPTER 18

# Genetic Basis of Acute Lung Injury

Hector R. Wong and Thomas P. Shanley

The influence of genetic variability on both health and disease is most evident in the classic mendelian disorders such as neurofibromatosis (autosomal dominant), cystic fibrosis (autosomal recessive), and Duchenne muscular dystrophy (X-linked recessive). In these disorders, there is a relatively unambiguous path leading from genotype to phenotype. Nevertheless, the phenotypes of classic mendelian disorders can be influenced by environmental factors, thereby leading to some degree of heterogeneity. The opposite situation exists for nonmendelian, multifactorial disorders such as acute lung injury (ALI): we understand a great deal about how environmental factors influence the development and outcome of ALI (e.g., sepsis, pneumonia, trauma, aspiration, ventilator-induced ALI, and transfusion-related ALI), but know much less about how genetics can influence the development and outcome of ALI.

One of the most common frustrations shared by physicians caring for patients with ALI is the observation that individuals undergoing seemingly similar biologic or physiologic insults and provided similar care can have such divergent outcomes, ranging from survival without sequelae to death. These experiences lend credence to the hypothesis that the genetics of an individual will interact with environmental factors (e.g., cause and medical care) to influence susceptibility to, propagation of, and resolution and final outcome of ALI. As such, studies aimed at elucidating the genetic contribution to ALI are complicated by phenotypic variation, incomplete penetrance, complicated patterns of heritability, and multiple variant mutations, which combine to create substantial heterogeneity among a population affected by ALI. Nevertheless, this type of disease process lends itself to the application of powerful investigative

tools, such as functional genomics and proteomics, outlined later.

One of the principal ways in which these investigative tools have been applied involves established animal models with ALI. Although this approach can generate an enormous amount of gene expression data, the results are unbiased in that the investigators do not limit their inquiry to a single gene or set of genes. This approach has been criticized for being hypothesis generating, rather than hypothesis driven; nevertheless, it has been used successfully to increase our knowledge of the gene expression profiles associated with and resulting from the biologic processes regulating lung inflammation and injury. Building on this preclinical science, these technologic advances in the field of functional genomics and proteomics have been increasingly applied to human patients with ALI.[1]

These studies not only led to important diagnostic and mechanistic insights, but also resulted in the establishment of an international investigative group committed to the goal of using functional genomics and proteomics as tools to advance our understanding of ALI. In January of 2002, the National Heart, Lung and Blood Institute (NHLBI) at the National Institutes of Health convened a working group to consider the most efficient and appropriate future direction of ALI-related research in the postgenomic era. In addition to reviewing the current available data, conference participants were charged with identifying major gaps in our understanding and suggesting promising avenues for investigation in the hope of charting a course for future research. Participants reported several broad areas with significant gaps in our mechanistic understanding of ALI, including the following: the specific responses of lung epithelium and endothelium; the regulation of apoptosis, necrosis, and fibrosis; the effect of mechanical forces on the lung; the role of the innate immune system; and the link between coagulation and inflammation as it pertains to lung injury.[2]

In the remainder of this chapter, we focus on three areas. First, we review some of the technology and approaches available to study the influence of genetics and genome-level responses on ALI. Second, we provide examples demonstrating that genetics and genomics influence the development and outcome of experimental ALI. Finally, we review the evolving literature suggesting that genetics and genomics influence clinical ALI. Although the distinction between ALI and acute respiratory distress syndrome (ARDS) is fully recognized, the term *ALI* is used throughout the remainder of this chapter for the sake of simplicity.

## TECHNOLOGY AND APPROACHES

### Large-Scale, High-Throughput Gene Expression Analysis

The field of genomics encompasses a radically different scientific paradigm: the study of entire genomes.[3] This paradigm attempts to take into account the vast complexity of biologic systems by simultaneously measuring and analyzing the expression patterns and interactions of thousands of gene products. The ability to sequence the entire genomes of several species,[4-7] including humans,[8,9] and the rapidly evolving field of bioinformatics[10] are two central forces that facilitate the field of genomics. Two other key components of the field are microarray technology and proteomics, which allow for the simultaneous analysis of thousands of gene products.

Several variations of microarray technology exist.[11] In general, microarray technology involves the immobilization of thousands of nucleic acid sequences, at specific locations of a solid support (nylon membranes or glass/silicone "chips"). The respective sequences can represent specific gene sequences (or partial gene sequences), expressed sequence tags (ESTs, representing genes of unknown function), or sequences representing gene polymorphisms. The nucleic acids (500 to 5000 base pairs) are robotically applied to the solid support by a process termed *spotting*, or an array of oligonucleotide probes (20 to 80 base pairs) is synthesized directly on the solid support. In either case, the resulting product is a high-density array of DNA sequences that can be used for large-scale analyses of a given genome.

Microarray technology has several high-throughput applications, including polymorphism analysis, gene discovery, and expression profiling.[11] Expression profiling may be the most immediately applicable for studying the genomics of ALI. When used for expression profiling, a microarray can be simply thought of as a large-scale Northern blot in which the steady-state messenger RNA (mRNA) levels of thousands of genes are analyzed simultaneously. In these types of experiments, total RNA is extracted from the tissue of choice (e.g., whole lung) and is reverse transcribed to the respective complementary DNAs (DNAs). During the process of reverse transcription, the cDNAs are either radiolabeled or fluorescence labeled and are subsequently applied to the microarray during a hybridization step. The microarray chip or membrane is then washed and scanned to measure the amount of hybridization that occurs between the labeled cDNAs (the "targets") and the nuclei acids (the "probes") that encompass the microarray. The resulting hybridization pattern provides a simultaneous mRNA expression profile of up to 30,000 genes.

Microarray technology measures mRNA expression patterns, which do not necessarily correlate with protein expression. Therefore, results of microarray analyses need to be confirmed and complemented by more traditional measurements of gene expression (e.g., Western blot, enzyme-linked immunosorbent assay [ELISA], real-time polymerase chain reaction [PCR]). A more powerful solution to this limitation is the field of proteomics, which allows for the systematic and large-scale analysis of protein expression.[12] Proteomics has now evolved to the point of achieving high-throughput capabilities on a scale that is relatively similar to that of microarray technology. Some of the key technologies in the field of proteomics are two-dimensional polyacrylamide gel electrophoresis (2D-PAGE), matrix-assisted laser desorption/ionization–time of flight (MALDI-TOF), surface-enhanced laser desorption ionization (SELDI-TOF), and mass spectroscopy.

Managing the unprecedented mass of data generated by these types of studies presents tremendous technical and administrative challenges to the research community. Two developments that directly address these issues are worth noting. First is the development of a proposed set of guidelines for presenting and exchanging microarray data. Minimum Information About a Microarray Experiment (MIAME) is a proposal describing the fundamental information that is required to allow for the interpretation and independent verification of microarray data, and it provides a set of standards for recording and reporting microarray data.[13-15] Second is the development of the Human Protein Reference Database (HPRD).[16] At the time of this writing, the HPRD catalogues more than 7500 human proteins with annotated data involving protein-protein interactions, post-translational modifications, enzyme-substrate relationships, disease associations, tissue expression, and subcellular localization. The HPRD is available to the public at the following web site: http://www.hprd.org.

The ability to study gene expression on such a large scale, and in a complementary fashion that combines microarray technology and proteomics, holds tremendous opportunities for developing a more comprehensive understanding of ALI. The complementary data derived from microarray and proteomics experiments can go beyond an expression analysis of the thousands of genes that are likely to be involved in a complex disease process such as ALI. Through the power of bioinformatics, expression patterns can also be organized into expression hierarchies of gene classes and can be mined to identify patterns of concerted gene expression (gene clusters) and gene interactions that are associated with the development ALI. These types of analyses hold the potential to identify novel genes and novel gene interactions involved in the pathophysiology of ALI.

## Laser Capture Microdissection

Another challenge involving microarray technology and proteomics is the heterogeneity of tissues being examined. When whole tissues are the source for RNA or protein extraction, the data derived from these samples can be confounded by a mixture of cell types that are likely to have differing genome-level responses to a given stimulus or disease process. Light capture microdissection (LCM) allows for the physical separation of specific cell types from a tissue sample, which can then be processed for RNA or protein extraction.[17] For example, if an investigator is specifically interested in alveolar cell responses in the setting of ALI, then a lung tissue sample from an experimental model of ALI could be subjected to LCM to isolate alveolar cells specifically. This type of approach is potentially much more powerful for addressing the question compared with extracting RNA or protein from whole lung.

## Polymorphisms

In general terms, a *polymorphism* is defined as a genetic variant. More specifically, a polymorphism consists of the regular occurrence (≥1%) in a population of two or more alleles at a particular chromosome location. An *allele* refers to one of two or more alternate forms of a gene. The functional consequences of a polymorphic gene are variable. In a few instances, the polymorphism leads to a change in protein function or expression and leads to a distinct phenotype. Somewhat more common are polymorphisms that do not lead to any alteration in protein function or expression, but rather are linked to a particular phenotype. The most commonly occurring polymorphisms, however, have no known effect on protein function or expression, and they have yet to be linked to any particular phenotype.

The most common and simplest type of polymorphism is generated by a single base change (substitution, deletion, or insertion) in either the coding region or the noncoding region of a given gene. These are referred to as *single nucleotide polymorphisms* (SNPs). At the time of this writing, almost 4 million SNPs have been reported in the human genome, and they are catalogued in a public database (http://www.ncbi.nlm.nih.gov/SNP/).

Because SNPs account of the majority of genetic variations among individuals, they have become a focus for investigating how the genetic background of the host can influence complex disease processes such as ALI. Since the late 1990's, many studies have linked SNPs with the development and outcome of severe sepsis or septic shock.[18] Because septic shock is a primary environmental factor leading to the development of ALI, it is highly plausible that some of these polymorphisms are also linked to the development and outcome of ALI. Specific polymorphisms linked to ALI are detailed in subsequent sections of this chapter. Further information linking specific SNPs with ALI can be found at the following web site: http://www.hopkins-genomics.org/ali/ali_info.html.

## Genetic Association Studies

When a genetic association study provides statistical evidence of an association or correlation between a particular gene allele (e.g., SNP) and a particular phenotype (e.g., ALI), this can be the result of three possible scenarios.[19] First, the gene allele can have functional consequences for protein function or expression that directly affects ALI. This situation is possible for certain forms of ALI, but it is highly unlikely that a single, common "ALI gene" will be discovered. Second, the gene allele can be linked (linkage disequilibrium) to another allele that is either functionally important in ALI or combines with other alleles to generate the ALI phenotype. This more complex scenario seems likely for a multifactorial and heterogenous condition such as ALI. The third scenario involves chance. If there is selection bias in the study population or if there are confounding factors that have not been identified or addressed, it may be possible to detect a "statistical" association when one does not truly exist (false-positive association).

The issue of false-positive genetic association studies can be addressed at several levels. For example, a well-performed, positive, replicate study by a different group of investigators using a different population set can add tremendous power to the validity of any preceding genetic association study. Although the requirement for replication has been debated, it still remains a valid benchmark for codifying links between polymorphic alleles and multifactorial disease processes.[20,21] When multiple studies have examined associations between a particular allele and a particular disease process, and the results are both positive and negative, then meta-analysis can play a role in addressing the issue of whether there is a valid genetic association.[22] Finally, published guidelines can assist in both the design and critique of genetic association studies (Box 18.1).[23]

## LABORATORY STUDIES

In the last few years, numerous investigators have systematically applied genomic approaches to cell and animal models of ALI. Yoneda and colleagues[24] examined the gene expression profiles (microarray analysis) associated with smoke- and hydrogen peroxide–induced injury and repair in human bronchial epithelial cells. Three phases of gene expression were noted. The first phase was characterized as an immediate response to oxidant injury and was associated with apoptosis- and mitogen-activated protein (MAP) kinase–related gene expression. The second phase, observed by 5 hours, was associated with induction of various stress proteins

(e.g., HSP-70) and ubiquitin, which were hypothesized to play a chaperone role for handling damaged intracellular macromolecules. The third phase, noted between 5 and 10 hours, was characterized by expression of genes involved in the reduction of oxidative stress (e.g., glutaredoxin) and enzymes responsible for tissue remodeling.

Birukov and colleagues[25] conducted gene expression profiling experiments in human lung endothelial cells subjected to cyclic stretch. These studies revealed that cyclic stretch regulates certain genes involved in endothelial cell signal transduction and genes involved in cytoskeleton and barrier function regulation. In addition, these investigators noted that many of these genes were expressed in an amplitude-dependent (i.e., increasing degrees of stretching) manner. Related to this line of investigation is the work of Copland and colleagues,[26] who examined gene expression profiles from whole rat adult lungs subjected to mechanical ventilation with high tidal volumes (25 mL/kg) and zero positive end-expiratory pressure, a strategy that readily induces ALI. These investigators noted the significant up-regulation of 10 genes and the significant suppression of 12 genes in the lungs subjected to high tidal volumes. Interestingly, none of the genes that were up-regulated in these experiments were found to be up-regulated in the in vitro studies of Birukov and colleagues outlined earlier. Although both studies generated biologically plausible results and provide a framework for further study, the discrepancy between the two gene lists illustrates how genomic studies are strongly influenced by experimental approach (in vitro versus in vivo), species (human versus rat), tissue source of RNA (endothelial cells versus whole lung), experimental model (stretching cultured cells versus subjecting the intact lung to high pressures and extreme stretching), and analytic approach.

Other notable examples of in vitro gene expression profile experiments related to ALI include the effect of keratinocyte growth factor on human airway epithelial cells[27] and the effect of the hepatic 3-methylglutaryl–coenzyme A reductase inhibitor, simvastatin, on human pulmonary artery endothelial cells.[28] These studies and the other in vitro studies discussed earlier are primarily descriptive and require thoughtful follow-up and confirmation. Nevertheless, they serve to illustrate the potential power and comprehensive nature of a genome-level approach to ALI.

Apart from the study by Copland and colleagues described earlier, other investigators have conducted genome-level expression profiles in animal models of ALI. One example is the work of McDowell and colleagues[29] involving a murine model of nickel-induced ALI. Using a microarray consisting of 8734 sequence-verified murine cDNAs, and RNA extracted from homogenized whole lungs, these investigators were able

---

**BOX 18-1**

**Summary of Proposed Guidelines for Designing and Critiquing Genetic Association Studies, with Adaptations for Acute Lung Injury**

- The heritability of the study phenotype should be established when possible. If this is not possible (e.g., in ALI), then the role of the study allele (candidate gene) in the given phenotype should have strong biologic plausibility.
- Case-control studies (likely to be the most frequently applied to ALI) must be well matched with regard to ethnic and geographic origin and other potentially confounding variables (e.g., initiating event for ALI).
- Validation should come in the form of a replicate study or functional studies in the laboratory setting.
- A hypothesis should be clearly stated to avoid post hoc analyses and multiple comparisons. In the case of post hoc analyses and multiple comparisons, appropriate statistical corrections for multiple testing should be performed.
- Associations are preferably reported as odds ratios and confidence limits.
- Because selective publication of positive findings leads to publication bias, mechanisms should exist to facilitate the publication of sound, negative genetic association studies.

ALI, acute lung injury.
From Cooper DN, Nussbaum RL, Krawczak M: Proposed guidelines for papers describing DNA polymorphism-disease associations. Hum Genet 2002;110:207–208.

to confirm the expression and repression of many genes (surfactant proteins [SPs], oxidative stress genes, hypoxia-related genes, cell proliferation–related genes, and genes involved in extracellular matrix repair) that are generally believed to be important in the pathophysiology of ALI. This finding is not trivial; it validates the potential reliability of applying microarray technology to in vivo models of ALI. In addition, these investigators were able to elucidate how these genes are expressed (or repressed) in relation to one another (temporal patterns) and found significant changes in genes previously not thought to be involved in the pathophysiology of ALI. Finally, this study also revealed significant changes in several ESTs with nominal homology to known human genes, thus providing the opportunity for discovering novel genes that play a role in ALI.

Another example is the work of Kaminski and colleagues,[30] who examined the gene expression profiles related to bleomycin-induced pulmonary inflammation and fibrosis in mice. A powerful strategy that was employed in these studies was to compare wild-type mice with mice carrying a null mutation for the epithelial-restricted integrin $\beta_6$ subunit ($\beta_6^{-/-}$). $\beta_6^{-/-}$ mice develop inflammation when treated with bleomycin, but they are protected from the fibrosis-inducing effects of bleomycin.[31] This approach revealed the expression of two distinct groups of genes associated with lung inflammation and fibrosis, as well as their temporal expression characteristics. Furthermore, the elucidation of a specific group of genes expressed in wild-type mice exposed to bleomycin, but not in the $\beta_6^{-/-}$ mice that are protected from fibrosis, allows for the potential identification of genes that mediate the fibrotic response of ALI.

Thus far, we have provided examples of microarray approaches in animal models of ALI. Another powerful experimental approach to studying the influence of genetics on ALI is based on the recognition that different strains of mice have variable susceptibility to stimuli that induce ALI. For example, the Leikauf laboratory provided evidence that genetic susceptibility to irritant-induced ALI in mice is inherited in a recessive manner.[32] This same laboratory investigated genetic susceptibility to ozone-induced ALI using a susceptible strain of mice (C57BL/6J) and a resistant strain of mice (A/J).[33,34] These two strains have sharply contrasting survival times when exposed to 10 ppm of ozone. Using quantitative trait locus analyses, these investigators identified a specific genetic region on the murine chromosome 11 with significant linkage to ozone susceptibility (Ali1), as well as a second region on chromosome 11 with a suggestion of linkage (Ali3).

In related experiments, Kleeberger and colleagues identified a quantitative trait locus for ozone susceptibility on murine chromosome 4.[35] This was achieved through linkage analysis of ozone-susceptible mice (C57BL/6J)

and ozone-resistant mice (C3H/HeJ). A potential candidate gene for ozone susceptibility in this locus is the Toll-like receptor 4 (Tlr4) gene, a key gene for innate immunity and host recognition of endotoxin. C3H/HeJ mice contain a polymorphism within the Tlr4 coding region that confers resistance to endotoxin. To test the role of Tlr4 in ozone susceptibility, these investigators exposed C3H/HeJ mice to ozone and compared the phenotype of these mice with that of the C3H/HeOuJ substrain (susceptible to endotoxin) exposed to ozone. These experiments revealed that the C3H/HeOuJ mice were more susceptible to ozone-mediated injury compared with the C3H/HeJ mice. Further, these investigators documented that ozone induced greater expression of lung Tlr4 mRNA levels in the C3H/HeOuJ substrain compared with the C3H/HeJ strain. Although an exact mechanism was not elucidated, these studies provide a strong rationale for investigating Tlr4 as a candidate gene for susceptibility to ozone-mediated ALI and suggest a commonality between susceptibility to ozone and susceptibility to endotoxin.

The final example of linkage analysis in the context of ALI involves susceptibility to hyperoxia. Cho and colleagues[36] searched for candidate genes in hyperoxia-mediated lung injury by comparing a strain of hyperoxia-susceptible mice (C57BL/6J) with a strain of hyperoxia-resistant mice (C3H/HeJ). Linkage analyses revealed a potential quantitative trait locus on murine chromosome 2. Subsequent comparative gene mapping yielded a potential candidate gene classified as nuclear factor (NF), erythroid derived 2, like 2 or Nrf2 (Nrf2/2), which encodes a transcription factor known as NRF2. The biologic plausibility of NRF2 in susceptibility to hyperoxia is evident by the demonstration that NRF2 regulates detoxifying enzymes related to electrophile toxicity, oxidant stress, and carcinogenesis,[37–40] and the demonstration that NRF2-null mice have increased toxicity in the setting of hyperoxia.[41] Consistent with these data, Cho and colleagues found that lung NRF2 mRNA expression was differentially regulated between the two strains of mice when exposed to hyperoxia and that the differential regulation correlated with phenotype.

## CLINICAL STUDIES

One of the first clinical studies attempting to associate a candidate gene with the incidence and outcome of ALI was predicated on the observation that the angiotensin-converting enzyme (ACE) contains a restriction fragment length polymorphism consisting of either the presence (insertion, I) or the absence (deletion, D) of a 287-base pair alu repeat sequence in intron 16 that was critical for regulating increased ACE activity.[42–43]

Because ACE was known to affect pulmonary vascular tone, epithelial cell survival, and fibroblast activation, it was hypothesized that allelic variation of this gene could be associated with the development and outcome of ALI.[44] Marshall and colleagues[44,45] compared caucusian patients with ALI (triggered principally by pneumonia, sepsis, or trauma) to patients with non-ALI respiratory failure, patients undergoing coronary artery bypass grafting, and to 1900 individuals from the general population. These investigators found the DD genotype frequency to be significantly increased in patients with ALI and was associated with increased mortality (54.5%, $P < .02$) as compared with the II (11.1%) and ID (27.9%) alleles.[44,45] This finding appeared independent of the ratio of the arterial partial pressure of oxygen to the fraction of inspired oxygen ($PaO_2/FiO_2$) among all three allelic combinations.

These observations support the concept that genetic factors may play a key role in both the development and the progression of ALI in humans. The goal of such studies is to broaden our mechanistic understanding of the pathobiology of ALI and, in so doing, identify novel therapeutic targets for either prevention or amelioration of ALI. With regard to targeting ACE, it is notable that in preclinical studies, ACE inhibition with enalapril attenuated tumor necrosis factor (TNF)–mediated activation of whole lung NF-κB and AP-1 signaling pathways,[46] which are known to contribute to ALI. These data, in combination with other observations regarding ACE regulation of pulmonary vasoconstriction,[47] epithelial cell viability,[48] and fibroproliferation,[49] provide biologic plausibility (see Box 18.1) that genetic variants of ACE expression may influence outcome in ALI.

Other clinical investigations into candidate ALI genes include evaluating the role of aquaporin (AQP). Aquaporins play an important role in water transport in several tissues including the lung. Various members of this family of proteins have been identified, such as AQP0, AQP1, AQP2, and AQP5. AQP1 is abundantly expressed on apical and basolateral membranes of pulmonary microvascular endothelial cells of the lung and is implicated in the regulation of lung vascular permeability.[50] In animal models of ALI, AQP1 was shown to be substantially increased, and, conversely, null mutations in AQP1 in both mice[51] and rare humans[52] were associated with protection from the development of lung edema fluid. $AQP1^{-/-}$ mice were not protected from acute lung edema formation triggered by an inflammatory stimulus.[53,54]

More recently, as part of their efforts at the HopGene Program in Genomics supported by the NHLBI, the Garcia and Brower laboratories identified two SNPs in the 3′-untranslated region of the *AQP1* gene at positions T525C and G578C (*http://www.hopkins-genomics.org/ali/abstracts/aqp1.html*). In these studies, a higher proportion of the C allele substitutions at both positions (525 and 578) were found in patients with sepsis as compared with controls, with a higher overall incidence of these "at-risk" C alleles found in African Americans. Data derived from these basic science and animal model investigations, in addition to clinical studies, support the concept that AQP1 plays a role in regulating pulmonary vascular permeability and that it is a candidate gene for ALI. Similar efforts to link polymorphisms in selected genes with ALI by this group are summarized on their web site and include identification of additional candidate genes such as migration inhibitory factor (*MIF*), the myosin light chain kinase (*MLCK*), and *CD14*, based on the presence of various polymorphisms among patients with ALI (*http://www.hopkins-genomics.org/ali/ali_snp.html*).

Another focus area for clinical investigation is the interaction between activation of the coagulation cascade and the development and course of ALI. A relationship between coagulation and inflammation has clearly been established.[55-57] In the setting of ALI, investigators showed that fibrin is readily deposited in the alveolar spaces of affected individuals, a phenomenon linked to imbalances between procoagulant and anticoagulant systems of the host that are reflected in both the circulation and alveolar compartment.[58,59] Numerous coagulation factors contain SNPs including fibrinogen, factor VIII, proteins C and S, antithrombin III, and plasminogen activator inhibitor-1 (PAI-1).[60] Although the impact of these SNPs has been investigated in many coagulation-related disorders (e.g., deep venous thromboembolism), few studies have fully determined their effect in ALI. Perhaps the best studied to date is an SNP in the promoter of PAI-1 in which either four or five guanines (G) are present, hence called 4G or 5G alleles. The 5G allele was associated with increased levels of PAI-1, and patients with this allele were at increased risk of shock or death from meningococcemia.[61] Additionally, the 4G allele was associated with increased PAI-1 circulating levels and mortality in trauma victims.[62] Importantly, patients who were homozygous for the 4G allele not only had the highest levels of PAI-1, but also had the highest levels of the proinflammatory cytokines, TNF, and interleukin-1 (IL-1). These findings suggest that SNPs of coagulation-related genes are likely to alter the clinical phenotype of patients and their subsequent development of critical illnesses (e.g., septic shock) that place them at risk for ALI.

Surfactant protein (Sp)–related polymorphisms have also been investigated with regard to genetic susceptibility to ALI. The SPs are categorized as A through D, with at least 19 polymorphisms identified among them.[63] The presence of the polymorphism C1580T results in a change from Thr to Ile within codon 131 of SP-B and has been found to be associated with significant differences among subgroups of patients with ALI.[63] An increased presence of this C allele in patients with ALI secondary to direct alveolar insults (e.g., pneumonia) suggested that this C allele may be a susceptibility factor in the development of ALI.[63] Following up on this report, Quasney and colleagues[64] demonstrated that the 1580 CC genotype was associated with the presence of ALI, septic shock, and the need for mechanical ventilation among 402 adults with community-acquired pneumonia. Although mortality rates did not differ among the genotypes (TT, 6.6%; TC, 4.4%; and CC, 10.2%), the study may not have been fully powered to examine the relationship between the CC genotype and mortality.

Another notable polymorphism has been localized to intron 4 of the SP-B gene, previously associated with neonatal respiratory distress syndrome.[65] Although most (~90%) caucusians carry the wild-type fragment, an increase in either insertion or deletion polymorphisms at intron 4 was observed in neonates with respiratory distress syndrome (29.3%) as compared with controls (16.8%).[66] Gong and colleagues[67] examined the presence of these polymorphisms in adults (n = 72) at risk for developing ALI. These investigators observed an increased odds ratio for developing ALI in women only who carried the variant SP-B gene as compared with women homozygous for the invariant gene, whereas no difference was discovered among men.[67] In addition to these observations, splicing mutations in the SP-C gene in children with chronic lung diseases of unknown origin were also identified, a finding suggesting that these genetic variants could be causally related to interstitial lung diseases.[68] It is likely, given the key physiologic and immunologic role of SPs in modulating lung homeostasis, that genetic factors influencing the expression and function of these proteins will have important phenotypic ramifications for the development and outcome of ALI.

Microarray technology was applied to the study of ALI using a human lung fibroblast model.[69,70] This study was based on the prior observation that pulmonary edema fluid from patients fulfilling criteria for ALI had a direct mitogenic effect on human lung fibroblasts.[69–71] In an attempt to identify other pathways activated in this process, cDNA microarray analyses were performed on human fibroblasts exposed to either ALI-induced pulmonary edema fluid or hydrostatic pulmonary edema fluid. Although several genes involved in inflammation, adhesion, and cell proliferation were initially found to be differentially increased, using strict criteria, six genes were observed to be at least twofold higher in human fibroblasts exposed to ALI-derived edema fluid, as compared with hydrostatic edema fluid stimulated cells.[70] Because many of these appeared to be related to IL-1 expression, IL-1 levels were measured and were noted to be ninefold higher in pulmonary edema fluid from patients with ALI. Furthermore, neutralization of IL-1 (by IL-1 receptor antagonist protein) attenuated not only the mitogenic activity, but also gene expression of

most of these differentially regulated genes, a finding suggesting that alveolar IL-1 activity may be an important modifier of the lung fibroproliferative response of ALI.

Another example of microarray technology application in lung injury involves lung biopsies from patients with interstitial lung disease as compared with controls.[72] Despite both etiologic and temporal heterogeneity among cases, by applying strict mathematical scoring, 164 genes were identified in the differential data set. The finding that many of these overlapped with a cluster of fibrosis-related genes from complementary mouse studies provided biologic plausibility. The metalloprotease martilysin (MMP-7) was among the most highly expressed genes found in the afflicted patients. Because of the numerous processes regulated by this protein, including extracellular matrix degradation, induction of TNF, and soluble Fas ligand expression, these studies identify MMP-7 as a possible target in ameliorating the fibroproliferative response during recovery from ALI.[72]

Proteomics has also been applied to the study of ALI using plasma and bronchoalveolar lavage (BAL) fluid from patients with ALI.[73] Two-dimensional gel electrophoresis (pI, 3 to 10; molecular weight, 10 to 200 kDa) was able to show approximately 300 spots on separation of the BAL fluid, and 158 of these were identified by mass spectroscopy (MALDI-TOF) sequencing. This allowed for comparisons of the BAL fluid and plasma proteome with simultaneous samples obtained from 12 control subjects.[73] It was notable that few proteins were uniquely expressed in the BAL fluid and that many were plasma proteins, findings consistent with the loss of the lung permeability barrier described in ALI. Additional proteins were noted to have undergone identifiable, post-translational modifications, as evidenced by lower-molecular-weight isoforms proposed by the investigators to be consistent with cleavage of proteins.[73] Although preliminarily descriptive, this publication demonstrates the exciting potential for the broad application of proteomic analysis in ALI.

## CONCLUSION

When considered as a whole, the application of these advanced molecular investigative tools is sure to advance the field of ALI research. Through multi-institutional collaboration and support from funding agencies, and with the participation of the biotechnology industry, novel insights are certain to provide the opportunity for predicting the onset of and response to ALI. The ultimate goal of these approaches is to discover novel therapeutic targets and approaches, to improve the outcomes of patients with ALI.

## REFERENCES

1. Villar J: Genetics and the pathogenesis of adult respiratory distress syndrome. Curr Opin Crit Care 2002;8:1–5.
2. Matthay MA, Zimmerman GA, Esmon C, et al: Future research directions in acute lung injury: Summary of a National Heart, Lung and Blood Institute working group. Am J Respir Crit Care Med 2003;167:1027–1035.
3. Steinmetz LM: Maximizing the potential of functional genomics. Nat Rev Genet 2004;3:190–201.
4. Adams MD, Celniker SE, Holt RA: The genome sequence of *Drosophila melanogaster*. Science 2000;287:2185–2195.
5. Parkhill J, Achtman M, James KD: Complete DNA sequence of a serogroup A strain of *Neisseria meningitidis*. Nature 2000;404:502–506.
6. Stover CK, Pham XQ, Erwin AL: Complete genome sequence of *Pseudomonas aeruginosa* PA01, an opportunistic pathogen. Nature 2000;406:959–964.
7. Watanabe TK, Bihoreau MT, McCarthy LC: A radiation hybrid map of the rat genome containing 5,255 markers. Nature 1999;22:27–36.
8. Venter JC, Adams MD, Myers EW: The sequence of the human genome. Science 2001;29:1304–1351.
9. Consortium IHGS: Initial sequencing and analysis of the human genome. Nature 2001;409:860–921.
10. Yu U, Lee SH, Kim YJ, Kim S: Bioinformatics in the post-genome era. J Biochem Mol Biol 2004;37:75–82.
11. Heller MJ: DNA microarray technology: Devices, systems, and applications. Annu Rev Biomed Eng 2002;4:129–153.
12. Weston A, Hood L: Systems biology, proteomics, and the future of health care: Toward predictive, preventative, and personalized medicine. J Proteome Res 2004;3:179–196.
13. Brazma A, Hingamp P, Quackenbush J, et al: Minimum information about a microarray experiment (MIAME): Toward standards for microarray data. Nat Genet 2001;29:365–371.
14. Becker KG: The sharing of cDNA microarray data. Nat Rev Neurosci 2001;2:438–440.
15. Ball CA, Sherlock G, Parkinson H, et al: Standards for microarray data. Science 2003;298:539.
16. Peri S, Navarro JD, Amanchy R, et al: Development of human protein reference database as an initial platform for approaching systems biology in humans. Genome Res 2003;13:2363–2371.
17. Emmert-Buck MR, Bonner RF, Smith PD, et al: Laser capture microdissection. Science 1996;274:998–1001.
18. Lin MT, Albertson TE: Genomic polymorphisms in sepsis. Crit Care Med 2004;32:569–579.
19. Cardon LR, Palmer LJ: Population stratification and spurious allelic association. Lancet 2003;361:598–604.
20. Colhoun HM, McKeigue PM, Smith GD: Problems of reporting genetic associations with complex outcomes. Lancet 2003;361:865–872.
21. Ioannidis JPA, Ntzani EE, Trikalinos TA, Contopoulos-Ioannidis GD: Replication validity of genetic association studies. Nat Genet 2001;29:306–309.
22. Lohmueller KE, Pearce CL, Pike M, et al: Meta-analysis of genetic association studies supports a contribution of common variants to susceptibility to common disease. Nat Genet 2003;33:177–182.
23. Cooper DN, Nussbaum RL, Krawczak M: Proposed guidelines for papers describing DNA polymorphism-disease associations. Hum Genet 2002;110:207–208.
24. Yoneda, K, Chang MM, Chmiel K, et al: Application of high-density DNA microarray to study smoke- and hydrogen peroxide-induced injury and repair in human bronchial epithelial cells. J Am Soc Nephrol 2003;14:S284–289.
25. Birukov KG, Jacobson JR, Flores AA, et al: Magnitude-dependent regulation of pulmonary endothelial cell barrier function by cyclic stretch. Am J Physiol 2003;285:L785–797.
26. Copland IB, Kavanagh BP, Engelberts D, et al: Early changes in lung gene expression due to high tidal volume. Am J Respir Crit Care Med 2003;168:1051–1059.
27. Prince LS, Karp PH, Moninger TO, Welsh MJ: KGF alters gene expression in human airway epithelia: Potential regulation of the inflammatory response. Physiol Genomics 2001;6:81–89.
28. Jacobson JR, Dudek SM, Birukov KG, et al: Cytoskeletal activation and altered gene expression in endothelial barrier regulation by simvastatin. Am J Respir Cell Mol Biol 2003;30:662–670.
29. McDowell SA, Gammon K, Bachurski DJ, et al: Differential gene expression in the initiation and progression of nickel-induced acute lung injury. Am J Respir Cell Mol Biol 2000;23:466–474.
30. Kaminski N, Allard JD, Pittet JF, et al: Global analysis of gene expression in pulmonary fibrosis reveals distinct programs regulating lung inflammation and fibrosis. Proc Natl Acad Sci U S A 2000;97:1778–1783.
31. Munger JS, Huang X, Kawakatsu H, et al: The integrin alpha v beta 6 binds and activates latent TGF beta 1: A mechanism for regulating pulmonary inflammation and fibrosis. Cell 1999;96:319–328.
32. Wesselkamper SC, Prows DR, Biswas P, et al: Genetic susceptibility to irritant-induced acute lung injury in mice. Am J Physiol 2000;279:L575–L582.
33. Prows DR, Shertzer HG, Daly MJ, et al: Genetic analysis of ozone-induced acute lung injury in sensitive and resistant strains of mice. Nat Genet 1997;17:471–474.
34. Prows DR, Daly MJ, Shertzer HG, Leikauf GD: Ozone-induced acute lung injury: Genetic analysis of F2 mice generated from A/J and C57Bl/6J strains. Am J Physiol 1999;277:L372–L380.
35. Kleeberger SR, Reddy S, Zhang LY, Jedlicka AE. Genetic susceptibility to ozone-induced lung hyperpermeability: Role of toll-like receptor 4. Am J Respir Cell Mol Biol 2000;22:620–627.
36. Cho HY, Jedlicka AE, Reddy SPM, et al: Linkage analysis of susceptibility to hyperoxia. Am J Respir Cell Mol Biol 2002;26:42–51.
37. Venugopal R, Jaiswal AK: Nrf1 and Nrf2 positively and c-Fos and Fra1 negatively regulate the human antioxidant response element–mediated expression of NAD(P)H:quinone oxidoreductase1 gene. Proc Natl Acad Sci U S A 1996;93:14960–14965.
38. Venugopal R, Jaiswal AK: Nrf2 and Nrf1 in association with Jun proteins regulate antioxidant response element-mediated expression and coordinated induction of genes encoding detoxifying enzymes. Oncogene 1998;17:3145–3156.
39. Xie T, Belinsky M, Xu Y, Jaiswal AK: ARE- and TRE-mediated regulation of gene expression: Response to xenobiotics and antioxidants. J Biol Chem 1995;270:6894–6900.
40. Jeyapaul J, Jaiswal AK: Nrf2 and c-Jun regulation of antioxidant response element (ARE)–mediated expression and induction of gamma-glutamylcysteine synthetase heavy subunit gene. Biochem Pharmacol 2000;59:1433–1439.
41. Cho HY, Jedlicka AE, Reddy SP, et al: Role of NRF2 in protection against hyperoxic lung injury in mice. Am J Respir Cell Mol Biol 2002;26:175–182.
42. Rigat B, Hubert C, Alhenc-Gelas F, et al: An insertion/deletion polymorphism in the angiotensin I–converting enzyme gene accounting for half the variance of serum enzyme levels. J Clin Invest 1990;86:1343–1346.

43. Tiret L, Rigat B, Visvikis S, et al: Evidence, from combined segregation and linkage analysis, that a variant of the angiotensin I–converting enzyme (ACE) gene controls plasma ACE levels. Am J Hum Genet 1992;51:197–205.

44. Marshall RP, Webb S, Bellingan GJ, et al: Angiotensin converting enzyme insertion/deletion polymorphism is associated with susceptibility and outcome in acute respiratory distress syndrome. Am J Respir Crit Care Med 2002;166:646–650.

45. Marshall RP, Webb S, Hill MR, et al: Genetic polymorphisms associated with susceptibility and outcome in ARDS. Chest 2002;121:68S–69S.

46. Ortiz LA, Champion HC, Lasky JA, et al: Enalapril protects mice from pulmonary hypertension by inhibiting TNF-mediated activation of NF-kappaB and AP-1. Am J Physiol 2002;282:L1209–1221.

47. Kiely DG, Cargill RI, Wheeldon NM, et al: Haemodynamic and endocrine effects of type 1 angiotensin II receptor blockade in patients with hypoxaemic cor pulmonale. Cardiovasc Res 1997;33:201–208.

48. Wang R, Zagariya A, Ibarra-Sunga O, et al: Angiotensin II induces apoptosis in human and rat alveolar epithelial cells. Am J Physiol 1999;276:L885–L889.

49. Marshall RP, Puddicombe A, Cookson WO, Laurent GJ: Adult familial cryptogenic fibrosing alveolitis in the United Kingdom. Thorax 2000;55:143–146.

50. King LS, Nielsen S, Agre P: Aquaporin-1 water channel protein in lung: Ontogeny, steroid-induced expression, and distribution in rat. J Clin Invest 1996;97:2183–2191.

51. Ma T, Fukuda N, Song Y, et al: Lung fluid transport in aquaporin-5 knockout mice. J Clin Invest 2000;105:93–100.

52. King LS, Nielsen S, Agre P, Brown RH: Decreased pulmonary vascular permeability in aquaporin-1-null humans. Proc Natl Acad Sci U S A 2002;99:1059–1063.

53. Song Y, Fukuda N, Bai C, et al: Role of aquaporins in alveolar fluid clearance in neonatal and adult lung, and in oedema formation following acute lung injury: Studies in transgenic aquaporin null mice. J Physiol 2000;525:771–779.

54. Song Y, Ma T, Matthay MA, Verkman AS: Role of aquaporin-4 in airspace-to-capillary water permeability in intact mouse lung measured by a novel gravimetric method. J Gen Physiol 2000;115:17–27.

55. Opal SM: Interactions between coagulation and inflammation. Scand J Infect Dis 2003;35:545–554.

56. Opal SM, Esmon CT: Bench-to-bedside review: Functional relationships between coagulation and the innate immune response and their respective roles in the pathogenesis of sepsis. Crit Care 2003;7:23–38.

57. van der Poll T: Coagulation and inflammation. J Endotoxin Res 2001;7:301–304.

58. Idell S, Peters J, James KK, et al: Local abnormalities of coagulation and fibrinolytic pathways that promote alveolar fibrin deposition in the lungs of baboons with diffuse alveolar damage. J Clin Invest 1989;84:181–193.

59. Seeger W, Hubel J, Klapettek K, et al: Procoagulant activity in bronchoalveolar lavage of severely traumatized patients: Relation to the development of acute respiratory distress. Thromb Res 1991;61:53–64.

60. Russell JA: Genetics of coagulation factors in acute lung injury. Crit Care Med 2003;31:S243–247.

61. Hermans PW, Hibberd ML, Booy R, et al: 4G/5G promoter polymorphism in the plasminogen-activator-inhibitor-1 gene and outcome of meningococcal disease: Meningococcal Research Group. Lancet 1999;354:556–560.

62. Menges T, Hermans PW, Little SG, et al: Plasminogen-activator-inhibitor-1 4G/5G promoter polymorphism and prognosis of severely injured patients. Lancet 2001;357:1096–1097.

63. Lin Z, Pearson C, Chinchilli V, et al: Polymorphisms of human SP-A, SP-B, and SP-D genes: Association of SP-B Thr131Ile with ARDS. Clin Genet 2000;58:181–191.

64. Quasney MW, Dahlmer MK, Kron GK, et al: Association between surfactant protein B + 1580 polymorphism and the risk of respiratory failure in adults with community-acquired pneumonia. Crit Care Med 2004;32:1115–1119.

65. Floros J, Veletza SV, Kotikalapudi P, et al: Dinucleotide repeats in the human surfactant protein-B gene and respiratory-distress syndrome. Biochem J 1995;305:583–590.

66. Veletza SV, Rogan PK, TenHave T, et al: Racial differences in allelic distribution at the human pulmonary surfactant protein B gene locus (SP-B). Exp Lung Res 1996;22:489–494.

67. Gong MN, Wei Z, Xu LL, et al: Polymorphism in the surfactant protein-B gene, gender, and the risk of direct pulmonary injury and ARDS. Chest 2004;125:203–211.

68. Nogee LM, Dunbar AE 3rd, Wert S, et al: Mutations in the surfactant protein C gene associated with interstitial lung disease. Chest 2002;121:20S–21S.

69. Olman MA, White KE, Ware LB, et al: Microarray analysis indicates that pulmonary edema fluid from patients with acute lung injury mediates inflammation, mitogen gene expression, and fibroblast proliferation through bioactive interleukin-1. Chest 2002;121:69S–70S.

70. Olman MA, White KE, Ware LB, et al: Pulmonary edema fluid from patients with early lung injury stimulates fibroblast proliferation through IL-1β–induced IL-6 expression. J Immunol 2004;172:2668–2677.

71. Pugin J, Verghese G, Widmer MC, Matthay MA: The alveolar space is the site of intense inflammatory and profibrotic reactions in the early phase of acute respiratory distress syndrome. Crit Care Med 1999;27:304–312.

72. Sheppard D: Roger S. Mitchell lecture: Uses of expression microarrays in studies of pulmonary fibrosis, asthma, acute lung injury, and emphysema. Chest 2002;121:21S–25S.

73. Bowler RP, Duda B, Chan ED, et al: Proteomic analysis of pulmonary edema fluid and plasma in patients with acute lung injury. Am J Physiol 2004;286:L1095–L1104.

# CHAPTER 19

# Cytokine Release

Jack J. Haitsma, Marcus J. Schultz, and Arthur S. Slutsky

Inflammation and increased endothelial permeability drive the pathogenesis of acute respiratory distress syndrome (ARDS). A characteristic feature of all inflammatory disorders is the excessive recruitment of leukocytes to the site of inflammation. During ARDS, an uncontrolled systemic inflammatory response involves activation of alveolar macrophages and sequestered neutrophils in the lung. Activation of the inflammation results in the release of a large number of messenger proteins, the so-called cytokines. The important role of cytokines in ARDS progression, outcome, and resolution has been observed in many studies, in which prolonged, higher levels of cytokines correlated with poor outcome.[1–4] Mechanical ventilation affects the level of inflammation and cytokine release.[5,6] In patients with ARDS who are ventilated with a lung-protective strategy (low tidal volume; high positive end-expiratory pressure [PEEP]), lower levels of inflammatory mediators were found.[6] These lower levels of inflammatory mediators correlated with lower levels of multiorgan failure and improved patient outcomes.[5]

Activation of cytokines in ARDS is also accompanied by activation of the coagulation pathway and vice versa.[7–9] In this chapter, we discuss how ventilation affects inflammation both in the lung and in other organs.

## NEUTROPHILS AND CYTOKINES

Neutrophils have been recognized as important contributors to the pathogenesis of ARDS. Because of the exaggerated systemic inflammatory response, leukocytes migrate into the pulmonary interstitium, and increased endothelial permeability leads to tissue edema.[10]

The disruption of the epithelial and endothelial barriers in the lungs is associated with a massive increase in epithelial and endothelial permeability, with accumulation of high-molecular-weight proteins. This occurs together with a marked influx of neutrophils, so neutrophils become the predominant leukocytes in the alveolar spaces. In a healthy lung, 90% or more of the air space cells are alveolar macrophages, fewer than 10% are lymphocytes, and only 1% to 2% are neutrophils. In patients with ARDS, this proportion shifts, and up to 90% of air space cells are neutrophils.

Activation and recruitment of neutrophils are accomplished by cytokines, which are low-molecular-weight soluble proteins (generally <30 kDa) that transmit signals between cells. Cytokines are produced by epithelial and mesenchymal cells (and many other cell types as well) and amplify the inflammatory responses in the lung and in other organs. Initial cytokine signals are amplified manyfold by target cells (cascades), such as epithelial cells, fibroblasts, and endothelial cells. Cytokines function in networks in which feedback occurs at many points to coordinate and regulate cytokine and cellular responses.[11] Chemokines are a family of mostly small (7- to 10-kDa), secreted proteins that function in leukocyte trafficking, recruiting, and recirculation and are characteristically basic heparin-binding proteins.

Apoptosis is a process of controlled cellular death whereby the activation of specific death-signaling pathways (receptor-ligand interaction, programmed cell death) leads to deletion of cells from tissue by nearby phagocytes. Apoptosis plays an important role in the immune system and tissue repair after injury. Apoptosis induced by Fas ligand (a proapoptotic molecule) is generally considered to be a noninflammatory process.

However, it has become clear that Fas ligand can actually induce proinflammatory cytokine responses, thus initiating acute inflammatory responses and tissue injury.[12] Neutrophil apoptosis plays an important role in the resolution of inflammation during ARDS and sepsis (Fig. 19.1).[13,14] A decrease in the clearance of apoptotic neutrophils or delayed apoptosis of neutrophils could prolong or exacerbate ARDS.[15–18] Teder and co-workers demonstrated that mice deficient in CD44 failed to clear apoptotic neutrophils, a characteristic that was associated with worsened inflammation and increased mortality.[19] However, CD44 can also increase the synthesis of chemokines such as interleukin-8 (IL-8) by enhanced clearance of the glycosaminoglycan hyaluronan.[20]

## CYTOKINES: INFLAMMATORY MEDIATORS

The observations that mechanical ventilation influences mediator levels and finally patient outcomes are substantiated by an extensive body of experimental data. Tremblay and colleagues demonstrated that injurious ventilation strategies could induce cytokine release.[21] Using an isolated nonperfused rat lung model, these investigators demonstrated that ventilation with high volumes (40 mL/kg body weight) and without PEEP resulted in increased levels of tumor necrosis factor-α (TNF-α), IL-1β, IL-6, macrophage inflammatory protein-2 (MIP-2), interferon-γ (IFN-γ), and IL-10, both in the presence of an inflammatory stimulus (lipopolysaccharide induced) and in a nonstimulated lung.[21] Ventilation in a noninflamed lung with a lower volume (15 mL/kg body weight) without PEEP increased only TNF-α and IL-1β, whereas all the foregoing cytokines (except IL-6 and IFN-γ) increased in the preinflamed lung (Fig. 19.2).[21] Adding a PEEP level of 10 cm $H_2O$ minimized this increase of cytokine release in both lung models.

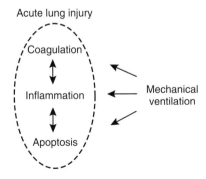

**Figure 19.1** Schematic view of the interdependence between inflammation and both coagulation and apoptosis in acute lung injury, all of which are affected by mechanical ventilation. See text for details.

Both alveolar macrophages[22] and lung epithelial cells[23] have been shown to produce cytokines following injurious ventilation. The observation that ventilation-induced cytokine release is dependent on the level of priming of the inflammatory milieu is corroborated by other studies.[22,24,25] In a similar set of experiments, Ricard and colleagues[24] found that IL-1β was increased fourfold without a prestimulus, whereas in the presence of a lipopolysaccharide (LPS) stimulus, the increase was almost 100-fold. However, these investigators failed to show any effect of ventilation on TNF-α release without a prestimulus. Similarly, Verbrugge and colleagues[25] could not demonstrate any release of TNF-α during different ventilation strategies in vivo in healthy lungs, although IL-6 and MIP-2 seemed to be more sensitive for ventilator-induced cytokine release.[26]

In contrast, numerous investigators have shown that ventilation of an inflamed lung results in cytokine release.[21,22,24,27,28] One of the proposed mechanisms for increased mediator levels found in injuriously ventilated lungs or in the serum of these animals is the loss of compartmentalization.[29–32] The concept of *compartmentalization* states that the inflammatory response remains compartmentalized in the area of the body where it is produced (i.e., in the alveolar space or in the systemic circulation).[29–31] Haitsma and associates[29] demonstrated that compartmentalization of TNF-α (a proinflammatory cytokine) is lost after ventilator-induced lung injury. This loss of compartmentalization is dependent on the amount of active surfactant present at the alveolar-capillary membrane.[30] Preserving the endogenous surfactant system with PEEP further reduces this loss of compartmentalization.[30] Alveolar capillary permeability plays a key role in maintaining compartmentalization.[32] In an isolated lung model, Tutor and colleagues[32] induced alveolar capillary permeability by pretreating the animals with α-naphthylthiourea (ANTU) intraperitoneally. The permeability changes observed after ANTU administration were similar to those observed during ARDS, characterized by an influx of proteins and an increased lung wet/dry ratio. These investigators also observed increases in airway pressures resulting from stiffening of these lungs. The increased alveolar capillary permeability resulted in loss of compartmentalization of TNF-α with leakage to the vascular site.[32] Permeability changes, whether already preexisting (ARDS) or ventilator induced or aggravated, can therefore result in decompartmentalization of an inflammatory response. Thus, mechanical ventilation can lead to increased cytokine release in susceptible lungs.

## ROLE OF VARIOUS CELL TYPES

In ARDS, the intense inflammatory process, with sequential activation of cytokines and chemokines and

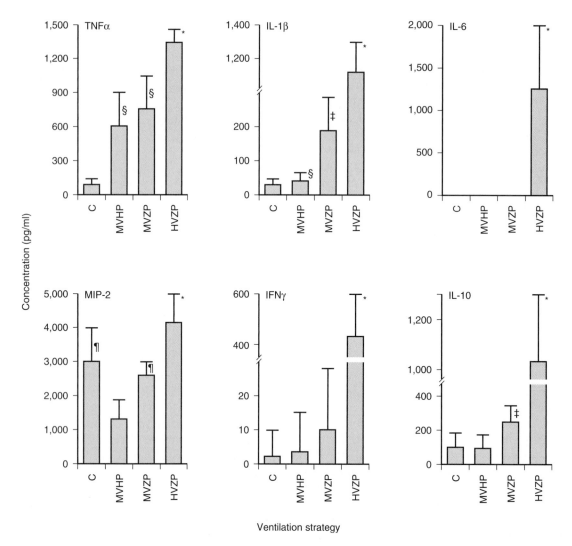

**Figure 19.2** Effect of ventilation strategy on lung lavage cytokine concentrations. Ex vivo rat lungs preinflamed with lipopolysaccharide (LPS) were ventilated for 2 hours with ventilatory strategies thought to be injurious (MVHP, medium-volume high positive end-expiratory pressure [PEEP]; MVZP, medium-volume zero PEEP; and HVZP, high-volume zero PEEP) and resulted in an increase in bronchoalveolar lavage (BAL) cytokines. A similar trend was seen for all cytokines, with the lowest levels in the control group C and the highest levels in the HVZP group. Although animals in the MVHP group exhibited similar end-expiratory distention, they had significantly lower BAL cytokine concentrations than did those in the HVZP group. *$P < 0.05$ vs. C, MVHP, MVZP; $P < .05$ versus C, MVHP; §$P < .05$ versus C; ‡, 0.05 vs. C, MVHP; ¶, 0.05 vs. C. (From Tremblay L, Valenza F, Ribeiro SP, et al: Injurious ventilatory strategies increase cytokines and c-fos m-RNA expression in an isolated rat lung model. J Clin Invest 1997;99:944–952.)

secretion of proteases, alters the inflammatory milieu in the lung and results in activation of several cell types in that organ.[33] Kawano and colleagues[34] demonstrated that rabbits who had their neutrophils depleted by nitrogen mustard had decreased ventilation-induced lung injury (superior oxygenation and less hyaline membrane formation) compared with a group in which the neutrophils were still present.

Alveolar macrophages have been reported to be very susceptible to mechanical stress.[35] Using a plastic lung model, several lung cells (alveolar macrophages, A549;

surrogate type II cells, monocyte-derived macrophages and promonocytic THP-1 cells; both as surrogates for alveolar macrophages) were subjected to cyclic strain resembling mechanical ventilation; the result was release of several key inflammatory mediators, such as TNF-α, IL-8, IL-6, and matrix metalloproteinase-9 (Fig. 19.3).[35]

Other cells such as endothelial cells, bronchial cells, and fibroblast failed to show a response in this model.[35] However, Vlahakis and colleagues[36] did show release of IL-8 in alveolar epithelial cells by stretching the cells for 48 hours. MIP-2 (a rodent homologue of IL-8) was also

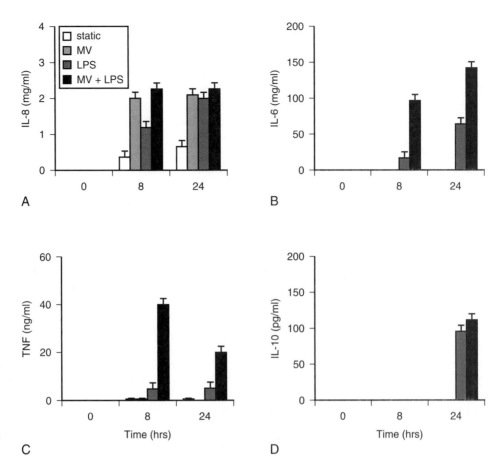

**Figure 19.3** Release of interleukin (IL)-8, IL-6, tumor necrosis factor-α (TNF), and IL-10 by human primary alveolar macrophages submitted to stretch (simulating mechanical ventilation (MV) for 8 and 24 hours in the absence and presence of lipopolysaccharide (LPS). Static control cells are macrophages plated on a similar Silastic membrane but not subjected to mechanical stress. Values are means ± SE. (From Pugin J, Dunn I, Jolliet P, et al: Activation of human macrophages by mechanical ventilation in vitro. Am J Physiol 1998;275:L1040–L1050.)

released by stretch in cultures of fetal rat lung cells, similar to LPS-induced release.[37] Stretch also resulted in apoptosis and necrosis of alveolar type II cells.[38] Two mechanisms of cellular damage were recognizable: necrosis peaked at 12 hours, followed by a peak in apoptosis between 18 and 24 hours suggesting membrane stress failure.[38]

Tschumperlin and associates[39] demonstrated that compressive stress shrinks the lateral intercellular space surrounding bronchial epithelial cells and triggers cellular signaling through autocrine binding of epidermal growth factor family ligands to the epidermal growth factor receptor. This important finding suggests that when the intercellular space is mechanically compressed, the corresponding volume decrease increases the concentration of ligands in this gap, and it also suggests that the increase in receptor signaling activity is primarily the result of the consequent changes in local ligand concentrations.[39]

Tremblay and colleagues[23] demonstrated the role of the pulmonary epithelium in cytokine networking within the lung. Using an ex vivo lung model, these investigators demonstrated both time-dependent and ventilation strategy–dependent release by epithelial cells of TNF-α and IL-6.[23] Especially in lungs allowed to collapse (no PEEP), widespread release of these cytokines was observed.[23] This finding suggests that cytokine release or production in the lung may be the result of the shear forces generated by the inhomogeneity of the lung injury, as observed in patients with ARDS.

## INTRACELLULAR PATHWAYS OF CYTOKINE RELEASE

Mechanical ventilation generates pressures on lung tissue and especially on lung cells. Depending on the extent of the physical forces applied, this stress may lead to activation of pulmonary cells through mechano-transduction[40] or as a result of rupture of membranes and tissue destruction.[41]

Although it is not clear how mechanical forces are converted to biochemical signals, several pathways have been suggested, such as stretch-sensitive channels, mechanoreceptors, deformation of the extracellular matrix-integrin cytoskeleton, and a reduction in intracellular space.[39,40,42] Activation of intracellular pathways has been studied more extensively. For example, stress-activated signaling cascades of the mitogen-activated protein kinase (MAPK)–dependent pathways[40,43,44] and activation of the transcription factor nuclear factor (NF)-κB have been shown to lead to subsequent release of proinflammatory mediators.[35,44–47]

MAPKs are a family of proline-targeted serine-threonine kinases that transduce environmental stimuli to the nucleus. Mammals express at least four distinctly regulated groups of MAPK: extracellular signal-related kinases (ERK)-1/2; c-Jun amino-terminal kinases (JNK1/2/3), also known as stress-activated protein kinases; p38 kinase; and ERK-5.[48] One major function of MAPK is activation of transcription factors such as ETS-like protein-1 (ELK-1), c-Jun, c-Fos, and activating transcription factor-2 (ATF-2), which control a wide variety of genes, many of which are involved in the regulation of inflammation and proliferation (Fig. 19.4). NF-κB is known to be a key transcription factor for maximal expression of many cytokines that are involved in the pathogenesis of lung inflammation.[40,49]

In patients with ARDS, increased activation of NF-κB expressed by alveolar macrophages has been observed,[50] and human macrophages subjected to cyclic changes in pressure have increased activation of NF-κB.[35] Held and co-workers[45] demonstrated that increased activation of NF-κB can be caused either by LPS or mechanical ventilation, and this activation resulted in release of several proinflammatory cytokines (MIP-2, IL-6, and TNF-α). In a follow-up study, Uhlig and colleagues[51] demonstrated that both ventilation and endotoxin promote proinflammatory responses by different pathways that converge at the level of NF-κB and that selective blockade of ventilation-induced mediator-release can be done without affecting the inflammatory response. In both alveolar macrophages and alveolar type II cells, NF-κB was activated by ventilation.[51]

MAPKs are activated by various forms of extracellular stress and may play an important role in the cellular responses to ventilation-induced mediator release. Uhlig and colleagues[44] demonstrated that ventilation of healthy rats with high inspiratory pressures triggered both MAPK and NF-κB pathways, which could contribute to the inflammatory response in the lung. Neutrophil infiltration, another hallmark of ventilator-induced lung injury, is also dependent on the MAPK pathway and more specifically the JNK pathway.[52] This activation of neutrophils also resulted in release of MIP-2.[52] The foregoing data clearly demonstrate that intracellular pathways are activated by ventilator-induced lung injury resulting in the release of cytokines.

## RELATIONSHIP BETWEEN INFLAMMATION AND COAGULOPATHY

A large body of evidence has demonstrated that coagulopathy is an important event in systemic inflammatory conditions such as sepsis.[53] During the initial phase of the inflammatory response, high levels of proinflammatory cytokines, such as TNF-α, IL-1, and IL-6, are released. Proinflammatory cytokines activate coagulation through tissue factor (TF) and attenuate fibrinolysis by stimulating the release of inhibitors of plasminogen activators (Fig. 19.5).[53] In addition, levels of the natural anticoagulants

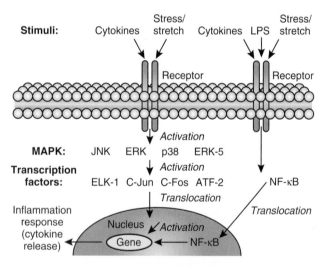

**Figure 19.4** Schematic representation showing how external stimuli (cytokine, stress/stretch, or lipopolysaccharide [LPS]) activate on one or more of the MAPK subfamilies (JNK, ERK, p38, and ERK-5) or the NF-κB pathway. Activation of the MAPK pathway can activate transcription factors (ELK-1, C-Fos, and ATF-2), which are subsequently translocated to the nucleus where they can induce transcription of early response genes. The results are an inflammatory and the production of cytokines. Activation of NF-κB by external stimuli results in translocation of this transcription factor to the nucleus and activation of gene transcription and finally in release of cytokines.

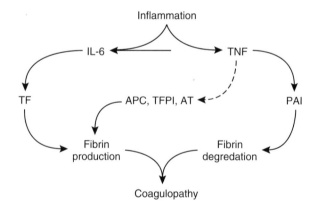

**Figure 19.5** Schematic view of the relation between inflammation and coagulopathy. With inflammation, proinflammatory cytokines are produced. Interleukin-6 (IL-6) activates coagulation, whereas tumor necrosis factor both inactivates natural inhibitors of coagulation and attenuates fibrinolysis. See text for details.

(activated protein C [APC], antithrombin [AT], and tissue factor pathway inhibitor [TFPI]) decline in sepsis because of decreased production and enhanced breakdown.[54] There is extensive cross-talk between inflammatory mediators and coagulation products, causing reciprocal modulation of their response (33). Similar processes are also observed in the lung.

In patients with ARDS or pneumonia, the activation of inflammation results in depressed fibrinolysis in the lung compartment.[55–57] We showed that the depressed alveolar fibrinolysis is in part mediated by mechanical ventilation, especially injurious ventilation,[58] again demonstrating the interaction between mechanical ventilation and inflammatory pathways. The effect of mechanical ventilation on cytokine release and coagulation disorders was also observed in the large multicenter ARDS Network trial.[59] In this study, lower tidal volumes reduced mortality compared with traditional tidal volumes.[59] In the lower–tidal volume arm of the trial, levels of IL-6 after 3 days of ventilation were lower, and the number of days without coagulation failure was significantly higher.[59]

## EFFECT OF INCREASED CYTOKINE LEVELS

Although a cardinal feature of ARDS is hypoxemia, patients who go on to die of ARDS usually do not succumb to severe hypoxemia, but rather die of multiorgan failure.[60,61] Slutsky and Tremblay[62,63] postulated that the ventilatory strategy used to ventilate ARDS patients may, in fact, be a cause of this late multiorgan failure. Data in support of this hypothesis were obtained by Ranieri and co-workers[5] in 2000 in a study in which they linked increased levels of serum inflammatory mediators to organ failure in patients suffering from ARDS. Higher serum levels of inflammatory mediators were observed in patients ventilated with conventional ventilation compared with patients treated with a lung-protective ventilation strategy consisting of higher levels of PEEP and smaller tidal volumes. Patients ventilated with the latter strategy had a decreased inflammatory response and subsequently had a lower incidence of organ failure.[5,6] Lavage fluid from the group ventilated with the conventional strategy led to activation of normal human polymorphonuclear leukocytes, a finding correlating with the inflammatory response seen in these patients.[64]

As discussed earlier, ventilation can induce mediator release, especially in susceptible (e.g., inflamed) lungs. Increased levels of cytokines in the serum were also observed in the ARDS Network trial, in which higher levels of IL-6, IL-8, and IL-10 were observed after 3 days of ventilation in the control arm compared with the reduced–tidal volume arm of the trial.[59,65] Similarly, the number of days without nonpulmonary

organ or system failure (circulatory, coagulation, and renal failure) was significantly higher in the group treated with lower tidal volumes.[59] Elevated plasma levels of soluble TNF receptors are also associated with higher morbidity and mortality in patients with acute lung injury.[66]

To investigate potential mechanisms leading to end-organ dysfunction, Imai and colleagues[67] used a rabbit acid-aspiration lung injury model. These investigators demonstrated that ventilation without PEEP and high tidal volume resulted in increased levels of end-organ epithelial cell apoptosis (injurious ventilation, 10.9%; noninjurious, 1.86%).[67] Renal tubular epithelial cells showed increased apoptosis, linking injurious ventilation with possible organ failure, as observed in many patients with ARDS.[67] This finding is in keeping with studies demonstrating that the kidneys are among the first organs to fail during multiorgan failure.[68] Plasma obtained from the rabbits that underwent the injurious ventilation strategy induced higher levels of apoptosis in cultured renal cells in vitro, a finding suggesting that circulating soluble factors associated with the injurious mechanical ventilation may be involved in this process.[67] Fas:Ig, a fusion protein that blocks soluble Fas ligand (a proapoptotic molecule), attenuated this induction of apoptosis in vitro. In plasma samples from patients included in a previous randomized controlled trial,[5,6] lower levels of soluble Fas ligand were found in the group ventilated with a lung-protective ventilation compared with the conventionally ventilated group.[67] These data link distant organ changes or failure and mechanical ventilation, as discussed in a review on renal failure and ventilation.[69] Gurkan and colleagues[70] showed similar results in mice, in which injurious ventilation resulted in increased levels of IL-6 in the kidney and liver after acid aspiration.

Injurious ventilation strategies, besides inducing an inflammatory response in the lung, down-regulate the peripheral immune response.[71] Vreugdenhil and colleagues[71] observed a decrease in MIP-2 and IL-10 production, splenocyte proliferation, splenic natural killer cell activity, and IFN-γ production during injurious ventilation. These data again demonstrated that, in addition to a local effect on the lung itself, injurious ventilation affects other cells and organs.[71]

Increased levels of inflammatory mediators correlate with the development of ARDS,[72] and high bronchoalveolar lavage levels of these mediators in ARDS lungs have been described in a number of studies.[4,73,74] Furthermore, persistent high levels of inflammatory mediators in the lung over time correlate with poor outcome.[3] Similarly, plasma levels of inflammatory mediators correlate with severity of ARDS and subsequent outcome.[3,75] Headley and co-workers[75] investigated the role of inflammatory plasma cytokines during infections and systemic inflammation and in the subsequent development and progression of ARDS. The final outcome in patients with ARDS correlated with the magnitude and duration of the host inflammatory response in the serum and was independent of the precipitating cause of ARDS or the occurrence of infections.[75] Similar observations were made in patients with multiple trauma in whom high concentrations of cytokines correlated with the development of ARDS and finally multiorgan failure.[76] We demonstrated that an injurious ventilatory strategy can result in loss of a compartmentalized inflammation response and can lead to increased serum levels of inflammatory mediators.[27,29,30] Loss of compartmentalization seems to be part of the inflammatory process, as is also observed in the early stage of community-acquired pneumonia.[77] Injury to alveolar capillary membrane resulting in increased permeability enhances the loss of compartmentalization.[32]

In healthy persons, no effects on plasma levels of mediators were observed during 1 hour of mechanical ventilation; even ventilation with high tidal volumes on PEEP did not result in higher cytokine levels compared with lung-protective ventilatory strategies.[78] A previously inflamed state seems to be important for the development of biotrauma, at least with the magnitude of tidal volumes that can be used in patients with normal lungs.[79] In inflamed lungs (patients with acute lung injury), Stüber and associates[80] switched ventilation strategies from high–tidal volume to lung-protective ventilation. High–tidal volume ventilation increased the release of cytokine in the plasma to baseline, whereas switching to a lung-protective strategy resulted in an immediate reduction in the levels of circulating inflammatory cytokines.[80]

Thus, in ARDS, there is an inflamed lung with increased levels of proinflammatory mediators, and ventilation itself can increase the amount of inflammatory mediators produced by the lung. When the barrier function of the alveolar-capillary membrane is lost because of the underlying disease process or secondary to increased alveolar-capillary permeability, the impact of the ventilatory strategy will result in leakage of mediators into the circulation (decompartmentalization). The subsequently increased levels of these mediators in the circulation correlate with multiorgan failure and, finally, mortality. The use of lung-protective ventilation in both experimental and clinical studies demonstrated a reduction in the inflammatory response, which, in turn, was associated with organ failure and mortality. Although increasing data support this hypothesis, further studies are needed to confirm this paradigm.

## REFERENCES

1. Bauer TT, Monton C, Torres A, et al: Comparison of systemic cytokine levels in patients with acute respiratory distress syndrome, severe pneumonia, and controls. Thorax 2000;55:46–52.
2. Meduri GU: Host defense response and outcome in ARDS. Chest 1997;112:1154–1158.
3. Meduri GU, Kohler G, Headley S, et al: Inflammatory cytokines in the BAL of patients with ARDS: Persistent elevation over time predicts poor outcome. Chest 1995;108:1303–1314.
4. Park WY, Goodman RB, Steinberg KP, et al: Cytokine balance in the lungs of patients with acute respiratory distress syndrome. Am J Respir Crit Care Med 2001;164:1896–1903.
5. Ranieri VM, Giunta F, Suter PM, et al: Mechanical ventilation as a mediator of multisystem organ failure in acute respiratory distress syndrome. JAMA 2000;284:43–44.
6. Ranieri VM, Suter PM, Tortorella C, et al: Effect of mechanical ventilation on inflammatory mediators in patients with acute respiratory distress syndrome: A randomized controlled trial. JAMA 1999;282:54–61.
7. Idell S: Coagulation, fibrinolysis, and fibrin deposition in acute lung injury. Crit Care Med 2003;31:S213–220.
8. Levi M, Schultz MJ, Rijneveld AW, et al: Bronchoalveolar coagulation and fibrinolysis in endotoxemia and pneumonia. Crit Care Med 2003;31:S238–S242.
9. Schultz MJ, Levi M, van der Poll T: Anticoagulant therapy for acute lung injury or pneumonia. Curr Drug Targets 2003;4:315–321.
10. Matthay MA, Zimmerman GA: Acute lung injury and the acute respiratory distress syndrome: Four decades of inquiry into pathogenesis and rational management. Am J Respir Cell Mol Biol 2005;33:319–327.
11. Martin TR: Lung cytokines and ARDS: Roger S. Mitchell Lecture. Chest 1999;116:2S–8S.
12. Park DR, Thomsen AR, Frevert CW, et al: Fas (CD95) induces proinflammatory cytokine responses by human monocytes and monocyte-derived macrophages. J Immunol 2003;170:6209–6216.
13. Cox G, Crossley J, Xing Z: Macrophage engulfment of apoptotic neutrophils contributes to the resolution of acute pulmonary inflammation in vivo. Am J Respir Cell Mol Biol 1995;12:232–237.
14. Hussain N, Wu F, Zhu L, et al: Neutrophil apoptosis during the development and resolution of oleic acid-induced acute lung injury in the rat. Am J Respir Cell Mol Biol 1998;19:867–874.
15. Li X, Shu R, Filippatos G, et al: Apoptosis in lung injury and remodeling. J Appl Physiol 2004;97:1535–1542.
16. Matute-Bello G, Liles WC, Radella F 2nd, et al: Modulation of neutrophil apoptosis by granulocyte colony-stimulating factor and granulocyte/macrophage colony-stimulating factor during the course of acute respiratory distress syndrome. Crit Care Med 2000;28:1–7.
17. Matute-Bello G, Liles WC, Steinberg KP, et al: Soluble Fas ligand induces epithelial cell apoptosis in humans with acute lung injury (ARDS). J Immunol 1999;163:2217–2225.
18. Matute-Bello G, Martin TR: Science review: Apoptosis in acute lung injury. Crit Care 2003;7:355–358.
19. Teder P, Vandivier RW, Jiang D, et al: Resolution of lung inflammation by CD44. Science 2002;296:155–158.
20. McKee CM, Penno MB, Cowman M, et al: Hyaluronan (HA) fragments induce chemokine gene expression in alveolar macrophages: The role of HA size and CD44. J Clin Invest 1996;98:2403–2413.
21. Tremblay L, Valenza F, Ribeiro SP, et al: Injurious ventilatory strategies increase cytokines and c-fos m-RNA expression in an isolated rat lung model. J Clin Invest 1997;99:944–952.
22. Whitehead TC, Zhang H, Mullen B, et al: Effect of mechanical ventilation on cytokine response to intratracheal lipopolysaccharide. Anesthesiology 2004;101:52–58.
23. Tremblay LN, Miatto D, Hamid Q, et al: Injurious ventilation induces widespread pulmonary epithelial expression of tumor necrosis factor-alpha and interleukin-6 messenger RNA. Crit Care Med 2002;30:1693–1700.

24. Ricard JD, Dreyfuss D, Saumon G: Production of inflammatory cytokines in ventilator-induced lung injury: A reappraisal. Am J Respir Crit Care Med 2001;163:1176–1180.

25. Verbrugge SJ, Uhlig S, Neggers SJ, et al: Different ventilation strategies affect lung function but do not increase tumor necrosis factor-alpha and prostacyclin production in lavaged rat lungs in vivo. Anesthesiology 1999;91:1834–1843.

26. Haitsma JJ, Uhlig S, Verbrugge SJ, et al: Injurious ventilation strategies cause systemic release of IL-6 and MIP-2 in rats in vivo. Clin Physiol Funct Imaging 2003;23:349–353.

27. Chiumello D, Pristine G, Slutsky AS: Mechanical ventilation affects local and systemic cytokines in an animal model of acute respiratory distress syndrome. Am J Respir Crit Care Med 1999;160:109–116.

28. van Kaam AH, Lutter R, Lachmann RA, et al: Effect of ventilation strategy and surfactant on inflammation in experimental pneumonia. Eur Respir J 2005;26:112–117.

29. Haitsma JJ, Uhlig S, Goggel R, et al: Ventilator-induced lung injury leads to loss of alveolar and systemic compartmentalization of tumor necrosis factor-alpha. Intensive Care Med 2000;26:1515–1522.

30. Haitsma JJ, Uhlig S, Lachmann U, et al: Exogenous surfactant reduces ventilator-induced decompartmentalization of tumor necrosis factor alpha in absence of positive end-expiratory pressure. Intensive Care Med 2002;28:1131–1137.

31. Nelson S, Bagby GJ, Bainton BG, et al: Compartmentalization of intraalveolar and systemic lipopolysaccharide-induced tumor necrosis factor and the pulmonary inflammatory response. J Infect Dis 1989;159:189–194.

32. Tutor JD, Mason CM, Dobard E, et al: Loss of compartmentalization of alveolar tumor necrosis factor after lung injury. Am J Respir Crit Care Med 1994;149:1107–1111.

33. Pugin J, Verghese G, Widmer MC, et al: The alveolar space is the site of intense inflammatory and profibrotic reactions in the early phase of acute respiratory distress syndrome. Crit Care Med 1999;27:304–312.

34. Kawano T, Mori S, Cybulsky M, et al: Effect of granulocyte depletion in a ventilated surfactant-depleted lung. J Appl Physiol 1987;62:27–33.

35. Pugin J, Dunn I, Jolliet P, et al: Activation of human macrophages by mechanical ventilation in vitro. Am J Physiol 1998;275:L1040–L1050.

36. Vlahakis NE, Schroeder MA, Limper AH, et al: Stretch induces cytokine release by alveolar epithelial cells in vitro. Am J Physiol 1999;277:L167–L173.

37. Mourgeon E, Isowa N, Keshavjee S, et al: Mechanical stretch stimulates macrophage inflammatory protein-2 secretion from fetal rat lung cells. Am J Physiol 2000;279:L699–706.

38. Hammerschmidt S, Kuhn H, Grasenack T, et al: Apoptosis and necrosis induced by cyclic mechanical stretching in alveolar type II cells. Am J Respir Cell Mol Biol 2004;30:396–402.

39. Tschumperlin DJ, Dai G, Maly IV, et al: Mechanotransduction through growth-factor shedding into the extracellular space. Nature 2004;429:83–86.

40. Dos Santos CC, Slutsky AS: Mechanisms of ventilator-induced lung injury: A perspective. J Appl Physiol 2000;89:1645–1655.

41. Uhlig S: Ventilation-induced lung injury and mechanotransduction: Stretching it too far? Am J Physiol 2002;282:L892–L896.

42. Liu M, Tanswell AK, Post M: Mechanical force-induced signal transduction in lung cells. Am J Physiol 1999;277:L667–683.

43. Kyriakis JM, Avruch J: Mammalian mitogen-activated protein kinase signal transduction pathways activated by stress and inflammation. Physiol Rev 2001;81:807–869.

44. Uhlig U, Haitsma JJ, Goldmann T, et al: Ventilation-induced activation of the mitogen-activated protein kinase pathway. Eur Respir J 2002;20:946–956.

45. Held HD, Boettcher S, Hamann L, et al: Ventilation-induced chemokine and cytokine release is associated with activation of nuclear factor-kappa B and is blocked by steroids. Am J Respir Crit Care Med 2001;163:711–716.

46. von Bethmann AN, Brasch F, Muller KM, et al: Prolonged hyperventilation is required for release of tumor necrosis factor alpha but not IL-6. Appl Cardiopulm Pathol 1996;6:171–177.

47. von Bethmann AN, Brasch F, Nusing R, et al: Hyperventilation induces release of cytokines from perfused mouse lung. Am J Respir Crit Care Med 1998;157:263–272.

48. Chang L, Karin M: Mammalian MAP kinase signalling cascades. Nature 2001;410:37–40.

49. Fan J, Ye RD, Malik AB: Transcriptional mechanisms of acute lung injury. Am J Physiol 2001;281:L1037–1050.

50. Schwartz MD, Moore EE, Moore FA, et al: Nuclear factor-kappa B is activated in alveolar macrophages from patients with acute respiratory distress syndrome. Crit Care Med 1996;24:1285–1292.

51. Uhlig U, Fehrenbach H, Lachmann RA, et al: Phosphoinositide 3-OH kinase inhibition prevents ventilation-induced lung cell activation. Am J Respir Crit Care Med 2004;169:201–208.

52. Li LF, Yu L, Quinn DA: Ventilation-induced neutrophil infiltration depends on c-Jun N-terminal kinase. Am J Respir Crit Care Med 2004;169:518–524.

53. Levi M, Ten Cate H: Disseminated intravascular coagulation. N Engl J Med 1999;341:586–592.

54. Fourrier F, Chopin C, Goudemand J, et al: Septic shock, multiple organ failure, and disseminated intravascular coagulation: Compared patterns of antithrombin III, protein C, and protein S deficiencies. Chest 1992;101:816–823.

55. Levi M, van der Poll T, Buller HR: Bidirectional relation between inflammation and coagulation. Circulation 2004;109:2698–2704.

56. Gunther A, Mosavi P, Heinemann S, et al: Alveolar fibrin formation caused by enhanced procoagulant and depressed fibrinolytic capacities in severe pneumonia: Comparison with the acute respiratory distress syndrome. Am J Respir Crit Care Med 2000;161:454–462.

57. Idell S, James KK, Levin EG, et al: Local abnormalities in coagulation and fibrinolytic pathways predispose to alveolar fibrin deposition in the adult respiratory distress syndrome. J Clin Invest 1989;84:695–705.

58. Dahlem P, Bos AP, Haitsma JJ, et al: Alveolar fibrinolytic capacity suppressed by injurious mechanical ventilation. Intensive Care Med 2005;31:724–732.

59. ARDS Network: Ventilation with lower tidal volumes as compared with traditional tidal volumes for acute lung injury and the acute respiratory distress syndrome. N Engl J Med 2000;342:1301–1308.

60. Esteban A, Anzueto A, Frutos F, et al: Characteristics and outcomes in adult patients receiving mechanical ventilation: A 28-day international study. JAMA 2002;287:345–355.

61. Ferring M, Vincent JL: Is outcome from ARDS related to the severity of respiratory failure? Eur Respir J 1997;10:1297–1300.

62. Slutsky AS, Tremblay LN: Multiple system organ failure: Is mechanical ventilation a contributing factor? Am J Respir Crit Care Med 1998;157:1721–1725.

63. Tremblay LN, Slutsky AS: Ventilator-induced injury: From barotrauma to biotrauma. Proc Assoc Am Physicians 1998;110:482–488.

64. Zhang H, Downey GP, Suter PM, et al: Conventional mechanical ventilation is associated with bronchoalveolar lavage-induced activation of polymorphonuclear leukocytes: A possible

mechanism to explain the systemic consequences of ventilator-induced lung injury in patients with ARDS. Anesthesiology 2002;97:1426–1433.

65. Parsons PE, Eisner MD, Thompson BT, et al: Lower tidal volume ventilation and plasma cytokine markers of inflammation in patients with acute lung injury. Crit Care Med 2005;33:1–6; discussion 230–232.

66. Parsons PE, Matthay MA, Ware LB, et al: Elevated plasma levels of soluble TNF receptors are associated with morbidity and mortality in patients with acute lung injury. Am J Physiol 2005;288:L426–L431.

67. Imai Y, Parodo J, Kajikawa O, et al: Injurious mechanical ventilation and end-organ epithelial cell apoptosis and organ dysfunction in an experimental model of acute respiratory distress syndrome. JAMA 2003;289: 2104–2112.

68. Wardle EN: Acute renal failure and multiorgan failure. Nephrol Dial Transplant 1994;4(Suppl):104–107.

69. Kuiper JW, Groeneveld AB, Slutsky AS, et al: Mechanical ventilation and acute renal failure. Crit Care Med 2005;33:1408–1415.

70. Gurkan OU, O'Donnell C, Brower R, et al: Differential effects of mechanical ventilatory strategy on lung injury and systemic organ inflammation in mice. Am J Physiol 2003;285:L710–718.

71. Vreugdenhil HA, Heijnen CJ, Plotz FB, et al: Mechanical ventilation of healthy rats suppresses peripheral immune function. Eur Respir J 2004;23:122–128.

72. Donnelly SC, Strieter RM, Kunkel SL, et al: Interleukin-8 and development of adult respiratory distress syndrome in at-risk patient groups. Lancet 1993;341:643–647.

73. Chollet-Martin S, Montravers P, Gibert C, et al: High levels of interleukin-8 in the blood and alveolar spaces of patients with pneumonia and adult respiratory distress syndrome. Infect Immun 1993;61:4553–4559.

74. Goodman RB, Strieter RM, Martin DP, et al: Inflammatory cytokines in patients with persistence of the acute respiratory distress syndrome. Am J Respir Crit Care Med 1996;154:602–611.

75. Headley AS, Tolley E, Meduri GU: Infections and the inflammatory response in acute respiratory distress syndrome. Chest 1997;111:1306–1321.

76. Roumen RM, Hendriks T, van der Ven-Jongekrijg J, et al: Cytokine patterns in patients after major vascular surgery, hemorrhagic shock, and severe blunt trauma: Relation with subsequent adult respiratory distress syndrome and multiple organ failure. Ann Surg 1993;218:769–776.

77. Dehoux MS, Boutten A, Ostinelli J, et al: Compartmentalized cytokine production within the human lung in unilateral pneumonia. Am J Respir Crit Care Med 1994;150:710–716.

78. Wrigge H, Zinserling J, Stuber F, et al: Effects of mechanical ventilation on release of cytokines into systemic circulation in patients with normal pulmonary function. Anesthesiology 2000;93:1413–1417.

79. Wrigge H, Uhlig U, Baumgarten G, et al: Mechanical ventilation strategies and inflammatory responses to cardiac surgery: A prospective randomized clinical trial. Intensive Care Med 2005;31:1379–1387.

80. Stüber F, Wrigge H, Schroeder S, et al: Kinetic and reversibility of mechanical ventilation-associated pulmonary and systemic inflammatory response in patients with acute lung injury. Intensive Care Med 2002;28:834–841.

# CHAPTER 20

# Lung Imaging in Acute Respiratory Distress Syndrome by Computed Tomography

Klaus Markstaller and Hans-Ulrich Kauczor

In routine clinical practice, respiratory therapy of acute respiratory distress syndrome (ARDS) is individualized according to clinical investigation, inspiratory and expiratory gas concentrations, airway pressures, and the oxygenation index (ratio of arterial oxygen tension to fraction of inspired oxygen [$PaO_2/FiO_2$]). These parameters summarize the effectiveness of the global system of lung ventilation and perfusion. Additional information is provided by assessment of the mixed venous oxygen concentration, cardiac output, dead space ventilation, oxygen carrying capacity, and intrapulmonary shunt fraction. Conventional chest radiography is frequently used for several reasons. First, the chest radiographic findings (i.e., bilateral infiltrates) are part of the definition of ARDS (Fig. 20.1). Second, chest radiography is routinely performed in the intensive care unit (ICU) to provide a regular, often daily documentation of the extent, severity, and distribution of infiltrates and atelectases, as well as complications such as pneumothorax or abscess (Fig. 20.2). Although computed tomography (CT) has much higher sensitivity and specificity for the depiction of regional disorders, it is not used regularly, mainly because it requires transport of the patient from the ICU to the CT suite in the radiology department. Thus, CT is performed if complications are suspected, ICU measurements reveal discrepant findings, and the chest radiograph is inconclusive (Fig. 20.3A). Typical CT findings are manifestations of barotraumas such as pneumothorax, interstitial emphysema, pneumomediastinum, inflammatory complications, pneumonia, abscess, empyema, fistula, and mediastinitis, as well as malpositions of tubes, drains, and catheters (Fig. 20.3B to D).

Ventilator-associated lung injury (VALI) is associated with cyclic recruitment and derecruitment phenomena during intermittent positive pressure ventilation (IPPV).[1,2] The challenge for the ICU physician is to minimize these effects by adapting the optimal respiratory parameters for each individual patient quickly and prospectively.

Experimental and clinical studies investigating new approaches to optimize ventilatory strategies usually

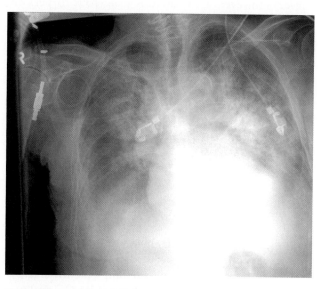

**Figure 20.1** Early exudative acute respiratory distress syndrome in a patient not yet intubated. Evident are bilateral alveolar infiltrates with perihilar preference, pleural effusion, and normal heart size.

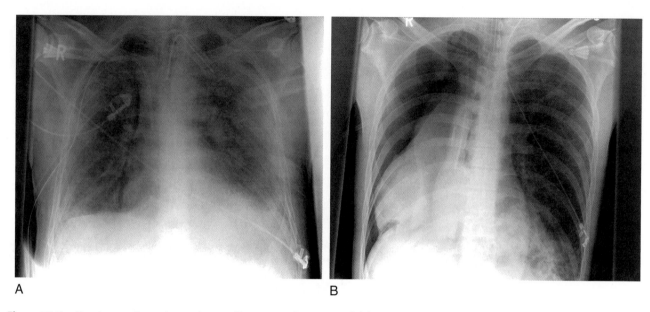

A                                                            B

**Figure 20.2**   Barotrauma in acute respiratory distress syndrome: small (*A*) and extensive (*B*) pneumothorax.

compare different airway pressures, inspiratory-to-expiratory time ratios, flow curves, and tidal volumes. However, other studies have demonstrated the importance of respiratory rate on the dynamic behavior of atelectasis and its cyclic collapse.[3]

Despite the multitude of studies that addressed an optimal positive end-expiratory pressure (PEEP) level, the best way to titrate PEEP is still controversial.[4] Traditionally, PEEP has been derived from the lower inflection point (LIP) of the static pressure-volume (PV) curve.[5] However, a PV curve is dangerous to perform and therefore is rarely applied in clinical practice. CT studies demonstrated that recruitment is not fixed to the LIP, but rather takes place over the whole PV curve.[6] Thus, the relevance of a PV curve for the respiratory therapy continues to be debated.

## LUNG IMAGING BY COMPUTED TOMOGRAPHY

Although ARDS was already described in the late 1960s and the first clinical CT scanners appeared in the mid-1970s, CT imaging was not recommended in ARDS until the mid-1980s. The common belief, based on findings from chest radiography, was that ARDS represented a homogeneous alteration of the lung parenchyma, but this concept was dramatically changed by CT findings. The application of CT revolutionized our knowledge about ARDS. The typical clinical course of ARDS, from the acute onset of respiratory insufficiency to complete

recovery or a fibrotic end stage, is reflected by a typical time course of pathologic stages that correspond to changes in radiologic patterns. To describe the morphologic CT findings accurately, appropriate terminology should be used:

*Ground-glass opacification* describes a hazy increase in lung attenuation with preservation of bronchial and vascular margins. *Consolidation* is consistent with a homogeneous increase in lung attenuation that obscures bronchovascular margins, and positive air bronchograms may be present, whereas *reticular patterns* are defined as innumerable interlacing line shadows that may be fine, intermediate, or coarse. The pathologic stages of ARDS are not sharply separated from each other, and transitions are fluent. Categorizations of the different phases (exudative, proliferative, and fibrotic), however, are parallel to the definitions derived from chest radiography.

In most cases, the very first chest radiograph of a patient with ARDS with acute onset of dyspnea and hypoxemia does not show any abnormalities. There is a time gap of approximately 12 hours between the onset of respiratory failure and the appearance of radiographic abnormalities characteristic of ARDS (Fig. 20.4). Because CT is much more sensitive, it demonstrates subtle ground-glass opacities with a predilection in the middle and perihilar or even peripheral subpleural regions of the lung if imaging is performed in this very early phase. Fluid leakage into the peripheral interstitium is minimal, but occasionally there are signs of interstitial edema, such as septal lines. Over time, the findings become more obvious and convert to patchy and ill-defined opacities. They have a more homogeneous

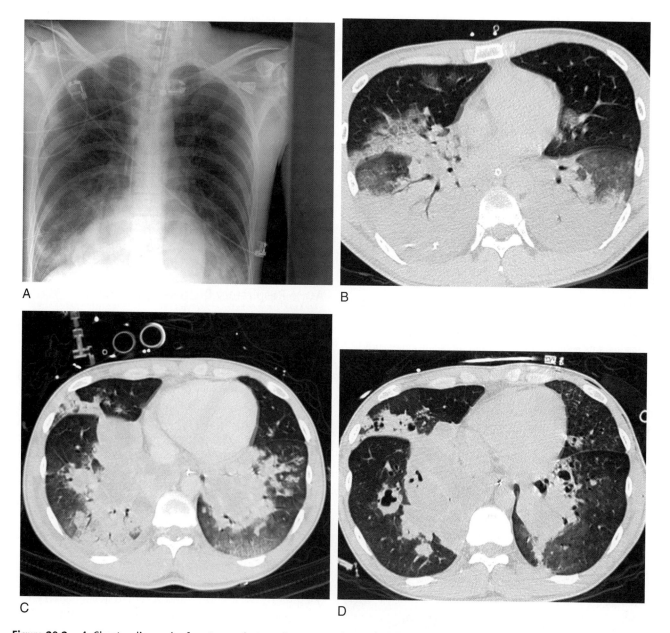

**Figure 20.3** *A,* Chest radiograph of acute respiratory distress syndrome (ARDS) with severe atelectasis in the lower lung fields. *B,* Computed tomography (CT) scan on the same day shows ARDS with severe atelectasis bilaterally with positive pneumobron-chograms. *C,* CT scan 4 days later: no change. *D,* CT scan another 8 days later: atelectasis is almost unchanged, but ventilator-associated lung injury with bilateral interstitial emphysema is evident.

appearance throughout both lungs, combined with broadening of the peribronchovascular interstitial tissue. These findings indicate transition to the exudative stage. The chest radiograph shows more ill-defined hazy opacities, and the vessels remain visible, probably because the disease is inhomogeneous and some lung areas remain aerated. As alveolar leakage and collapse progress, the opacities become denser and more homogeneous. Positive air bronchograms may become a prominent feature. They are helpful in differentiating the increased permeability

edema encountered in ARDS from edema caused by cardiac failure. At CT, ground-glass opacities and consolidations with a patchy, peripheral distribution are the leading patterns (Fig. 20.5). The patchiness of mild or moderate ARDS is much better revealed on CT scans than on plain radiographs. It may reflect the heterogeneous nature of the disease, as well as subsequent differences in local compliance and aeration reflecting the respirator settings. The nondependent lung regions often have a normal or ground-glass appearance, and the

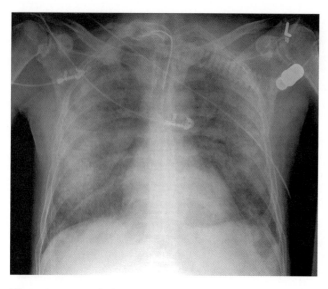

**Figure 20.4** Exudative acute respiratory distress syndrome in an intubated patient. Evident are typical bilateral alveolar infiltrates with a reticulonodular appearance and positive pneumobronchograms resulting from intermittent positive pressure ventilation with high mean airway pressures.

dependent and dorsal lung regions exhibit some consolidations. Thus, an anteroposterior and a cephalocaudal gradient of lung attenuation may be observed. These findings are frequently accompanied by CT-demonstrated pleural effusions. Depending on the severity of ARDS, massive air space consolidations and alveolar infiltrations of both lungs may develop. Later, the consolidations become inhomogeneous and develop a reticular pattern.

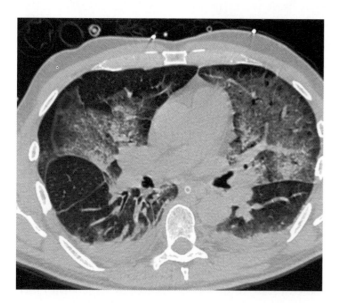

**Figure 20.5** Pulmonary acute respiratory distress syndrome with infiltrates in nondependent lung areas, little atelectasis in dependent lung areas, and small pleural effusions.

The development of persistent patchy spots may correspond to secondary pneumonia, an important hint for recognizing this frequent complication. However, radiologic morphology is often constant without secondary supervening infection.

After a week, the exudative or alveolar phase of ARDS turns into the organizing and proliferative phase. The overall lung density decreases as the consolidations give way to a mixture of ground-glass opacities and parenchymal distortion that later evolve into a coarser reticular, partly bubbly pattern resulting from the development of fibrosis (Fig. 20.6). Cysts may form, ranging from a few millimeters to several centimeters in diameter. These cysts can be subpleural or deep in the parenchyma. Rupture of a cyst can cause pneumothorax or pneumomediastinum.

## Pulmonary Versus Extrapulmonary Acute Respiratory Distress Syndrome

CT imaging can be helpful in identifying the cause of ARDS (i.e., pulmonary or extrapulmonary ARDS). In the early phase, pulmonary and extrapulmonary ARDS cases can be differentiated morphologically. Extrapulmonary ARDS shows a typical, rather symmetric distribution of normally aerated lung parenchyma, ground-glass opacities, and dorsal consolidations, whereas intrapulmonary ARDS has a more asymmetric morphology with a combination of dense consolidations and ground-glass opacities. These results were described in several studies, but most of these studies suffered from a small sample size and from heterogeneous conditions that limit their value.[7–9]

## Impact of Computed Tomography on Current Clinical Practice

Despite the well-known and accepted advantages of CT, its application in patients with ARDS is still not routine. Obstacles to this technique are the potential risks associated with the transport of a critically ill patient to the radiology facility, cost calculations, and radiation dose. In some centers with a modern infrastructure, CT is part of the routine clinical protocol. There are even dedicated, mobile CT scanners available in some centers with a high caseload of patients with ARDS. In general, the application of CT imaging in ARDS is rising, and CT is more frequently used in patients from the ICU. The indication for CT imaging of an ICU patient is the clinical dilemma of a deteriorating case of ARDS or one that is not improving. Obviously, in such a devastating state, the whole procedure, including transport, change of ventilation regimen, apnea phase, and contrast media administration, poses an imminent challenge. Thus, some controversy still exists regarding the optimal clinical indications for CT in patients with ARDS.[10,11]

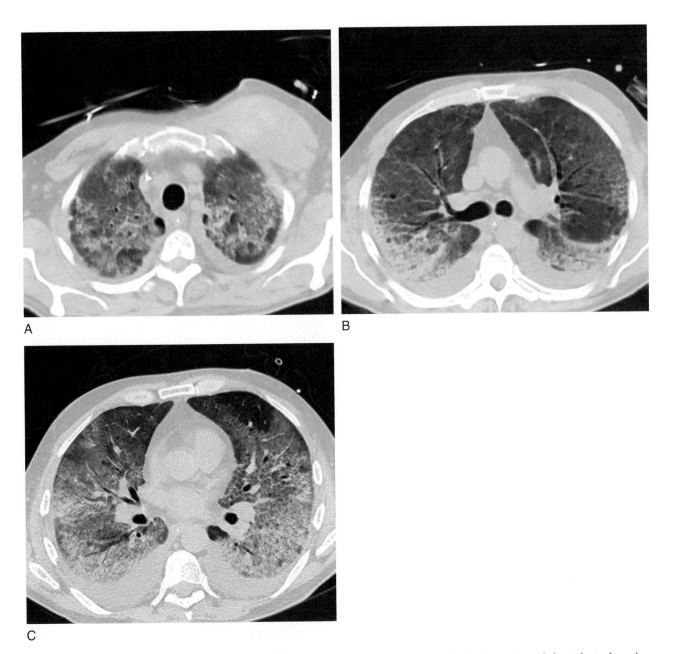

**Figure 20.6** *A* to *C*, Proliferative acute respiratory distress syndrome with a patchy and reticular pattern. Little atelectasis and small pleural effusions are noted bilaterally. The clearly visible and broad peripheral airways are the result of intermittent positive pressure ventilation with high mean airway pressures.

With regard to the difficulties in image interpretation, CT scanning of patients with respiratory failure right at the onset of the disease (i.e., right before admission to the ICU) significantly enhances the diagnostic and therapeutic impact of this technique. It also facilitates the interpretation of repeated CT scans during the clinical course because the development of ARDS, complications, and preexisting disorders as well as the evaluation of treatment effects (e.g., ventilatory parameters during IPPV) can be much better assessed.

The most frequent ventilator-related complications are barotrauma and volutrauma with overdistention of the lung, pneumothorax, and pneumomediastinum. Sometimes, these findings are very subtle and difficult to depict by chest radiography. CT is very helpful in this phase, because atelectasis and complications can be detected much more easily and with greater confidence.

The main problem in the radiologic classification of patients with ARDS is the heterogeneity of the disease. Thus, the effects of individual measures are very difficult to ascertain for both radiologists and ICU physicians. The best results can be expected only after careful selection and characterization of subgroups.

Gattinoni and colleagues[12] recently demonstrated that the potential to recruit the lung can be assessed in the clinical scenario by CT, and patients with ARDS can be divided into recruiters and nonrecruiters. These investigators showed that a higher amount of recruitable lung correlated with poorer gas exchange and lung compliance, as well as significantly lower survival rates.[12] This study was the first to show the potential of CT imaging to predict the outcome in ARDS in the clinical setting.

## Long-Term Findings

In many survivors of ARDS, reticular or cystic patterns prevail. There seems to be a relationship between artificial respiration and fibrosis, air cysts, and bronchiectasis. Because cyclic recruitment and collapse, as well as overdistention of lung regions, are responsible for lung damage, these areas are prone to the development of fibrosis or air cysts. The most dependent (posterior) lung areas, usually not recruitable by IPPV, and not exposed to cyclic recruitment or derecruitment and toxic $FiO_2$ levels, do not tend to develop fibrosis later. The nondependent anterior areas (i.e., areas of the lung that are cyclically recruited or overdistended) show fibrosis significantly more frequently and in a more pronounced manner.[13] The severity of morphologic alterations is associated with higher inspiratory peak pressures (>30 mm Hg), longer exposure to higher oxygen

concentrations ($FiO_2 > 0.7$),[13] and the longer duration of mechanical ventilation.[14]

## Routine Clinical Protocols

There are no general standard CT scan protocols for patients with ARDS. A contrast-enhanced spiral CT with contiguous 5-mm slices is helpful to obtain a global overview. For the minute evaluation of the lung parenchyma, a classic high-resolution CT (HRCT) scan with a 1-mm slice thickness at a 10-mm interval is recommended. With multidetector CT (MDCT) now more widely available, volume scanning at high resolution is becoming a reality. Thus, the advantages of spiral CT and HRCT can be combined within a single scan using several reconstruction algorithms. This means that contrast-enhanced slices that are less than 3 mm thick and that are reconstructed from a 1-mm collimation acquisition with a lung kernel are appropriate. Obviously, thoracic motion resulting from the patient's breathing is associated with severe degradation of image quality that hampers image interpretation. It is mandatory to acquire the CT scans during a breath-hold. For adequate image interpretation, the applied positive airway pressure has to be taken into account (Fig. 20.7). Accurate assessment of recruitment, atelectasis, alveolar collapse, consolidation, and risk of barotrauma is feasible only when airway pressures are known. If particular breathing maneuvers are performed directly before or during CT scanning, functional evaluation will be achievable (see later).

Porcine Lavage-ARDS/PCV, I:E = 1:1, RR = 10/min, $FiO_2$ = 1.0

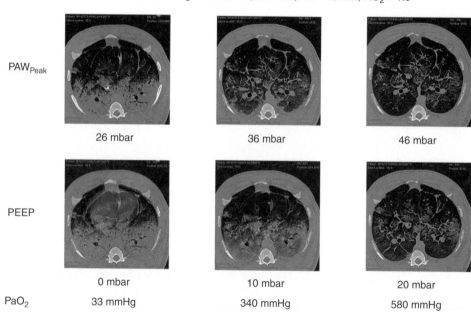

| | | | |
|---|---|---|---|
| PAW$_{Peak}$ | 26 mbar | 36 mbar | 46 mbar |
| PEEP | 0 mbar | 10 mbar | 20 mbar |
| PaO$_2$ | 33 mmHg | 340 mmHg | 580 mmHg |

**Figure 20.7** The effect of increasing airway pressures on the recruitment of atelectasis in porcine lavage acute respiratory distress syndrome.

## Quantitative Image Analysis in Computed Tomography

Four different influences contribute to radiation absorption in CT (at functional residual capacity): air (~60%), blood (~15%), water (interstitial, alveolar, and intracellular, ~20%), and solid tissue (~5%).[15] A lung acinus comprises approximately 2000 alveoli at a volume of approximately 16 to 22 mm³. The volume of a CT voxel is defined by the slice thickness and the CT matrix, such as 0.56 mm³ with the following imaging parameters for CT: 1-mm slice thickness, matrix 512 × 512, voxel dimensions of 0.75 × 0.75 × 1 mm, summarizing over approximately 50 alveoli. Whereas the CT voxel does not change in size and position during ventilation, the lung acinus does.[16] In addition, the content of air, edema, vessels, septa, collapsed alveoli, and aerated alveoli of the imaged lung voxel will vary during the respiratory cycle.

Obviously, CT does not attain the spatial resolution to image individual alveoli. Thus, changes in lung density at inspiration versus expiration do not necessarily represent real alveolar collapse and recruitment. The dominating mechanism, which is responsible for VALI and also for the beneficial effect of lung protective ventilation, is debated because evidence indicated that high-density areas in CT may reflect water flooded alveoli next to aerated alveoli.[17] Obviously, this theory also puts the contributing factors for VALI into a new light. Further studies are needed to prove whether CT shows atelectatic collapse and recruitment, which may be the dominating pathomechanism of VALI. Nevertheless, quantitative CT is worth pursuing to monitor response to different ventilator settings. Different density parameters for quantitative CT studies have been developed and presented over the past few years.

### Mean Lung Density

Mean lung density (MLD) represents a single-number descriptor summarizing all pixels of a transversal lung slice or a predefined region of interest (ROI). It is implemented in nearly every image postprocessing software. However, this parameter does not distinguish among air, water, or tissue within the observed lung structure.[16] The contribution of these factors to MLD can be estimated only by a density histogram of the analyzed ROI.[18,19]

### Air-Tissue Content

Because air has a density of −1000 HU in CT, any density value less than 0 HU allows the determination of its specific air fraction. Thus, a density of −600 HU in a pixel reflects 60% air in that pixel. As the exact dimensions of a voxel are known, the total amount of air in milliliters can be calculated easily.[10] This parameter offers a very comprehensible number (i.e., milliliters of air). Compared with MLD, the calculated amount of air will vary during respiration (because the transversal lung slice [i.e., the pixel number] will vary), even if the MLD remains unchanged. However, the limitations of a single-number descriptor still apply: comparable to MLD, this parameter is not able to distinguish the amount of atelectatic lung, poorly aerated lung, overinflated lung, or airways within a lung slice or an ROI. This discrimination can be reached only with a density histogram of the observed ROI, which is cumbersome for a large number of CT images.

### Functional Lung Compartments by Hounsfield Unit Ranges

Predefined density ranges are specifically assigned to different functional lung compartments (e.g., atelectasis or ventilated or overinflated lung). Several specific density ranges were related to these functional lung compartments by different authors and in different species, disorders, and imaging parameters.[20–22] Dedicated software tools are available, which planimetrically calculate the respective lung area (in square centimeters) of each of these density ranges. To allow for interindividual comparison of the data, the respective lung area of a density range is usually given as a fraction of the total lung area.[23,24]

These density parameters for quantitative image analysis require an automatic lung segmentation tool to postprocess a high number of images.[25] Software tools have been developed that use expert anatomic knowledge to detect the lung accurately and subsequently calculate any kind of density measurements in this area (Fig. 20.8).

### Dynamic Lung Imaging

Clearly, imaging of the lungs by standard HRCT, spiral CT, or multislice CT during breath-hold maneuvers does not reflect the dynamic behavior of lung ventilation and perfusion during the respiratory cycle. Pulmonary ventilation is determined regionally by local resistance and compliance. At the same time, lung perfusion is influenced by gravity, airway pressures, and atelectasis. The following newer imaging techniques address lung ventilation and perfusion with high temporal and regional resolution for regional ventilation-perfusion analysis: (1) dynamic CT (dCT), which offers high temporal and spatial resolution and allows for visualization of the effect of artificial ventilation on different functional lung compartments as atelectasis, ventilated lung area, and overinflated lung area;[19,23] and (2) electrical impedance tomography, which is a bedside technique capable of visualizing differences in lung aeration during artificial ventilation.[26]

Impaired gas exchange in ARDS is caused by insufficient gas exchange area in the lung, either as a result of inadequate ventilation or because of maldistribution of pulmonary

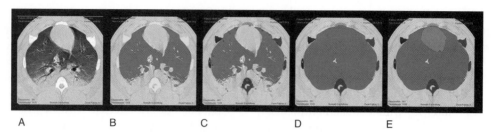

**Figure 20.8** Illustration of an automatic segmentation tool in a porcine lavage acute respiratory distress syndrome (ARDS) image. *A,* Computed tomography image of porcine lavage ARDS with high amount of atelectasis in the dependent parts of the lungs. *B,* Detection of bones (density based on morphologic opening and closing algorithms). *C,* Anatomic classification of bones by means of implemented expert anatomic knowledge (color-coded depiction of the sternum, the left and right ribs, and the spinal column). *D,* Segmentation of lung parenchyma using an interpolation curve. *E,* Detection of the heart using morphologic opening and closing algorithms and subtraction of the heart area from the pulmonary area.

perfusion (ventilation-perfusion mismatch). Some studies showed a close correlation among the volume of lung tissue as measured by CT, impairment of $Pao_2$, and increase in pulmonary artery pressure.[27] Redistribution of pulmonary blood flow toward the upper lobes and uneven distribution of pulmonary edema have been considered possible causes for the more pronounced excess lung tissue in the upper lobes observed at expiratory CT when compared with healthy subjects.[10] Determination of pulmonary blood flow by electrocardiographically triggered CT is highly dependent on the normalization factors applied in the postprocessing algorithm.[28] Another reason for this finding may be a selection bias with different ARDS morphologies (lobar attenuations, diffuse attenuations, patchy attenuations).

## Functional Lung Imaging by Dynamic Computed Tomography

dCT was originally developed for cardiac perfusion imaging. More recently, this imaging modality has been applied to visualize recruitment and derecruitment processes in acute lung injury. dCT uses a continuous rotation of the x-ray tube at a fixed table position. Thus, it is limited to a single slice (two-dimensional over time). Minimal slice thickness and a high-resolution reconstruction algorithm (e.g., a matrix of $512 \times 512$) yield maximal spatial resolution. Modern CT scanners reach a complete rotation of the x-ray tube in less than 500 milliseconds, and raw data acquired within a 270-degree rotation of the x-ray tube are already sufficient to reconstruct an image. Once the raw data of a 270-degree scan have been acquired, additional raw data of only 50 degrees of the x-ray tube rotation are used to reconstruct a subsequent image (sliding-window reconstruction technique). This algorithm allows a temporal increment of 100 milliseconds in dCT image series. Respiratory motion can now be visualized over several respiratory cycles.

The total scan duration is limited by the random access memory capacity of the scanner for raw data storage and the performance of the x-ray tube. Obviously, the scan duration should be as short as possible, to minimize radiation exposure.

Several experimental studies have been presented, with the aim of quantifying lung aeration and recruitment during dCT imaging. The following sections give an overview of this research area.

### Image-Based Analysis of Pulmonary Shunt Fraction

Studies using the multiple inert gas elimination technique (MIGET) suggested that the total amount of atelectasis should be the major contributing factor to oxygenation impairment resulting from the intrapulmonary shunt fraction in ARDS. Studies using CT imaging tried to correlate the intrapulmonary shunt fraction with the image-derived amount of atelectasis. However, these studies reported controversial results.

Whereas the atelectatic lung area correlated positively with the calculated shunt fraction by the MIGET during expiratory breath-hold,[29,30] other authors showed a correlation at inspiratory, but not expiratory, breath-holds.[19] Obviously, a breath-hold does not reflect the pathologic or physiologic situation during IPPV. dCT offers temporal resolution high enough to follow the respiratory cycle during uninterrupted IPPV. Using this novel technique, a positive correlation of the mean atelectatic lung area during IPPV and the calculated shunt fraction measured by arterial and mixed-venous blood gases has been shown (Fig. 20.9).[24,31]

### Assessment of Alveolar Recruitment

Studies on lung recruitment performed with CT imaging showed that recruitment takes place over the whole inspiration process (i.e., independent of the lower infection point and upper inflection point as determined by the static PV curve).[6,32] In an experimental animal model of lavaged

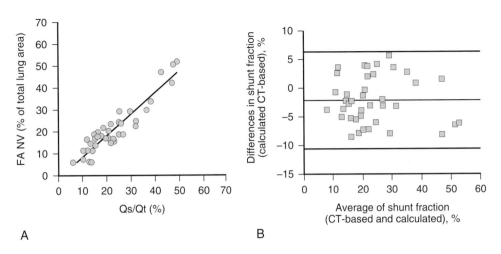

**Figure 20.9** Linear correlation (*A*) and Bland Altman analysis (*B*) of mean nonventilated lung area shunt fraction determined by blood gas analyses in porcine subjects. (From David M, Karmrodt J, Bletz C, et al: Analysis of atelectasis, ventilated, and hyperinflated lung during mechanical ventilation by dynamic CT. Chest 2005;128:3757–3770.)

lungs, higher PEEP levels, as suggested by the LIP, were shown to prevent end-expiratory lung collapse.[31]

## Calculation of Pulmonary Time Constants

Time constants (Tc) are usually measured by spirometry and allow the adaption of inspiration: expiration time and the respiratory rate in artificial ventilation. Functional lung imaging by dCT offers the possibility to determine Tc of recruitment processes even on a regional basis. This would be of interest in a diseased lung with an inhomogeneous distribution of ventilation. In some studies, regional Tc of lung aeration derived from dCT imaging have been assessed using MLD or predefined density ranges in healthy lungs and in different ARDS animal models.[19,23]

This imaging technique also has been applied in anesthetized volunteers[33] and in patients with ARDS.[34] Compared with conventional lung function, discrimination of different Tc and localization of the respective functional compartments, which respond differently to changes in airway pressure, are feasible. No prospective trial has been performed up to now, hence no data are available to judge the importance of this technique for optimizing respiratory therapy.

## Four-Dimensional Computed Tomography

Newer volumetric CT scanners offer dynamic imaging of the lung in three dimensions. Thus, it is a three-dimensional over time (four-dimensional) acquisition. Whether a representative ARDS lung section exists to describe the disease process in the whole organ is also debated.[4,35-39] In experimental ARDS, investigators have shown that quantitative image analysis in a supradiaphragmatic slice gives a reliable estimate of whole lung ventilation.[40]

However, there is no doubt that real four-dimensional acquisition should be used when it is available. Because ARDS is not a homogeneous disease, it is important to analyze the functional characteristics of the residual ventilated and perfused "baby" lung as well as to assess the atelectatic regions for complications or features that differentiate pulmonary from extrapulmonary ARDS. Easley and colleagues[41] compared different animal models of acute lung injury by MDCT imaging, gated to the respiratory cycle. These investigators found substantial differences in lung volumes and blood flow distribution with this imaging technique and related their findings to varying activation of hypoxic pulmonary vasoconstriction.[41]

Four-dimensional CT can be done by either prospective or retrospective gating. Image quality in gated images is comparable to imaging during breath-hold.[42] Thus, high-quality imaging is possible even during uninterrupted respiration. Different devices can be used as a trigger, such as a pneumatic belt, a charge-coupled device (CCD) camera, or an input from the ventilator. A recent study showed the superiority of respiratory gating by a CCD camera compared with a laser sensor.[43]

## Limitations of Dynamic Computed Tomography

One limitation of dCT is the relatively high radiation exposure, which has been estimated to approximately 50 mGy for a 10-second single-slice dCT scan in humans.[37] Furthermore, transport of ICU patients to the CT scanner is demanding in sophisticated transport ventilators, requires continuous invasive monitoring and labor, and greatly increases the costs of therapy.

Studies aiming at functional CT analysis for visualization of respiratory settings were often limited to a single slice approximately 1 cm above the diaphragm that covered a large cross-sectional lung area. Sometimes, three slices at different positions were examined. Although these slices were thought to be representative, the inhomogeneous distribution of ventilation in the diseased lung has to be taken into consideration.[35] The main advantage of this technique is the limited radiation exposure compared with protocols scanning the whole lung volume. Low-dose CT offers another possibility for reducing radiation exposure during functional CT analyses.

Developments related to the introduction of MDCT will improve spatial resolution and will minimize acquisition time but increase radiation exposure. Dedicated MDCT low-dose protocols have already been developed and tested in animal experiments. Although subjective image quality was rated inferior for low-dose as compared with standard-dose scans because pixel noise was doubled, exact information about extent, localization, and distribution of lung opacities was equally well provided by low-dose MDCT.[36] Thus, low-dose protocols offer a reasonable opportunity to reduce radiation exposure significantly for ICU patients.

## CONCLUSION

CT plays an indispensable role in the imaging approach to structure and function of the lung in ARDS. ARDS is characterized by a marked increase in lung tissue and a massive loss of aeration. In the beginning of the disease, alveolar and interstitial edema corresponds to ground-glass opacities. During the later course of ARDS, widespread consolidations (atelectasis) develop. Proliferation leads to fibrotic changes, which also represent the final, healed state.

CT also has an impact on the optimization of the ventilatory parameters. Lung imaging by CT allows for accurate assessment of the volumes of gas and lung tissue and functional lung compartments (e.g., atelectasis and overdistended lung). However, quantitative analysis requires dedicated postprocessing of the CT images (i.e., delineation of lung parenchyma and calculation of overdistended, normally aerated, poorly aerated, and nonaerated lung regions). dCT provides visualization of recruitment and collapse during the respiratory cycle as well as the basis for the calculation of regional lung function, such as lung compliance, shunt fraction, or Tc. CT can support the selection of optimal airway pressures such as plateau pressure and PEEP. Whereas conventional breath-hold CT already has been proven to serve as a predictor of survival by differentiation of recruiters and nonrecruiters, dCT algorithms have to be tested in prospective trials in the near future.

## REFERENCES

1. American Thoracic Society, European Society of Intensive Care Medicine, Société de Réanimation Langue Française. International consensus conferences in intensive care medicine: Ventilator-associated lung injury in ARDS. Intensive Care Med 1999;25:1444–1452.
2. Acute Respiratory Distress Syndrome Network: Ventilation with lower tidal volumes as compared with traditional tidal volumes for acute lung injury and the acute respiratory distress syndrome. N Engl J Med 2000;342:1301–1308.
3. Baumgardner JE, Markstaller K, Pfeiffer B, et al: Effects of respiratory rate, plateau pressure, and positive end-expiratory pressure on $PaO_2$ oscillations after saline lavage. Am J Respir Crit Care Med 2002;166:1556–1562.
4. Brunet F, Jeanbourquin D, Monchi M, et al: Should mechanical ventilation be optimized to blood gases, lung mechanics, or thoracic CT scan? Am J Respir Crit Care Med 1995;152:524–530.
5. Amato MB, Barbas CS, Medeiros DM, et al: Effect of a protective-ventilation strategy on mortality in the acute respiratory distress syndrome. N Engl J Med 1998;338:347–354.
6. Pelosi P, Goldner M, McKibben A, et al: Recruitment and derecruitment during acute respiratory failure: An experimental study. Am J Respir Crit Care Med 2001;164:122–130.
7. Winer-Muram H, Steiner R, Gurney J, et al: Ventilator-associated pneumonia in patients with adult respiratory distress syndrome: CT evaluation. Radiology 1998;208:193–199.
8. Goodman L, Fumagalli R, Tagliabue P, et al: Adult respiratory distress syndrome due to pulmonary and extrapulmonary causes: CT, clinical, and functional correlation. Radiology 1999;213:545–552.
9. Desai S, Wells A, Rubens M, et al: Acute respiratory distress syndrome: CT abnormalities at long-term follow up. Radiology 1999;210:29–35.
10. Puybasset L, Cluzel P, Gusman P, et al: Regional distribution of gas and tissue in acute respiratory distress syndrome. I. Consequences for lung morphology: CT Scan ARDS Study Group. Intensive Care Med 2000;26:857–869.
11. Desai S, Wells A, Suntharalingam G, et al: Acute respiratory distress syndrome caused by pulmonary and extrapulmonary injury: A comparative CT study. Radiology 2001;218:689–693.
12. Gattinoni L, Caironi P, Cressoni M, et al: Lung recruitment in patients with the acute respiratory distress syndrome. N Engl J Med 2006;354:1775–1786.
13. Nobauer-Huhmann I, Eibenberger K, Schaefer-Prokop C, et al: Changes in lung parenchyma after acute respiratory distress syndrome (ARDS): Assessment with high-resolution computed tomography. Eur Radiol 2001;11:2436–2443.
14. Treggiari M, Romand J, Martin J, Suter P: Air cysts and bronchiectasis prevail in nondependent areas in severe acute respiratory distress syndrome: A computed tomographic study of ventilator-associated changes. Crit Care Med 2002;30:1747–1752.
15. Benumof J: Anesthesia for Thoracic Surgery. Philadelphia: WB Saunders, 1995, p 29.
16. Gattinoni L, Caironi P, Pelosi P, Goodman LR: What has computed tomography taught us about the acute respiratory distress syndrome? Am J Respir Crit Care Med 2001;164:1701–1711.
17. Hubmayr RD: Perspective on lung injury and recruitment: A skeptical look at the opening and collapse story. Am J Respir Crit Care Med 2002;165:1647–1653.
18. Neumann P, Berglund JE, Mondejar EF, et al: Effect of different pressure levels on the dynamics of lung collapse and recruitment in oleic-acid–induced lung injury. Am J Respir Crit Care Med 1998;158:1636–1643.
19. Neumann P, Berglund JE, Mondejar EF, et al: Dynamics of lung collapse and recruitment during prolonged breathing in porcine lung injury. J Appl Physiol 1998;85:1533–1543.

20. Dambrosio M, Roupie E, Mollet JJ, et al: Effects of positive end-expiratory pressure and different tidal volumes on alveolar recruitment and hyperinflation. Anesthesiology 1997;87:495–503.

21. Markstaller K, Kauczor HU, Eberle B, et al: [Multi-rotation CT during continuous ventilation: Comparison of different density areas in healthy lungs and in the ARDS lavage model]. Rofo 1999;170:575–580.

22. Vieira SR, Puybasset L, Richecoeur J, et al: A lung computed tomographic assessment of positive end-expiratory pressure-induced lung overdistension. Am J Respir Crit Care Med 1998;158:1571–1577.

23. Markstaller K, Eberle B, Kauczor HU, et al: Temporal dynamics of lung aeration determined by dynamic CT in a porcine model of ARDS. Br J Anaesth 2001;87:459–468.

24. Markstaller K, Kauczor HU, Weiler N, et al: Lung density distribution in dynamic CT correlates with oxygenation in ventilated pigs with lavage ARDS. Br J Anaesth 2003;91:699–708.

25. Markstaller K, Arnold M, Dobrich M, et al: [A software tool for automatic image-based ventilation analysis using dynamic chest CT-scanning in healthy and in ARDS lungs]. Rofo 2001;173:830–835.

26. Frerichs I: Electrical impedance tomography (EIT) in applications related to lung and ventilation: A review of experimental and clinical activities. Physiol Meas 2000;21:R1–R21.

27. Gattinoni L, Pesenti A, Bombino M, et al: Relationships between lung computed tomographic density, gas exchange, and PEEP in acute respiratory failure. Anesthesiology 1988;69:824–832.

28. Chon D, Beck KC, Larsen RL, et al: Regional pulmonary blood flow in dogs by 4D–x-ray CT. J Appl Physiol 2006;101:1451–1465.

29. Tokics L, Hedenstierna G, Strandberg A, et al: Lung collapse and gas exchange during general anesthesia: Effects of spontaneous breathing, muscle paralysis, and positive end-expiratory pressure. Anesthesiology 1987;66:157–167.

30. Tokics L, Hedenstierna G, Svensson L, et al: V/Q distribution and correlation to atelectasis in anesthetized paralyzed humans. J Appl Physiol 1996;81:1822–1833.

31. David M, Karmrodt J, Bletz C, et al: Analysis of atelectasis, ventilated, and hyperinflated lung during mechanical ventilation by dynamic CT. Chest 2005;128:3757–3770.

32. Crotti S, Mascheroni D, Caironi P, et al: Recruitment and derecruitment during acute respiratory failure: A clinical study. Am J Respir Crit Care Med 2001;164:131–140.

33. Rothen HU, Neumann P, Berglund JE, et al: Dynamics of re-expansion of atelectasis during general anaesthesia. Br J Anaesth 1999;82:551–556.

34. Karmrodt J, Markstaller K, Doebrich M, et al: Determination of different coexisting pulmonary time constants in human ARDS by dynamic CT. Intensive Care Med 2002;28:S141.

35. Lu Q, Malbouisson LM, Mourgeon E, et al: Assessment of PEEP-induced reopening of collapsed lung regions in acute lung injury: Are one or three CT sections representative of the entire lung? Intensive Care Med 2001;27:1504–1510.

36. Wildberger J, Max M, Wein B, et al: Low-dose multislice spiral computed tomography in acute lung injury: Animal experience. Invest Radiol 2003;38:9–16.

37. Heussel CP, Hafner B, Lill J, et al: Paired inspiratory/expiratory spiral CT and continuous respiration cine CT in the diagnosis of tracheal instability. Eur Radiol 2001;11:982–989.

38. Tagliabue P, Giannatelli F, Vedovati S, et al: Lung CT scan in ARDS: Are three sections representative of the entire lung? Intensive Care Med 1998;24(Suppl 1):93.

39. Gattinoni L, Bombino M, Pelosi P, et al: Lung structure and function in different stages of severe adult respiratory distress syndrome. JAMA 1994;271:1772–1779.

40. Bletz C, Markstaller K, Karmrodt J, et al: [Quantification of atelectases in artificial respiration: Spiral-CT versus dynamic single-slice CT]. Rofo 2004;176:409–416.

41. Easley RB, Fuld MK, Fernandez-Bustamante A, et al: Mechanism of hypoxemia in acute lung injury evaluated by multidetector-row CT. Acad Radiol 2006;13:916–921.

42. Saba OI, Chon D, Beck K, et al: Static versus prospective gated non-breath hold volumetric MDCT imaging of the lungs. Acad Radiol 2005;12:1371–1384.

43. Zaporozhan J, Ley S, Unterhinninghofen R, et al: Free-breathing three-dimensional computed tomography of the lung using prospective respiratory gating: Charge-coupled device camera and laser sensor device in an animal experiment. Invest Radiol 2006;41:468–475.

# CHAPTER 21

# Flexible Bronchoscopy in Mechanically Ventilated Patients

Irene Perillo, Mark J. Utell, and Gary Dudek

Bronchoscopy provides the physician with a tool to examine the larynx and the tracheobronchial tree in both clinically stable and critically ill, mechanically ventilated patients. This technique has been widely used since its introduction into clinical practice, first with the rigid bronchoscope and more recently with the introduction of the flexible fiberoptic bronchoscope. Flexible bronchoscopy is versatile, easy to use, and better tolerated than rigid bronchoscopy in critically ill patients.[1] It primarily serves a diagnostic role because it assists in understanding the causes, complications, and consequences of acute respiratory failure. Secretions are collected from the airways for microbiologic and cytologic examination, and tissue is sampled from the bronchus, parenchyma, or lymph node for histologic examination. Bronchoscopy is also used as a therapeutic tool, for example, to remove mucus plugs or to control massive hemoptysis. Table 21.1 lists the indications for bronchoscopy.

In this chapter, we first review the special technical requirements for bronchoscopy in ventilated patients. We next consider indications for the procedure in critically ill patients and examine diagnostic approaches. Finally, we explore potential therapeutic indications but also point out the limitations of bronchoscopy in this group of patients. We assume that the reader is familiar with the normal anatomy of the tracheobronchial tree, as has been reviewed in the literature by Athul Mehta[2] and Ko Pen Wang.[1]

## INSTRUMENT

The flexible bronchoscope has three components: the bundle of optical fibers, a longitudinal channel for suction and biopsy, and a mechanism to flex the distal tip. The proximal end contains the videocassette recorder button, camera button, deflection control lever, suction control valve, suction nipple, and electrical connector for video equipment. The instrument channel inlet is the site for instilling anesthetics or saline or for inserting brushes, biopsy forceps, and catheters. The external diameter of available flexible bronchoscopes ranges from 2.7 to 6.2 mm. The length of the insertion cord is 600 mm, and the diameter of the working channel varies from 1.2 to 6.0 mm. The distal end can be flexed upward and downward to a maximum of 180 and 130 degrees, respectively.

## TECHNIQUE

### Preparation of the Patient

Bronchoscopy in ventilated patients raises several unique issues. The most important consideration is ensuring adequate ventilation and oxygenation throughout the procedure. In mechanically ventilated patients, the

**Table 21-1  Indications for Flexible Bronchoscopy**

Evaluation of infiltrates
    Infectious
    Noninfectious
Airway control
    Fiberoptic intubation
    Percutaneous tracheostomy
Foreign body extraction
Mediastinal adenopathy
Massive hemoptysis
Central airway obstruction

bronchoscope is introduced through an endotracheal or tracheostomy tube. It causes airway obstruction when it is introduced into the artificial airway, and it can decrease oxygenation and ventilation.[1] A bronchoscope can occupy as much as 51% of the cross-sectional area of an endotracheal or tracheostomy tube, depending on its size.[1] This increases resistance to flow and leads to increased positive end-expiratory pressure, which can result in barotrauma.[1] To ensure adequate oxygenation, the inspired oxygen concentration should be increased to 100%, and the oxygen saturation should be monitored with a continuous pulse oximeter. We always place a bite block in the patient's mouth to prevent accidental biting or damage by teeth or gums to the fiberoptic scope.

## Mode of Ventilation

Before bronchoscopy, it may be appropriate to change the mode of ventilation. Several different modes of ventilation are now available, varying from volume cycle to pressure control modes. Some studies have looked at the diagnostic and therapeutic usefulness as well as the safety of flexible bronchoscopy in critically ill patients,[3,4] and all these studies have shown that flexible bronchoscopy is safe to use in critically ill patients who require mechanical ventilation. Unfortunately, no studies are available that compare the safety of the different modes of mechanical ventilation during bronchoscopy. However, from a technical perspective, a volume cycle mode delivers the tidal volume in a square wave pattern, whereas a pressure cycle mode delivers it in a decelerating wave pattern. Because airway pressures increase once the bronchoscope is placed into the airway, the decelerating waveform may be better tolerated by the patient. In either mode, the peak pressure limits must be increased during the procedure to maintain a tidal volume of at least 6 to 8 mL/kg.

One potential problem during bronchoscopy, as a result of the high pressures, is that the artificial airway can dislodge. Therefore, it is necessary before and during the procedure to check that the endotracheal or tracheostomy tube is tightly secured. Occasionally, an additional person is necessary to hold the endotracheal tube to ensure that it does not dislodge.

## Sedation and Anesthesia

Although the need for sedation before or during bronchoscopy is frequently debated, this is not an issue in mechanically ventilated patients because they routinely require sedation and pain medication. The choice of medication will depend predominantly on the patient's hemodynamic stability. Benzodiazepines, narcotics, and anesthetics all cause some degree of respiratory and myocardial depression. When used together, they act synergistically, and thus caution and careful monitoring are necessary, especially in critically ill patients.

In our experience, lorazepam for sedation and fentanyl for pain control are the agents of choice in mechanically ventilated patients. During bronchoscopy, boluses of lorazepam (0.044 mg/kg, with a maximum dose of 2 mg) and fentanyl (25 to 100 µg) are given to maintain patient comfort and hemodynamic stability. Lorazepam is preferable to midazolam because it is cheaper. However, boluses of midazolam (2 to 4 mg) are useful to control patient agitation quickly because this agent has a quicker onset of action (1 to 3 minutes) than lorazepam (15 to 20 minutes). Jones and colleagues[5] showed that benzodiazepines, specifically midazolam, are safe to use during bronchoscopy.

Fentanyl is a synthetic intravenous narcotic that is often coadministered with benzodiazepines, most commonly midazolam. It is frequently used because of its rapid onset of action (60 to 90 seconds) and short half-life (2 to 4 hours). During bronchoscopy, fentanyl enhances sedation, blunts airway reflexes, and suppresses coughing.

Propofol is a general anesthetic that has a rapid onset of action (10 to 50 seconds) and a very short duration of action (3 to 10 minutes) because it is rapidly metabolized. It is frequently used for sedation or induction and maintenance of anesthesia. It is a phenol derivative and is lipid soluble, formulated in a white aqueous emulsion containing soybean oil and purified egg phosphatidyl glycerol. Its extremely short duration of action makes it very useful in the operating room, but its propensity to cause hypotension limits its use in critically ill patients with unstable blood pressure.

Another potentially valuable group of drugs, the neuromuscular blocking agents, has not been studied during bronchoscopy in mechanically ventilated patients. Neuromuscular blocking agents must be used cautiously in the critically ill because of the risk of critical care polyneuropathy. In our experience, there is a specific but limited role for these agents because they provide paralysis and thus total control of ventilation and elimination of cough.

This class of medications can be used in patients with high inspired fraction of oxygen requirements or patients who are extremely agitated but in whom the use of narcotics or sedatives is contraindicated as a result of hypotension. Neuromuscular blocking agents should always be combined with benzodiazepines for patient comfort and to decrease anxiety. We prefer to use atracurium or cis-atracurium because of its quick onset (2 to 3 minutes) and short duration of action (20 to 35 minutes).

Typically, 1% to 2% lidocaine liquid is instilled into the airway to blunt cough and to minimize airway reflexes. Lidocaine has a wide margin of safety, fast onset of action, and prolonged duration of action.[6] The maximum safe dose is 7.1 mg/kg, but we generally start with 4.5 mg/kg; 1 to 2 mL can be instilled at the main carina and before intubation of any secondary bronchus. Although uncommon, adverse effects include seizures and arrhythmias, and the risk of toxicity is increased in liver disease.

### Positioning of the Patient

Before bronchoscopy, the patient should be placed in a recumbent position, with the head of the bed at a 30-degree angle to minimize the risk of aspiration. The placement of the bronchoscopist depends on the size of the room, the location of the ventilator, the length of the bronchoscope, and the site of electrical connectors for video equipment. The goal is to select a comfortable position for the patient and the bronchoscopist while at the same time ensuring the safety and stability of the endotracheal or tracheostomy tube.

### Method of Insertion

The flexible bronchoscope can be inserted through a nasotracheal, orotracheal, or tracheostomy tube in the mechanically ventilated patient. Regardless of the method, the bronchoscopist must ensure that the diameter of the artificial airway will permit easy passage of the flexible bronchoscope. In addition, a swivel adapter is attached to the endotracheal tube or tracheostomy to minimize air leaks, to maintain ventilation and oxygenation, and to avoid forceful expulsion of respiratory secretions.

Most flexible bronchoscopes pass through endotracheal or tracheostomy tubes with inner diameters of 7.0 mm or larger. It is good practice to check the ease of passage of the flexible bronchoscope routinely by inserting the scope into a separate endotracheal or tracheostomy tube with the same diameter as in the patient. Adequate lubrication with either lidocaine jelly or Cetacaine spray will facilitate easier movement of the flexible bronchoscope through an endotracheal tube or tracheostomy.

These agents can be applied topically on the bronchoscope or instilled directly into the artificial airway. In our experience, Cetacaine spray is preferable to lidocaine jelly because it has better lubricating capability and does not obstruct vision. In addition, the high airflow through the airway dries the lidocaine jelly, thus possibly making it difficult to pass the bronchoscope in and out of the artificial airway.

## DIAGNOSTIC ROLE

Fiberoptic bronchoscopy is most frequently used as a diagnostic tool in the intensive care unit. It has been applied to numerous common clinical scenarios such as ventilator-associated pneumonia (VAP), pulmonary infiltrates in immunocompromised patients, and acute respiratory distress syndrome (ARDS) of unknown origin. Other potential uses include inspection of lower airway to evaluate the cause of lung collapse or atelectasis, evaluation of mediastinal disease, and investigation of upper airway disorders causing respiratory failure or complicating other established disease processes.

VAP remains a difficult and often elusive diagnosis because fever, leukocytosis, purulent tracheal secretions, and pulmonary infiltrates are frequent occurrences in the intensive care unit, as are noninfectious reasons for these infiltrates. Meduri and Chastre[7] are, in large part, responsible for the validation and evaluation of bronchoscopic techniques capable of differentiating infectious from noninfectious pulmonary infiltrates in mechanically ventilated individuals. Both protected specimen brush (PSB) cultures and bronchoalveolar lavage (BAL) cultures have proven useful in this context. When obtaining these samples, care must be taken to avoid contamination of the bronchoscope's working channel with tracheal secretions to maximize the sensitivity of the test. This is usually accomplished by advancing the bronchoscope into the lung segment of interest with suction disconnected. Once in position, a PSB or BAL sample can be obtained. The resultant specimen is then quantitatively cultured. It is generally accepted that growth of 1000 or more colony forming units/mL on a PSB specimen or 10,000 or more colony forming units/mL on a BAL specimen is consistent with pneumonia. This undertaking can be labor intensive, and quantitative culture capabilities are not universally available; as a result, some investigators recommend the use of clinical decision tools as a more generally applicable approach to the diagnosis of VAP.[8] Largely in response to this controversy, Fagon and Chastre[9] compared clinical diagnosis with invasive diagnosis in a randomized trial involving 413 patients in 31 intensive care units in France. Those patients receiving invasive evaluation demonstrated significantly more antibiotic-free days at 14 and 28 days following enrollment ($P < .001$). A decrease mortality was also seen at 14 days ($P = .022$) for the invasive diagnostic arm of the study. However, a mortality advantage at 28 days in this group could be demonstrated only by multivariate analysis.[9] This reduction in mortality was greatest when the onset of VAP occurred after 4 days of intubation. Moreover, both a mortality advantage and more antibiotic-free days were seen with invasive evaluation in patients receiving antibiotics at the time of bronchoscopy.

A related indication for fiberoptic bronchoscopy in mechanically ventilated patients is the evaluation of pulmonary infiltrates in immunocompromised patients. This group is more heterogeneous as a consequence of diverse forms of immunosuppression, which include the acquired immunodeficiency syndrome (AIDS), chemotherapy-induced neutropenia, bone marrow transplantation, and solid organ transplantation (especially lung transplantation). BAL carries the least risk of complications and is generally the first means of sample acquisition attempted. The yield of BAL is greatest in patients with AIDS, in whom the sensitivity for *Pneumocystis carinii* pneumonia (PCP) is as high as 86% to 97%,[10] owing to the large number of organisms associated with this form of immunosuppression. The number of organisms is less in patients receiving PCP prophylaxis or in patients with non-AIDS immunosuppression. The sensitivity of BAL consequently falls, but it can be improved by multilobe sampling targeting areas of greatest radiographic abnormality.[11] Related opportunistic infections are also associated with lower BAL sensitivities and include cytomegalovirus (CMV) pneumonia and invasive aspergillosis. The former diagnosis is best made by observation of CMV cells with inclusions, because culture positivity without disease is not uncommon. The sensitivity of BAL culture in the diagnosis of aspergillosis varies from 23% to 40%; however, the observation of hyphae on fungal stain improves BAL sensitivity to 58% to 64%.[12] An overall diagnostic yield of 49% has been reported for BAL in the neutropenic and bone marrow transplant population. However, the high mortality rate of these patients in respiratory failure (71% if neutropenic, 93% if bone marrow transplant recipient) is unaltered by these results.[13]

Tissue examination can improve diagnostic sensitivity, although the potential morbidities associated with transbronchial biopsy (TBBx) or open lung biopsy have resulted in a trend toward empirical therapy in individuals requiring mechanical ventilation who have a nondiagnostic BAL result. Interest in the use of TBBx despite the potential risks has increased, especially in lung transplant recipients, in whom rejection and infection are competing clinical concerns. Furthermore, TBBx carries a sensitivity (70% to 90%) and specificity (90% to 100%)

for rejection sufficient to warrant the potential risks of bleeding and pneumothorax in this patient population.[12] In lung transplant centers, increasing experience with fluoroscopically guided TBBx in ventilated patients has led to its use in patients who are not transplant recipients.

O'Brien and colleagues[14] reported their experience in 71 patients with diffuse infiltrates, respiratory failure requiring mechanical ventilation, and nondiagnostic BAL. Forty eight percent of these patients were lung transplant recipients, and 52% had a wide range of other diagnoses, including 24% who were considered immunocompromised. Fourteen percent of these patients developed pneumothorax requiring tube thoracostomy, and the incidence was higher among patients who were not lung transplant recipients (19%). Also noted was a 7% incidence of bleeding more than 30 mL. All these hemorrhages responded to bronchoscopic tamponade or 1:100,000 epinephrine instillation. An overall mortality rate of 21% included no deaths related to TBBx. A specific histologic diagnosis was obtained in 37% of the lung transplant recipients, in 30% of the nonimmunocompromised patients, and in 35% of the immunocompromised patients who were not transplant recipients. These results prompted management changes in 59% of immunocompromised patients who were not transplant recipients and in 60% of the remaining nontransplant patients, whereas management changes were seen in only 26% of the lung transplant group. The magnitude of the management changes, especially among the non–lung transplant patient cohort, suggests that TBBx is a useful technique in mechanically ventilated patients.

Unexplained ARDS represents another category of ventilated patients who may benefit from bronchoscopic evaluation. Infection is frequently presumed to underlie the development of this form of lung injury. At times, unexpected primary lung infections such as miliary tuberculosis, hantavirus infection, herpes simplex, varicella-zoster, PCP, and CMV infection can be found on BAL specimens. Evaluation of BAL cell differentials may provide diagnostic clues such as relative eosinophilia (>15%), which can suggest such disorders as acute eosinophilic pneumonia, Churg-Strauss syndrome, or drug-induced lung disease.[15] Cytologic evaluation may be helpful in cases of bronchoalveolar cell carcinoma, lymphangitic carcinoma, or pulmonary lymphoma. Diffuse alveolar hemorrhage can be diagnosed by a progressively more hemorrhagic lavage return and can be seen as a complication of bone marrow transplantation or collagen vascular disease. Alveolar hemorrhage can also be representative of primary disorders such as Goodpasture's syndrome, Wegener's granulomatosis, or primary pulmonary hemosiderosis. Bronchoscopy is less useful in defining idiopathic inflammatory lung diseases such as cryptogenic organizing pneumonia or acute interstitial pneumonitis because lung biopsy, usually by video-assisted thoracic surgery, is required for diagnostic confirmation. Nevertheless, bronchoscopy can exclude infection in these disorders, as it can in the fibroproliferative phase of ARDS, and can permit the safe application of corticosteroid therapy.

Use of a fiberoptic bronchoscope for evaluation of upper airway disease has been very important in our practice not only in determining the presence of laryngeal edema complicating prolonged intubation but also in identifying unsuspected causes of respiratory failure such as epiglottitis or laryngeal injury resulting from uncontrolled gastroesophageal reflux disease. Repeated upper airway endoscopy can then be very useful in timing extubation attempts as well as facilitation reintubation if stridor persists.

Fiberoptic bronchoscopy is also useful for evaluation of the lower airways. Frequently, atelectasis or lung collapse can occur in ventilated patients. The causes vary and can include mucus plugs, foreign bodies, endobronchial lesions, and external compression of the airway from mediastinal adenopathy or a lung mass. Direct visualization of the affected airway or lung segment is the best way to differentiate among the different causes. For a tissue diagnosis, an endobronchial lesion can be sampled for biopsy with a brush or forceps. Needle aspiration with either a 22-gauge needle or a 19-gauge needle can also be used to obtain tissue samples. Therapeutic procedures, discussed later in the chapter, may be performed to restore airway patency.

The causative identification of mediastinal adenopathy in the ventilated patient has traditionally been the purview of mediastinoscopy. The development of transbronchial needle aspiration biopsy techniques expanded the diagnostic potential of the flexible bronchoscope in the outpatient arena, but concerns for mediastinal dissection of air in patients receiving positive pressure ventilation delayed application of this technique in the intensive care unit. Ghamande and associates[16] reviewed their experience using both 22-gauge and 19-gauge needles in eight mechanically ventilated patients. A diagnosis was obtained in five of eight (63%) patients, and no complications occurred, thereby substantiating the safety of this technique in patients receiving mechanical ventilation.

## THERAPEUTIC ROLE

In patients with respiratory failure requiring mechanical ventilatory support, the role of fiberoptic bronchoscopy is largely diagnostic. Nevertheless, there are instances in which bronchoscopy can provide valuable interventional capability to facilitate management of patients with respiratory failure. Some of these techniques have been shown to facilitate weaning from mechanical ventilation directly.[6,17,18] Table 21.2 summarizes several areas of concern faced by clinicians treating patients in respiratory failure for whom fiberoptic bronchoscopy can play a vital therapeutic role.

### Airway Control

Even before mechanical ventilation begins, one must be able to establish a stable artificial airway. Although this is usually accomplished by placement of an endotracheal tube using direct laryngoscopy, situations such as facial trauma, an unstable cervical spine, or concerns for upper airway obstruction (neoplasm, laryngeal edema, epiglottitis, morbid obesity) may preclude the safe implementation of this approach. In these situations, fiberoptically guided intubation in awake patients can be performed either transorally or transnasally.[19] Mild intravenous sedation with midazolam and fentanyl can be provided to facilitate the procedure while maintaining spontaneous ventilation. Topical anesthesia of the oropharynx and larynx with nebulized 2% lidocaine minimizes cough and laryngospasm, which can be seen with transglottic passage of a flexible bronchoscope. An appropriately sized endotracheal tube is placed over the insertion tube of the bronchoscope. Once the bronchoscope has been adequately positioned in the middle or lower trachea, the endotracheal tube can be advanced over the bronchoscope with a slight twisting motion to avoid engagement of the epiglottis. The endotracheal position of the endotracheal tube can then be visually confirmed, and the bronchoscope can be removed. This process is aided by liberal lubrication of the endotracheal tube lumen using Cetacaine spray.

If prolonged mechanical ventilation is required, tracheostomy placement is used to prevent laryngeal injury, which can accompany prolonged endotracheal tube use. Percutaneous bedside placement of a tracheostomy tube is becoming more common. This technique requires a small neck incision, after which a needle is placed through the anterior trachea, two to three cartilaginous rings below the cricoid cartilage. A "J"-tipped guidewire is then inserted through the needle into the trachea, and then dilators and the tracheostomy tube can be paced using the Seldinger technique. Obviously, the existing endotracheal tube must be withdrawn sufficiently to permit this tracheal access while maintaining ventilation. Similarly, care must be taken to prevent puncture of the posterior membranous trachea and to ensure intratracheal rather than paratracheal positioning of the guidewire, dilators, and tracheostomy tube. This is best accomplished by continuous visual monitoring of the tracheal lumen using a fiberoptic bronchoscope whose tip is maintained just inside the distal endotracheal tube lumen to protect the bronchoscope from inadvertent puncture.[20]

**Table 21-2  Therapeutic Role of Flexible Bronchoscopy**

| Indications | Equipment |
|---|---|
| Fiberoptic intubation | Diagnostic FB, endotracheal tube[19] |
| Percutaneous tracheostomy | Diagnostic FB, percutaneous tracheostomy kit[20] |
| Endobronchial foreign body extraction | Diagnostic FB with forceps, Fogarty catheter, Dormia basket, fishnet basket[21,22] Therapeutic FB with cryotherapy probe[13,24] Streptokinase (1000 U/mL)[25] |
| Massive hemoptysis | Diagnostic or therapeutic FB: Cold epinephrine solution 1:10,000–1:100,000[30] 4-Fr–7-Fr, 14-Fr Fogarty catheter DLC[29] |
| Bronchopleural fistula | Diagnostic FB with: Fogarty catheter/surgery[31] DLC/fibrin glue[32] DLC/tetracycline/blood patch[33] DLC/ethanol[34] |
| Central airway obstruction | Therapeutic FB with: Laser coagulation[36,37] Electrocautery probe and snare[38] Cryotherapy probe[40] Argon plasma coagulator[39] Photofrin/laser[6] |

DLC, dual-lumen balloon-tipped catheter; FB, flexible bronchoscope.

## Foreign Body Extraction

The issue of foreign body aspiration is commonly associated with respiratory failure in adults. Situations that raise concern for the presence of endotracheal foreign bodies in mechanically ventilated adults include the following: trauma involving missing teeth or dental appliances; survival after cardiac arrest, especially if emesis accompanies the event; and burn injury, whose victims can develop soot plugs capable of significantly hindering mechanical ventilation.[21] In these instances, flexible bronchoscopy is both diagnostic and therapeutic because lavage, suction, biopsy forceps, and foreign body retrieval baskets can all be used through the working channel of the bronchoscope to remove the foreign matter.[22] Soft vegetable material, thick mucus, and blood clots can often prove quite frustrating to remove because these materials cannot be grasped by the forceps or basket and are too viscous to be suctioned. Use of a cryotherapy probe through the bronchoscope's working channel offers the unique advantage of being able to freeze these substances to the probe, thus allowing for their removal as a unit with the bronchoscope and probe.[23,24]

A unique "foreign body" obstruction can be seen following the administration of anticoagulants or thrombolytic agents in patients with acute myocardial infarction or pulmonary embolus whose course becomes complicated by subsequent hemoptysis. Although the bleeding frequently stops with discontinuation of the foregoing therapies, the airways may become obstructed by organized thrombus. This can be difficult and tedious to remove by ordinary bronchoscopic methods. A cryotherapy probe can be helpful if it is available. Intrabronchial instillation of streptokinase (1000 U/mL) in 5- to 10-mL aliquots has been demonstrated to dissolve a thrombus sufficiently to allow its removal with suction and biopsy forceps and thereby permit normalization of mechanical ventilation.[25]

Bronchoscopy for atelectasis in the ventilated patient without a history suggestive of foreign body aspiration is less clearly beneficial. In the setting of acute lobar atelectasis, bronchoscopic intervention has been shown to be no more effective than standard respiratory therapy technique.[26] Bronchoscopy for secretion removal has therefore generally been reserved for multilobar or whole lung atelectasis, particularly if it is refractory to respiratory therapy–directed attempts to achieve reexpansion. The patient with a burn injury may represent an exception because the bronchoscopic removal of soot plugs is frequently performed. Although the findings of airway injury and carbonaceous debris can predict respiratory complications, no data suggest that bronchoscopic removal of this material, as opposed to early ventilatory support and aggressive respiratory therapy, will alter the patient's respiratory course.[27,28]

## Massive Hemoptysis

*Massive hemoptysis* has been defined by some authors as the volume of blood expectorated in 24 hours, with criteria ranging from 100 to 1000 mL. Others choose to define this condition by its physiologic manifestations such as respiratory failure, shock, or the need for transfusion therapy.[29] Massive hemoptysis in the intensive care unit most often manifests with threatened or actual respiratory failure regardless of the volume of blood expectorated. This condition constitutes an urgent need for fiberoptic bronchoscopic evaluation in an attempt to localize the source of the hemorrhage and, secondarily, to determine its cause. The bronchoscope can then be used to help control bleeding as well as to protect uninvolved lung from blood aspiration. Dupree and colleagues[30] reported the efficacious use of cold saline lavage containing epinephrine in a concentration of 1:10,000 to 1:100,000 administered through a flexible bronchoscope into the offending airway. Control was achieved in 6 of 7 cases following 1 to 20 bronchoscopic interventions.

Airway protection can also be afforded in this setting using bronchoscopic guidance. Should the right mainstem bronchus prove to be the source of persistent hemorrhage, an endotracheal tube can be advanced over the bronchoscope into the left mainstem bronchus to permit unilateral lung ventilation. In a similar manner, if the left lung is the source of bleeding, a 14-French Fogarty catheter can be guided alongside an existing endotracheal tube and positioned in the left mainstem bronchus, where balloon inflation can occlude this airway and thus permit secure right lung ventilation. In addition, should a more distal bleeding site be confirmed, smaller (5-French) balloon-tipped catheters can be paced through the working channel of the bronchoscope to occlude lobar bronchi to achieve stabilization. Once the patient is thus stabilized, further surgical or angiographic measures to control hemoptysis can be entertained.[29]

## Bronchopleural Fistula

Mechanical ventilation is occasionally associated with pneumothorax development but, fortunately, not with persistent bronchopleural fistula. When this does occur as a consequence of pneumonia or prior lung surgery, chest tube thoracotomy is often able to manage the air leak, reexpand the lung, and thus seal the fistula. When the air leak is large, however, the lung cannot be completely reexpanded, and alveolar ventilation can be significantly impaired by loss of tidal volume through the chest tube.

Surgical intervention is often necessary in this case. When patients are too unstable to consider operative intervention, bronchoscopic intervention can be used. A 4- to 5-French Fogarty catheter can be inserted through the bronchoscope's working channel such that lobar and even segmental bronchi can be serially occluded to determine the effect on air leak through the chest tube. This approach isolates the lobe or segment responsible for the fistula. A separate catheter can then be advanced alongside the endotracheal tube into the culprit airway to seal the fistula, thereby improving ventilation sufficiently to permit surgical repair of the fistula.[31] If the patient is not a surgical candidate as a result of other comorbidities, closure of the culprit airway can be attempted with fibrin glue,[32] tetracycline/blood patch instillation,[33] or absolute ethanol injection.[34]

## Central Airway Obstruction/Postobstructive Pneumonia

Mechanical ventilatory support is at times used to treat individuals with respiratory failure resulting from central airway obstruction with or without postobstructive pneumonia. Most of these obstructions are neoplastic. In cases of respiratory failure caused by high-grade tracheal or bilateral mainstem obstruction, further management is best undertaken by rigid bronchoscopy, which provides maximum airway control and can most quickly establish an adequate airway.[13,35] When the situation is less urgent and an endotracheal tube can adequately control the airway, fiberoptic bronchoscopic intervention is possible.

In the setting of an exophytic primary or metastatic endobronchial neoplasm for which surgery is contraindicated, airway patency can be restored with tissue ablative techniques such as laser photocoagulation,[36,37] electrocautery,[38] argon plasma coagulation,[39] cryotherapy,[40] and photodynamic therapy.[6] The use of laser, electrocautery, and argon plasma coagulation has been associated with airway fire when oxygen concentrations are greater than 40%; this risk can limit the utility of these techniques unless oxygen concentrations lower than 40% can be tolerated, at least for short periods during device activation. Cryotherapy avoids this potential complication; however, tissue destruction occurs at a slower pace than with "hot" therapies, and longer procedure times and often repeated procedures are therefore necessary.

Electrocautery, argon plasma coagulation, and cryotherapy have the advantage of easy portability and can thus be performed in the intensive care unit. All modalities have approximately equivalent success rates of 70% to 80%.[35] Endobronchial bleeding (50 to 250 mL) is the most common complication, and an increased risk of airway perforation is noted with laser use.

The presence of extrinsic airway obstruction is not amenable to ablative therapies unless an endobronchial component is also present. In patients with otherwise unresectable neoplastic disease with extrinsic airway obstruction and respiratory failure, the use of self-expandable metal stents has been shown to facilitate rapid weaning from mechanical ventilation.[7,18] These devices are deployed over a wire positioned through and beyond the stenotic airway using a fiberoptic bronchoscope. Accurate placement of the stent is aided by simultaneous use of fluoroscopy, which can also help direct bronchoplastic stent dilatation if needed. Using these techniques, Saad and associates[17] reported 14 of 16 ventilator-dependent patients weaned, whereas Shaffer and Allen[18] reported similar success in 7 of 8 patients. As suggested by Unger,[41] this expensive technology, coupled with short anticipated survival of this patient population after extubation, raises a serious ethical and financial dilemma for clinicians. Intervention in this setting requires thoughtful deliberation on a case-by-case basis.

## Future Technologies

Several newer technologies are likely to assist significantly in the planning and execution of therapeutic bronchoscopic procedures in mechanically ventilated patients. Sixteen- and 64-head computed tomography scanners are capable of data acquisition sufficient to portray endobronchial anatomy in exquisite detail, thus allowing both virtual bronchoscopic examination and three-dimensional renderings of the airway with surrounding mediastinal structures. At present, this is proving most useful in defining the length and nature of an airway obstruction, as well as in assessing the patency of the airway distal to the obstruction. This information is vital in planning maneuvers to alleviate the obstruction and in helping to determine the potential utility of doing so.[42]

Endobronchial ultrasound probes are now available that can be passed through the working channel of a flexible bronchoscope. These ultrasound data can also provide information on the length and nature of an obstructing lesion and can help to assess the normality of the airway distally. In addition, significant detail of the airway wall is visible. It is possible to determine either the preservation or loss of supporting cartilaginous rings, which will determine the need for airway stenting should the obstructing lesion prove to be endoscopically resectable.[43]

## CONCLUSION

It can be seen by this discussion that flexible bronchoscopy has a significant role to play in mechanically ventilated patients. This procedure can be performed safely and at the bedside in most instances. The role of bronchoscopy is largely diagnostic, with applicability of most procedural techniques common to outpatient diagnostic bronchoscopy. It is of particular value in the evaluation of VAP and in pulmonary infiltrative processes associated with a variety of immunocompromised states. In addition, there is an ever-increasing role for therapeutic intervention in the critical care setting ranging from establishment of a secure airway to management of endobronchial obstruction. Newer technologies such as virtual bronchoscopy and endobronchial ultrasound will enhance the application of currently available therapeutic techniques and may help suggest future, yet to be conceived, interventional strategies.

## REFERENCES

1. Wang KP, Mehta AC, Turner JF: Flexible Bronchoscopy, 2nd ed. Malden, MA: Blackwell, 2004.
2. Prakash UBS: Bronchoscopy. New York, Raven Press, 1994.
3. Turner JS, Willcox PA, Hayhurst MD, et al: Fiberoptic bronchoscopy in the intensive care unit: A prospective study of 147 procedures in 107 patients. Crit Care Med 1994;22:259–264.
4. Trouillet JL, Guiguet M, Gibert C, et al: Fiberoptic bronchoscopy in ventilated patients. Chest 1990;97:927–933.
5. Jones AM, O'Driscoll R: Do all patients require supplemental oxygen during flexible bronchoscopy? Chest 2001;119:1906–1909.
6. Shah SK, Ost D: Photodynamic therapy: A case series demonstrating its role in patients receiving mechanical ventilation. Chest 2000;118:1419–1423.
7. Meduri GU, Chastre J: The standardization of bronchoscopic techniques for ventilator-associated pneumonia. Chest 1992;102(Suppl 1):557S–564S.
8. Niederman MS, Torres A, Summer W: Invasive diagnostic testing is not needed routinely to manage ventilator-associated pneumonia. Am J Respir Crit Care 1994;150:565–569.
9. Fagon JY, Chastre J, Wolff M, et al: Invasive and non-invasive strategies for management of ventilator-associated pneumonia. Ann Intern Med 2000;132:621–603.
10. Golden JA, Klatt EC, Koss MN, et al: Bronchoalveolar lavage as the exclusive diagnostic modality for *Pneumocystis carinii* and cytomegalovirus pulmonary infections in acquired immunodeficiency syndrome. Chest 1986;90:18–22.
11. Yung RC, Weinacker AB, Steiger DJ, et al: Upper and middle lobe bronchoalveolar lavage to diagnose *Pneumocystis* pneumonia. Am Rev Respir Dis 1993;148:1563–1566.
12. Dakin J, Griffiths M: The pulmonary physician in critical care: Pulmonary investigations for acute respiratory. Thorax 2002;57:79–85.
13. Gruson D, Hilbert G, Valentino R, et al: Utility of fiberoptic bronchoscopy in neutropenic patients admitted to the intensive

care unit with pulmonary infiltrates. Crit Care Med 2000;28:2224–2230.

14. O'Brien JD, Ettinger NA, Shevlin D, Kollef MH: Safety and yield of transbronchial biopsy in mechanically ventilated patients. Crit Care Med 1997;25:440–446.

15. Allen JN, Davis WB, Pacht ER: Diagnostic significance of increased bronchoalveolar lavage fluid eosinophils. Am Rev Respir Dis 1990;142:642–647.

16. Ghamande S, Rafanan A, Dweik R, et al: Role of transbronchial needle aspiration in patients receiving mechanical ventilation. Chest 2002;121:985–989.

17. Saad CP, Murthy S, Krizmanich G, et al: Self-expandable metallic airway stents and flexible bronchoscopy: Long term outcomes analysis. Chest 2003;124:1993–1999.

18. Shaffer JP, Allen JN: The use of expandable metal stents to facilitate extubation in patients with large airway obstruction. Chest 1998;114:1378–1382.

19. George E, Haspel KL: The difficult airway. Int Anesthesiol Clin 2000;38:47–63.

20. Rogers S, Puyana JC: Bedside percutaneous tracheostomy in the critically ill patient. Int Anesthesiol Clin 2000;38:95–110.

21. Marquette CH, Martinot A: Foreign body removal in adults and children. In Bolliger CT, Mathur PN (eds): Interventional Bronchoscopy: Progress in Respiratory Research, vol 30. Basel, Karger, 2000, pp 96–107.

22. Mehta AC, Rafanan AL: Extraction of airway foreign body in adults. J Bronchol 2001;8:123–131.

23. Sheski FD, Mathur PN: Endobronchial cryotherapy for benign tracheobronchial lesions. Chest 1998;114:261S–262S.

24. Thommi G, McLeay M: Cryobronchoscopy in the management of foreign body in the tracheobronchial tree. Chest 1998;114:303S.

25. Vajo Z, Parish J: Endobronchial thrombolysis with streptokinase for airway obstruction due to blood clots. Mayo Clin Proc 1996;71:595–596.

26. Marini J, Pierson D, Hudson L: Acute lobar atelectasis: A prospective comparison of bronchoscopy and respiratory therapy. Am Rev Respir Dis 1979;119:971–978.

27. Clark CJ, Reid WH, Telfer ABM, et al: Respiratory injury in the burned patient. Anaesthesia 1983;38:35–39.

28. Kkoo AK, Lee ST, Poh WT: Tracheobronchial cytology in inhalation injury. J Trauma 1997;42:81–85.

29. Dweik RA, Stoller JK: Role of bronchoscopy in massive hemoptysis. Clin Chest Med 1999;20:89–105.

30. Dupree HJ, Lewejohann JC, Gleiss J, et al: Fiberoptic bronchoscopy of intubated patients with life threatening hemoptysis. West J Surg 2001;25:104–107.

31. McCormick BA, Wilson LH, Berrisford RG: Bronchopleural fistula complicating group A beta-haemolytic streptococcal pneumonia: Use of a Fogarty embolectomy catheter for selective bronchial blockade. Intensive Care Med 1999;25:535–537.

32. Torre M, Quaini E, Ravini M, et al: 1987: Endoscopic gluing of bronchopleural fistula. Updated in 1994. Ann Thorac Surg 1994;58:901–902.

33. Martin WR, Siefkin AD, Allen R: Closure of bronchopleural fistula with bronchoscopic instillation of tetracycline. Chest 1991;99:1040–1042.

34. Takaoka K, Inoue S, Ohira S: Central bronchopleural fistulas closed by bronchoscopic injection of absolute ethanol. Chest 2002;122:374–378.

35. Seijo LM, Sterman DH: Interventional pulmonology. N Engl J Med 2001;344:740–748.

36. Chan AL, Juarez MM, Albertson TE, et al: Laser treatment of endobronchial renal cell carcinoma. J Bronchol 2004;11: 92–97.

37. Stanopoulos IT, Beamis JF Jr, Martinez FJ, et al: Laser bronchoscopy in respiratory failure from malignant airway obstruction. Crit Care Med 1993;21:386–391.

38. Coulter TD, Mehta AC: The heat is on: Impact of endobronchial electrocautery on the need for Nd-YAG laser photoresection. Chest 2000;118:516–521.

39. Morice RC, Ece T, Ece F: Endobronchial argon plasma coagulation for treatment of hemoptysis and neoplastic airway obstruction. Chest 2001;119:781–787.

40. Sheski FD, Mathur PN: Cryotherapy, electrocautery, and brachytherapy. Clin Chest Med 1999;20:123–138.

41. Unger M: Tracheobronchial stents, stunts, and medical ethics revisited. Chest 1996;110:1155–1160.

42. McLennan G, Hoffman EA, Swift RD, et al: Virtual bronchoscopic assessment of major airway obstructions. Proc Soc Photo Opt Instrum Eng 1999;3660: 313–320.

43. Nakamura Y, Endo C, Sato M, et al: A new technique for endobronchial ultrasonography and comparison of two ultrasonic probes. Chest 2004;126:192–197.

## SUGGESTED READINGS

Colt, HG, Morris JF: Fiberoptic bronchoscopy without premedication. Chest 1990;96:1327–1330.

Diacon AH, Bolliger CT: Functional evaluation before and after interventional bronchoscopy in patients with malignant central airway obstruction. Monaldi Arch Chest Dis 2001;56: 67–73.

Fulkerson WJ: Fiberoptic bronchoscopy. N Engl J Med 1984;311:511–514.

Greig J H, Cooper SM, Kasimbazi HJN, et al: Sedation for fiberoptic bronchoscopy. Respir Med 1995;89:53–56.

Olopade CO, Prakash UBS: Bronchoscopy in the critical-care unit. Mayo Clin Proc 1989;64:1255–1263.

Shelley MP, Wilson P, Norman J: Sedation for fiberoptic bronchoscopy. Thorax 1989;44:769–775.

Williams T, Brooks T, Ward C: The role of atropine premedication in fiberoptic bronchoscopy using intravenous midazolam sedation. Chest 1998;113:1394–1398.

# SECTION 3

# MECHANICAL VENTILATION

# CHAPTER 22

# Basic Modes of Mechanical Ventilation

Yuh-Chin T. Huang and Jaspal Singh

Mechanical ventilation has evolved substantially since the days of the polio epidemics. Negative pressure ventilators that were used during that time have been replaced by positive pressure ventilators. The analog display has been replaced by digital technology. Almost all ventilators in the modern era are now driven by advanced computer algorithms that enable clinicians to change almost any parameter. The advances in ventilator technology have created a unique professional specialist in allied health care, the respiratory care practitioner, whose main function is to help manage the ventilators and the intricacies of mechanical ventilation. Despite these major advances, many of the physical principles that govern the delivery of gas during mechanical ventilation have remained the same. It is thus important for clinicians to understand these basic principles.

Mechanical ventilation is primarily a form of supportive care and *does not treat the underlying illness.* Mechanical ventilation should support two very important physiologic goals: (1) normalizing arterial blood gas and acid-base imbalance by providing adequate ventilation and oxygenation through the use of volumes and positive pressures, and (2) decreasing the patient's work of breathing by unloading respiratory muscles in a synchronous manner.

When instituting mechanical ventilation, one should recognize the primary gas exchange derangement of the patient. Patients whose primary problem is hypoxemia, such as those with congestive heart failure or acute respiratory distress syndrome (ARDS), will require more attention to ventilator parameters that improve oxygenation (fraction of inspired oxygen [$FiO_2$], positive end-expiratory pressure [PEEP], mean airway pressure).

On the contrary, patients who have hypercapnic respiratory failure, such as those with acute exacerbations of chronic obstructive pulmonary disease (COPD), drug overdose, or neuromuscular diseases, mainly need attention to the delivery of adequate ventilation. There are also patients who are intubated merely for airway protection (e.g., seizure, altered mental status, and anesthesia). In these patients, mechanical ventilation is instituted simply to maintain the patient's normal breathing capacity. Because many of these patients have relatively normal lungs, mechanical ventilation can usually be discontinued quickly once the underlying conditions that compromise the integrity of the airways are adequately treated.

This chapter focuses on four basic modes of mechanical ventilation that are commonly used in clinical practice. These four modes are volume assist-control (VAC), pressure assist-control (VAC), pressure support ventilation (PSV), and synchronized intermittent mandatory ventilation (SIMV).

## TERMINOLOGY

We first discuss the physical parameters used in these modes of ventilation. The parameters that are set by clinicians are sometimes called *independent variables,* which specify ventilator output. The parameters measured by the ventilators are called *dependent variables.* It is essential for those who are taking care of mechanically ventilated patients to discriminate between these two variables during daily rounds, to ensure accurate assessment of patients' progress. Commonly used variables are defined as follows:

- Tidal volume ($V_T$): The amount of air delivered to the patient per breath. It is customarily expressed in milliliters.
- Respiratory rate/frequency (f): The number of breaths per minute. This can be from the ventilator, the patient, or both. It has a unit of breaths/minute.
- Minute ventilation ($V_E$): The product of $V_T$ and respiratory frequency ($V_T \cdot f$). It is usually expressed in liters/minute.
- Peak airway pressure (Paw): The pressure that is required to deliver the $V_T$ to the patient. It has a unit of centimeters of water (cm $H_2O$).
- Plateau pressure (Pplat): The pressure that is needed to distend the lung. This pressure can only be obtained by applying an end-inspiratory pause. It also has a unit of cm $H_2O$.
- Peak inspiratory flow: The highest flow that is used to deliver $V_T$ to the patient during inspiratory phase. It is usually measured in liters/minute.
- Mean airway pressure: The time-weighted average pressure during the respiratory cycle. It is expressed in cm $H_2O$.
- Inspiratory time: The amount of time (in seconds) it takes to deliver $V_T$.
- Positive end-expiratory pressure (PEEP): The amount of positive pressure that is maintained at end-expiration. It is expressed in cm $H_2O$.
- Fraction of inspired oxygen ($FiO_2$): The concentration of $O_2$ in the inspired gas, usually between 0.21 (room air) and 1.0 (100% $O_2$).

## MECHANISMS OF MECHANICAL VENTILATORY SUPPORT

Next, one needs to understand how ventilators deliver breaths to the patient. Mechanical ventilatory support can be either total support (controlled mechanical ventilation [CMV]) or partial support (assisted mechanical ventilation [AMV]). In total support, the ventilator does all the work during ventilation. This situation may occur in patients under general anesthesia or in those who are comatose, in whom the ventilator provides all the work needed to trigger and deliver breaths. In partial support, the ventilator simply assists the patient during breathing. In most cases, the ventilator assists a breath initiated by the patient by delivering the volume through a flow-targeted or a pressure-targeted mechanism. In today's ventilators, however, total support and partial support are frequently present in one mode (e.g., assist-control), and whether the breaths are assisted breaths or control breaths can be

recognized by the presence or absence of the patient's trigger effort. Paying attention to the number of assisted breaths relative to the number of controlled breaths may help to determine the integrity of the central nervous system and the depth of sedation when changes to the ventilator setting are being considered. There are four phases during each ventilatory cycle: trigger phase (breath initiation), flow delivery phase, cycle phase (breath termination), and expiratory phase (Fig. 22.1).

Breaths can be initiated during the trigger phase by three mechanisms: (1) *machine timer*, in which breaths are initiated by a timer in the machine set by the clinician; (2) *pressure change* (pressure trigger), in which patient effort pulls the airway/circuit pressure negative, and machine breaths are initiated when this pressure drop exceeds the set negative pressure threshold (pressure sensitivity); and (3) *flow change* (flow trigger), in which patient effort draws flow from the circuit, and machine breaths are initiated when flow into the patient exceeds the set flow threshold (flow sensitivity).

Once the breath is triggered, the inspiratory valve in the ventilator opens, and the flow is delivered. The flow delivery is governed by a target or limit set by the clinician for the ventilator during inspiration. There are two commonly used targets or limits (1) *flow target*, which is a flow rate and pattern set by the clinician; airway pressure thus varies; and (2) *pressure target*, which is an inspiratory pressure limit set by the clinician; flow and volume thus vary.

The flow delivery phase is followed by the cycle phase, during which the machine terminates a breath by any of four commonly used cycle-off criteria: (1) *volume*, in which a breath is terminated when a target volume is achieved; (2) *time*, in which a breath is terminated when a set inspiratory time is achieved; (3) *flow*, in which a breath is terminated when inspiratory flow has fallen to a set level; and (4) *pressure*, in which a breath is terminated when a set inspiratory pressure is achieved.

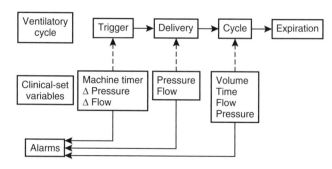

**Figure 22.1** The four phases of each ventilatory cycle (see text for detail). Depending on the mode, the clinician sets different variables (independent variables) for each phase except the expiratory phase, which is passive. Each ventilatory cycle is also monitored by built-in alarm systems that can detect any ventilator output variables (measured parameters) that fall outside the preset limits.

These four cycle-off mechanisms are also commonly used to classify mechanical ventilation into volume-cycled, time-cycled, flow-cycled, and pressure-cycled, respectively.

The cycle phase is then followed by expiration, which is mostly passive and depends on lung recoil pressure (compliance) and airway/circuit resistance. The product of compliance and airway resistance is called the *time constant* (Tc). Patients with a long Tc (e.g., COPD and asthma) will need a longer expiratory time to empty the lung completely, whereas patients with a short Tc (e.g., ARDS, pulmonary fibrosis) can empty the lung quickly. Sometimes the patient may use accessory muscles to actively exhale the gas. This is seen frequently during acute exacerbations of COPD and asthma.

## BASIC MODES OF MECHANICAL VENTILATION

The following sections discuss four commonly used modes of mechanical ventilation: VAC, PAC, PSV, and SIMV. The characteristics of these four basic modes are summarized in Table 22.1.

## Volume Assist-Control Mode

In the VAC mode, a breath can be initiated by the machine timer (control mode) or by the patient (assist mode) (Fig. 22.2). The $V_T$ is then delivered by a flow-targeted mechanism (i.e., a fixed flow set by the clinician) until a preset $V_T$ is reached. The ventilator terminates the breath (volume cycle-off) and allows expiration to proceed. The clinician sets respiratory rate, $V_T$, and peak inspiratory flow, in addition to $FiO_2$ and PEEP. The dependent variables are pressures (Paw and Plat). The inspiratory time (Ti) is determined by the ratio of $V_T$ and inspiratory flow (Ti = $V_T$/flow rate). Patients who are placed on the VAC mode breathe at a respiratory rate that is at least equal to the set rate, and each breath (whether it is machine trigger or patient trigger) has the same $V_T$. Thus, if a patient stops triggering the breath, he or she will receive at least a $V_E$ that is equal to the preset rate times the $V_T$. One other advantage of this mode is that patients can be fully rested on the

**Table 22-1** Characteristics of Volume Assist-Control, Pressure Assist-Control, Pressure Support Ventilation, and Synchronized Intermittent Mandatory Ventilation

| Modes | Description | Advantages | Disadvantages |
|---|---|---|---|
| VAC | Delivers $V_T$ that is machine or patient triggered, flow targeted, and at a frequency that at least equals the preset rate; each breath is terminated by a preset $V_T$ (volume cycle-off) | Guaranteed $V_E$ | Not easy to monitor plateau pressure<br>May be uncomfortable in patients who require high inspiratory flow |
| PAC | Delivers $V_T$ that is machine or patient triggered, pressure targeted, and at a frequency that at least equals the preset rate; each breath is terminated by a preset Ti (time cycle-off) | Pressure limiting<br>Patient comfort | No guaranteed $V_T$ or $V_E$ |
| PSV | Delivers $V_T$ that is patient triggered and pressure targeted; each breath is terminated by preset inspiratory flow (flow cycle-off); $V_T$, Ti, and frequency are determined by the patient | Patient comfort<br>Better patient-ventilator synchrony | No guaranteed $V_E$<br>Inadequate for patients with unreliable respiratory drive |
| SIMV | Delivers synchronized breaths at preset $V_T$ that is machine triggered, flow or pressure targeted, and at a preset frequency; patients can breathe spontaneously with or without PSV between machine breaths | Guaranteed $V_E$ | Increased work of breathing<br>Less capable of changing $V_E$ as patient's status changes<br>May prolong weaning |

PAC, pressure assist-control; PSV, pressure support ventilation; SIMV, synchronized intermittent mandatory ventilation; Ti, inspiratory time; VAC, volume assist-control; $V_E$, minute ventilation; $V_T$, tidal volume.

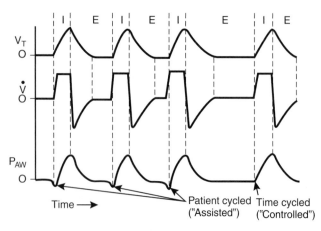

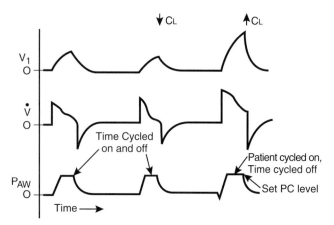

**Figure 22.2** Volume assist-control (VAC) mode. The first three breaths are assisted breaths, as shown by the drop in airway pressure (Paw) at the beginning of each breath. The fourth breath is a controlled breath. The volume is delivered by a fixed flow (flow-targeted), and the breath is terminated when a preset tidal volume (VT) is reached (volume cycle-off). Note that the assisted breath and the controlled breath have the same VT. Expiration (E) then follows. I, inspiration; V, flow. (Adapted from MacIntyre NR: Graphical Analysis of Flow, Pressure and Volume during Mechanical Ventilation, 3rd ed. Yorba Linda, CA: Bear Medical System, 1991.)

**Figure 22.3** Pressure assist-control (PAC) mode. The first two breaths are controlled breaths, and the third breath is an assisted breath, as shown by the drop in airway pressure (Paw) at the beginning of the breath. The volume is delivered by a pressure-targeted mechanism with a decelerating flow pattern. The airway pressure (Paw) is maintained at the set pressure control (PC) level until a set inspiratory time is reached (time cycled off). Expiration then follows. When the lung compliance (CL) decreases (second breath), the tidal volume (VT) decreases. When CL increases (third breath), VT increases. Note that Paw is maintained by varying the flow pattern when lung mechanics change. (Adapted from MacIntyre NR: Graphical Analysis of Flow, Pressure and Volume during Mechanical Ventilation, 3rd ed. Yorba Linda, CA: Bear Medical System, 1991.)

ventilator, except for triggering, assuming that the peak inspiratory flow is adequate. The problem of this mode is that patients tend to hyperventilate as they come out of deep sedation, thereby resulting in hypocapnia and respiratory alkalosis. In addition, patients who demand high inspiratory flow may "fight" the ventilator if the flow rate is set too low.

## Pressure Assist-Control Mode

The PAC mode is also called pressure controlled mode (Fig. 22.3). In the PAC mode, a breath can be initiated by the machine timer (control mode) or by the patient (assist mode). The VT is delivered by a pressure-targeted mechanism (i.e., an inspiratory pressure set by the clinician). The ventilator continues to deliver the breath until a preset Ti is reached (time cycle-off). The breath is then terminated, and expiration follows. The clinician sets respiratory rate, inspiratory pressure, and Ti, in addition to FiO2 and PEEP. The flow waveform is always decelerating in the PAC mode because the flow slows as it reaches the pressure limit. The dependent variables are VT and inspiratory flow. Patients who are placed on PAC mode breathe at a respiratory rate that is at least equal to the set rate, and each breath has the same preset inspiratory pressure. The magnitude of VT, however, depends on the resistance and compliance of the respiratory system and, sometimes, on Ti. Thus, if a patient stops triggering the breath, he or she will continue to breathe at a rate

that is at least equal to the preset rate, but the VE will vary depending on the VT the patient receives. Like the VAC mode, the PAC mode can fully rest patients, except for triggering. One major advantage of the PAC mode compared with the VAC mode is that the Pplat can be more easily regulated, an important consideration in patients with ARDS during ventilation using the lung protective strategy. Decelerating flow patterns in PAC improve the distribution of ventilation in a lung with heterogeneous mechanical properties (as in acute lung injury).[1] The PAC mode is also useful in patients who are ventilated using a cuffless endotracheal tube (e.g., neonates and children and patients with bronchopleural fistula). Under these conditions, the PAC mode continues to attempt to pressurize the airway for the duration of the Ti despite the volume loss through the leak. In addition, because of the high variable inspiratory flow needed to deliver the volume, the PAC mode may be more comfortable for some patients who have strong respiratory drive and demand high flow that cannot be satisfied by the fixed flow in the VAC mode.[2,3]

## Pressure Support Ventilation Mode

In the PSV mode, all breaths are initiated by the patient (Fig. 22.4). The VT is delivered by a pressure-targeted mechanism (i.e., an inspiratory pressure set by the clinician).

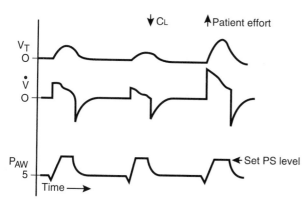

**Figure 22.4** Pressure support ventilation (PSV). Each breath is patient triggered, as shown by the drop in airway pressure (Paw) at the initiation of the breath. The volume is delivered by a mechanism that targets a set pressure level (pressure targeted). The breath is terminated when the inspiratory flow has decreased to a preset level. Expiration then follows. When the lung compliance (CL) decreases (second breath), the tidal volume (VT) decreases. When CL increases (third breath), VT increases. Note that Paw is maintained by varying the flow pattern when lung mechanics change. (Adapted from MacIntyre NR: Graphical Analysis of Flow, Pressure and Volume during Mechanical Ventilation, 3rd ed. Yorba Linda, CA: Bear Medical System, 1991.)

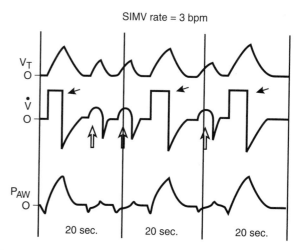

**Figure 22.5** Synchronized intermittent mandatory ventilation (SIMV). Three IMV breaths are shown (*arrows*). Each IMV breath is synchronized with the patient's breathing effort, as shown by the drop in airway pressure (Paw) at the initiation of each breath. The example shows volume SIMV in which each IMV breath is flow targeted, volume cycled-off. Unassisted spontaneous breaths (*black arrows*) are interspersed between IMV breaths. (Adapted from MacIntyre NR: Graphical Analysis of Flow, Pressure and Volume during Mechanical Ventilation, 3rd ed. Yorba Linda, CA: Bear Medical System, 1991.)

The ventilator continues to deliver the breath until the inspiratory flow has decreased to a specific level (e.g., at 25% of the peak inspiratory flow) (flow cycle-off). Expiration then follows. Because each breath on the PSV mode is initiated by the patient, it is very important to ensure that the patient has reliable breathing effort before being placed on the PSV mode. Otherwise, hypoventilation or apnea may occur. The magnitude of VT delivered may differ from breath to breath, depending on lung mechanics and the patient's respiratory drive. One of the major advantages of the PSV mode is that it allows the patient to determine the rate, the duration of inspiration, and the size of VT. This may enhance patient-ventilator synchrony and provide patient comfort.[4] As the patient recovers, the clinician can determine how much work the ventilator can take from the patient by altering the pressure support level, thus making this a very attractive mode for weaning. PSV can also be added to another mode (e.g., SIMV) to support spontaneous breaths, as discussed later.

## Synchronized Intermittent Mandatory Ventilation

In the IMV mode, machine-triggered (mandatory) breaths are delivered at a preset frequency by a flow-targeted volume-cycled (volume IMV) or pressure-targeted time-cycled (pressure IMV) mechanism (Fig. 22.5). Between mandatory breaths, the patient can breathe spontaneously. There are two problems with the original design of the IMV mode: (1) it is possible for the patient

and the ventilator to inspire in series, thus "stacking" one breath on top of another and leading to high airway pressures; and (2) the workload of spontaneous breaths remains quite high because the patient still has to open a demand valve and inspire without assistance through an endotracheal tube. The first problem has been addressed by fitting a sensor in the ventilator to detect and synchronize the patient's spontaneous breaths (up to the mandatory rate) in a manner similar to the assist-control mode. The "S" in SIMV thus denotes the ability of this mode to synchronize the mandatory breath with the patient's own inspiratory effort. The synchronization decreases the conflicts between the patient's breathing efforts and mandatory machine breaths. The second problem of increased work of breathing during spontaneous breaths is solved by introducing pressure support for the spontaneous breaths. Thus, in the SIMV mode, the patient receives three types of breaths: the control (mandatory) breaths that are flow targeted volume-cycled or pressure targeted time-cycled (as in pressure IMV mode), assisted (synchronized) breaths that are also flow targeted volume cycled or pressure targeted time cycled, and spontaneous breaths that can be pressure supported. In clinical practice, SIMV and PSV are frequently combined and are prescribed as one setting (SIMV/PSV). The IMV mode was initially developed as a method of partial ventilatory support to facilitate liberation from mechanical ventilation. The demand valve placed in the breathing system allows the patient to breathe spontaneously while also receiving mandatory breaths. As the patient's respiratory function improves, the number of mandatory breaths is decreased. The patient can be extubated when he or she is breathing with minimal mandatory breaths. Large clinical trials, however, show that SIMV is associated with a higher number of weaning failures compared with PSV,[5] and SIMV tends to liberate patients more slowly from mechanical ventilation than PSV or T-piece methods.[6]

## PRESSURE VERSUS VOLUME MODES

There has been an ongoing debate about whether pressure modes or volume modes are superior. In reality, if set up appropriately, both modes are likely equivalent in supporting gas exchange, hemodynamics, and pulmonary mechanics. As discussed earlier, one advantage of pressure modes is that the clinician can easily regulate inspiratory pressure in patients who need a protective lung strategy (e.g., patients with ARDS). It is also easier to adjust Ti and thus the inspiratory-expiratory (I:E) ratio in the PAC mode in patients who need to maintain high mean airway pressure for oxygenation. In addition, pressure modes (PAV and PSV) provide higher initial flow to meet the strong demands in some critically ill patients compared with volume modes (VAC and SIMV).[4] This approach improves patient-ventilator synchrony and decreases inspiratory work of breathing.[2,3]

Conversely, volume modes have the ability to deliver a constant VT and guarantee VE regardless of changes in lung mechanics. However, because the airway pressure is a dependent variable, it may not be as easy to monitor the alveolar pressure in patients with ARDS because an inspiratory pause maneuver needs to be performed to obtain the Pplat. The fixed flow used to deliver the VT also may be inadequate in some patients who have high flow demand.

## SETTING UP THE VENTILATOR MODE FOR THE PATIENT

A clinician should ask the following questions when selecting and setting up a ventilator mode:

1. *What are the objectives for mechanical ventilation?* Generally, the first objectives are to improve gas exchange and to correct acid-base imbalance, but sometimes the goal is merely to support patients for airway protection or inconsistent central respiratory drive (e.g., seizure, stroke, or drug overdose). An additional objective in patients with acute respiratory failure is to unload respiratory muscles and relieve respiratory distress. These objectives should be achieved with special attention to minimizing injury associated with mechanical ventilation, including $O_2$ toxicity and lung overstretch (ventilator-induced lung injury). Common conditions requiring mechanical ventilatory support and primary physiologic derangements associated with these conditions are listed in Table 22.2.

2. *Does the patient have a reliable central respiratory drive?* In general, partial support modes (e.g., PSV) can be safely applied to patients who have adequate central respiratory drive to support ventilation. In patients who have a tendency for apnea (e.g., patients with drug overdose, brainstem stroke), a mode that provides guaranteed VE is preferable (assist-control or IMV). Patients who are deeply sedated and possibly paralyzed also fall into the latter category. The patient's ability to initiate a breath ("trigger the ventilator") should be reevaluated before one switches from assist-control modes to PSV.

3. *What are the patient's acute disease processes and comorbid conditions?* In general, patients who have restrictive diseases and are in hypoxemic respiratory failure (e.g., ARDS, pulmonary edema, diffuse pneumonia) may require higher $FiO_2$ and PEEP to support oxygenation. Their VE requirement is usually higher and may be supported by using higher respiratory rates (20 to 25/minute) and lower VT. On the contrary, patients with obstructive lung disease or hypercapnic respiratory failure (e.g., status asthmaticus, severe COPD) usually do not require high $FiO_2$. High PEEP should be avoided because it may cause lung overinflation and barotrauma. The only exception is when the patient has developed a trigger problem resulting from intrinsic PEEP caused by airway obstruction. In this case, extrinsic PEEP can be carefully titrated to improve trigger sensitivity. The main treatments in this case, however, are effective bronchodilation and adequate expiratory time. It is important to reassess the presence of intrinsic PEEP, the trigger sensitivity, and the level of extrinsic PEEP frequently as the disease evolves. One should also ensure a maximum expiratory time so that the lung can empty the VT adequately, thus minimizing intrinsic PEEP. Therefore, if a control rate is needed for a deeply sedated patient with airway obstruction, a lower rate is preferable (8 to 15/minute).

4. *How does the patient's underlying disease respond to treatment?* Patients who receive mechanical ventilation should be assessed frequently to determine whether the current ventilator settings remain appropriate because the diseases or conditions that prompt the initiation of mechanical ventilation may change rapidly. If a patient's respiratory status is worsening, more machine support may be needed. In contrast,

**Table 22-2**  Common Conditions Requiring Mechanical Ventilatory Support and Primary Physiologic Derangements Associated with These Conditions*

| Clinical Conditions | Primary Physiologic Derangements |
| --- | --- |
| Severe pneumonia | Hypoxemia, increased work of breathing |
| Sepsis/acute respiratory distress syndrome | Hypoxemia, low compliance, increased work of breathing, metabolic acidosis |
| Cardiogenic pulmonary edema | Hypoxemia, increased work of breathing, low compliance |
| Pulmonary embolism | Hypoxemia |
| Status asthmaticus | Increased work of breathing, increased airway resistance |
| Exacerbation of chronic obstructive pulmonary disease | Hypercapnia, hypoxemia, increased work of breathing, increased airway resistance |
| Drug overdose | Hypercapnia, apnea, metabolic acidosis |
| Severe neuromuscular diseases | Hypercapnia, apnea |
| Restrictive chest wall diseases (kyphosis/scoliosis, multiple sclerosis) | Low compliance (stiff chest wall) |
| Head trauma | Apnea, airway patency |
| Chest wall trauma | Hypoxemia, airway patency, asynchronous chest wall (flail chest) |
| Seizure | Airway patency, metabolic acidosis |

*In hypoxemic respiratory failure, hypercapnia may ensue at a late stage.

if the patient is improving rapidly, machine support should be decreased to keep pace with the changing demands of the patient. Many patients become uncomfortable with excessive ventilatory support when their respiratory status is improving. If the ventilator settings are not accommodating, the patient may "fight" the ventilator. This, in turn, may lead to excessive sedation and may prolong ventilator weaning and intensive care unit stay.[7] Thus, always "fit your ventilator to the patient, not the patient to the ventilator."

## DIAGNOSTICS DURING MECHANICAL VENTILATION

The following are simple bedside diagnostic guidelines for patients receiving basic modes of mechanical ventilation.

A. $V_T$
   a. In volume modes (VAC and IMV), the $V_T$ usually is set at 6 to 8 mL/kg of ideal body weight. For patients with ARDS or similar bilateral alveolar processes, the lower end of the $V_T$ (6 mL/kg) should always be used as long as the patient can tolerate it.[8] Most ventilators measure exhaled $V_T$. If there is a significant decrease in the measured $V_T$ compared with the set $V_T$, one needs to check for leaks in the ventilator circuit, including the cuff and tubing. Patients with a chest tube may also have lower measured $V_T$ if there is a lung leak and a portion of the $V_T$ is lost through the chest tube (e.g., in bronchopleural fistula).
   b. In pressure modes (PAC, PSV), a decrease in $V_T$ may indicate increases in airway resistance or decreases in lung compliance or both (see Figs. 22.3 and 22.4). This can happen in

patients who develop bronchospasm, mucus plugging, barotrauma, or pulmonary edema. Migration of the endotracheal tube into the right mainstem bronchus may also decrease $V_T$ because it decreases lung compliance. An increase in $V_T$ may be associated with improvement in underlying respiratory conditions. Occasionally, patients may have very strong respiratory drive and may generate high $V_T$ even at low pressure support.

B. Respiratory rate

a. In general, one should use a higher rate for patients with hypoxemic respiratory failure (20 to 25 breaths/minute) and a lower rate for patients with hypercapnic respiratory failure (8 to 15 breaths/minute). Patients with severe metabolic acidosis may also require a higher rate and $V_E$ to compensate.

b. The development of a high respiratory rate (tachypnea) in a patient who is previously stable may be associated with anxiety, worsening of respiratory conditions, development of complications (e.g., nosocomial pneumonia, sepsis, acute lung injury, fever), or inappropriate ventilator settings. A quick assessment for these latter conditions should be performed before tachypnea is attributed to anxiety. During the assessment, one also needs to pay attention to the development of intrinsic PEEP because the expiratory time tends to be shortened when respiratory rate increases.

c. A low respiratory rate usually is associated with loss of respiratory drive, as seen in deep sedation or the development of acute neurologic events. In these situations, a backup rate may be added to ensure minimum $V_E$ in case the patient develops apnea. This is especially important if the patient is receiving only PSV.

C. Oxygenation

a. When the patient is intubated for hypoxemic respiratory failure, an $FiO_2$ of 1.0 is usually prescribed initially. The $FiO_2$ can be adjusted to maintain an arterial partial pressure of $O_2$ ($PaO_2$) of 60 mm Hg or higher and an $O_2$ saturation of at least 90%.

b. When the $PaO_2$ decreases acutely, one should look for causes of ventilation-perfusion mismatch or shunt. Common causes of acute hypoxemia in mechanically ventilated patients include nosocomial pneumonia, sepsis, pulmonary edema, acute lung injury, pulmonary embolism, and atelectasis/lung collapse. $PaO_2$ can be increased by increasing $FiO_2$ unless a large shunt is present. In patients with ARDS,

pulmonary edema, or diffuse lung parenchymal diseases, increasing PEEP also improves oxygenation. The effect of increasing $V_T$ and respiratory rate (and hence $V_E$) on oxygenation is quite small.

D. Inspiratory flow rate

a. In volume modes (VAC and IMV), the inspiratory flow rate is usually set at 40 to 90 L/minute. If the patient has high inspiratory flow demands, the inspiratory flow can be increased up to 90 to 120 L/minute. In these patients, higher flow rates may improve comfort, decrease inspiratory work, and, if they slow the respiratory rate, decrease intrinsic PEEP. Increases in inspiratory flow rate invariably result in increased Paw, which may trigger high-pressure alarms. If this happens or if the patient is still not comfortable, one can try pressure modes (PAC or PSV). The pressure modes usually provide much higher initial inspiratory flow than the volume modes while limiting the airway pressure.

b. Volume modes (VAC, IMV) typically show a square flow pattern because of the fixed inspiratory flow rate, whereas pressure modes (PAC, PSV) usually employ a decelerating flow pattern. Modern ventilators allow clinicians to set the flow patterns even in the volume modes. A decelerating flow pattern is associated with lower inspiratory pressure.[1]

E. Paw and Pplat

a. In volume modes, increases in Paw are associated with increased airway resistance or decreased respiratory system compliance. One can measure Pplat using an inspiratory pause function at end-inspiration to differentiate the two conditions. If increased airway resistance is the cause of increased Paw (e.g., bronchospasm, mucus plugging), the Pplat will be unchanged. If decreased respiratory system compliance is the cause (e.g., pneumothorax, pulmonary edema), the Pplat will increase.

b. In pressure modes, because pressures are limiting, changes in airway resistance or respiratory system compliance are not associated with airway pressure changes. Rather, the $V_T$ will decrease (see Figs. 22.3 and 22.4).

F. Trigger sensitivity

a. If the ventilator uses pressure trigger, the trigger sensitivity is usually set at −0.5 to −1.5 cm $H_2O$. If flow is the trigger mechanism, the trigger sensitivity is usually set at 1 to 3 L/minute. If the trigger is too sensitive, excessive numbers of breaths may be delivered inadvertently. At worst, the machine may even self-cycle. If the trigger is too insensitive, it may result in increased work of breathing. Both situations can cause patient's discomfort and anxiety and may lead to patient-ventilator dyssynchrony.

b. The recognition of patient-ventilator dyssynchrony resulting from inappropriate triggering is important and can be facilitated by observing the patient's chest wall movement and analyzing the pressure and flow waveforms. The most common cause of trigger insensitivity is the intrinsic PEEP. One should always be vigilant about the presence of intrinsic PEEP and, if present, minimize it.

## CONCLUSIONS

Mechanical ventilators have become more sophisticated, but the basic physical principles involved in gas delivery by the ventilators are unchanged. The four modes discussed in this chapter employ these basic principles and are available in all ventilators in the modern era. Understanding how to use these basic modes not only allows the clinicians to manage critically ill patients more effectively but also provides a foundation for using the more advanced modes of mechanical ventilation discussed later in this book.

## REFERENCES

1. Munoz JJ, Guerrero E, Escalante JL, et al: Pressure-controlled ventilation versus controlled mechanical ventilation with decelerating inspiratory flow. Crit Care Med 1993;21: 1143–1148.
2. Cinnella G, Conti G, Lofaso F, et al: Effects of assisted ventilation on the work of breathing: Volume-controlled versus pressure-controlled ventilation. Am J Respir Crit Care Med 1996;153:1025–1033.
3. Kallet RH, Campbell AR, Alonso JA, et al: The effects of pressure control versus volume control assisted ventilation on patient work of breathing in acute lung injury and acute respiratory distress syndrome. Respir Care 2000;45: 1085–1096.
4. MacIntyre NR, McConnell R, Cheng KC, Sane A: Patient-ventilator flow dyssynchrony: Flow-limited versus pressure-limited breaths. Crit Care Med 1997;25:1671–1677.
5. Brochard L, Rauss A, Benito S, et al: Comparison of three methods of gradual withdrawal from ventilatory support during weaning from mechanical ventilation. Am J Respir Crit Care Med 1994;150:896–903.
6. Esteban A, Frutos F, Tobin MJ, et al: A comparison of four methods of weaning patients from mechanical ventilation: Spanish Lung Failure Collaborative Group. N Engl J Med 1995;332:345–350.
7. Kress JP, Pohlman AS, O'Connor MF, Hall JB: Daily interruption of sedative infusions in critically ill patients undergoing mechanical ventilation. N Engl J Med 2000;342: 1471–1477.
8. Acute Respiratory Distress Syndrome Network: Ventilation with lower tidal volumes as compared with traditional tidal volumes for acute lung injury and the acute respiratory distress syndrome. N Engl J Med 2000;342:1301–1308.

# CHAPTER 23

# Inverse Ratio Ventilation

Christian Putensen

Today's lung protective ventilatory strategies use a tidal volume ($V_T$) of not more than 6 mL/kg ideal body weight, which has been shown to result in a better outcome when compared with a $V_T$ of 12 mL/kg ideal body weight in patients with acute respiratory distress syndrome (ARDS).[1] During ventilation with small $V_T$, a respiratory rate (RR) up to a maximum of 35 breaths/minute with inspiratory-to-expiratory (I:E) ratios ranging from 1:3 to 1:1 has been recommended to provide alveolar ventilation that minimizes hypercapnia and respiratory acidosis.[1]

In healthy patients breathing for themselves, the ratio of the time spent in inspiration to that in expiration is about 1:2.[2] Therefore, traditionally the I:E ratio has been usually set at 1:2 or 1:1.5 to approximate the normal physiology of inspiration and expiration.

Alternative strategies using lower inflating pressures were initially developed to treat infants with hyaline membrane disease. Reynolds noted in these infants that alveolar recruitment and hence arterial oxygenation could be improved by using low rates of 30 to 40 breaths/minute and long I:E ratios.[2,3] In some infants, improvements in arterial oxygenation were seen when inspiratory times exceeded expiratory times (inversed I:E ratios). In inverse ratio ventilation (IRV), the inspiration time is prolonged, thereby increasing mean airway pressures and allowing the use of lower airway pressure limits. As neonatal ventilation became more widely used in nurseries in the late 1970s, this strategy was frequently used, even though the evidence of efficacy was based on small numbers with improved arterial blood gases as the primary outcome.

In the early 1980s, this ventilation strategy was adopted for adult patients with ARDS to improve severe arterial hypoxemia.[4,5] In the past 25 years, IRV has been used increasingly as an alternative ventilation technique in adult patients with ARDS[4,6–27] to improve oxygenation at lower than conventional peak airway pressure.

## APPLICATION

IRV can be delivered using pressure controlled, time-cycled ventilation (PC-IRV) (5) or volume controlled, time-cycled ventilation (VC-IRV).[4]

### Volume Controlled Inverse Ratio Ventilation

Lengthening the inspiratory time to I:E ratios exceeding 1:1 can be accomplished with VC-IRV either by providing a very slow inspiratory flow or by adding an additional end-inspiratory pause and holding the alveoli inflated for a period of time.[4,28,29] A decelerating flow pattern is seldom used during VC-IRV.[28] When recruitment of initially collapsed lung units or filling of units with long time constants occurs during an end-inspiratory pause, interfilling from areas of different time constants will occur (pendelluft) because no additional fresh gas will be delivered with VC-IRV (Fig. 23.1).[4,28] For an equivalent $V_T$, I:E ratio, and respiratory system impedance, an inspiratory pause results in a greater mean airway pressure than a slow flow insufflation of the lungs. Although a slow inspiratory flow decreases peak airway pressure, this does not necessarily reduce alveolar pressures.

An effect of longer inspiratory times is the potential for incomplete lung emptying resulting from short expiratory times.[4,7,10–12,16,28,30] Under this condition, the lung cannot return to its normal recoil volume, and intrinsic positive end-expiratory pressure (PEEPi) develops.[4,7,10–12,16,28,30] During ongoing mechanical

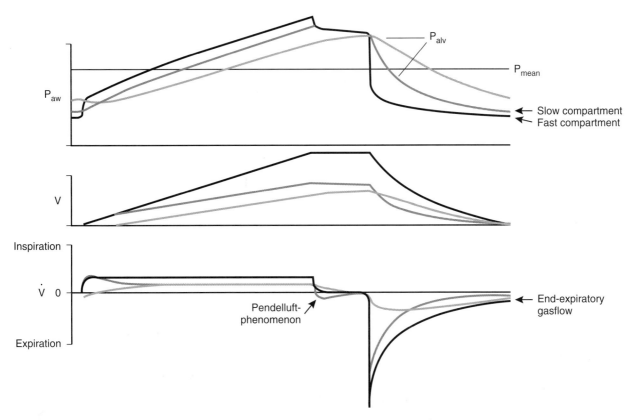

**Figure 23.1** Computer simulation of airway pressure (Paw), volume (V), and gas flow (V) for the respiratory system: a fast and a slow lung compartment for short release time during volume controlled inverse ratio ventilation (IRV). Prolonged inspiratory time with a constant gas flow results in an equilibration of alveolar and airway opening pressure of the slow compartment. Consequent to opening of lung units, gas is distributed from fast to slow compartments during the plateau phase (pendelluft). Expiration in the slow compartment is not completed at end-expiration, as indicated by end-expiratory gas flow, which is associated with intrinsic positive end-expiratory pressure (PEEP).

ventilation, PEEPi may be indicated by the presence of an end-expiratory gas flow.[4,28,31] When this occurs, a fixed $V_T$ will result in higher peak, plateau, and mean airway pressures. Increased plateau pressures may cause overinflation of initially well-ventilated lung areas.[32] Changes in respiratory mechanics, $V_T$, RR, or I:E ratio can significantly alter PEEPi and can thereby contribute to increased plateau pressure.[11]

Advantages claimed for the use of VC-IRV are the delivery of a guaranteed $V_T$, the setting of the inspiratory flow pattern, and the reduction of peak airway pressures (Table 23.1).[4,28,31] A major disadvantage of VC-IRV is that airway pressures may exceed the desired level when, for example, changes in respiratory mechanics lead to an unrecognized increase in PEEPi.[28] Therefore, careful monitoring and continuous display of airway pressures and expiratory flow are recommended during VC-IRV.

## Pressure Controlled Inverse Ratio Ventilation

Prolonging inspiratory time to I:E ratios exceeding 1:1 with PC-IRV results in a square-wave pressure to the airway and a decelerating inspiratory gas flow holding the alveoli inflated for a period of time.[6,7,16,18,19,21,28,33–35]

Flow initially enters the lung rapidly to reach the preset airway pressure as quickly as possible (Fig. 23.2). Alveoli that are open and fill fast receive the greatest amount of gas flow and reach equilibrium with the preset pressure more quickly than slow compartments.[28,31] This may explain why dynamic computed tomography (CT) reveals more overinflated units in nondependent lung slices with PC-IRV.[36] As the open alveoli fill and their pressure reaches equilibrium with the preset pressure, flow decelerates as slow compartments continue to fill with gas (see Fig. 23.2). Flow into the lung continues until the preset pressure reaches equilibrium with alveolar pressure throughout all lung units, as indicated by deceleration of the flow pattern to zero.[31] The ventilator constantly adjusts gas flow so that inspiratory pressure is maintained during the entire set inspiratory time. When recruitment of initially collapsed lung units or filling of units with long time constants occurs during prolonged inspiration, additional fresh gas is delivered with PC-IRV (see Fig. 23.2).[28,31] An effect of longer inspiratory times during PC-IRV is always an increase in the mean airway pressure without altering preset inspiratory pressure.

$V_T$ depends mainly on respiratory compliance and resistance and on the difference between the preset

**Table 23-1**  Advantages and Disadvantages of Volume Controlled Inverse Ratio Ventilation

| Advantages | Disadvantages |
|---|---|
| Guaranteed tidal volume and minute ventilation | Peak and plateau pressure may vary with changes in intrinsic positive end-expiratory pressure |
| Preset flow pattern | Peak and plateau pressure may vary with changes in respiratory system compliance resulting from recruitment or derecruitment |
| Allows low inspiratory gas flows | Peak and plateau pressure may vary considerably and must be monitored carefully to avoid overdistention of lung units<br>Recruitment of lung areas causes delivery of additional gas as well as redistribution of gas from well-ventilated to initially nonventilated lung units (pendelluft)<br>Requires deep sedation |

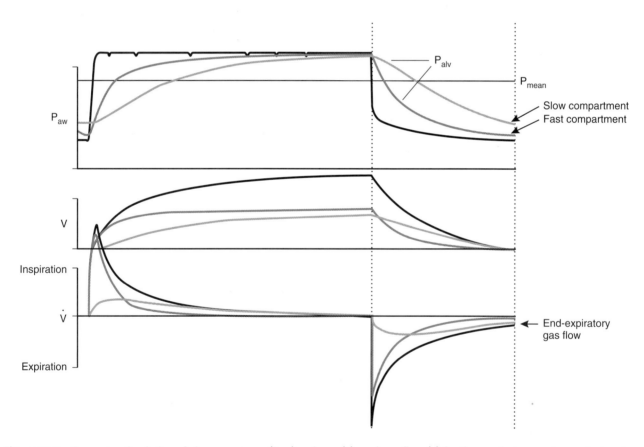

**Figure 23.2**  Computer simulation of airway pressure (Paw), volume (V), and gas flow (V̇) for the respiratory system: a fast and a slow lung compartment for short release time during pressure controlled inverse ratio ventilation (IRV). Prolonged inspiratory time allows completed insufflation of the slow compartment. Expiration in the slow compartment is not completed at end-expiration, as indicated by end-expiratory gas flow, which is associated with intrinsic positive end-expiratory pressure (PEEP).

pressure levels.[28,31] Therefore, any level of PEEPi exerts a direct and possibly undetected opposing pressure, resulting in a smaller alveolar pressure amplitude; consequently, alveolar ventilation decreases and arterial carbon dioxide tension ($PaCO_2$) increases.[31]

The potential advantage of PC-IRV is that airway pressures do not exceed the preset level (Table 23.2). Major disadvantages of PC-IRV include inconstant $V_T$ and hence minute ventilation when, for example, changes in respiratory mechanics lead to an unrecognized increase in PEEPi. Therefore, careful monitoring and continuous display of $V_T$ and expiratory flow are recommended during PC-IRV.

## PRINCIPLES

Lengthening inspiratory time at a constant RR may result in increased mean airway pressure, end-inspiratory pause, and PEEPi. The potential advantage of IRV has been attributed to one of these results or a combination of them.[4,6–22,24,28,31]

### Intrinsic Positive End-Expiratory Pressure

PEEPi occurs when regional or total expiration remains incomplete within the expiratory time available.[24,37] This dynamic phenomenon depends on the respiratory mechanics and on the setting of $V_T$ and the RR and I:E ratio, which determine expiratory time.[38] Thus, PEEPi can be caused by high $V_T$, by short expiratory time, or by high respiratory time constants, or a combination

of these.[7,11,24,37,39,40] Because the time constant is equal to resistance times compliance, high time constants are caused by high airway resistance or compliance, which may occur on a regional basis (e.g., in slow compartments), as well as for the whole respiratory system.[4,31,38] Elevation in airway resistance also can be caused by the design of the ventilator circuit (e.g., narrow tubes, slow PEEP valves).[38]

In inhomogeneous lungs, different PEEPi may occur.[4] It is evident that mainly the slower compartments profit from PEEPi. In ARDS-affected lungs, there is generally a preponderance of fast compartments. Nevertheless, evidence indicates that regional airway and tissue resistances may also be elevated.[41] In large part, this may reflect a decrease in the number of functioning alveoli corresponding to a smaller aerated lung, rather than any alteration in the caliber of airways during ARDS.[41] Although this point is controversial, poorly aerated lung units may have longer time constants than well-aerated lung regions.[42]

A major problem during IRV is that changes in PEEPi (e.g., resulting from altered respiratory mechanics) may not be immediately clinically evident. A remaining terminal flow at the end of expiration indicates that a certain PEEPi exists, but it does not quantify the amount.[4,31] To quantify static PEEPi maneuvers that discontinue mechanical ventilations are required.[43] Static PEEPi represents the average value of PEEPi within a nonhomogeneous lung after equilibration among lung units with differing time constants during end-expiratory occlusion maneuvers of 3 to 5 seconds (Fig. 23.3).[44] The total PEEP (PEEPtotal) applied is the sum of external PEEP and PEEPi.

**Table 23-2   Advantages and Disadvantages of Pressure Controlled Inverse Ratio Ventilation**

| Advantages | Disadvantages |
|---|---|
| Preset airway pressure allows precise control of the peak distending pressure | Tidal volume may vary with changes in intrinsic PEEP |
| Increase in intrinsic PEEP will not result in increased plateau pressures | Tidal volume may vary with changes in respiratory system compliance owing to recruitment or derecruitment |
| Recruited lung units receive additional gas volume | Minute ventilation may vary considerably and must be monitored carefully |
| May be tolerated with lighter deep sedation | Greater shear forces have been postulated (?) |

PEEP, positive end-expiratory pressure.

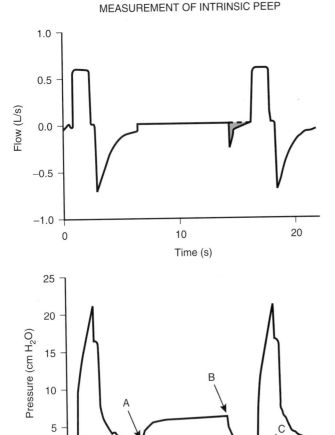

MEASUREMENT OF INTRINSIC PEEP

**Figure 23.3** Measurement of intrinsic positive end-expiratory pressure (PEEPi) performed by the occlusion technique. At end-expiration, the airway is occluded with a valve (A). The pressure measured at this moment is the preset extrinsic PEEP (A). Then, redistribution of gas increases at end-expiration (B). The pressure difference between A and B represents PEEPi. When the valve is opened and expiration occurs (C), the shaded area under the flow curve equals the change in end-expiratory lung volume caused by PEEPi.

## Mean Airway Pressure

During positive pressure ventilation of a passive subject, mean airway pressure is the pressure measured at the airway opening, averaged over the entire ventilatory cycle. Prolongation of inspiratory time and occurrence of PEEPi increase mean airway pressure during IRV.[4,6,8–10,14,37] An increase in mean airway pressure elevates mean alveolar pressure by a variable amount, depending mainly on the ventilated volume and the relative differences of resistances during expiration and inspiration.[28,41] Mean airway pressure is also a major

determinant of the transpulmonary pressure, which is the difference between alveolar and pleural pressures.[45]

During insufflation, a sufficiently high transpulmonary pressure has to be generated to open airways and to recruit nonventilated alveoli, thereby reducing intrapulmonary shunting of blood and improving arterial oxygenation.[45,46] Observations in patients with ARDS confirmed that recruitment of nonventilated alveoli occurs along the whole pressure volume curve.[46] However, to prevent recollapse of these airways and alveoli, a minimum level of transpulmonary pressure has to be maintained during expiration.[46,47] Therefore, during IRV, elevation in mean airway pressure is a major determinant of oxygenation because it increases transpulmonary pressure and thus promotes alveolar recruitment.[24,48,49]

Because the normal lungs are inflated to total lung capacity with transpulmonary pressures of approximately 35 cm $H_2O$, the consensus is that peak transpulmonary pressures exceeding 35 cm $H_2O$ may significantly increase the risk of lung tissue injury. Experimental models indicate that transpulmonary pressures of 30 to 50 cm $H_2O$ provoke diffuse lung edema and injury and increase the incidence of barotrauma.[50,51] In one study using extremely large VT of 15 to 20 mL/kg, pneumothoraces occurred in 23% of the IRV attempts.[9] Thus, during IRV, an increase in mean airway pressure to recruit nonaerated alveoli has to be carefully balanced against the risk of overdistending and injuring already well-aerated regions in the inhomogeneously injured lungs in ARDS.

## Sustained Insufflation and End-Inspiratory Pause

Sustained elevations in airway pressure have been claimed to recruit lung units more effectively than transient increases.[52–54] Investigators have suggested that nonaerated alveoli may require sustained high airway pressures to open. In fact, sustained inflation pressures applied during recruitment maneuvers could be demonstrated to be advantageous to recruit nonaerated lung units in the early phase of ARDS.[55] Furthermore, some lung units with long ventilatory time constants may require a prolonged inspiratory time to inflate completely. Although this point is controversial, poorly aerated lung units may have longer time constants and therefore may benefit from prolonged inspiratory times. Based on current knowledge, sustained inflation during IRV should be used only in the early phase of ARDS, when lung units are still recruitable.

Prolonged inspiration may be accomplished using different flow patterns. The decelerating flow pattern during PC-IRV is believed to provide better gas distribution than continuous low-flow inflation during VC-IRV.[52–54] The high flow rates generated in the beginning of inspiration during PC-IRV are claimed to result in greater shear forces because gas in this phase is primarily distributed to the well-aerated alveoli, whereas ventilation of collapsed alveoli and units with long ventilatory time constants may start later. In contrast, low flow rates that can be set during VC-IRV are suggested to lower shear forces between different aerated lung units.[56] However, no data are currently available to support these suggested advantages of PC-IRV or VC-IRV.

## VENTILATORY SETTING

### Setting Ventilation Pressures and Tidal Volumes

Mechanical ventilation with PEEP titrated to more than the lower inflection pressure of a static pressure-volume curve and a low $V_T$ is thought to prevent tidal alveolar collapse at end-expiration and overdistention of lung units at end-inspiration in patients with ARDS.[1] This lung protective strategy causes improvement in lung compliance, venous admixture, and arterial oxygen tension ($PaO_2$) without causing cardiovascular impairment in ARDS.[1] Mechanical ventilation using $V_T$ of not more than 6 mL/kg ideal body weight has been shown to result in a better outcome when compared with a $V_T$ of 12 mL/kg ideal body weight in patients with ARDS.[1] In these patients, plateau pressure was limited to 30 cm $H_2O$ during mechanical ventilation using $V_T$ of not more than 6 mL/kg ideal body weight because plateau pressure independently predicts mortality when $V_T$ is held constant.[1] Based on these results, $V_T$ of not more than 6 mL/kg ideal body weight should be used, whereas airway pressure levels during IRV should be titrated to prevent end-expiratory alveolar collapse and tidal alveolar overdistention.

The PEEPtotal applied is the sum of external and PEEPi and should at least be kept at a level sufficient to prevent recollapse of the alveoli at risk.[46,47,49] The shortening of the expiratory time consequent to the higher RR frequently used with low $V_T$ may generate substantial PEEPi and may lead to an unrecognized increase in PEEPtotal.[39,57] Therefore, regular determination of PEEPi using an end-expiratory occlusion technique is recommended.[43] If PEEPtotal exceeds the desired level, reduction of the external PEEP or of PEEPi by prolonging the expiratory time may be required. However, in this situation, external PEEP and PEEPi may not be equipotent in recruiting the lungs and in improving gas exchange.[16]

### Setting Respiratory Rate and Inspiratory-to-Expiratory Ratio

During conventional lung protective ventilation using $V_T$ of not more than 6 mL/kg ideal body weight, an RR up to a maximum of 35 breaths/minute with I:E ratios ranging from 1:3 to 1:1 has been recommended to provide adequate alveolar ventilation and to minimize hypercapnia and respiratory acidosis.[1] Setting the RR to 35 breaths/minute and the I:E ratio to 1:1 results in an expiration time of 0.85 seconds, which has been demonstrated to generate PEEPi in patients with ARDS.[39,57]

During IRV, I:E ratios from 1.5:1 to 4:1 are used.[4,6–22,24,28,31] Setting the RR to 35 breaths/minute and increasing the I:E ratio to 4:1 result in an extremely short expiration time of 0.35 seconds. Therefore, a lower RR is generally required to allow expiratory times that do not result in extremely high levels of PEEPi. If the expiratory time is shorter than four times the time constant of the lungs (time constant = compliance × resistance), alveolar pressure will not equilibrate at external PEEP, and PEEPi will result.[39,43,57] At a fixed I:E ratio, already small alterations in the RR may significantly change PEEPi.

During PC-IRV, the duration of the inspiratory pressure level needs to allow at least complete inflation of the lungs, as indicated by an end-inspiratory phase of no flow.[28,58] During VC-IRV, the constant inspiratory gas flow should be reduced to a level allowing a small inspiratory pause,[4,28,29] to guarantee complete application of $V_T$.

## ANALGESIA AND SEDATION

Analgesia and sedation are used not only to ensure satisfactory pain relief and anxiolysis but also to help the patient adapt to mechanical ventilation.[38] The long inspiratory phase of IRV usually makes this technique incompatible with spontaneous breathing, and respiratory depressants or muscle relaxants frequently must be administered to ensure patient acceptance.[12] Thus, the levels of analgesia and sedation required during IRV are equivalent to a Ramsay score between 4 and 5 (i.e., a deeply sedated patient unable to respond when spoken to and who has no sensation of pain).[12]

Suppressing spontaneous breathing during IRV can be achieved by hyperventilation, sedation, or muscle relaxation. Hyperventilation in conjunction with respiratory alkalosis may result in a drop in cardiac output, cerebral vasoconstriction, increased oxygen consumption, bronchoconstriction, and alveolar ventilation-perfusion mismatch.[59,60] Analgesia and sedation sufficient to suppress respiratory efforts is known to cause significant cardiovascular depression.[61] In addition, it may take longer for the patient to wake up, and weaning may be prolonged following the long-term use of sedatives and analgesics.[62] Using muscle relaxants to facilitate adaptation with IRV has been frequently recommended when high doses of sedatives and analgesics do not provide adequate adaptation of the patient to IRV.

Airway pressure release ventilation (APRV) provides a pressure pattern identical to PC-IRV by switching between the two continuous positive airway pressure levels while allowing spontaneous breathing in any phase of the ventilator cycle.[63] Reports on the favorable effects of APRV support the concept of PC-IRV.[64] In fact, APRV incorporates the characteristics of PC-IRV, spontaneous breathing, and partial ventilatory support into one technique with potentially widespread applicability.

## Ventilation Distribution

The change in the I:E ratio from the conventional 1:2 to 2:1 up to 4:1 was claimed to improve alveolar gas mixing, ventilation distribution, and alveolar recruitment and thereby gas exchange.[15,58] IRV is usually provided in the PC-IRV mode, which results in an early rapid increase in airway pressure and inspiratory flow. This rapid flow increase was thought to open up closed airways, and the prolonged inspiratory phase was claimed to promote alveolar recruitment.[28,58]

Although the foregoing may be possible mechanisms, the main effect is more likely to be interruption of expiration by the short expiratory time. This causes PEEPi that should keep the alveoli recruited. When compared with conventional mechanical ventilation using extrinsic PEEP of the same magnitude as that produced intrinsically by IRV, IRV had no advantage.[16]

CT imaging of patients with ARDS has demonstrated radiographic densities corresponding to alveolar collapse localized primarily in the dependent lung regions; this alveolar collapse correlates with intrapulmonary shunting and accounts for the observed arterial hypoxemia.[65] Formation of radiographic densities has been attributed to alveolar collapse caused by superimposed pressure on the lung and a cephalad shift of the diaphragm most notable in dependent lung areas.[66] Because of the long inspiratory time in conjunction with the short expiratory time, IRV was postulated to promote aeration of poorly aerated lung units that may have longer time constants. However, this concept was not supported by CT observations in experimentally induced lung injury. Investigators demonstrated that, during IRV, the upper, already well-aerated lung regions become even more aerated, whereas poorly or nonaerated lung units localized in the dependent lung regions were less aerated when compared with conventional mechanical ventilation with essentially the same mean airway pressure and extrinsic PEEP or PEEPi.[30,32,36] Distribution of pulmonary blood flow, assessed by injection of radioactive microspheres, showed no consistent difference between IRV and conventional mechanical ventilation, but intrapulmonary shunt, assessed by a multiple inert gas elimination technique, increased during IRV.[16]

In patients with ARDS, conversion from volume controlled time-cycled mechanical ventilation to PC-IRV or VC-IRV has been frequently observed to improve compliance and arterial oxygenation and to decrease the ratio of dead space ($V_D$) to $V_T$ and $Paco_2$.[4,6-10,13,14,17,21,26,29,35] However, this oxygenation improvement may be accounted for either by recruitment of lung units or by redirected blood flow within the injured lung. In the latter circumstance, $Paco_2$ may increase. When recruitment is the explanation for improved oxygenation, carbon dioxide exchange is not compromised and may even improve, a finding reflecting increased alveolar ventilation.[67] Other investigations did not find any improvement in pulmonary mechanics or gas exchange during IRV.[14,16,20,25,40] Based on these data, it may be concluded that IRV may improve ventilation of initially poorly or nonventilated alveoli only in selected patients with severe ARDS.

## Gas Exchange

The change in the I:E ratio from the conventional 1:2 to 2:1 up to 4:1 was initially reported to improve arterial oxygenation, sometimes dramatically.[4,6-10,13,14,17,21,26,29,35] However, all these observations were made when conventional mechanical ventilation and IRV were compared with different levels of PEEPtotal and mean airway pressures.

Zavala and co-workers observed that VC-IRV and PC-IRV did not provide any short-term improvement of intrapulmonary shunting and gas exchange when compared with conventional mechanical ventilation with PEEP at similar levels of PEEPtotal, $V_T$, RR, and inspiratory fraction of oxygen.[16] These results are in agreement with those of previous studies,[14] which showed that IRV did not improve arterial oxygenation compared with conventional mechanical ventilation with PEEP, when the comparison was made at equal levels of PEEPtotal, with the other ventilator settings kept constant. Comparably, Lessard and co-workers, in a study of nine patients with ARDS, found that PC-IRV and VC-IRV at 2:1 and 3:1 showed no additional benefit in respiratory mechanics and arterial oxygenation over ventilation with a 1:2 ratio.[25]

Armstrong and MacIntyre compared conventional mechanical ventilation PC-IRV using identical $V_T$ and PEEP values while avoiding generation of PEEPi during IRV.[13] Thus, the effect of prolonged inspiratory times to increase mean airway pressure in the absence of PEEPi was investigated. Armstrong and MacIntyre demonstrated that arterial oxygenation is primarily a function of mean airway pressure, and longer inspiratory times can be used to improve arterial oxygenation.[13] In contrast, Mercat and co-workers demonstrated, in patients with ARDS, that prolongation of inspiratory pressure in the absence of a significant increase in PEEPi does not consistently improve arterial oxygenation but may enhance carbon dioxide elimination.[24]

Clinical observations indicate that IRV does not improve gas exchange in all patients with severe ARDS despite mean airway pressure increases.[14,25] Apparently, improvement of arterial oxygenation requires recruitment of previously nonventilated lung areas during IRV. When arterial oxygenation increases because of recruitment, the $PaCO_2$ decreases primarily because of increased alveolar ventilation, because part of the minute ventilation is delivered to the newly recruited and perfused lung regions.[67] This mechanism may explain why most studies found improved oxygenation and enhanced efficacy of ventilation with reduction in $V_D/V_T$ and $PaCO_2$.[7,10,14,24,53] In contrast, when an increase in mean airway pressure during IRV results in overdistention of well-aerated lung units, redistribution of pulmonary blood flow to poorly or nonventilated lung units may even deteriorate arterial oxygenation and increase $PaCO_2$.[9,13,19,26,40] Clinical studies in patients with ARDS show that IRV does not necessarily lead to instant improvement in gas exchange, but rather leads to a continuous improvement in oxygenation over time.[4,12]

## Cardiovascular Effects

Application of positive pressure ventilation generates an increase in airway pressure and, therefore, in intrathoracic pressure, which, in turn, reduces venous return to the heart.[68] In normovolemic and hypovolemic patients, this produces a reduction in right and left ventricular filling and results in decreased stroke volume, cardiac output, and oxygen delivery ($DO_2$).[68] To normalize systemic blood flow during mechanical ventilation, intravascular volume often needs to be increased, or the cardiovascular system needs pharmacologic support.

Elevation of mean airway pressure resulting from prolongation of inspiratory time with or without PEEPi increases intrathoracic pressure and thereby decreases venous return to the heart, as well as right and left ventricular filling, cardiac output, and $DO_2$.[69] Clinical studies showed that IRV, with or without PEEPi, decreases cardiac index.[7,10,14,29,40] It is possible to select I:E ratios that improve gas exchange without adverse cardiocirculatory consequences.[7] In 10 patients with severe ARDS who were ventilated with IRV, Cole and co-workers observed a decrease in cardiac index with I:E ratios of 4:1, but not with ratios of 1.7:1 or 1.1:1.[7] Similarly, other investigators did not see severe cardiocirculatory instability when converting conventional ventilation to IRV with I:E ratios of 2:1.[6,17,25]

## Oxygen Supply and Demand Balance

A decrease in cardiac index and improvement of arterial oxygenation during IRV may not improve or may even deteriorate the relationship between tissue oxygen supply and demand.[7,10,14,29] Then IRV can have a negative effect on the perfusion and functioning of extrathoracic organ systems.[20,23] Increased $DO_2$ with unchanged oxygen consumption indicates an improved tissue oxygen supply and demand balance, as reflected by a decrease in oxygen extraction rate and higher central or mixed venous oxygen saturation. Therefore, careful monitoring of central or mixed venous oxygen saturation is recommended during IRV.

## CLINICAL ADVANTAGES

Based on physiologic findings, IRV may be advantageous in recruiting atelectasis and thereby in improving pulmonary gas exchange, even in patients with severe ARDS who are treated with conventional mechanical ventilation and high PEEP and inspiratory oxygen fraction.[15,27]

## LIMITATIONS

It is obvious that IRV is strictly contraindicated in obstructive lung diseases (e.g., acute bronchial asthma and chronic obstructive pulmonary disease) because of the risk of further deterioration of the already increased lung volume.[28,38] In these patients, IRV is expected to cause further filling of overdistended lung units. In small-caliber airways, the short expiration and prolonged expiratory time constants result in extreme PEEPi caused by gas trapping. Excessive air trapping and hyperinflation of these lung units may exacerbate the potential for alveolar rupture.

Because increases in transalveolar pressure are caused by higher mean airway pressures, the concomitant rise in intrathoracic pressure may contribute to deterioration of cardiovascular function during IRV.[10,16,29] Therefore, in the presence of improved arterial oxygenation, reduction of systemic blood flow may not necessarily result in better $DO_2$.

Incompatibility with spontaneous breathing is a major limitation of IRV. The long inspiratory phase of IRV usually is incompatible with spontaneous breathing because deep sedation and sometimes muscle paralysis are needed to ensure patient acceptance. Therefore, use of IRV is limited to patients who do not require deep sedation for the management of their underlying disease. An increased need for sedation during IRV may not help to reduce the doses of vasopressors and positive inotropes, while maintaining cardiovascular function stable, and probably does not shorten the duration of ventilator support.[61] An alternative to PC-IRV is APRV, which provides a long inspiratory phase with continuous positive airway pressure (CPAP) and therefore allows unrestricted spontaneous breathing in any phase of the mechanical ventilator cycle.[64]

## INDICATIONS

Based on published data, IRV should be restricted to patients with severe ARDS and profound hypoxemia, despite conventional mechanical ventilation with high PEEP and inspiratory oxygen fraction, and deep sedation for the management of their underlying disease.[15,27]

## REFERENCES

1. Acute Respiratory Distress Syndrome Network: Ventilation with lower tidal volumes as compared with traditional tidal volumes for acute lung injury and the acute respiratory distress syndrome. N Engl J Med 2000;342:1301–1308.

2. Reynolds EO: Effect of alterations in mechanical ventilator settings on pulmonary gas exchange in hyaline membrane disease. Arch Dis Child 1971;46:152–159.

3. Reynolds EO: Pressure waveform and ventilator settings for mechanical ventilation in severe hyaline membrane disease. Int Anesthesiol Clin 1974;12:259–280.

4. Baum M, Benzer H, Mutz N, et al: [Inversed ratio ventilation (IRV): Role of the respiratory time ratio in artificial respiration in ARDS]. Anaesthesist 1980;29:592–596.

5. Lachmann B, Schairer W, Armbruster S, et al: Effects of different inspiratory/expiratory (I/E) ratios and PEEP-ventilation on blood gases and hemodynamics in dogs with severe respiratory distress syndrome (RDS). Adv Exp Med Biol 1989;248:769–777.

6. Abraham E, Yoshihara G: Cardiorespiratory effects of pressure controlled inverse ratio ventilation in severe respiratory failure. Chest 1989;96:1356–1359.

7. Cole AG, Weller SF, Sykes MK: Inverse ratio ventilation compared with PEEP in adult respiratory failure. Intensive Care Med 1984;10:227–232.

8. Gurevitch MJ, Van DJ, Young ES, Jackson K: Improved oxygenation and lower peak airway pressure in severe adult respiratory distress syndrome: Treatment with inverse ratio ventilation. Chest 1986;89:211–213.

9. Tharratt RS, Allen RP, Albertson TE: Pressure controlled inverse ratio ventilation in severe adult respiratory failure. Chest 1988;94:755–762.

10. Mercat A, Graini L, Teboul JL, et al: Cardiorespiratory effects of pressure-controlled ventilation with and without inverse ratio in the adult respiratory distress syndrome. Chest 1993;104:871–875.

11. Valta P, Takala J: Volume-controlled inverse ratio ventilation: Effect on dynamic hyperinflation and auto-PEEP. Acta Anaesthesiol Scand 1993;37:323–328.

12. Sydow M, Burchardi H, Ephraim E, et al: Long-term effects of two different ventilatory modes on oxygenation in acute lung injury: Comparison of airway pressure release ventilation and volume-controlled inverse ratio ventilation. Am J Respir Crit Care Med 1994;149:1550–1556.

13. Armstrong BW Jr, MacIntyre NR: Pressure-controlled, inverse ratio ventilation that avoids air trapping in the adult respiratory distress syndrome. Crit Care Med 1995;23:279–285.

14. Mercat A, Titiriga M, Anguel N, et al: Inverse ratio ventilation (I/E = 2/1) in acute respiratory distress syndrome: A six-hour controlled study. Am J Respir Crit Care Med 1997;155:1637–1642.

15. Falke KJ: Randomized clinical trial of pressure-controlled inverse ratio ventilation and extracorporeal $CO_2$ removal for adult respiratory distress syndrome. Am J Respir Crit Care Med 1997;156:1016–1017.

16. Zavala E, Ferrer M, Polese G, et al: Effect of inverse I:E ratio ventilation on pulmonary gas exchange in acute respiratory distress syndrome. Anesthesiology 1998;88:35–42.

17. Gore DC: Hemodynamic and ventilatory effects associated with increasing inverse inspiratory-expiratory ventilation. J Trauma 1998;45:268–272.

18. Okamoto K, Kukita I, Hamaguchi M, et al: Combination of inhaled nitric oxide therapy and inverse ratio ventilation in patients with sepsis-associated acute respiratory distress syndrome. Artif Organs 2000;24:902–908.

19. Smith RP, Fletcher R: Pressure-controlled inverse ratio ventilation after cardiac surgery. Eur J Anaesthesiol 2001;18:401–406.

20. Huang CC, Shih MJ, Tsai YH, et al: Effects of inverse ratio ventilation versus positive end-expiratory pressure on gas exchange and gastric intramucosal $PCO_2$ and pH under constant mean airway pressure in acute respiratory distress syndrome. Anesthesiology 2001;95:1182–1188.

21. Wang SH, Wei TS: The outcome of early pressure-controlled inverse ratio ventilation on patients with severe acute respiratory distress syndrome in surgical intensive care unit. Am J Surg 2002;183:151–155.

22. Tripathi M, Pandey RK, Dwivedi S: Pressure controlled inverse ratio ventilation in acute respiratory distress syndrome patients. J Postgrad Med 2002;48:34–36.

23. Taplu A, Gokmen N, Erbayraktar S, et al: Effects of pressure- and volume-controlled inverse ratio ventilation on haemodynamic variables, intracranial pressure and cerebral perfusion pressure in rabbits: A model of subarachnoid haemorrhage under isoflurane anaesthesia. Eur J Anaesthesiol 2003;20:690–696.

24. Mercat A, Diehl JL, Michard F, et al: Extending inspiratory time in acute respiratory distress syndrome. Crit Care Med 2001;29:40–44.

25. Lessard MR, Guerot E, Lorino H, et al: Effects of pressure-controlled with different I:E ratios versus volume-controlled ventilation on respiratory mechanics, gas exchange, and hemodynamics in patients with adult respiratory distress syndrome. Anesthesiology 1994;80:983–991.

26. Lain DC, DiBenedetto R, Morris SL, et al: Pressure control inverse ratio ventilation as a method to reduce peak inspiratory pressure and provide adequate ventilation and oxygenation. Chest 1989;95:1081–1088.

27. Morris AH, Wallace CJ, Menlove RL, et al: Randomized clinical trial of pressure-controlled inverse ratio ventilation and extracorporeal $CO_2$ removal for adult respiratory distress syndrome. Am J Respir Crit Care Med 1994;149: 295–305.

28. Marcy TW, Marini JJ: Inverse ratio ventilation in ARDS: Rationale and implementation. Chest 1991;100:494–504.

29. Duma S, Baum M, Benzer H, et al: [Inversed ratio ventilation (IRV) following cardiosurgical procedures]. Anaesthesist 1982;31:549–556.

30. Ludwigs U, Klingstedt C, Baehrendtz S, et al: Volume-controlled inverse ratio ventilation in oleic acid induced lung injury: Effects on gas exchange, hemodynamics, and computed tomographic lung density. Chest 1995;108:804–809.

31. Marik PE, Krikorian J: Pressure-controlled ventilation in ARDS: A practical approach. Chest 1997;112:1102–1106.

32. Neumann P, Berglund JE, Andersson LG, et al: Effects of inverse ratio ventilation and positive end-expiratory pressure in oleic acid-induced lung injury. Am J Respir Crit Care Med 2000;161:1537–1545.

33. Lachmann B, Grossmann G, Freyse J, Robertson B: Lung-thorax compliance in the artificially ventilated premature rabbit neonate

in relation to variations in inspiration:expiration ratio. Pediatr Res 1981;15:833–838.

34. Lachmann B, Schairer W, Armbruster S, et al: Effects of different inspiratory/expiratory (I/E) ratios and PEEP-ventilation on blood gases and hemodynamics in dogs with severe respiratory distress syndrome (RDS). Adv Exp Med Biol 1989;248:769–777.

35. McCarthy MC, Cline AL, Lemmon GW, Peoples JB: Pressure control inverse ratio ventilation in the treatment of adult respiratory distress syndrome in patients with blunt chest trauma. Am Surg 1999;65:1027–1030.

36. Edibam C, Rutten AJ, Collins DV, Bersten AD: Effect of inspiratory flow pattern and inspiratory to expiratory ratio on nonlinear elastic behavior in patients with acute lung injury. Am J Respir Crit Care Med 2003;167:702–707.

37. Yanos J, Watling SM, Verhey J: The physiologic effects of inverse ratio ventilation. Chest 1998;114:834–838.

38. Burchardi H: New strategies in mechanical ventilation for acute lung injury. Eur Respir J 1996;9:1063–1072.

39. Richard JC, Brochard L, Breton L, et al: Influence of respiratory rate on gas trapping during low volume ventilation of patients with acute lung injury. Intensive Care Med 2002;28:1078–1083.

40. Markstrom AM, Lichtwarck-Aschoff M, Hedlund AJ, et al: Under open lung conditions inverse ratio ventilation causes intrinsic PEEP and hemodynamic impairment. Ups J Med Sci 1996;101:257–271.

41. Pelosi P, Cereda M, Foti G, et al: Alterations of lung and chest wall mechanics in patients with acute lung injury: Effects of positive end-expiratory pressure. Am J Respir Crit Care Med 1995;152:531–537.

42. Broseghini C, Brandolese R, Poggi R, et al: Respiratory resistance and intrinsic positive end-expiratory pressure (PEEPi) in patients with the adult respiratory distress syndrome (ARDS). Eur Respir J 1988;1:726–731.

43. Pepe PE, Marini JJ: Occult positive end-expiratory pressure in mechanically ventilated patients with airflow obstruction: The auto-PEEP effect. Am Rev Respir Dis 1982;126:166–170.

44. Rossi A, Gottfried SB, Zocchi L, et al: Measurement of static compliance of the total respiratory system in patients with acute respiratory failure during mechanical ventilation: The effect of intrinsic positive end-expiratory pressure. Am Rev Respir Dis 1985;131:672–677.

45. Gattinoni L, Vagginelli F, Chiumello D, et al: Physiologic rationale for ventilator setting in acute lung injury/acute respiratory distress syndrome patients. Crit Care Med 2003;31:S300–S304.

46. Crotti S, Mascheroni D, Caironi P, et al: Recruitment and derecruitment during acute respiratory failure: A clinical study. Am J Respir Crit Care Med 2001;164:131–140.

47. Gattinoni L, Pelosi P, Crotti S, Valenza F: Effects of positive end-expiratory pressure on regional distribution of tidal volume and recruitment in adult respiratory distress syndrome. Am J Respir Crit Care Med 1995;151:1807–1814.

48. Berman LS, Downs JB, Van EA, Delhagen D: Inspiration: expiration ratio: Is mean airway pressure the difference? Crit Care Med 1981;9:775–777.

49. Gattinoni L, Chiumello D, Carlesso E, Valenza F: Bench-to-bedside review: Chest wall elastance in acute lung injury/acute respiratory distress syndrome patients. Crit Care 2004;8:350–355.

50. Dreyfuss D, Soler P, Basset G, Saumon G: High inflation pressure pulmonary edema: Respective effects of high airway pressure, high tidal volume, and positive end-expiratory pressure. Am Rev Respir Dis 1988;137:1159–1164.

51. Dreyfuss D, Soler P, Saumon G: Mechanical ventilation-induced pulmonary edema. Interaction with previous lung alterations. Am J Respir Crit Care Med 1995;151:1568–1575.

52. Modell HI, Cheney FW: Effects of inspiratory flow pattern on gas exchange in normal and abnormal lungs. J Appl Physiol 1979;46:1103–1107.

53. Knelson JH, Howatt WF, DeMuth GR: Effect of respiratory pattern on alveolar gas exchange. J Appl Physiol 1970;29:328–331.

54. Al-Saady N, Bennett ED: Decelerating inspiratory flow waveform improves lung mechanics and gas exchange in patients on intermittent positive-pressure ventilation. Intensive Care Med 1985;11:68–75.

55. Grasso S, Mascia L, Del Turco M, et al: Effects of recruiting maneuvers in patients with acute respiratory distress syndrome ventilated with protective ventilatory strategy. Anesthesiology 2002;96:795–802.

56. Ludwigs U, Philip A, Robertson B, Hedenstierna G: Pulmonary epithelial permeability: An animal study of inverse ratio ventilation and conventional mechanical ventilation. Chest 1996;110:486–493.

57. de Durante G, del Turco M, Rustichini L, et al: ARDSNet lower tidal volume ventilatory strategy may generate intrinsic positive end-expiratory pressure in patients with acute respiratory distress syndrome. Am J Respir Crit Care Med 2002;165:1271–1274.

58. Gurevitch MJ: Pressure-controlled inverse ratio ventilation: What have we learned? Chest 1993;104:664–665.

59. Domino KB, Lu Y, Eisenstein BL, Hlastala MP: Hypocapnia worsens arterial blood oxygenation and increases VA/Q heterogeneity in canine pulmonary edema. Anesthesiology 1993;78:91–99.

60. Culpepper JA, Rinaldo JE, Rogers RM: Effect of mechanical ventilator mode on tendency towards respiratory alkalosis. Am Rev Respir Dis 1985;132:1075–1077.

61. Putensen C, Zech S, Wrigge H, et al: Long-term effects of spontaneous breathing during ventilatory support in patients with acute lung injury. Am J Respir Crit Care Med 2001;164:43–49.

62. Kress JP, Pohlman AS, O'Connor MF, Hall JB: Daily interruption of sedative infusions in critically ill patients undergoing mechanical ventilation. N Engl J Med 2000;342:1471–1477.

63. Stock MC, Downs JB: Airway pressure release ventilation. Crit Care Med 1987;15:462-466.

64. Putensen C, Mutz NJ, Putensen-Himmer G, Zinserling J: Spontaneous breathing during ventilatory support improves ventilation-perfusion distributions in patients with acute respiratory distress syndrome. Am J Respir Crit Care Med 1999;159:1241–1248.

65. Gattinoni L, Presenti A, Torresin A, et al: Adult respiratory distress syndrome profiles by computed tomography. J Thorac Imaging 1986;1:25–30.

66. Puybasset L, Cluzel P, Chao N, et al: A computed tomography scan assessment of regional lung volume in acute lung injury: The CT Scan ARDS Study Group. Am J Respir Crit Care Med 1998;158:1644–1655.

67. Pelosi P, Cadringher P, Bottino N, et al: Sigh in acute respiratory distress syndrome. Am J Respir Crit Care Med 1999;159:872–880.

68. Pinsky MR: The effects of mechanical ventilation on the cardiovascular system. Crit Care Clin 1990;6:663–678.

69. Downs JB, Douglas ME, Sanfelippo PM, Stanford W: Ventilatory pattern, intrapleural pressure, and cardiac output. Anesth Analg 1977;56:88–96.

# CHAPTER 24

# Airway Pressure Release Ventilation

Christian Putensen

Although introduced as weaning techniques, partial ventilator support modes have become standard methods for primary mechanical ventilator support in critically ill patients with pulmonary dysfunction.[1]

## PRINCIPLES

Airway pressure release ventilation (APRV) ventilates by time-cycled switching between two pressure levels in a high-flow or demand valve continuous positive airway pressure (CPAP) circuit; therefore, APRV allows unrestricted spontaneous breathing in any phase of the mechanical ventilator cycle (Fig. 24.1).[2,3] The degree of ventilator support with APRV is determined by the duration of both CPAP levels and the mechanically delivered tidal volume ($V_T$).[2,3] $V_T$ depends mainly on respiratory compliance and the difference between CPAP levels. In principle, changes in ventilatory demand do not alter the level of mechanical support during APRV. When spontaneous breathing is absent, APRV resembles conventional pressure controlled, time-cycled mechanical ventilation.[2–4]

Biphasic positive airway pressure,[2] bilevel airway pressure, and intermittent mandatory pressure release ventilation (IMPRV)[5] are closely related to APRV. Biphasic positive airway pressure is identical to APRV, except that no restrictions are imposed on the duration of the low CPAP level (release pressure).[2] Based on the initial description, APRV the low CPAP level (release time) for 1.5 seconds or less.[3,6]

## MODIFICATIONS

### Synchronized Airway Pressure Release Ventilation

Asynchronous interferences between spontaneous and mechanical ventilation may increase the work of breathing and reduce alveolar ventilation during APRV.[7] Switching between the two CPAP levels synchronized to spontaneous inspiration or expiration has been incorporated into all commercially available demand valve APRV circuits. Trigger windows of 0.25 to 0.30 second are usually used, to allow synchronization of switching between the two CPAP levels to spontaneous breathing efforts. Data observed in an experimental model mimicking spontaneous ventilation indicated that spontaneous inspiration synchronized to restoration of the high CPAP level, but not spontaneous expiration synchronized with pressure release, may be beneficial.[7] Currently, clinical data on the advantage of synchronized APRV are lacking. Patient-triggered mechanical cycles

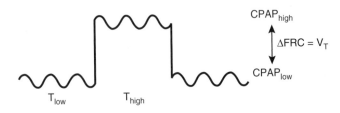

**Figure 24.1** Principle of airway pressure release ventilation.

during intermittent mandatory ventilation (IMV) have not been demonstrated to be advantageous for patients.[8] Comparably, no clinical study demonstrated that synchronized APRV prevents asynchronous interferences between spontaneous and mechanical breaths.[7]

Synchronization during APRV may result in inconstant durations of high and low CPAP. Therefore, to maintain a constant mean airway pressure over time, commercial ventilators often use algorithms to vary the durations of the CPAP levels during synchronized APRV.

## Combination with Other Partial Ventilatory Support Modalities

Most commercially available ventilators offer APRV in combination with other partial ventilatory support modalities, such as APRV in combination with pressure support ventilation (PSV) and APRV in combination with automatic tube compensation (ATC).[9]

## Intermittent Mandatory Pressure Release Ventilation

During IMPRV, spontaneous inspiratory efforts on the high CPAP level are assisted with PSV during APRV.[5] Breath-to-breath inspiratory support, synchronization of mechanical breaths to spontaneous breathing, and increase in airway pressure to more than the high CPAP level are the differences between IMPRV and APRV. IMPRV has been demonstrated in patients with acute respiratory failure to provide adequate ventilatory support compared with spontaneous breathing with CPAP.[5] Results of comparisons between IMPRV and other modalities of ventilatory support are not available.

## Airway Pressure Release Ventilation in Combination with Pressure Support Ventilation

Some commercially available ventilators allow assistance of spontaneous inspiratory efforts on the low CPAP level with PSV during APRV. It remains doubtful whether breath-to-breath ventilatory support during short pressure release is of any advantage. Currently, clinical and experimental data are lacking that demonstrate increased ventilatory efficacy by assisting spontaneous breathing on the low CPAP level with PSV during APRV.[10]

## Airway Pressure Release Ventilation in Combination with Automatic Tube Compensation

ATC compensates for endotracheal tube resistance. The ventilator increases airway pressure during inspiration, reduces it during expiration, and aims to keep the tracheal pressure constant and independent of tube resistance. When spontaneous breathing is assisted with ATC during APRV, considerable inspiratory muscle unloading and increased alveolar ventilation can be accomplished without decreasing functional residual capacity or worsening pulmonary gas exchange.[9] Apparently, the transient lowering of airway pressures during expiration with ATC does not promote alveolar collapse or worsen gas exchange when superimposed on APRV.[9] Therefore, in selected patients, APRV combined with ATC may be useful to decrease the work of breathing imposed by the resistance of the endotracheal tube.

Very few of the combinations of APRV with ventilator modalities have been shown to be clinically advantageous.[9] Applying pressure supported breaths with PSV or ATC on the high CPAP level during APRV may result in peak airway pressures associated with significant overdistention of the lungs. Therefore, pressure limits have to be set extremely carefully when using APRV in combination with PSV or APRV in combination with ATC, and airway pressures should not exceed 35 cm $H_2O$. Furthermore, it remains doubtful whether simply combining different modalities of ventilation results in additive positive effects.[11] In contrast, the possibility cannot be ruled out that proven physiologic effects of one modality of ventilatory support may be minimized or even abolished by combining it with another method.

## VENTILATORY SETTING

### Setting Ventilation Pressures and Tidal Volumes

Mechanical ventilation with positive end-expiratory airway pressure titrated above the lower inflection pressure of a static pressure-volume curve and a low $V_T$ is thought to prevent tidal alveolar collapse at end-expiration and overdistention of lung units at end-inspiration in patients with acute respiratory distress syndrome (ARDS).[12] This lung protective strategy causes improvement in lung compliance, venous admixture, and arterial oxygen tension ($Pao_2$) without causing cardiovascular impairment in ARDS.[12] Mechanical ventilation using $V_T$ of not more than 6 mL/kg ideal body weight has been shown to result in a better outcome when compared with a $V_T$ of 12 mL/kg ideal body weight in patients with ARDS.[12,13] Based on these results, CPAP levels during APRV should be titrated to prevent end-expiratory alveolar collapse and tidal alveolar overdistention.[12,13] When CPAP levels during APRV were adjusted in patients with ARDS according to a lung protective strategy, spontaneous breathing led to improved cardiorespiratory function without affecting total oxygen consumption secondary to the work of breathing.[14] Moreover, pulmonary compliance should be greatest in this range of airway pressures, and, thus, a small change in transpulmonary

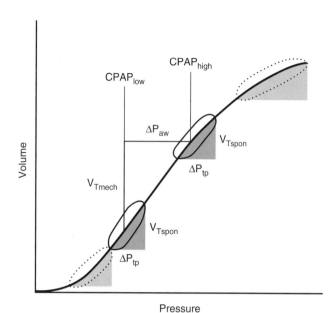

**Figure 24.2** During airway pressure release ventilation (APRV), both continuous positive airway pressure (CPAP) levels should be titrated to result in the highest compliance. A small transpulmonary pressure change allows normal tidal breathing, whereas the elastic work of breathing (*shaded area*) is minimal. CPAP levels that are too high or too low (*dashed line*) will result in an unnecessary increase in the elastic work of breathing (*shaded area*).

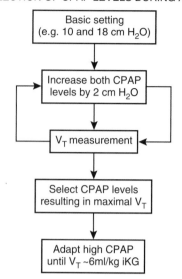

**Figure 24.3** Selection of continuous positive airway pressure (CPAP) levels during airway pressure release ventilation (APRV).

pressure will achieve normal tidal breathing with minimal elastic work of breathing (Fig. 24.2).[15] Because APRV does not provide assistance on every inspiratory effort, the CPAP levels need to be carefully adjusted to achieve efficient spontaneous ventilation with minimal work of breathing.

In clinical practice, increasing the CPAP levels by 2 cm $H_2O$ until a maximal VT is observed facilitates pressure settings during APRV (Fig. 24.3). However, VT should not be more than 6 mL/kg ideal body weight during APRV.

## Setting Times

The duration of the high CPAP level needs to allow at least complete inflation of the lungs, as indicated by an end-inspiratory phase of no flow when spontaneous breathing is absent. Spontaneous breathing occurs normally on the high CPAP level. Thus, duration of the high CPAP level should be adjusted so that it is long enough to allow spontaneous breathing. If the release time is shorter than four times the time constant of the lungs (time constant = compliance × resistance), alveolar pressure will not equilibrate at low CPAP level, and intrinsic positive end-expiratory pressure (PEEPi) will result.[16,17] Incomplete expiration and the likelihood of PEEPi are indicated by gas flow at end-expiration (Fig. 24.4).

In the presence of PEEPi, alveolar pressure amplitude is reduced; consequently, alveolar ventilation decreases, and arterial carbon dioxide tension ($Paco_2$) increases. To date, data do not indicate that PEEPi is superior to external PEEP in preventing derecruitment of the lungs. Thus, the duration of the low CPAP level should be adjusted to allow complete expiration to the resting lung volume.

## Traditional Concepts of Setting Airway Pressure Release Ventilation

Traditionally, high CPAP levels that were soon released to near-ambient pressure were suggested during APRV. Depending on the time constant of the lungs, short release times may result in PEEPi.[16] Clinical studies demonstrate that external PEEP is not superior to PEEPi in restoring gas exchange in mechanically ventilated patients with acute lung injury (ALI).[18] Not surprisingly, in patients with ARDS, atelectasis formation was increased when high CPAP levels were released within 1 to 1.5 seconds to near-ambient pressure during APRV.[19] Using this concept, VT greater than 6 mL/kg ideal body weight was accepted during APRV. Based on available scientific and clinical data, adjusting ventilator settings during APRV should not be recommended.

## ANALGESIA AND SEDATION

Suppression of spontaneous breathing during conventional mechanical ventilation (CMV) can be achieved by

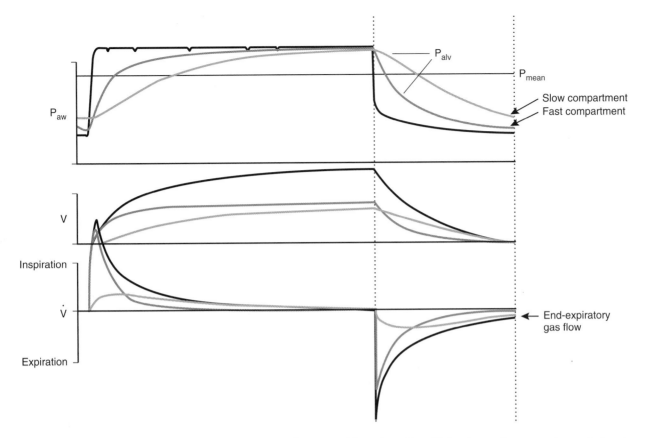

**Figure 24.4** Computer simulation of airway pressure (Paw), volume (V), and gas flow (V̇) for the respiratory system: a fast and a slow lung compartment for short release time. Expiration in the slow compartment is not completed at end-expiration, as indicated by end-expiratory gas flow, which is associated with intrinsic positive end-expiratory pressure (PEEP).

hyperventilation, sedation, or muscle relaxation. Hyperventilation in conjunction with respiratory alkalosis may result in a drop in cardiac output, cerebral vasoconstriction, increased oxygen consumption, bronchoconstriction, and alveolar ventilation-perfusion (VA/Q) mismatch.[20–22] Analgesia and sedation sufficient to suppress respiratory efforts are known to cause significant cardiovascular depression.[23] In addition, it may take longer for the patient to wake up following the long-term use of sedatives and analgesics.[24] Using muscle relaxants to facilitate adaptation with CMV is also open to question. Increasing numbers of reports claim that long-term deep sedation and application of muscle relaxants during CMV in the intensive care unit can lead to muscular atrophy, damage to the neuromuscular end plate, and other muscle function disorders and can therefore delay or even prevent weaning from mechanical ventilation.[25–27]

Analgesia and sedation are used not only to ensure satisfactory pain relief and anxiolysis but also to help the patient adapt to mechanical ventilation.[28] The level of analgesia and sedation required during CMV is equivalent to a Ramsay score between 4 and 5 (i.e., a deeply sedated patient unable to respond when spoken to and who has no sensation of pain). During APRV, a Ramsay score between 2 and 3 can be targeted (i.e., an awake, responsive, and cooperative patient).[23]

In nearly 600 patients after cardiac surgery,[29] and in patients with multiple injuries,[23] maintenance of spontaneous breathing during APRV led to less consumption of analgesics and sedatives as compared with initial use of CMV followed by weaning with partial ventilator support. Higher doses of analgesics and sedatives used exclusively to adapt patients to CMV required higher doses of vasopressors and positive inotropes to maintain stable cardiovascular function compared with spontaneous breathing during APRV.[23] Higher doses of analgesics and sedatives used in patients managed with CMV are associated with the use of higher doses of vasopressors and inotropic agents to maintain stable cardiovascular function.[23] Compared with an initial period of CMV followed by weaning, maintenance of spontaneous breathing with APRV is associated with significantly fewer days of ventilator support, earlier extubation, and a shorter stay in the intensive care unit.[23] These findings may be explained by a lower level of sedation required during APRV.

## PHYSIOLOGIC EFFECTS

### Ventilation Distribution

Radiologic studies demonstrate that ventilation is distributed differently during pure spontaneous breathing and CMV.[30] During spontaneous breathing, the posterior muscular sections of the diaphragm move more than the anterior tendon plate.[30] Consequently, in patients in the supine position, the dependent lung regions tend to be better ventilated during spontaneous breathing (Fig. 24.5). If the diaphragm is relaxed, it will be moved by the weight of the abdominal cavity, and the intra-abdominal pressure toward the cranium and the mechanical $V_T$ will be distributed more to the anterior, nondependent, and less perfused lung regions.[31] When compared with spontaneous breathing, this leads, both in patients with healthy lungs and in patients undergoing mechanical ventilation, to lung areas in the dorsal lung regions close to the diaphragm that are less ventilated or atelectatic. Investigators have demonstrated that the posterior muscular sections of the diaphragm move more than the anterior tendon plate when large breaths or sighs are present during spontaneous breathing.[32]

Computed tomography (CT) of patients with ARDS demonstrated radiographic densities corresponding to alveolar collapse localized primarily in the dependent lung regions that correlated with intrapulmonary shunting and accounted entirely for the observed arterial hypoxemia.[33] Formation of radiographic densities has been attributed to alveolar collapse caused by superimposed pressure on the lung and a cephalad shift of the diaphragm most evident in dependent lung areas during CMV.[34] The cephalad shift of the diaphragm may be even more pronounced in patients with extrapulmonary-induced ARDS, in whom an increase in intra-abdominal pressure is invariably observed. Persistent spontaneous breathing has been considered to improve distribution of ventilation to dependent lung areas and thereby $V_A/Q$ matching, presumably by the opposition of diaphragmatic contraction and alveolar compression.[14,30] This concept is supported by CT observations in anesthetized patients that contractions of the diaphragm induced by phrenic nerve stimulation favor distribution of ventilation to dependent, well-perfused lung areas and decrease atelectasis formation.[35]

Spontaneous breathing with APRV in experimentally induced lung injury was associated with less atelectasis formation in end-expiratory spiral CT findings in whole lungs and in CT scans above the diaphragm (Fig. 24.6).[36] Although other inspiratory muscles may contribute to improvement in aeration during spontaneous breathing, the craniocaudal gradient in aeration, aeration differences, and the marked differences in aeration in regions close to the diaphragm between APRV with and without spontaneous breathing suggest a predominant role of diaphragmatic contractions on the observed aeration differences.[36] Spontaneous breathing resulted in significant improvement of end-expiratory lung volume in experimental lung injury.[36] Experimental data suggested that recruitment of dependent lung areas may be caused essentially by an increase in transpulmonary pressure resulting from the decrease of pleural pressure with spontaneous breathing during APRV.[37]

### Pulmonary Gas Exchange

In patients with ARDS, APRV with spontaneous breathing of 10% to 30% of the total minute ventilation ($V_E$) accounted for an improvement in $V_A/Q$ matching, intrapulmonary shunting, and arterial oxygenation.[14] These results confirmed earlier investigations in animals with induced lung injury demonstrating improvement in intrapulmonary shunt and arterial oxygenation during spontaneous breathing with APRV.[4,38] An increase in arterial oxygenation in conjunction with greater pulmonary compliance indicated recruitment of previously nonventilated lung areas. Clinical studies in patients with ARDS showed that spontaneous breathing during APRV

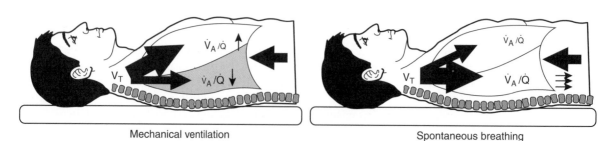

**Figure 24.5** Distribution of ventilation during pure mechanical and spontaneous ventilation.

APRV *with* spontaneous breathing       APRV *without* spontaneous breathing

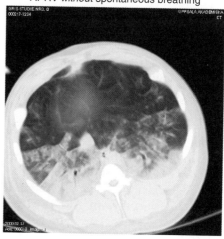

**Figure 24.6** Computed tomography scan of a lung region above the diaphragm at end-expiration in oleic acid–induced lung injury with and without spontaneous breathing during airway pressure release ventilation (APRV). Atelectasis formation is reduced with spontaneous breathing.

does not necessarily lead to instant improvement in gas exchange but rather in a continuous improvement in oxygenation within 24 hours after the start of spontaneous breathing.[39]

In patients at risk of developing ARDS, maintained spontaneous breathing with APRV resulted in lower venous admixture and better arterial blood oxygenation over an observation period of more than 10 days as compared with CMV with subsequent weaning.[23] These results show that, even in patients requiring ventilatory support, maintained spontaneous breathing can counteract progressive deterioration in pulmonary gas exchange.

## Cardiovascular Effects

Application of a mechanical ventilator breath generates an increase in airway pressure and therefore in intrathoracic pressure, which, in turn, reduces venous return to the heart. In normovolemic and hypovolemic patients, this produces a reduction in right and left ventricular filling and decreases stroke volume, cardiac output, and oxygen delivery ($DO_2$).[40] To normalize systemic blood flow during mechanical ventilation, intravascular volume often needs to be increased, or the cardiovascular system needs pharmacologic support. Reducing mechanical ventilation to a level that provides adequate support for existing spontaneous breathing should help to reduce the cardiovascular side effects of ventilator support.[41]

Periodic reduction of intrathoracic pressure resulting from maintained spontaneous breathing during mechanical ventilator support promotes venous return to the heart and right and left ventricular filling, thereby increasing cardiac output and $DO_2$.[42] Experimental[4,38,43] and clinical[14,39,44] studies showed that during APRV with spontaneous breathing of 10% to 40% of total $V_E$ at unchanged $V_E$ or airway pressure limits, this results in an increase in cardiac index. A simultaneous rise in right ventricular end-diastolic volume during spontaneous breathing with APRV indicates improved venous return to the heart.[14] In addition, the outflow from the right ventricle, which depends mainly on the lung volume, the major determinant of pulmonary vascular resistance, may benefit from a decrease in intrathoracic pressure during APRV.[14]

Patients with left ventricular dysfunction may not benefit from augmentation of venous return to the heart and increased left ventricular afterload as a result of reduced intrathoracic pressure. Thus, switching abruptly from CMV to PSV with simultaneous reduction in airway pressure has been demonstrated to result in decompensation of existing cardiac insufficiency.[45] Räsänen and colleagues[46] showed the need for adequate ventilator support and CPAP levels in patients with respiratory and cardiogenic failure. Provided spontaneous breathing receives adequate support and sufficient CPAP levels are applied, maintenance of spontaneous breathing during APRV should not prove disadvantageous and is not contraindicated per se in patients with ventricular dysfunction.[46,47]

## Oxygen Supply and Demand Balance

Increase in cardiac index and $PaO_2$ during APRV improved the relationship between tissue oxygen supply and demand because oxygen consumption remained unchanged despite the work of spontaneous breathing. In accordance with previous experimental[4] and clinical findings,[14,39,48] total oxygen consumption is not measurably altered by adequately supported spontaneous breathing in patients with low lung compliance. Increased $DO_2$ with unchanged oxygen consumption indicates an improved tissue oxygen supply and demand balance, as reflected by a decrease in oxygen extraction rate and higher mixed venous $PO_2$.

## Organ Perfusion

By reducing cardiac index and venous return to the heart, CMV can have a negative effect on the perfusion and functioning of extrathoracic organ systems. Because of the periodic fall in intrathoracic pressure during spontaneous inspiration, an increase in venous return and cardiac index should significantly improve organ perfusion and function during partial ventilatory support. In patients with ARDS, spontaneous breathing with IMV leads to an increase in glomerular filtration rate and sodium excretion.[49] Compatible with these results in patients with ARDS, kidney perfusion and glomerular filtration rate improve during spontaneous breathing with APRV.[50] Thus, maintained spontaneous breathing may be favorable for the perfusion and function of the kidney in patients requiring ventilatory support as a result of severe pulmonary dysfunction.

Preliminary data in patients requiring ventilatory support for ALI suggest that maintained spontaneous breathing may be beneficial for liver function. These clinical data are supported by experimental observations using colored microspheres in pigs with oleic acid–induced lung injury demonstrating improved perfusion of the splanchnic area.[51]

## COMPARISON WITH OTHER VENTILATORY MODALITIES

### Airway Pressure Release Ventilation Versus Pressure Support Ventilation

APRV and PSV were compared in 24 patients with ALI/ARDS using equal $V_E$ or airway pressure limits. Because insufflation during PSV is flow cycled, alveolar end-inspiratory pressure may not reach the preset pressure level. Thus, in patients with reduced lung compliance, equal airway pressure limits result in lower $V_T$ during PSV compared with APRV and require a compensatory increase in respiratory rate during PSV to maintain alveolar ventilation. To deliver APRV and PSV with comparable $V_T$ at an acceptable respiratory rate, the pressure support level has to be increased during PSV.[14]

In contrast to spontaneous breathing with APRV, assisted inspiration with PSV did not produce significant improvement in intrapulmonary shunt, gas exchange, and cardiac output when compared with CMV.[14] Apparently, the spontaneous contribution on a mechanically assisted breath was not sufficient to counteract the $V_A/Q$ maldistribution and cardiovascular depression of positive pressure lung insufflations. One possible explanation may be that inspiration is terminated by the decrease in gas flow at the end of inspiration during PSV, and this, in turn, may reduce ventilation in areas of the lung with a slow time constant.

### Airway Pressure Release Ventilation Versus Intermittent Mandatory Ventilation

In a randomized, multicenter trial in 52 patients with ALI, APRV with lower peak airway pressures resulted in better alveolar ventilation and equal arterial oxygenation when compared with IMV.[52] Not surprisingly, a similar trial in 58 patients with ALI supported these findings but could not show a difference in mortality between the ventilator modalities.[53] In 8 patients recovering from open heart surgery, APRV provided adequate ventilation with lower airway pressures and dead space ventilation than IMV or PSV.[54] Arterial oxygenation was not different among the tested modalities.

## CLINICAL ADVANTAGES

Based on physiologic findings, APRV is advantageous for recruiting atelectasis adjacent to the diaphragm and thereby for improving pulmonary gas exchange in patients with ALI and ARDS, as well as after major surgery.[14,23,29,39] Because the increase in transalveolar pressure is localized to the areas near the diaphragm and is caused by a decrease in intrapleural pressure, the concomitant decrease in intrathoracic pressure contributes to improved cardiovascular function.[14,23,44] Areas of atelectasis not adjacent to the diaphragm may not be successfully recruited by spontaneous breathing during APRV.[55] The reduced requirement for sedation during APRV helps to decrease the doses of vasopressors and positive inotropes, while maintaining stable cardiovascular function, and shortens the duration of ventilator support.[23] Therefore, the use of APRV has to be limited to patients who do not require deep sedation for the management of their underlying disease (e.g., cerebral edema with increased intracranial pressure).

## LIMITATIONS

When airway pressure release occurs during spontaneous inspiration and when restoration of CPAP occurs during spontaneous expiration, ventilation may be impaired because spontaneous and ventilator efforts oppose each other. Given that a reduction in ventilatory efficiency, as indicated by a decrease in alveolar ventilation and an increase in work of breathing, may result from asynchrony, synchronized APRV and sedation may be required in these rare cases.[7]

APRV does not provide breath-to-breath assistance of spontaneous inspiration. Several investigations demonstrated that, in a patient who is difficult to wean, separation from mechanical ventilation may be prolonged when using IMV and shortened with breath-to-breath assistance of inspiratory efforts during PSV.[56] Thus, APRV may not be advantageous in patients who are difficult to wean from mechanical ventilation.

## INDICATIONS

Based on the current literature, APRV is indicated in patients with ALI and ARDS, as well as after major surgery, to recruit atelectasis adjacent to the diaphragm and to restore pulmonary gas exchange while improving cardiovascular and extrathoracic organ function.

## CONTRAINDICATIONS

Because lower levels of sedation (Ramsay score of 2 to 3) are used during APRV to allow spontaneous breathing, APRV should not be used in patients who require deep sedation for management of their underlying disease (e.g., cerebral edema with increased intracranial pressure). APRV has not been investigated in patients with obstructive lung disease or neuromuscular disease. In principle, a short release time would not be beneficial in patients with obstructive lung disease and long expiratory time constants of the lungs. Currently, the use of APRV in patients with obstructive lung disease or neuromuscular disease is not supported by clinical research.

## CONCLUSIONS

Small, randomized, controlled studies suggested that spontaneous breathing during ventilator support should not be suppressed even in patients with severe pulmonary dysfunction if no contraindications (e.g., increased intracranial pressure) are present. Improvements in pulmonary gas exchange, systemic blood flow, and oxygen supply to the tissues, as observed when spontaneous breathing was allowed during ventilator support, are reflected in clinical improvement of the patient's condition. Maintaining spontaneous breathing with APRV may help to decrease days on ventilator support and time of stay in the intensive care unit. In the future, large-scale, randomized, multicenter investigations will be warranted

to evaluate the validity outcome results with APRV in critically ill patients.

Although CMV followed by weaning with partial ventilator support is still considered standard in ventilation therapy, spontaneous breathing with APRV should be reconsidered in view of available data. Today's standard practice should be to maintain spontaneous breathing from the very beginning of ventilatory support and to adapt ventilator support continuously to the patient's individual needs.

## REFERENCES

1. Downs JB, Stock MC, Tabeling B: Intermittent mandatory ventilation (IMV): A primary ventilatory support mode. Ann Chir Gynaecol 1982;196(Suppl):57–63.
2. Baum M, Benzer H, Putensen C, Koller W: Biphasic positive airway pressure (BIPAP): A new form of augmented ventilation. Anaesthesist 1989;38:452–458.
3. Stock MC, Downs JB: Airway pressure release ventilation. Crit Care Med 1987;15:462–466.
4. Putensen C, Räsänen J, Lopez FA: Ventilation-perfusion distributions during mechanical ventilation with superimposed spontaneous breathing in canine lung injury. Am J Respir Crit Care Med 1994;150:101–108.
5. Rouby JJ, Ben Ameur M, Jawish D: Continuous positive airway pressure (CPAP) vs. intermittent mandatory pressure release ventilation (IMPRV) in patients with acute respiratory failure. Intensive Care Med 1992;18:69–75.
6. Garner W, Downs JB, Stock MC: Airway pressure release ventilation (APRV): A human trial. Chest 1988;94:779–781.
7. Putensen C, Leon MA, Putensen-Himmer G: Timing of pressure release affects power of breathing and minute ventilation during airway pressure release ventilation. Crit Care Med 1994;22:872–878.
8. Heenan TJ, Downs JB, Douglas ME, et al: Intermittent mandatory ventilation: Is synchronization important? Chest 1980;77:598–602.
9. Wrigge H, Zinserling J, Hering R, et al: Cardiorespiratory effects of automatic tube compensation during airway pressure release ventilation in patients with acute lung injury. Anesthesiology 2001;95:382–389.
10. Putensen C, Hering R, Wrigge H: Controlled versus assisted mechanical ventilation. Curr Opin Crit Care 2002;8:51–57.
11. Räsänen J: IMPRV: Synchronized APRV, or more? Intensive Care Med 1992;18:65–66.
12. Amato MB, Barbas CS, Medeiros DM, et al: Effect of a protective-ventilation strategy on mortality in the acute respiratory distress syndrome. N Engl J Med 1998;338:347–354.
13. ARDS Network: Ventilation with lower tidal volumes as compared with traditional tidal volumes for acute lung injury and the acute respiratory distress syndrome: The Acute Respiratory Distress Syndrome Network. N Engl J Med 2000;342:1301–1308.
14. Putensen C, Mutz NJ, Putensen-Himmer G, Zinserling J: Spontaneous breathing during ventilatory support improves ventilation-perfusion distributions in patients with acute respiratory distress syndrome. Am J Respir Crit Care Med 1999;159:1241–1248.
15. Katz JA, Marks JD: Inspiratory work with and without continuous positive airway pressure in patients with acute respiratory failure. Anesthesiology 1985;63:598–607.

16. Martin LD, Wetzel RC: Airway pressure release ventilation in a neonatal lamb model of acute lung injury. Crit Care Med 1991;19:373–378.

17. Neumann P, Golisch W, Strohmeyer A, et al: Influence of different release times on spontaneous breathing pattern during airway pressure release ventilation. Intensive Care Med 2002;28:1742–1749.

18. Zavala E, Ferrer M, Polese G, et al: Effect of inverse I:E ratio ventilation on pulmonary gas exchange in acute respiratory distress syndrome. Anesthesiology 1998;88:35–42.

19. Cane RD, Peruzzi WT: Airway pressure release ventilation in severe acute respiratory failure. Chest 1991;100:460–463.

20. Hudson LD, Hurlow RS, Craig KC, Pierson DJ: Does intermittent mandatory ventilation correct respiratory alkalosis in patients receiving assisted mechanical ventilation? Am Rev Respir Dis 1985;132:1071–1074.

21. Domino KB, Lu Y, Eisenstein BL, Hlastala MP: Hypocapnia worsens arterial blood oxygenation and increases VA/Q heterogeneity in canine pulmonary edema. Anesthesiology 1993;78:91–99.

22. Culpepper JA, Rinaldo JE, Rogers RM: Effect of mechanical ventilator mode on tendency towards respiratory alkalosis. Am Rev Respir Dis 1985;132:1075–1077.

23. Putensen C, Zech S, Wrigge H, et al: Long-term effects of spontaneous breathing during ventilatory support in patients with acute lung injury. Am J Respir Crit Care Med 2001;164:43–49.

24. Kress JP, Pohlman AS, O'Connor MF, Hall JB: Daily interruption of sedative infusions in critically ill patients undergoing mechanical ventilation. N Engl J Med 2000;342:1471–1477.

25. Hsiang JK, Chesnut RM, Crisp CB, et al: Early, routine paralysis for intracranial pressure control in severe head injury: Is it necessary? Crit Care Med 1994;22:1471–1476.

26. Hansen-Flaschen JH, Brazinsky S, Basile C, Lanken PN: Use of sedating drugs and neuromuscular blocking agents in patients requiring mechanical ventilation for respiratory failure: A national survey. JAMA 1991;266:2870–2875.

27. Rossiter A, Souney PF, McGowan S, Carvajal P: Pancuronium-induced prolonged neuromuscular blockade. Crit Care Med 1991;19:1583–1587.

28. Burchardi H, Rathgeber J, Sydow M: The concept of analgo-sedation depends on the concept of mechanical ventilation. In Vincent JL (ed): Yearbook of Intensive Care and Emergency Medicine. New York: Springer-Verlag, 1995, pp 155–164.

29. Rathgeber J, Schorn B, Falk V, et al: The influence of controlled mandatory ventilation (CMV), intermittent mandatory ventilation (IMV) and biphasic intermittent positive airway pressure (BIPAP) on duration of intubation and consumption of analgesics and sedatives: A prospective analysis in 596 patients following adult cardiac surgery. Eur J Anaesthesiol 1997;14:576–582.

30. Froese AB, Bryan AC: Effects of anesthesia and paralysis on diaphragmatic mechanics in man. Anesthesiology 1974;41:242–255.

31. Reber A, Nylund U, Hedenstierna G: Position and shape of the diaphragm: Implications for atelectasis formation. Anaesthesia 1998;53:1054–1061.

32. Kleinman BS, Frey K, VanDrunen M, et al: Motion of the diaphragm in patients with chronic obstructive pulmonary disease while spontaneously breathing versus during positive pressure breathing after anesthesia and neuromuscular blockade. Anesthesiology 2002;97:298–305.

33. Gattinoni L, Presenti A, Torresin A, et al: Adult respiratory distress syndrome profiles by computed tomography. J Thorac Imaging 1986;1:25–30.

34. Puybasset L, Cluzel P, Chao N, et al: A computed tomography scan assessment of regional lung volume in acute lung injury: The CT Scan ARDS Study Group. Am J Respir Crit Care Med 1998;158:1644–1655.

35. Hedenstierna G, Tokics L, Lundquist H, et al: Phrenic nerve stimulation during halothane anesthesia: Effects of atelectasis. Anesthesiology 1994;80:751–760.

36. Wrigge H, Zinserling J, Neumann P, et al: Spontaneous breathing improves lung aeration in oleic acid–induced lung injury. Anesthesiology 2003;99:376–384.

37. Henzler D, Dembinski R, Bensberg R, et al: Ventilation with biphasic positive airway pressure in experimental lung injury: Influence of transpulmonary pressure on gas exchange and haemodynamics. Intensive Care Med 2004;30:935–943.

38. Putensen C, Räsänen J, Lopez FA: Effect of interfacing between spontaneous breathing and mechanical cycles on the ventilation-perfusion distribution in canine lung injury. Anesthesiology 1994;81:921–930.

39. Sydow M, Burchardi H, Ephraim E, Zielmann S: Long-term effects of two different ventilatory modes on oxygenation in acute lung injury: Comparison of airway pressure release ventilation and volume-controlled inverse ratio ventilation. Am J Respir Crit Care Med 1994;149:1550–1556.

40. Pinsky MR: Determinants of pulmonary arterial flow variation during respiration. J Appl Physiol 1984;56:1237–1245.

41. Kirby RR, Perry JC, Calderwood HW, Ruiz BC: Cardiorespiratory effects of high positive end-expiratory pressure. Anesthesiology 1975;43:533–539.

42. Downs JB, Douglas ME, Sanfelippo PM, et al: Ventilatory pattern, intrapleural pressure, and cardiac output. Anesth Analg 1977;56:88–96.

43. Falkenhain SK, Reilley TE: Improvement in cardiac output during airway pressure release ventilation. Crit Care Med 1992;20:1358–1360.

44. Kaplan LJ, Bailey H, Formosa V: Airway pressure release ventilation increases cardiac performance in patients with acute lung injury/adult respiratory distress syndrome. Crit Care 2001;5:221–226.

45. Lemaire F, Teboul JL, Cinotti L, et al: Acute left ventricular dysfunction during unsuccessful weaning from mechanical ventilation. Anesthesiology 1988;69:171–179.

46. Räsänen J, Heikkila J, Downs J, et al: Continuous positive airway pressure by face mask in acute cardiogenic pulmonary edema. Am J Cardiol 1985;55:296–300.

47. Nikki P, Räsänen J, Tahvanainen J, Makelainen A: Ventilatory pattern in respiratory failure arising from acute myocardial infarction. I. Respiratory and hemodynamic effects of IMV4 vs IPPV12 and PEEP0 vs PEEP10. Crit Care Med 1982;10:75–78.

48. Staudinger T, Kordova H, Roggla M, et al: Comparison of oxygen cost of breathing with pressure-support ventilation and biphasic intermittent positive airway pressure ventilation. Crit Care Med 1998;26:1518–1522.

49. Steinhoff H, Falke K, Schwarzhoff W: Enhanced renal function associated with intermittent mandatory ventilation in acute respiratory failure. Intensive Care Med 1982;8:69–74.

50. Hering R, Peters D, Zinserling J, et al: Effects of spontaneous breathing during airway pressure release ventilation on renal perfusion and function in patients with acute lung injury. Intensive Care Med 2002;28:1426–1433.

51. Hering R, Viehofer A, Zinserling J, et al: Effects of spontaneous breathing during airway pressure release ventilation on intestinal blood flow in experimental lung injury. Anesthesiology 2003;99:1137–1144.

52. Räsänen J, Cane RD, Downs JB, et al: Airway pressure release ventilation during acute lung injury: A prospective multicenter trial. Crit Care Med 1991;19:1234–1241.

53. Varpula T, Valta P, Niemi R, et al: Airway pressure release ventilation as a primary ventilatory mode in acute respiratory distress syndrome. Acta Anaesthesiol Scand 2004;48:722–731.

54. Valentine DD, Hammond MD, Downs JB, et al: Distribution of ventilation and perfusion with different modes of mechanical ventilation. Am Rev Respir Dis 1991;143:1262–1266.

55. Neumann P, Wrigge H, Zinserling J, et al: Spontaneous breathing affects the spatial ventilation and perfusion distribution during mechanical ventilatory support. Crit Care Med 2005;33:1090–1095.

56. Brochard L, Rauss A, Benito S, et al: Comparison of three methods of gradual withdrawal from ventilatory support during weaning from mechanical ventilation. Am J Respir Crit Care Med 1994;150:896–903.

# CHAPTER 25

# Open Lung Management

Miranda D. Reis, Diederik Gommers, and Burkhard Lachmann

Open lung management is a ventilation strategy aimed at preventing atelectasis and thereby preserving surfactant function.[1] The first part of this chapter describes why the lung should be opened, the second part describes methods of opening the lung, and the last part outlines the effects of this strategy on other organ systems.

## WHY SHOULD WE OPEN UP THE LUNG?

Mechanical ventilation has become a lifesaving therapy for patients with impaired pulmonary function. However, experience has shown that certain modes of mechanical ventilation may be associated with related adverse effects, such as decreases in lung compliance and gas exchange, atelectasis, pulmonary edema, pneumonitis, and fibrosis. Many of these pathophysiologic changes seen in ventilated patients are logically attributed to the ventilation strategies and are therefore called ventilator-induced lung injury (VILI). Components of VILI are biotrauma, volutrauma, barotrauma, and atelect-trauma.[2] Volutrauma, barotrauma, and atelect-trauma can be seen as mechanical injury to the lung; biotrauma reflects pulmonary and systemic inflammation caused by mediators originating from the ventilated lung.

### Biotrauma

The term *biotrauma* describes the process by which mechanical stress resulting from mechanical ventilation creates an inflammatory process.[3] Investigators have demonstrated that ventilation with high inspiratory pressures stretches alveolar epithelial cells and thus triggers an inflammatory process.[4]

Cytokine production and the cellular inflammatory response to mechanical ventilation cause not only local injury; the local reaction spills over into the systemic circulation and results in end-organ apoptosis.[2] In particular, renal, and small intestine epithelial apoptosis was seen in experimental lung injury during injurious ventilation.[5] Besides end-organ damage, injurious ventilation is a predisposing factor to bacterial translocation from the lung into the systemic circulation.[6,7]

### Effect of Open Lung Management on Biotrauma

Although the exact pathways to biotrauma are unclear, it is widely appreciated that biotrauma originates from the mechanical stress at the alveolocapillary wall.[2,3,8–10] Limiting stress to the alveolocapillary wall by avoiding end-expiratory collapse has resulted in reduced levels of biochemical markers (purines) from damaged cells after high-pressure ventilation. From these results, one can conclude that shear stress is more damaging to the lung than overdistention.[11] These findings were supported by studies by van Kaam and associates,[12] who demonstrated that application of OLM in surfactant-depleted piglets resulted in a reduction of inflammatory cells and interleukin-8 (IL-8) in a bronchoalveolar lavage sample, in comparison with animals ventilated with low positive end-expiratory pressure (PEEP). Stuber and colleagues[13] showed that serum IL-6 concentrations increased 2 hours after a change from a lung protective ventilation strategy to an injurious strategy in an experimental model.

Moreover, this IL-6 increase was reversed in 2 hours when the injurious strategy was again reversed to the protective ventilation strategy.[13] Moreover, clinical data show that OLM reduces interleukin release. In cardiac surgical patients, serum IL-8 concentrations were decreased when OLM was compared with conventional ventilation.[14] In addition, serum IL-8 concentrations normalized earlier when patients were ventilated with OLM. In the OLM-treated group, serum IL-8 concentrations normalized 24 hours after aortic cross-clamp release. In the group receiving conventional ventilation, serum IL-8 concentrations did not normalize after 72 hours. Ventilation with OLM also minimizes alveolar and systemic decompartmentalization of inflammatory mediators[15] and reduces bacterial translocation.[7] Ranieri and colleagues[16] confirmed these experimental data in patients suffering from acute respiratory distress syndrome (ARDS). In these patients, cytokine levels were attenuated by a ventilation strategy minimizing overdistention.[16] Amato and colleagues[17] later demonstrated a reduction in mortality when OLM was applied to patients suffering from severe ARDS. At present, extensive evidence seems to indicate that ventilation strategies aiming at avoiding atelect-trauma, as in OLM, indeed reduce biotrauma to the lung and probably also decrease the systemic inflammatory response and even mortality.

## Mechanotrauma

In the past, VILI and the accompanying high airway pressures were automatically associated with clinical barotrauma, defined as the appearance of air leaks. However, in 1975, Kirby and associates[18] showed that very high airway pressures ($\leq 140$ cm $H_2O$) did not lead to increased mortality. Nevertheless, in 1994, the American-European consensus conference[19] recommended that plateau pressure should not exceed the arbitrary pressure limit of 35 cm $H_2O$, thus limiting the risk of barotrauma. Boussarsar and colleagues[20] again emphasized the risk of barotrauma when plateau pressures higher than 35 cm $H_2O$ are applied. The adverse consequences of these macroscopic events are usually immediately obvious; only recently have more subtle physiologic and morphologic alterations resulting from barotrauma been recognized, as mentioned in the previous section.

To explore the role of tidal volume and peak inspiratory pressure (PIP) in lung injury further, Dreyfuss and colleagues[21] applied high inspiratory pressures in combination with high volumes in an experimental model and found the following: (1) high pressures together with high tidal volume resulted in increased alveolar permeability; (2) combining low pressure with high volume (iron lung ventilation) resulted in increased alveolar permeability; and (3) when high pressure was associated with low tidal volume (chest wall strapping), the alveolar

permeability of the study group did not differ from the control group.

Avoiding alveolar overdistention by limiting tidal volume is optimal in a homogeneous lung. In an atelectatic lung, however, alveolar overdistention is not prevented by small tidal volume ventilation because of the baby lung effect, as explained in the following paragraph.

Atelectasis is a common occurrence in spontaneously breathing humans and is also present after endotracheal intubation, even in healthy lungs in volume controlled ventilation.[22–27] Depending on the amount of collapsed lung tissue, even small tidal volumes (e.g., 6 mL/kg) will increase severalfold the actual tidal volume delivered to the open lung areas, thereby leading to the so-called baby lung. For example, when 75% of the lung is collapsed, the applied volume to the open part of the lung will be 24 mL/kg.

The pioneering work of Mead and colleagues[28] demonstrated that forces acting on lung tissue in nonuniformly expanded lungs are not simply applied transpulmonary pressures. Shear forces acting on the fragile alveolar membrane in atelectatic regions predominate because of the pulmonary interdependence of the alveoli. Transpulmonary pressures of 30 cm $H_2O$ result in shear forces between atelectatic and normal lung areas of 140 cm $H_2O$. These shear forces, rather than end-inspiratory overstretching, may be the reason for epithelial disruption and the loss of barrier function of the alveolar epithelium. Epithelial disruption leads to high-permeability edema with washout or dilution of the surfactant or inactivation of the surfactant by plasma components,[29] as described in Chapter 12. This surfactant impairment causes an increase of atelectasis, increased formation of edema, and impairment of local host defense.[2] Indeed, investigators have found that abnormalities of surfactant already occur in patients at risk of developing ARDS, a finding suggesting that these abnormalities, occurring in VILI, precede ARDS.[30]

### Effect of Open Lung Management on Mechanotrauma

Preventing atelectasis by applying OLM preserves lung mechanics, attenuates mechanotrauma, and thereby reduces mortality during ventilation.[31–33] In an experimental study, in vivo microscopic images were made and alveolar instability was seen when recruitment was followed by inadequate PEEP, whereas with adequate PEEP after recruitment (the OLM philosophy), alveoli were very stable.[34] Indeed, no atelectasis was demonstrated by computed tomography in anesthetized healthy children who were treated with OLM.[27] In patients with severe chest trauma, OLM significantly reduced the amount of atelectasis, as assessed by computed tomography examinations.[35] In addition, OLM reduces protein leakage into the alveolus, which inactivates the surfactant system.[32] An impaired surfactant system, in turn, increases shear forces, which increase mechanotrauma, thereby inducing a vicious cycle. By ventilating with OLM and thus reducing atelectasis, VILI can be reduced,[36] or may even be prevented, as shown in cardiac surgical patients.[37] In this latter study, it was shown that early application of OLM significantly increased functional residual capacity (FRC) *after* extubation, compared with conventional ventilation.[37] This increased FRC was maintained up to 5 days after extubation. In addition, compared with conventional ventilation, the occurrence of hypoxemia after extubation was also significantly reduced up to 3 days after extubation. In this study, we concluded that application of OLM during and after cardiac surgery protected the lung against additional postoperative lung injury.[37]

## HOW TO VENTILATE WITH OPEN LUNG MANAGEMENT

The basic principle is demonstrated in the pressure-volume curve in Figure 25.1. In this figure, Po is the pressure that is needed to open the lung. Once the lung has been opened, we can operate in the area between D and C to keep the lung open (see Fig. 25.1). If the pressure decreases to less than the closing pressure (Pc), the lung will collapse again.[1] This principle of OLM has three steps: (1) finding the Po and the collapse pressure for the patient's lung, (2) opening the lung, and (3) keeping the lung open (Fig. 25.2). The Po is reached

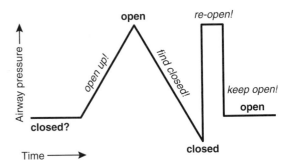

**Figure 25.2**  Schematic representation of the opening procedure for collapsed lungs. The *exclamation marks* show the treatment goal of each specific intervention. The words printed bold indicate the achieved state of the lung. At the beginning, the precise amount of collapsed lung tissue is not known.

with PIP, and the collapse pressure is determined by PEEP.[1]

### Monitoring an Open Lung

In OLM, opening or closure of lung units is monitored by gas exchange.[1] However, while doing this one should note that determining lung collapse by gas exchange assumes a minimal extrapulmonary shunt. The Po is found when the arterial oxygen tension ($PaO_2$) reaches its maximum value and does not increase any further with increasing the airway pressure.[1] Usually, a ratio of $PaO_2$ to fraction of inspired oxygen ($FiO_2$) that is greater than 50 kPa can be obtained, but in consolidated or fibrotic lungs, this ratio may be lower. Therefore, ideally blood gas is monitored continuously. An alternate solution is setting the $FiO_2$ at a level at which peripheral saturation is between 90% and 95% before performing a recruitment maneuver. During a recruitment maneuver, PIP is increased until oxygen saturation as measured using pulse oximetry ($SaO_2$) reaches its maximum value. If $SpO_2$ has reached 99% to 100%, then $FiO_2$ is lowered again, and a new recruitment maneuver is performed until $SpO_2$ reaches its maximum value once again. $SpO_2$ is a less exact parameter than $PaO_2$ in determining Po.

### Opening the Lung: Theory

The lung is opened with a recruitment maneuver in a pressure controlled ventilation mode. Different recruitment maneuvers all reach a certain PIP for a few seconds, but they vary in driving pressure (defined as PIP minus total PEEP). Recruitment strategies that reach high PIP using high driving pressures usually generate a high tidal volume (>12 mL/kg). Other recruitment strategies maintain a normal driving pressure; then a PIP sufficient to recruit the lung is achieved by increasing PEEP levels with a constant driving pressure. Strategies using a low

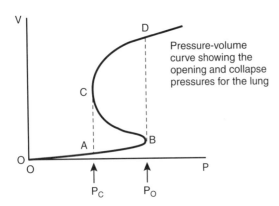

**Figure 25.1**  In this theoretical pressure-volume curve, Po is the pressure needed to open the lung. Once the lung has been opened, we can operate in the area between D and C to keep the lung open. If the pressure decreases to less than the closing pressure (Pc), the lung will collapse again. This principle of open lung management consists of three steps: (1) finding the Po and the collapsing pressure of the patient's lung, (2) opening the lung, and (3) keeping the lung open.

driving pressure produce sufficient levels of PIP by generating high intrinsic PEEP levels. Therefore, the respiratory rate is increased (usually between 80 and 150/minute), as is inspiratory time (usually 50% to 80%). With this recruitment strategy, tidal volume remains low (usually 2 to 4 mL/kg) as intrinsic PEEP increases by increasing PIP. Strategies using no driving pressure use an inspiratory hold on the desired PIP to open the lung.

In one study, recruitment by pressure controlled ventilation using high driving pressures seemed superior to other recruitment maneuvers.[38] Lim and colleagues[38] compared three recruitment maneuvers: (1) high driving pressures, (2) low driving pressure and incremental PEEP, and (3) inspiratory hold. Unfortunately, because these recruitment strategies were performed with different PIP levels and various ventilation modes, the results of this study are difficult to interpret. Comparisons of well-standardized recruitment maneuvers are currently lacking. In our experience, strategies using pressure controlled ventilation with low driving pressure have the best results in opening atelectatic lung regions, and they may also have a lower complication rate. Again, recruitment maneuvers are brief increments of PIP, only 5 to 15 seconds long.

## Opening the Lung: Practical Considerations

Three different methods are used to open the lung. These recruitment maneuvers should not be performed in patients with hypovolemia. Preferentially, hypovolemia is monitored in relation to the respiratory cycle. During hypovolemia, systolic arterial pressure decreases by more than 5 mm Hg during inspiration.[39,40] Hypovolemia can also be monitored using transesophageal echocardiography: a 35% collapse of the vena cava superior during inspiration indicates hypovolemia.[41,42] The inferior vena cava can also be used as a discriminator of hypovolemia: an 18% increase of the diameter of the vena cava inferior indicates hypovolemia. When hypovolemia is present, but fluid administration is not desirable for clinical reasons, α-mimetic or β-mimetic agents should be used to avoid a large decrease of cardiac output during a recruitment maneuver. During the recruitment maneuver, attention is given to the heart rate and the arterial pressure. A decrease in arterial pressure is normal and is usually self-limiting. Minimal arterial pressures accepted during a recruitment maneuver should be decided on a case-by-case basis. A recruitment maneuver can be performed with (1) high tidal volume, (2) normal tidal volume, or (3) low tidal volume.

Whichever strategy is used, however, all recruitment maneuvers require a sufficient level of PEEP before they are initiated. PEEP does not recruit atelectatic regions, but rather keeps open only what was recruited during inspiratory pressures. While recruiting the lung with high tidal volume, the respiratory rate is set between 6 and 10/minute, PEEP is set at between 10 and 14 cm $H_2O$, and the inspiratory-to-expiratory (I:E) ratio is 1:1. PIP is now gradually increased in approximately 3 seconds to 40 cm $H_2O$ for three breaths and is then gradually decreased in approximately 3 seconds to PIP, thus obtaining a tidal volume of approximately 6 mL/kg. If the lung is not open yet (see the earlier discussion of monitoring an open lung), PIP is increased by 5 cm $H_2O$. In several OLM studies in cardiac surgical patients, we used a maximal recruitment pressure of 60 cm $H_2O$. However, the maximal pressure that can be used safely to open the lung differs in each patient, especially in patients with ARDS. Higher recruitment pressures may still be safe in patients with severe ARDS.

While recruiting the lung with normal tidal volume, the respiratory rate is set at between 20 and 40/minute, PEEP is set at between 10 and 14 cm $H_2O$, the I:E ratio is 1:1, and a driving pressure is used to obtain a tidal volume of 6 mL/kg. During recruitment, the driving pressure is kept constant, and PEEP set on the ventilator is gradually increased in approximately 3 seconds until PIP reaches 40 to 60 cm $H_2O$ for a few seconds; then PEEP is again gradually decreased in 3 seconds to the original setting. This maneuver is easily accomplished with ventilators in which PIP is set as an inspiratory pressure greater than PEEP. If actual PIP is set on the ventilator, both PEEP and PIP have to be increased to maintain a constant driving pressure. In this case, PEEP is increased by 5 cm $H_2O$, then followed by PIP of 5 cm $H_2O$, and this is repeated until PIP is at the desired value. If the lung is not open yet (see the earlier discussion of monitoring an open lung), PIP is increased by 5 cm $H_2O$.

While recruiting the lung with low tidal volume, PEEP is set at 10 to 14 cm $H_2O$, the respiratory rate is set between 40 and 150/minute, and the I:E ratio is up to 4:1. PIP is gradually increased in 3 seconds up to 40 to 60 cm $H_2O$ for a few seconds and is then gradually decreased in 3 seconds to the previous setting. The respiratory rate and the I:E ratio are again restored to the previous setting. During the recruitment maneuver, care is taken to keep tidal volume at less than 6 mL/kg.

## Setting the Positive End-Expiratory Pressure: Practical Considerations

Before a recruitment maneuver, PEEP is set normally between 10 and 25 cm $H_2O$. The lung remains open after a recruitment maneuver if oxygenation does not decrease after this maneuver. If oxygenation does not diminish, PEEP is gradually lowered by 1 cm $H_2O$ until a decrease in oxygenation does occur. This pressure is the Pc. Then PEEP is set 2 cm higher than the Pc, and the last performed recruitment procedure is repeated.

In most patients, decreasing oxygenation over a certain period is usually caused by PEEP that is too low. This sequence is repeated until oxygenation is stable after a recruitment procedure. However, if lung distensibility is improving as a result of this procedure, deterioration of oxygenation and circulation is caused by PEEP that is too high, and in this case, PEEP should be reduced. If oxygenation does decrease after a recruitment procedure, PEEP is increased by 2 cm $H_2O$, and the last performed recruitment procedure is repeated.

## Keeping the Lung Open: Theory

After a recruitment maneuver, the lung is ventilated in a pressure controlled mode with sufficient PEEP levels to keep the lung open: just higher than Pc (see Fig. 25.1). The ventilator is set to obtain (1) the lowest possible airway pressure and (2) the lowest possible driving pressure and tidal volume.[43] Ideally, the driving pressure is less than 15 cm $H_2O$ with a tidal volume between 4 and 6 mL/kg. This is to avoid possible shear forces and to ensure proper elimination of carbon dioxide ($CO_2$) from the lung. $CO_2$ elimination while ventilating with low tidal volume can be improved by optimizing respiratory rate and inspiratory time. The respiratory rate can be increased as long as the inspiratory flow reaches zero. If the inspiratory flow does not reach zero, a less than optimal tidal volume for the given driving pressure will be delivered. This will result in inappropriate $CO_2$ elimination. With an increasing respiratory rate, if inspiratory flow is interrupted prematurely, the respiratory rate can be increased if inspiration time is increased. While inspiration time increases, expiration time decreases, with a possible increase in intrinsic PEEP. Then external PEEP is lowered to keep total PEEP constant. Intrinsic PEEP probably offers the best $CO_2$ elimination.[44] When six patients with ARDS described by Lachmann and associates[33] were compared with 28 patients described by Amato and colleagues,[17] $CO_2$ elimination was better in the group described by Lachmann and colleagues.[33] Thus, driving pressures were lower, but intrinsic PEEP was higher (Fig. 25.3). Although these two studies are difficult to compare, this finding may suggest that intrinsic PEEP results in improved $CO_2$ elimination. The optimal division of total PEEP into intrinsic and static PEEP is often different in each patient and is most effectively made on a trial-and-error basis. The best parameter to control $CO_2$ elimination is the breath-to-breath $CO_2$ minute production, measured in the airway adapter because there is a delay before arterial $CO_2$ starts to change.

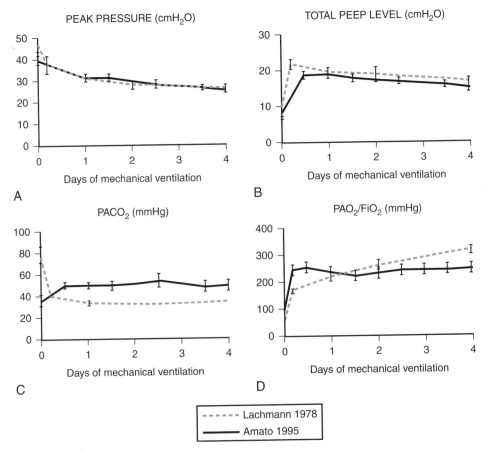

**Figure 25.3** Examples of two studies of protective mechanical ventilation. The open lung concept applied in patients with acute respiratory distress syndrome by Lachmann and associates[33] and by Amato and colleagues.[17] Carbon dioxide elimination is greater in Lachmann's group than in Amato's group, probably because of the use of more intrinsic positive end-expiratory pressure (PEEP) in Lachmann's group. (From Vazquez de Anda GF, Lachmann B: Protecting the lung during mechanical ventilation with the open lung concept. Acta Anaesthesiol Scand 1998;42:63–66.)

## Complications

When OLM is used with caution, no complications are expected. In a study by our group in cardiac surgical patients, no increment in pneumothorax was observed, and the rate of myocardial infarction was not increased when patients were ventilated with OLM.[45] In addition, Scheiter and colleagues[46] did not observe an increased rate of pneumothorax while using ventilation with OLM in patients with severe chest trauma. In both studies, recruitment maneuvers were performed with low driving pressures, as described earlier. We speculate that the risk for pneumothorax is increased when recruitment maneuvers are used with high driving pressures.

## CASE STUDY

A 52-year-old man, complaining of severe dyspnea, had severe aortic valve stenosis and mitral valve regurgitation resulting from annulus dilatation. He was scheduled for mitral valve repair and aortic valve replacement. The mitral valve repair was difficult, and on the third consecutive pump run, the mitral valve was replaced. The total aortic occlusion time was 4 hours and 10 minutes, with nearly 5 hours on cardiopulmonary bypass, without the use of corticosteroids. In the intensive care unit, the patient's gas exchange was poor: a $PaO_2/FiO_2$ ratio of 35 kPa was achieved using volume controlled ventilation and 8 cm $H_2O$ PEEP with a tidal volume of 9 mL/kg. The intensive care specialists decided to change the ventilator strategy. The lung was recruited several times, and at a pressure of 50 cm $H_2O$, the lung was opened. The lung was kept open at 10 cm $H_2O$ PEEP. $PaO_2/FiO_2$ increased to 76 kPa. Ventilation was maintained with a respiratory rate of 40/minute to preserve a low tidal volume of 5 mL/kg with adequate $CO_2$ removal. Five hours and 20 minutes after arrival in the intensive care unit, the patient could be extubated. The next morning, the patient did not need additional oxygen to maintain peripheral oxygen saturation at more than 90%, and oxygen was removed. FRC was measured on the first day after operation, and it was 77% of the preoperative value. Normally, FRC is reduced by approximately 40% to 50% on the first postoperative day.[47] On the fifth postoperative day, FRC was even increased to 86% of the preoperative value. On the sixth postoperative day, the patient was discharged.

## EFFECT OF OPEN LUNG MANAGEMENT ON DIFFERENT ORGAN SYSTEMS

OLM has the potential to affect other organ systems. The effects on circulation, splanchnic perfusion, renal function, and intracerebral pressure are described in the following sections.

## Circulation

Preload reduction is the main effect of ventilation with OLM on the circulatory system.[45] The effect of OLM on left ventricular contractility depends on global left ventricular function. If left ventricular function is good, then increasing the intrathoracic pressure will not affect left ventricular contractility.[48] However, in left ventricular failure, an increment of intrathoracic pressure leads to an increment of left ventricular contractility.[48] A possible mechanism for this phenomenon is a reduction in left ventricular afterload during increased intrathoracic pressure.[48] This ventricular afterload is defined as transmural pressure. While ventilating with high PEEP levels, intraventricular pressure (as reflected by systemic arterial pressure) is not increased, but extraventricular pressure (as reflected by pleural pressure) is increased. This leads to decreased transmural pressure and thus to decreased left ventricular afterload. Left ventricular function does not improve indefinitely during progressively increasing PEEP levels: left ventricular function is dependent on right ventricular function. At high PEEP levels, increased right ventricular afterload has been reported.[49–52] This change impairs left ventricular preload in two ways: (1) by impeding blood flow from right to left and (2) by enlarging the right ventricle during diastole. Because the heart is housed in a common pericardial sac, an increment of right ventricular volume is at the expense of left ventricular volume, a mechanism called *ventricular interdependence*.[53–55]

We found that, after a recruitment maneuver, high PEEP levels do not increase right ventricular afterload in cardiac surgical patients.[45] This study confirmed the results of Dyhr and colleagues[56] and van den Berg and colleagues,[57] who found that cardiac output was not affected by high PEEP after a recruitment maneuver in cardiac surgical patients. These findings can probably be explained by the use of low tidal volumes during ventilation with OLM. Vieillard-Baron and colleagues[58] found that tidal volume and not PEEP determined right ventricular afterload in patients with ARDS. These results were confirmed by our group.[59] Twenty-eight cardiac surgical patients were enrolled in a crossover study comparing right ventricular afterload during OLM and conventional ventilation. In this study, right ventricular afterload was assessed with Doppler echocardiography of the pulmonary artery. During expiration, no increased afterload was found in the OLM-treated group compared with patients receiving conventional ventilation.[59] During inspiration, however, lower right ventricular afterload was found during OLM ventilation compared with conventional ventilation.[59] This effect of OLM on right ventricular afterload is probably the result of the avoidance of atelectasis and the use of low tidal volumes, despite the use of relatively high PEEP levels.

High PEEP, also during OLM, does decrease right ventricular preload. In the study conducted by our group[45] and another study by Dyhr and colleagues,[56] patients were volume loaded. In volume-loaded cardiac surgical patients, van der Berg[57] suggested that, because of caudal displacement of the diaphragm, fluid is squeezed out of the liver. This would counterbalance right ventricular preload reduction during high PEEP ventilation. We found that during ventilation with OLM, more fluids were needed to keep the right ventricular end-diastolic volume constant.[45] These fluids were especially needed during the first hours after initiation of ventilation with OLM.[45] The long-term effect of ventilation with OLM on fluid administration is not yet known.

## Splanchnic Perfusion

Splanchnic oxygenation and hepatic performance during ventilation with OLM are not yet known. However, splanchnic and hepatic performance is not dependent on PEEP but rather on cardiac output.[60-62] During a recruitment maneuver, splanchnic, hepatic, and splenic flow is decreased, but this decrease is transient,[63] if it occurs at all.[60] When cardiac output after high PEEP was restored, splanchnic flow, perfusion, and metabolism were unaltered.[60] Moreover, hepatic flow and metabolism were restored when a PEEP-induced decrease in cardiac output was reversed by fluid administration.[61] Aneman and colleagues[64] increased PEEP from 0 to 10 cm $H_2O$ and observed a decrease in splanchnic perfusion. These authors did not measure cardiac output and therefore could not restore a potential PEEP-induced decrease in cardiac output. As stated previously, a PEEP-induced decrease in cardiac output usually originates in a reduction of preload. To avoid a PEEP-induced decrease in cardiac output, patients have to be volume loaded when they are treated with an OLM ventilation strategy.

## Renal Function

The influence of ventilation with OLM on renal function is not yet known. However, PEEP-induced renal abnormalities include a decrease in urine output and probably also a decrease in renal blood flow and glomerular filtration rate.[65] These PEEP-induced renal abnormalities could be caused by (1) cardiovascular changes, (2) intrarenal changes, (3) hormonal changes, and (4) activation of inflammatory mediators. Correcting the PEEP-induced preload decrement may correct all observed PEEP-induced renal abnormalities.[65,66]

PEEP-induced circulatory changes may affect renal function by a decrease in renal blood flow. As shown by

Dyhr and colleagues[56] and by our group,[45] cardiac output is not affected by ventilation with OLM in volume-loaded patients. These results confirmed the work by Priebe and colleagues,[67] who found that fluid resuscitation restored PEEP-induced renal abnormalities.

PEEP-induced intrarenal changes may consist of redistribution of intrarenal blood flow from cortical to juxtamedullary nephrons.[68] However, in a later study using a radioactive microsphere technique, no intrarenal blood flow redistribution was observed during high PEEP.[67]

PEEP-induced hormonal alterations consist of changes in antidiuretic hormone (ADH), sympathetic tone, and atrial natriuretic peptide (ANP). An increase in ADH concentration during PEEP is induced by relative intravascular volume depletion. However, ADH concentrations did not correlate with the observed changes in urine production associated with PEEP.[65] The second PEEP-induced hormonal change concerns sympathetic tone. Sympathetic denervation prevented PEEP-induced decreases in renal blood flow, glomerular filtration rate, and urinary output in dogs.[65] Again, when renal blood flow is maintained, PEEP-induced sympathetic stimulation was reversed.[65] The third hormonal change by PEEP is the release of ANP. This substance is released by the atria in response to increased transmural pressure and has potent diuretic and natriuretic properties.[65] During PEEP administration, transmural atrial pressure decreases, as do ANP concentrations.[65] However, volume loading compensating for PEEP-induced preload decrement was reported to restore atrial transmural pressure. When atrial transmural pressure was restored by fluid resuscitation, sodium excretion and urine output normalized.[69]

Inflammatory mediator release induced by mechanical ventilation[70] may cause epithelial apoptosis in kidney tissue.[5] Lung protective ventilation strategies, using high PEEP and low tidal volumes, may reduce inflammatory mediator release.[16] In addition, the use of ventilation with OLM leads to a decrease in inflammatory mediators.[36] Serum inflammatory mediator release was significantly attenuated by application of ventilation with OLM in cardiac surgical patients.[14] Therefore, it can be speculated that ventilation with OLM may attenuate renal failure in patients suffering from ARDS. Further investigation is needed.

## Intracranial Pressure

High PEEP levels, as used during OLM, probably do not increase intracranial pressure (ICP) in either the normal brain or the injured brain. Ventilation with OLM using PEEP levels up to 15 cm $H_2O$ did not increase ICP in severe brain injury,[71] whereas the recruitment maneuver itself did cause a short and transient increment of ICP.[72] Moreover, when high PEEP was used without recruitment maneuvers, ICP did not increase with PEEP levels up to 15 cm $H_2O$.[73] In patients with acute stroke, high PEEP can be used without increasing the ICP.[74] Only McGuire and colleagues[75] found a significant increase of ICP during PEEP at levels greater than 10 cm $H_2O$. However, ICP increased only 0.8 mm Hg when PEEP was increased from 5 to 15 cm $H_2O$. Cerebral perfusion pressure (ICP minus mean arterial pressure) increased, instead of decreasing, by 2.7 mm Hg.

Toung and colleagues[76] gave two possible explanations for the lack of effect of PEEP on ICP. First, because of the head-elevated position of patients with brain injury, venous pressure in the jugular veins outside the thorax is low. However, intrathoracic pressure is high as a result of the elevated PEEP levels, thereby compressing jugular veins at the thoracic inlet. Second, all cerebral venous blood flows into the vertebral venous plexus during high intrathoracic pressure.[77] This vertebral venous plexus drains through the spinal canal into the inferior vena cava, instead of into the superior vena cava. Because these venous plexus do not directly connect to the superior vena cava, they are not subject to immediate intrathoracic pressure variations.[76] According to this view, it is important for patients who have brain injury to be maintained in a 30-degree position, especially during ventilation at high PEEP levels. Instead, when the head is at heart level, the jugular vein does not collapse, thus transmitting the intrathoracic pressure to the ICP. This was also seen in experimental work of Toung and colleagues.[76] When the head was at heart level, ICP increased linearly with increased PEEP levels. When the head was positioned well above the level of the heart, however, ICP did not increase with PEEP. Patients who have sustained brain injury must be fluid resuscitated to avoid preload reduction during ventilation with OLM. Preload reduction lowers cardiac output, decreases mean arterial pressure, and thus decreases cerebral perfusion pressure.

The effect of OLM on other organ systems is limited to a decrease in cardiac output based on preload reduction. Recruitment maneuvers transiently affect other organ systems such as the circulation and ICP. Normalizing cardiac output by fluid resuscitation counterbalances the potential negative effects of the application of OLM on other organ systems.

## CONCLUSION

Ventilation with OLM searches for an optimized gas exchange at the lowest possible pressure amplitude (tidal volume <6 mL/kg) at the lowest possible mean airway pressure. It is initiated by sufficient levels of PEEP, followed by a recruitment maneuver. A successful recruitment maneuver is characterized by a maximal

$PaO_2$ that does not increase further if PIP is increased. Usually, this corresponds to a $PaO_2/FiO_2$ ratio greater than 50 kPa. The PEEP level is sufficient if $PaO_2$ does not decrease after a recruitment maneuver. During a recruitment maneuver as well as during ventilation, tidal volumes are best kept low.

Ventilation with OLM is usually accompanied by preload reduction. Counterbalancing this preload reduction with fluid therapy counteracts almost all the negative effects of OLM on other organ systems.

## REFERENCES

1. Lachmann B. Open up the lung and keep the lung open. Intensive Care Med 1992;18:319–321.
2. Pinhu L, Whitehead T, Evans T, et al: Ventilator-associated lung injury. Lancet 2003;361:332–340.
3. Dos Santos CC, Slutsky AS. Invited review: Mechanisms of ventilator-induced lung injury. A perspective. J Appl Physiol 2000;89:1645–1655.
4. Uhlig U, Haitsma JJ, Goldmann T, et al: Ventilation-induced activation of the mitogen-activated protein kinase pathway. Eur Respir J 2002;20:946–956.
5. Imai Y, Parodo J, Kajikawa O, et al: Injurious mechanical ventilation and end-organ epithelial cell apoptosis and organ dysfunction in an experimental model of acute respiratory distress syndrome. JAMA 2003;289:2104–2112.
6. Lin CY, Zhang H, Cheng KC, et al: Mechanical ventilation may increase susceptibility to the development of bacteremia. Crit Care Med 2003;31:1429–1434.
7. Verbrugge SJ, Sorm V, van't Veen A, et al: Lung overinflation without positive end-expiratory pressure promotes bacteremia after experimental Klebsiella pneumoniae inoculation. Intensive Care Med 1998;24:172–177.
8. Liu M, Tanswell AK, Post M: Mechanical force-induced signal transduction in lung cells. Am J Physiol 1999;277:L667–L683.
9. Ricard JD, Dreyfuss D, Saumon G: Ventilator-induced lung injury. Curr Opin Crit Care 2002;8:12–20.
10. Pugin J: Molecular mechanisms of lung cell activation induced by cyclic stretch. Crit Care Med 2003;31(Suppl):S200–S206.
11. Verbrugge SJ, de Jong JW, Keijzer E, et al: Purine in bronchoalveolar lavage fluid as a marker of ventilation-induced lung injury. Crit Care Med 1999;27:779–783.
12. van Kaam AH, Dik WA, Haitsma JJ, et al: Application of the open-lung concept during positive-pressure ventilation reduces pulmonary inflammation in newborn piglets. Biol Neonate 2003;83:273–280.
13. Stuber F, Wrigge H, Schroeder S, et al: Kinetic and reversibility of mechanical ventilation-associated pulmonary and systemic inflammatory response in patients with acute lung injury. Intensive Care Med 2002;28:834–841.
14. Reis Miranda D, Gommers D, Struijs A, et al: Ventilation according to the open lung concept attenuates pulmonary inflammatory response in cardiac surgery. Eur J Cardiothorac Surg 2005;28:889–895.
15. Haitsma JJ, Uhlig S, Goggel R, et al: Ventilator-induced lung injury leads to loss of alveolar and systemic compartmentalization of tumor necrosis factor-alpha. Intensive Care Med 2000;26:1515–1522.
16. Ranieri VM, Suter PM, Tortorella C, et al: Effect of mechanical ventilation on inflammatory mediators in patients with acute

respiratory distress syndrome: A randomized controlled trial. JAMA 1999;282:54–61.

17. Amato MB, Barbas CS, Medeiros DM, et al: Effect of a protective-ventilation strategy on mortality in the acute respiratory distress syndrome. N Engl J Med 1998;338:347–354.

18. Kirby RR, Downs JB, Civetta JM, et al: High level positive end expiratory pressure (PEEP) in acute respiratory insufficiency. Chest 1975;67:156–163.

19. Slutsky AS: Consensus conference on mechanical ventilation: January 28–30, 1993 at Northbrook, Illinois. Part 2. Intensive Care Med 1994;20:150–162.

20. Boussarsar M, Thierry G, Jaber S, et al: Relationship between ventilatory settings and barotrauma in the acute respiratory distress syndrome. Intensive Care Med 2002;28:406–413.

21. Dreyfuss D, Soler P, Basset G, et al: High inflation pressure pulmonary edema: Respective effects of high airway pressure, high tidal volume, and positive end-expiratory pressure. Am Rev Respir Dis 1988;137:1159–1164.

22. Gunnarsson L, Tokics L, Gustavsson H, et al: Influence of age on atelectasis formation and gas exchange impairment during general anaesthesia. Br J Anaesth 1991;66:423–432.

23. Hedenstierna G, Tokics L, Strandberg A, et al: Correlation of gas exchange impairment to development of atelectasis during anaesthesia and muscle paralysis. Acta Anaesthesiol Scand 1986;30:183–191.

24. Jensen AG, Kalman SH, Eintrei C, et al: Atelectasis and oxygenation in major surgery with either propofol with or without nitrous oxide or isoflurane anaesthesia. Anaesthesia 1993;48:1094–1096.

25. Rothen HU, Sporre B, Engberg G, et al: Influence of gas composition on recurrence of atelectasis after a reexpansion maneuver during general anesthesia. Anesthesiology 1995;82:832–842.

26. Tenling A, Hachenberg T, Tyden H, et al: Atelectasis and gas exchange after cardiac surgery. Anesthesiology 1998;89:371–378.

27. Tusman G, Bohm SH, Tempra A, et al: Effects of recruitment maneuver on atelectasis in anesthetized children. Anesthesiology 2003;98:14–22.

28. Mead J, Takishima T, Leith D: Stress distribution in lungs: A model of pulmonary elasticity. J Appl Physiol 1970;28:596–608.

29. Seeger W, Gunther A, Walmrath HD, et al: Alveolar surfactant and adult respiratory distress syndrome: Pathogenetic role and therapeutic prospects. Clin Invest 1993;71:177–190.

30. Verbrugge SJC, Lachmann B: Surfactant replacement therapy in experimental and clinical studies. Appl Cardiopulm Pathophysiol 1998;7:237–250.

31. Hartog A, Gommers D, Verbrugge SJ, et al: Maintaining high lung volume during surfactant depletion attenuates the decrease in lung function. Intensive Care Med 1997;23:S13.

32. Hartog A, Vazquez de Anda GF, Gommers D, et al: At surfactant deficiency, application of "the open lung concept" prevents protein leakage and attenuates changes in lung mechanics. Crit Care Med 2000;28:1450–1454.

33. Lachmann B, Danzmann E, Haendly B, et al: Ventilator settings and gas exchange in respiratory distress syndrome. In Prakash O (ed): *Applied Physiology in Clinical Respiratory Care*. The Hague: Martinus Nijhoff, 1982, pp 141–176.

34. Halter JM, Steinberg JM, Schiller HJ, et al: Positive end-expiratory pressure after a recruitment maneuver prevents both alveolar collapse and recruitment/derecruitment. Am J Respir Crit Care Med 2003;167:1620–1626.

35. Schreiter D, Reske A, Scheibner L, et al: [The open lung concept: Clinical application in severe thoracic trauma]. Chirurg 2002;73:353–359.

36. van Kaam AH, de Jaegere A, Haitsma JJ, et al: Positive pressure ventilation with the open lung concept optimizes gas exchange and reduces ventilator-induced lung injury in newborn piglets. Pediatr Res 2003;53:245–253.

37. Reis Miranda D, Struijs A, Koetsier P, et al: Open lung ventilation improves functional residual capacity after extubation in cardiac surgery. Crit Care Med 2005;33:2253–2258.

38. Lim SC, Adams AB, Simonson DA, et al: Intercomparison of recruitment maneuver efficacy in three models of acute lung injury. Crit Care Med 2004;32:2371–2377.

39. Pizov R, Cohen M, Weiss Y, et al: Positive end-expiratory pressure-induced hemodynamic changes are reflected in the arterial pressure waveform. Crit Care Med 1996;24:1381–1387.

40. Preisman S, Pfeiffer U, Lieberman N, et al: New monitors of intravascular volume: A comparison of arterial pressure waveform analysis and the intrathoracic blood volume. Intensive Care Med 1997;23:651–657.

41. Vieillard-Baron A, Augarde R, Prin S, et al: Influence of superior vena caval zone condition on cyclic changes in right ventricular outflow during respiratory support. Anesthesiology 2001;95:1083–1088.

42. Vieillard-Baron A, Chergui K, Rabiller A, et al: Superior vena caval collapsibility as a gauge of volume status in ventilated septic patients. Intensive Care Med 2004;30:1734–1739.

43. Verbrugge SJ, Lachmann B: Mechanisms of ventilation-induced lung injury: Physiological rationale to prevent it. Monaldi Arch Chest Dis 1999;54:22–37.

44. Vazquez de Anda GF, Lachmann B: Protecting the lung during mechanical ventilation with the open lung concept. Acta Anaesthesiol Scand 1998;42:63–66.

45. Reis Miranda D, Gommers D, Struijs A, et al: The open lung concept: Effects on right ventricular afterload after cardiac surgery. Br J Anaesth 2004;93:327–332.

46. Schreiter D, Reske A, Stichert B, et al: Alveolar recruitment in combination with sufficient positive end-expiratory pressure increases oxygenation and lung aeration in patients with severe chest trauma. Crit Care Med 2004;32:968–975.

47. Nicholson DJ, Kowalski SE, Hamilton GA, et al: Postoperative pulmonary function in coronary artery bypass graft surgery patients undergoing early tracheal extubation: A comparison between short-term mechanical ventilation and early extubation. J Cardiothorac Vasc Anesth 2002;16:27–31.

48. Denault AY, Gorcsan J III, Pinsky MR: Dynamic effects of positive-pressure ventilation on canine left ventricular pressure-volume relations. J Appl Physiol 2001;91:298–308.

49. Biondi JW, Schulman DS, Soufer R, et al: The effect of incremental positive end-expiratory pressure on right ventricular hemodynamics and ejection fraction. Anesth Analg 1988;67:144–151.

50. Spackman DR, Kellow N, White SA, et al: High frequency jet ventilation and gas trapping. Br J Anaesth 1999;83:708–714.

51. Dambrosio M, Fiore G, Brienza N, et al: Right ventricular myocardial function in ARF patients: PEEP as a challenge for the right heart. Intensive Care Med 1996;22:772–780.

52. Schmitt JM, Vieillard-Baron A, Augarde R, et al: Positive end-expiratory pressure titration in acute respiratory distress syndrome patients: Impact on right ventricular outflow impedance evaluated by pulmonary artery Doppler flow velocity measurements. Crit Care Med 2001;29:1154–1158.

53. Jardin F, Farcot JC, Boisante L, et al: Influence of positive end-expiratory pressure on left ventricular performance. N Engl J Med 1981;304:387–392.

54. Jardin F: Ventricular interdependence: How does it impact on hemodynamic evaluation in clinical practice? Intensive Care Med 2003;29:361–363.

55. Vieillard-Baron A, Schmitt JM, Augarde R, et al: Acute cor pulmonale in acute respiratory distress syndrome submitted to protective ventilation: Incidence, clinical implications, and prognosis. Crit Care Med 2001;29:1551–1555.

56. Dyhr T, Laursen N, Larsson A: Effects of lung recruitment maneuver and positive end-expiratory pressure on lung volume, respiratory mechanics and alveolar gas mixing in patients ventilated after cardiac surgery. Acta Anaesthesiol Scand 2002;46:717–725.

57. van den Berg PC, Jansen JR, Pinsky MR: Effect of positive pressure on venous return in volume-loaded cardiac surgical patients. J Appl Physiol 2002;92:1223–1231.

58. Vieillard-Baron A, Loubieres Y, Schmitt JM, et al: Cyclic changes in right ventricular output impedance during mechanical ventilation. J Appl Physiol 1999;87:1644–1650.

59. Reis Miranda D, Klompe L, Mekel J, et al: Open lung ventilation does not increase right ventricular outflow impedance: An echo-Doppler study. Crit Care Med 2006;34:2555–2560.

60. Kiefer P, Nunes S, Kosonen P, et al: Effect of positive end-expiratory pressure on splanchnic perfusion in acute lung injury. Intensive Care Med 2000;26:376–383.

61. Matuschak GM, Pinsky MR, Rogers RM: Effects of positive end-expiratory pressure on hepatic blood flow and performance. J Appl Physiol 1987;62:1377–1383.

62. Lehtipalo S, Biber B, Frojse R, et al: Effects of dopexamine and positive end-expiratory pressure on intestinal blood flow and oxygenation: The perfusion pressure perspective. Chest 2003;124:688–698.

63. Nunes S, Rothen HU, Brander L, et al: Changes in splanchnic circulation during an alveolar recruitment maneuver in healthy porcine lungs. Anesth Analg 2004;98:1432–1438.

64. Aneman A, Eisenhofer G, Fandriks L, et al: Splanchnic circulation and regional sympathetic outflow during perioperative PEEP ventilation in humans. Br J Anaesth 1999;82:838–842.

65. Pannu N, Mehta RL: Effect of mechanical ventilation on the kidney. Best Pract Res Clin Anaesthesiol 2004;18:189–203.

66. Pannu N, Mehta RL: Mechanical ventilation and renal function: An area for concern? Am J Kidney Dis 2002;39:616–624.

67. Priebe HJ, Heimann JC, Hedley-Whyte J: Mechanisms of renal dysfunction during positive end-expiratory pressure ventilation. J Appl Physiol 1981;50:643–649.

68. Hall SV, Johnson EE, Hedley-Whyte J: Renal hemodynamics and function with continuous positive-pressure ventilation in dogs. Anesthesiology 1974;41:452–461.

69. Ramamoorthy C, Rooney MW, Dries DJ, et al: Aggressive hydration during continuous positive-pressure ventilation restores atrial transmural pressure, plasma atrial natriuretic peptide concentrations, and renal function. Crit Care Med 1992;20:1014–1019.

70. Zhang H, Downey GP, Suter PM, et al: Conventional mechanical ventilation is associated with bronchoalveolar lavage-induced activation of polymorphonuclear leukocytes: A possible mechanism to explain the systemic consequences of ventilator-induced lung injury in patients with ARDS. Anesthesiology 2002;97:1426–1433.

71. Wolf S, Schurer L, Trost HA, et al: The safety of the open lung approach in neurosurgical patients. Acta Neurochir 2002; 81(Suppl):99–101.

72. Bein T, Kuhr LP, Bele S, et al: Lung recruitment maneuver in patients with cerebral injury: Effects on intracranial pressure and cerebral metabolism. Intensive Care Med 2002;28:554–558.

73. Huynh T, Messer M, Sing RF, et al: Positive end-expiratory pressure alters intracranial and cerebral perfusion pressure in severe traumatic brain injury. J Trauma 2002;53:488–492.

74. Georgiadis D, Schwarz S, Baumgartner RW, et al: Influence of positive end-expiratory pressure on intracranial pressure and cerebral perfusion pressure in patients with acute stroke. Stroke 2001;32:2088–2092.

75. McGuire G, Crossley D, Richards J, et al: Effects of varying levels of positive end-expiratory pressure on intracranial pressure and cerebral perfusion pressure. Crit Care Med 1997;25:1059–1062.

76. Toung TJ, Aizawa H, Traystman RJ: Effects of positive end-expiratory pressure ventilation on cerebral venous pressure with head elevation in dogs. J Appl Physiol 2000;88:655–661.

77. Eckenhoff JE: The physiologic significance of the vertebral venous plexus. Surg Gynecol Obstet 1970;131:72–78.

# CHAPTER 26

# Liquid Ventilation

Jürgen P. Meinhardt and Michael Quintel

Attempts to improve the outcome of acute lung injury (ALI) and acute respiratory distress syndrome (ARDS) remain major challenges in contemporary critical care medicine. Both ALI and ARDS represent the final common pathway of widely independent, simultaneously operating cellular and humoral mediator systems and cascades.[1] Apparently, numerous and heterogeneous diseases as well as extrinsic factors are related to the development and progression of ALI and ARDS. Primary (pulmonary) and secondary (extrapulmonary) types of ARDS, including their reaction to different therapeutic interventions, may represent epiphenomena of different respiratory mechanics rather than expressing a real relationship with the underlying disease process. Certainly, the most important finding of the last decade was our increasing knowledge about the iatrogenic consequences of ventilatory treatment, including volutrauma, atelect-trauma, and biotrauma.[2] The concept of minimizing the iatrogenic consequences of conventional mechanical ventilation represents the background for the development and investigation of alternative treatment strategies such as high-frequency oscillation ventilation (HFOV), extracorporeal lung support, pulmonary application of surfactant, and liquid ventilation. This chapter focuses on the intrapulmonary application of liquids to establish liquid ventilation in its different forms.

## HISTORICAL BACKGROUND

The physiologic implications of liquid filling in mammalian lungs, such as in the fetal stage, have occupied researchers for thousands of years. Early knowledge of pulmonary physiology was gained indirectly through the pathophysiology of drowning and pulmonary edema. In ancient times, the role of the lungs as "gas exchange units" was not understood. Galen believed that the lungs of drowning mammals took up water until the overfill of stomach and intestines caused the death of the organism.[3] In 1819, the French pulmonologist René Laënnec, who also invented the stethoscope, noted that "the lung liquid fill impairs the permeability of gases."[4] In 1873, the physiologist Gabriel-Constant Colin, of Lyon, France, tried to establish a model to measure the pulmonary volume accurately by filling the organs with water. However, he found that the fast resorption of hypo-oncotic solutions caused systematic errors in the resulting volumes.[5]

The devastating experiences with war gas poisoning during World War I forced Winternitz and Smith, in 1920, to investigate the effects of pulmonary lavage with isotonic saline solution.[6] Subsequently, in 1929, the Swiss physiologist von Neergard found, as an incidental effect of his experiments on pulmonary surface tension, that filling of the lungs with saline solution dramatically improved static pulmonary compliance.[7] Furthermore, pulmonary filling with saline solution became an instrument to investigate pulmonary physiology in the following decades.

Eliminating the liquid-gas interface, the effects of surface-active forces on alveolar morphology and function were studied and investigated.[8] The liquid-filled lung became the base of J.B. West's work on determinants of intrapulmonary ventilation-perfusion matching.[4] In 1962, Kylstra and associates demonstrated the general practicability of mammalian liquid ventilation with hyperbaric oxygenated saline solutions.[9] However, a still low amount of dissolved oxygen as well as the poor diffusion coefficient of saline solution for carbon dioxide and the increased viscosity compared with air caused hypercapnia and acidosis, and animals survived only for very short periods.[10] Thereafter, the intrapulmonary use of saline solution was limited to bronchopulmonary lavage and mobilization of secretions. The idea of "liquid breathing" forced the search for other liquid compounds better suited to intrapulmonary application. For example, oxygenated silicone oil was used; however, its viscosity and toxicity precluded its further use.[10] Finally, in 1966, Clark and Gollan, in a pioneer study, demonstrated the survival of spontaneously breathing mice that had been submerged for 1 hour in a normobarically oxygenated perfluorocarbon (PFC) solution (tetrahydrofuran, FX 80) and were thus "breathing" an organic fluid.[11]

## PHYSICAL AND CHEMICAL PROPERTIES OF PERFLUOROCARBONS

PFCs are a relatively homogeneous group of perfluorinated compounds not present in nature. With increased knowledge and improvements in chemical synthesis techniques, a series of aliphatic and cyclic compounds have been isolated. Table 26.1 gives an overview of PFCs of medical importance. The chemical and physical properties of PFC compounds are determined by their chain length and the branching of carbon chains as well as the degree of fluorination or substitution with other halogens. PFCs are characterized by chemical inertness and stability. They are inflammable and noncorrosive; furthermore, they are electrically isolating and have high thermic stability. At room temperature, most compounds are liquids, except for some solid-state chemicals such as polytetrafluoroethylene (Teflon). Liquid PFCs are clear and odorless, and their relatively high vapor pressure causes a high evaporation rate into the atmosphere. However, because of their chemical inertness, they have little effect on the ozone layer, thus marking an important distinction from the chlorofluorocarbons (CFCs) as well as other halogenated hydrocarbons.

Because of the complex synthesis and separation processes, first-generation PFCs were mixtures of different compounds; in contrast, modern PFCs demonstrate high purity (see Table 26.1). PFCs are in widespread use for dielectric isolation in large-scale technical facilities and for direct-contact cooling in microelectronics. Nevertheless, chemical production is limited to certain aliphatic PFCs with a defined carbon chain length in the range of 6 to 10. Because exposure to elementary fluorine or fluoride is highly toxic, medical use is limited to PFCs with an extraordinary high grade of purification.

Sterilization of liquids is performed by filtration over normal commercially available bacteria filters or by autoclaving. In review articles, investigators have ascertained the medically important characteristics of PFCs.[12,13] An overview of the physiologic mechanisms of PFCs, based on the chemical and physical properties of these substances, is displayed in Table 26.2.

In 1974, Shaffer and colleagues demonstrated the practicability of full total or tidal liquid ventilation (TLV) in intubated and sedated dogs with a ventilation system based on diaphragmatic pumps proposed by Moskowitz in 1970.[14,15] In 1976, Shaffer and associates also reported on liquid ventilation in a neonatal model of pulmonal immaturity.[16] In 1978, the first description of partial liquid ventilation (PLV) was published; this technique was performed as pulmonary lavage with consecutive gas ventilation.[17] By the late 1970s, studies focusing on experimental models of prematurity, congenital diaphragmatic hernia (CDH), meconium aspiration, and persistent pulmonary hypertension of the newborn (PPNH) were published.[18] Furthermore, animal models of pulmonary injury by saline washout and intravenous application of oleic acid were used to attempt to show the beneficial effects of liquid ventilation.[19,20]

The first pulmonary application of PFCs in humans was reported by Puchetti and colleagues 1984 in Italy.[21] These investigators used a Rimar 101 solution for unilateral pulmonary lavage in four adult patients with ARDS.[21] In 1989, the first use of PFCs for TLV in human neonates was reported by Greenspan and colleagues.[22] In a lavage-type system, these investigators connected a PFC-filled reservoir to the endotracheal tube, and inspiration and expiration were performed by manually changing the level of the reservoir in relation to the patient. In this setup, the driving force consisted of the gravity difference between the lung and the reservoir.[22]

The principle of PLV as used today was first described by Fuhrman and colleagues in 1991.[23] It is based on a combination of PFC filling of the lungs up to the measured or estimated functional residual capacity (FRC) and a gas tidal volume similar to that usually used for conventional gas ventilation. While investigating TLV in pigs, these authors discovered the possibility of ventilating a PFC-filled lung with a conventional gas ventilator, and they attributed this to PFC-assisted gas exchange (PAGE).[23] In consequence, largely independent of species, liquid FRC has been defined in the range of 20 to 30 mL/kg body weight.[12] In terms of nomenclature, PAGE was soon replaced by PLV, to describe more generally the pulmonary application of PFCs during conventional mechanical ventilation.

Although almost all early research on the pulmonary use of PFCs was performed as TLV, PLV quickly became widely accepted, for several reasons. First, PLV is less

**Table 26-1    Overview of Chemical Properties of Perfluorocarbons with Medical Importance Compared with Water**

| Chemical Nomenclature | Trade Name | Molecular Mass (g/mol) | Boiling Point (°C) | Melting Point (°C) | Density (kg/L) | Dynamic Kinematic Surface Viscosity (mPas [at 25°C]) | Surface Tension (mN/m) | Diffusion Coefficient (dyne/cm) | Vapor Pressure (mbar) | Oxygen Solubility* (vol %) | Carbon Dioxide Solubility* (vol %) |
|---|---|---|---|---|---|---|---|---|---|---|---|
| Water | | 18 | 100 | 0 | 1 | 1 | 72 | | 47 | 3 | 57 |
| PFC mixtures | FC-77 | | 97 | | 1.78 | 0.8 | 15 | 8.5 | 85 | 50 | 198 |
| (first-generation PFCs) | RM-101<br>FC-75 | 416<br>416 | 101<br>102 | | 1.77<br>1.78 | 0.82<br>0.82 | 15<br>15 | 6.9<br>6.9 | 64<br>64 | 52<br>52 | 160<br>160 |
| Perfluoro-n-propane | | 188 | −36 | −183 | 1.35 | | | | 790 | | |
| Perfluoro-n-butane | | 238 | −2 | | 1.52 | | | | 280 | | |
| Perfluoro-n-pentane | | 288 | 29 | −120 | 1.60 | 0.47 | 9.4 | | 862 | | 205 |
| Perfluoromethylcyclopentane | | 300 | 48 | −70 | 1.71 | 1.05 | 12.6 | | 368 | | |
| Perfluoro-n-hexane | | 338 | 57 | −90 | 1.68 | 0.66 | 11.1 | | 294 | 57 | 55 |
| Perfluoromethylcyclohexane | | 350 | 76 | −30 | 1.79 | 1.56 | 15.4 | | 141 | 57 | |
| Perfluoro-1,3-dimethylcyclohexane | | 400 | 102 | −70 | 1.83 | 1.92 | 16.6 | | 48 | 28.6 | 109 |
| Perfluorooctane | | 438 | 104 | | 1.78 | 1.4 | 14 | | 43 | 48–52 | |
| Perfluorodecaline (cis-+transisomer) | | 462 | 142 | 10 | 1.92 | 5.53 | 17.6 | | 8.8 | 24–44 | 93 |
| Perfluoromethyldecaline | | 512 | 155 | −70 | 1.93 | 6.41 | 18.5 | | 2.9 | 22 | 82 |
| Perfluoroperhydrofluorene | | 574 | 194 | −40 | 1.98 | 9.58 | 19.7 | | <1 | | |
| Perfluoroperhydrophenanthrene | | 624 | 215 | −20 | 2.03 | 28.4 | 19 | | <1 | 22 | 82 |
| Perfluoro-octylbromide | Perflubron | 499 | 141 | 4 | 1.93 | 2.11 | 18.2 | 2.7 | 10.5 | 49 | 210 |
| Perfluoro-1,3,5,-trimethylcyclohexane | PP 4 | | 128 | −68 | 1.89 | | | | 9.6 | | |

*At room temperature and mean atmospheric pressure. Values for empty spaces are currently unknown.
PFC, perfluorocarbon.

**Table 26-2   Mechanisms of Liquid Ventilation**

| | |
|---|---|
| 1  High physical solubility for gases according to Henry's law linear to partial pressure<br>Low cohesive energy of PFC molecules | Transportation of oxygen and carbon dioxide along a gradient over the alveolocapillary membrane[36,98–103] |
| 2  High specific weight | Gravity-dependent recruitment of consolidated lung areas, tamponade effect, liquid PEEP, consecutive reduction of intra-alveolar edema and redistribution of pulmonary blood flow, reduction of ventilation-perfusion mismatch[92,104] |
| 3  No mixing with chemically polar compounds | Separation of aqueous solutions, such as pulmonary secretions, and possibility of suctioning |
| 4  High biocompatibility<br>No metabolism | Phagocytosis of PFC in defined particle size (0.1–0.3 μm) in the reticuloendothelial system and storage in macrophages[105]<br>Accumulation in relevant concentration in fatty tissues, brain, liver, and kidney[106]<br>Transitory changes in hepatic enzymatic activity at cytochrome P-450 and arylesterase[107]<br>Excretion >99% per exhalation |
| 5  Low surface tension | Surfactant-like activities not impaired by mediators in the alveolar edema fluid[32,108,109] |
| 6  Positive diffusion coefficient as an indicator for interactions at physical borderlines | Wide dispersion of PFC in the lungs[110,111] |
| 7  Physical barrier | Tamponade effect, prevention of alveolar accumulation of secretions and bacterial debris, reduction in migration of inflammatory cells[112,113] |
| 8  High kinematic viscosity | Sufficient rheologic characteristics as a liquid breathing medium[72,114] |
| 9  High vapor pressure | Balance between pulmonary accumulation and loss of substance by evaporation[56,57,115–117] |
| 10  Anti-inflammatory and immunomodulatory effects | Reduced inflammatory response of the lungs, inhibition of acute lung injury–induced activation of neutrophils, reduction in tumor necrosis factor-α–induced production of interleukin-8 by alveolar epithelium[35]<br>Reduction of myeloperoxidase activity[106] |

PFC, perfluorocarbons.

complex and more practical. It can be performed while using the "usual" gas ventilator, and no additional technical devices and sophisticated monitoring are required. Additionally, early TLV research used first-generation PFCs with poor purification grades and shifting composition of compounds, thereby resulting in inconstant physiologic effects. The admixture of fluorine radicals and fluorides frequently interacted with the pulmonary endothelium.[24] Coincident with the first description of PLV, PFCs of high purity and with constant composition became available. A further improvement was achieved when perfluoro-octylbromide (PFOB, perflubron;

Alliance Pharmaceutical Corp., San Diego, CA) was licensed by the National Institutes of Health for human use in phase II/III studies.

## EVOLUTION OF PARTIAL LIQUID VENTILATION

The introduction of PLV marked a turning point in the history of liquid ventilation. After demonstration of general applicability of this new technique, investigations attempted to show the safety and efficacy of PLV in different models of ALI in several species. In 1995, the safe clinical use of PLV was proven in patients with ARDS who also had extracorporeal membrane oxygenation (ECMO) backup.[19] Simultaneously, animal experiments showed improvements in arterial oxygenation ($PaO_2$) in the supine as well as the prone position,[25] in the alveolar-arterial oxygen partial pressure difference, in intrapulmonary shunt ratio, and, in mixed venous oxygen saturation. Additionally, investigators demonstrated a dose-dependent prevalent distribution of PFCs to dependent lung areas, with a marked trend toward a more homogeneous distribution at higher liquid volumes.[26] However, later, more detailed studies revealed that, at least at positive end-expiratory pressure (PEEP) levels of 5 cm $H_2O$, the most dependent parts of the lungs, even while using 30 mL perflubron/kg body weight, are still not reached with adequate amounts of PFC to "liquid recruit" these areas totally[27] (Fig. 26.1). Additionally, while using PFC sampling techniques as well as magnetic resonance imaging, investigators demonstrated that oxygen content in the PFC liquid followed a gravity-dependent distribution pattern and showed the highest amounts of oxygen in the least dependent parts of the lungs.[28,29] Using microsphere techniques, the redistribution of pulmonary blood flow toward the upper, less dependent lung regions was shown.[30] Furthermore, strong regional differences in blood flow between apical and basal lung regions were found in PLV.[31] Animal studies elucidated histologic and morphometric changes during PLV and were able to show a marked reduction in alveolar damage as well as improvements in the diffuse alveolar damage score with increased alveolar diameter and reduced septal thickness and capillary diameter.[26] These effects were attributed to the washout and dilution of proinflammatory mediators as well as to the inherent anti-inflammatory properties of PFCs.[24,32–35]

The concept of liquid ventilating inhomogeneously injured lungs and thus potentially reaching fast recruitment and more homogeneous distribution of ventilation was so fascinating that initial research focused more on the effects of PLV than on practical considerations of PFC dosage and ventilation of the patient. The FRC dosing dogma may even, in combination with non-adapted tidal volumes and PEEP levels, have caused barotrauma and overdistention of nondependent gas-ventilated lung areas and may thus have induced ventilator-associated lung injury (Cox R, personal communication). Meanwhile, numerous studies on dosage and ventilator settings in PLV were published; however, studies that rigorously compare the effects of different settings are still lacking. Volume and pressure controlled modes have been applied, without showing a significant advantage of either mode.[36] Although initially the influence of PEEP was considered poor, as a result of the "PEEP in a bottle" effect of the PFCs, later studies revealed the relationship between PEEP and gas exchange as well as the respiratory mechanics during PLV.[37] Investigators showed that instilling PFC markedly decreases the lower inflection point (LIP), which can be determined from the pressure-volume curve. Although a maximum is reached with 10 mL PFC/kg body weight, a further increase in the amount of PFC applied does not lead to a further decrease of the LIP that can be determined. Setting the PEEP level 1 cm $H_2O$ higher than the LIP does induce a marked increase in oxygenation when compared with a PEEP level of 5 cm $H_2O$.[38] A further increase in PEEP, but not a further increase in the amount of PFC applied, does improve oxygenation. In one study, the increase in total PEEP caused by a higher intrinsic PEEP led to similar effects while using inversed inspiratory-to-expiratory ratios.[39]

Most studies on the hemodynamic effects of PLV showed no significant influence even with doses of 30 mL/kg body weight, when normovolemia and unaltered cardiac function were present.[37,40] In addition, thermodilution and double-indicator cardiac output measurement techniques have been shown to be accurate even in liquid-filled lungs.[41]

Additional measures such as the intrapulmonary application of surfactant and prostaglandins or the

VCV

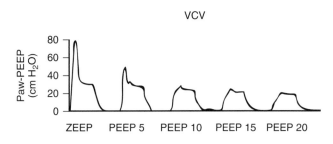

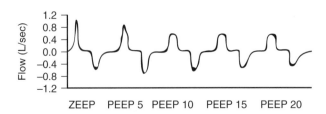

**Figure 26.1** Effect of increasing positive end-expiratory pressure (PEEP) on airway pressure during volume controlled ventilation in partial liquid ventilation (PLV). (From Ferreyra G, Goddon S, Fujino Y, Kacmaerk RM: The relationship between gas delivery patterns and the lower inflection point of the pressure-volume curve during partial liquid ventilation. Chest 2000;117:191–198.)

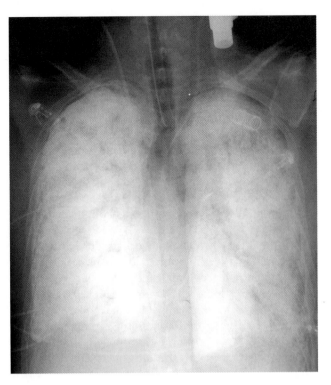

inhalation of nitric oxide in combination with PLV have been studied. Results have not been conclusive. HFOV was investigated as an alternative ventilation mode in several studies, which showed the applicability and safety of the combination of PLV and HFOV.[42-44]

In 1996, Hirschl and colleagues reported the results of the first phase I study, which was performed in 10 adult patients who had severe ARDS mostly secondary to pneumonia.[45] PLV was started while these patients were receiving extracorporeal lung support.[45] Six of these patients were weaned from extracorporeal lung support, and five survived. In 1995, a multicenter phase II randomized controlled trial in adult patients was launched and approved by the Food and Drug Administration.[46] Results of this study were first published in abstract form in 1995.[46] The study, using an FRC-based dosage regimen over a 3-day period, clearly demonstrated the safety of PLV, and no major adverse events were reported. PLV caused significant improvements in static pulmonary compliance and oxygenation, thus allowing a reduction of the fraction of inspired oxygen. However, with regard to the primary end point of the study, no reduction in ventilator-free days was reported when PLV was compared with conventional gas ventilation.[47] A post hoc subgroup analysis revealed significantly faster discontinuation from mechanical ventilation and a trend toward an increase in the number of ventilator-free days at 28 days after inclusion (8.9 versus 4.1), as well as a lower mortality rate during PLV (25.6 versus 36.8%) among patients less than 55 years of age. Problems related to the study design were patient selection, full FRC-based dosing, inconsistent handling of PFC instillation among the different study centers, and the use of a mandatory volume controlled ventilation mode in all patients. In 1998, a phase III multicenter study was started in 50 centers, with a phase II dose finding component comparing two different volumes of perflubron (10 mL/kg body weight versus 20 mL/kg body weight; i.e., carina semi-FRC level versus laryngeal level) against a conventionally treated control group (Fig. 26.2).

This study was terminated after an interim analysis including 311 adult patients in November 2001, when neither the primary end point for improvement in ventilator-free days nor the secondary end point for improvement in 28-day mortality was met. Moreover, the study failed to demonstrate any advantages of PLV when compared with conventional mechanical ventilation. However, it showed that, in a large population of patients, PLV can be performed safely at both dosages. Analysis of these data shows that the gap between the positive results obtained in numerous laboratory studies and the lack of clinical proof for the advantages of PLV is striking. It is likely that too many questions regarding type of ventilation, optimal PEEP settings, dosage and redosing interval, and identification of patients who would

**Figure 26.2** Native chest radiograph of an adult patient with acute respiratory distress syndrome and partial liquid ventilation: anteroposterior, 120 kV; lung fill, 10 mL/kg body weight perflubron.

probably benefit from PLV were unresolved when the clinical study was started. Other effects and potential side effects of PLV are still not clearly elucidated. This is particularly true for the effects on the alveolar level.[48] Little is known about the regional distribution of oxygenation and deoxygenation and the mechanisms through which gas exchange in the inhomogeneously distributed PFC is realized.[49] Additionally there is a lack of knowledge about the effects of PLV on pulmonary fibrosis in late-stage ARDS[50] and about the possible use of PLV in the intermediate and long term.[51] Although potential sequelae of intrapulmonary PFC use have been evaluated in numerous studies, up to now only reticuloendothelial system storage has been demonstrated.[52] In summary, some evidence indicates that a promising therapeutic approach to treat acute lung failure was buried before it was born.

## PERFLUOROCARBON INHALATION

Several reports on the inhalational use of PFC as a vapor or aerosol for enhancement of pulmonary function in experimental lung injury have been published by different investigators.[53-58] Nevertheless, the underlying mode of action remains unclear. Given the physical conditions such as body temperature and vapor pressure of PFC compounds, the aggregate state in the lungs is balanced between liquid and gaseous. However, this balance is largely influenced by the unequal distribution of the substance in inhomogeneously aerated lungs.

In a study applying 18 volume percent of perfluorohexane in an oleic acid model of ALI, significant improvements in static and dynamic pulmonary compliance were found, far beyond the extent and duration of the PFC vapor use.[57] In contrast, in another study using PF 5080 in a saline washout model, no significant changes in $PaO_2$ and pulmonal compliance were detected.[59]

Because these studies, among others, differ in the type and amount of PFC vapor, and because results are strongly contradictory, no clear statement about the value of this treatment option is possible at present. In a randomized trial comparing the inhalational effects of PFCs on lung function, four different compounds with high and low vapor pressures were applied; a measurable impact on gas exchange and lung mechanics was only found in the perfluorohexane group.[60] However, PFCs as aerosols or vapor represent another interesting approach to their application in injured lungs, including the potential use of PFCs as vehicles for the intrapulmonary application of drugs.

## RENAISSANCE OF TOTAL LIQUID VENTILATION

Although TLV represented the initial starting point of PFC use for ventilatory support, further improvements in TLV technology lagged in the 1990s. Investigators realized that a TLV device was technically limited, and the physiologic effects such as expiratory flow limitations and resulting choked-flow phenomena were not sufficiently understood.[61–64] Subsequently, TLV itself was implicated as a cause of alterations in acid-base balance, perpetuated by a reduction in cardiac stroke volume.[65] However, TLV research was continued by a small group of investigators who considered the possibility of effects by far exceeding those of PLV, such as more pronounced improvements in pulmonary compliance and elastance by elimination of the intrapulmonary liquid-gas interface. Distinctive improvements in the pulmonary pressure-volume relationship are noted when liquid tidal volume is applied in addition to liquid FRC.[66,67] Furthermore, in TLV, ventilation-perfusion inequalities are reduced to a significant extent when compared with PLV.[12,66] For these reasons, investigators have long assumed that TLV is capable of reducing barotrauma in the injured lung and may be a helpful mode in the prevention of

ventilator-induced lung injury, if only the technical realization were possible.[68]

Efforts to automate the TLV process and to establish an option for long-term use led to the development of different pump-driven systems. Diaphragmatic or bellows pumps,[14,15] centrifugal pumps,[69] and roller pumps[66,70] were applied. Deriving from extracorporeal circulation, those systems showed technical characteristics mimicking physiologic blood flow conditions by providing unidirectional, pulsatile, or continuous flow patterns.[71] Nevertheless, their applicability for TLV use has been discouraging, because these systems are counter to the bidirectional nature of breathing and therefore require extensive servoregulated valve systems. These liquid delivery systems are prone to flow irregularities owing to positive or negative acceleration,[71] and they produce insufficient tidal volumes as a result of inadequate volume control. Additionally, in roller pumps, maximum flow is limited to approximately 15 to 20 L/minute, thus causing consecutive problems in maximum flow as required in larger individuals. Therefore, in most studies, these pump systems were used exclusively for liquid inspiration, whereas expiration was performed passively by draining the liquid by gravity from the lungs after decoupling through a valve system over a siphon mechanism.[66]

In open systems, expiratory driving forces of the breathing liquid consist of the elastic recoil force of the thoracopulmonary system in combination with the height difference between lung and reservoir,[72] counterbalanced by the physical limitation of maximum flow speed of PFCs in the branching bronchial tree.[73] Such systems are unstable regarding height changes and are poorly applicable to clinical practice. Therefore, combined with the viscosity of PFCs and choked-flow phenomena, passive liquid drainage from the lungs is limited, thus restricting the ventilatory rate and causing hypercapnia, acidosis, and cardiocirculatory depression.[65,69,74] These side effects are caused to a greater extent by the inadequacy of the ventilatory systems when compared with TLV per se and have prevented the use of this technique in ALI.[65,75,76] Although investigators showed that the application of TLV in an oleic acid lung injury model led to improvements in static compliance, an ECMO backup was used in this study, and therefore results from gas exchange were not representative.[77,78] Furthermore, no large-scale trials in animals with a body weight of more than 20 kg have been performed.

In 1999, the double-piston pump system for use in TLV was introduced, based on two parallel operating cylinder-piston circuits, interconnected by a reservoir and driven by a linear motor.[79] Thus, it was recognized that a closed-loop liquid ventilation system with active expiration is mandatory, because optimization of expiratory flow profiles is the key to TLV, to avoid a drift in

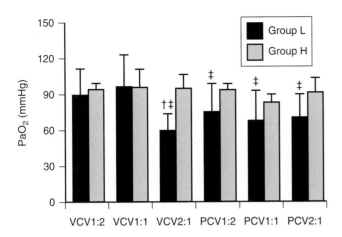

**Figure 26.3** Lower inflection point (LIP) during partial liquid ventilation (PLV). (From Fujino Y, Goddon S, Chiche JD, et al: Partial liquid ventilation ventilates better than gas ventilation. Am J Respir Crit Care Med 2000;162:650–657.)

pulmonary liquid FRC. In Figure 26.3, the homogeneous distribution of liquid volumes during this process is shown. Applying this system, the earlier assumption of a relationship between TLV and acidotic conditions was disproved, and stable blood gas conditions were possible over longer time intervals.[70,79] Elaborated control software allows control of system components, such as adjustment of alarm limits and feedback to the system, for example by reducing inspiratory flow when a limit is met.[80] These characteristics add up to an integrative ventilatory system providing sophisticated online monitoring and control of ventilatory patterns. Because of the stability of ventilatory parameters, continuous hemodynamic and cardiopulmonary measurements are possible in TLV.[81–83] Furthermore, for the first time, TLV has been performed in a non–neonatal oleic acid model of ALI and in a model of late-stage ARDS fibrosis caused by bleomycin.[84] The double-piston principle of TLV provides the secure use of this technique over longer periods with stable ventilatory parameters and physiologic effects.

## FUTURE PERSPECTIVES

Perflubron has been the perfluorochemical of choice for performing liquid ventilation[85] in a multitude of animal studies as well as in human trials, including two randomized controlled trials. However, large numbers of PFCs are available, with marked differences in physical and chemical properties and in their resulting effects when applied to the lungs. Taking the demands of different application forms into account, it seems questionable whether the ideal PFC has been identified. Moreover, with increasing

knowledge and extended applications, it seems unlikely that only one optimal PFC exists. Early experience with alternative PFCs for PLV has been published.[86] For TLV, many different substances have been used over the last 30 years.[12,15,87]

The PLV technique experienced a major setback when clinical studies were stopped in 2001 when they demonstrated no difference with regard to outcome and other parameters such as ventilator-free days in a 28-day period in patients with ARDS. However, the study design and the time point remained debatable, and research groups continued to investigate PLV to address open questions as optimal dosing and redosing, optimal ventilator modes and settings, and the role of ventilatory adjuncts such as prone positioning (Fig. 26.4).

Another innovative approach in the evolution of perfluorochemicals is their role as carriers for the pulmonary application of drugs, by either mixing or chemically attaching substances to the PFC, the latter being nearly obviated for most drugs by the chemical structure of PFCs. In this field, semifluorinated alkanes may play a role in the future. Mixed gentamicin,[88] suprarenin and atropine,[89] nitric oxide,[90–94] prostaglandin $E_2$,[95] activated protein C,[96] and halothane[97] have already been investigated in animal studies. The topical pulmonary application of other antibiotics, vasoactive drugs, steroids, and antineoplastic agents (e.g., methotrexate) has not yet been performed, but it has become possible as a result of increasing knowledge and technical improvements.

Besides genuine lung injury, further applications, such as temperature regulation of the central body

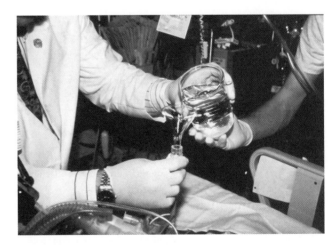

**Figure 26.4** Photograph of the first adult human perfluorocarbon use for partial liquid ventilation. Perflubron filling of the lungs through an endotracheal tube performed in 1996 at the University of Michigan Medical Center, Ann Arbor, Michigan. (Adapted from Hirschl RB, Conrad S, Kaiser R, et al: Partial liquid ventilation in adult patients with ARDS: A multicenter phase I-II trial. Adult PLV Study Group. Ann Surg 1998;228:692–700.)

compartment and anticancer therapy, may be conceivable for TLV.[52] Temperature control may be performable for the maintenance of isothermy, especially in neonates and preterm infants or in septic patients, and for hyperthermia in subdiaphragmatic tumors while providing normal core temperature. Adjuvant antineoplastic treatments could consist of the topical application of drugs, hyperoxygenation of pulmonary tumors, and preconditioning for chemotherapy or radiotherapy. The value of liquid-filled lungs for cardiopulmonary resuscitation with regard to oxygenation and transthoracic pressure transfer has not yet been determined.

Despite the widespread increase in knowledge, liquid ventilation in its different forms is still an area with many unanswered questions. The unfavorable results of two prospective randomized controlled trials mark a major drawback in the clinical application of PLV as well as in the number of ongoing or planned studies. This trend is consistent with a marked reduction of research support in the field of liquid ventilation. Therefore, conclusive results cannot be expected in the near future for PLV, TLV, or PFC inhalation. Further research will be necessary to gain new insights and thus perhaps to allow a return of PFC use to the clinical setting.

## REFERENCES

1. Gattinoni L, et al: Acute respiratory distress syndrome, the critical care paradigm: What we learned and what we forgot. Curr Opin Crit Care 2004;10:272–278.
2. Putensen C, Wrigge H: Ventilator-associated systemic inflammation in acute lung injury. Intensive Care Med 2000;26:1411–1413.
3. Metken S: Die letzte Reise. Munich: Hugendubel Verlag, 1984.
4. West JB: *Respiratory Physiology: People and Ideas.* New York: Oxford University Press, 1996.
5. Colin GC: On adsorption in airways. In Traité de Physiologie Comparée des Animaux. Paris: Baillière, 1873, pp 108–111.
6. Winternitz MC, Smith GH: Preliminary studies in intratracheal therapy. In Winternitz MC (ed): *Pathology of War Gas Poisoning.* New Haven, CT: Yale University Press, 1920, pp 144–160.
7. von Neergard K: Neue Auffassungen ueber einen Grundbegriff der Atemmechanik: Die Retraktionskraft der Lunge, abhaengig von der Oberflaechenspannung in den Alveolen. Z Gesamte Exp Med 1929;66:373–394.
8. Clements JA: Surface tension on lungs extracts. Proc Soc Exp Biol Med 1957;95:170–172.
9. Kylstra JA: Required properties of a liquid for respiration. Fed Proc 1970;29:1724.
10. Kylstra JA, Paganelli CV, Lanphier EH: Pulmonary gas exchange in dogs ventilated with hyperbarically oxygenated liquid. J Appl Physiol 1966;21:177–184.
11. Clark C, Gollan F: Survival of mammals breathing organic liquids equilibrated with oxygen at atmospheric pressure. J Appl Physiol 1966;21:1755–1756.
12. Quintel M, Meinhardt J, Waschke KF: [Partial liquid ventilation]. Anaesthesist 1998;47:479–489.
13. Shaffer TH: A brief review: Liquid ventilation. Undersea Biomed Res 1987;14:169–179.
14. Moskowitz GD: A mechanical respirator for control of liquid breathing. Fed Proc 1970;29:1751–1752.
15. Shaffer TH, Moskowitz GD: Demand-controlled liquid ventilation of the lungs. J Appl Physiol 1974;36:208–213.
16. Shaffer TH, et al: Gaseous exchange and acid-base balance in premature lambs during liquid ventilation since birth. Pediatr Res 1976;10:227–231.
17. Shaffer TH, et al: Pulmonary lavage in preterm lambs. Pediatr Res 1978;12:695–698.
18. Quintel M, Meinhardt J, Waschke K: Partielle Fluessigkeitsventilation [Partial liquid ventilation]. Anaesthesist 1998;47:479–489.
19. Hirschl RB, et al: Development and application of a simplified liquid ventilator. Crit Care Med 1995;23:157–163.
20. Jackson JC, et al: Full-tidal liquid ventilation with perfluorocarbon for prevention of lung injury in newborn non-human primates. Artif Cells Blood Substit Immobil Biotechnol 1994;22:1121–1132.
21. Puchetti V, et al: Liquid ventilation in man: First clinical experiences on pulmonary unilateral washing using fluorocarbon liquid [abstract]. In Fourth World Congress for Bronchology. 1984, p 115.
22. Greenspan JS, et al: Liquid ventilation of preterm baby [letter]. Lancet 1989;2:1095.
23. Fuhrman BP, Paczan PR, DeFrancisis M: Perfluorocarbon-associated gas exchange. Crit Care Med 1991;19:712–722.
24. Rotta AT, et al: Partial liquid ventilation with perflubron attenuates in vivo oxidative damage to proteins and lipids. Crit Care Med 2000;28:202–208.
25. Max M, et al: Combining partial liquid ventilation and prone position in experimental acute lung injury. Anesthesiology 1999;91:796–803.
26. Quintel M, et al: Effects of partial liquid ventilation on lung injury in a model of acute respiratory failure: A histologic and morphometric analysis. Crit Care Med 1998;26:833–843.
27. Luecke T, et al: End-expiratory lung volumes and density distribution patterns during partial liquid ventilation in healthy and oleic acid–injured sheep: A computed tomography study. Crit Care Med 2003;31:2190–2197.
28. Uchida T, et al: Relationship between airway pressure and the distribution of gas-liquid interface during partial liquid ventilation in the oleic acid lung injury model: Fluorine-19 magnetic resonance imaging study. Crit Care Med 2000;28:2904–2908.
29. Heussel CP, et al: Measurements of alveolar pO2 using 19F-MRI in partial liquid ventilation. Invest Radiol 2003;38:635–641.
30. Morris KP, et al: Distribution of pulmonary blood flow in the perfluorocarbon-filled lung. Intensive Care Med 2000;26:756–763.
31. Doctor A, et al: Pulmonary blood flow distribution during partial liquid ventilation. J Appl Physiol 1998;84:1540–1550.
32. Croce MA, et al: Partial liquid ventilation decreases the inflammatory response in the alveolar environment of trauma patients. J Trauma 1998;45:273–280; discussion 280–282.
33. Colton DM, et al: Neutrophil accumulation is reduced during partial liquid ventilation. Crit Care Med 1998;26:1716–1724.
34. Rotta AT, et al: Perfluorooctyl bromide (perflubron) attenuates oxidative injury to biological and nonbiological systems. Pediatr Crit Care Med 2003;4:233–238.
35. Baba A, et al: Perfluorocarbon blocks tumor necrosis factor-alpha–induced interleukin-8 release from alveolar epithelial cells in vitro. Crit Care Med 2000;28:1113–1118.

36. Fujino Y, Goddon S, Chiche JD, et al: Partial liquid ventilation ventilates better than gas ventilation. Am J Respir Crit Care Med 2000;162:650–657.

37. Manaligod JM, et al: Variations in end-expiratory pressure during partial liquid ventilation: Impact on gas exchange, lung compliance, and end-expiratory lung volume. Chest 2000;117:184–190.

38. Kirmse M, et al: Positive end-expiratory pressure improves gas exchange and pulmonary mechanics during partial liquid ventilation. Am J Respir Crit Care Med 1998;158:1550–1556.

39. Fujino Y, et al: The effect of mode, inspiratory time, and positive end-expiratory pressure on partial liquid ventilation. Am J Respir Crit Care Med 1999;159:1087–1095.

40. Degraeuwe PL, et al: Effect of perfluorochemical liquid ventilation on cardiac output and blood pressure variability in neonatal piglets with respiratory insufficiency. Pediatr Pulmonol 2000;30:114–124.

41. Houmes RJ, et al: Hemodynamic effects of partial liquid ventilation with perfluorocarbon in acute lung injury. Intensive Care Med 1995;21:966–972.

42. Gothberg S, et al: High-frequency oscillatory ventilation and partial liquid ventilation after acute lung injury in premature lambs with respiratory distress syndrome. Crit Care Med 2000;28:2450–2456.

43. Uchida T, et al: Inhaled nitric oxide during partial liquid ventilation shifts pulmonary blood flow to the non-dependent lung regions. Intensive Care Med 2000;26:764–769.

44. Leach CL, Morin III FC, Fuhrman BP: Efficacy and pharmacokinetics of nitric oxide inhalation during partial liquid ventilation with perflubron (Liquivent) [abstract]. Pediatr Res 1994;37:160A.

45. Hirschl RB, Pranikoff T, Wise C, et al: Initial experience with partial liquid ventilation in adult patients with the acute respiratory distress syndrome. JAMA 1996 275:383–389.

46. Hirschl RB, Pranikoff T, Gauger P, et al: Liquid ventilation in adults, children, and full-term neonates. Lancet 1995;346:1201–1202.

47. Hirschl RB, Conrad S, Kaiser R, et al: Partial liquid ventilation in adult patients with ARDS: A multicenter phase I-II trial. Adult PLV Study Group. Ann Surg 1998;228:692–700.

48. Shaffer TH, Wolfson MR, Greenspan JS: Liquid ventilation: Current status. Pediatr Rev (Online) 1999;20:e134–e142.

49. Max M, et al: Time-dependency of improvements in arterial oxygenation during partial liquid ventilation in experimental acute respiratory distress syndrome. Crit Care (Lond) 2000;4:114–119.

50. Hood CI, Modell JH: A morphologic study of long-term retention of fluorocarbon after liquid ventilation. Chest 2000;118:1436–1440.

51. Degraeuwe PL, Vos GD, Blanco CE: Perfluorochemical liquid ventilation: From the animal laboratory to the intensive care unit. Int J Artif Organs 1995;18:674–683.

52. Shaffer TH, Wolfson MR, Clark LC Jr: Liquid ventilation. Pediatr Pulmonol 1992;14:102–109.

53. von der Hardt K, et al: Comparison of aerosol therapy with different perfluorocarbons in surfactant-depleted animals. Crit Care Med 2004;32:1200–1206.

54. Bleyl JU, et al: Changes in pulmonary function and oxygenation during application of perfluorocarbon vapor in healthy and oleic acid–injured animals. Crit Care Med 2002;30:1340–1347.

55. Ragaller M, et al: [From isoflurane to perfluorohexane? Perfluorocarbons: Therapeutic strategies in acute lung failure]. Anaesthesist 2000;49:291–301.

56. Warner DO: Vaporized perfluorocarbon: Taking the "liquid" out of liquid ventilation. Anesthesiology 1999;91:340–342.

57. Bleyl JU, et al: Vaporized perfluorocarbon improves oxygenation and pulmonary function in an ovine model of acute respiratory distress syndrome. Anesthesiology 1999;91:461–469.

58. Sass DJ, et al: Gas embolism due to intravenous FC 80 liquid fluorocarbon. J Appl Physiol 1976;40:745–751.

59. Kelly KP, Stenson BJ, Drummond GB: Randomised comparison of partial liquid ventilation, nebulised perfluorocarbon, porcine surfactant, artificial surfactant, and combined treatments on oxygenation, lung mechanics, and survival in rabbits after saline lung lavage. Intensive Care Med 2000;26:1523–1530.

60. Meinhardt JP, Schmittner M, Herrmann P, et al: Comparison of different inhalational perfluorocarbons in a rabbit model of acute lung injury. ASAIO J 2005;51:85–91.

61. Baba Y, et al: Assessment of the development of choked flow during total liquid ventilation. Crit Care Med 2004;32:201–208.

62. Dawson SV, Elliott EA: Use of the choke point in the prediction of flow limitation in elastic tubes. Fed Proc 1980;39:2765–2770.

63. Elliott EA, Dawson SV: Test of wave-speed theory of flow limitation in elastic tubes. J Appl Physiol 1977;43:516–522.

64. Mead J: Expiratory flow limitation: A physiologist's point of view. Fed Proc 1980;39:2771–2775.

65. Lowe C, et al: Liquid ventilation: Cardiovascular adjustments with secondary hyperlactatemia and acidosis. J Appl Physiol 1979;47:1051–1057.

66. Hirschl RB, et al: Evaluation of gas exchange, pulmonary compliance, and lung injury during total and partial liquid ventilation in the acute respiratory distress syndrome. Crit Care Med 1996;24:1001–1008.

67. Meinhardt JP, et al: Comparison of static airway pressures during total liquid ventilation while applying different expiratory modes and time patterns. ASAIO J 2004;50:68–75.

68. Shaffer TH, Wolfson MR: Liquid ventilation: An alternative ventilation strategy for management of neonatal respiratory distress. Eur J Pediatr 1996;155(Suppl 2):S30–S34.

69. Harris DJ, et al: Liquid ventilation in dogs: An apparatus for normobaric and hyperbaric studies. J Appl Physiol 1983;54:1141–1148.

70. Stavis RL, et al: Physiologic, biochemical, and histologic correlates associated with tidal liquid ventilation. Pediatr Res 1998;43:132–138.

71. Zwischenberger JB, Bartlett RH: ECMO: *Extracorporeal Cardiopulmonary Support in Critical Care*. Ann Arbor, MI: Extracorporeal Life Support Organization, 1995, p 680.

72. La Rocca J, Perez Fontan JJ: Effect of liquid inflation on the viscoelastic behavior of the lungs in developing piglets. J Appl Physiol 1994;77:1653–1658.

73. Lambert RK: A new computational model for expiratory flow from nonhomogeneous human lungs. J Biomech Eng 1989;111:200–205.

74. Koen PA, Wolfson MR, Shaffer TH: Fluorocarbon ventilation: Maximal expiratory flows and $CO_2$ elimination. Pediatr Res 1988;24:291–296.

75. Curtis SE, Fuhrman BP, Howland DF: Airway and alveolar pressures during perfluorocarbon breathing in infant lambs. J Appl Physiol 1990;68:2322–2328.

76. Shaffer TH, et al: Cardiopulmonary function in very preterm lambs during liquid ventilation. Pediatr Res 1983;17:680–684.

77. Richman PS, Wolfson MR, Shaffer TH: Lung lavage with oxygenated perfluorochemical liquid in acute lung injury. Crit Care Med 1993;21:768–774.

78. Hirschl RB: A liquid panacea for failing lungs. Nat Med 1996;2:1195–1196.

79. Meinhardt J, Quintel M, Hirschl R: Development and application of a double piston configured total liquid ventilation device. Am J Respir Crit Care Med 1999;159:A79.

80. Herrmann P, et al: Entwicklung eines PC-gestützten Systems zur totalen Flüssigkeitsventilation mit Perfluorcarbonen in der experimentellen Intensivmedizin. In Jamle R, Jaschinski H (eds): *Virtuelle Instrumente in der Praxis.* Heidelberg: Hüthig Verlag, 2000, pp 313–320.

81. Aresta F, et al: Pulmonary vascular resistance in total liquid ventilated rabbits. Am J Respir Crit Care Med 2000;161:A550.

82. Meinhardt J, Quintel M, van Ackern K: Influence of I:E ratio on cardiac index during partial liquid ventilation in a sheep model of acute lung injury. Intensive Care Med 1999;25(Suppl 1):S199.

83. Meinhardt J, et al: Comparison of static airway pressures during total liquid ventilation while applying different expiratory modes and time patterns. Am J Respir Crit Care Med 1999;159:A79.

84. Meinhardt JP, et al: Temporary elevation in static pulmonary compliance in bleomycin lung-injured, total liquid ventilated rabbits. Intensive Care Med 2000;26(Suppl 3):S287.

85. Weers JG: A physiochemical evaluation of perfluorochemicals for oxygen transport applications. J Fluorine Chem 1993;64:73–93.

86. Al-Rahmani A, Awad K, Miller TF, et al: Effects of partial liquid ventilation with perfluorodecalin in the juvenile rabbit lung after saline injury. Crit Care Med 2000;28:1459–1464.

87. Hirschl RB: Liquid ventilation in the setting of respiratory failure. ASAIO J 1998;44:231–233.

88. Cullen AB, et al: Intra-tracheal delivery strategy of gentamicin with partial liquid ventilation. Respir Med 1999;93:770–778.

89. Wolfson MR, Greenspan JS, Shaffer TH: Pulmonary administration of vasoactive substances by perfluorochemical ventilation. Pediatrics 1996;97:449–455.

90. Kaisers U, Rossaint R: Nitric oxide in partial liquid ventilation: Better matching ventilation to perfusion in ARDS? [editorial]. Intensive Care Med 1997;23:139–140.

91. Hartog A, et al: Partial liquid ventilation and inhaled nitric oxide have a cumulative effect in improving arterial oxygenation in experimental ARDS. Adv Exp Med Biol 1997;428:281–283.

92. Max M, et al: Effect of PEEP and inhaled nitric oxide on pulmonary gas exchange during gaseous and partial liquid ventilation with small volumes of perfluorocarbon. Acta Anaesthesiol Scand 2000;44:383–390.

93. Uchida T, et al: Inhaled nitric oxide during partial liquid ventilation shifts pulmonary blood flow to the non-dependent lung regions. Intensive Care Med 2000;26:764–769.

94. Wilcox DT, et al: Perfluorocarbon associated gas exchange (PAGE) and nitric oxide in the lamb with congenital diaphragmatic hernia model [abstract]. Pediatr Res 1994;35:260A.

95. Nakazawa K, et al: Pulmonary administration of prostacyclin (PGI$_2$) during partial liquid ventilation in an oleic acid–induced lung injury: Inhalation of aerosol or intratracheal instillation? Intensive Care Med 2001;27:243–250.

96. Riesmeier A, et al: Histological effects of intrapulmonary application of APC and PP4 during PLV in a rabbit model of acute lung injury [abstract]. Eur J Anaesth 2004;21.

97. Kimless-Garber DB, et al: Halothane administration during liquid ventilation. Respir Med 1997;91:255–262.

98. Newth CJ: Ventilation techniques including liquid ventilation. Pediatr Pulmonol 2004;26(Suppl):125–126.

99. Laukemper-Ostendorf S, Scholz A, Burger K, et al: 19F-MRI of perflubron for measurement of oxygen partial pressure in porcine lungs during partial liquid ventilation. Magn Reson Med 2002;47:82–89.

100. Cox CA, et al: Liquid ventilation: Gas exchange, perfluorochemical uptake, and biodistribution in an acute lung injury. Pediatr Crit Care Med 2002;3:288–296.

101. Suh GY, et al: Partial liquid ventilation shows dose-dependent increase in oxygenation with PEEP and decreases lung injury associated with mechanical ventilation. J Crit Care 2000;15:103–112.

102. Cheifetz IM, et al: Liquid ventilation improves pulmonary function and cardiac output in a neonatal swine model of cardiopulmonary bypass. J Thorac Cardiovasc Surg 1998;115:528–535.

103. Parent AC, Overbeck MC, Hirschl RB: Oxygen dynamics during partial liquid ventilation in a sheep model of severe respiratory failure. Surgery 1997;121: 320–327.

104. Wong DH: Liquid ventilation: More than "PEEP in a bottle"? Crit Care Med 1999;27:1052–1053.

105. Lowe KC: Synthetic oxygen transport fluids based on perfluorochemicals: Applications in medicine and biology. Vox Sang 1991;60:129–140.

106. Rotta AT, Steinhorn DM: Partial liquid ventilation reduces pulmonary neutrophil accumulation in an experimental model of systemic endotoxemia and acute lung injury. Crit Care Med 1998;26:1707–1715.

107. Armstrong FH, Shaw ST, Lowe KC: Effects of emulsified perfluorochemicals on rat liver aryl esterase activity. Br J Pharmacol 1990;99:300P.

108. Merz U, et al: Partial liquid ventilation reduces release of leukotriene B4 and interleukin-6 in bronchoalveolar lavage in surfactant-depleted newborn pigs. Pediatr Res 2002;51:183–189.

109. Baba A, et al: Perfluorocarbon blocks tumor necrosis factor-alpha–induced interleukin-8 release from alveolar epithelial cells in vitro. Crit Care Med 2000;28:1113–1118.

110. Quintel M, et al: Electron beam tomography (EBT) based volume measurements in healthy and oleic acid injured adult sheep lungs during partial liquid ventilation (PLV). Am J Respir Crit Care Med 1999;159:A901.

111. Quintel M, et al: Computer tomographic assessment of perfluorocarbon and gas distribution during partial liquid ventilation for acute respiratory failure. Am J Respir Crit Care Med 1998;158:249–255.

112. Quintel M, Meinhardt J, Waschke KF: [Partial liquid ventilation]. Anaesthesist 1998;47:479–489.

113. Meinhardt JP, et al: [Liquid ventilation: Historic developments and future trends]. Anaesthesiol Intensivmed 2002;43:147–159.

114. Rosenzweig J, Jensen OE: Capillary-elastic instabilities of liquid-lined lung airways. J Biomech Eng 2002;124: 650–655.

115. Trevisanuto D, et al: Positive end-expiratory pressure modulates perfluorochemical evaporation from the lungs. Biol Neonate 2003;84:53–58.

116. Davies MW, Dunster KR: Effect of perfluorocarbon (perfluorooctyl bromide) vapor on tidal volume measurement during partial liquid ventilation. Crit Care Med 2002;30:1123–1125.

117. Rich PB, et al: Prolonged partial liquid ventilation in spontaneously breathing awake animals. Crit Care Med 1999;27:941–945.

# CHAPTER 27

# Extracorporeal Life Support in Acute Respiratory Distress Syndrome

Sven Bercker, Thilo Busch, and Udo Kaisers

Acute respiratory distress syndrome (ARDS) is characterized by pulmonary and endothelial inflammation, which induces (1) edema as a result of increased permeability of the lung, (2) loss and dysfunction of surfactant with atelectasis and reduction in pulmonary compliance, (3) hypoxemia as a result of ventilation-perfusion mismatch associated with intrapulmonary right-to-left shunt (Qs/Qt), and (4) pulmonary hypertension.[1] Conventional treatment of this syndrome in the intensive care unit is based on lung protective mechanical ventilation with adequate positive end-expiratory pressure (PEEP). In a large, randomized controlled trial, the use of low tidal volumes was demonstrated to improve survival significantly in patients with ARDS.[2] However, mechanical ventilation with low tidal volumes is often insufficient to reverse severe hypoxemia immediately, and further adjunctive conventional therapies such as recruitment maneuvers,[3] prone positioning,[4] and negative fluid balance[5] are required. If these measures fail to improve gas exchange, then selective pulmonary vasodilation with inhaled nitric oxide or inhaled prostaglandins is used in specialized centers.[6] In the most severe cases of refractory hypoxemia, extracorporeal gas exchange using membrane lungs provides an ultimate rescue treatment in patients with ARDS.

## HISTORICAL BACKGROUND

The first attempts to establish extracorporeal life support (ECLS) were performed to allow surgery on the resting heart. After extensive experimental research in the 1950s, it was Gibbon who first described extracorporeal oxygenation and carbon dioxide ($CO_2$) removal using a bubble oxygenator during short-term application in cardiac surgery.[7] Extracorporeal membrane oxygenation (ECMO) for prolonged support became feasible with the development of new types of oxygenators using silicone rubber membranes to separate blood from oxygen.[8] Five years after the first description of ARDS, by Ashbaugh and colleagues,[9] a 22-year-old patient with ARDS was treated with prolonged extracorporeal oxygenation.[10] Soon after this report, Bartlett and colleagues described the first ECMO treatment in a newborn.[11] As a member of Kolobov's group, Gattinoni published results from a larger population of patients with ARDS who were treated with low-frequency positive pressure ventilation combined with extracorporeal carbon dioxide removal (LFPPV- $ECCO_2R$).[12] This concept combined low-flow venovenous ECMO and specific ventilator settings to achieve apneic oxygenation through the patient's natural lung, along with $CO_2$ removal through the extracorporeal system. Based on these encouraging results, attempts were made to show the beneficial effects of ECMO compared with conventional therapy of ARDS. In a randomized controlled study, Morris and colleagues treated a group of patients with venovenous ECMO combined with inverse ratio ventilation (IRV) and compared this group with a control group treated with positive pressure ventilation alone. No significant differences in survival rate could be demonstrated,[13] although overall survival in both groups was considerably increased when compared with the results of the earlier arteriovenous US ECMO trial in 1979.[14]

An ongoing British randomized controlled study (the CESAR Trial), with more than 150 patients currently enrolled, is designed to investigate the impact of ECMO on patient outcome, as well as cost effectiveness.[15] However, there is already evidence of the effectiveness of ECMO in neonates, particularly those with severe cases of infant respiratory distress syndrome (IRDS).[16,17] Recently, a meta-analysis confirmed the beneficial effects of this technique in neonates.[18]

## TERMINOLOGY

Numerous terms have come into use to describe systems of extracorporeal oxygenation and $CO_2$ removal. In the literature, these terms are not always used consistently.

*Extracorporeal membrane oxygenation* (ECMO) was originally introduced in the 1970s as a high-flow venoarterial bypass system and is now commonly used to denote pump driven extracorporeal gas exchange in general.[14]

*Extracorporeal $CO_2$ removal* (ECCO$_2$R) is used to underline the importance of the elimination of $CO_2$, provided by a low-flow venovenous bypass technique.[19]

*Partial extracorporeal $CO_2$ removal* (PECOR) was introduced to define partial $CO_2$ removal.[20]

*Extracorporeal lung assist* (ECLA) initially described a low-flow venovenous bypass system, primarily used in patients treated without mechanical ventilation.[21]

*Extracorporeal life support* (ECLS) was proposed by Zwischenberger and Bartlett[22] as a general term to define prolonged temporary support of heart or lung function.

*Arteriovenous $CO_2$ removal* (AVCO$_2$R) describes a passive pumpless system for extracorporeal $CO_2$ elimination.[23] The term pumpless ECLA (PECLA) is often used synonymously.

## RATIONALE FOR USE

Because ECLS/ECMO provides a rescue option for sufficient arterial oxygenation and $CO_2$ removal, theoretically without any supplementary pulmonary gas exchange, it plays an important role as an emergency procedure in patients with ARDS and life-threatening hypoxemia. This role is underlined by the *fast entry criteria* in most centers; the general assumption is that severe hypoxemia is refractory to conventional ventilatory strategies for several hours. As mentioned previously, earlier studies failed to show evidence that ECMO improved outcome in patients with ARDS. A major dilemma in studying the beneficial effects of extracorporeal techniques in comparison with conventional treatment in controlled trials is that it is ethically problematic to refuse potentially lifesaving therapies because of randomization. This issue has been debated extensively in the literature.[24]

Pulmonary fibroproliferation has been identified as a major cause of mortality.[25] It has been estimated that approximately 60% of patients with ARDS fail to improve early and show signs of fibrosis in the later course of their disease.[26] After failure of systemic high-dose corticosteroid therapy in ARDS, Meduri and colleagues treated selected cohorts with ARDS and proven fibroproliferation with dexamethasone and demonstrated beneficial effects.[27] However, it still remains unclear which mechanisms contribute to the fibrotic damage of the lung. Among septic mediators identified as contributors to this process through activation of fibroblasts, it has become evident that shear stress during aggressive ventilator therapy precedes ventilator-induced lung injury.[28,29] Investigators have convincingly shown that, during ventilatory support, reducing tidal volumes improves outcomes in patients with ARDS.[2] Furthermore, oxygen toxicity is still considered to play a role in ARDS-related lung injury. In experimental studies, high concentrations of oxygen induced pulmonary and endothelial damage, with a subsequent increase in fatality rates. The extent to which high concentrations of oxygen are toxic to the injured lung remains controversial. Because of the differences in study designs, clinical results are inconsistent.[30,31]

ECMO has been demonstrated to take over oxygenation and $CO_2$ removal, to a certain extent, that otherwise would require ventilatory settings that would aggravate lung injury. In particular, ECMO allows significant reductions in fraction of inspired oxygen (Fio$_2$), airway pressures, and tidal volumes. This concept of lung rest has provided the rationale for ECMO *slow entry criteria* in some centers. The need for early reduction of Fio$_2$ is widely accepted; however, it has currently not been determined how effective $CO_2$ removal alone would be.[24]

In fact, the decision to treat a patient with an extracorporeal device to provide oxygenation or to remove $CO_2$ is still based on expert knowledge, with the result that entry criteria differ among ECMO centers.

## ENTRY CRITERIA

Entry criteria differ significantly among centers. There are typically modifications of the fast and slow entry criteria, as described in the early prospective trial by Zapol and colleagues.[14] In this study, fast entry criteria included severe hypoxemia with a high Qs/Qt ratio refractory to conventional treatment. Entry criteria differ because of particular therapeutic strategies for severe gas exchange disorders; therefore, no generally accepted and distinct revision of entry criteria for ECMO has been published. The current entry criteria of the Berlin ARDS center, published in 1997, are listed in Table 27.1.[32]

Because different centers use different criteria for acceptance of patients with ARDS and for entry to ECMO, reported survival rates should be interpreted with caution. Attempts have been made to bring together rational entry criteria. As a result of the variety of parameters influencing the entry decision, establishment of a knowledge-based computer system has been proposed, according to the fuzzy set theory.[33] Most patients with severe respiratory failure have to be transported to specialized ARDS/ECMO centers. During transportation of the patient, a process that frequently takes hours, adequate gas exchange has to be maintained. Some experts have even recommended transporting patients on ECMO if it is not possible to stabilize gas exchange and hemodynamics at a satisfactory level on site.[34] Appropriate equipment is commercially available, and a review of 100 cases of mobile ECMO demonstrated that this can be performed safely by an experienced team.[35] The use of ECMO in patients with ARDS has been decreasing during the last few years, probably because of improved conventional treatment strategies and the availability of adjunctive therapies such as inhaled nitric oxide.[6] Currently, ECMO is primarily used as a rescue treatment for refractory hypoxemia in ARDS if these adjunctive options fail.

## PUMPS AND OXYGENATORS

In ECLS, roller pumps and centrifugal pumps are used. Both techniques have theoretical advantages in terms of complications and biocompatibility. Roller pumps may induce high arterial pressure levels, thereby leading to disruption of connections, as well as negative venous pressure levels, with the risk of endothelial damage in the cannulated veins. These potential complications emphasize the need for thorough pressure monitoring and regulation. Centrifugal pumps act through a spinning rotor to generate blood flow. This technique avoids high pressures in the case of distal circuit occlusion, but it may induce shear stress and turbulence to blood cells that may lead to hemolysis and thromboembolic complications. In fact, the roller pump was preferred in a 2002 survey among US neonatal ECMO centers; 95% of those surveyed claimed to use those devices.[36] In centers specializing in ECMO treatment in adults, the use of centrifugal pumps seems to be standard practice.

Since the first application of extracorporeal circulation in 1954,[7] efforts have been made to develop efficient oxygenators. Two different basic techniques have been used: bubble oxygenators, operating with direct contact between blood and gas; and membrane oxygenators. The application of bubble oxygenators is limited to a few hours because these devices damage blood cells. Bubble oxygenators were replaced by membrane oxygenators, which were significantly improved in oxygenation performance: up to more than 200 mL oxygen/minute/$m^2$.[37] Today, heparin-coated silicone membrane oxygenators as well as hollow fiber oxygenators are in use for ECMO in patients with ARDS. Although many oxygenators are available from different manufacturers, the basic principle is similar: blood flows into a manifold region of the oxygenator, from which point it is distributed among the microporous fibers of the device. Oxygen is conducted in the opposite direction through the fibers, and oxygenation and $CO_2$ removal are provided by diffusion (Fig. 27.1).[38] Advances in oxygenator development will

| Table 27-1 Entry Criteria for Extracorporeal Membrane Oxygenation | |
|---|---|
| Fast entry criteria | $Pao_2/Fio_2 < 50$ mm Hg at PEEP $\geq 10$ cm $H_2O$ despite maximum therapy >2 hr |
| Slow entry criteria | $Pao_2/Fio_2 < 150$ mm Hg at PEEP $\geq 10$ cm $H_2O$, Qs/Qt $\geq 30\%$, EVLW $\geq 15$ mL/kg, Cstat $\leq 30$ mL/cm $H_2O$ or recurrent barotrauma, despite maximum therapy >48 hr |

Cstat, static compliance; EVLW, extravascular lung water; $Pao_2/Fio_2$, ratio of arterial oxygen tension to inspired fraction of oxygen; PEEP, positive end-expiratory pressure; Qs/Qt, intrapulmonary right-to-left shunt.
Adapted from Lewandowski K, Rossaint R, Pappert D, et al: High survival rate in 122 ARDS patients managed according to a clinical algorithm including extracorporeal membrane oxygenation. Intensive Care Med 1997;23:819–835.

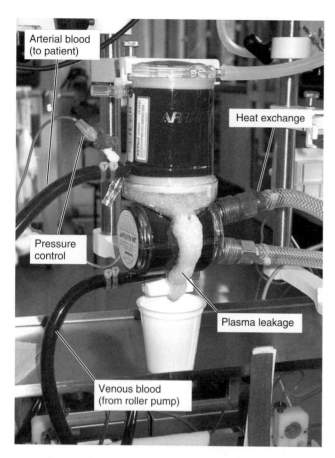

**Figure 27.1** Oxygenator with plasma leakage in a patient with acute respiratory distress syndrome who was undergoing extracorporeal membrane oxygenation (ECMO). Transmembranous pressure gradients often increase during extracorporeal lung assist, impair gas exchange properties, and terminate the function of the oxygenator.

aim to reduce shear stress on blood cells, blood side pressure, and priming volume while maximizing gas transfer. The common problem of plasma leakage depends on the type of the oxygenator and appears to be additionally influenced by the inflammatory status of the patient.[39]

## PROCEDURE

In the typical low-flow venovenous bypass frequently used at present, as in our ECMO center,[32] venous blood is drained through two heparin-coated, wire-reinforced catheters that are percutaneously inserted from both sides of the groin area into the inferior vena cava and are then connected by a Y-piece. The oxygenated blood is returned to the superior vena cava through a heparin-coated, wire-reinforced catheter, which is also advanced percutaneously through the right internal jugular vein.

A femorojugular venovenous bypass is established using a near-occlusive roller pump and a hollow fiber oxygenator. For safety reasons, a parallel configuration of two oxygenators is established if gas exchange of the patient's lung is marginal. All internal surfaces of the extracorporeal system, including the membrane oxygenators, tubing, and connectors, are coated with covalently bound heparin. Before connection to the patient, the system is primed with packed red blood cells and fresh frozen plasma at a ratio of 2:1. The gas phase of the oxygenator is initially flushed with dry pure oxygen. The gas flow rate is adjusted to the intended arterial $CO_2$ tension level. Oxygenation is accomplished both through the mechanically ventilated lung of the patient and by arterializing the circulating blood through the membrane oxygenators. This ECMO technique is just one possible approach; some centers use modifications of this circuit (Fig. 27.2).[40]

In our center, the mean duration of ECMO treatment is 12 days. Analyzing data from 60 ECMO-treated patients, the additional mean costs per treatment were 35,000 ($42,000 US). The average survival rate to discharge from the hospital was 60% in our series. This finding was confirmed by a study by Hemilla and colleagues, who reported a 52% survival rate in 225 ECMO-treated patients.[41] In our opinion, these favorable results in a patient population with an otherwise high risk of mortality fully justify the additional costs of treatment.

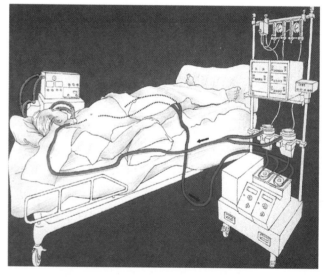

**Figure 27.2** Extracorporeal membrane oxygenation (ECMO) circuit presenting a venovenous system: blood is passively drained from both femoral veins and then is pumped through oxygenators using occlusive roller pumps back into the upper caval vein, thus providing prepulmonary oxygenation. Note that the patient still requires mechanical ventilation to maintain adequate gas exchange.

## OTHER EXTRACORPOREAL AND INTRAVASCULAR SUPPORT SYSTEMS

Because ECMO is a costly and labor-intensive procedure requiring significant intensive care unit resources including substantial amounts of blood transfusions, attempts have been made to develop less invasive techniques for extracorporeal gas exchange. Intravascular devices such as the IVOX system promised to have explicit advantages concerning nursing and the risk of septic complications, however, failed to demonstrate sufficient $O_2$ transfer.[42] Several systems are recently under development and their future clinical value still has to be determined.[43] An important approach was the invention of pumpless ECLA, usually established as an arteriovenous system.[23] To establish PECLA, usually arterial and venous cannulas are inserted into the groin area using Seldinger's technique. When cannulas are established and flooded with blood, the prefilled membrane is connected, and the bypass is set up for the procedure.

Although such systems show adequate capability to remove $CO_2$, they usually do not contribute sufficiently to oxygenation. Therefore, the term *extracorporeal arteriovenous $CO_2$ removal* (EAVCO_2R) is also used.[23] In some patients, impairments in oxygen content during PECLA treatment have been reported.[44] Because oxygenation through the extracorporeal membrane is highly dependent on the patient's cardiac output and on arterial blood pressure, flow impairments and hypotension significantly limit the efficacy of the system. However, in several studies, PECLA turned out to be safe and easy to establish for effective $CO_2$ removal.[23] These characteristics provide arguments that whenever $CO_2$ removal is essential to restore pH and to provide cardiocirculatory stability in patients' ARDS, PECLA should be considered an effective treatment option (Fig. 27.3).

## COMPLICATIONS

The most important contraindications for ECMO in our center are a fatal illness underlying ARDS, severe immunosuppression, irreversible brain damage, and acute and severe bleeding. Chronic lung diseases are considered relative contraindications, and ECMO is very rarely used as a bridge to lung transplantation.[45]

Complications of extracorporeal circuits can be either technical or patient related. In an analysis of 255 patients with ARDS who were undergoing ECMO treatment, the most frequent technical problems were associated with cannulas, oxygenator failure, clots in the circuit, air in the circuit, pump failure, tubing rupture, and heat

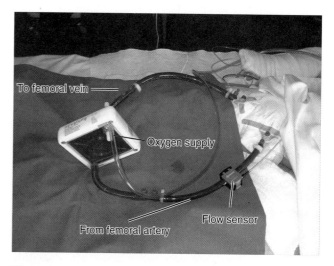

**Figure 27.3** Pumpless extracorporeal lung assist (PECLA) with arterial and venous cannula both in the right groin area. The novel polymethylpenthene membrane in this system increases plasma leakage resistance and allows a higher gas flow rate with increased carbon dioxide elimination.

exchanger malfunction. None of these complications were significantly correlated to survival or to length of stay.[41] The most frequent cause of patient-related hemorrhage was cannula site bleeding. Other factors associated with mortality were cerebral infarction, the need for renal replacement therapy, cardiac and pulmonary complications such as pneumothorax and pulmonary hemorrhage, new infections, severe acidosis, and thromboembolic complications.

Bleeding is mainly affected by underlying septic conditions, by the need for systemic heparinization, and by activation of coagulation through blood contact to a huge surface of synthetic material. The introduction of surface-heparinized circuits has reduced the need for blood transfusions and may thus have improved bleeding-related mortality.[46] Anticoagulation during ECMO is normally monitored using bedside activated clotting time (ACT, Hemochrom); it should be maintained at an ACT of 120 to 160 seconds. However, the decision regarding heparin dosage should be based on activated partial thromboplastin time (aPTT) measurements (55 to 80 seconds).[47] Before ECMO Start, heparin should initially be administered as an intravenous bolus of 5 to 10 U/kg, followed by an infusion of 500 to 1000 U/hour adjusted according to the patient's ACT. Fresh frozen plasma and antithrombin III (ATIII) are frequently administered during ECMO to maintain ATIII plasma levels greater than 70%.

Balancing anticoagulation between bleeding and thrombosis is a challenging task during prolonged ECMO. Treatment strategies for thrombotic complications depend on the location of the clots. Inflow-cannula clots are the most difficult to treat. Single case reports demonstrated that clots in sites at risk of imminent or apparent pulmonary embolism were successfully treated with systemic thrombolytic therapy.[48]

## MECHANICAL VENTILATION AND PRONE POSITIONING DURING EXTRACORPOREAL MEMBRANE OXYGENATION

Mechanical ventilation during ECMO should aim simultaneously at preventing alveolar collapse and at reducing lung damage resulting from ventilator-induced lung injury. Currently, no data exist to define an optimal ventilator strategy for lung rest, but low tidal volumes and low peak pressure levels are presumably most advantageous. To prevent alveolar collapse, an adequate level of PEEP has to be maintained.

No evidence-based data exist concerning the beneficial effects of prone positioning on clinical outcome during ECMO. Although an actual randomized controlled trial failed to demonstrate increased survival related to prone positioning in ARDS,[4] most centers adhere to this protocol. Prone positioning during ECMO therapy may provide recruitment of atelectatic lung areas and may thus improve gas exchange and hasten the drainage of secretions. A strong argument against this procedure is that it may pose a risk for accidental dislocation of cannulas. In an analysis of 962 positional changes in pediatric patients who were undergoing ECMO, no severe complications were reported, but as the authors stated, safe application of this approach requires an experienced team.[49]

In our center, mechanical ventilation during ECMO therapy is maintained with PEEP levels of 10 to 16 cm $H_2O$, low tidal volume ventilation (5 to 6 mL/kg body weight), a respiratory rate of 12 breaths/minute, and an inspiratory-to-expiratory ratio of 1:1. Prone positioning is performed for time intervals of 6 to 8 hours, preferentially at night, if it contributes to improved gas exchange (Fig. 27.4).

## CONCLUSION

In patients with ARDS and severe refractory hypoxemia, ECMO provides a feasible option for rescue treatment. The development of novel materials with optimized gas exchange capabilities has increased oxygenation efficacy, along with reducing the risk of bleeding complications. Currently, pumpless arteriovenous ECLA systems, mainly for the removal of $CO_2$, are clinically under evaluation. In view of favorable survival rates in patients with an otherwise high risk of mortality, the additional costs of ECMO treatment appear to be fully justified.

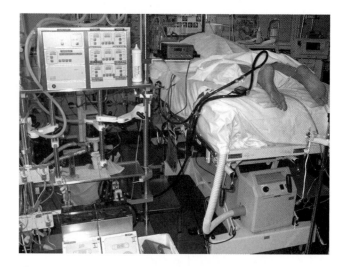

**Figure 27.4** Prone position during extracorporeal membrane oxygenation (ECMO). Despite complex instrumentation of the patient with ECMO, tubing and standard monitoring, as well as positional maneuvers, can be safely performed by an experienced intensive care unit team.

## REFERENCES

1. Ware LB, Matthay MA: The acute respiratory distress syndrome. N Engl J Med 2000;342:1334–1349.
2. Acute Respiratory Distress Syndrome Network: Ventilation with lower tidal volumes as compared with traditional tidal volumes for acute lung injury and the acute respiratory distress syndrome. N Engl J Med 2000;342:1301–1308.
3. Oczenski W, Hormann C, et al: Recruitment maneuvers during prone positioning in patients with acute respiratory distress syndrome. Crit Care Med 2005;33:54–61.
4. Gattinoni L, Tognoni G, et al: Effect of prone positioning on the survival of patients with acute respiratory failure. N Engl J Med 2001;345:568–573.
5. Martin GS, Moss M, et al: A randomized, controlled trial of furosemide with or without albumin in hypoproteinemic patients with acute lung injury. Crit Care Med 2005;33:1681–1687.
6. Kaisers U, Busch T, et al: Modulation of pulmonary vascular tone in ARDS. In Matthay M (ed): *Lung Biology in Health and Disease.* New York: Marcel Dekker, 2003, vol 179, pp 465–508.
7. Gibbon J: The application of a mechanical heart and lung apparatus to cardiac surgery. Minn Med 1954;37:171–180.
8. Kolobov T, Zapol W, et al: Partial extracorporeal gas exchange in alert newborn lambs with a membrane artificial lung perfused via an A-V shunt for periods up to 96 hours. Trans Am Soc Artif Intern Organs 1968;14:328–334.
9. Ashbaugh DG, Bigelow DB, et al: Acute respiratory distress in adults. Lancet 1967;2:319–323.
10. Hill JD, O'Brien TG, et al: Prolonged extracorporeal oxygenation for acute post-traumatic respiratory failure (shock-lung syndrome): Use of the Bramson membrane lung. N Engl J Med 1972;286:629–634.
11. Bartlett RH, Gazzaniga AB, et al: Extracorporeal membrane oxygenation (ECMO) cardiopulmonary support in infancy. Trans Am Soc Artif Intern Organs 1976;22:80–93.
12. Gattinoni L, Agostoni A, et al: Treatment of acute respiratory failure with low-frequency positive-pressure ventilation and extracorporeal removal of $CO_2$. Lancet 1980;2:292–294.

13. Morris AH, Wallace CJ, et al: Randomized clinical trial of pressure-controlled inverse ratio ventilation and extracorporeal CO$_2$ removal for adult respiratory distress syndrome. Am J Respir Crit Care Med 1994;149:295–305.

14. Zapol WM, Snider MT, et al: Extracorporeal membrane oxygenation in severe acute respiratory failure: A randomized prospective study. JAMA 1979;242:2193–2196.

15. www.cesar-trial.org.

16. UK Collaborative ECMO Trail Group: UK collaborative randomised trial of neonatal extracorporeal membrane oxygenation. Lancet 1996;348:75–82.

17. Bennett CC, Johnson A, et al: UK collaborative randomised trial of neonatal extracorporeal membrane oxygenation: Follow-up to age of 4 years. Lancet 2001;357:1094–1096.

18. Elbourne D, Field D, Mugford M: Extracorporeal membrane oxygenation for severe respiratory failure in newborn infants. Cochrane Rev 2005;2.

19. Kolobow T, Gattinoni L, et al: Control of breathing using an extracorporeal membrane lung. Anesthesiology 1977;46:138–141.

20. Marcolin R, Mascheroni D, et al: Ventilatory impact of partial extracorporeal CO$_2$ removal (PECOR) in ARF patients. Trans Am Soc Artif Intern Organs 1986;32:508–510.

21. Terasaki H, Nogami T, et al: Extracorporeal lung assist without endotracheal intubation and mechanical ventilation [letter]. Crit Care Med 1987;15:84–85.

22. Zwischenberger J, Bartlett RH: An introduction to extracorporeal life support. In Zwischenberger J, Bartlett RH (eds): *ECMO: Extracorporeal Cardiopulmonary Support in Critical Care.* Ann Arbor, MI: Extracorporeal Life Support Organization, 1995, pp 11–13.

23. Conrad SA, Zwischenberger JB, et al: Total extracorporeal arteriovenous carbon dioxide removal in acute respiratory failure: A phase I clinical study. Intensive Care Med 2001;27:1340–1351.

24. Lantos JD: Was the UK collaborative ECMO trial ethical? Paediatr Perinatol Epidemiol 1997;11:264–268.

25. Zapol WM, Trelstad RL, et al: Pulmonary fibrosis in severe acute respiratory failure. Am Rev Respir Dis 1979;119:547–554.

26. Marshall RP, Bellingan G, et al: Fibroproliferation occurs early in the acute respiratory distress syndrome and impacts on outcome. Am J Respir Crit Care Med 2000;162:1783–1788.

27. Meduri GU, Chinn AJ, et al: Corticosteroid rescue treatment of progressive fibroproliferation in late ARDS: Patterns of response and predictors of outcome. Chest 1994;105:1516–1527.

28. Kumar A, Pontoppidan H, et al: Pulmonary barotrauma during mechanical ventilation. Crit Care Med 1973;1:181–186.

29. Dreyfuss D, Saumon G: Ventilator-induced lung injury: Lessons from experimental studies. Am J Respir Crit Care Med 1998;157:294–323.

30. Gillbe CE, Salt JC, et al: Pulmonary function after prolonged mechanical ventilation with high concentrations of oxygen. Thorax 1980;35:907–913.

31. Register SD, Downs JB, et al: Is 50% oxygen harmful? Crit Care Med 1987;15:598–601.

32. Lewandowski K, Rossaint R, Pappert D, et al: High survival rate in 122 ARDS patients managed according to a clinical algorithm including extracorporeal membrane oxygenation. Intensive Care Med 1997;23:819–835.

33. Steltzer H, Fridrich P, et al: Definition of severity and compiling of entry criteria in patients undergoing ECLA: The use of a fuzzy logic expert system. Acta Anaesthesiol Scand 1996;109(Suppl):125–126.

34. Rossaint R, Pappert D, et al: Extracorporeal membrane oxygenation for transport of hypoxaemic patients with severe ARDS. Br J Anaesth 1997;78:241–246.

35. Foley DS, Pranikoff T, et al: A review of 100 patients transported on extracorporeal life support. ASAIO J 2002;48:612–619.

36. Lawson DS, Walczak R, et al: North American neonatal extracorporeal membrane oxygenation (ECMO) devices: 2002 survey results. J Extra Corpor Technol 2004;36:16–21.

37. Leonard RJ: The transition from the bubble oxygenator to the microporous membrane oxygenator. Perfusion 2003;18:179–183.

38. Hirschl RB: Devices. In Zwischenberger J, Bartlett RH (eds): *ECMO: Extracorporeal Cardiopulmonary Support in Critical Care.* Ann Arbor, MI: Extracorporeal Life Support Organization, 1995, pp 159–190.

39. Meyns B, Vercaemst L, et al: Plasma leakage of oxygenators in ECMO depends on the type of oxygenator and on patient variables. Int J Artif Organs 2000;28:30–34.

40. Lewandowski K: Extracorporeal membrane oxygenation for severe acute respiratory failure. Crit Care 2000;4:156–168.

41. Hemmila MR, Rowe SA, et al: Extracorporeal life support for severe acute respiratory distress syndrome in adults. Ann Surg 2004;240:595–605.

42. Brunet F, Mira JP, et al: Permissive hypercapnia and intravascular oxygenator in the treatment of patients with ARDS. Artif Organs 1994;18:826–832.

43. Hattler BG, Lund LW, et al: A respiratory gas exchange catheter: In vitro and in vivo tests in large animals. J Thorac Cardiovasc Surg 2002;124:520–530.

44. Reng M, Philipp A, et al: Pumpless extracorporeal lung assist and adult respiratory distress syndrome. Lancet 2000;356:219–220.

45. Jurmann MJ, Schaefers HJ, Demertzis S, et al: Emergency lung transplantation after extracorporeal membrane oxygenation. ASAIO J 1993;39:M448–M452.

46. Knoch M, Kollen B, et al: Progress in veno-venous long-term bypass techniques for the treatment of ARDS: Controlled clinical trial with the heparin-coated bypass circuit. Int J Artif Organs 1992;15:103–108.

47. Uziel L, Cugno M, et al: Physiopathology and management of coagulation during long-term extracorporeal respiratory assistance. Int J Artif Organs 1990;13:280–287.

48. Foehre B, Deja M, et al: Systemic lysis during ECMO: A case report [abstract]. Int J Artif Organs 2003;26:672.

49. Haefner SM, Bratton SL, et al: Complications of intermittent prone positioning in pediatric patients receiving extracorporeal membrane oxygenation for respiratory failure. Chest 2003;123:1589–1594.

SECTION **4**

# SPECIAL SITUATIONS FOR VENTILATORY SUPPORT

# CHAPTER 28

# Prehospital Care

Anthony F.T. Brown and Jeffrey Lipman

The prehospital arena is a hostile environment. It requires expertise and training to traverse appropriately, and it should be regarded as an important component of care before a critically ill or injured patient's arrival in hospital. Critical care patients the world over are moved every day as primary, secondary, or tertiary transfers. This chapter deals with what is required to perform these transfers safely and expediently.

*Primary transfers* move the patient from the scene to the first recognized medical facility, by road, helicopter, or occasionally fixed wing aircraft. *Secondary transfers* take patients from the initial receiving facility to a higher level of medical care such as from a remote or rural hospital to an urban or regional facility, again by road, helicopter, or fixed wing aircraft. This may now include jets and commercial airliners. *Tertiary transfers* move patients by similar means to a specialist center usually available only in one or two hospitals such as a burn unit, transplant unit, or spinal injuries unit.

The foregoing transfers are all based on clinical need. However, patient transfers are increasingly being made as a result of resource limitations and access issues alone, such as the temporary lack of a critical care bed in a designated higher-level facility. This practice occurs despite the knowledge that it is associated with a delay to intensive care unit (ICU) admission and a prolonged length of stay in the ICU and hospital.[1] Finally, critical care patients may be flown internationally to be repatriated to their country of origin.

Whatever term is preferred for this interfacility movement of patients, whether transit care medicine, transit intensive care, retrieval medicine, prehospital transport, or interhospital transfer, the basic tenets of this specialized care are the same.[2] The underlying requirements to move any patient, including one who is critically ill, include multidisciplinary cooperation across hospitals, health departments and even regions, and crew selection, training, and rostering. Dedicated equipment and innovative technology are necessary, as are careful vehicle selection, availability, and maintenance. Finally, agreed patterns of referral, clinical organization with clearly demarcated lines of responsibility, and a best practice quality assurance program looking carefully at the varied facets of care as well as cost effectiveness are essential. All these features are integral to success, irrespective of the affluence of the system.[2–5]

Some organizations have enshrined many of the concepts that relate to the movement or transfer of critical care patients by publishing guidelines, such as in the United States, or minimum standards, as in Australasia, that emphasize that this specialized movement of patients has inherent risks and hazards.[3,4,6] What is clear is that the use of inexperienced physicians, unsuitable equipment, inappropriate vehicles, untrained air crew, and ad hoc arrangements is unacceptable, because both morbidity and mortality are increased for patients and staff alike.[7,8] Additional special considerations are needed to move pediatric patients safely, whether these patients are neonates, infants, children, or adolescents.[9–12]

This chapter focuses on the whole process of prehospital care during the transport of critically ill adult patients and covers vehicle choice and coordination, pressurized cabin flight, equipment and monitoring, staffing, training, and quality assurance and makes some general conclusions. Aspects concerned with the movement of patients within a hospital facility, or intrahospital transport, are dealt with separately in Chapter 31.

## VEHICLE CHOICE AND COORDINATION

Whenever a critical care patient is transported from one facility to another, it is essential that the level of care during every phase of this transport is ideally never less than, and in many cases can and should exceed, the level of care of the referring institution.[13-15] This includes moving the patient within the hospital to the ambulance and in the ambulance to the airport, in the case of fixed wing transfers, or to a helipad remote from a hospital when one is not physically part of the building. Alternatively, where the helipad is hospital based, access to and from this area must also be included, whether the patient is traveling on a custom-designed trolley or in a registered ambulance. There must be no hiatus in the quality of patient care monitoring, or an equipment malfunction at any stage of care, however brief.[3]

The broad types of transport vehicle used are ground ambulance, rotary wing aircraft or helicopter, and fixed wing aircraft. Ground ambulances may be used for primary responses to a scene, to transfer patients to a second vehicle, or between facilities as in the secondary or tertiary transfer. Overall, they provide the majority of emergency medical systems (EMS) systems trips. Rotary wing craft or helicopters may be used either as primary response vehicles to remote areas or as secondary or tertiary transport vehicles. Finally, fixed wing craft are used for secondary or tertiary transfers and for international repatriation.[16] They are most commonly small turbo prop aircraft, but can include small executive jets and occasionally commercial airliners.

### Coordination or Dispatch of Care

The choice and availability of vehicle crew and the dispatch and estimated arrival times should be coordinated through a designated coordination or dispatch center, staffed 24 hours per day. The *single-point contact principle* of the referring physician making just a single telephone call to a predesignated number linking him or her to a transport service specialist should be all that is needed to activate the entire transfer system. The specialist contacted then arranges and coordinates all the different facets of care from that point. Under no circumstances should the referring physician be expected to make multiple phone calls to different hospital specialties or to have to find a bed at an appropriate level of care. The physician's only priority in these conditions is the optimal provision of initial clinical care to the sick or injured patient who requires transfer.[3,4,17] Clear lines of communication must be maintained to exchange clinical information and advice and to update the patient's general condition or response to treatment as time passes before the retrieval team's arrival. The coordination center should also inform the transferring hospital of the estimated time of arrival of the critical care retrieval team. In turn, salient local information such as the weather, exact patient location, particularly in a prehospital primary mission, and the type of vehicle and crew meeting the retrieval team are relayed back, when an ambulance transfer is needed to the referring hospital or scene site.[3,4,17]

### Road Transport

Road ambulances are used when transfer distances are short in high-density populations or when adverse weather prevents helicopter transport. Trips of 30 minutes one way, even up to 60 minutes in less densely populated areas, are preferable. Beyond 1 hour, ambulances become uncomfortable, and long trips may inappropriately deprive a local area of its EMS vehicle for a considerable period of time. This period includes the time taken to unload and return; if prolonged, it is unjustified if an alternative such as a helicopter is available.

Ambulance crew make up and training vary from a single-driver crew, a driver and basic ambulance officer (Basic Life Support trained), a driver and advanced or paramedic ambulance officer Advanced Life Support (ALS) trained, to an ALS-trained driver and officer. Ambulance vehicle configuration can be single stretcher or dual stretcher and may include minimum equipment[16] right up to critical care–designated vehicles with built-in oxygen, multiple power outlets, and monitoring and ventilation devices.[13,14,18]

Whichever type of ambulance is used, it must provide sufficient seating for the accompanying transfer team, with suitable lap-shoulder strap seat belts, secure equipment stowage, adequate lighting, and a locking system for the patient's transport stretcher. There is no longer any justification for the unsafe practice of carrying loose bags and equipment, unrestrained medical attendants, or an unsecured stretcher because all may become lethal secondary missiles in the event of a crash. Alternatively, unsecured delicate equipment may simply fail.[16] Therefore, advance planning and communication about the number of medical crew, the type and amount of equipment to be carried, and the stretcher system used are essential, particularly when arriving in a remote or unfamiliar area.[4] Again, the coordination center is responsible for relaying this information to the transferring facility about the retrieval team sent.

Finally, all road ambulances as part of the regular EMS service should meet local designated construction and maintenance specifications,[3,4,16] whether or not the vehicle is dedicated to interhospital transport and remains sidelined between trips. The type and level of training of vehicle crew will depend on local demand and fiscal constraints and are discussed later.[17]

## Helicopter Rotary Wing Craft

Helicopters have become increasingly common in inter-hospital transfers, usually for distances from 50 to 250 km. In addition, helicopters provide a rapid response to primary scenes in remote, rugged, or inaccessible terrain.[15,19]

Many different makes of helicopter are used, with many different funding models that may include sponsoring company logos painted on the cabin. Various crewing combinations are available, although for critical care transfers a minimum of two dedicated medical personnel is required, usually including a physician or at least an ALS critical care–trained nurse or paramedic.[14,16]

The advantages a helicopter offers include speed; many travel in excess of 200 km/hour or 125 mph (Box 28-1). Helicopters provide door-to-door transport, which avoids multiple or secondary handling in a road vehicle. They can also access remote terrain including wilderness areas or flooded hospital access roads. Finally, helicopters allow low-level flying capability that does not require cabin pressurization, and most have a dedicated aeromedical configuration. This would normally include power outlets that facilitate power saving of battery-operated devices, an on-board oxygen supply, and direct radio or mobile telephone communications to the coordination center and receiving hospital.[15–17,19–21] The adage espoused as long ago as the Korean War that "A man dies in a period of time, not over a distance of miles" is as prescient now as then.[22]

There are, however, real dangers and inherent difficulties with the overzealous use of helicopters in EMS, whether for primary or interhospital transfer, basic care, or critical care (Box 28-2). Helicopters are costly to run and have frequent maintenance requirements compared with road or fixed wing craft. They have several different operating profiles. These include single or twin engines, instrument flight rules (IFR), or non-IFR visual flight rules (VFR) capability and appropriate levels of pilot training. Helicopters should ideally have a dedicated flight crew member in addition to the pilot, rather than be pilot-only operated (excluding the medical crew).

---

**BOX 28-1**

### Advantages of Helicopters in Aeromedical Transfers

Speed: 125 mph or 200 kph
Door-to-door transport
Difficult or remote access capability
No cabin pressurization
Dedicated aeromedical configuration
    Power, oxygen, stretcher system, communications

*kph, kilometers per hour; mph, miles per hour.*

---

**BOX 28-2**

### Disadvantages of Helicopters in Aeromedical Transfers

Cost: $1500 or more per hour
Frequent down time for maintenance
Variable flying profiles
    Single or twin engine
    Instrument flight rules (IFR) or visual flight rules (VFR)
Noise and vibration
    Crew discomfort
    Flight path restrictions
Injury risk from main and tail rotor blades
Stabilization and packaging of patient prior to departure
    Requires time and expertise
Risk of crashing greater than non–emergency medical services helicopters

---

They are noisy and subject to vibration inside, and external noise creates flight restrictions in urban areas. They may be cramped, and they also have strict maximum weight restrictions that depend on the travel distance and ambient temperature. There are danger zones around the main and tail rotor blades, which not only may injure persons in the area, but also, if anything is sucked into or hits the rotors, will instantly incapacitate the helicopter. Unfortunately, medical helicopters crash with considerably higher frequency than non-EMS helicopter services, possibly related to flying for a perceived overriding medical precedent. Accident crash statistics repeatedly highlight pilot difficulties with helicopters used in the VFR mode flying in darkness or inclement weather.

There are additional, often unrecognized, time delay considerations to take into account when using helicopters. These include callout response time, rotor engine startup and shutdown times that run to several minutes, and additional patient preparation time. Thus, to prepare a critical care patient for safe interhospital air transfer, it is mandatory to spend time at the referring hospital in stabilizing the patient, to preempt any problems that may otherwise occur in flight. Access to the patient's airway and to all monitoring and resuscitation equipment is much more difficult in flight than on the ground. Although time is of the essence, the methodical predeparture process of interventional stabilization is essential and should not be rushed unnecessarily. All these times must be accounted for when estimating the total mission time, rather than only considering the direct flying time.[14,16,17,20] Thus, a 30-minute flight time may compound to a return mission time of more than 3 hours.[20] Finally, different types of rotary wing aircraft may be needed, depending on whether most flights are prehospital transports or primary, rather than interhospital, transports. No one ideal aircraft exists for all conditions.[20]

It has been frustratingly difficult to prove that helicopter transport unequivocally saves lives in the pre-hospital arena when compared with road transportation or whether it significantly reduces overall adverse clinical event rates, although the relevant comparative data are admittedly limited.[15,17,20] In regard to cost effectiveness, cost efficiency, cost containment, or lost cost opportunity, the high expense of running a helicopter service is influenced by sponsorship deals, reimbursement to the hospital for care provided by insurance or private medical coverage, and the use of existing hospital staff, rather than a separately funded, stand-alone service. When considering local area needs, residents may be biased by the public visibility of a helicopter, by anxiety reduction from the knowledge that a helicopter is available, and by knowing that a helicopter reduces regional health care inequities. However, limited study work does indicate that community perceptions of value in terms of willingness to pay for a helicopter ambulance service compare highly favorably with the option of paying for more heart operations or more hip replacements.[23]

## Fixed Wing Aircraft

Fixed wing aircraft are the preferred method of transport of critical care patients when distances exceed 250 km or 150 miles, roughly equivalent to 60 to 90 minutes of flying time in a helicopter. In addition, these aircraft are able to fly in poorer weather conditions, and, effectively, there is no real upper limit to the distance they can travel internationally or even across sparsely populated areas in large countries such as Australia or Canada.[24]

Various aircraft have been used, from twin turbo prop craft such as the Beechcraft Super King Air (Raytheon Aircraft Company, Wichita, KS) with a wide fuselage door for ease of patient loading, to smaller executive jets such as the Learjet (Bombardier Aerospace, Inc., Montreal, Canada), right up to long-haul commercial airliners or wide-bodied military aircraft designed for mass casualty transport.[17] Trips involve additional transport of the patient by road ambulance to and from the airport. All aircraft should incorporate some type of stretcher loading and transferring system, as well as using dedicated air crew. There should be on-board oxygen and power supply outlets, usually DC, secure but accessible baggage stowage areas, and an air-to ground communication system. An excellent description of one such configured dedicated intensive care fixed wing aircraft is given by Gilligan and associates[25] (Box 28-3).

Fixed wing aircraft that are capable of traveling long distances require cabin pressurization, generally equivalent to a cabin altitude pressure in the range from 5000 to 8000 feet, corresponding to barometric pressures of 632 to 565 mm Hg, respectively.[26] It is actually possible to pressurize an aircraft to sea level or 1 atm or 760 mm Hg

---

**BOX 28-3**

### Example of a Fixed Wing Airborne Intensive Care Facility

Medical fittings
    Dual stretcher accommodation and loading device
    Medical oxygen/suction
    Monitoring, defibrillator
Portable resuscitation equipment
    Ventilator
    Defibrillator
    Monitor and reserve monitor
    Infusion pumps
    Resuscitation equipment
    Neonatal incubator

*From Gilligan JE, Goon P, Maughan G, et al: An airborne intensive care facility (fixed wing). Anaesth Intensive Care 1996;24:245–253.*

to transport certain patients, for instance, patients with decompression illness, air embolism, or other barotraumas, or simply to vary cabin pressure according to the particular cardiorespiratory status of the patient. The disadvantage of this approach is that it requires flying at a lower altitude, which reduces airspeed, increases fuel costs and consumption, exposes the aircraft to more weather turbulence, and is usually restricted to small aircraft over limited distances of up to 1500 km or 950 miles.[25,26]

## PRESSURIZED CABIN FLIGHT

Several fundamental aeromedical considerations are particular to pressurized cabin flight, such as hypobaric conditions, and some features are common to all aircraft, such as humidity and vibration, noise and space restrictions, and medical crew fatigue (Boxes 28-4 and 28-5).

---

**BOX 28-4**

### Pressurized Cabin Flight: Hypobaric Consequences

Gas expansion
    Expansion of pneumothorax
    Atelectasis
    Endotracheal cuff expansion
    Arterial gas embolism
    Increased abdominal compartment pressures
    Deterioration of (unrecognized) decompression illness
Hypoxia
Changes in lung function
    Reduced forced vital capacity
    Increased residual volume

## BOX 28-5

**Other Pressurized Cabin Flight Aeromedical Considerations**

Humidity and vibration
    Drying of secretions
    Equipment failure
Noise and space restriction
    Communication difficulty
    Stethoscope no value
    Lack of stowage and equipment mounting points
Medical crew fatigue
    Hypoxia
    Dehydration
    Hypothermia or hyperthermia
    Noise, cramped conditions
    Disturbed sleep patterns, jet lag
    Mental and logistics exhaustion

## Hypobaric Conditions

Special considerations that must be taken into account when transporting a patient in a pressurized cabin aircraft include the effects of gas expansion both on the patient and on the medical equipment, as well as hypobaric hypoxia.

### Gas Expansion

Gas expansion is governed by Boyle's law, which dictates that the change in volume of a gas is inversely proportional to the change in pressure of that gas at a constant temperature. Thus, at 8000 feet, gas expands by a factor of 1.35 compared with sea level; this increases the size of an undrained pneumothorax by 34.5% and allows tension characteristics to develop[26,27] (see Box 28-4) In addition, trapped gas may lead to the expansion of bullae causing atelectasis of adjacent lung and even lung rupture. Increased abdominal compartment pressure may cause respiratory and vascular compromise and a change or worsening of lung parenchymal compliance. Systemic arterial gas embolism may occur from underlying lung disease. Finally, the deterioration of unrecognized decompression illness in a patient who has recently been diving with compressed air cylinders (SCUBA) is a well-recognized problem.[26,27] Box 28-4 highlights these consequences.

Equipment is similarly affected by gas expansion. Thus, gas in the endotracheal tube expands, potentially leading to tracheal mucosal ischemia, occasionally cuff rupture, and, rarely, tracheal rupture.[27] In addition, gas expansion alters the tidal volume ($V_T$) delivered by a volume-cycled ventilator unless the ventilator has been fitted with an altitude compensation device, which is uncommon.

### Hypobaric Hypoxia

Although the fraction of inspired oxygen ($FiO_2$) of air remains constant at 0.21 (21%), the partial pressure of oxygen in ambient air declines progressively in proportion to the barometric pressure at altitude. Thus, a patient requiring a high-flow, reservoir face mask delivering 70% oxygen at sea level will actually need 97% oxygen at 8000 feet just to maintain an equivalent inspired partial pressure of oxygen.[26]

This does not take into account the effect of added positive end-expiratory pressure (PEEP), but no reliable data accurately determine appropriate changes needed in the $FiO_2$ for varying amounts of PEEP applied at altitude. The balance between the therapeutic changes in alveolar recruitment and distention and the deleterious hemodynamic effects of PEEP, with their consequent impact on oxygen delivery at height, compared with sea level, is unpredictable.[26] Even in healthy subjects, changes in pulmonary function, such as reduced forced vital capacity and increased residual volume, occur at moderate altitude.[28] Suffice it to say, supplemental oxygen is essential in most ill patients transported by pressurized aircraft.

Mechanical ventilation will therefore be necessary in the patient with respiratory compromise if inappropriately high $FiO_2$ requirements and an increased work of breathing are present on the ground or are predicted in flight. The basic tenets of ventilation to limit alveolar stress should be applied similar to the principles in the ICU, thereby limiting excess barotrauma or volutrauma.[29] Whether PEEP should be applied routinely or prophylactically in mechanically ventilated patients traveling at altitude, as supported by animal experiments, and the way in which to use PEEP most safely and efficaciously, particularly in acute respiratory distress syndrome (ARDS), requires further prospective human outcome data.[26,30] A reduction in barometric pressure alone causes a reduction in the arterial partial pressure of oxygen in the mechanically ventilated patient independent of any effects of PEEP.[31] The exact mechanisms responsible for this are unclear but include pulmonary interstitial edema, regional changes in lung parenchymal compliance, blood flow redistribution, and pulmonary vasoconstriction.

### Humidity and Vibration

Warmed cabin air taken from the ambient atmosphere contains minimal water vapor or humidity, thus leading to drying of sections. Vibration caused by mechanical aircraft functions including the engines or from air turbulence may be uncomfortable and tiring, and it may also interfere with medical equipment in flight.[16,27]

## Noise and Space Restriction

Noise contributes to communication difficulties, as well as rendering common medical devices such as the stethoscope unhelpful. Noise also mandates visible as well as audible alarms on medical monitoring equipment and an efficient ergonomic layout of the cabin to maximize equipment and patient visibility.[27] Other space considerations include the need for adequate stowage space, comfortable crew seating with enough leg room and appropriate lighting, and crash-worthy mounting points for all medical equipment, as well as hooks for intravenous fluid or invasive monitoring pressure bags.

## Medical Crew Fatigue

The transport of a critical care patient is physically and mentally exhausting, and it may be the only time that a clinician is truly "alone" looking after a sick patient with just one other medical care provider, without immediate backup. Fatigue is multifactorial and is contributed to by hypobaric hypoxia, dehydration, ambient cabin hyperthermia or hypothermia, noise, disturbed sleep patterns and jet lag, cramped conditions, constant vibration, equipment malfunction, communication and logistics challenges, and sheer mental taxation. One hour of work in the air should be considered equivalent to 2 hours of similar care on the ground. Recognition of the increased demands and fatigue of flying is legislated for by governments, with restricted continuous hours of service for air crew, but often no such consideration is given to the attendant medical staff.

## EQUIPMENT AND MONITORING

Important issues to consider when planning for prehospital care include the types and choice of transport ventilation available and respiratory monitoring in particular, in addition to other types of monitoring and general equipment.

### Transport Ventilation

No ideal transport ventilator is capable of reproducing the standard sophistication of the hospital-based intensive care ventilator. The special needs of a transport ventilator include requirements that it be small, lightweight (4 to 5 kg), robust, reliable, and portable, whether it is oxygen or battery driven. In addition, the ventilator should be economical of oxygen and power and versatile by offering a similar range of ventilation modes, yet simple to operate in the high-stress and complex environment of critical care transport.[32]

It is therefore no surprise to find that one of the most common forms of mechanical ventilation during transport in the United States is actually manual ventilation, usually with a self-inflating bag device, either alone or in combination with some form of small transport ventilator device.[8,32] This approach is most commonly used in the prehospital or primary transfer scenario and when transport times are less than 20 minutes. What is surprising is the overall degree of variability seen in practice. As recently as 1998, some transport agencies in the United States still relied exclusively on manual ventilation, with or without a transport ventilator, in all helicopter or fixed wing interfacility transfers.[8] In addition, although the use of pulse oximetry was almost universal, quantitative end-tidal carbon dioxide ($ETCO_2$) monitoring was only used in a little over half, with just a qualitative $CO_2$ detector or no $CO_2$ monitoring used in the remainder.[8] Although no established national standards of care governing the use of transport ventilators over manual ventilation were available at that time, and no standardization of monitoring adjuncts, the more recent publication of clinical guidelines in the United States should improve adherence to new recommended standards of care.[3,4] The different forms of transport ventilation may be considered as either manual ventilation or mechanical ventilation, and the types of mechanical ventilation include automatic resuscitators, simple transport ventilators, and sophisticated transport ventilators.

### Manual Ventilation

Self-inflating manual bag ventilation of adult critical care patients remains common, alone or combined with some form of transport ventilator. However, significant disadvantages are seen with manual ventilation, particularly unintentional respiratory alkalosis, variable $V_T$, and excessive inspiratory pressures of up to 80 cm $H_2O$.[27,32] Although oxygenation may be maintained at high levels, these excessive pressures may still lead to cardiac arrhythmias, hypotension, and barotrauma.[33] The argument that the caregiver can feel changes in the patient's lung compliance at all times, particularly in children, and may therefore intervene accordingly is countered by the fact that this member of the transport team is completely occupied and is unable to provide further assistance.[9]

Manual ventilation is also subject to limitation from operator fatigue.[34] Clearly, the underlying severity and cause of the critical illness will determine the extent of any resulting clinical morbidity. This would be expected in the patient with a major head injury who is intolerant of systemic hypotension or excessive intracranial vasoconstriction or in the patient who is predisposed to the development of ARDS with the risk of ventilator-associated lung injury.[14]

The common practice of disconnecting a transport ventilator to move a patient onto a stretcher or into an ambulance is not recommended, particularly if the patient requires high levels of PEEP, because changing from mechanical to manual ventilation will alter mean airway pressure. This may result in a sudden loss of functional residual capacity, with rapidly resulting but sustained hypoxemia, as well as cardiovascular compromise.[14]

Self-inflating manual bag ventilation is also commonly used in pediatric transport because of its simplicity, portability, and reliability. However, just as in adults, it may cause greater changes in ventilatory parameters compared with a pediatric transport ventilator. Although one tertiary pediatric intensive care service stated that this did not lead to clinical outcome differences, their transport times were only 8 to 12 minutes, and the study sample was small, with just 49 patients split evenly between manual or transport ventilator.[11] Power calculations revealed that the study size was inadequate to detect a significant difference, and the results of this study could not be generalized to other situations.

There is, however, one universal indication for the self-inflating manual bag device. It is to keep one such device checked and assembled with the patient at all times, in the event the transport ventilator fails unexpectedly.

## Mechanical Ventilation

Readers are directed to the review by Austin and colleagues for comprehensive information comparing a variety of transport ventilators with complete data on their capabilities, intended use, performance, size, weight, power and oxygen requirements, and manufacturer contact details.[32] In addition, Wheeler and colleagues discuss the ventilated pediatric patient in depth.[9] Finally, there is a comprehensive 2004 buyer's guide freely available on the Internet with an extensive review of mechanical ventilators with all their specifications in table form, complete with the manufacturer's details.[35]

**Automatic Resuscitators** Austin and associates classified the automatic resuscitator as intended for use in the prehospital arena by medical personnel of limited respiratory care expertise.[32] These models, which include the Ambu Matic (Ambu, Inc., Linthicum, MD), VAR Models RT or RC (Vortran Medical Technology 1, Inc., Sacremento, CA), Oxylator EM-100 or FR 300 (Lifesaving Systems, Inc., Roswell, GA), and the paraPAC Responder (Pneupac, Waukesha, WI), provide controlled ventilation with a fixed $FiO_2$, have simple controls for breath rate and $V_T$, have fixed pressure-limiting valves, and are time or flow cycled, although some are pressure cycled. All are solely pneumatically powered and have minimal or no monitoring capability, thus necessitating close clinical patient care. The disadvantages of the automatic resuscitator include a $V_T$ that varies according to lung compliance and the risk of hypoventilation in pressure cycling with poor lung compliance. However, these deficiencies are more than compensated for by the simplicity and compactness of these devices.[32]

**Simple Transport Ventilators** Austin and colleagues classified these devices as primarily intended for prehospital use by medical personnel with some respiratory care expertise.[32] These ventilators offer a broader range of breath rate and $V_T$ adjustment, and they may allow spontaneous breathing in suitable patients, although this mode is not commonly recommended in critical care patients. In addition, these ventilators include some alarms and provide a variable two-setting $FiO_2$, with a capacity for PEEP either internally or, less ideally, through an external valve. Models include the Auto Vent 2000 or 3000 (Allied Healthcare Products, Inc., St Louis, MO), paraPAC Medic (Pneupac, Waukesha, WI), and Uni-Vent 706 (Impact Instrumentation, Inc., West Caldwell, NJ). Intermittent mandatory ventilation (IMV) breaths may be time triggered, flow or pressure limited, and time cycled. Spontaneous breaths may be pressure triggered, pressure limited, and pressure cycled. Inspiratory-to-expiratory (I:E) combinations may be preset to suit the typical standard adult, child, or infant, cardiopulmonary resuscitation, or hyperventilation modes.[32] In a 1995 study, paramedics showed that they were able to use even the more sophisticated of these devices effectively compared with bag-valve manual devices.[36]

**Sophisticated Transport Ventilators** Austin and associates classified these ventilators as designed to be used for interfacility transport by medical personnel experts in respiratory care.[32] These devices try to offer many of the features found on standard intensive care ventilators. These ideally have a demand valve for spontaneous breathing, built-in PEEP or continuous positive airway pressure (CPAP), PEEP-compensated triggering, variable $FiO_2$ capability, and a full complement of built-in monitoring and alarm features. Many models are available and are constantly changing. They include the Avian (Bird Products Corporation, Palm Springs, CA), Crossvent 3 or 4 (Bio-Med Devices, Inc., Guilford, CT), 1C-2A, $iVent_{201}$ (VersaMed, Inc., Hackensack, NJ), LTV 1000 (Pulmonetics Systems, Inc., Minneapolis, MN), MVP-10 (Bio-Med Devices, Inc., Guilford, CT), Oxylog 2000 and 3000 (Draeger Medical, Inc., Telford, PA), paraPAC Transport (Pneupac, Waukesha, WI), and Uni-Vent 750 or 754 (Impact Instrumentation, Inc., West Caldwell, NJ).

These models range from those now considered low end, such as the MVP-10 (Bio-Med Devices, Inc., Guilford, CT) or the Oxylog 2000 (Draeger Medical, Inc., Telford, PA), to the more complex Avian

(Bird Products Corporation, Palm Springs, CA), which is pneumatically powered, microprocessor controlled, time or pressure triggered, pressure limited, and time cycled capable of controlled mandatory ventilation, assisted mandatory ventilation (AMV), synchronized IMV (SIMV), CPAP, and external PEEP. At the high end are now the Oxylog 3000 (Draeger Medical, Inc., Telford, PA), LTV 1000 (Pulmonetics Systems, Inc., Minneapolis, MN), Crossvent 4 (Bio-Med Devices, Inc., Guilford, CT), and Uni-Vent 754 (Impact Instrumentation, Inc., West Caldwell, NJ). The Uni-Vent 754 is an electrically powered flow or pressure controller that is pressure, time, or manually triggered and time or pressure cycled; it contains an internal compressor and oxygen blender and is capable of delivering AMV, SIMV, CPAP, pressure triggered PEEP, compensated $V_T$ sensitivity, sigh, and PEEP. Sophisticated displays and alarms and a proven track record have added to its popularity.[32]

This wide array of transport ventilators available must be tempered against several considerations. These include their cost, intended use, complexity of the interface that determines the medical personnel training required, the ability to ventilate adults as well as children or infants, and their alarms or displays. In addition, the degree of ancillary patient monitoring, the transport vehicle layout, and the overall training and expertise of the transport team will contribute just as much to patient outcome as simply choosing to purchase the most sophisticated transport ventilator. Thus, Gilligan and colleagues described the successful use of a relatively simple ventilator, the Oxylog (Draeger Medical Australia Pty., Ltd.), over distances up to 1300 km in a medically dedicated Beechcraft Super King Air B200C (Raytheon Aircraft Company, Wichita, KS) in 2000 missions between 1987 and 1992, during which 40% of patients were ventilator dependent.[25] The Oxylog is a time cycled, constant volume, rate determined, pressure limited, fixed I:E (1:1.5), two-setting $Fio_2$ (0.5 or 1.0) ventilator.

Whichever transport ventilator is chosen, it is important to assess its actual performance in the field, because surprising and significant variations from claimed performance and designated settings for $V_T$ delivery, triggering ease, trapped volume and PEEP effect may occur either in laboratory testing or in the clinical arena.[37–39]

## Respiratory Monitoring

There are generally accepted basic minimum requirements for respiratory monitoring, as well as the need for $ETCO_2$ monitoring and other ventilator-based monitoring.

### Minimum Requirements

A variety of respiratory monitoring equipment are necessary, as dictated by the type of mission performed. Considerations include primary scene transport or secondary or tertiary interhospital transfer, whether the patient is manually ventilated or ventilated using a transport ventilator, and the expected mission duration time. Absolute minimum requirements are a pulse oximeter, a noninvasive blood pressure monitor, and a continuous electrocardiographic (ECG) trace.[3,8,20,27]

### End-Tidal Carbon Dioxide Monitoring

The use of continuous $ETCO_2$ monitoring in the ventilated patient is inconsistent in some EMS services or may be absent. Some systems instead utilize simple disposable $CO_2$ detectors that undergo a cyclic color change, but these are of value only in determining correct endotracheal tube placement. Other EMS services make no measurement of exhaled $CO_2$ at all.[8] The measurement of $ETCO_2$ has been clearly shown to improve the maintenance of optimum $ETCO_2$ levels, designed to reflect ideal arterial partial $CO_2$ pressure ($Paco_2$) targets such as during the normoventilation of the major trauma victim.[40] Otherwise, huge variations in $Paco_2$ values from 16 to 86 mm Hg on admission to hospital are seen in the manually ventilated patient.[40]

The use of $ETCO_2$ measurements is essential in the critically ill ventilated patient. Continuous $ETCO_2$ monitoring has become the recommended standard of care in Australasia for all patients receiving mechanical ventilation.[4] In addition, it is recommended "in selected patients, based on clinical status" in North American guidelines.[2,3] However, it does have some limitations. $ETCO_2$ measurements alone cannot indicate increased alveolar dead space from reduced cardiac output with decreased alveolar perfusion or maldistribution or from segmental pulmonary blood flow occlusion.[9,40,41] Another important consideration in the interpretation of $ETCO_2$ monitoring is that $ETCO_2$ measurements are unpredictably lower at the usual reduced cabin altitude of approximately 6000 feet in pressurized aircraft. This may be as much as a 1% reduction in the $ETCO_2$ reading, without any change in the minute ventilation of the patient. This situation can reliably be avoided only by pressurizing the cabin to sea level, with all its inherent disadvantages.[25]

### Ventilator-Based Monitoring

Minimum ventilator-based monitoring, such as $V_T$, rate or minute ventilation, inspiratory pressure, and PEEP, and low-pressure (disconnect) and high-pressure alarms are essential in the transport of the critical care patient.[18] Other parameters such as exhaled $V_T$, ventilator battery status, and oxygen supply status will depend on the sophistication and type of ventilator used. All add to the ability of trained crew to respond rapidly and effectively to avoid or solve critical incidents during transport.[27]

## Other Monitoring and Equipment

Monitoring protocols and equipment will depend on the type of transfer performed and its expected duration. All equipment chosen for use in transport must be evaluated with regard to weight, size, reliability and durability, battery life, oxygen requirement, ease of visibility, particularly in high ambient light conditions such as direct sun, and the ability to operate at variable ambient temperatures or degrees of vibration and in a reduced pressure environment.

Safety and ergonomic considerations mandate that all bulky equipment in continuous use should be attached to the patient's stretcher, usually screwed to a frame or bridge placed over the patient's torso. Although this clearly reduces access to the patient in flight, it is unacceptable to balance on a stretcher unsecured heavy items of equipment that should all be adequately fixed.[4] In addition, the use of a bridge allows the patient, complete with monitoring and therapeutic equipment, to be lifted and moved as a single unit. Finally, all the equipment carried must comply with local and federal aviation regulatory requirements and must be suitable for the spectrum of age groups likely to be attended from neonatal and pediatric to adult, as well as extra tall and the obese patients. Additional items may be categorized in equipment groups for respiratory support, circulatory support, miscellaneous use, and point-of-care testing.

## Respiratory Support

This group includes manual and mechanical ventilator systems and appropriate respiratory monitoring, as discussed earlier. Other essential items to be carried include oxygen masks, oral or nasopharyngeal airways, and intubation equipment, including a range of laryngoscope blades and handles. Difficult intubation adjuncts such as the gum elastic bougie, airway exchange catheter, laryngeal mask airway, and emergency surgical airway kit are essential. Finally, thoracic (pleural) drainage equipment incorporating one-way valves, such as the Heimlich valve, and suction equipment are required, as well as adequate oxygen supplies to last the duration of the intended mission, and in addition a range of valves and fittings for international travel.[3,4,9,14]

Readers are directed to detailed reviews of airway management techniques to refamiliarize themselves with the variety and optimal use of airway adjuncts available and their advantages and disadvantages. It is absolutely essential that medical flight crew members are trained and competent in the use of all the airway equipment carried.[42–44] Endotracheal intubation of a critical care patient in the controlled environment of a hospital resuscitation area is unable to foreshadow the challenges faced in the prehospital arena. A patient trapped upside down in a car with a crumpled passenger compartment, in the dark, with extraneous noise from rescue equipment compressors, crackling radios, and passing sirens is an altogether different prospect. So is the patient with his or her head jammed up against a cabin bulkhead lying under an equipment-laden bridge on a compact, narrow stretcher who suddenly loses his or her airway. Even the most accomplished articles published on the management of the difficult airway are no substitute for medical crew training, expertise, and practical experience in caring for the critically ill or injured patient before arrival at the hospital.[45]

The importance of spending adequate preparation time on the ground before departure, time aimed at predicting and preempting every conceivable airway, respiratory, and cardiovascular problem, cannot be emphasized enough. Thus, before leaving, the airway must be secured against possible adverse events that may arise during transport, however unlikely.[3,46,47] Despite its established role in routine anesthesia and in the failed intubation drill, the laryngeal mask airway has not been accepted as a recommended method of airway management in the transport of the critically ill or injured patient.[2,3]

## Circulatory Support

This group of equipment must again be carefully selected for its suitability in transport care. Compact monitors are now available with high-visibility displays for ECG traces, pulse oximetry, noninvasive blood pressure, and $ETCO_2$ capnography. These monitors also have multiple invasive monitoring channels, which can display real-time readings of intra-arterial pressure, central venous pressure, pulmonary artery pressure, intracranial pressure, and internal temperature. The monitors may be combined with a portable pacer-defibrillator as one unit, or the pacer-defibrillator may be carried separately. Intravenous fluids must be run through an infusion pump or a syringe driver, all of which are now available as compact multichannel devices. There should be the capacity to run simultaneous infusions with an adequate battery life for the complete trip. It is critical for these devices to be reliable. Failure of a vasopressor or inotrope infusion is just as catastrophic as failure of respiratory equipment. A range of intravenous cannulas, infusion sets, stopcocks, syringes, swabs, tape, tourniquets, and preferably a needle-less system of drug port injection are essential.[3,4,14] Finally, a Sharps disposable container for glass ampules and biohazard refuse bags is required.

## Miscellaneous Support

The exact details of this group will depend on the types of transport missions undertaken, but this equipment should include nasogastric tubes and drainage systems, urinary catheter and bag systems, suitable dressings, splints and spinal immobilization devices, surgical instrument sets, thermal insulation, gloves, goggles, scissors, a torch, a clip-board, and mobile communication devices.[3,4,14] A stethoscope is traditional but is limited by background noise, although electronic damping or white-noise blocking systems are now available for stethoscopes and communication head sets.

## Point-of-Care Testing

Point-of-care testing has become commonplace at the bedside with advances in medical technology and is a vast improvement on carrying only blood glucose analysis strips. Many hematologic and biochemical tests are now available that measure sodium, potassium, chloride, urea (or blood urea nitrogen), creatinine, glucose, hematocrit, and hemoglobin, as well as ionized calcium, lactate, prothrombin time, cardiac troponin, and pH, $Po_2$, and $Pco_2$. Modern portable point-of-care testing clinical analyzers integrate biochemical and silicon chip technologies in self-calibrating, disposable cartridges, such as used in the i-STAT System (Abbott Laboratories, Abbott Park, IL). This system measures assays using potentiometric, amperometric, or conductometric circuits. Several other portable laboratory analyzer systems, some using immunoradiometric assays, are available for implementation in critical care patients.[13,14,16,27] These may even be integrated into a customized "smart stretcher" such as the LSTAT patient care platform (Integrated Medical Systems, Inc., Signal Hill, CA), which includes a ventilator, infusion devices, and laboratory facilities in an all-in-one critical care transport system. Concepts such as these clearly have commercial appeal in military or civilian environments where total weight is not so important.[16]

## Critical Care Pharmacy

A comprehensive critical care pharmacy must be taken, ranging from cardiac drugs, sedatives, and muscle relaxants to anticonvulsants, bronchodilators, narcotics, and even antivenom. The safe storage, carriage, and recording of scheduled or restricted drugs in particular must be scrupulous. Clear advice should be sought about the carriage of all drugs before crossing national boundaries or visiting international destinations even if just "in transit." These drugs can be carried with the other equipment discussed in special transport bags with multiple pockets and compartments such as the Thomas Pack (Emergency Medical Products, Inc., Waukesha, WI).

## STAFFING, TRAINING, AND QUALITY ASSURANCE

The final considerations in prehospital care include staffing arrangements, training, ethical issues, and medical control.

## Staffing Arrangements

Considerable debate exists in the literature about the relative benefits of various staffing arrangements for transporting patients. This debate mainly centers on the need for a physician, rather than an ICU-trained paramedic or nurse.[13,17] The key is to match the flight crew with the site, complexity, and duration of the transport and to the extent of stabilization interventions expected before departure. These recommendations are limited in the primary prehospital scenario, in which immediate transport to the nearest appropriate medical facility is needed, as compared with interhospital transfer, in which careful preparation and packaging of the patient are necessary before departure.

## Training

Specific training in both theory and practice of prehospital and aviation medicine is essential. Task-specific crewing involves matching the seniority, training, and expertise of the crew to the expected complexity of the transport. The other basic tenet of care for the critically ill patient is to replicate the ICU's standards as closely as possible. A minimum of two medical personnel should accompany a critically ill patient, in addition to the standard road ambulance, helicopter, or fixed wing vehicle's crew.[2,3] Additional expertise and special training are required for neonatal and pediatric transport medical teams.[9,10,12]

The highest quality of training for prehospital or interhospital work is paramount. Transporting critically ill patients increases their risk of morbidity and mortality, and staff must be prepared for the hostile, dangerous, and unpredictable prehospital arenas they enter.[3,13,14,17,18,48] Medical crew should be chosen with broad hospital critical care experience and adaptable leadership skills, yet they must be able to work within variable team structures and be safe unsupervised.

Specific aspects of this additional training include transport vehicle familiarity, monitoring and equipment familiarity, communication skills, and command and control procedures. In addition, it is essential medical staff know the local geography, the usual regional patterns of medical referrals and the relevant medical policies and procedures, and safety and emergency procedure drills. Interpersonal and team skills are necessary, as is an acceptable level of physical fitness.[3,4,17,48,49]

## Ethics

Medical staff must also understand a particular set of ethics that relate to individual character or virtue and teamwork.[50] The ethical principles regarding teamwork and its barriers as well as virtue-based ethics may all be taught and learned in preparation for caring for patients before arrival at the hospital. The respect for patient autonomy now demands that informed consent is obtained from the competent patient or guardian for every patient transport. In the case of the incompetent patient, consent is obtained from the patient's legally authorized representative.[3,50] A frank discussion of the risks and benefits of patient transfer must now occur and must be documented in the medical case notes.[51] When time-critical emergencies preclude the acquisition of consent, documentation of the reasons for not obtaining consent and the indications for transfer must be stated instead. Some countries, such as the United States, have federal or state laws governing the practice of interhospital patient transfer. Thus, the Emergency Medical Treatment and Active Labor Act (EMTALA), which is periodically updated from the 1986 Consolidated Omnibus Budget Reconciliation Act (COBRA) and 1990 COBRA amendments, clearly defines the legal responsibilities of both the referring and receiving facilities and their practitioners. This law places unique ethical and legal constraints on EMS services.[3,50] Clearly, these essential legislative requirements must now be incorporated into standard training procedures.

### Medical Control

Whatever the composition of the crew used in the transport of critical care patients, physician input, overview, and leadership are essential in the planning, development, evaluation, and continuous improvement of each component of the system. On-line medical direction provides immediately available clinical advice direct to the medical crew in the field or at the transferring hospital 24 hours a day. Additional expert critical care advice may be obtained from intensive care, emergency medicine, or anesthetic specialists according to local staffing and practice.

Off-line medical direction is strictly organizational, with responsibility for the standards, policies and procedures, training and credentialing, and quality assurance, such as continuous quality improvement, critical incident monitoring, root cause analysis, and open or closed feedback for every mission. Readers are referred to an excellent interfacility transfer algorithm, "Guidelines for the Inter- and Intrahospital Transport of Critically Ill Patients," by Warren and colleagues.[3] The apparent simplicity of this algorithm belies the underlying complexity of the entire process of the transportation of patients before arrival at the hospital.[3]

## CONCLUSIONS

The prehospital care of critically ill patients, whether they are moved from the scene to the first point of medical contact or transported from one health care facility to another, is a complex process demanding careful team selection and training and the highest standards of care. National guidelines and minimum standards for both adult and pediatric patients and a plethora of published research are now available on which to base systems of care.

Transport ventilators are just one small facet of the overall care process. The fact that they must meet the competing requirements of being small, robust, and reliable yet be able to deal with sometimes difficult, even extreme, physiologic derangements in the critically ill patient is an ongoing struggle. The adage that "There is no patient too sick to transport, only those too ill to leave behind" has set a serious challenge. Transport ventilators may eventually be able to reproduce other modern ventilator functions that use higher mean alveolar pressure to counteract poor pulmonary compliance, decelerating flow patterns to recruit those collapsed alveoli with longer inflation time constants, and PEEP to splint alveoli at end-expiration. These goals have to be achieved at the same time as avoiding volume shear force and pressure trauma or ventilator-associated lung injury, particularly to the noninvolved alveoli.

These are the goals of the ideal transport ventilator. No such ventilator currently exists, but newer portable models are approaching many of these capabilities. However, performance variations in flight under reduced cabin pressures, which are often unpredictable and poorly quantified in the literature, serve only to increase the sophistication and demands made on these ventilators.

Whether future high-end ventilator technology using computer feedback linked to smart real-time central monitoring, effective portable noninvasive ventilators, or portable imaging techniques such as ultrasound will make a significant difference to the clinical course of individual patients remains to be seen. Only by viewing the system as a whole and by measuring system outcomes can the true overall worth of the prehospital care provided be evaluated and thus continually improved.

## REFERENCES

1. Duke GJ, Green JV: Outcome of critically ill patients undergoing interhospital transfer. Med J Aust 2001;174:122–125.
2. Nagappan R: Transit care medicine: A critical link. Crit Care Med 2004;32:305–306.
3. Warren J, Fromm RE Jr, Orr RA, et al: Guidelines for the inter- and intrahospital transport of critically ill patients. Crit Care Med 2004;32:256–262.
4. Australasian College for Emergency Medicine, Joint Faculty of Intensive Care Medicine, Australian and New Zealand College of Anaesthetists: Minimum standards for transport of critically ill patients. Emerg Med (Fremantle) 2003;15:197–201.

5. American College of Emergency Physicians: Appropriate utilization of air medical transport in the out-of-hospital setting. Ann Emerg Med 1999;34:420.

6. Day S, McCloskey K, Orr R, et al: Pediatric interhospital critical care transport: Consensus of a national leadership conference. Pediatrics 1991;88:696–704.

7. Bellingan G, Olivier T, Batson S, Webb A: Comparison of a specialist retrieval team with current United Kingdom practice for the transport of critically ill patients. Intensive Care Med 2000;26:740–744.

8. Perez L, Klofas E, Wise L: Oxygenation/ventilation of transported intubated adult patients: A national survey of organizational practices. Air Med J 2000;19: 55–58.

9. Wheeler DS, Poss WB: Transport of the mechanically ventilated pediatric patient. Respir Care Clin N Am 2002;8: 83–104.

10. Gausche M, Seidel JS: Out-of-hospital care of pediatric patients. Pediatr Clin North Am 1999;46:1305–1327.

11. Dockery WK, Futterman C, Keller SR, et al: A comparison of manual and mechanical ventilation during pediatric transport. Crit Care Med 1999;27:802–806.

12. Edge WE, Kanter RK, Weigle CG, Walsh RF: Reduction of morbidity in interhospital transport by specialized pediatric staff. Crit Care Med 1994;22:1186–1191.

13. Gebremichael M, Borg U, Habashi NM, et al: Interhospital transport of the extremely ill patient: The mobile intensive care unit. Crit Care Med 2000;28:79–85.

14. Reynolds HN, Habashi NM, Cottingham CA, et al: Interhospital transport of the adult mechanically ventilated patient. Respir Care Clin N Am 2002;8:37–50.

15. Cameron PA, Zalstein S: Transport of the critically ill. Med J Aust 1998;169:610–611.

16. Fromm RE Jr, Varon J: Critical care transport. Crit Care Clin 2000;16:695–705.

17. Flabouris A, Seppelt I: Optimal interhospital transport systems for the critically ill. In Vincent JL (ed): *Yearbook of Intensive Care and Emergency Medicine 2001*. Berlin: Springer-Verlag, 2001, pp 647–660.

18. Uusaro A, Parviainen I, Takala J, Ruokonen E: Safe long-distance interhospital ground transfer of critically ill patients with acute severe unstable respiratory and circulatory failure. Intensive Care Med 2002;28:1122–1125.

19. Havill JH, Hyde PR, Forrest C: Transport of the critically ill patient: An example of an integrated model. N Z Med J 1995;108:378–380.

20. Munford BJ: What is the right helicopter for air medical scene response? Injury 2003;34:800–803.

21. Nagappan R, Barker J, Riddell T, et al: Helicopter in transit care of the critically ill: The Whangarei experience. N Z Med J 2000;113:303–305.

22. Driscoll RS: U.S. Army medical helicopters in the Korean War: New York Chapter History of Military Medicine Award. Mil Med 2001;166:290–296.

23. Olsen JA, Donaldson C: Helicopters, hearts and hips: Using willingness to pay to set priorities for public sector health care programmes. Soc Sci Med 1998;46:1–12.

24. Topley D: An international Critical Care Air Transport flight: Intervening in the Korean airline crash. Aviat Space Environ Med 1998;69:806–807.

25. Gilligan JE, Goon P, Maughan G, et al: An airborne intensive care facility (fixed wing). Anaesth Intensive Care 1996;24:245–253.

26. Chang D-M: Intensive care air transport: The sky is the limit; or is it? Crit Care Med 2001;29:2227–2230.

27. Beninati W, Jones KD: Mechanical ventilation during long-range air transport. Respir Care Clin N Am 2002;8: 51–65.

28. Dillard TA, Rajagopal KR, Slivka WA, et al: Lung function during moderate hypobaric hypoxia in normal subjects and patients with chronic obstructive pulmonary disease. Aviat Space Environ Med 1998;69: 979–985.

29. Tremblay L, Valenza F, Ribeiro SP, et al: Injurious ventilatory strategies increase cytokines and c-fos m-RNA expression in an isolated rat lung model. J Clin Invest 1997;99:944–952.

30. Lawless N, Tobias S, Mayorga MA: $FiO_2$ and positive end-expiratory pressure as compensation for altitude-induced hypoxemia in an acute respiratory distress syndrome model: Implications for air transportation of critically ill patients. Crit Care Med 2001;29:2149–2155.

31. Saltzman AR, Grant BJ, Aquilina AT, et al: Ventilatory criteria for aeromedical evacuation. Aviat Space Environ Med 1987;58:958–963.

32. Austin PN, Campbell RS, Johannigman JA, Branson RD: Transport ventilators. Respir Care Clin N Am 2002;8: 119–150.

33. Miyoshi E, Fujino Y, Mashimo T, Nishimura M: Performance of transport ventilator with patient-triggered ventilation. Chest 2000;118:1109–1115.

34. Beyer AJ 3rd, Land G, Zaritsky A: Nonphysician transport of intubated pediatric patients: A system evaluation. Crit Care Med 1992;20:961–966.

35. 2004 Ventilator Buyers Guide: http://www.advanceformrc.com/resources/MR010104_p61VentBuyguide.pdf. Accessed April 3, 2004.

36. Johannigman JA, Branson RD, Johnson DJ, et al: Out-of-hospital ventilation: Bag-valve devices vs transport ventilators. Acad Emerg Med 1995;2:719–724.

37. Zanetta G, Robert D, Guerin C: Evaluation of ventilators used during transport of ICU patients: A bench study. Intensive Care Med 2002;28:443–451.

38. Breton L, Minaret G, Aboab J, Richard JC: Fractional inspired oxygen on transport ventilators: An important determinant of volume delivery during assist control ventilation with high resistive load. Intensive Care Med 2002;28: 1181.

39. Guerin C: Reply to the letter "Fractional inspired oxygen on transport ventilators: An important determinant of volume delivery during assist control ventilation with high resistive load." Intensive Care Med 2002; 28:1182.

40. Helm M, Schuster R, Hauke J, Lampl L: Tight control of prehospital ventilation by capnography in major trauma victims. Br J Anaesth 2003;90:327–332.

41. Russell GB, Graybeal JM: Reliability of the arterial to end-tidal carbon dioxide gradient in mechanically ventilated patients with multisystem trauma. J Trauma 1994;36: 317–322.

42. Nolan JD: Prehospital and resuscitative airway care: Should the gold standard be reassessed? Curr Opin Crit Care 2001;7:413–421.

43. Idris AH, Gabrielli A: Advances in airway management. Emerg Med Clin North Am 2002;20:843–857.

44. Shuster M, Nolan J, Barnes TA: Airway and ventilation management. Cardiol Clin 2002;20:23–35.

45. Butler KH, Clyne B: Management of the difficult airway: Alternative airway techniques and adjuncts. Emerg Med Clin North Am 2003;21:259–289.

46. Sing RF, Rotondo MF, Zonies DH, et al: Rapid sequence induction for intubation by an aeromedical transport team: A critical analysis. Am J Emerg Med 1998;16:598–602.
47. Ricard-Hibon A, Chollet C, Belpomme V, et al: Epidemiology of adverse effects of prehospital sedation analgesia. Am J Emerg Med 2003;21:461–466.
48. Manji M, Bion JF: Transporting critically ill patients. Intensive Care Med 1995;21:781–783.
49. Crommett JW, McCabe D, Holcomb JB: Training for the transport of mechanically ventilated patients. Respir Care Clin N Am 2002;8:105–118.
50. Larkin GL, Fowler RL: Essential ethics for EMS: Cardinal virtues and core principles. Emerg Med Clin North Am 2002;20:887–911.
51. ACEP Board of Directors: Appropriate interhospital patient transfer. Ann Emerg Med 2004;43:685–686.

# CHAPTER 29

# Mechanical Ventilation During General Anesthesia

Hans Ulrich Rothen

During general anesthesia, mechanical ventilation has two principal aims:

- To provide oxygenation of arterial blood. In combination with an appropriate amount of oxygen transport capacity in blood and an intact hemodynamic system, this will allow for adequate delivery of oxygen to peripheral tissues and organs. Some evidence indicates that aiming at what could be called "supranormal" oxygenation of blood may even have some beneficial effects in the perioperative period, as discussed in the first part of this chapter.
- To secure appropriate alveolar ventilation to allow for adequate carbon dioxide ($CO_2$) elimination. To assume the latter, again an intact hemodynamic system is required.

Mechanical ventilation per se usually causes some derangement of pulmonary gas exchange and thus impedes perfect oxygenation of blood and maximal $CO_2$ elimination. The pathophysiologic background of this phenomenon is discussed in more detail in the second part of this chapter. In the third part, advantages and risks of possible measures to improve gas exchange are presented.

Even though volume controlled mechanical ventilation is probably the type of respiratory support most often used during general anesthesia, other modes are available, too. They are discussed in detail in Chapters 22 to 27. Therefore, only a few additional comments are given in this chapter. Finally, a few specific clinical problems, such as mechanical ventilation during laparoscopic surgery or in obese patients, are discussed in the final sections of this chapter.

What is the base of knowledge of the presented material? The amount of information available is huge. For example, a search in a biomedical bibliographic database,[1] such as MEDLINE, using the keywords "anesthesia" and "respiration, artificial" revealed 3872 references (Table 29.1), and the combination of "anesthesia" and "pulmonary gas exchange" resulted in 861 hits. Thus, one could conclude that the amount of information available worldwide is overwhelming and can hardly be summarized in a brief chapter. Conversely, we may choose a much more rigid approach to summarize knowledge, such as by using scientific strategies to reduce bias in collection, appraisal, and interpretation of relevant studies. Such a tool would be a systematic review on perioperative pulmonary function. Unfortunately, no such review has yet been presented in the medical literature.[2] Further, the number of prospective randomized studies in the present field of interest is small. Therefore, the following discussion is primarily based on pathophysiologic studies and on what may be called "expert opinion."

## WHAT ARE THE IMPLICATIONS OF IMPAIRED GAS EXCHANGE IN THE PERIOPERATIVE PERIOD?

Pulmonary function is altered both by surgery and by general anesthesia with mechanical ventilation. Accordingly, pulmonary gas exchange is regularly impaired in the perioperative period. Even though

**Table 29-1  Search in a Biomedical Bibliographic Database***

|  | Anesthesia | Respiration, Artificial | Ventilators, Mechanical | Respiratory Physiology | Pulmonary Gas Exchange | Ventilation-Perfusion Ratio | Atelectasis |
|---|---|---|---|---|---|---|---|
| Anesthesia | 171,812 | | | | | | |
| Respiration, artificial | 3872 | 36,090 | | | | | |
| Ventilators, mechanical | 718 | 1752 | 5510 | | | | |
| Respiratory physiology | 8580 | 9217 | 1121 | 135,826 | | | |
| Pulmonary gas exchange | 861 | 2345 | 186 | 14,656 | 14,953 | | |
| Ventilation-perfusion ratio | 297 | 527 | 62 | 5159 | 5124 | 5235 | |
| Atelectasis | 526 | 712 | 43 | 1042 | 280 | 153 | 6893 |

*MEDLINE was accessed on November 21, 2004, using the tool "PubMed search" in ProCite for Windows, Version 5.0. For each search, a single keyword or a combination of two keywords was used. The number of citations resulting from each search is given.

cyanosis is an unreliable indicator of hypoxemia,[3] impaired gas exchange was described in the 1940s and 1950s.[4,5] Using a three-compartment model, a marked increase of dead space, compensated by intubation and an increase in alveolar-arterial oxygen tension difference ($PA\text{-}aO_2$), was described at that time.[6] After introduction of pulse oximetry as a technique to monitor oxygenation of arterial blood ($SpO_2$), moderate hypoxemia, defined as $SpO_2$ of 85% to 90%, was observed in approximately half of all adults undergoing elective surgery.[7] Such hypoxemia lasted up to 30 minutes. Probably even more important, in that single-blind, observational study, about one fifth of all patients suffered from severe hypoxemia (defined as $SpO_2 <81\%$) for up to 5 minutes. Similar findings were described during transport after general anesthesia,[8] in the postanesthesia care unit,[9] later in the postoperative course,[10] and in children.[11]

Certainly, today's routine monitoring of oxygenation helps to detect such problems at an early stage and to take appropriate measures. Still, impaired oxygenation remains a relevant problem. For example, in the postoperative period, electrocardiographic abnormalities[12] and delirium[13] have been linked to hypoxemia. In this context, delirium may be an independent predictor of mortality in mechanically ventilated patients in the intensive care unit.[14] Further, elderly patients who were hypoxemic in

the perioperative period were more likely to suffer myocardial ischemia than those without hypoxemia.[15] Conversely, hypoxemia and hypotension were not significant risk factors for postoperative cognitive dysfunction in elderly patients.[10] Finally, pulmonary complications are associated with longer hospital stay,[16] and general anesthesia and type of surgery are elements of a postoperative risk index for predicting postoperative pneumonia after major noncardiac surgery.[17]

Improving oxygenation to "supranormal" levels has been shown to have possibly beneficial effects. Thus, supplemental oxygen augments antimicrobial and proinflammatory responses of alveolar macrophages.[18] If administered in the immediate perioperative period, supplemental oxygen may reduce the incidence of surgical wound infections,[19] even though conflicting results have been presented.[20] Supplemental intraoperative oxygen may be effective in preventing postoperative nausea and vomiting after gynecologic laparoscopy and in other types of surgery.[21,22] However, no reduction of postoperative nausea and vomiting was found in other studies.[23,24] Moreover, as described in Chapters 5 and 37, because of oxygen toxicity, such therapy also may have adverse effects. Indeed, no large-scale prospective randomized trial aiming at a more general primary outcome, such as long-term survival rate or mortality at

6 and 12 months after the intervention, has been undertaken thus far. Therefore, the question of whether supplemental intraoperative or perioperative oxygen (or hyperoxia) results in an overall benefit remains unanswered. In this context, the concentration of oxygen in inspiratory gas and the partial pressure of oxygen in arterial blood ($PaO_2$) are just two components in the complex cascade involved in optimal delivery of oxygen to peripheral tissue and organs.[25]

In summary, impaired or inadequate oxygenation in the perioperative period is an important clinical problem, resulting in morbidity and possibly mortality. Thus, an analysis of the mechanisms causing deterioration in gas exchange during general anesthesia with mechanical ventilation and measures to improve oxygenation are relevant for daily clinical practice.

## MECHANISMS OF IMPAIRED GAS EXCHANGE DURING GENERAL ANESTHESIA WITH MECHANICAL VENTILATION

### Ventilation-Perfusion Mismatch

Pulmonary ventilation and perfusion, including mismatch between ventilation and perfusion, are discussed in Chapters 9 and 10. Therefore, only changes in ventilation-perfusion (V/Q) distribution during general anesthesia with mechanical ventilation are discussed briefly in the following text.

Soon after its introduction as a research tool, the multiple inert gas elimination technique (MIGET) began to be used to analyze changes of V/Q distribution during general anesthesia.[26,27] In young, healthy volunteers, both ventilation and perfusion are distributed to wider ranges (as measured by an increase in the standard deviation of the logarithmic distribution of ventilation [log SDV] and perfusion [log SDQ]) after induction of general anesthesia with muscle paralysis (Fig. 29.1). In some subjects, there is a marked increase in pulmonary shunt up to 25% of cardiac output. In addition to this increase in log SDV and log SDQ, an increase in perfusion to lung regions with low V/Q distribution after induction of anesthesia was found in several studies using MIGET.[28–30] An even more marked impairment of V/Q distribution may be present in older patients.[29,31] Similarly, a marked V/Q mismatch was found in patients undergoing both coronary artery bypass grafting and surgery for mitral valve disease.[32]

What causes such V/Q mismatch? On the one hand, there are changes in functional residual capacity (FRC) and ventilation distribution. Several studies have shown that the FRC is reduced by about 20% during general anesthesia, as compared with the awake state.[33,34] This reduction in FRC, in turn, is caused by a cranial shift of the diaphragm (probably mostly of its dependent parts[35,36]),

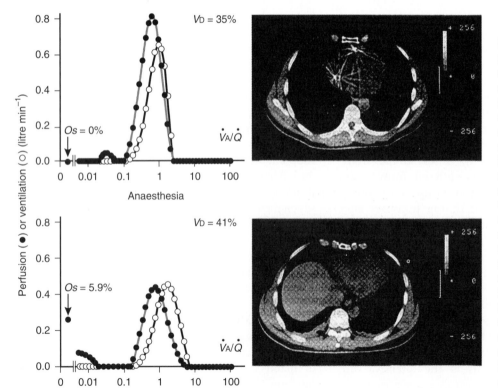

**Figure 29.1** Ventilation-perfusion ($\dot{V}A/\dot{Q}$) distribution and computed tomography in a supine subject. *Left*, $\dot{V}A/\dot{Q}$ distribution in the awake (*top*) and anesthetized (*bottom*) subject. Note the appearance of pulmonary shunt and an increase in $\dot{V}A/\dot{Q}$ mismatch during general anesthesia with mechanical ventilation. *Right*, Computed tomography of the chest, taken just above the top of the right diaphragm. Note the appearance of densities in the dependent lung regions during anesthesia. (Redrawn from Gunnarsson L, Tokics L, Gustavsson H, et al: Influence of age on atelectasis formation and gas exchange impairment during general anaesthesia. Br J Anaesth 1991;66: 423–432.)

and a change in the rib cage configuration.[37] The extent of such changes depends on the type of anesthetic used, and whether muscle relaxation is added or not. With inhalation anesthetics, rib cage contribution to normal tidal breathing is reduced[38] or unchanged.[39] On the other hand, ketamine increases rib cage contribution[40] or at least keeps the contribution unchanged.[41] An additional factor, probably relevant for the decrease in FRC, is the change in intrathoracic blood volume.[42] As a result of all these changes, regional ventilation will change, too. In general, during spontaneous breathing, there is some gravity-dependent distribution of ventilation, with an increase in regional ventilation from nondependent to dependent lung regions.[43–45] There is also a marked gravity-independent inhomogeneity of regional ventilation.[46,47] With induction of anesthesia and muscle paralysis, there is a marked change in ventilation distribution,[23] caused at least in part by a change in position and movement of the diaphragm (see also later). During normal tidal breathing, inspiratory gas predominantly goes to nondependent lung regions, whereas dependent regions are less ventilated.[48]

Besides the change in ventilation distribution, there is also a change in the distribution of pulmonary blood flow.[49] In addition, increased intrathoracic pressure, as present during positive pressure ventilation, for example, may reduce cardiac output and affect pulmonary vascular resistance.[50,51] This may result in decrease of blood flow to lung regions where intra-alveolar pressure is higher than the intravascular pressure (zone I according to West and colleagues[51]). Other models of lung perfusion have been presented.[52–54] Despite such uncertainty, it is fair to state that there is probably also some change in distribution of pulmonary perfusion with induction of general anesthesia and mechanical ventilation. The net result will then be the well-documented impairment in V/Q distribution.[55]

As compared with general anesthesia, regional anesthesia usually results in markedly less impairment of V/Q distribution.[30,56,57] Accordingly, this topic is not discussed here in detail.

In summary, there is a marked change in V/Q distribution with induction of general anesthesia. Probably, changes in ventilation distribution contribute more to this than changes in perfusion distribution. The net result is an increase in V/Q mismatch and pulmonary shunt.

## Atelectasis

### General Findings

Besides V/Q mismatch, probably an even more important cause of impaired gas exchange appears to be atelectasis.[58,59] The Greek words ατελεσ (*ateles*) and εκτασισ (*ektasis*) signify "incomplete/imperfect" and "extension/ expansion," respectively. Strictly speaking, this refers only to incomplete expansion of lung tissue in the newborn. However, the term *atelectasis* usually is used more loosely, as in this chapter, to describe collapse of lung tissue in general.

Even though the concept of progressive atelectasis during mechanical ventilation and in the postoperative period was proposed a long time ago,[60–62] researchers were not able to confirm this hypothesis by conventional chest radiography.[63] Only when computed tomography of the chest was introduced into clinical practice could atelectasis be demonstrated, first in children[64] and soon after in adults as well.[65] Atelectasis causes pulmonary shunt and thus clearly contributes to the impairment of gas exchange during general anesthesia. Furthermore, in animal models, atelectasis stimulates alveolar macrophages to produce inflammatory mediators such as interleukin-1 and tumor necrosis factor-$\alpha$,[66] results in decreased function of surfactant,[67] or causes vascular leak and right ventricular failure.[68] Whether such effects are present in humans and whether they contribute to morbidity or mortality remain to be analyzed.

Atelectasis appears immediately with induction of anesthesia and is present both during spontaneous breathing and after muscle paralysis, regardless of whether intravenous or inhalational anesthetics are used.[69,70] The only exception to this is ketamine.[71] It has been estimated that in adults with healthy lungs, 20% to 25% of the lung tissue in basal regions (i.e., adjacent to the diaphragm) or roughly 15% of the entire lung may be atelectatic.[69] This results in true pulmonary shunt, as measured by MIGET. A regression equation, based on a total of 45 patients, has been calculated (modified from reference 31):

$$\text{Shunt (\% CO)} = 1.7 + 0.8 \bullet \text{atelectasis (\%)};$$
$$r = 0.81, P < .01$$

Where shunt is pulmonary shunt, expressed as a percentage of cardiac output (CO), and atelectasis is measured as a percentage of the total pulmonary area just above the diaphragm.

During general anesthesia with mechanical ventilation, a pulmonary shunt of 5% to 10% of cardiac output is found in adults.[30,31] Shunt does not increase with age, whereas regions with poor ventilation in relation to their perfusion (low V/Q; see later) show a dependency on age.[31] In obese patients, larger atelectatic areas are present than in lean ones[30,72] (see also later). Finally, patients with chronic obstructive pulmonary disease (COPD) may show less or even no atelectasis.[73]

In summary, atelectasis is found in 85% to 90% of anesthetized adults. Atelectasis causes pulmonary shunt. It thus appears that the early formation of atelectasis and the increase in pulmonary shunt are unavoidable adverse effects of anesthesia.

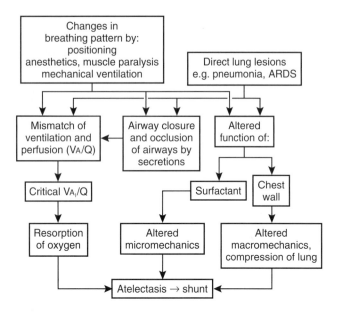

**Figure 29.2** Changes in pulmonary physiology resulting in atelectasis and pulmonary shunt. For details, see text.

## Causes of Atelectasis Formation

Three possible mechanisms may cause atelectasis:[58,59,74] absorption of gas trapped by occluded airways, compression of lung tissue, and impaired function of surfactant (Fig. 29.2).

**Gas Resorption** Investigators have long known that a lung unit will ultimately collapse if it is not ventilated.[75–77] Accordingly, if induction of anesthesia results in an increased number of lung units with poor or no ventilation, and if such lung units are filled with an easily resorbed gas, lung collapse may result.[78] Indeed, even short periods of breathing 100% oxygen near the residual volume may cause atelectasis.[79] Thus, an increased inspired fraction of oxygen ($FiO_2$) may promote atelectasis formation if there is a concomitant increase in low V/Q (e.g., caused by a decrease in FRC).[80,81]

**Compression Atelectasis** The diaphragm separates two spaces with different pressures as well as vertical pressure gradients. Thus, the end-expiratory intrathoracic pressure normally is lower than the abdominal pressure. The vertical pressure gradient in the pleural space of the awake subject is 0.2 to 0.4 cm $H_2O$/cm, whereas this gradient approximates 1 cm $H_2O$/cm in the abdomen.[82] If the diaphragm no longer acts as a rigid wall between these two spaces, the abdominal pressure will be transferred into the thoracic cavity, thus increasing the pleural pressure in dependent lung regions. This process could result in compression atelectasis. Indirect evidence of this is the finding in one investigation that no atelectasis developed during anesthesia with ketamine,[71] a drug known to maintain respiratory muscle tone and rib cage function. Moreover,

a cephalad shift with anesthesia and muscle paralysis was found in several investigations.[30,83] Conversely, tensing the diaphragm by phrenic nerve stimulation reduces the amount of atelectasis at isovolumic conditions.[84]

**Surfactant** The function of surfactant may be impeded by anesthesia.[85] Furthermore, a lack of intermittent deep breaths, as is usual during mechanical ventilation, may result in decreased content of active forms of alveolar surfactant. In addition, atelectasis per se may cause impaired function of surfactant.[67] This decreased function results in reduced alveolar stability and causes alveolar collapse. In addition, decreased function may contribute to liquid bridging in the airway lumen and may cause airway closure.[86] For further details, see Chapter 12.

In summary, atelectasis is present immediately after induction of anesthesia. Gas resorption, compression of lung regions, and altered function of surfactant may all contribute to the formation of atelectasis. Probably, resorption and compression are the two mechanisms most commonly involved in the perioperative formation of atelectasis.

### Attenuation of Hypoxic Pulmonary Vasoconstriction

Because atelectasis is present during anesthesia, the attenuation of hypoxic pulmonary vasoconstriction (HPV)[87–89] may contribute to impairment in gas exchange by increasing pulmonary shunt. Such attenuation in general can be found with inhalational anesthetics,[90,91] and it is less prominent or even absent with intravenous anesthetics.[92] However, this effect is relevant only if there is a V/Q mismatch or shunt; it does not cause any disturbances in an otherwise normally functioning lung.

### Airway Closure

In addition to the mechanisms discussed earlier, airway closure may contribute to ventilation inhomogeneity in the lung. Airway closure was initially demonstrated in awake subjects and was shown to increase in magnitude with age.[93] However, there is not complete agreement over the extent of airway closure in anesthetized subjects and its influence on gas exchange in the anesthetized subject.[94–98] Intermittent closure of airways can be expected to reduce the ventilation of dependent lung regions. Such lung units may then become low V/Q units (i.e., units with a low V/Q ratio) if perfusion is maintained or not reduced to the same extent as ventilation. Overall, close to 75% of impairment of the arterial oxygenation can be explained by a combination of atelectasis and airway closure, according to the following equation:[98]

$$PaO_2 \text{ (mm Hg)} = 218 - 22 \bullet \ln \text{atelectasis (cm}^2\text{)}$$
$$- 0.06 \bullet (CV\text{-}ERV) \text{ (mL)};$$
$$r = 0.86, P < .001$$

Where (CV-ERV) indicates the amount of airway closure occurring above FRC, CV is closing volume, ERV is expiratory reserve volume, and atelectasis is measured as the area of collapsed lung tissue just above the diaphragm (ln, natural logarithm).

## IMPROVING GAS EXCHANGE

### Change in Fraction of Oxygen in Inspiratory Gas

#### Increasing Fraction of Inspired Oxygen

Increasing $FiO_2$ when there is acute deterioration in oxygenation is certainly accepted standard practice. Selecting an $FiO_2$ high enough to attain a minimal or appropriate level of $PaO_2$ seems trivial. However, there are no clear guidelines about a minimal $PaO_2$. Usually, a threshold of 60 mm Hg for $PaO_2$ (or 90% for $SpO_2$) is cited, but depending on the specific circumstances, much lower levels are compatible with survival. For example, it was estimated that at the summit of Mt. Everest, $PaO_2$ may be as low as 30 mm Hg, whereas estimated $PaCO_2$ is 11 mm Hg.[99] Conversely, as briefly discussed earlier, hypoxemia during anesthesia clearly may result in an adverse outcome. Aiming at a supranormal $PaO_2$ may possibly even be beneficial. Accordingly, an increase in $FiO_2$ during general anesthesia with mechanical ventilation from the normal level of 0.21 up to 0.3 to 0.5 is considered standard practice by many clinicians.

In certain situations, an increase in $FiO_2$ greater than the previously mentioned levels may be advisable. In an animal model, investigators showed that, in acute normovolemic hemodilution down to a "critical" hemoglobin concentration, an $FiO_2$ of 1.0 may be beneficial in terms of short-term survival.[100] Similar findings were also presented in severe hemorrhagic shock.[101] In a very different clinical setting (i.e., severe brain damage in humans), at least in short-term studies, an increase of $FiO_2$ again to 1.0 may have beneficial effects (decrease in tissue lactate[102]).

In summary, the use of higher than normal $FiO_2$ values is standard practice. Selecting an appropriate level of $FiO_2$ is primarily based on clinical judgment, rather than on firm scientific data. For further details, see also Chapter 37.

### Adverse Effects of High Fraction of Inspired Oxygen

**Formation of Atelectasis**  If a lung unit has a low V/Q ratio, it may eventually collapse. The V/Q at which such collapse occurs at a specific level of $FiO_2$ has been called *critical V/Q*.[78] The higher the amount of well-resorbed gas (e.g., oxygen) in the inspiratory gas mixture, the higher the critical V/Q ratio. In elderly patients, during spontaneous breathing of 100% oxygen, a pulmonary shunt of more than 10% caused by collapse of lung units has been found.[103] Similarly, breathing 100% oxygen immediately before extubation may promote formation of atelectasis.[104] This may result in impaired gas exchange after extubation.[105] Accordingly, avoiding 100% oxygen during induction of general anesthesia may prevent the early formation of atelectasis.[80]

Once lung units are atelectatic, a much higher transpulmonary pressure is needed to reopen the unit than is commonly used during mechanical ventilation using normal tidal breathing. This is discussed in more detail later.

**Oxygen Toxicity**  Even though recent research has focused mostly on mechanically induced lung injury, oxygen itself may also damage the lungs. This is discussed in Chapter 5 and therefore is mentioned only briefly here. Toxic effects of oxygen were described long ago.[106] In general, it is assumed that the use of $FiO_2$ lower than 0.5 to 0.6 at atmospheric pressure may be considered safe. If applied for less than 24 hours, even higher levels of oxygen may be used. This statement, however, is based on clinical data that were presented in the early 1970s.[107,108]

Exposure of the lungs to high concentrations of oxygen may result in increased production of reactive oxygen species ($O_2^-$, $H_2O_2$, and $OH^-$) and may lead to oxidative stress.[109] At low levels, reactive oxygen species regulate cell growth and cell adaptation; high levels of reactive oxygen species, however, may result in cell damage or even cell death.[110] The extent of injury depends on the amount of oxygen added and the duration of exposure.[111,112] If this occurs in combination with another injury, more damage may result. For example, acid aspiration increases the sequelae of high $FiO_2$.[113] Moreover, the use of high concentrations of oxygen was found to increase mortality from pneumonia in an animal model.[114] Finally, using increased $FiO_2$ together with bleomycin may result in more lung damage than if a decreased $FiO_2$ is used.[115]

In summary, even though an increase in $FiO_2$ is considered mandatory during acute hypoxemia, adverse effects of oxygen have to be kept in mind during prolonged use. The pragmatic guidelines established many years ago probably will be refined when recent findings in animal research (and in a few observational studies in humans) are transferred to the clinical environment.

### Prevention and Treatment of Atelectasis

Various procedures can prevent atelectasis or reopen collapsed tissue.[58,59] The procedures discussed in the following sections include minimization of pulmonary gas resorption, recruitment maneuvers, positive end-expiratory pressure (PEEP), and maintenance or restoration of respiratory muscle tone.

## Avoidance of High Fraction of Inspired Oxygen

As discussed previously, collapse caused by gas resorption may be present in a lung unit if there is a total cessation of gas flow to this unit (thus resulting in trapped gas) or if the expired ventilation of this lung unit falls to zero (critical V/Q[78]). Accordingly, avoidance of the preoxygenation procedure during induction of anesthesia may eliminate the formation of atelectasis.[80,116] Although it is obvious that lowering the $FiO_2$ can increase the risk of hypoxemia in a difficult and prolonged intubation,[117] recent findings call for a reevaluation of the currently implemented standard procedures for inducing anesthesia.[118]

After recruitment of a collapsed lung (see later), ventilation of the lungs with pure oxygen results in rapid reappearance of atelectasis.[81,119] When, conversely, 40% oxygen in nitrogen is used for ventilation of the lungs, atelectasis reappears slowly, and 40 minutes after recruitment only 20% of the initial atelectasis is found[81] (see Fig. 29.5). Thus, ventilation during anesthesia should be performed with a moderate $FiO_2$ in nitrogen (e.g., 0.3 to 0.4), and $FiO_2$ should be increased only if arterial oxygenation or oxygen delivery is compromised. Further, if the lungs are ventilated with high $FiO_2$, the use of PEEP should be considered (see later). Because studies on the effect of $FiO_2$ on postoperative atelectasis and gas exchange show variable results,[104,105,120,121] no general clinical guidelines can be formulated at present.

In summary, avoiding a high concentration of oxygen during induction and ongoing anesthesia may prevent the formation of atelectasis. However, because no data exist on the effect of such an approach on long-term outcome, no further recommendations are possible.

## Recruitment Maneuver

To reopen collapsed lung tissue in the supine adult subject during general anesthesia with mechanical ventilation, a high airway pressure is needed (see also Chapter 25). For example (Fig. 29.3, *left*), at inflation to an airway pressure of 30 cm $H_2O$, the amount of atelectasis can be reduced to approximately half of the initial value. To reopen all collapsed lung tissue completely, inflation up to an airway pressure of 40 cm $H_2O$ is required.[30] Such a large inflation and subsequent expiration down to −20 cm $H_2O$ corresponds to vital capacity, as measured during spontaneous breathing with the patient awake,[30] and thus also may be called the *vital capacity maneuver*.[119] Repeated inflation of the lung to an airway pressure of 30 cm $H_2O$ only results in minor further opening of lung tissue after the first maneuver (Fig. 29.3, *right*). With sustained inflation to an airway pressure of 40 cm $H_2O$, a time constant of 2.6 seconds for the exponential decrease in amount of atelectasis was found[122] (Fig. 29.4). Thus, in adults with healthy lungs, inflation of the lungs to 40 cm $H_2O$ maintained for no more than 7 to 8 seconds may reexpand all previously collapsed lung tissue. Whether the time constant is different in patients with pulmonary disease remains to be shown. Moreover, instead of using an exponential equation,[122] other mathematical models may possibly more adequately

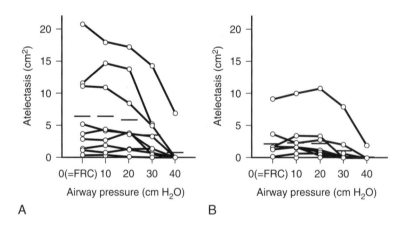

A

B

**Figure 29.3** Reexpansion of collapsed lung tissue by sustained inflation of the lungs. *Left,* Stepwise inflation of the lungs. Between each step, the lungs were ventilated during 3 to 5 minutes at a tidal volume of 9 mL/kg body weight and zero end-expiratory pressure (ZEEP). During the reexpansion maneuver, the end-inspiratory pressure, as indicated on the x-axis, was kept for 15 seconds. Atelectasis was measured as dense lung areas (−100 to +100 HU) in a computed tomography scan in a transverse plane 0 to 1 cm above the top of the right diaphragm. Individual values and mean are given. *Right,* Same procedure as described earlier. However, repeated inflation of the lungs to an end-inspiratory of 30 cm $H_2O$ is used for recruitment of collapsed lung (see x-axis). (From Rothen HU, Sporre B, Engberg G, et al: Re-expansion of atelectasis during general anaesthesia: A computed tomography study. Br J Anaesth 1993;71:788–795.)

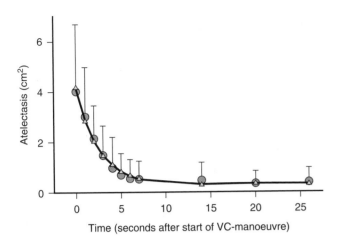

**Figure 29.4** Change over time during a recruitment maneuver: atelectasis during a vital capacity maneuver. Atelectasis is measured as described in Figure 29.3. Also shown is a curve with negative exponential decay, fitted to individual data according to the following:

atelectasis $(cm^2) = a + y_0 \bullet e^{(time(s)/\tau)}$,

$\tau$ (time constant) = 2.6 seconds (95% CI, 1.8 to 4.3 seconds), $a = 0.3\ cm^2$, $y_0 = 3.9\ cm^2$.

(From Rothen HU, Neumann P, Berglund JE, et al: Dynamics of re-expansion of atelectasis during general anaesthesia. Br J Anaesth 1999;82:551–556.)

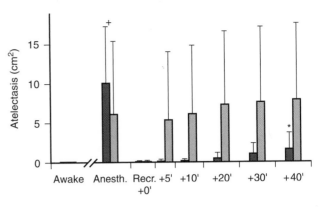

**Figure 29.5** Recurrence of atelectasis after a recruitment maneuver: atelectasis in the awake, supine subject after induction of anesthesia and after a recruitment maneuver. *Hatched bars*, $Fio_2 = 0.4$ after recruitment; *open bars*, $Fio_2 = 1.0$ after recruitment. Atelectasis is measured as described in Figure 29.3. (From Rothen HU, Sporre B, Engberg G, et al: Influence of gas composition on recurrence of atelectasis after a reexpansion maneuver during general anesthesia. Anesthesiology 1995;82:832–842.)

describe reexpansion of collapsed lung units.[123,124] The pressure necessary to reopen collapsed alveoli is markedly higher than the pressure needed to reopen collapsed airways.[125,126] Thus, during normal tidal breathing, airways may collapse during expiration and reopen during inspiration (airway closure; see earlier), whereas collapsed alveoli remain unchanged throughout the respiratory cycle.

Another type of recruitment maneuver, using a stepwise increase in PEEP, has been described.[127] Whether this technique is superior to the vital capacity maneuver has not yet been studied. To reexpand collapsed lung tissue, manual hyperinflation of the lungs also may be used,[128,129] although the estimation of tidal volume from the reservoir bag may be erroneous.[130] In addition, any disconnection from the ventilator may expose the lung to zero end-expiratory pressure (ZEEP), thus causing renewed collapse after attempted reexpansion.

A recruitment maneuver may also be effective during cardiac surgery[121,131] and during general anesthesia in children.[132] A similar approach may be successful in adults with respiratory failure.[133,134]

In anesthetized adults with healthy lungs, a recruitment maneuver reduces the amount of atelectasis and pulmonary shunt (Fig. 29.5) and, despite a concomitant increase in perfusion to poorly ventilated lung units (low V/Q ratio), may result in a small but significant reduction of $P_{A-a}O_2$ for at least 40 minutes.[135] Alveolar recruitment also improves ventilatory efficiency, as measured by $CO_2$ elimination.[136] In addition, a single deep breath may result in release of surfactant,[137] thus contributing to improved alveolar stability and preventing lung collapse. Finally, reducing atelectasis attenuated bacterial growth and translocation in an animal model of pneumonia.[138] However, a recruitment maneuver also may have adverse effects. For example, in patients with septic shock, a recruitment maneuver may cause hemodynamic derangement.[139] The extent of these changes seems to be related to the cardiovascular state before the procedure. In patients with cerebral injury, a recruitment maneuver may result in deterioration of cerebral hemodynamics.[140] Moreover, in one study in an animal model, despite recovery of systemic circulation within a few minutes, splanchnic, renal, and portal blood flows remained slightly reduced during the short period of observation,[141] and the authors cautioned that this decrease could present a risk in conditions with markedly compromised circulatory reserves. Finally, in patients with COPD, anesthesia causes only a small amount of atelectasis, and impaired oxygenation is primarily caused by V/Q mismatch.[73] Under such circumstances, any further expansion of lung tissue may be of limited value or may even be harmful because of possible regional overinflation. Thus, as with any therapeutic measure, before performing a recruitment maneuver one should carefully weigh the assumed benefits and possible risks.[142]

In summary, a recruitment maneuver should be considered if atelectasis is suspected as a cause of a relevant impairment of gas exchange during general anesthesia with mechanical ventilation. Until further data are available, the choice between a sustained inflation (time constant $\approx 3$ seconds, end-inspiratory pressure $\approx 40$ cm $H_2O$) and a stepwise inflation to reexpand collapsed lung tissue will depend mostly on personal experience and on the equipment available.

### Positive End-Expiratory Pressure

Another approach to reopen collapsed lung is PEEP. If used in patients with healthy lungs, PEEP reduces the amount of atelectasis, but it has a variable effect on pulmonary shunt and often results in increased dead space.[143] Further, atelectasis redevelops within a few minutes after cessation of PEEP.[84] Thus, if sustained reopening of atelectasis and reduction of pulmonary shunt are the main goals of a therapeutic measure, a vital capacity maneuver may be more appropriate than PEEP,[135] although direct comparison of these two procedures is lacking.

After a recruitment maneuver, PEEP significantly reduces the rate of renewed lung collapse even if a high $FiO_2$ is used.[144-146] This technique corresponds to the so-called open lung concept, as described in a landmark article by Lachmann.[147] PEEP may also be used to prevent formation of atelectasis and to prolong the time of nonhypoxic apnea during induction of anesthesia.[148,149]

### Maintenance of Muscle Tone

The use of an anesthetic that allows maintenance of respiratory muscle tone probably will prevent formation of atelectasis. As discussed previously, ketamine neither impairs muscle tone and nor causes atelectasis. However, if this anesthetic is combined with muscle paralysis, atelectasis will also develop.[71]

### Effect of Anesthetic Techniques and Postoperative Care

In this section, the effects of anesthetic techniques and postoperative care on pulmonary morbidity are briefly discussed. This topic is dealt with in more detail elsewhere in this book. Therefore, only brief comments are given here.

Indeed, there is no clear evidence that V/Q mismatch and atelectasis are the only causes of postoperative hypoxemic events in the majority of cases. Many concomitant factors have to be considered, such as respiratory depression from residual effects of anesthetic drugs, the type and anatomic site of surgery (i.e., change in lung mechanics), and hemodynamic impairment.[150]

Residual neuromuscular block still has to be considered as a risk factor for postoperative pulmonary complications.[151] Moreover, the appropriate use of analgesic techniques may influence pulmonary outcome. In a comparison of epidural local anesthetics, epidural opioids, or patient-controlled analgesia with systemic opioids, favorable effects were found in terms of pulmonary morbidity for the former methods.[152-154]

A meta-analysis showed that appropriate positioning in the postoperative period may help to improve postoperative pulmonary function.[155] Unfortunately, the studies that were included in the meta-analysis were quite heterogeneous, thereby preventing any generalization.

## FEATURES OF RESPIRATORS USED DURING GENERAL ANESTHESIA

### Respiratory Circuit

In contrast to mechanical ventilators used in the intensive care unit, respirators used for mechanical ventilation during general anesthesia often have a circular system. Even though numerous variations of the circular arrangement are possible, the general components are identical and include (1) fresh gas inflow, (2) inspiratory and expiratory tubes, (3) a Y-piece connector, (4) inspiratory and expiratory unidirectional valves, (5) an overflow valve, (6) $CO_2$ absorbent, and (7) a reservoir bag.[156] Presumed advantages of the circular system include the prevention of operating room pollution, the conservation of respiratory moisture and heat, and the relative stability of inspiratory gas concentrations. Only a few articles have addressed specific problems such as criteria for the choice[157] or performance of anesthesia respirators.[158-160]

### Comparing Various Modes of Mechanical Ventilation

In addition to conventional modes of mechanical ventilation, such as constant volume or constant pressure ventilation,[156] modern ventilatory equipment allows for more patient-adapted respiratory support. For example, biphasic intermittent positive airway pressure may reduce the duration of intubation and the need for analgesics or sedatives.[161] Similarly, nasal bilevel positive airway pressure can be used to provide adequate respiratory support during surgery of the lower abdomen or the lower extremities.[162] Moreover, intermittent continuous positive airway pressure (CPAP) results in a decrease in alveolar dead space and thus in improved efficiency of ventilation.[163]

In patients with the laryngeal mask airway, spontaneous breathing is the mode used most often.[164] However, because gas exchange may be less effective than with positive pressure ventilation,[165] the use of pressure support ventilation may be considered.[166] Pressure support ventilation provides more effective gas exchange than spontaneous breathing while preserving leak fraction and hemodynamic homeostasis. Whether newer modes of mechanical ventilation, such as variable ventilation[167] or neural control of mechanical ventilation,[168] will gain any place in mechanical ventilation during general anesthesia remains speculative.

## SPECIFIC SITUATIONS

### Obese Patients

Obesity is an important risk factor for impaired oxygenation and pulmonary complications in the perioperative period[26,169,170] (Fig. 29.6). A major cause is the reduction of FRC in obese patients, a change that is even more marked in the supine position and after induction of anesthesia.[33,77,171] Accordingly, the combined effect of compression of dependent lung regions and gas resorption in lung units with low V/Q ratio or airway closure results, on average, in a considerable amount of atelectasis[30,72,172] (Fig. 29.7), present even in the postoperative period.[72] These changes probably also explain the shorter time to desaturation during induction of anesthesia, as observed in morbidly obese patients.[173]

All measures to prevent or treat atelectasis, as discussed previously, may also be used in obese patients. Accordingly, CPAP/PEEP may be considered to prevent formation of atelectasis during induction of anesthesia.[174,175] Whether an $FiO_2$ lower than standard (1.0) during this procedure is beneficial remains to be shown.[118] PEEP also improves oxygenation during ongoing anesthesia with mechanical ventilation, and a recruitment maneuver should be used as discussed earlier.[176,177] Moreover, appropriate positioning of the patient should be used whenever possible.[178,179]

Obese patients often also have coexisting problems, such as obstructive sleep apnea,[180] cardiovascular disease with right and left ventricular impairment (obesity cardiomyopathy),[181] insulin resistance or diabetes mellitus,[182] and impaired perioperative tissue oxygenation.[183] All these problems should be taken into account when caring for the obese patient.

### Laparoscopic Surgery

Laparoscopic surgery has multiple benefits, such as less impairment in postoperative pulmonary dysfunction,

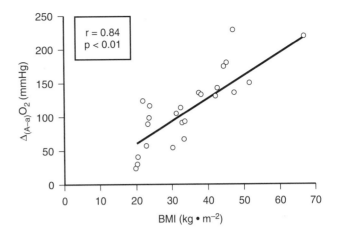

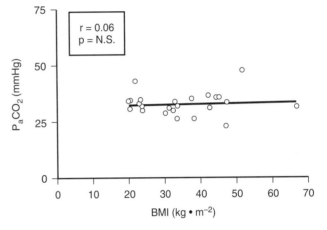

**Figure 29.6** Arterial blood gas in obese patients during general anesthesia. Obese patients have a marked impairment of oxygenation, whereas carbon dioxide can be kept normal during general anesthesia with mechanical ventilation. There is a linear correlation between the alveolar-arterial oxygen tension difference ($P_{A}$-$aO_2$) and body mass index (BMI, r = 0.84, $P < .01$). (From Pelosi P, Croci M, Ravagnan I, et al: The effects of body mass on lung volumes, respiratory mechanics, and gas exchange during general anesthesia. Anesth Analg 1998;87:654–660.)

quicker recovery, and shorter hospital stay.[184] Despite these advantages, marked intraoperative cardiorespiratory dysfunction may occur in a subgroup of patients. Accordingly, appropriate monitoring and a thorough understanding of pathophysiologic changes that occur during such procedures are needed.

The major ventilatory problems during laparoscopic surgery are related to the cardiopulmonary effects of pneumoperitoneum.[185,186] The most prominent changes concerning the respiratory system are cephalad displacement of the diaphragm, followed by reduction of the FRC and derangement of gas exchange.[187] In addition, the compliance of the respiratory system is decreased by

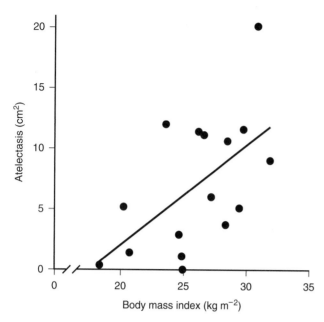

**Figure 29.7** Body mass index versus atelectasis during general anaesthesia. Obese patients have more atelectasis (r = 0.66, *P* = .006). (From Rothen HU, Sporre B, Engberg G, et al: Re-expansion of atelectasis during general anaesthesia: A computed tomography study. Br J Anaesth 1993;71:788–795.)

up to 50%.[188] These effects further are modified by the positioning of the patient during surgical procedures[189] and by obesity.[190]

Patients with cardiopulmonary disease may have an increased $P_{A-a}CO_2$; end-tidal $CO_2$ pressure ($PETCO_2$) may thus be misleading.[189,191,192] Besides absorption of $CO_2$ (with consecutively increased pulmonary elimination of $CO_2$,[192,193] V/Q mismatch and an increase in pulmonary shunt are possible mechanisms. Dead space ventilation, however, was found to be unchanged in most studies.[194,195]

Respiratory complications that can occur during laparoscopic surgery using $CO_2$ insufflation include $CO_2$ emphysema, pneumothorax, pneumomediastinum and pneumopericardium, and gas embolism. Gasless laparoscopy may be considered to reduce the risk of occurrence of such complications.[196]

## Lung Surgery and One-Lung Ventilation

During general anesthesia, gas exchange impairment in patients with severe COPD is primarily the result of a marked increase in low V/Q ratio and an increased log SDQ; there is, however, only a minimal amount of atelectasis.[73] Accordingly, PEEP should be used only at moderate levels (if at all), and a recruitment maneuver is probably only rarely indicated. However, if a patient has

no COPD, these techniques may be used,[197] based on the pathophysiologic principles discussed earlier.

Discussing the numerous techniques available for isolating one lung from ventilation[198] is beyond the scope of this chapter. Tidal volume should be adjusted when changing from two-lung to one-lung ventilation (OLV), to avoid overdistention of the ventilated lung.

OLV results in worsened gas exchange, caused by an obligatory increase in pulmonary shunt. With normal autoregulation, blood flow to the nonventilated lung may be reduced by HPV (see also earlier). With respect to attenuation of HPV, the choice of anesthetic is probably of minor importance. For example, no difference in alteration of arterial oxygenation was found between desflurane and isoflurane during OLV.[199,200] In addition, the use of inhaled nitric oxide as a selective pulmonary vasodilator failed to improve oxygenation during OLV.[201] Conversely, systemic vasodilators such as nitroprusside and glyceryl trinitrate inhibit HPV. Overall, the clinical role of HPV remains unclear.[202]

In cases of severe hypoxemia during OLV, there are three main options. Parallel to checking for the correct placement and patency of the artificial airways (e.g., blockers), a first possibility is to increase $FiO_2$ back to 1.0. The second option is to expand the nonventilated lung smoothly with 100% oxygen and to use a CPAP of 5 to 10 cm $H_2O$ thereafter.[203] A third option is to use PEEP during ventilation of the dependent lung.[204] However, whether this approach is beneficial depends on the underlying pulmonary disease because PEEP may divert blood flow from the ventilated to the nonventilated lung, and application of 100% oxygen to the nonventilated lung may abolish HPV. Thus, no uniform recommendations can be made. Rather, the ventilatory settings have to be tailored individually.[205] In any case, clamping the pulmonary artery to the nonventilated lung effectively removes any shunt caused by this lung.

Patients scheduled for lung surgery often have preexisting lung disease and therefore have an increased perioperative risk.[206] A discussion of preoperative risk assessment is beyond the scope of this chapter. However, it may be appropriate to mention the beneficial effect of a preoperative smoking intervention on postoperative complications,[207] as well as the preoperative use of bronchodilators and measures to loosen or remove secretions, when appropriate.

## CONCLUSION

In summary, pulmonary function is regularly altered both by surgery and by general anesthesia with mechanical ventilation. There is a marked increase in V/Q mismatch and pulmonary shunt with induction of anesthesia.

In addition, atelectasis is found in most anesthetized adults and causes pulmonary shunt. It thus appears that the early formation of atelectasis and the increase in pulmonary shunt are unavoidable adverse effects of anesthesia. In general, obese patients have more atelectasis than lean ones or patients with COPD. Using PEEP during induction of anesthesia and avoiding a very high $Fio_2$ during induction and maintenance of anesthesia may prevent the formation of atelectasis.

A recruitment maneuver should be considered if atelectasis is suspected as cause of a relevant impairment of gas exchange during anesthesia. Until further data are available, the choice between a sustained and a stepwise inflation to reexpand collapsed lung tissue depends mostly on personal experience and available equipment. To impede renewed lung collapse, the use of PEEP should be considered. In the postoperative period, appropriate positioning helps to improve pulmonary function.

Although some modes of ventilatory support may be superior in terms of pathophysiologic changes, no randomized controlled trial has yet been published, to show advantages of a specific modality over others in terms of long-term outcome. Nonetheless, appropriate monitoring and a thorough understanding of pathophysiologic changes that occur during specific procedures such as laparoscopic surgery or thoracic surgery with OLV are prerequisites for adequate care of patients during general anesthesia with mechanical ventilation.

The author of this chapter wishes to acknowledge Göran Hedenstierna (Department of Clinical Sciences, University Hospital, Uppsala, Sweden) for mentoring and most generous support.

## REFERENCES

1. Rothen HU, Grossenbacher F: How to perform a search in the biomedical literature. In Zbinden AM, Thomson D (eds): *Conducting Research in Anaesthesia and Intensive Care Medicine.* Oxford: Butterworth & Heinemann, 2001, pp 1–20.

2. Choi PT, Halpern SH, Malik N, et al: Examining the evidence in anesthesia literature: A critical appraisal of systematic reviews. Anesth Analg 2001;92:700–709.

3. Comroe JH, Botelho S: The unreliability of cyanosis in the recognition of arterial anoxemia. Am J Med Sci 1947;214:1–6.

4. Maier HC, Cournand A: Studies of the arterial oxygen saturation in the postoperative period after pulmonary resection. Surgery 1943;13:199–213.

5. Campbell EJ, Nunn JF, Peckett BW: A comparison of artificial ventilation and spontaneous respiration with particular reference to ventilation-bloodflow relationships. Br J Anaesth 1958;30:166–175.

6. Riley RL, Cournand A: "Ideal" alveolar air and the analysis of ventilation-perfusion relationships in the lungs. J Appl Physiol 1949;1:825–847.

7. Moller JT, Johannessen NW, Berg H, et al: Hypoxaemia during anaesthesia: An observer study. Br J Anaesth 1991;66:437–444.

8. Mathes DD, Conaway MR, Ross WT: Ambulatory surgery: Room air versus nasal cannula oxygen during transport after general anesthesia. Anesth Analg 2001;93:917–921.

9. Daley MD, Norman PH, Sandler AN: Hypoxaemia in adults in the post-anaesthesia care unit. Can Anaesth Soc J 1991;38:740–746.

10. Moller JT, Cluitmans P, Rasmussen LS, et al: Long-term postoperative cognitive dysfunction in the elderly ISPOCD1 study: ISPOCD investigators. International Study of Post-Operative Cognitive Dysfunction. Lancet 1998;351:857–861.

11. Coté CJ, Goldstein EA, Coté MA, et al: A single-blind study of pulse oximetry in children. Anesthesiology 1988;68:184–188.

12. Rosenberg J, Rasmussen V, von Jessen F, et al: Late postoperative episodic and constant hypoxaemia and associated ECG abnormalities. Br J Anaesth 1990;65:684–691.

13. Aakerlund L P, Rosenberg J: Postoperative delirium: Treatment with supplemental oxygen. Br J Anaesth 1994;72:286–290.

14. Ely EW, Shintani A, Truman B, et al: Delirium as a predictor of mortality in mechanically ventilated patients in the intensive care unit. JAMA 2004;291:1753–1762.

15. Gill NP, Wright B, Reilly CS: Relationship between hypoxaemic and cardiac ischaemic events in the perioperative period. Br J Anaesth 1992;68:471–473.

16. Lawrence VA, Hilsenbeck SG, Mulrow CD, et al: Incidence and hospital stay for cardiac and pulmonary complications after abdominal surgery. J Gen Intern Med 1995;10:671–678.

17. Arozullah AM, Khuri SF, Henderson WG, et al: Development and validation of a multifactorial risk index for predicting postoperative pneumonia after major noncardiac surgery. Ann Intern Med 2001;135:847–857.

18. Kotani N, Hashimoto H, Sessler DI, et al: Supplemental intraoperative oxygen augments antimicrobial and proinflammatory responses of alveolar macrophages. Anesthesiology 2000;93:15–25.

19. Greif R, Akca O, Horn EP, et al: Supplemental perioperative oxygen to reduce the incidence of surgical-wound infection: Outcomes Research Group. N Engl J Med 2000;342:161–167.

20. Pryor KO, Fahey TJ 3rd, Lien CA, et al: Surgical site infection and the routine use of perioperative hyperoxia in a general surgical population: A randomized controlled trial. JAMA 2004;291:79–87.

21. Goll V, Akca O, Greif R, et al: Ondansetron is no more effective than supplemental intraoperative oxygen for prevention of postoperative nausea and vomiting. Anesth Analg 2001;92:112–117.

22. Greif R, Laciny S, Rapf B, et al: Supplemental oxygen reduces the incidence of postoperative nausea and vomiting. Anesthesiology 1999;91:1246–1252.

23. Purhonen S, Turunen M, Ruohoaho UM, et al: Supplemental oxygen does not reduce the incidence of postoperative nausea and vomiting after ambulatory gynecologic laparoscopy. Anesth Analg 2003;96:91–96.

24. Joris JL, Poth NJ, Djamadar AM: Supplemental oxygen does not reduce postoperative nausea and vomiting after thyroidectomy. Br J Anaesth 2003;91:857–861.

25. Rivers E, Nguyen B, Havstad S, et al: Early goal-directed therapy in the treatment of severe sepsis and septic shock. N Engl J Med 2001;345:1368–1377.

26. Prutow RJ, Dueck R, Davies NJH, et al: Shunt development in young adult surgical patients due to inhalation anesthesia. Anesthesiology 1982;57:A477.

27. Rehder K, Knopp TJ, Sessler AD, et al: Ventilation-perfusion relationship in young healthy awake and anesthetized-paralyzed man. J Appl Physiol 1979;47:745–753.

28. Bindslev L, Hedenstierna G, Santesson J, et al: Ventilation-perfusion distribution during inhalation anaesthesia: Effects of spontaneous breathing, mechanical ventilation and positive end-expiratory pressure. Acta Anaesthesiol Scand 1981;25:360–371.

29. Dueck R, Young I, Clausen J, et al: Altered distribution of pulmonary ventilation and blood flow following induction of inhalation anesthesia. Anesthesiology 1980;52:113–125.

30. Rothen HU, Sporre B, Engberg G, et al: Re-expansion of atelectasis during general anaesthesia: A computed tomography study. Br J Anaesth 1993;71:788–795.

31. Gunnarsson L, Tokics L, Gustavsson H, et al: Influence of age on atelectasis formation and gas exchange impairment during general anaesthesia. Br J Anaesth 1991;66:423–432.

32. Hachenberg T, Mollhoff T, Holst D, et al: The ventilation-perfusion relation and gas exchange in mitral valve disease and coronary artery disease: Implications for anesthesia, extracorporeal circulation, and cardiac surgery. Anesthesiology 1997;86:809–817.

33. Hedenstierna G, Santesson J: Breathing mechanics, dead space and gas exchange in the extremely obese, breathing spontaneously and during anaesthesia with intermittent positive pressure ventilation. Acta Anaesthesiol Scand 1976;20:248–254.

34. Wahba RW: Perioperative functional residual capacity. Can J Anaesth 1991;38:384–400.

35. Froese AB, Bryan AC: Effects of anesthesia and paralysis on diaphragmatic mechanics in man. Anesthesiology 1974;41:242–255.

36. Warner DO, Warner MA, Ritman EL: Human chest wall function while awake and during halothane anaesthesia. I. Quiet breathing. Anesthesiology 1995;82:6–19.

37. Morton CP, Drummond GB: Change in chest wall dimensions on induction of anaesthesia: A reappraisal. Br J Anaesth 1994;73:135–139.

38. Jones JG, Faithfull D, Jordan C, et al: Rib cage movement during halothane anaesthesia in man. Br J Anaesth 1979;51:399–407.

39. Lumb AB, Petros AJ, Nunn JF: Rib cage contribution to resting and carbon dioxide stimulated ventilation during 1 MAC isoflurane anaesthesia. Br J Anaesth 1991;67:712–721.

40. Mankikian B, Cantineau JP, Sartene R, et al: Ventilatory pattern and chest wall mechanics during ketamine anesthesia in humans. Anesthesiology 1986;65:492–499.

41. Morel DR, Forster A, Gemperle M: Noninvasive evaluation of breathing pattern and thoraco-abdominal motion following the infusion of ketamine or droperidol in humans. Anesthesiology 1986;65:392–398.

42. Hedenstierna G, Strandberg A, Brismar B, et al: Functional residual capacity, thoracoabdominal dimensions, and central blood volume during general anesthesia with muscle paralysis and mechanical ventilation. Anesthesiology 1985;62:247–254.

43. Darquenne C, Paiva M, Prisk GK: Effect of gravity on aerosol dispersion and deposition in the human lung after periods of breath holding. J Appl Physiol 2000;89:1787–1792.

44. Milic-Emili J, Henderson JAM, Dolovich MB, et al: Regional distribution of inspired gas in the lung. J Appl Physiol 1966;21:749–759.

45. West JB: Regional differences in gas exchange in the lung of erect man. J Appl Physiol 1962;17:893–898.

46. Altemeier WA, McKinney S, Glenny RW: Fractal nature of regional ventilation distribution. J Appl Physiol 2000;88:1551–1557.

47. Verbanck S, Linnarsson D, Prisk GK, et al: Specific ventilation distribution in microgravity. J Appl Physiol 1996;80:1458–1465.

48. Tokics L, Hedenstierna G, Svensson L, et al: V/Q distribution and correlation to atelectasis in anesthetized paralyzed humans. J Appl Physiol 1996;81:1822–1833.

49. Landmark SJ, Knopp TJ, Rehder K, et al: Regional pulmonary perfusion and V/Q in awake and anesthetized-paralyzed man. J Appl Physiol 1977;43:993–1000.

50. Permutt S, Bromberger-Barnea B, Bane HN: Alveolar pressure, pulmonary venous pressure and the vascular waterfall. Med Thorac 1962;19:239–260.

51. West JB, Dollery CT, Naimark A: Distribution of blood flow in isolated lung: Relation to vascular and alveolar pressures. J Appl Physiol 1964;19:713–724.

52. Glenny RW, Robertson HT: Fractal modeling of pulmonary blood flow heterogeneity. J Appl Physiol 1991;70:1024–1030.

53. Hakim TS, Dean GW, Lisbona R: Effect of body posture on spatial distribution of pulmonary blood flow. J Appl Physiol 1988;64:1160–1170.

54. Walther SM, Domino KB, Glenny RW, et al: Pulmonary blood flow distribution in sheep: Effects of anesthesia, mechanical ventilation, and change in posture. Anesthesiology 1997;87:335–342.

55. Hedenstierna G: Contribution of multiple inert gas elimination technique to pulmonary medicine. 6. Ventilation-perfusion relationships during anaesthesia. Thorax 1995;50:85–91.

56. McCarthy GS: The effect of thoracic extradural analgesia on pulmonary gas distribution, functional residual capacity and airway closure. Br J Anaesth 1976;48:243–248.

57. Reber A, Bein T, Högman M, et al: Lung aeration and pulmonary gas exchange during lumbar epidural anaesthesia and in the lithotomy position in elderly patients. Anaesthesia 1998;53:854–861.

58. Hedenstierna G, Rothen HU: Atelectasis formation during anesthesia: Causes and measures to prevent it. J Clin Monit Comput 2000;16:329–335.

59. Magnusson L, Spahn DR: New concepts of atelectasis during general anaesthesia. Br J Anaesth 2003;91:61–72.

60. Bendixen HH, Hedley-Whyte J, Laver MB: Impaired oxygenation in surgical patients during general anesthesia with controlled ventilation. N Engl J Med 1963;269:991–996.

61. Hamilton WK, McDonald JS, Fischer HW, et al: Postoperative respiratory complications: A comparison of arterial gas tensions, radiographs and physical examination. Anesthesiology 1964;25:607–612.

62. Pasteur W: Active lobar collapse of the lung after abdominal operations. Lancet 1910;2:1080–1083.

63. Prys-Roberts C, Nunn JF, Dobson RH, et al: Radiologically undetectable pulmonary collapse in the supine position. Lancet 1967;2:399–401.

64. Damgaard-Pedersen K, Qvist T: Pediatric pulmonary CT-scanning: Anaesthesia-induced changes. Pediatr Radiol 1980;9:145–148.

65. Brismar B, Hedenstierna G, Lundquist H, et al: Pulmonary densities during anesthesia with muscular relaxation: A proposal of atelectasis. Anesthesiology 1985;62:422–428.

66. Kisala JM, Ayala A, Stephan RN, et al: A model of pulmonary atelectasis in rats: Activation of alveolar macrophage and cytokine release. Am J Physiol 1993;264:610–614.

67. Froese AB, McCulloch PR, Sugiura M, et al: Optimizing alveolar expansion prolongs the effectiveness of exogenous surfactant therapy in the adult rabbit. Am Rev Respir Dis 1993;148:569–577.

68. Duggan M, McCaul CL, McNamara PJ, et al: Atelectasis causes vascular leak and lethal right ventricular failure in uninjured rat lungs. Am J Respir Crit Care Med 2003;167:1633–1640.

69. Lundquist H, Hedenstierna G, Strandberg Å, et al: CT-assessment of dependent lung densities in man during general anaesthesia. Acta Radiol 1995;36:626–632.

70. Warner DO, Warner MA, Ritman EL: Atelectasis and chest wall shape during halothane anesthesia. Anesthesiology 1996;85:49–59.

71. Tokics L, Strandberg A, Brismar B, et al: Computerized tomography of the chest and gas exchange measurements during ketamine anaesthesia. Acta Anaesthesiol Scand 1987;31:684–692.

72. Eichenberger A, Proietti S, Wicky S, et al: Morbid obesity and postoperative pulmonary atelectasis: An underestimated problem. Anesth Analg 2002;95:1788–1792.

73. Gunnarsson L, Tokics L, Lundquist H, et al: Chronic obstructive pulmonary disease and anaesthesia: Formation of atelectasis and gas exchange impairment. Eur Respir J 1991;4:1106–1116.

74. Rahn H, Farhi LE: Gaseous environment and atelectasis. Fed Proc 1963;22:1035–1041.

75. Joyce CJ, Williams AB: Kinetics of absorption atelectasis during anesthesia: A mathematical model. J Appl Physiol 1999;86:116–1125.

76. Lichtheim L. Archiv für Experimentelle Pathologie and Pharmacologie 1879;10:54–100.

77. Volhard F: Ueber künstliche Atmung durch Ventilation der Trachea und eine einfache Vorrichtung zur rhythmischen künstlichen Atmung. Munch Med Wochenschr 1908;55:219–211.

78. Dantzker DR, Wagner PD, West JB: Instability of lung units with low VA/Q ratios during $O_2$ breathing. J Appl Physiol 1975;38:886–895.

79. Nunn JF, Coleman AJ, Sachithanandan T, et al: Hypoxaemia and atelectasis produced by forced expiration. Br J Anaesth 1965;37:3–12.

80. Rothen HU, Sporre B, Engberg G, et al: Prevention of atelectasis during general anaesthesia. Lancet 1995;345:1387–1391.

81. Rothen HU, Sporre B, Engberg G, et al: Influence of gas composition on recurrence of atelectasis after a reexpansion maneuver during general anesthesia. Anesthesiology 1995;82:832–842.

82. Agostoni E: Mechanics of the pleural space. Physiol Rev 1972;52:57–128.

83. Reber A, Nylund U, Hedenstierna G: Position and shape of the diaphragm: Implications for atelectasis formation. Anaesthesia 1998;53:1054–1061.

84. Hedenstierna G, Tokics L, Lundquist H, et al: Phrenic nerve stimulation during halothane anesthesia: Effects of atelectasis. Anesthesiology 1994;80:751–760.

85. Wollmer P, Schairer W, Bos JA, et al: Pulmonary clearance of 99mTc-DTPA during halothane anaesthesia. Acta Anaesthesiol Scand 1990;34:572–575.

86. Otis DR Jr, Johnson M, Pedley TJ, et al: Role of pulmonary surfactant in airway closure: A computational study. J Appl Physiol 1993;75:1323–1333.

87. Marshall BE, Hanson CW, Frasch F, et al: Role of hypoxic pulmonary vasoconstriction in pulmonary gas exchange and blood flow distribution. 2. Pathophysiology. Intensive Care Med 1994;20:379–389.

88. Moudgil R, Michelakis ED, Archer SL: Hypoxic pulmonary vasoconstriction. J Appl Physiol 2005;98:390–403.

89. van Euler US, Liljestrand G: Observation on the pulmonary arterial blood pressure in the cat. Acta Physiol Scand 1946;12:302–318.

90. Sykes MK, Loh L, Seed RF, et al: The effect of inhalational anaesthetics on hypoxic pulmonary vasoconstriction and pulmonary vascular resistance in the perfused lungs of the dog and cat. Br J Anaesth 1972;44:776–788.

91. Thilenius OG: Effect of anesthesia on response of pulmonary circulation of dogs to acute hypoxia. J Appl Physiol 1966;21:901–904.

92. Marshall BE: Anesthetic influences on the pulmonary circulation. In Hand ST, Sperry RJ (eds): *Anesthesia and the Lung 1989:*

*Developments in Critical Care Medicine and Anaesthesiology.* New York: Springer, 1989, pp 69–77.

93. Anthonisen NR, Danson J, Robertson PC, et al: Airway closure as a function of age. Respir Physiol 1969;70:58–65.

94. Bergman NA, Tien YK: Contribution of the closure of pulmonary units to impaired oxygenation during anesthesia. Anesthesiology 1983;59:395–401.

95. Gilmour I, Burnham M, Craig DB: Closing capacity measurement during general anesthesia. Anesthesiology 1976;45:477–482.

96. Hedenstierna G, McCarthy G, Bergström M: Airway closure during mechanical ventilation. Anesthesiology 1976;44:114–123.

97. Juno J, Marsh HM, Knopp TJ, et al: Closing capacity in awake and anesthetized-paralyzed man. J Appl Physiol 1978;44:238–244.

98. Rothen HU, Sporre B, Engberg G, et al: Airway closure, atelectasis and gas exchange during general anaesthesia. Br J Anaesth 1998;81:681–686.

99. Wagner PD, Sutton JR, Reeves JT, et al: Operation Everest II: Pulmonary gas exchange during a simulated ascent of Mt. Everest. J Appl Physiol 1987;63:2348–2359.

100. Meier J, Kemming GI, Kisch-Wedel H, et al: Hyperoxic ventilation reduces 6-hour mortality at the critical hemoglobin concentration. Anesthesiology 2004;100:70–76.

101. Meier J, Kemming GI, Kisch-Wedel H, et al: Hyperoxic ventilation reduces six-hour mortality after partial fluid resuscitation from hemorrhagic shock. Shock 2004;22:240–247.

102. Reinert M, Barth A, Rothen HU, et al: Effects of cerebral perfusion pressure and increased fraction of inspired oxygen on brain tissue oxygen, lactate and glucose in patients with severe head injury. Acta Neurochir 2003;145:341–349.

103. Wagner PD, Laravuso RB, Uhl RR, et al: Continuous distributions of ventilation-perfusion ratios in normal subjects breathing air and 100 percent $O_2$. J Clin Invest 1974;54:54–68.

104. Benoit Z, Wicky S, Fischer JF, et al: The effect of increased $F_{IO_2}$ before tracheal extubation on postoperative atelectasis. Anesth Analg 2002;95:1777–1781.

105. Loeckinger A, Kleinsasser A, Keller C, et al: Administration of oxygen before tracheal extubation worsens gas exchange after general anesthesia in a pig model. Anesth Analg 2002;95:1772–1776.

106. Clark JM, Lambertsen CJ: Pulmonary oxygen toxicity: A review. Pharmacol Rev 1971;23:37–133.

107. Singer MM, Wright F, Stanley LK, et al: Oxygen toxicity in man: A prospective study in patients after open-heart surgery. N Engl J Med 1970;283:1473–1478.

108. Winter PM, Smith G: The toxicity of oxygen. Anesthesiology 1972;37:210–241.

109. Pagano A, Barazzone-Argiroffo C: Alveolar cell death in hyperoxia-induced lung injury. Ann N Y Acad Sci 2003;1010:405–416.

110. Lum H, Roebuck KA: Oxidant stress and endothelial cell dysfunction. Am J Physiol 2001;280:C719–C741.

111. Chow CW, Herrera Abreu MT, Suzuki T, et al: Oxidative stress and acute lung injury. Am J Respir Cell Mol Biol 2003;29:427–431.

112. Mantell LL, Lee PJ: Signal transduction pathways in hyperoxia-induced lung cell death. Mol Genet Metab 2000;71:359–370.

113. Knight PR, Kurek C, Davidson BA, et al: Acid aspiration increases sensitivity to increased ambient oxygen concentrations. Am J Physiol 2000;278:1240–1247.

114. Tateda K, Deng JC, Moore TA, et al: Hyperoxia mediates acute lung injury and increased lethality in murine *Legionella* pneumonia: The role of apoptosis. J Immunol 2003;170:4209–4216.

115. Berend N: Protective effect of hypoxia on bleomycin lung toxicity in the rat. Am Rev Respir Dis 1984;130:307–308.

116. Reber A, Engberg G, Wegenius G, et al: Lung aeration: The effect of pre-oxygenation and hyperoxygenation during total intravenous anaesthesia. Anesthesia 1996;51:733–737.

117. Benumof JL: Preoxygenation: Best method for both efficacy and efficiency. Anesthesiology 1999;91:603–605.

118. Edmark L, Kostova-Aherdan K, Enlund M, et al: Optimal oxygen concentration during induction of general anesthesia. Anesthesiology 2003;98:28–33.

119. Magnusson L, Zemgulis V, Tenling A, et al: Use of a vital capacity maneuver to prevent atelectasis after cardiopulmonary bypass: An experimental study. Anesthesiology 1998;88:134–142.

120. Akca O, Podolsky A, Eisenhuber E, et al: Comparable postoperative pulmonary atelectasis in patients given 30% or 80% oxygen during and 2 hours after colon resection. Anesthesiology 1999;91:991–998.

121. Murphy GS, Szokol JW, Curran RD, et al: Influence of a vital capacity maneuver on pulmonary gas exchange after cardiopulmonary bypass. J Cardiothorac Vasc Anesth 2001;15:336–340.

122. Rothen HU, Neumann P, Berglund JE, et al: Dynamics of re-expansion of atelectasis during general anaesthesia. Br J Anaesth 1999;82:551–556.

123. Hantos Z, Tolnai J, Asztalos T, et al: Acoustic evidence of airway opening during recruitment in excised dog lungs. J Appl Physiol 2004;97:592–598.

124. Markstaller K, Eberle B, Kauczor HU, et al: Temporal dynamics of lung aeration determined by dynamic CT in a porcine model of ARDS. Br J Anaesth 2001;87:459–468.

125. Naureckas ET, Dawson CA, Gerber BS, et al: Airway reopening pressure in isolated rat lungs. J Appl Physiol 1994;76:1372–1377.

126. Tiddens HA, Hofhuis W, Bogaard JM, et al: Compliance, hysteresis, and collapsibility of human small airways. Am J Respir Crit Care Med 1999;160:1110–1118.

127. Tusman G, Böhm SH, Vazquez de Anda GF, et al: Alveolar recruitment strategy improves arterial oxygenation during general anaesthesia. Br J Anaesth 1999;82:8–13.

128. Shambauch GE, Harrison WG, Farrell JI: Treatment of the respiratory paralysis of poliomyelitis in a respiratory chamber. JAMA 1930;94:1371–1373.

129. Tweed WA, Phua WT, Chong KY, et al: Tidal volume, lung hyperinflation and arterial oxygenation during general anesthesia. Anaesth Intensive Care 1993;21:806–810.

130. Kulkarni PR, Lumb AB, Platt MW, et al: Estimation of tidal volume from the reservoir bag: A laboratory study. Anaesthesia 1992;47:936–938.

131. Tenling A, Hachenberg T, Tydén H, et al: Atelectasis and gas exchange after cardiac surgery. Anesthesiology 1998;89:371–378.

132. Tusman G, Böhm SH, Tempra A, et al: Effects of recruitment maneuver on atelectasis in anesthetized children. Anesthesiology 2003;98:14–22.

133. Lapinsky SE, Aubin M, Metha S, et al: Safety and efficacy of a sustained inflation for alveolar recruitment in adults with respiratory failure. Intensive Care Med 1999;25:1297–1301.

134. Pelosi P, Cardingher P, Bottino N, et al: Sigh in acute respiratory distress syndrome. Am J Respir Crit Care Med 1999;159:872–880.

135. Rothen HU, Sporre B, Engberg G, et al: Reexpansion of atelectasis during general anaesthesia may have a prolonged effect. Acta Anaesthesiol Scand 1995;39:118–125.

136. Tusman G, Böhm SH, Suarez-Sipmann F, et al: Alveolar recruitment improves ventilatory efficiency of the lungs during anesthesia. Can J Anaesth 2004;51:723–727.

137. Nicholas TE, Power JH, Barr HA: The pulmonary consequences of a deep breath. Respir Physiol 1982;49:315–324.

138. van Kaam AH, Lachmann RA, Herting E, et al: Reducing atelectasis attenuates bacterial growth and translocation in experimental pneumonia. Am J Respir Crit Care Med 2004;169:1046–1053.

139. Jellema WT, Groeneveld AB, van Goudoever J, et al: Hemodynamic effects of intermittent manual lung hyperinflation in patients with septic shock. Heart Lung 2000;29:356–366.

140. Bein T, Kuhr L P, Bele S, et al: Lung recruitment maneuver in patients with cerebral injury: Effects on intracranial pressure and cerebral metabolism. Intensive Care Med 2002;28:554–558.

141. Nunes S, Rothen HU, Brander L, et al: Changes in splanchnic circulation during an alveolar recruitment maneuver in healthy porcine lungs. Anesth Analg 2004;98:1432–1438.

142. Oczenski W, Schwarz S, Fitzgerald RD: Vital capacity manoeuvre in general anaesthesia: Useful or useless? Eur J Anaesthesiol 2004;21:253–259.

143. Tokics L, Hedenstierna G, Strandberg Å, et al: Lung collapse and gas exchange during general anesthesia: Effects of spontaneous breathing, muscle paralysis, and positive end-expiratory pressure. Anesthesiology 1987;66:157–167.

144. Dyhr T, Laursen N, Larsson A: Effects of lung recruitment maneuver and positive end-expiratory pressure on lung volume, respiratory mechanics and alveolar gas mixing in patients ventilated after cardiac surgery. Acta Anaesthesiol Scand 2002;46:717–725.

145. Dyhr T, Nygards E, Laursen N, et al: Both lung recruitment maneuver and PEEP are needed to increase oxygenation and lung volume after cardiac surgery. Acta Anaesthesiol Scand 2004;48:187–197.

146. Neumann P, Rothen HU, Berglund JE, et al: Positive end-expiratory pressure prevents atelectasis during general anaesthesia even in the presence of a high inspired oxygen concentration. Acta Anaesthiol Scand 1999;43:295–301.

147. Lachmann B: Open up the lung and keep the lung open. Intensive Care Med 1992;18:319–321.

148. Herriger A, Frascarolo P, Spahn DR, et al: The effect of positive airway pressure during pre-oxygenation and induction of anaesthesia upon duration of non-hypoxic apnoea. Anaesthesia 2004;59:243–247.

149. Rusca M, Proietti S, Schnyder P, et al: Prevention of atelectasis formation during induction of general anesthesia. Anesth Analg 2003;97:1835–1839.

150. Kehlet H: Multimodal approach to control postoperative pathophysiology and rehabilitation. Br J Anaesth 1997;78:606–617.

151. Berg H, Roed J, Viby-Mogensen J, et al: Residual neuromuscular block is a risk factor for postoperative pulmonary complications: A prospective, randomised, and blinded study of postoperative pulmonary complications after atracurium, vecuronium and pancuronium. Acta Anaesthesiol Scand 1997;4:1095–1103.

152. Ballantyne JC, Carr DB, deFerranti S, et al: The comparative effects of postoperative analgesic therapies on pulmonary outcome: Cumulative meta-analyses of randomized, controlled trials. Anesth Analg 1998;86:598–612.

153. Rodgers A, Walker N, Schug S, et al: Reduction of postoperative mortality and morbidity with epidural or spinal anaesthesia: Results from overview of randomised trials. BMJ 2000;321:1493.

154. Walder B, Schafer M, Henzi I, et al: Efficacy and safety of patient-controlled opioid analgesia for acute postoperative pain: A quantitative systematic review. Acta Anaesthesiol Scand 2001;45:795–804.

155. Nielsen KG, Holte K, Kehlet H: Effects of posture on postoperative pulmonary function. Acta Anaesthesiol Scand 2003;47:1270–1275.

156. Otteni JC, Beydon L, Cazalaà JB, et al: Anesthesia ventilators. Ann Fr Anesth Reanim 1997;16:895–907.

157. Otteni JC, Ancellin J, Cazalaà JB, et al: Ventilators for anesthesia: Models available in France. Criteria for choice. Ann Fr Anesth Reanim 1995;14:13–28.

158. Jaber S, Langlais N, Fumagalli B, et al: Laboratory bench testing of six new anaesthesia ventilators. Ann Fr Anesth Reanim 2000;19:16–22.

159. Klemenzson GK, Perouansky M: Contemporary anesthesia ventilators incur a significant "oxygen cost." Can J Anaesth 2004;51:616–620.

160. Stayer SA, Bent ST, Skjonsby BS, et al: Pressure control ventilation: Three anesthesia ventilators compared using an infant lung model. Anesth Analg 2000;91:1145–1150.

161. Rathgeber J, Schorn B, Falk V, et al: The influence of controlled mandatory ventilation (CMV), intermittent mandatory ventilation (IMV) and biphasic intermittent positive airway pressure (BIPAP) on duration of intubation and consumption of analgesics and sedatives: A prospective analysis in 596 patients following adult cardiac surgery. Eur J Anaesthesiol 1997;14:576–582.

162. Iwama H: Application of nasal bi-level positive airway pressure to respiratory support during combined epidural-propofol anesthesia. J Clin Anesth 2002;14:24–33.

163. Bratzke E, Downs JB, Smith RA: Intermittent CPAP: A new mode of ventilation during general anesthesia. Anesthesiology 1998;89:334–340.

164. Verghese C, Brimacombe JR: Survey of laryngeal mask airway usage in 11,910 patients: Safety and efficacy for conventional and nonconventional usage. Anesth Analg 1996;82:129–133.

165. Keller C, Sparr HJ, Luber TJ, et al: Patient outcomes with positive pressure versus spontaneous ventilation in non-paralysed adults with the laryngeal mask. Can J Anaesth 1998;45:564–567.

166. Brimacombe J, Keller C, Hormann C: Pressure support ventilation versus continuous positive airway pressure with the laryngeal mask airway: A randomized crossover study of anesthetized adult patients. Anesthesiology 2000;92:1621–1623.

167. Boker A, Haberman CJ, Girling L, et al: Variable ventilation improves perioperative lung function in patients undergoing abdominal aortic aneurysmectomy. Anesthesiology 2004;100:608–616.

168. Sinderby C, Navalesi P, Beck J, et al: Neural control of mechanical ventilation in respiratory failure. Nat Med 1999;5:1433–1436.

169. Brooks-Brunn JA: Predictors of postoperative pulmonary complications following abdominal surgery. Chest 1997;111:564–571.

170. Vaughan RW, Wise L: Intraoperative arterial oxygenation in obese patients. Ann Surg 1976;184:35–42.

171. Pelosi P, Croci M, Ravagnan I, et al: The effects of body mass on lung volumes, respiratory mechanics, and gas exchange during general anesthesia. Anesth Analg 1998;87:654–660.

172. Strandberg A, Tokics L, Brismar B, et al: Constitutional factors promoting development of atelectasis during anaesthesia. Acta Anaesthesiol Scand 1987;31:21–24.

173. Berthoud MC, Peacock JE, Reilly CS: Effectiveness of preoxygenation in morbidly obese patients. Br J Anaesth 1991;67:464–466.

174. Coussa M, Proietti S, Schnyder P, et al: Prevention of atelectasis formation during the induction of general anesthesia in morbidly obese patients. Anesth Analg 2004;98:1491–1495.

175. Cressey DM, Berthoud MC, Reilly CS: Effectiveness of continuous positive airway pressure to enhance pre-oxygenation in morbidly obese women. Anaesthesia 2001;56:680–684.

176. Pelosi P, Ravagnan I, Giurati G, et al: Positive end-expiratory pressure improves respiratory function in obese but not in normal subjects during anesthesia and paralysis. Anesthesiology 1999;91:1221–1231.

177. Yoshino J, Akata T, Takahashi S: Intraoperative changes in arterial oxygenation during volume-controlled mechanical ventilation in modestly obese patients undergoing laparotomies with general anesthesia. Acta Anaesthesiol Scand 2003;47:742–750.

178. Mynster T, Jensen LM, Jensen FG, et al: The effect of posture on late postoperative oxygenation. Anaesthesia 1996;51:225–227.

179. Vaughan RW, Bauer S, Wise L: Effect of position (semirecumbent versus supine) on postoperative oxygenation in markedly obese subjects. Anesth Analg 1976;55:37–41.

180. Young T, Peppard PE, Gottlieb DJ: Epidemiology of obstructive sleep apnea: A population health perspective. Am J Respir Crit Care Med 2002;165:1217–1239.

181. Kenchaiah S, Evans JC, Levy D, et al: Obesity and the risk of heart failure. N Engl J Med 2002;347:305–313.

182. van den Berghe G, Wouters P, Weekers F, et al: Intensive insulin therapy in the critically ill patients. N Engl J Med 2001;345:1359–1367.

183. Kabon B, Nagele A, Reddy D, et al: Obesity decreases perioperative tissue oxygenation. Anesthesiology 2004;100:274–280.

184. McMahon AJ, Fischbacher CM, Frame SH, et al: Impact of laparoscopic cholecystectomy: A population-based study. Lancet 2000;356:1632–1637.

185. Sharma KC, Brandstetter RD, Brensilver JM, et al: Cardiopulmonary physiology and pathophysiology as a consequence of laparoscopic surgery. Chest 1996;110:810–815.

186. Wahba RW, Béïque F, Kleiman SJ: Cardiopulmonary function and laparoscopic cholecystectomy. Can J Anaesth 1995;42:51–63.

187. Wittgen CM, Andrus CH, Fitzgerald SD, et al: Analysis of the hemodynamic and ventilatory effects of laparoscopic cholecystectomy. Arch Surg 1991;126:997–1000.

188. Kendall AP, Bhatt S, Oh TE: Pulmonary consequences of carbon dioxide insufflation for laparoscopic cholecystectomies. Anaesthesia 1995;50:286–289.

189. Mäkinen MT, Yli-Hankala A: Respiratory compliance during laparoscopic hiatal and inguinal hernia repair. Can J Anaesth 1998;45:865–870.

190. Sprung J, Whalley DG, Falcone T, et al: The impact of morbid obesity, pneumoperitoneum, and posture on respiratory system mechanics and oxygenation during laparoscopy. Anesth Analg 2002;94:1345–1350.

191. Hirvonen EA, Nuutinen LS, Kauko M: Ventilatory effects, blood gas changes, and oxygen consumption during laparoscopic hysterectomy. Anesth Analg 1995;80:961–966.

192. Mullett CE, Viale JP, Sagnard PE, et al: Pulmonary $CO_2$ elimination during surgical procedures using intra- or extraperitoneal $CO_2$ insufflation. Anesth Analg 1993;76:622–626.

193. Leighton TA, Liu SY, Bongard FS: Comparative cardiopulmonary effects of carbon dioxide versus helium pneumoperitoneum. Surgery 1993;113:527–531.

194. Andersson L, Lagerstrand L, Thorne A, et al: Effect of $CO_2$ pneumoperitoneum on ventilation-perfusion relationships during laparoscopic cholecystectomy. Acta Anaesthesiol Scand 2002;46:552–560.

195. Bures E, Fusciardi J, Lanquetot H, et al: Ventilatory effects of laparoscopic cholecystectomy. Acta Anaesthesiol Scand 1996;40:566–573.

196. Lindgren L, Koivusalo AM, Kellokumpu I: Conventional pneumoperitoneum compared with abdominal wall lift for laparoscopic cholecystectomy. Br J Anaesth 1995;75:567–572.

197. Tusman G, Böhm SH, Melkun F, et al: Alveolar recruitment strategy increases arterial oxygenation during one-lung ventilation. Ann Thorac Surg 2002;73:1204–1209.

198. Campos JH: Current techniques for perioperative lung isolation in adults. Anesthesiology 2002;97:1295–1301.

199. Pagel PS, Fu JL, Damask MC, et al: Desflurane and isoflurane produce similar alterations in systemic and pulmonary hemodynamics and arterial oxygenation in patients undergoing one-lung ventilation during thoracotomy. Anesth Analg 1998;87:800–807.

200. Schwarzkopf K, Schreiber T, Bauer R, et al: The effects of increasing concentrations of isoflurane and desflurane on pulmonary perfusion and systemic oxygenation during one-lung ventilation in pigs. Anesth Analg 2001;93:1434–1438.

201. Schwarzkopf K, Klein U, Schreiber T, et al: Oxygenation during one-lung ventilation: The effects of inhaled nitric oxide and increasing levels of inspired fraction of oxygen. Anesth Analg 2001;92:842–847.

202. Friedlander M, Sandler A, Kavanagh B, et al: Is hypoxic pulmonary vasoconstriction important during single lung ventilation in the lateral decubitus position? Can J Anaesth 1994;41:26–30.

203. Capan LM, Turndorf H, Patel C, et al: Optimization of arterial oxygenation during one-lung anesthesia. Anesth Analg 1980;59:847–851.

204. Hedenstierna G, Santesson J, Bindslev L: Regional differences in lung function during anaesthesia and intensive care: Clinical implications. Acta Anaesthesiol Scand 1982;26: 429–434.

205. Valenza F: Mechanical ventilation during thoracic anesthesia. Minerva Anestesiol 1999;65:263–266.

206. Kroenke L, Lawrence VA, Theroux JF, et al: Operative risk in patients with severe obstructive pulmonary disease. Arch Intern Med 1992;152:967–791.

207. Moller AM, Villebro N, Pedersen T, et al: Effect of preoperative smoking intervention on postoperative complications: A randomised clinical trial. Lancet 2002;359: 114–117.

## SUGGESTED READINGS

Celebi S, Koner O, Menda F, et al: The pulmonary and hemodynamic effects of two different recruitment maneuvers after cardiac surgery. Anesth Analg 2007;104:384–90.

Claesson J, Lehtipalo S, Bergstrand U, et al: Negative mesenteric effects of lung recruitment maneuvers in oleic acid lung injury are transient and short lasting. Crit Care Med 2007;35:230–8.

Duggan M, Kavanagh BP: Pulmonary atelectasis: a pathogenic perioperative entity. Anesthesiology 2005;102:838–54.

Miranda DR, Gommers D, Papadakos PJ, et al: Mechanical ventilation affects pulmonary inflammation in cardiac surgery patients: the role of the open-lung concept. J Cardiothorac Vasc Anesth 2007;21:279–84.

Mutch WA, Harms S, Ruth Graham M, et al: Biologically variable or naturally noisy mechanical ventilation recruits atelectatic lung. Am J Respir Crit Care Med 2000; 162:319–323.

Pasquina P, Tramer MR, Granier JM, et al: Respiratory physiotherapy to prevent pulmonary complications after abdominal surgery: a systematic review. Chest 2006; 130:1887–99.

Rehder K, Sessler AD, Rodarte JR: Regional intrapulmonary gas distribution in awake and anesthetized-paralyzed man. J Appl Physiol 1977;42:391–402.

Squadrone V, Coha M, Cerutti E, et al. Continuous Positive Airway Pressure for treatment of Postoperative Hypoxaemia: A Randomized Controlled Trial. JAMA 2005;293:589–595.

Tenling A, Joachimsson PO, Tyden H, et al: Thoracic epidural anesthesia as an adjunct to general anesthesia for cardiac surgery: Effects on ventilation-perfusion relationships. J Cardiothorac Vasc Anesth 1999;13:258–264.

Tsuchida S, Engelberts D, Peltekova V, et al: Atelectasis causes alveolar injury in nonatelectatic lung regions. Am J Respir Crit Care Med 2006; 174:279–89.

Von Ungern-Sternberg BS, Regli A, Schneider MC, et al: Effect of obesity and site of surgery on perioperative lung volumes. Br J Anaesth 2004;92:202–207.

# CHAPTER 30

# Independent Lung Ventilation and Bronchopleural Fistula

Sanjeev V. Chhangani

Independent lung ventilation (ILV) is the cornerstone of thoracic anesthesia. Since its introduction in thoracic surgery in 1931, the application of ILV has expanded within the field of thoracic anesthesia and surgery to include critical care medicine.

In 1931, Gale and Waters[1] first described ILV using a single-lumen endobronchial tube placed in the main bronchus. This allowed selective ventilation of the unaffected lung and prevented contralateral drainage of purulent secretion from the affected lung. Since the 1930s, the ability to provide lung isolation and ILV evolved from a single-lumen tube (SLT) and bronchial blocker (BB) to double-lumen tubes (DLTs). The greatest limitation of SLT and BB use was the ability to ventilate only the unaffected lung. In 1949, Carlens introduced a double-lumen catheter that allowed ILV of both lungs. This advance was a landmark in the evolution of thoracic anesthesia. Since that time, coupled with the use of fiberoptic bronchoscope, double-lumen endobronchial tubes (DLTs) have undergone significant refinements in design and shape to reduce airway mucosal injury, to allow safe placement in either the right or left main bronchus, and to provide effective ILV.

For many years, DLTs and ILV were used in the perioperative period for thoracic anesthesia and surgery, to allow deflation of one lung for surgical access and to protect the dependent lung from potentially fatal purulent or malignant secretions or blood from the nondependent lung. In 1976, Glass and colleagues[2] first reported the use of ILV in a critical care setting. Since that time, the application of ILV has broadened to a wide range of perioperative and critical care conditions and ventilation techniques.

## INDICATIONS AND RATIONALE

Indications for ILV have expanded from traditional isolation of the healthy lung from pus, blood, or air to include various surgical (pulmonary and nonpulmonary) and nonsurgical (critical care) conditions (Table 30.1). In the surgical setting, ILV offers distinct advantages to both anesthesiologists and surgeons. Using this technique, the anesthesiologist maintains full control of anesthetic concentration and gas exchange in a single lung. The untoward effects of the pneumothorax problem invariably associated with intrapulmonary procedures can be managed with positive pressure ventilation. For the surgeon, this technique provides better exposure and exploration of the operative field with minimal trauma to the ipsilateral lung. In the critical care setting, ILV is a therapeutic option whenever there is a large discrepancy between the optimal gas exchange and lung mechanics of the two lungs, such as in patients with predominantly unilateral or asymmetric bilateral lung disease. In one institution familiar with ILV, it was used in approximately 0.5% of all mechanically

**Table 30-1   Indications for Independent Lung Ventilation**

| Thoracic Anesthesia and Surgery | Anatomic Indications | Physiologic Indications |
|---|---|---|
| **Video-Assisted Thoracoscopy**<br>Diagnostic<br>　Lung and pleural biopsy<br>　Mediastinal masses<br>　Pericardial biopsy and effusion<br>Therapeutic<br>　Decortication, pleurodesis<br>　Drainage of pleural effusions<br>　Lobectomy and wedge resection<br>　Lung volume reduction<br>　Sympathectomy<br>　Chylothorax<br>　Patent ductus arteriosus ligation<br>　Transmyocardial laser<br>　　revascularization<br>　Pericardial stripping | Massive hemoptysis<br>Whole lung lavage<br>　Pulmonary alveolar proteinosis<br>　Asthma<br>　Cystic fibrosis<br>　Chronic bronchitis<br>　Dust inhalation<br>　Radioactive dust<br>　Silica<br>Secretions<br>　Purulent<br>　Malignant | Unilateral lung injury<br>　Aspiration<br>　Lung contusion<br>　Pneumonia<br>　Unilateral lung edema<br>　Unilateral atelectasis<br>　Unilateral bronchospasm<br>Bronchopleural fistula<br>Single-lung<br>Bilateral symmetric lung<br>　disease (failing<br>　conventional ventilation)<br>Acute respiratory distress<br>　syndrome<br>　Bilateral aspiration |
| **Relative Indications**<br>Lobectomy (right upper lobe)<br>Pneumonectomy<br>Thoracic aortic aneurysm repair<br>Esophagectomy<br>Anterior thoracic spine surgery | | |

ventilated patients. Although infrequently required in the critical care setting, ILV can be potentially lifesaving.

## PHYSIOLOGIC CONSIDERATIONS

Physiologic considerations for ILV include those for thoracic anesthesia and surgery as well as those relevant to critical care.

### Thoracic Anesthesia and Surgery

In thoracic anesthesia, one-lung ventilation (OLV) is used, so only a single (nonoperative) lung is ventilated. The primary effects of OLV are to reduce the surface area over which respiratory gas exchange may take place and to create an obligatory right-to-left intrapulmonary shunt (35% to 50%). In most thoracic operations, the nondependent, nonventilated lung is collapsed while the patient is in the lateral decubitus position. Keeping the overall ventilation constant when changing to OLV naturally increases the portion of the peak airway pressure resulting from compliance, with the amount depending on the particular pressure-volume curve. However, there is more than sufficient volume capacity for a single lung to receive the total tidal volume ($V_T$) used during

anesthesia. As stated previously, the obligatory intrapulmonary shunt associated with OLV increases the alveolar-arterial oxygen ($A$-$aO_2$) gradient, and despite hypoxic pulmonary vasoconstriction, the development of life-threatening hypoxemia (oxygen saturation as measured using pulse oximetry [$SpO_2$] <90%) during OLV is a real possibility. The distribution of pulmonary blood flow and the pressure differential between two lungs and the lung volume represent important factors affecting oxygenation during thoracic anesthesia and surgery. Strategies to reduce intrapulmonary shunt and thereby to maintain adequate arterial oxygen tension during OLV in thoracic anesthesia and surgery include titrating inspired oxygen concentration ($FiO_2$) to maintain an $SpO_2$ greater than 90%, application of nondependent lung continuous positive airway pressure (CPAP) using 100% oxygen, and using lung protective ventilation with positive end-expiratory pressure (PEEP) to the dependent (ventilated) lung.

### Critical Care

More often than not, ILV in critical care is utilized to achieve physiologic lung separation whereby each lung is ventilated as an independent unit after one side is isolated from the other. The rationale for ILV in this setting is based on the premise that different ventilator strategies can be used on each side because of asymmetric lung disease with different airway resistance and lung compliance. Respiratory failure in patients with severe asymmetric or unilateral lung disease may not respond to the conventional modes of ventilator support, which apply their volume and pressure characteristics indiscriminately to all lung regions. In this case, $V_T$ is mostly distributed to the normal or less diseased lung, possibly resulting in overinflation and parenchymal lung injury owing to volutrauma and barotrauma. At the same time, PEEP is transmitted to alveolar capillaries and acts as a Starling resistor, resulting in reduced perfusion of the normal or less diseased lung and diversion of a share of pulmonary perfusion to the diseased lung. The net effects of PEEP in asymmetric or unilateral lung disease are increases in ventilation-perfusion (V/Q) mismatching and in intrapulmonary shunt, thereby worsening gas exchange. Under such circumstances, ILV has been utilized to improve V/Q matching of each lung. Therefore, a proposed indication for ILV is the demonstration of a paradoxical PEEP effect: a fall in arterial oxygen tension ($PaO_2$) and an increase in shunt resulting from redistribution of pulmonary blood flow associated with increasing two-lung PEEP. The decision to institute ILV in critical care in the management of hypoxemia refractory to conventional modes of ventilation must be carefully weighed against the skills of the intensive care specialist in establishing lung isolation as well as the ability of the patient to tolerate the procedure.

# DEVICES AND TECHNIQUES OF LUNG ISOLATION

Effective lung isolation is central to the conduct of ILV. Currently, there are many intubation devices for ILV. These include DLTs, BBs, and SLTs advanced into the desired main bronchus. Although there are several devices for isolating a lung, the most common is the DLT, which allows independent ventilation (or lack of) to each lung. The advantages and limitations of different lung isolation devices are listed in Table 30.2.

## Endobronchial Intubation

Endobronchial intubation using a DLT represents the most common and definitive method of providing lung isolation for ILV. The modern DLT has evolved from the rubber Carlens tube with a carinal hook to the present Robertshaw design. Disposable left DLTs with carinal hooks are available but are not in widespread use because most practitioners position their tubes with bronchoscopy and prefer the Robertshaw design. The current choices of DLT are the polyvinyl chloride (PVC)

type, such as those made by Mallinckrodt (Broncho-Cath EB tube, Nellcor, Pleasanton, CA), Sheridan (Sheridan, Argyle, NY), and Rusch (Duluth, GA) and the silicone type (Silbroncho, Vitaid, Williamsville, NY). The left-sided Broncho-Cath, manufactured by Mallinckrodt, is the most popular DLT in the United States. Current disposable DLTs are latex free and have high-volume, low-pressure tracheal and bronchial cuffs and radiopaque marking. By convention, the bronchial cuff is blue, to permit easy identification by fiberoptic bronchoscopy. The current DLTs have a far lower resistance to airflow than the older versions. The resistances of these newer DLTs for the spontaneously breathing patient compare favorably with those of commonly used sizes of SLTs.

## Double-Lumen Tube Sizes

The DLTs used in current practice are clear, disposable PVC devices of Robertshaw design, available as right- and left-sided tubes in French sizes (related to the external circumference of the tube; 1 Fr = 1/3 mm). Adult DLTs commonly come in sizes 35, 37, 39, and 41 Fr. Some manufacturers also provide sizes 26, 28, 32 (Rusch), and 33 Fr (Silbroncho, Vitaid). Left-sided DLTs are most commonly used because of the greater margin of safety in positioning them in the left main bronchus (left main bronchus, 5 cm, versus right main bronchus, 2.5 cm). An appropriately sized DLT for an individual patient fits through the glottic opening, the trachea, and the mainstem bronchus with only a small air leak when the cuff is deflated and provides a good seal with the bronchus when the cuff is inflated in the range of its resting volume. The resting bronchial cuff volume is defined as the smallest cuff volume beyond which a 0.5-mL increase results in an increase in cuff pressure greater than 10 mm Hg. This bronchial cuff volume varies slightly with the tube size and manufacturer, but it is in the range of 1 to 3 mL for most commonly used adult DLTs.

Various parameters (height, weight, and gender) were studied to predict the correct size of a DLT for an individual patient, but the prediction was imprecise. One method of choosing DLT size is based on the size of the tracheal diameter as determined from the chest radiograph or computed tomography (CT) scan. A left bronchial-to-tracheal width ratio of 0.75 for men and 0.77 for women using chest CT has been reported. The goal is to select a DLT with a bronchial end that is 1 to 2 mm smaller in its outer diameter than the diameter of the intubated bronchus, to allow for the size of the deflated cuff. A simple and useful technique recommended by Slinger is based on the patient's height, as follows: male patients taller than 5'7", 41 Fr, male patients shorter than 5'7", 39 Fr, and male patients shorter than 5'4", 37 Fr or less; female patients taller

**Table 30-2    Devices for Lung Isolation**

| | Advantages | Limitations |
|---|---|---|
| **Double-Lumen Endobronchial Tube (DLT)** <br> Sizes: <br> Left: 26, 28, 32, 33, 35, 37, 39, 41 French <br> Pediatric: <40 kKg: 28 French (L) <br> >40 Kg: 35 French (L) <br> Right: 35, 37, 39, 41 French | Ease of selective lung treatment (e.g., suction, CPAP, PEEP) <br> Ease of rapid conversion from two-lung to one-lung ventilation and vice versa | Contraindicated in the presence of distorted tracheobronchial tree along the path of insertion <br> Requires changing of single-lumen tube for postoperative care in intensive care unit |
| **Bronchial Blockers** <br> Univent Tube <br>   Adult (6.0–9.0 mm) <br>   Pediatric sizes (3.5 mm, 4.5 mm) <br> Uniblocker is only available in one size (9 French) for use with an ETT ≥8.0 mm <br> Wire-guided bronchial blocker (Arndt) for use with an ETT ≥8.0 mm <br>   Spherical balloon (5, 7, 9 French) <br>   Elliptic balloon (9 French) | Ease of insertion, especially with difficult intubation <br> No need to change tubes at the end of surgery <br> Can apply CPAP and HFJV to bronchial blocker <br> Can be used selectively to block an individual lobe or segment | Slow deflation times with narrow bronchial blocker lumen <br> High-pressure, smooth surface bronchial blocker cuff may become dislodged easily <br> Inability to suction the operative lung effectively, increasing risk for spillover to other side <br> Inability to apply conventional mechanical ventilation |
| **Endobronchial Intubation with Single-Lumen Tube** <br> Small size: 6 or 7 mm internal diameter | Rapidity and ease of insertion and positioning | Inability to apply selective treatment to diseased lung (e.g., CPAP or suction) <br> Less secure <br> Hypoxemia may be a problem with right lung intubation |

CPAP, continuous positive airway pressure; ETT, endotracheal tube; HFJV, high-frequency jet ventilation; PEEP, positive end-expiratory pressure.

than 5′4″, 37 Fr, female patients shorter than 5′4″, 35 Fr, and female patients shorter than 5′0″, 32 Fr. It is important to identify a DLT that is too large (unable to fit bronchial lumen into the mainstem bronchus or forms an airtight seal with cuff deflated) or too small (requires >3 mL of air in the bronchial cuff to create a seal) for an individual patient.

## Placement and Positioning of Double-Lumen Tubes

As with the tube size, there is no consensus among anesthesiologists on the optimal method to place a DLT. One prospective, randomized study compared the success rates of lung isolation devices among anesthesiologists with limited experience in thoracic anesthesia. Up to 40% of the participants failed to place the lung isolation device successfully. The most critical factor in successful placement was the anesthesiologist's knowledge of endoscopic bronchial anatomy. *A DLT should not be positioned or utilized unless a suitable fiberoptic bronchoscope is available.* Our method of placement and positioning of DLT, as described later, emphasizes the importance of recognizing airway anatomy using a fiberoptic bronchoscope and eliminates variability described in the literature. Figure 30.1 shows positioning

of the right- and left-sided DLT along with illustrations of the corresponding fiberoptic endoscopic bronchial anatomy.

After ensuring adequate oxygenation, anesthesia, and relaxation, the following sequence is used for placement of a DLT:

1. A Macintosh blade may be preferred for laryngoscopy, because it provides more room for manipulation of the tube within the pharynx.
2. The tube is placed into the pharynx with the concavity of the distal tip facing anteriorly.
3. Once the distal tip is through the vocal cords, the stylet is removed, and the tube is gently rotated 90 degrees so that the bronchial lumen and distal concavity are facing the side to be intubated. Keeping the laryngoscope in place during this maneuver will assist in passing the tube.
4. The tube is then gently advanced until the tracheal cuff is well below the vocal cords. The tracheal cuff is inflated and tracheal placement confirmed by the presence of breath sounds and end-tidal carbon dioxide ($ETCO_2$) by auscultation and capnography, respectively.

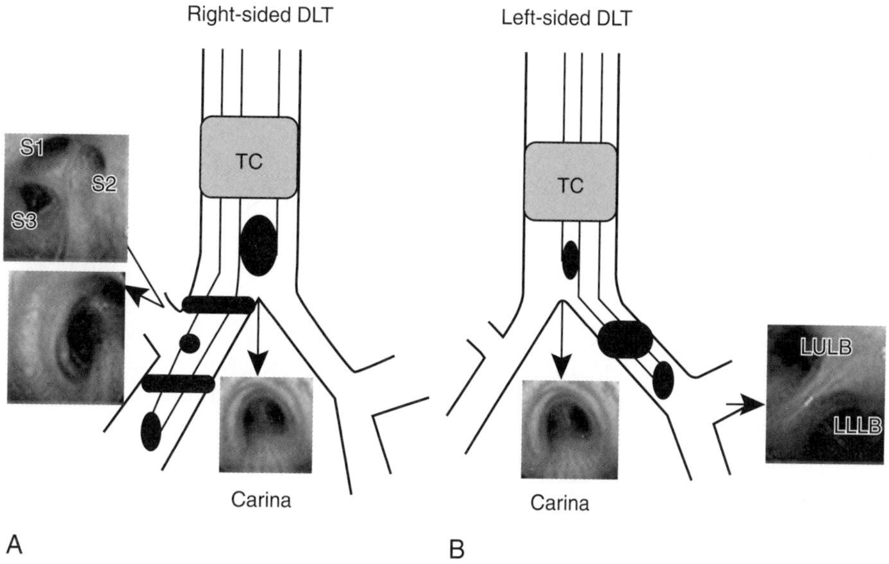

**Figure 30.1** Schematic drawings of right-sided (*A*) and left-sided (*B*) double-lumen tube positioning using fiberoptic bronchoscopy. The corresponding airway anatomy is illustrated. The right upper lobe opening and its classic trifurcation (S1, S2, S3) are seen. The bronchial cuff is blue. LLLB, left lower lobe bronchus; LULB, left upper lobe bronchus; TC, tracheal cuff.

5. Fiberoptic bronchoscopy is performed through the bronchial lumen first, with the anteroposterior orientation of the airway anatomy confirmed by identifying tracheal rings anteriorly and membranous portion posteriorly, and the carina is visualized.

6. The bronchial lumen is then passed into the desired bronchus under vision utilizing fiberoptic bronchoscopy. Before advancing the tube, the tracheal cuff must be deflated to prevent mucosal injury.

7. The depth of the bronchial lumen is controlled with the fiberoptic bronchoscope to place the tip of the left-sided tube above the left mainstem bifurcation and to position the side hole on the bronchial lumen of the right-sided tube at the level of the right upper lobe orifice. Because of the tendency for carinal shift and upward DLT movement with lateral positioning, it is recommended to keep the bronchial cuff at least 1 cm inside the mainstem bronchus before turning the patient laterally. The tracheal and bronchial cuffs are inflated with recommended volumes of air. A "Just-seal" technique has been described using an air bubble method (end point: no air bubbles when non-ventilated outer end is immersed under water) or capnography (end point: no $ETCO_2$ movement when nonventilated outer end is connected to capnograph tubing) to prevent overinflation or underinflation of the bronchial cuff.

8. Final placement is confirmed by looking through the tracheal lumen.

9. A fiberoptic bronchoscope must be immediately available during the entire period of intubation with a DLT.

### Methods of Tube Placement Confirmation

After tube placement, accurate anatomic position and adequate functional separation of the lungs need to be ascertained. The following methods can be used to confirm and troubleshoot the position of the DLT:

1. Fiberoptic bronchoscopy: This technique allows direct visualization of the airway anatomy and confirms the location of the bronchial cuff within the mainstem bronchus. It is also helpful in diagnosing and repositioning a malpositioned DLT. A fiberoptic bronchoscope must be immediately available throughout the entire period of intubation with a DLT.

2. Radiologic studies: A chest radiograph is usually obtained to follow the course of lung disease in a critically ill patient. Radiopaque marking on the DLT allows assessment of the depth of bronchial lumen within the mainstem bronchus.

3. Assessment of functional separation of lungs: It is important to ensure that the bronchial cuff is not overinflated or underinflated. An overinflated cuff is more likely to be herniated into the carina, or it may result in tracheobronchial ischemic complications or even rupture. Conversely, an underinflated cuff may result in air leak or spillover and contamination of the contralateral lung. A "Just-seal" technique has been described using an air bubble method (end point: no air bubbles when outer end of nonventilated lumen is immersed under water) or capnography (end point: no $ETCO_2$ movement when outer end of nonventilated lumen is connected to capnograph tubing) to prevent overinflation or underinflation of the bronchial cuff.

### MODES AND TECHNIQUES

Numerous modes and techniques for ILV are available.

## One-Lung Ventilation

In OLV, one lung is mechanically ventilated while the other lung is either occluded or open to the atmosphere. This option is used mainly in thoracic anesthesia and surgery to keep the operative (nondependent) lung collapsed and immobile. It may also be used in patients with bronchopleural fistula (BPF) to prevent all air leaks and for selective airway protection if secretions from the affected lung prevent any useful ventilation (e.g., massive hemoptysis). OLV can be achieved using a DLT with mechanical ventilation applied to only one lumen. It can also be achieved using a Univent tube or an independent BB placed through an SLT, by advancing the BB and inflating its balloon in the mainstem or lobar bronchus of the side to be collapsed or by advancing an SLT alone into the mainstem bronchus to the side to be ventilated.

OLV creates an obligatory shunt in the collapsed lung. Despite hypoxic pulmonary vasoconstriction in the nonventilated lung, it still receives some blood flow. When combined with V/Q mismatch in the dependent lung (decreased lung volume and atelectasis owing to the effects of general anesthesia and paralysis and compression by the mediastinum and abdominal contents), this blood flow can result in a total shunt of up to 30% to 50% and can lower the overall $PaO_2$ during OLV. Strategies to improve oxygenation during OLV include the use of $FiO_2$ of 1.0 and selective PEEP to dependent lung ventilation. Application of selective low levels of PEEP to the dependent (ventilated) lung, especially in patients with normal spirometry, may improve oxygenation by recruiting alveoli and enhancing lung compliance. This approach is thought to be superior to lung recruitment using a large $V_T$, which is associated with a repeated "shearing" effect and higher peak airway pressure. Excessive PEEP to the dependent lung may worsen hypoxemia during OLV by decreasing cardiac output and increasing intrinsic PEEP and thus causing hyperinflation and diversion of blood flow away from the ventilated lung.

## Volume Controlled versus Pressure Controlled Ventilation

Volume controlled ventilation (VCV) is traditionally used in patients during OLV. I use an $FiO_2$ of 1.0, a $V_T$ of 8 mL/kg, and a respiratory rate (RR) adjusted to maintain pH within normal range during OLV. The use of VT much greater than 10 mL/kg may adversely affect oxygenation. With VCV, pressure is the dependent variable, and the peak airway pressure varies depending on the changing lung compliance and flow resistance. A modest increase in airway pressure is observed after switching from two-lung ventilation to OLV using VCV. Excessive airway pressure may lead to barotrauma and an increase in the vascular resistance in the dependent lung. This may increase the shunt flow through nondependent (nonventilated) lung by diverting blood to it. The final result of excessive airway pressure in the dependent (ventilated) lung is a decrease in $PaO_2$.

With pressure controlled ventilation (PCV), $V_T$ is the dependent variable, which rises or falls depending on lung compliance. The salutary effects of PCV on oxygenation and peak airway pressure result from decelerating inspiratory flow, longer mean inflation pressure, and fewer "shearing" forces. When compared with VCV, most patients showed better oxygenation with PCV during OLV. Tugrul and colleagues[3] studied 48 patients undergoing thoracotomy requiring OLV. The patients were randomized to PCV or VCV mode to deliver a $V_T$ of 10 mL/kg. The peak airway pressure and plateau pressure (Pplat) were significantly lower and the mean $PaO_2$ higher in the PCV-treated group.

## Inspiratory-to-Expiratory Ratio and End-Inspiratory Pause

The inspiratory-to-expiratory (I:E) ratio during mechanical ventilation is generally kept at 1:2. However, patients with significant airflow obstruction should be allowed I:E ratios from 1:2.5 to 1:4 to minimize dynamic hyperinflation or intrinsic PEEP. End-inspiratory pause (EIP) is characterized by a period of no flow occurring at the end of inspiration. EIP shortens expiratory time, and this may promote development of intrinsic PEEP in patients with chronic obstructive pulmonary disease (COPD). Bardoczky examined the effects of EIP of different duration on pulmonary mechanics and gas exchange during OLV for thoracic surgery. It was found that changing the duration of EIP from 0% to 30% of total inspiration time resulted in a significant increase in intrinsic PEEP and a significant decrease in $PaO_2$. $PaO_2$ showed an inverse relationship with the duration of EIP and with the magnitude of intrinsic PEEP. Arterial carbon dioxide tension ($PaCO_2$) did not change significantly with EIP. It seems plausible that the effect of EIP on $PaO_2$ is similar to that of external PEEP on oxygenation in the patients with COPD during OLV: a reduction in $PaO_2$. The effect of EIP on oxygenation in healthy lungs undergoing OLV remains to be examined.

## Nondependent Lung Continuous Positive Airway Pressure

Although much attention is given to the ventilator management of the dependent lung during OLV, it is important to consider selective treatment of the nondependent (nonventilated) lung in an attempt to improve oxygenation. The nondependent lung may present unique operative and anatomic considerations that must be taken into account when selecting a management plan.

The primary effects of OLV are to reduce the area over which respiratory gas exchange may take place and to create an obligatory right-to-left intrapulmonary shunt through the nonventilated atelectatic lung. The amount of blood flowing through the collapsed lung determines the extent of shunt and final $PaO_2$. Hypoxemia during OLV occurs in 7% to 10% of cases despite adequate cardiac output and dependent lung ventilation. Usually, hypoxemia can be readily corrected by application of 100% oxygen CPAP to the nondependent nonventilated lung. Even low levels of nonventilated lung CPAP (2 to 5 cm $H_2O$) are as efficacious as high levels (>10 cm $H_2O$) and cause less distention, less surgical interference, and no hemodynamic effects. The nondependent lung CPAP must be applied during the deflation phase because the critical pressures needed to reopen atelectatic alveoli fully are much greater. This technique has several advantages and dangers. When the chest is open, CPAP partially inflates the lung that the surgeon is operating on, and this may make the procedure more difficult, especially during thoracoscopy. Because this lung is not being ventilated, in open chest procedures it is usually possible for the surgeon gently to retract the portion of the lung that is obstructing the field. The use of CPAP can be dangerous if the pressure is allowed to build to a greater level than desired. This is particularly true when the chest is closed and the overexpanded lung cannot be directly observed.

### High-Frequency Jet Ventilation

Nonventilated lung high-frequency jet ventilation (HFJV) may be considered when the application of CPAP is either impractical or hazardous during OLV. Some of the indications for nonventilated lung HFJV include BPF, surgery of the major airways, and acute respiratory distress syndrome (ARDS). HFJV utilizes delivery of oxygen using small VT (<2 mL/kg) at very fast rates (100 to 400 breaths/minute). Gas exchange during HFJV occurs by several mechanisms: mass movement, enhanced molecular diffusion, coaxial gas flow, and pendelluft movement. Theoretical advantages of nonventilated lung HFJV include the ability to deliver small VT through a small cannula, lower peak and mean airway pressures, and much smaller inflation and deflation movements of the lung. However, hyperinflation and barotraumas resulting from the development of intrinsic PEEP and drying of the airway mucosa by the high gas flows represent some of the risks associated with this modality.

## SYNCHRONIZED VERSUS ASYNCHRONIZED INDEPENDENT LUNG VENTILATION

Synchronized ILV (SILV) consists of synchronous initiation of inspiration into each lung. Each lung must necessarily have the same RR, but it may have different VT, PEEP, and inspiratory flow. The respiratory cycle can either be in phase or 180 degrees out of phase. There is less flexibility in manipulation of ventilator settings with SILV. SILV may be achieved by a variety of techniques, as described in the following sections.

### Single Ventilator with Modified Circuits

A single ventilator is linked to a twin circuit with devices that create different flows into each circuit. Placing variable resistances in each inspiratory limb divides the inspiratory flow from the ventilator in a variable manner. Both the resistance in the circuit and the impedance in the lung determine the flow and VT that each lung receives. The resistance in the circuit can be adjusted based on the desired VT measured from each circuit. Separate PEEP in each circuit may be achieved by placing expiratory flow controllers in expiratory limbs. Alternative single-ventilator systems have been described, but they are all subject to several disadvantages: leaks and disconnections from different attachments in the circuits, limited adjustments of different ventilator parameters, and inadequate monitoring of each lung parameter.

### Two Ventilators in Synchronized Mode

ILV may be achieved by the synchronous delivery of VT to each lung by using two ventilators that have been synchronized mechanically or electronically (slaving second ventilator to the primary master ventilator). The setting of each ventilator is limited by the same RR set on both ventilators. The respiratory cycle of each ventilator has to be completed before the next breath is delivered. This method allows for different VT, PEEP, ratio of duration of inspiration to expiration, and inspiratory flow combinations.

Asynchronous ILV (AILV) consists of completely independent ventilatory techniques applied to each lung using two separate ventilators. Lack of synchronization between the two lungs offers the greatest flexibility of technique and appears to have no disadvantages compared with SILV. Triggering of inspired breaths is not an issue because patients are usually sedated and many are paralyzed. Each ventilator can be set according to the different disorders and mechanical characteristics of each lung. AILV permits delivery of different RR, VT, inspiratory flow, I:E ratio, and PEEP to each lung. Considerable improvement in respiratory function and gas exchange without hemodynamic compromise has been reported with AILV. The use of AILV intermittent positive pressure ventilation applied to nondependent lung using small VT (1 mL/kg) and rapid RR (20 breaths/minute) was described as a solution to refractory hypoxemia during chest surgery. AILV may be administered using either single-mode or dual-mode mechanical ventilation.

## SINGLE-MODE VERSUS DUAL-MODE INDEPENDENT LUNG VENTILATION

Many variations of ventilation modes in AILV have been described. Both lungs may be ventilated using a similar mode (single-mode, conventional, or unconventional) or different modes (dual-mode, conventional, or unconventional) of ventilation. Evidence of the superiority of one mode over another is lacking in the literature. Whatever mode is chosen, consideration must be given to lung protective strategy to protect the normal lung, to prevent complications, and to allow the healing process by lowering mechanical stress during ventilation.

Various modes have been described, as follows:

1. PCV or VCV to both lungs with selective PEEP to each lung.
2. PCV or VCV with selective PEEP to one lung and HFJV to the other.
3. PCV or VCV with selective PEEP to one lung and CPAP to the other.
4. Selective CPAP to both lungs.
5. High-frequency oscillatory ventilation (HFOV) to both lungs.
6. Airway pressure release ventilation (APRV) to one lung and CPAP to the other.

With the PCV mode, $V_T$ is the dependent variable. Ventilation is determined by the inspiratory pressure rise, $\Delta P$ (calculated as Pinsp – PEEP), I:E ratio, and the lung compliance. As a lung protective strategy, the PCV mode may limit alveolar overdistention and potential volutrauma. However, dynamic changes in lung mechanics may result in undesirable changes in $V_T$ or excessive air trapping in patients with emphysema or COPD. With the VCV mode, pressure is the dependent variable, and the peak airway pressure varies depending on the changing lung compliance and flow resistance. Applying the evidence from ventilatory strategy in ARDS to severe asymmetric or unilateral lung injury, the ventilator setting in ILV should be chosen to avoid high plateau airway pressure.

High-frequency ventilation has been shown to be efficacious in patients with severe hypoxemic respiratory failure and minimal underlying parenchymal disease, such as patients with trauma or proximal BPF and postsurgical patients. High-frequency ventilation utilizes delivery of oxygen with very small $V_T$ (<2 mL/kg) at very fast RR (100 to 400 breaths/minute) and increased mean airway pressure to recruit atelectatic lung units and to maintain lung volume at higher than a critical opening pressure. A potential advantage of this technique is lower mean lung volumes, which may reduce pulmonary vascular resistance and dead space. However, hyperinflation and barotraumas resulting from the development of intrinsic PEEP and drying of the airway mucosa by high gas flows represent some of the risks associated with this modality.

APRV can be described as CPAP with regular, brief, intermittent releases in airway pressure. The CPAP level facilitates oxygenation and the timed releases aid in carbon dioxide removal. APRV achieves exhalation by releasing airway pressure from a high preset CPAP to a lower preset pressure in a time-cycled fashion. When the airway pressure release valve closes, the high preset pressure inflates the lung. The high preset pressure is set equal to Pplat and is titrated to the oxygenation goal. The low preset pressure, usually set at zero, accelerates the expiratory flow of gas and facilitates resumption of the high preset pressure as soon as possible. The high timed release, initially set at 4 to 6 seconds, determines the duration of inspiration. The patient is allowed to breathe spontaneously during the high timed release and at a higher CPAP level. Automatic tube compensation (ATC), a feature available in most modern ventilators, can be switched on to decrease the resistive work of breathing from artificial airway. The low timed release, initially set at 50% to 75% of peak expiratory flow rate, determines the duration of exhalation and maintains lung volume. The benefits of APRV include lung recruitment, facilitation of spontaneous breathing, and improvement in V/Q matching and gas exchange, as well as increase in venous return and cardiac output.

## MONITORING

Just separating and independently ventilating the two lungs are not enough. Evaluation of the effectiveness of ILV and of the severity of the pulmonary dysfunction and monitoring of the course of the lung disease require sequential measurements of pulmonary mechanics, ventilation, and gas exchange parameters. Baseline data should be obtained immediately after placement of the DLT. The parameters discussed in the following sections may be monitored during ILV to assess ILV's effectiveness, to assess resolution of lung injury, and to determine the timing of the weaning process.

### Gas Exchange

Arterial blood gases and $PaO_2/FiO_2$ ratios are monitored to assess the efficiency of ventilation and oxygenation during mechanical ventilation. Improvement in $SpO_2$ or $PaO_2/FiO_2$ is used to titrate $FiO_2$ rapidly down to less than toxic levels. Permissive hypercapnia must be tolerated as long as pH and oxygenation are physiologically acceptable. In time, an improvement in gas exchange indicates the effectiveness of ventilator intervention and an improvement in lung disease.

## Hemodynamics

Cardiopulmonary interactions between those induced by disease process and ventilatory intervention may result in hemodynamic compromise and therefore must be aggressively monitored during the acute phase of critical illness. An intra-arterial catheter allows direct and beat-to-beat measurement of systemic blood pressure. A pulmonary artery catheter may be helpful to assess cardiac output, shunt fraction, and intracardiac filling pressures and may help to guide fluid and vasoactive therapy. Alternatively, less invasive means to assess and help manage hemodynamics include central venous pressure and central venous oximetry monitoring coupled with cardiac output and stroke volume variation derived from arterial pressure waveform using FloTrac (Edwards Lifesciences, Irvine, CA).

## Lung Mechanics

Although most modern ventilators are capable of providing a wide range of spirometric, airway pressure and flow, and static and dynamic compliance measurements, simple measures of lung mechanics should be chosen that are easily measured and reproducible. These measurements must from be made from each lung as a guide to quantification of asymmetric lung pathophysiology and titration of ventilatory therapy.

*V$_T$ and Pplat:* Exhaled V$_T$ must be carefully monitored for each lung. Pplat is measured at the end of inspiration by holding the end-inspiratory knob for 2 seconds. Traditionally, equal V$_T$ in two lungs is the widely used setting for ILV. However, this practice may lead to levels of Pplat higher than 30 cm $H_2O$ in the diseased lung because of inhomogeneity and unequal compliance between the two lungs. Therefore, to prevent overinflation of the normal lung and to protect the diseased lung from high Pplat, the V$_T$ for each lung must be adjusted to maintain Pplat lower than a safe threshold value for barotrauma (<30 cm $H_2O$). A diminishing difference in V$_T$ between the two lungs may be an indication of resolution of lung disease and time to initiate weaning.

*Static compliance:* Static compliance for each lung can be computed as V$_T$/(Pplat – EEP). End-expiratory pressure (EEP) is measured by holding the end-expiratory knob for 2 seconds. For the same mechanism explained earlier, keeping the same V$_T$ in both lungs during ILV, there is a significant difference in Pplat and static compliance between the normal lung and the diseased lung.

*EEP and PEEP:* Different disorders (e.g., normal versus ARDS and emphysema versus single-lung transplant) and varying ventilator settings in the two lungs may result in different degrees of EEP (intrinsic PEEP) between the two lungs. Inspiratory flow, I:E ratio, V$_T$, and external PEEP must be adjusted accordingly to prevent hyperinflation of the normal lung.

## End-Tidal Carbon Dioxide

A difference in ETCO$_2$ between normal and diseased lung is observed during ILV. ETCO$_2$ is found to be lower in the diseased lung when using the same V$_T$ for both lungs during ILV. The reason is inhomogeneity related to the lung injury (e.g., pulmonary contusion) with coexistence of less diseased, more compliant areas and more diseased, less compliant areas within the same lung resulting in variable ratios of overinflated (high V/Q) and underinflated (low V/Q) parenchymal areas. Equalization of ETCO$_2$ between the two lungs may indicate improvement in disease and time to initiate weaning.

## Radiologic Studies

Radiologic studies, such as chest radiographs and thoracic CT scans, are commonly used during the course of ILV to evaluate asymmetric lung disease, to investigate complications, and to follow the patient's course.

In summary, during ILV, in the damaged lung (e.g., pulmonary contusion), together with improvement in lung disease, the Pplat developed by a given V$_T$ is reduced, whereas shunting is reduced and ETCO$_2$ is increased.

## WEANING

Most patients can be quickly weaned from OLV and extubated in the operating room at the conclusion of thoracic surgery. Adherence to routine extubation criteria after general anesthesia and consideration of the patient's limitations in preoperative pulmonary function may help to improve extubation success.

Weaning from ILV should be considered when the patient's respiratory function shows continuous improvement and adequate oxygenation using relatively low levels of PEEP and oxygen concentration. Because of limited experience with ILV, there are no generally accepted criteria for initiation of weaning. In general, conventional mechanical ventilation (CMV) may be attempted when the difference between the lung mechanics on the two sides is minimal, thus indicating resolution of the lung disorder. For example, weaning from ILV may be initiated when there is little or no difference in $V_T$ (<100 mL), static compliance (<20%), and $ETCO_2$ between the two lungs. For this reason, it is extremely important to monitor individual lung behavior during ILV.

## CLINICAL APPLICATIONS

Whereas clinical physiologic justification and methods of lung separation seem established, clearly established guidelines for initiation and choice of ILV are lacking. Although most patients requiring ventilatory support can be managed satisfactorily with CMV, ILV may be useful in situations in which patients may benefit from lung separation for anatomic or physiologic reasons. A strategy for initiation of ILV is shown in Figure 30.2. Common indications for ILV can be conveniently grouped into three categories: thoracic anesthesia and surgery, anatomic (watertight) lung separation, and physiologic (airtight) lung separation.

### Thoracic Anesthesia and Surgery

Indications for ILV during thoracic anesthesia and surgery have expanded from traditional isolation of the healthy lung from pus or blood to include various pulmonary and nonpulmonary surgical procedures by providing better operating conditions through a limited incision. Common indications for ILV in thoracic anesthesia and surgery are listed in Table 30.1. Although OLV is required during surgery, ILV may be required before and, if applicable, after the surgical procedure.

In OLV in thoracic anesthesia, only a single (nonoperative) lung is ventilated. Although there are several techniques for isolating a lung, the most common is the use of a DLT that allows independent ventilation (or lack of) each lung. The advantages and limitations of different devices used for lung isolation are listed in Table 30.2. When DLT intubation is difficult, OLV can be delivered using a BB, either incorporated within the SLT (Univent tube) or placed separately through an SLT. The narrow lumen of the BB enables lung inflation using CPAP or HFJV but does not allow conventional ILV. OLV may be delivered to either lung, but repositioning of the BB is required. If ILV is no longer required postoperatively, the BB is either retracted within the wall of the Univent tube or is removed from the normal SLT.

Most thoracic procedures are performed in lateral decubitus position. Careful attention must be paid to prevent direct pressure on dependent bony prominences as well as on the neurovascular bundle in the dependent axilla. In modern practice, despite the availability of better endobronchial tubes, fiberoptic bronchoscopy, and adequate cardiac output, hypoxemia during OLV remains a clinical problem. Several factors have been identified preoperatively that predict a patient's risk of developing hypoxemia during OLV (Box 30-1). Therefore, a strategic plan to maximize oxygenation can be developed based on data available before initiation of OLV. Close communication with the surgeon is extremely important to arrive at a plan that is safe for the patient. The strategies to maximize oxygenation during OLV are described in the following sections.

### Ventilator Strategy

It is difficult to recommend one ventilation method that is ideal for all. Proper placement of the DLT or BB should be confirmed using fiberoptic bronchoscope immediately before initiation of OLV. In general, during OLV, a $V_T$ of 8 to 10 mL/kg with an $FiO_2$ of 1.0, an RR adjusted to keep pH >7.30, and an I:E ratio of 1:2 (longer exhalation time for patients with COPD/emphysema) provide adequate minute ventilation in most patients. Patients with good elastic recoil and normal pulmonary function may benefit from 5 cm $H_2O$ PEEP applied to the dependent lung. The choice of VCV versus PCV mode of ventilation is based on individual patient characteristics. Any sudden changes in peak airway pressures or $V_T$ should be investigated for malposition of the DLT or BB using fiberoptic bronchoscope. For this reason, the fiberoptic bronchoscope is kept in the operating room until the case is completed and the patient is extubated in the operating room. Careful attention is given to tracheobronchial hygiene by suctioning secretions and blood and using bronchodilators delivered by a metered dose inhaler. In most instances, low levels (2 to 5 cm $H_2O$) of nondependent CPAP using 100% oxygen may readily correct hypoxemia. Sequential increase in nondependent CPAP and dependent PEEP may be used in small increments to treat persistent hypoxemia. Nonventilated HFJV may be considered when the application of CPAP is either impractical or hazardous. AILV using intermittent positive pressure ventilation to the nondependent lung has been described as a solution to refractory hypoxemia during chest surgery. Selective placement of a BB into a lobar bronchus may reduce the amount of atelectatic lung and shunt. Finally, the surgeon may be able to interrupt the blood flow to the nonventilated lung by applying a ligature around the pulmonary artery supplying the part or whole of the nonventilated lung, depending on the surgical procedure.

### Pharmacologic Strategy

Maintaining adequate cardiac output during OLV is as important as maintaining adequate dependent lung

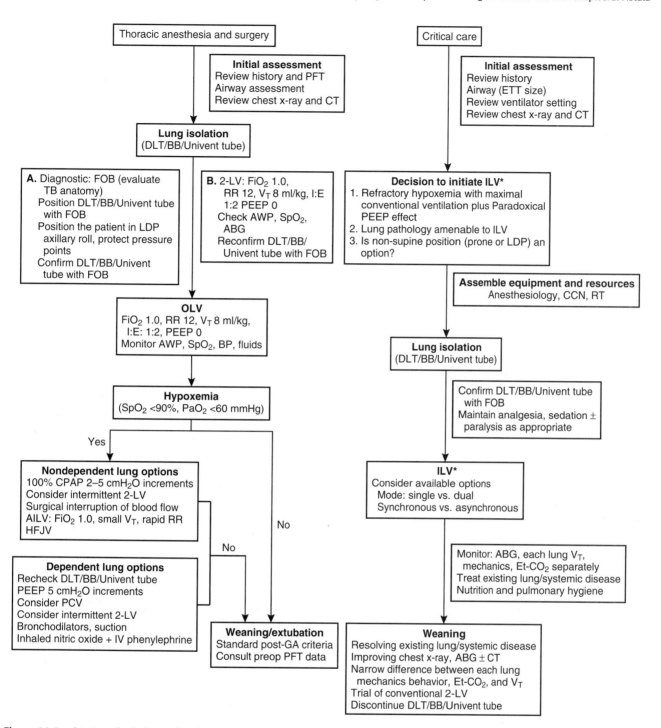

**Figure 30.2** Strategy for independent lung ventilation. See text for details. 2-LV, two-lung ventilation; ABG, arterial blood gas; BB, bronchial blocker; CT, computed tomography scan; DLT, double-lumen tube; Et-CO$_2$, end-tidal carbon dioxide; ETT, endotracheal tube; FOB, fiberoptic bronchoscopy; GA, general anesthesia; ILV, independent lung ventilation; IV, intravenous; LDP, lateral decubitus; OLV, one-lung ventilation; PCV, pressure controlled ventilation; PEEP, positive end-expiratory pressure; PFT, pulmonary function test; RR, respiratory rate; V$_T$, tidal volume.

ventilation in maximizing oxygenation. Patients with low cardiac output resulting from right ventricular dysfunction or high PEEP may benefit from an inotrope (e.g., dobutamine). Careful attention to fluid replacement is important in avoiding fluid overload. Invasive monitoring of cardiac filling pressures, cardiac output, and mixed venous oxygen saturation is required in only a few patients. Pulmonary circulation can be modulated by administration of selective pulmonary vasodilator and vasoconstrictor agents. The combination of inhaled nitric oxide (a selective pulmonary vasodilator) 5 to 20 ppm to the ventilated lung and an intravenous infusion of almitrine (a pulmonary vasoconstrictor) can restore $PaO_2$ during OLV to levels close to those during two-lung ventilation, although the complexity of this therapy limits its routine clinical use.

## ANATOMIC REASONS FOR INDEPENDENT LUNG VENTILATION

Current major indications for selective airway protection (anatomic lung separation) are protection of a healthy lung from purulent or malignant secretions and airway protection during unilateral whole lung lavage or massive hemoptysis. Because these diseases compromise lung function, such a watertight seal produced by anatomic separation is almost invariably combined with ILV.

### Lung Protection from Secretions

Purulent abscess, empyema, bronchiectasis, cavitating tuberculosis, and cavitating malignant disease are uncommon, as is thoracic surgery for these indications. However, when these situations arise, the spread of copious amounts of infective or malignant secretions to the contralateral, normal lung is associated with considerable risk. As well as being necessary for thoracic surgery, a DLT provides an important protective role for the normal lung, which is placed in the dependent position and is at risk of receiving the often copious secretions draining from the cavities in the nondependent lung. Furthermore, because of the asymmetric nature of the lung disease, ILV is sometimes required both during surgery and postoperatively.

Although now rarely needed or reported for this purpose, a DLT with or without ILV may still have an occasional role in the prevention or spread of purulent material following cavity or abscess rupture in the absence of thoracic surgery. However, viscous or tenacious secretions may not drain as well through the narrower lumen of a DLT, and a standard SLT may be a more appealing alternative.

### Massive Hemoptysis

Massive hemoptysis is an emergency with a high mortality rate. Prompt intervention with ILV can be lifesaving until definitive therapy can be instituted. Common causes include tuberculosis, bronchiectasis, pulmonary carcinoma, mycetoma, and cystic fibrosis. The source of bleeding is usually the bronchial arterial system. Iatrogenic causes are uncommon but include Swan-Ganz catheter balloon rupture of the pulmonary artery and transbronchial lung biopsy. Death usually occurs from acute asphyxia and is related to the rate and volume of blood loss and the patient's underlying condition. Factors increasing risk of death include preexisting pulmonary insufficiency, obtundation from any cause, poor cough, and coagulopathy.

Management of massive hemoptysis consists of general measures, diagnosing the site of bleeding, isolating the bleeding site, and controlling the bleeding. The patient should be given 100% oxygen and placed in the head-down lateral decubitus position with the side of suspected bleeding downward. Blood should be sent for coagulation screening and crossmatching, wide-bore intravenous access should be established, and resuscitation and suction equipment should be kept in close proximity.

Numerous alternatives exist for isolation and control of the bleeding, and the choice depends on the rate of bleeding, the ready availability of the technique, and the skill of the personnel involved:

1. Fiberoptic bronchoscopy and Fogarty catheter placement: These procedures can be performed in a patient with a moderate rate of bleeding and who may or may not be intubated. Fiberoptic bronchoscopy can allow accurate localization of bleeding and placement of a Fogarty catheter in a bronchial segment or subsegment. They also allow lavage with iced isotonic saline solution for identification and control of hemorrhage and instillation of dilute epinephrine if bleeding is from a proximal airway lesion.

2. Rigid bronchoscopy: This is more suitable when blood loss is massive, because of better suction, better visual access, and better airway control. It also allows placement of a Fogarty catheter, iced saline lavage, epinephrine instillation, and diathermy.

3. Endotracheal intubation: Placement of an endotracheal tube (usual size, 6 to 7 mm) may be required when bleeding is so rapid that acute asphyxia-related arrest is imminent. Under this circumstance, the endotracheal tube is advanced beyond the carina (usually into the right main bronchus) and OLV is begun. If blood does not flow out of the endotracheal tube (implying bleeding from the contralateral side), the cuff is inflated, and the endotracheal tube is left in place. If bleeding continues through the endotracheal tube, a Fogarty catheter is passed, the main bronchus is occluded, and the endotracheal tube is withdrawn to the trachea to ventilate the contralateral side. Selective intubation has the advantage of reliable protection of the nonbleeding lung and disadvantage of permitting OLV only and excluding the bleeding lung from endobronchial procedures and suctioning. Bleeding must then be controlled by balloon tamponade or bronchial angiography and embolization.

4. DLT placement: DLT insertion is an alternative that isolates the lungs but preserves access to them. A DLT enables lateralizing of the bleeding site, protects the nonbleeding lung from aspiration of blood, allows ILV, which is usually necessary, allows application of PEEP to the bleeding lung, which may reduce bleeding, and allows suctioning and endobronchial therapeutic procedures on the bleeding lung without compromising the healthy lung. A left-sided DLT is preferred.

Once the bleeding lung or segment has been isolated, the bleeding must be controlled. Correction of any coagulopathy and time may be all that is required. Whenever bronchial arterial bleeding is the probable cause, bronchial angiography may be performed to localize and embolize the bleeding site. Continued major bleeding that is not controlled by the foregoing measures requires urgent surgical resection. ILV is usually required because of higher impedance in the bleeding lung and because of the need to perform a procedure on that lung. Most commonly, a single ventilator with a Y-connection to the DLT is used to ventilate the healthy lung.

## Whole Lung Lavage

*Pulmonary alveolar proteinosis* was first described in 1958. Soon thereafter, bronchopulmonary lavage became established as the major form of treatment for this condition. Pulmonary alveolar proteinosis is a condition of unknown origin that may be associated with systemic disease or hematologic malignancy but most commonly arises de novo. Its clinical course varies from asymptomatic to minimally symptomatic, to progressive respiratory insufficiency, and eventually to remission in some cases. The decision to undertake whole lung lavage is based not on the presence of the disease, but rather on the progression of the disease and on the symptomatic state.

*Asthma*, refractory to treatment, may cause occlusion of a significant number of small airways with tenacious, inspissated secretions that may persist despite aggressive treatment. Bronchial lavage was first reported for this condition in 1964, and since then there have been reports of its use not only in asthma, but also in *cystic fibrosis* and *chronic bronchitis*. The goal of lavage under these conditions is to remove the inspissated secretions and to hydrate those secretions that are not washed out, to aid their subsequent expectoration. The success of this procedure is related to the amount of bronchial cast removed. *Radioactive dust inhalation* has also been reported as an indication for whole lung lavage to remove particulate radioactive material that would otherwise remain and injure the host.

### Procedure

To minimize hypoxemia during the procedure, the most severely affected lung should be lavaged first. That lung can be identified by chest radiographic appearance, V/Q lung scan, and bronchospirometry during OLV to each lung using a DLT in the supine position.

The procedure is usually performed with inhalational anesthesia, neuromuscular paralysis, and a left-sided DLT. Complete lung isolation to prevent spillage of fluid from the lavaged lung into the ventilated lung is essential. Before lavage, both lungs must be oxygenated with 100% oxygen. This maximizes gas exchange in the lung to be ventilated and eliminates nitrogen from the lung to be lavaged. Residual air, dominated by nitrogen, may prevent lavage fluid from reaching some sections of the lung, whereas oxygen retained in the lung is rapidly absorbed, thereby allowing entry of lavage fluid. Isotonic saline solution warmed to body temperature is then infused through wide-bore tubing into the lung to be lavaged from a gravitational height 30 cm above the midaxillary line in volumes compatible with compliance of the lung (500 to 1000 mL). Efflux of fluid may be begun, as soon as fluid influx is complete, by placing the drainage tube below the patient and percussion and vibration to the hemithorax. The total fluid exchange may range from 10 to 50 L and should be continued until the efflux fluid is relatively clear.

The choice of body position is important and is related to the mechanism of hypoxemia and to the risk of fluid spillage during the procedure. Placing the patient in the lateral decubitus position with the lavaged lung in the dependent position minimizes the risk from fluid leakage during the procedure; however, it also maximizes blood flow to the nonventilated lung during lung emptying and hence increases the risk of hypoxemia. Placing the lavaged lung in the nondependent position would minimize desaturation during the lavage phase. However, most clinicians regard the risk of fluid spillage in this position as unacceptably high and thus favor the supine position. Leakage of fluid into the ventilated lung is a feared complication and is recognized by desaturation, fluid in the lumen of the ventilated lung, and air bubbles in the lavage efflux. This complication mandates stopping the lavage procedure, rechecking the DLT position and placing the patient in the lateral decubitus position with the lavaged side down, and suctioning both lungs.

At the conclusion of lavage, double-lung ventilation should be recommenced with the DLT in situ using a single ventilator and a bifurcated circuit. If oxygenation is satisfactory, the patient may be weaned and extubated or reintubated with an SLT for weaning to occur in the intensive care unit. If oxygenation is unsatisfactory as a result of asymmetric lung disease, then ILV may need to be initiated. Up to 1000 mL of saline solution may be retained in the lavaged lung, and although this solution is rapidly absorbed, lung function may not improve for several hours or days. The procedure is then repeated on the second lung, usually after an interval of 2 to 3 days.

## PHYSIOLOGIC REASONS FOR INDEPENDENT LUNG VENTILATION

Physiologic lung separation (airtight seal) may be necessary when a different ventilatory strategy to each lung is applied because of differences in lung mechanics and disease processes between the two lungs. Indications for physiologic lung separation include BPF, unilateral or asymmetric lung disease (parenchymal injury, unilateral atelectasis, single-lung transplant, and unilateral bronchospasm), and bilateral symmetric lung disease.

### Bronchopleural Fistula

BPF represents a persistent communication between the bronchial tree and the pleural space. Approximately two thirds of BPFs are related to the surgical procedures; the remaining one third of these fistulas are caused by tuberculosis, trauma, necrotizing pneumonia, lung abscess, ARDS, and iatrogenic injury to lung from inappropriate mechanical ventilation and central venous cannulation. Persistent BPF often leads to infection of the pleural space. Regardless of the cause, BPF is associated with significant mortality, ranging from 18% to 67%.

Patients with BPF may require mechanical ventilation and chest tube placement. Massive air leak (1 to 16 L/minute) from BPF during mechanical ventilation may produce respiratory insufficiency from loss of VT through the BPF and sometimes tension pneumothorax leading to respiratory or circulatory collapse. Management goals are to relieve tension pneumothorax, if present, and to facilitate healing and subsequent closure of the BPF while maintaining adequate gas exchange.

Management of BPF includes antibiotics, pleural sclerosing agents, surgical control of air leaks at thoracotomy, chest tube drainage with underwater seal with suction, conventional ventilation strategies to reduce air leakage, positioning of the patient, HFJV, a variety of bronchoscopic occlusion techniques, and ILV. Chest tube management is a crucial first step in the control of BPF. Chest tubes must be adequate in number and diameter. Because flow varies exponentially to a power of the radius, the internal diameter of the chest tube is an important consideration. A short chest tube with a large internal diameter allows maximal flow. The drainage system connected to the chest tube also affects maximal flow rate. Commercially available chest tube drainage systems can handle flow rates up to 35 L/minute. Ideally, maximum flow capacity should approximate or exceed the percentage of VT lost to the BPF multiplied by inspiratory flow. With massive air leaks, more than one underwater seal drainage system may be required.

The ventilatory strategy for conventional positive pressure ventilation is directed toward lowering both alveolar and airway pressures, especially if dynamic hyperinflation is present. The amount of the air leak through a BPF is proportional to the mean airway pressure, which is determined by minute ventilation, inspiratory flow, and PEEP. Inspiratory flow is controversial, because increasing it may reduce air leakage by decreasing the duration of inspiration, but proximal air leaks may be aggravated by the increase in peak airway pressure that occurs when inspiratory flow is increased. Peak inspiratory pressure greater than 30 cm $H_2O$ has been associated with greater air leak. Dennis and colleagues showed the adverse effects of PEEP on air leak. Increasing PEEP from 0 to 16 cm $H_2O$ significantly increased air leak, whereas increasing peak airway pressure from 10 to 30 cm $H_2O$ did not increase air leak. In addition, PEEP of 6 cm $H_2O$ or greater was associated with a greater percentage of air leak than any level of peak inspiratory pressure.

HFJV alone appears to benefit patients with a proximal BPF and otherwise normal lungs. However, reported successes of HFJV in patients with parenchymal lung disease, in whom BPFs are usually peripheral, are variable. There are many reports of ILV use in the management of BPF. Conditions in which ILV has been used for BPF include pneumonia with or without underlying chronic airflow obstruction, ARDS, trauma, pulmonary contusion, emphysema, and thoracic surgery. Most of these patients had air leaks exceeding 50% of $V_T$, lung collapse despite multiple chest tube insertions, and hypercapnic acidosis and hypoxemia despite attempts at optimizing CMV. It is unclear whether ventilatory mode or SILV, as opposed to AILV, makes a significant difference in BPF.

The most common form of ILV utilized for BPF is AILV using two ventilators with conventional ventilation on both sides, but lower $V_T$, lower RR, or no PEEP used for the lung with the BPF. Various other combinations of ILV have been reported: CPAP to the nonfistulous lung and HFJV to the side with the BPF, CPAP or T-piece to the fistula side and APRV to the opposite side, and HFJV to the fistula side and conventional ventilation to the other side. The overall survival is approximately 50%, mostly dependent on the prognosis of the underlying disease.

## Unilateral or Asymmetric Lung Disease

Three major examples of unilateral or asymmetric lung disease when ILV may be indicated are unilateral parenchymal injury, unilateral atelectasis, and unilateral airway obstruction.

### Unilateral Parenchymal Injury

In almost 50% of cases, ILV is used in patients with thoracic trauma who have unilateral lung contusion. For ILV to be indicated, the unilateral lung injury usually results in asymmetric lung compliance, a large shunt through the injured lung, and severe hypoxemia that is generally refractory to standard mechanical ventilation strategies, including PEEP and high $FiO_2$. Under these circumstances, the net effect of increasing PEEP is a paradoxical decline in $PaO_2$ combined with reduced cardiac output and hence reduced oxygen delivery.

The prime objective of ILV under these circumstances is differential PEEP, although various ventilatory patterns (e.g., differential $V_T$, RR, CPAP, Pplat, HFJV) have been applied to achieve a similar effect, to optimize gas exchange, and to minimize barotrauma. PEEP applied to the diseased lung can be applied at a higher level than would be tolerated if applied to both lungs and can improve oxygenation both by alveolar recruitment in that lung and by diverting blood flow to the more normal lung. PEEP may be titrated to the diseased lung during ILV using gas exchange criteria, pressure-volume (compliance) curve until a predetermined inflection point is reached, until compliance or $V_T$ is about equal on the two sides, or by using $ETCO_2$ to monitor pulmonary response. PEEP may or may not be required in the contralateral lung, depending on its involvement in the disease process, the adequacy of gas exchange after

PEEP is added to the affected lung, and the effect of application of PEEP to the contralateral lung on circulation. Equal $V_T$ to both lungs is most commonly used and has been shown to improve gas exchange during ILV. However, $V_T$ to the affected lung may need to be reduced if excessive pressure results in that lung. AILV appears to have no disadvantages when compared with SILV.

### Unilateral Atelectasis

Unilateral atelectasis that has failed to respond to standard mechanical ventilatory support, bronchoscopy, or both is another indication for ILV. Selective high-level PEEP or CPAP ($\leq 80$ cm $H_2O$) may be required to open the atelectatic lung without the risk of overinflation of the contralateral lung and generalized elevation in intrathoracic pressure.

### Unilateral Airway Obstruction

Unilateral airway obstruction may occur following single-lung transplant, mechanical or chemical insult to one lung in a patient with asthma, or partial occlusion of one of the major bronchi. Under these circumstances, standard mechanical ventilation can result in dynamic hyperinflation and a high level of intrinsic PEEP in the lung with airway obstruction. This process can elevate intrathoracic pressure, reduce cardiac output, and compress the other lung. This effect is similar to the effect of bilateral PEEP in unilateral parenchymal injury, except PEEP (intrinsic) is occurring in only one lung. Under these circumstances, to allow deflation of one lung while meeting the patient's ventilatory requirements, greatly reduced minute ventilation (reduced RR and $V_T$) must be applied to the obstructed side.

### Single-Lung Transplantation

Single-lung transplantation is a popular alternative to double-lung transplantation, especially in patients more than 50 years of age. The most common indications for single-lung transplantation are chronic airflow obstruction and pulmonary fibrosis. Bronchiectasis, cystic fibrosis, bilateral bullous lung disease, and severe pulmonary vascular disease are contraindications to single-lung transplantation. The functional outcome is sufficient to improve quality of life substantially following single-lung transplantation, and there is no difference in maximum work capacity and maximum oxygen consumption between single- and double-lung transplantation.

ILV has been used successfully to treat native lung hyperinflation as a complication of single-lung transplantation for emphysema or chronic airflow obstruction. Single-lung transplantation may be complicated postoperatively by a difference in compliance between native and donor lungs (2.7:1), a difference that may be exacerbated by transplant lung injury, infection, or rejection.

The nontransplanted (native) lung with severe chronic airflow obstruction undergoes progressive dynamic hyperinflation during CMV, just as both lungs would have during CMV before transplantation. This is compounded by high compliance in the native lung and normal or low compliance in the transplanted lung, which selectively redistributes ventilation to the native lung and further promotes the unilateral dynamic hyperinflation, mediastinal shift, and compression of the transplanted lung with consequent impairment of gas exchange and hemodynamic compromise. Factors that increase the risk of this problem are the severity of airflow obstruction in the native lung, the size of the transplanted lung, and preoperative or intraoperative injury to the donor lung. Injury to a transplanted lung has three effects. First, it usually necessitates mechanical ventilation with increased ventilatory requirement (minute ventilation or PEEP), which increases the degree of dynamic hyperinflation in the native lung. Second, it increases the propensity for collapse in the transplanted lung. Third, impaired function in the transplanted lung results in more hypoxia from redistribution of blood flow into that lung from dynamic hyperinflation in the native lung. Resumption of spontaneous ventilation may minimize dynamic hyperinflation and reduce the need for ILV in these patients.

AILV is commonly instituted in this situation using CMV to the transplanted lung and CPAP or spontaneous ventilation to the native lung. The donor lung commonly requires PEEP at a sufficient level to expand collapsed lobes and improve oxygenation, a VT sufficiently low to keep Pplat lower than 30 cm $H_2O$ and avoid stress injury to the lung, and RR high enough for adequate carbon dioxide elimination without causing flow limitation in the donor lung. The native lung may be mechanically ventilated using small VT (<4 mL/kg), high inspiratory flow (70 to 100 L/minute), and low RR (2 to 10 breaths/minute). The dynamic hyperinflation can be assessed by measuring EEP (intrinsic PEEP), by measuring total exhaled volume from the native lung during 30- to 60-second apnea, or by observing flow pattern of exhaled gas. Bronchodilator treatment must be maximized in these patients. Withdrawal of ILV can be initiated when function in the transplanted lung improves and its ventilatory requirements decrease. Some patients may require tracheostomy and prolonged ILV with DLT. In a large series reported by Mitchell and colleagues[4] of patients undergoing single-lung transplantation for emphysema, 10% of patients required ILV to treat dynamic hyperinflation. The median duration of ILV was 14 days. One-year survival in patients who required ILV was 54%.

### Bilateral Symmetric Lung Disease

Acute bilateral lung disease (e.g., ARDS) often manifests with diffuse, uniform, and symmetric patterns on chest radiographs. However, a thoracic CT scan of these patients shows inhomogeneity with basal predominance. Many of these changes may result from supine position and the effect of gravity and weight of the mediastinum to produce lung collapse in the dependent zones.

The application of ILV under these circumstances, although controversial, is based on two principles. First, there may be differences in compliance, V/Q ratios, and gas exchange between the two lungs that are not evident by plain radiologic studies. Second, placing a patient in the lateral decubitus position may induce gravitational differences between the two lungs that previously existed within each lung in the supine position. In acute bilateral lung disease, the changes in V/Q and V/Q mismatch in the lateral decubitus position are similar to those in patients with normal lungs. When combined with placement of the patient in the lateral decubitus position and application of equal VT to each lung and selective PEEP to the dependent lung, ILV has been shown to improve shunt fraction, arterial oxygenation, cardiac output, and oxygen delivery in patients with acute bilateral lung disease.

## COMPLICATIONS AND CHALLENGES

Any decision to institute ILV must account for available resources, the expertise required in DLT/BB insertion, skilled critical care nursing and respiratory staff, and ready availability of specialized monitoring and fiberoptic bronchoscopy. Initiation of ILV should be carefully planned, and all involved with patient care must be well versed in the indications and the process. Many of the complications and challenges with ILV are related to DLT intubation.

### Lung Isolation Device–Related Complications

The limitations of lung isolation devices are listed in Table 30.2. It is occasionally necessary to provide OLV in patients with known or anticipated difficult airway by history or physical examination. The possible options for these patients include fiberoptically guiding intubation with DLT, securing the airway with an SLT first and then exchanging it for DLT over a tube exchanger, placing a BB or Univent tube, and advancing an uncut SLT into the desired mainstem bronchus. The optimal choice depends on the patient, the indication for OLV, and the skills of the intubator.

The modern PVC DLTs are generally safer than the older types made from rubber. Iatrogenic injury has been reported to occur in 0.5 to 2 per 1000 cases with DLT. Most of the complications of DLT are related to high bronchial cuff pressures. Bronchial ischemia and stenosis, pneumothorax, pneumomediastinum, and subcutaneous emphysema have been reported. The risk factors increasing the likelihood of complications or bronchial rupture can be grouped as tube related (traumatic intubation, overinflated cuff, oversized tube, and prolonged intubation), patient related (underlying malignancy, infection, long-term steroid use, and prior tracheobronchial surgery), or operator related (lack of knowledge of fiberoptic tracheobronchial anatomy). The recommendations to reduce the risk of complications include anticipation of difficult endobronchial intubation on clinical examination and review of chest radiograph and CT scan, use of an appropriately sized tube, inflation of the bronchial cuff to less than its resting volume (<3 mL), deflation of the bronchial and tracheal cuff before moving the patient or the DLT, avoidance of nitrous oxide during anesthesia (nitrous oxide 70% can increase the bronchial cuff volume from 5 to 16 mL intraoperatively and has been associated with bronchial cuff rupture), and gentle handling of the airway.

Movement and malpositioning of DLTs are far more common, especially with blind insertion and when turning the patient. Precise positioning of a DLT is most reliably achieved using a fiberoptic bronchoscope. Right upper lobe occlusion can occur in 10% to 90% of cases. Three critical malpositions of DLTs have been described: the left endobronchial limb blocking the left upper or lower lobe, the right endobronchial limb blocking the right upper lobe, and intratracheal dislocation of more than half of the bronchial cuff. Fiberoptic bronchoscopy is used to resolve this problem quickly.

Even though lumen diameter has considerably improved with the PVC tubes, difficult suction access, retained secretions, and lumen blockage remain problems and can lead to difficult ventilation and the need to change the DLT. Rare inclusion of a DLT or the wire loop of a wire-guided BB in the tracheobronchial sutures has been reported.

### One-Lung Ventilation

In spite of the routine use of fiberoptic bronchoscopy to position DLTs and limiting inspired concentrations of volatile agents, hypoxemia during OLV remains a significant clinical problem. The incidence of hypoxemia during OLV is reported to be between 7% and 10% of cases. A strategy that maximizes V/Q matching while minimizing resistance to blood flows in the dependent (ventilated) lung and maximizes the pulmonary vascular resistance while minimizing the shunt in the nondependent (nonventilated) lung may reduce intraoperative hypoxemia during OLV. Such a strategy is described earlier. Rare complications include cardiovascular collapse after induced DLT displacement of a mediastinal tumor into the mediastinal vessels and exsanguination following

inclusion of the DLT in sutures during pneumonectomy with subsequent vessel laceration when the DLT was removed.

### Independent Lung Ventilation

When ILV is continued for some time, certain difficulties related to the care of patients arise. Head movement, movement of the patient, and routine turning of the patient all threaten DLT position and can lead to loss of lung isolation or lobe occlusion. Frequent bronchoscopy may be required to maintain DLT position. Running two ventilators requires additional space, oxygen, air, and suction outlets, and standard bedside flow charts are usually inadequate. There are significant increases in nursing time requirement and workload.

## CONCLUSION

Advances in thoracic anesthesia, surgery, and critical care have expanded the application of ILV in a wide range of perioperative and critical care conditions utilizing a variety of techniques. Effective lung isolation is the cornerstone of successful ILV. Appreciating the details of different lung isolation devices and tracheobronchial anatomy and developing expertise in fiberoptic bronchoscopy will improve success in providing effective lung isolation even in the most challenging circumstances.

Up to now, no clear guidelines have been established for initiating and qualifying the need for ILV in critical care. The current data are confined to case reports and series with no prospective, randomized trials. Outcome and mortality data are lacking and remain areas for future clinical research. A general strategy for initiating ILV is presented in Figure 30.2. Although most patients requiring ventilatory support in critical care can be managed satisfactorily with CMV, ILV may be potentially lifesaving in clinical situations in which lung separation for anatomic or physiologic reasons may be beneficial. Any decision to institute ILV must account for available resources, the expertise required in DLT/BB insertion, skilled critical care nursing and respiratory staff, ready availability of specialized monitoring and fiberoptic bronchoscopy, and the ability of the patient to tolerate the procedure.

## REFERENCES

1. Gale JW, Waters RM: Closed endobronchial anesthesia in thoracic surgery: Preliminary report. J Thorac Surg 1931;1:432.
2. Glass DD, Tonnesen AS, Gabel JC, et al: Therapy of unilateral pulmonary insufficiency with a double lumen endotracheal tube. Crit Care Med 1976;4:323–326.

3. Tugrul M, Camci E, Karadeniz H, et al: Comparison of volume controlled with pressure controlled ventilation during one-lung anesthesia. Br J Anaesth 1997;79:306–310.
4. Mitchell JB, Shaw ADS, Donald S, et al: Differential lung ventilation after single-lung transplantation for emphysema. J Cardiothorac Anesth 2002;16:459–462.

## SELECTED READINGS

Adoumie R, Sshennib H, Brown R, et al: Differential lung ventilation beyond the operating room. J Thorac Cardiovasc Surg 1993;105:229–333.

Anantham D, Jagadesan R, Tiew P: Clinical review: Independent lung ventilation in critical care. Crit Care 2005;9:594–600.

Benumof JL: Conventional and differential lung management of one-lung ventilation. In Benumof JL (ed): *Anesthesia for Thoracic Surgery*, 2nd ed. Philadelphia: WB Saunders, 1994, pp 406–431.

Benumof JL: High-frequency and high-flow apneic ventilation during thoracic surgery. In Benumof JL (ed): *Anesthesia for Thoracic Surgery*, 2nd ed. Philadelphia: WB Saunders, 1994, pp 432–452.

Blanch L, Fernandez R, Artigas A: The expiratory capnogram in mechanically ventilated patients. In Vincent JL (ed): *Update in Intensive Care and Emergency Medicine*. New York: Springer, 1993.

Campos JH, Hallam EA, Van Natta T, et al: Devices for lung isolation used by anesthesiologists with limited thoracic experience: Comparison of double-lumen endotracheal tube, Univent torque control blocker, and Arndt wire-guided endobronchial blocker. Anesthesiology 2006;104:261–266.

Carlon GC, Kahn R, Howland WS, et al: Acute life-threatening ventilation perfusion inequality: An indication for independent lung ventilation. Crit Care Med 1978;6:380–383.

Chhangani SV: Ventilation techniques for 1-lung anesthesia. Semin Anesth 2002;3:196–203.

Cinella G, Dambrosio M, Brienza N, et al: Compliance and capnography monitoring during independent lung ventilation: Report of two cases. Anesthesiology 2000;93:275–278.

Cinnella G, Dambrosio M, Giuliani R, et al: Independent lung ventilation in patients with unilateral pulmonary contusion: Monitoring with compliance and EtCO$_2$. Intensive Care Med 2001;27:1860–1867.

Darwish RS, Gilbert TB, Fahy BG: Management of a bronchopleural fistula using differential lung airway pressure release ventilation. J Cardiothorac Anesth 2003;17:744–746.

Geiger K: Differential lung ventilation. Int Anesthesiol Clin 1983;21:83–96.

Graciano AL, Barton P, Luckett PM, et al: Feasibility of asynchronous independent lung high-frequency oscillatory ventilation in the management of acute hypoxemic respiratory failure: A case report. Crit Care Med 2000;28:3075–3077.

Gattinoni L, Presenti A, Avelli L, et al: Pressure-volume curve of total respiratory system in acute respiratory failure: Computed tomography scan study. Am Rev Respir Dis 1987;136:730–736.

Hurford WE, Alfille PH: A quality improvement study of the placement and complications of double-lumen endobronchial tubes. J Cardiothorac Anesth 1993;7:517–520.

Massard G, Rouge C, Dabbagh A: Tracheobronchial lacerations after intubation and tracheostomy. Ann Thorac Surg 1996;61:1983–1987.

Micha S, Yaacov G, Yuval W, et al: Asynchronous independent intermittent positive pressure ventilation as a solution to refractory hypoxemia during chest surgery. Anesthesiology 2002;97:743–745.

Moutafis M, Liu N, Dalibon N, et al: The effect of inhaled nitric oxide and its combination with intravenous almitrine on PaO$_2$ during one-lung ventilation in patients undergoing thoracoscopic procedures. Anesth Analg 1997;85:1130–1135.

Ost D, Corbridge T: Independent lung ventilation. Clin Chest Med 1996;17:591–603.

Peden CJ, Galizia EJ, Smith RB: Bronchial trauma secondary to intubation with PVC double-lumen tube. J R Soc Med 1992;85:705–706.

Plotz FB, Hassing MBF, Sibarani-Ponsen RD, et al: Differential HFO and CMV for independent lung ventilation in a pediatric patient. Intensive Care Med 2003;29:1855.

Scherer R: Independent lung ventilation. Intensive Care World 1989;6:27–31.

Siegel JH, Stoklosa JC, Borg U, et al: Quantification of asymmetric lung pathophysiology as a guide to the use of simultaneous independent lung ventilation in posttraumatic and septic adult respiratory distress syndrome. Ann Surg 1985;202:425–443.

Slinger PD, Suissa S, Triolet W: Predicting arterial oxygenation during one-lung anesthesia. Can J Anesth 1992;39:1030–1035.

Slinger P: Lung isolation in thoracic anesthesia. Can J Anesth 2001;48:R1–R10.

Slinger P, Kruger M, McRae K, et al: Relation of static compliance curve and positive end-expiratory pressure to oxygenation during one-lung ventilation. Anesthesiology 2001;95:1096–1102.

Spragg RG, Benumof JL, Alfrey DD: New method for performance of unilateral lung lavage. Anesthesiology 1982;57:535–538.

Stow PJ, Grant J: asynchronous independent lung ventilation. Anaesthesia 1985;40:163–166.

Trew F, Warren BR, Potter WA: Differential ventilation in the lungs of man. Crit Care Med 1976;4:112.

# CHAPTER 31

# Intrahospital Transport of the Ventilator-Supported Patient

Helmar Wauer and Steffen Wolf

Patient transportation occurs in three situations: prehospital transport, interhospital transport, and intrahospital transport. The focus of this chapter is on intrahospital transportation. The transport of mechanically ventilated patients to other departments within the hospital, for diagnostic or therapeutic interventions, is common. This form of transport is often underappreciated in its complexity and potential risks for complications.

Transfer within the hospital of the ventilated patient can be short, such as from the operation room to the intensive care unit (ICU), or it can take hours, such as for diagnostic procedures or therapeutic interventions (e.g., endoscopic retrograde cholangiopancreatography). Equipment and staffing needed for intrahospital transport vary by hospital, by clinical service, and by patient. Intrahospital transport of the critically ill patient from intensive care areas of the hospital (e.g., ICU, emergency departments, operating theaters, and recovery rooms) typically involves areas not designed for the delivery of such care (e.g., radiology department).

Regardless of duration, transportation staff members need to be aware of the potential risks for the patient while outside the intensive care areas. A structured approach, with a checklist, should be implemented before every transfer. Safe transportation of the critically ill patient requires accurate assessment and stabilization of the patient before displacement. There should be appropriate planning of transport and optimal use of communications resources. Safe transportation requires an appropriately trained workforce with essential equipment, as well as an effective liaison among referring, transporting, and receiving staff members.

## INCIDENCE

Although absolute numbers of intrahospital transfers are not available in the literature, one can assume that at least 15% of ICU patients are transported during a year.[1] The number of transports seems to depend on the ICU profile. Trauma patients and children need more frequent transportation for diagnostic reasons compared with patients from internal ICUs. During a 3-month period, 103 transports were necessary among 56 patients of a shock trauma unit.[2] Hurst and associates reported on 100 transports for diagnostic purposes among 81 trauma patients.[3] In another report, 180 transports were performed from a 50-bed ICU of 139 children during a 4-month period.[4] From our own experience in two different ICUs during in the first 10 months of 2004, we had to perform 445 intrahospital transfers of 962 patients admitted at our neurosurgical ICU, whereas 470 such transfers were needed of 690 patients in our trauma and postoperative ICUs.

## RATIONALE

The mechanically ventilated ICU patient is usually transported either for diagnostic procedures or for surgical interventions.[1] Mechanical ventilation is administered to these patients for different reasons, including impaired pulmonary function or deficient respiratory mechanics, or both, or deep analgesic sedation (e.g., treatment of elevated intracranial pressure).

## ADVERSE EVENTS

Adverse events during transport of critically ill patients can be attributed to the following:

Equipment failures: Examples include lead disconnections, loss of battery power, loss of intravenous access, accidental extubation, occlusion of the endotracheal tube, and exhaustion of oxygen supply.

Patient-related disorders: Examples include worsening hypotension and hypoxemia.

When is an event adverse, however? What are transport-related complications? How are they defined? Descriptions vary from nonspecific definitions[1] to clearly fixed cardiovascular values.[2] Adverse events are mostly unexpected or unplanned, associated with transportation, and potentially detrimental to the stability of the patient, and they often require medical intervention.[1]

In a group of 27 patients with head injury (35 transfers for diagnostic procedures or to the operating room), adverse events were observed in 51%.[5] These events included hypotension (systolic blood pressure <90 mm Hg in 8.6%), hypoxia (oxygen saturation <90% in 5.7%), and increased intracranial pressure (42.9%, including 17% of cases with a pressure increase of >30 mm Hg). However, similar events were recorded in 60% of patients during the 4 hours before transportation and in 66% thereafter. After transportation, newly abnormal physiologic values were obtained in 17 patients. Although extensive data have accumulated with respect to adverse events while patients are absent from the ICU, less is known about the long-term effects of such events.

Rates of reported adverse events during intrahospital transportation of critically ill patients range from 5.9% to 84%.[1–3,5–8] Typical hazards and complications are listed in Box 31-1. In some reports,[1–5,7] the overall incidence of adverse events during intrahospital transport has ranged from 6% to 71.1%.[1–3,5,7,9–13] The first indications that intrahospital transportation potentially put the patient at risk were provided in the early 1970s, when arrhythmias were encountered in up to 84% of transfers of patients with high-risk cardiac disease; these patients required emergency therapy in 44% of cases.[8] Another investigator observed significant complications such as bleeding and hypotension in 7 of 33 patients transported from the operating room to the ICU.[14]

These rates of adverse events are clearly much higher than would be observed in an unselected population of critically ill patients. In an evaluation of 127 intrahospital

---

> **BOX 31-1**
>
> **Typical Hazards and Complications of Transport**
>
> - Hyperventilation during manual ventilation may cause respiratory alkalosis, cardiac dysrhythmias, and hypotension.
> - Loss of positive end-expiratory pressure may result in hypoxemia or shock.
> - Changes in a patient's composure may result in hypotension, hypercarbia, and hypoxemia.
> - Tachycardia and other dysrhythmias have been associated with transport.
> - Equipment failure can result in inaccurate data or loss of monitoring capabilities.
> - Inadvertent disconnection of intravenous access for pharmacologic agents may result in hemodynamic instability.
> - Movement may cause disconnection from ventilatory support and respiratory compromise.
> - Movement may result in accidental extubation.
> - Movement may result in accidental removal of vascular access.
> - Loss of oxygen supply may lead to hypoxemia.
> - Ventilator-associated pneumonia has been associated with transport.

---

transfers in ICU patients, Smith and colleagues reported that 24% of these patients were in worse condition after transfer.[15]

Whether the adverse events observed can be attributed to the transport itself or are related to the impaired physiologic state of critically ill patients irrespective of their location has been assessed in few studies, and the findings have been controversial. Wallen and colleagues compared patients over a period of 1 to 2 hours before intrahospital transfer for diagnostic purposes and then again during the transfer.[4] In most of the published data, an exact estimation of the severity of complications is missing, and definitions of adverse events are not consistent. However, the incidence of major life-threatening adverse events requiring intervention (e.g., administration of vasoactive drugs, fluid boluses, or cardiopulmonary resuscitation), as well as those related to the disconnection of ventilators or intravenous or intraarterial lines, may be as high as 8%.[1,4,7,12]

Obviously, death may occur during intrahospital transport,[14] but most studies have reported no fatalities in this situation.[1,2,4,5,8,9,13,15] Several studies have reported before-and-after variations concerning oxygen saturation and end-tidal carbon dioxide pressure ($PETCO_2$).[16–18] One study included a score for severity of illness (PRISM).[16] The case mix was inadequately reported in one study,[17] and it was omitted.[18]

## Respiratory System

The most common respiratory complications and adverse events during intrahospital transport are related to dysfunctions of ventilation, oxygenation, and ventilator equipment. These events occur in up to 29% of intrahospital transfers and they include a change in respiratory rate in 20% of patients, with consecutive hypercapnia and hypocapnia and a fall in arterial oxygen saturation in 2% to 17%.[2,3] In one study,[3] no change of arterial carbon dioxide tension ($PaCO_2$) or of pH was found during transport. In a prospective observational study, the prolonged effects of respiratory function after intrahospital transports of mechanically ventilated patients were addressed.[19]

In a study by Kollef and colleagues, 273 mechanically ventilated ICU patients had to be transported for miscellaneous reasons. The incidence of pneumonia was 24.4%, compared with 4.4% in patients of similar severity of illness who had not been transported.[20] In 49 transported patients, gas exchange significantly decreased from a ratio of fraction of inspired oxygen to arterial oxygen tension ($FiO_2/PaO_2$ ratio) of 267 mm Hg at baseline to 220 mm Hg 1 hour after transportation, an effect that lasted at least for the next 24 hours. A fall in $FiO_2/PaO_2$ of more than 20% from baseline was noted 1 hour after transport in 42.8%, and in 12.2% of patients this was still found 24 hours after transportation. However, the increased rate of complications may be attributed to the selection of patients requiring transportation for diagnostic or therapeutic purposes.

## Cardiac and Circulatory System

In a prospective study of 50 adult high-risk cardiac patients who underwent intrahospital transport, arrhythmias were found in 84%, 52% of whom required emergency treatment.[8] In addition, Insel and colleagues showed a higher incidence of hemodynamic changes necessitating therapeutic intervention when intrahospital transport involved transfers from the operating room to the ICU compared with patients transported from the ICU to diagnostic procedures.[11] An earlier report compared the transport of postoperative patients from the operating room to the ICU with that of patients transferred from the ICU for diagnostic tests. No complications and hemodynamic deterioration were noted in the latter group, whereas the postoperative patients were subject to hypotension, hypertension, or arrhythmias in 44% of cases. These findings suggest that transport from the operating room to the ICU involves a population of high-risk patients who need optimal equipment and logistics, whereas transfer from the ICU is associated with better preparation for transport or even the decision not to transfer a patient with impaired organ function.

In a study of trauma patients transported for diagnostic studies, a change in blood pressure (>20 mm Hg) and heart rate (>20 beats/minute) was observed in 40% and 21% of transports, respectively.[2] This change is similar to findings in other investigations (Box 31-2).[3] Although the overall incidence of complications was low in the study of Szem and colleagues, these investigators reported three cases of cardiac arrest and one case of pneumothorax that required chest tube placement.[1] Furthermore, in medical patients, electrocardiographic changes may occur that cannot be seen with standard electrocardiographic monitoring.[21]

In several studies, cardiocirculatory adverse events were noted in 0% to 47% of patients.[1,2,9,13] In particular, hypotension (a fall in systolic blood pressure ≥40 mm Hg) and arrhythmias were predominant in mechanically ventilated patients in a combined medical and surgical ICU.[9]

## Technical Adverse Events

In 125 transports of ventilated and nonventilated patients reported in a study by Smith and co-workers,[7] adverse events occurred in 34% of cases. Most of these events were related to the equipment or to the monitoring itself. Electrocardiographic lead disconnection (23%), monitor power failure (14%), a combination of both (10%), intravenous line and vasoactive drug infusion disconnection (9% and 5%, respectively), and disconnection from the ventilator (3%) were the most frequent problems. Adverse events occurred mainly at the destination site either before or during the procedure, but not during the transfer. In a study by Wallen and colleagues, equipment-related adverse events occurred in 10% of patients transported.[4] These events

---

**BOX 31-2**

**Pretransport Technical Checklist**

The monitors function properly and the alarm limits are set appropriately.
The manual resuscitator bag functions properly.
The ventilator (if used) functions properly, and the respiratory variables and alarms are set appropriately.
The suction device functions properly.
Oxygen and air cylinders are full.
A spare oxygen cylinder is available.
Airway apparatus and intubation equipment are available and working.
An adequate power supply (fully charged) and backup are available.
Patient notes, imaging films, and necessary forms are available.
Infusion pumps for drug infusions are available and have appropriate alarms.

included malfunction of equipment, loss of nasogastric tubes or chest tubes, and problems related to endotracheal tubes or intravenous lines.

## RISK STRATIFICATION IN TRANSPORT

Risk stratification can be used to determine outcomes in correlation to the severity of illness. Szem and co-workers stratified patients into low-risk and high-risk groups based on treatment regimens at the time of transport.[1] Treatments in the high-risk groups included any of the following: positive end-expiratory pressure (PEEP) of more than 5 cm $H_2O$, inotropic support with dobutamine, and vasopressor support with norepinephrine. Subgroups were created based on whether patients were receiving one, two, or all three modalities. Mortality in the low-risk group did not differ from that of the nontransported control group. Mortality in the high-risk group was higher; however, this seemed to be the result of an unexpected low mortality in the control group. Wallen and colleagues found that the duration of transport and the therapeutic intervention severity score (TISS) were significantly correlated with the occurrence of physiologic deterioration or with the requirement of major interventions, and the prevalence of major therapeutic interventions was more than three times higher in ventilated patients than in nonventilated patients.[4] Andrews and co-workers found that, in patients with severe head injuries, the overall injury severity score was found to be the only predictor for the development of adverse effects during transport.[5]

Waydhas pointed out the following: "The overall yield of diagnostic procedures that require a transport of critically ill patients in terms of a direct and consecutive change of therapy is at least 25% and may be as high as 70%, provided that the decision to perform a specific procedure is based on criteria similar to the ones used in those studies. Unfortunately, little information was provided by investigators regarding why a specific procedure had been done and whether alternative methods would have been available. In summary, the efficiency of transports in trauma and surgical patients, and in search of a septic focus, a source of bleeding, or the identification and follow-up of injuries appears to be moderate to fairly high, indicating a good risk:benefit ratio, as long as restrictive criteria are used to order those procedures."[22]

## TRANSPORT ALTERNATIVES

In light of the previously mentioned risk-to-benefit ratio and the development of highly sophisticated bedside tools for diagnostic purposes (e.g., ultrasound devices, mobile endoscopic units), the first question to ask is whether the trip is truly necessary. Although many diagnostic studies require transfer to the area where the equipment is located, a more portable alternative can sometimes be brought to the patient's bedside. Indeck and associates reviewed 103 consecutive transports from the shock trauma unit to diagnostic areas and found that 68% of patients experienced serious physiologic changes, whereas only 25 (24%) of the transports resulted in significant changes to the patient's management.[2]

## METHODS OF VENTILATION DURING TRANSPORT

The way in which the patient will be ventilated during transport as well as during the procedure needs to be evaluated before any equipment is assembled. The patient's current ventilator settings may necessitate the use of one modality of ventilation over another. Currently, the options for ventilation during transportation are the following: (1) manual ventilation using a manual resuscitation device (MRD) with supplemental oxygen, (2) mechanical ventilation using a transport ventilator, and (3) mechanical ventilation using the patient's current critical care ventilator. Each option has benefits and concerns that need to be further evaluated.

### Manual versus Mechanical Ventilation

The use of an MRD to ventilate a ventilator-dependent patient during intrahospital transfer has been shown to be a safe alternative, provided the staff members responsible for ventilation approximate the minute ventilation and the $FiO_2$ as dictated by pretransport ventilation.[13] The use of a spirometer to monitor volumes during transport reduces the risk of inadvertent hypoventilation or hyperventilation.[17] The variability of volumes delivered with manual ventilation, especially when one hand, as opposed to two, is used for squeezing the MRD, should be appreciated.[23] Use of an MRD with a supplemental oxygen supply allows one to ventilate with an increased $FiO_2$ ($FiO_2$ of ≤1.0). During short-term transports, this approach will not put the patient at risk; on the contrary, it ensures the patient's safety, but it will require additional oxygen should the duration of the transport be extended. In neonates, an $FiO_2$ greater than 0.6 may be counterproductive, thus requiring an MRD with an adjustable $FiO_2$.

Three studies compared manual with mechanical ventilation for intrahospital transportation. The first study, a randomized controlled trial in postoperative pediatric cardiosurgical patients, showed that manually ventilated patients were at risk of hyperventilation. $PaCO_2$ decreased from $32\pm1.6$ to $26\pm1.4$ mm Hg.[16] Apart from this finding, the results of manual ventilation appeared comparable to those of portable mechanical ventilation. Gervais and colleagues came to similar conclusions in adults; $PaCO_2$ dropped significantly in the manually ventilated group from $41\pm2$ to $34\pm2$ mm Hg ($P < .01$), with a consecutive increase in pH.[17] The use of a volumeter adequately reduced the risk for hyperventilation.[16] Although many patients tolerated this mild hyperventilation, supraventricular tachycardia did occur in 2 of 14 patients.[24]

Modern ventilators can be superior to manual ventilation. In a small study, Nakamura and colleagues found that 5 of 11 patients had significant deterioration in the $PaO_2/FiO_2$ ratio, whereas only 1 of 11 in the ventilator-treated group showed a similar decline.[24]

## Requirements for Mechanical Ventilators

Many authors have recommended the use of a mechanical ventilator for intrahospital transportation, because there can be significant variability in the $PaCO_2$, $ETCO_2$, and arterial pH[9,13,25] when transport ventilation with an MRD is compared with the use of a mechanical ventilator. The ability to monitor minute ventilation fosters stable $PaCO_2$ and arterial pH values.

Mechanical ventilation for intrahospital transfers can be accomplished by using either a ventilator designed specifically for transportation or, if the duration of the transport is short, the patient's critical care ventilator. Transport ventilators were reviewed extensively by Branson.[26] Even though many additional products have been made available since the publication of Branson's article, the same evaluation methods should be applied to any transport ventilator. The optimal transport ventilator should provide all ventilatory patterns and features that are standard for patients in the critical care unit. This list includes intermittent mandatory ventilation as well as pressure support ventilation in both pressure-controlled and volume-controlled ventilation modes. In addition, $FiO_2$ should be adjustable, especially for transportation of premature neonates at risk of developing retinopathy. The ventilator should also provide an adjustable PEEP (ideally as an integral part of the ventilator as opposed to an external valve) and programmable alarms for tidal volume ($V_T$), minute ventilation, inspiratory peak pressures, and disconnection. In addition, the size and weight of the unit, the battery life, the amount of gas consumption, and the ease of cleaning and reassembling the device should be taken into account. Ideally, the transport ventilator has been evaluated in a laboratory for a variety of resistances and compliances applied to the test lung, and flow and volume meters

have been evaluated for clinical application. Heinrichs and colleagues showed that variation of $V_T$ with a transport ventilator under less than ideal conditions may jeopardize the patient's condition.[27]

Evaluations of some transport ventilators, released since Branson's study,[26] have shown less variability than encountered by Heinrichs and associates.[27-29] A study by Campbell and colleagues identified that spontaneous breathing while a patient is connected to a transport ventilator superimposes significant breathing work to the patient,[28] and there may be a shortage of power supply by different types of mechanical ventilation.[30] This information should be considered when selecting and operating a transport ventilator. Alternatively, the patient's critical care ventilator can be used for transportation. Elaborate transport units have been developed to facilitate the use of existing ventilators for intrahospital transport.[31,32] These transport units have backup gas sources and power sources that allow extended transportation. Most newer ventilators for use in the ICU have internal batteries capable of powering the ventilator for a period ranging from 30 minutes to 2.5 hours and provide internal mechanisms to decrease gas waste by adding environmental gas.

In patients with impairments of gas exchange or lung function, the ideal ventilatory pattern is coercive. Therefore, ventilators used during transport of these patients must reliably and efficiently manage numerous respiratory conditions to maintain adequate oxygenation and ventilation.[2,19] The ventilators used for this purpose may be either ICU ventilators or less sophisticated machines.[5] Comparative studies regarding portable ventilators have been published.[29,33,34]

In an experimental study, a single protocol was used to compare five portable ventilators with three ICU devices.[35] The main findings of this study were as follows:

1. $V_T$ delivery was better achieved with the three ICU ventilators than with any of the portable ventilators.
2. The lowest trapped volume was obtained with two portable ventilators.
3. The triggering system performance was poor for Oxylog 2000 (Dräger Medical, Telford, PA) but good or excellent for Osiris 2 (Taema SA, Cedex, France) and for the three ICU ventilators.
4. Performance was more homogeneous among the ICU ventilators than among the portable ventilators.

These were experimental in vitro findings, however. They cannot be transferred directly to in vivo conditions and should be applied with caution to the ICU patient in respiratory failure.

The adjusted $V_T$ was imperfectly delivered under baseline conditions from four portable ventilators. With increased resistance and reduced compliance, the delivery of $V_T$ was reduced relative to the baseline in most cases.

These changes were neither statistically nor clinically significant; thus, $V_T$ delivery remained sufficient in this condition, which simulated disturbances of respiratory mechanics commonly observed in acute respiratory failure in the ICU.[36-38] When resistance was markedly increased, however, the reduction of $V_T$ from the portable ventilators was clinically relevant.

Furthermore, Zanetta and colleagues found significant gas trapping, along with its deleterious effects.[35] These investigators concluded that the portable ventilators behave differently from one another in delivering $V_T$, in offering resistance during expiration, and in activating the triggering system. Specifically, one transport ventilator was not recommended. Substantial differences were also found between portable ventilators and the ICU machines, and these differences should be taken into account when these small ventilators are used during patient transportation.

Whichever method of transporting critically ill mechanically ventilated patients is chosen, the monitoring of minute ventilation and airway pressure, as well as all hemodynamic and oxygenation variables, should be as extensive as that employed in the critical care area. Additionally, regardless of the method of ventilation selected, the transport team must assess the need to humidify inspired gases. If humidification is desired because of the patient's condition or the duration of the transport, a heat and moisture exchanger can be used for the duration of the transport.

In summary, intrahospital transport is a complex maneuver involving multiple personnel who must be well trained to monitor for, recognize, and treat critical changes occurring during transport of the ventilator-dependent patient. An automatically activated device to monitor oxygen supply pressure and to warn of low pressure should be fitted to the oxygen supply. When an automatic ventilator is in use, a device capable of issuing a prompt warning of a breathing system disconnection, ventilator failure, or high pressure in the breathing system should also be in continuous operation. Equipment to monitor and continually display the electrocardiogram must be available for every critically ill patient during transport.

## MONITORING DURING TRANSPORT

Many authors have recommended the use of a mechanical ventilator for intrahospital transportation, because $Pa_{CO_2}$, $ETCO_2$, and arterial pH can vary significantly when transport ventilation with an MRD is compared with the use of a mechanical ventilator.[3,9,13] The ability to control minute ventilation and to monitor for fluctuations of this value allows more stable $Pa_{CO_2}$ levels and arterial pH values. Although the technology exists to monitor blood gases in transport with a portable blood gas analyzer,[39] a more practical approach is to monitor $ETCO_2$ by capnography.[40,41] The use of capnography in conjunction with an MRD or mechanical ventilator may facilitate a more optimal level of ventilation when direct assessment of spirometry is not available.

It is worth noting briefly another practice, which involves the use of mobile bedside monitor units, as opposed to standard procedures for intrahospital transportation. Because studies of this topic have been limited to clinical descriptions, with no definition or systematic evaluation of adverse events,[8,42-44] these practices are not reviewed further here.

The clinical significance of the hyperventilation observed in manually ventilated patients during intrahospital transportation has yet to be determined. Mechanical ventilation was associated with respiratory alkalosis when ventilatory settings were inaccurate. No adverse effect (i.e., morbidity) was observed as a result of the method of ventilation. Use of a volumeter when manually ventilating a patient reduced the risk of hyperventilation. However, these studies were underpowered to detect significant mortality differences.

Another issue is the type of monitoring required for the duration of the transfer. The incidence of complications during intrahospital transfer is well documented, with alterations to blood gas and pH values, as well as a loss of airway and alterations in hemodynamic stability (including cardiac arrest), occurring at a significant rate.[9,17,45] Monitoring of the patient during transport should be at least as extensive as that within the ICU and perhaps, in the case of minute ventilation and oxygenation, more extensive. This may mean that additional respiratory monitoring, such as capnography and volume measurement by spirometry, should be made available for the duration of transport in addition to the electrocardiogram, invasive pressure monitoring, and oximetry currently in use.[6,17,46]

## RECOMMENDATIONS FOR INTRAHOSPITAL TRANSPORT

The transport itself must be justified. The benefits of the proposed interventions must outweigh the risks of moving the critically ill patient and those posed by the interventions themselves. The transport of critically ill patients to procedures or tests outside the ICU is potentially hazardous, and the transport process must be organized and efficient. To provide for this transport, the considerations and protocols discussed in the following sections need to be addressed, and checklists should be used to ensure optimal transfers.

## Pretransport Considerations

The hospital should prepare an intrahospital transport protocol for critically ill patients and should ensure that all relevant transport staff members are familiar with it. When a different team at a receiving location will assume responsibility for the patient's management after arrival, the continuity of patient care will be ensured by communication between and among physicians and nurses, to review the patient's condition and current treatment plan. This communication should occur each time the responsibility for the patient's care is transferred. Before transport, the receiving location should confirm that it is ready to receive the patient for an immediate procedure or test. All pieces of equipment must be checked, and notes and imaging films must be collected. A sample checklist is given in Box 31-3. Individual responsibilities for checking equipment must be defined.

## Accompanying Personnel

Having a well-defined team of personnel familiar with the intricacies of intrahospital transport reduces the incidence of complications.[1,4,47] The level of critical support necessary for the duration of transport and for the severity of the patient's condition at the time of transport should dictate the number and qualifications of personnel required.[1,4] Specialized transport teams characteristically receive consistently high levels of training and experience in the transportation of critically ill patients,[47-49] compared with teams assembled in an impromptu manner.

Safe transport requires the deployment of appropriately trained staff with essential equipment, as well as effective liaison among referring, transporting, and receiving staff. A minimum of two staff members should accompany a critically ill patient. One is usually a nurse with a competency-based orientation who meets standards for critical care nurses. The second person is a physician, well trained in difficult airway management and Advanced Cardiac Life Support, as well as in critical care. Only if the receiving location provides appropriately trained personnel and only if the circumstances are acceptable to both parties may patient care be transferred. Each team must be familiar with the equipment and must be experienced with securing of the airway, ventilation of the lungs, resuscitation, and other anticipated emergency procedures.

## Equipment and Drugs

Equipment and pharmacologic agents should be adequate in amount for each transport. The duration of transport and the patient's condition need to be taken into account. Drugs to allow management of general emergencies should always be available. Additional drugs should be added, depending on specific circumstances (e.g., specific antiarrhythmic agents, antibiotic dosage due during transport). When choosing equipment, the following considerations are important: size, weight, battery life, durability, ability to fit to trolley railings, ability to function under conditions of vibration, and ease of use in poor light and cramped spaces. Equipment should be adequately restrained and continuously and conveniently available to the operator. Equipment should be dedicated for transport use only, if possible. The availability of backup equipment may be desirable in certain circumstances. Boxes 31-4 through 31-6 provide checklists for essential equipment and drugs used in intrahospital transport.

---

### BOX 31-3

**Checklist for Respiratory Support Equipment**

Oxygen, masks
Self-inflating hand ventilating assembly with PEEP valve, appropriately sized for the patient transported (adult, child, neonate)
Stethoscope
Suction equipment of appropriate standard
Intubation set
Cricothyroidotomy set
Emergency pleural drainage equipment
Pulse oximeter
End tidal carbon dioxide monitor for ventilated patients
Portable ventilator
   With disconnection alarm (PEEP ability desirable)
   With tidal volume control
   With control of respiratory rate
   With monitoring of airway pressures
   Optional with adjustable inspired fraction of oxygen

PEEP, positive end-expiratory pressure.

---

### BOX 31-4

**Checklist for Circulatory Support Equipment**

Monitor/defibrillator/external pacer
Noninvasive blood pressure measuring device with appropriately sized cuffs
Vascular cannulas, peripheral and central
Intravenous fluids and pressure set (adequate for duration of transport)
Infusion pumps
Arterial cannulas and arterial monitoring device (if indicated)
Syringes and needles
External pacing equipment (e.g., postoperative cardiac cases)

---

## BOX 31-5

### Checklist for Other Equipment

Nasogastric tube and bag
Urinary catheter and bag
Gloves
Restraints

## Patient Status

The final preparation of the patient should be made before the actual move, with conscious anticipation of clinical needs. Administering appropriate doses of muscle relaxants or sedatives, replacing near-empty inotropic and other intravenous solutions with fresh bags, and emptying drainage bags are essential before transportation. The patient must be reassessed before transport begins, especially after monitoring equipment and the transport ventilator (if used) are in use. Transport preparations must not preempt the patient's care. Therefore, always check to ensure that the patient's airway is secured and patent, that ventilation is adequate, that respiratory variables are appropriate, that all equipment alarms are switched on, and that the patient is hemodynamically stable. Vital signs must be displayed on transport monitors and have to be clearly visible to transport staff. PEEP/continuous positive airway pressure (if set) and $FiO_2$ levels must be correct. All drains (urinary, wound, or underwater seal) must be functioning and secured, and underwater seal drains must not be

## BOX 31-6

### Checklist for Drugs

Pharmacologic agents that assist the management of the following emergencies should always be available:
    Cardiac arrest
    Intubation
    Hypotension and hypertension
    Agitation and pain
    Cardiac dysrhythmia
    Anaphylaxis
    Bronchospasm
    Hypoglycemia and hyperglycemia
    Seizures
In specific circumstances, it may be necessary to be able to treat the following during transport:
    Raised intracranial pressure
    Uterine atony
    Adrenal dysfunction
    Narcotic depression

clamped. Venous access must be adequate and patent. Intravenous drips and infusion pumps must be functioning properly.

The transferring personnel should be familiar with the patient's history, condition, and special requirements, to allow appropriate planning and anticipation of problems unique to the patient. Always reassess the patient immediately before leaving, with all transport equipment attached and functioning. In adults and children, a default $FiO_2$ of 1.0 generally is used. However, the oxygen concentration must be precisely regulated for neonates and for those patients with congenital heart disease who have single-ventricle physiology or are dependent on a right-to-left shunt to maintain systemic blood flow.

For patients requiring mechanical ventilation, equipment available at the receiving location should ideally be capable of delivering ventilatory support equivalent to that delivered at the patient's original location. In mechanically ventilated patients, endotracheal tube position is noted and secured before transport, and the adequacy of oxygenation and ventilation is reconfirmed. Occasionally, patients may require modes of ventilation or ventilator settings not reproducible at the receiving location or during transportation. Under these circumstances, staff members at the original location must try alternate modes of mechanical ventilation before transport, to ensure acceptability and patient stability with this therapy.

Contraindications for transport are considered before the transfer is begun and should preclude the procedure if the risks outweigh the benefits. These contraindications include, for example, an inability to provide adequate oxygenation and ventilation during transport either by manual ventilation or by portable ventilator, an inability to maintain acceptable hemodynamic performance during transport, an inability to monitor the patient's cardiopulmonary status adequately during transport, and an inability to maintain airway control during transport. Transport should not be undertaken unless all the necessary members of the transport team are present.

### In-Transit Procedures

The best route should be planned. Lifts should be secured or reserved beforehand. Adequate communication facilities during transit and at the destination must be available. The status of the patient must be checked at intervals, especially if the journey takes considerable time. Any change in the patient's condition, an unexpected event, or a critical incident must be acted on immediately. All critically ill patients being transported within the hospital receive the same level of basic physiologic monitoring during transport as they had in the ICU.

This includes, at a minimum, continuous electrocardiographic monitoring, continuous pulse oximetry, and periodic measurement of blood pressure, pulse rate, and respiratory rate. In addition, selected patients may benefit from capnography or from continuous intraarterial blood pressure, pulmonary artery pressure, or intracranial pressure monitoring. Special circumstances may warrant intermittent cardiac output or pulmonary artery occlusion pressure measurements. An automatically activated device to monitor oxygen supply pressure and to warn of low pressure should be fitted to the oxygen supply. When an automatic ventilator is in use, a device capable of warning promptly of a breathing system disconnection, ventilator failure, or high pressure in the breathing system should be in continuous operation. The patient's circulation must be monitored frequently and at clinically appropriate intervals by detection of the arterial pulse and measurement of the arterial blood pressure. Ventilatory function should be assessed at frequent and clinically appropriate intervals. The patient's oxygenation should be assessed often and at clinically appropriate intervals by observation and by pulse oximetry. Some modern transportation systems have all the essential devices stored in a space-saving and clearly arranged manner on a specially designed stretcher (Fig. 31.1). The use of such a system can shorten preparation time and transport time and may require fewer transport team members.[50]

## Arrival Procedures

On arrival at the destination, the receiving monitoring, ventilation, gas, suction, and power facilities are checked if the patient is to be transferred from the transport facilities. The patient must be assessed when the new monitors, ventilators (if used), and gas and power supplies are

established. If another team assumes responsibility of care, the patient is transferred to the new team leader. The transport staff must remain with the patient until the receiving team is fully ready to take over the patient's care.

## Documentation

The clinical record should document the patient's clinical status during transport until transfer occurs at the destination. Basic requirements are similar for intrahospital and interhospital transport. Interhospital transport may, however, require more careful planning, a greater variety of drugs, greater attention to items such as available battery life of equipment, availability of essential gases for life support systems, backup equipment, consideration of transport vehicles drawbacks, and knowledge of the effects of altitude.

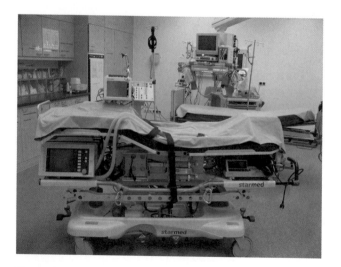

**Figure 31.1**  Example of a transportation system.

## REFERENCES

1. Szem JW, Hydo LJ, Fischer E, et al: High-risk intrahospital transport of critically ill patients: Safety and outcome of the necessary "road trip." Crit Care Med 1995;23:1660–1666.
2. Indeck M, Peterson S, Smith J, Brotman S: Risk, cost, and benefit of transporting ICU patients for special studies. J Trauma 1988;28:1020–1025.
3. Hurst JM, Davis K Jr, Johnson DJ, et al: Cost and complications during in-hospital transport of critically ill patients: A prospective cohort study. J Trauma 1992;33:582–585.
4. Wallen E, Venkataraman ST, Grosso MJ, et al: Intrahospital transport of critically ill pediatric patients. Crit Care Med 1995;23:1588–1595.
5. Andrews PJ, Piper IR, Dearden NM, Miller JD: Secondary insults during intrahospital transport of head-injured patients. Lancet 1990;335:327–330.
6. Kalisch BJ, Kalisch PA, Burns SM, et al: Intrahospital transport of neuro ICU patients. J Neurosci Nurs 1995;27:69–77.
7. Smith I, Fleming S, Cernaianu A: Mishaps during transport from the intensive care unit. Crit Care Med 1990;18:278–281.
8. Taylor JO, Chulay, Landers CF, et al: Monitoring high-risk cardiac patients during transportation in hospital. Lancet 1970;2:1205–1208.
9. Braman SS, Dunn SM, Amico CA, Millman RP: Complications of intrahospital transport in critically ill patients. Ann Intern Med 1987;107:469–473.
10. Evans A, Winslow EH: Oxygen saturation and hemodynamic response in critically ill, mechanically ventilated adults during intrahospital transport. Am J Crit Care 1995;4:106–111.
11. Insel J, Weissman C, Kemper M, et al: Cardiovascular changes during transport of critically ill and postoperative patients. Crit Care Med 1986;14:539–542.
12. Stearley HE: Patients' outcomes: Intrahospital transportation and monitoring of critically ill patients by a specially trained ICU nursing staff. Am J Crit Care 1998;7:282–287.
13. Weg JG, Haas CF: Safe intrahospital transport of critically ill ventilator-dependent patients. Chest 1989;96:631–635.
14. Waddell G: Movement of critically ill patients within hospital. BMJ 1975;2:417–419.

15. Smith SC, Clarke TA, Matthews TG, et al: Transportation of newborn infants. Ir Med J 1990;83:152–153.
16. Dockery WK, Futterman C, Keller SR, et al: A comparison of manual and mechanical ventilation during pediatric transport. Crit Care Med 1999;27:802–806.
17. Gervais HW, Eberle B, Konietzke D, et al: Comparison of blood gases of ventilated patients during transport. Crit Care Med 1987;15:761–763.
18. Hurst JM, Davis K Jr, Branson RD, Johannigman JA: Comparison of blood gases during transport using two methods of ventilatory support. J Trauma 1989;29:1637–1640.
19. Waydhas C, Schneck G, Duswald KH: Deterioration of respiratory function after intra-hospital transport of critically ill surgical patients. Intensive Care Med 1995;21:784–789.
20. Kollef MH, Von Harz B, Prentice D, et al: Patient transport from intensive care increases the risk of developing ventilator-associated pneumonia. Chest 1997;112:765–773.
21. Carson KJ, Drew BJ: Electrocardiographic changes in critically ill adults during intrahospital transport. Prog Cardiovasc Nurs 1994;9:4–12.
22. Waydhas C: Intrahospital transport of critically ill patients. Crit Care 1999;3:R83–R89.
23. Hess DGG: The effects of two-hand versus one-hand ventilation on volumes delivered during bag-valve ventilation at various resistances and compliances. Respir Care 1987;32:1025–1028.
24. Nakamura T, Fujino Y, Uchiyama A, et al: Intrahospital transport of critically ill patients using ventilator with patient-triggering function. Chest 2003;123:159–164.
25. Evans W, Capelle SC, Edelstone DI: Lack of a critical cardiac output and critical systemic oxygen delivery during low cardiac output in the third trimester in the pregnant sheep. Am J Obstet Gynecol 1996;175:222–228.
26. Branson RD: Intrahospital transport of critically ill, mechanically ventilated patients. Respir Care 1992;37:775–793.
27. Heinrichs W, Mertzlufft F, Dick W: Accuracy of delivered versus preset minute ventilation of portable emergency ventilators. Crit Care Med 1989;17:682–685.
28. Campbell RS, Paul N, Johannigman JA, et al: Comparison of the imposed work of breathing of 9 portable ventilators [abstract]. Crit Care Med 1999;27:A107.
29. Johannigman JA, Branson RD, Campbell R, Hurst JM: Laboratory and clinical evaluation of the MAX transport ventilator. Respir Care 1990;35:952–959.
30. Campbell RS, Johannigman JA, Branson RD, et al: Battery duration of portable ventilators: Effects of control variable, positive end-expiratory pressure, and inspired oxygen concentration. Respir Care 2002;47:1173–1183.
31. Barton AC, Tuttle-Newhall JE, Szalados JE: Portable power supply for continuous mechanical ventilation during intrahospital transport of critically ill patients with ARDS. Chest 1997;112:560–563.
32. Murphy EJ, Desautels DA, Modell JH: A compact headboard and ventilator transport system. Crit Care Med 1978;6:387–388.
33. Campbell RS, Davis K Jr, Johnson DJ, et al: Laboratory and clinical evaluation of the impact Uni-Vent 750 portable ventilator. Respir Care 1992;37:29–36.
34. McGough EK, Banner MJ, Melker RJ: Variations in tidal volume with portable transport ventilators. Respir Care 1992;37:233–239.
35. Zanetta G, Robert D, Guerin C: Evaluation of ventilators used during transport of ICU patients: A bench study. Intensive Care Med 2002;28:443–451.
36. Bernasconi M, Ploysongsang Y, Gottfried SB, et al: Respiratory compliance and resistance in mechanically ventilated patients with acute respiratory failure. Intensive Care Med 1988;14:547–553.
37. Broseghini C, Brandolese R, Poggi R, et al: Respiratory mechanics during the first day of mechanical ventilation in patients with pulmonary edema and chronic airway obstruction. Am Rev Respir Dis 1988;138:355–361.
38. East TD, Andriano KP, Pace NL: Computer-controlled optimization of positive end-expiratory pressure. Crit Care Med 1986;14:792–797.
39. Bhatia N, Silver P, Quinn C, Sagy M: Evaluation of a portable blood gas analyzer for pediatric interhospital transport. J Emerg Med 1998;16:871–874.
40. Palmon SC, Liu M, Moore LE, Kirsch JR: Capnography facilitates tight control of ventilation during transport. Crit Care Med 1996;24:608–611.
41. Tobias JD, Lynch A, Garrett J: Alterations of end-tidal carbon dioxide during the intrahospital transport of children. Pediatr Emerg Care 1996;12:249–251.
42. Hanning CD, Gilmour DG, Hothersal AP, et al: Movement of the critically ill within hospital. Intensive Care Med 1978;4:137–143.
43. Holst D, Rudolph P, Wendt M: Mobile workstation for anaesthesia and intensive-care medicine. Lancet 2000;355:1431–1432.
44. Link J, Krause H, Wagner W, Papadopoulos G: Intrahospital transport of critically ill patients. Crit Care Med 1990;18:1427–1429.
45. Singer M, Vermaat J, Hall G, et al: Hemodynamic effects of manual hyperinflation in critically ill mechanically ventilated patients. Chest 1994;106:1182–1187.
46. Brokalaki HJ, Brokalakis JD, Digenis GE, et al: Intrahospital transportation: Monitoring and risks. Intensive Crit Care Nurs 1996;12:183–186.
47. Edge WE, Kanter RK, Weigle CG, Walsh RF: Reduction of morbidity in interhospital transport by specialized pediatric staff. Crit Care Med 1994;22:1186–1191.
48. Bellingan G, Olivier T, Batson S, Webb A: Comparison of a specialist retrieval team with current United Kingdom practice for the transport of critically ill patients. Intensive Care Med 2000;26:740–744.
49. Leslie AJ, Stephenson TJ: Audit of neonatal intensive care transport: Closing the loop. Acta Paediatr 1997;86:1253–1256.
50. Velmahos GC, Demetriades D, Ghilardi M, et al: Life support for trauma and transport: A mobile ICU for safe in-hospital transport of critically injured patients. J Am Coll Surg 2004;199:62–68.

# CHAPTER 32

# Air Embolism and Diving Injury

Robert A. van Hulst, Claus-Martin Muth, and Peter Radermacher

Air embolism is a potentially life-threatening complication of many medical and surgical procedures.[1,2] It may also occur as a result of various diagnostic and surgical procedures when air is accidentally infused into the systemic circulation.[3] Air bubbles that occlude the brain vasculature may cause acute neurologic events such as coma, disorientation, focal sensory deficits, or motor deficits.[4] Another problem faced by clinicians is cerebral air embolism (CAE), which occurs in divers and in compressed air workers as a result of rapid ascent.[5] In addition, arterial air embolism can lead to various cardiovascular symptoms, regardless of the underlying cause.[1,6] Table 32.1 shows an overview of documented cases of clinical gas embolism.

In most cases, "gas" embolism is, in fact, air embolism, although the medical use of other gases such as carbon dioxide, nitrous oxide, nitrogen, and helium can also result in embolism.[7-9] In an experimental setting, the effects of air emboli differ greatly, depending on whether they are venous or arterial and on the organs where the emboli finally lodge.[10] Although air bubbles can reach any organ, occlusion of the cerebral and cardiac circulation is particularly deleterious because these systems are highly vulnerable to hypoxia.

## CLASSIFICATION

### Diving-Related Embolism

Air embolism resulting from pulmonary barotrauma is an ongoing cause of concern in all types of diving operations.[11] In diving, pulmonary conditions associated with bronchial obstruction are hazardous, particularly during ascent, even when all the usual precautions are taken.[12] Air embolism is the clinical manifestation of Boyle's law as it affects the lung and is the result of overdistention and rupture of the alveoli by expanding gases during ascent. Normally, intrapulmonary and environmental pressures are equalized by exhalation during ascent. A change in pressure of approximately 70 mm Hg is sufficient to cause pulmonary barotrauma.[13,14] Thus, a full inspiration with compressed air at 1 m underwater could theoretically lead to pulmonary barotrauma.

### Venous Air Embolism

Venous air emboli most often occur in patients during the insertion, maintenance, or removal of a central venous catheter.[15,16] In a review of the literature, Heckmann and colleagues discussed 26 cases in which most venous air emboli occurred during a subclavian or jugular vein catheterization procedure.[3] Embolism can also occur as a result of lung trauma induced by mechanical ventilation.[17,18] Bricker and colleagues used transesophageal echocardiography in patients who required mechanical ventilation with positive end-expiratory pressure and found continuous venous air embolism in five of the eight patients with lung trauma.[19] These investigators concluded the occurrence of venous air embolism is relatively high in patients with pulmonary barotrauma associated with increased ventilatory pressures and that venous emboli may contribute to cardiovascular instability and may exacerbate lung injury in critically ill patients. In gynecologic surgical and diagnostic procedures, venous air embolism is a rare and unexpected complication.[20,21]

**Table 32-1   An Overview of Documented Cases of Clinical Gas Embolism**

**Surgery**
Neurosurgery, especially upright
Liver transplantation
Laparoscopic surgery
Prostatectomy

**Orthopedics**
Hip replacement
Arthroscopy

**Thoracic Surgery**
Open heart surgery
Intraaortic balloon pump
Cardiac ablation

**Gynecology**
Hysterectomy
Cesarean section

**Anesthesiology**
Central line placement
Epidural catheter placement
Cardiopulmonary
   resuscitation
Positive pressure ventilation

**Pulmonary Medicine**
Percutaneous lung biopsy
Bronchoscopy
Chest/lung trauma

**Internal Medicine**
Hemodialysis
Percutaneous lithotripsy
Gastrointestinal endoscopy
Cardiology: angiographic studies and procedures

**Radiology**
Infusion computed tomography scanning

**Otolaryngology**
Laser (neodymium:yttrium-aluminum-garnet) surgery
   on the larynx and trachea/bronchi

**Miscellaneous**
Blast injuries
Self-induced (suicide) injury
Orogenital sex
Scuba diving
Hydrogen peroxide irrigation/ingestion
Dental implants

Laparoscopy using carbon dioxide can also lead to a venous carbon dioxide embolism.[8] Finally, during neurosurgery air may enter the veins, especially when patients are in the sitting position.[22]

## Paradoxical Embolism

In principle, every venous gas embolism has the potential to develop into an arterial gas embolism; when this happens, it is called a *paradoxical embolism*.[23] A paradoxical embolism occurs when the filter capacity for air bubbles of the pulmonary capillary bed is exceeded, and gas bubbles shunt from the venous side to the arterial side of the circulation. Transcardiac passage of venous gas bubbles can also occur in the presence of any right-to-left shunt, including a patent foramen ovale.[24] The application of positive end-expiratory pressure during mechanical ventilation,[25] Valsalva maneuvers,[26] and coughing[27] can increase the interatrial movement of bubbles in patients with atrial shunts.

In divers, a shunt from the right atrium to the left atrium can cause bubbles that have formed during decompression to pass directly to the left side of the heart and into the arterial circulation, thus bypassing the pulmonary filter.[28,29] It is believed that the presence of a patent foramen ovale may be a risk factor for the development of decompression illness,[30] particularly decompression illness occurring early (within minutes after exiting the water) and with cerebral signs and symptoms out of proportion to the dive stress. A consensus opinion on the approach to a patent foramen ovale as a risk factor for decompression illness has not been reached.[31,32]

## Arterial Gas Embolism

Arterial gas embolism causes ischemia in the organ in which the air bubbles are trapped. Although air bubbles can reach any organ, occlusion of the cerebral and cardiac circulation is particularly deleterious because these systems are highly vulnerable to hypoxia.

## Coronary Air Embolism

A key article on coronary air embolism was published in 1949 by Durant and colleagues, who noted the main symptoms: temporary ischemia of the myocardium, short periods (<5 minutes) of hypertensive crisis, and ventricular fibrillation.[33] Coronary air embolism has been studied by intracoronary injection of a bolus of air that led to a serious depression of heart function.[34] In a study of dogs, a 28% mortality rate was reported for an air dose of 0.02 mL/kg, whereas surviving animals showed recovery of heart function within 15 minutes. Other studies of coronary air embolism showed that depression of regional myocardial function could pass

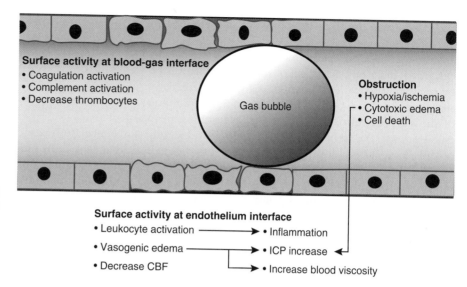

**Surface activity at blood-gas interface**
• Coagulation activation
• Complement activation
• Decrease thrombocytes

Gas bubble

**Obstruction**
• Hypoxia/ischemia
• Cytotoxic edema
• Cell death

**Figure 32.1** Bubble obstruction in a cerebral vessel. Three levels of inter-action are present: (1) the bubble interacts with the blood; (2) there is a reaction with the endothelium; (3) the obstruction leads to distal hypoxia and ischemia, finally resulting in neuronal cell death. CBF,: cerebral blood flow; ICP, intracranial pressure.

**Surface activity at endothelium interface**
• Leukocyte activation ⟶ • Inflammation
• Vasogenic edema ⟶ • ICP increase
• Decrease CBF ⟶ • Increase blood viscosity

unnoticed on the basis of hemodynamic measurements. Air bubbles with a volume of 2 μL/kg injected in the coronary artery did not change systemic hemodynamics, whereas significant changes were found in systolic segment shortening, a finding suggesting depressed myocardial function with silent ischemia.[34,35]

## Cerebral Air Embolism

CAE is a serious hazard: when bubbles occlude the brain vasculature (Fig. 32.1), intracranial pressure (ICP) increases,[7] and an extremely nonhomogeneous distribution of blood flow in the brain causes hyperemia and ischemia.[36-39] The pathophysiology of CAE mainly depends on the air bubble size. Microbubbles may irritate the vascular wall and lead to an instantaneous breakdown of the blood-brain barrier.[40] In some cases, however, these tiny bubbles are rapidly absorbed and only briefly interrupt cerebral arteriolar flow.[41] A good correlation has been found between cerebral blood flow and brain function after gas embolism by small bubbles at a maximum size of 250 μm.[36,42,43] The passage of an air bubble obstructs local blood flow, but flow normalizes after disappearance of the bubbles. However, normalization is often only temporary, and blood flow may subsequently decrease to levels lower than those required to maintain neuronal function and survival.[43-45] An explanation for this mechanism was suggested by Dexter and Hindman, who calculated that the absorption of large air emboli may take several hours, which is long enough to cause primary ischemic injury with diffuse brain edema leading to raised ICP.[46] This finding was later confirmed by our group in an experimental study showing that after a large air embolism ICP increased from 12 to 52 mm Hg within 2 hours after embolization, with severely detrimental effects on brain oxygenation and glucose metabolism.[47]

## EFFECTS ON BLOOD-BRAIN BARRIER

The presence of bubbles and their contact with the endothelium of the blood-brain barrier lead to activation and adhesion of polymorphonuclear leukocytes in the damaged area of the brain[48] (see Fig. 32.1). Brain swelling and inflammation may therefore play a stronger role in the occurrence of infarction by air emboli than they do in other forms of cerebral ischemia.[49] Leukocytes have been implicated in the progressive fall in cerebral blood flow and decreased cerebral function in animal models of gas embolism.[42,50] Various plasma proteins, including the coagulation system, complement, and kinins, are also activated by bubbles.[51-54] Coagulopathies are common in animal models of air embolism but are extremely rare in humans.[55]

## DIAGNOSIS OF CEREBRAL AIR EMBOLISM

The greatest risks for a cerebral arterial gas embolism are cardiac surgery with cardiopulmonary bypass,[56,57] hip replacement,[58,59] craniotomy performed with the patient in a sitting position,[60,61] and cesarean section.[21] All these procedures have an incised vascular bed and a hydrostatic gradient favoring the intravascular entry of gas.[2] In most of these patients, the diagnosis of CAE is made during recovery from anesthesia, when neurologic symptoms become evident. Air embolism can manifest in many ways, depending on the patient's position, the volume and type of gas, the size of the bubbles, and the rapidity of gas entry into the arteries.

For the clinician, pathognomonic signs have been described, including detection of air in the retinal vessels by ophthalmoscopic examination and the occurrence of sharply defined areas of pallor on the tongue. Marbling of the skin may also occur, presumably resulting from embolism of the skin vessels; this sign is especially notable in superiorly located parts of the body because the distribution of air within the circulation is determined by the principle of air buoyancy.[33] Pulmonary symptoms such as chest pain, dyspnea, and tachypnea may occur. Neurologic symptoms and signs include dizziness, chest pain, paresthesias, convulsions, paralysis, nausea, visual disturbances, and headache. Sporadic or continued seizure activity may also occur. Approximately 50% of the patients have some history of unconsciousness at some time.[4,62,63] Anesthesia and analgesics alter the symptoms and may complicate evaluation of the patient's clinical status. In addition to neurologic signs, patients may have circulatory collapse, evidence of lung rupture, and a variety of pain syndromes.[63]

The diagnosis of CAE should be made when there are central neurologic changes and the circumstances are such that a gas embolism could have occurred. However, because definite confirmation of the diagnosis is not always easy, anesthesiologists and surgeons should be aware of the risk of an embolic event during medical procedures. Ultrasound techniques such as transthoracic and transesophageal echocardiography during surgery can visualize intravenous or intracardiac bubbles.[64,65] Direct perioperative monitoring of cardiorespiratory parameters by the anesthesiologist may also detect emboli; for example, a sudden decrease in end-tidal carbon dioxide by capnography or a sudden increase in pulmonary artery pressure may be a sign of air embolism during surgery.[66]

### Radiographic Techniques

Animal studies[67,68] and several clinical case reports have used computed tomography (CT) to demonstrate the presence of CAE.[69–75] Conversely, Hodgson and colleagues studied 47 divers with neurologic or pulmonary symptoms by CT scanning and were unable to show any evidence of CAE in any of the divers.[76] Brain magnetic resonance imaging (MRI) in CAE may show local edema, but in two such cases, even the MRI scan was normal.[77] A review of the studies using CT, MRI, and single-photon emission CT (SPECT) allows us to conclude that, at present, no single imaging technique has sufficient accuracy to warrant its use for diagnostic purposes; therefore, clinical evaluation is still preferred for the assessment of CAE.[78] Although radiographic investigations may support or confirm the diagnosis of CAE, they cannot be used to rule it out definitively.

## THERAPY

Immediate treatment aims to interrupt the intervention that caused the embolic event. If indicated in a comatose patient, cardiopulmonary resuscitation and endotracheal intubation should also be performed as quickly as possible to maintain adequate oxygenation and ventilation.[4] Administration of oxygen is important, not only to treat hypoxia and hypoxemia, but also to decrease air bubble size by establishing a diffusion gradient that favors the elimination of gas from the bubbles.[2,79] Although hyperventilation is recommended,[80] investigators demonstrated in pigs that hypocapnia and hyperoxygenation do not improve cerebral functional parameters as characterized by, for example, ICP and brain lactate levels.[81] Systemic hypertension for a short period following bubble entrapment in the cerebral circulation is usual.[6,33] A short period of hypertension is therapeutic because it facilitates bubble redistribution through the arterioles to the capillaries and into the veins. Although supranormal blood pressure has been promoted,[80] in some animal models prolonged hypertension leading to increased ICP compromised the neurologic outcome, as characterized by electroencephalographic and other neurophysiologic parameters.[42,82] Far worse is progressive hypotension. A fall in blood pressure results in both increased bubble entrapment and, given that the autoregulation is lost,[45] causes cerebral blood flow to fall to levels lower than those required for normal neuronal function. Therefore, the primary treatment goal is to maintain normal blood pressure.[2]

### Adjuvant Drug Therapy

In the 1980s, Bove stated that the use of drugs in the treatment of CAE is often empirical and controversial, and it varies among different centers and countries.[83] Twenty-five years later, this statement is still valid.[84]

**Intravenous Fluids** Hemoconcentration has been reported in CAE,[85–87] and posttreatment residual symptoms have been correlated with the degree of hemoconcentration.[65] Therefore, fluid administration is advantageous in patients with CAE, to achieve normovolemia. For a diver, fluid replacement is particularly important because, as a result of immersion, there is already diuresis-induced hemoconcentration and, eventually, hypovolemia that affect off-gassing of inert gases in decompression illness in a negative way. For hemodilution, colloid solutions are preferred because it is believed that crystalloids may promote cerebral edema. However, there is no scientific proof that colloids are superior to crystalloids in focal brain edema,[88] so no clear rationale supports the use of one over the other,[89] although hydroxyethyl starch (HES) may offer some advantages (see later). In animals, even moderate hemodilution to a hematocrit of 30% has been shown to reduce neurologic damage.[90]

**Glucose** Neurologic traumas can be worsened by hyperglycemia,[91,92] probably resulting from increased production of lactate, which leads to intracellular acidosis. Because a small amount of glucose (e.g., 5% dextrose solution), even in the absence of significant hyperglycemia, may worsen the neurologic outcome,[93] it is advised to avoid use of glucose-containing solutions in the acute phase of CAE.[84] Electrolyte solutions containing lactate have a buffer effect and avoid the potential risk of hyperchloremic acidosis unless another anion is present in the solution. Furthermore, lactate is a metabolic substrate that has possibly protective effects in the brain, as shown in animal and human studies.[94–96]

**Albumin** Albumin is the natural colloid in human blood. It formerly played a role in colloid infusion therapy. However, it has been replaced by artificial colloids for various reasons, starting with the possibility of transmitting infectious diseases such as variant Creutzfeldt-Jakob disease.[97] This acquired and fatal human prion disease apparently results from exposure to the bovine spongiform encephalopathy (BSE) agent through human blood donations.

**Gelatin** Gelatin solutions are prepared from bovine collagen. Of all the colloid preparations, gelatin solutions have the highest incidence of allergic reactions.[98] Furthermore, there is a very small but real risk of transmission of BSE. For these reasons, as well as its relatively short duration of action and its small volume effect, gelatin is no longer recommended for clinical use.

**Hydroxyethyl Starch** HES is a clinically well-tolerated complex polysaccharide.[89] It is available in multiple preparations, each with different pharmacologic characteristics based on concentration, molecular weight, degree of substitution, and C2/C6 hydroxyethylation ratio. Although HES has shown a protective effect with reductions in infarct size and improved outcome in experimental models of ischemic injury in both central nervous system and peripheral tissues,[99] results of its use in clinical stroke trials, of interest because of the relation to cerebral arterial gas embolism, have been controversial. This may relate to the time window of administration of the preparation relative to the onset of vessel occlusion, as well as the pharmacologic characteristics of the particular HES preparation. Nevertheless, clinical interest in HES still remains, particularly in situations of elevated ICP. Strong evidence indicates that HES has beneficial effects on ischemic brain injury, although its mechanism of action remains unclear.

**Hypertonic Saline** Hypertonic saline (HS) has been advocated as a hyperosmolar agent for the treatment of cerebral edema, especially after traumatic brain injury, because HS solutions theoretically are better osmotic agents than mannitol. Furthermore, several case series and randomized clinical trials demonstrated improved outcome with HS therapy in traumatic brain injury.[100] Therefore, investigators have hypothesized that HS therapy could be beneficial in cerebral ischemia and stroke. In contrast, HS-induced hypernatremia and hyperosmolality may alter tissue outcome by leading to significant hypernatremia, which can increase tissue damage after vascular occlusion and focal cerebral ischemia; it has also been demonstrated that continuous HS therapy worsens infarct volume after transient focal ischemia.[101] Thus, caution is advised in the use of HS for patients who experience an ischemic insult. The combination of HS and colloid solution, such as HS with HES (HS-HES), used in small-volume resuscitation, may combine the advantages and minimize the side effects,[102,103] but this still is a matter of further research.

**Dextran** Dextran solutions were used in the past,[104] and although they may offer some advantages (e.g., improvement of the microcirculation, antisludging effects),[105] these benefits are small compared with the potential risks of acute volume overload, lung congestion, and anaphylaxis.[83,84] Therefore, dextran solutions are no longer routinely used.

**Barbiturates** CAE often causes generalized seizures that may not respond to benzodiazepines.[80] In such cases, barbiturates are recommended. Barbiturates have the advantage of reducing cerebral oxygen consumption and lowering ICP as well as inhibiting the release of endogenous catecholamines, with resulting cerebral protection after ischemia.[106,107] Intravenous phenytoin is also recommended because it protects against further convulsions during hyperbaric treatment.[108]

**Aminophylline** This drug is theoretically useful for pulmonary symptoms such as chest pain, tachypnea, and dyspnea in venous air embolism. Aminophylline is contraindicated, however, because it leads to dilatation of the pulmonary vasculature and results in increased release of trapped bubbles into the systemic circulation.[109]

**Heparin** Heparin is advocated because of its protective effect against platelet clumping, but reports on its use are not consistent. For example, a single case report of heparin that was given to a patient with neurologic symptoms indicated neither adverse nor beneficial effects.[110] In animal studies, administration of heparin alone showed no benefit in CAE,[84] whereas a combined regimen of indomethacin, prostaglandin $I_2$ (prostacyclin), and heparin resulted in a better neurophysiologic outcome in rabbits.[111] However, investigators demonstrated that, given prophylactically, heparin decreased neurologic impairment in an animal model of severe CAE.[112]

**Steroids** CAE initially induces increased transudation of fluid across a damaged blood-brain barrier (vasogenic edema) and later causes swelling of cells that no longer have sufficient energy to maintain osmotic integrity (cytotoxic edema).[113,114] Formerly, cerebral edema in CAE was treated with corticosteroids,[115,116] but because later studies showed that corticosteroids increased ischemic injury as a result of vessel occlusion,[117,118] the use of these drugs is no longer recommended.

**Lidocaine** McDermott and colleagues demonstrated in cats that lidocaine may depress the rise of blood pressure and ICP and may improve recovery of the somatosensory evoked potential following CAE.[119] Results of other animal studies showed that lidocaine reduces infarct size,[120] preserves cerebral blood flow,[118,121,122] reduces cerebral edema,[121] and preserves neuroelectrical function.[118,120,122,123] These results in brain-injured animals showed that lidocaine improves cerebral function. This finding was later confirmed in the clinical situation by Mitchell and colleagues, who reported significantly fewer postoperative cognitive deficits in patients who had undergone valve replacement and who had received lidocaine for 48 hours from the beginning of the surgical procedure.[124]

**Fluorocarbons** These carbon-fluorine compounds are characterized by a high gas-dissolving capacity (oxygen, carbon dioxide, inert gases), low viscosity, and chemical and biologic inertness.[125] Thus, intravenous administration of these agents in doses sufficient to increase the transport of these gases should both increase tissue oxygen delivery and shrink gas bubbles as a result of the higher diffusion gradient. Animal studies demonstrated a reduction in mortality in gas embolism,[126–128] a reduction in brain infarct size,[129] an improvement in cardiovascular function after air embolization,[130] and less vascular damage in the retina.[131] More studies on perfluorocarbons are needed to prove their efficacy and safety in humans, particularly with regard to oxygen toxicity.[84]

## Hyperbaric Oxygen Therapy

Hyperbaric oxygen ($HBO_2$) has been advocated as therapy for CAE.[132–135] $HBO_2$ diminishes the volume of intravascular bubbles by enhancing the ambient pressure; the increase in the partial pressure of oxygen favors denitrogenation of the cerebral tissue and diminishes the cerebral edema, and $HBO_2$ increases the partial pressure of dissolved oxygen in the blood and thus allows better oxygenation of ischemic tissue.[136,137] These physiologic modes of action seem entirely sufficient to warrant the application of $HBO_2$ in CAE, despite the lack of prospective clinical studies confirming its efficacy.[138] These findings also imply that, in a clinical study on CAE, the inclusion of an untreated patient control group would be unethical.[4] Conversely, the main criticism of the use of $HBO_2$ is that no prospective randomized trials have been conducted to prove its utility,[138,139] and only a few animal studies have shown the benefits of $HBO_2$ therapy in CAE.[140–144] However, in a pig model of CAE, our group showed that $HBO_2$ treatment after 3 minutes and after 60 minutes improved brain parameters, characterized by ICP, brain oxygenation, and brain lactate, compared with the natural progression of severe CAE.[145]

### Clinical Reports

Table 32.2 presents an overview of studies that have described reports of patients with air embolism; these studies included divers, submariners, and clinical patients. Although patients with many different iatrogenic types of gas embolism have been treated with $HBO_2$, the numbers of patients are still small. A general conclusion is that the results have been better when the time to treatment was as short as possible, although some patients were treated after a delay of as long as 48 hours.[146–148] Murphy and colleagues reported that after $HBO_2$ therapy in 16 patients, 8 had complete relief of CAE symptoms, 5 patients had partial relief, and 3 had no benefit.[149] In a study of 34 patients by Takahashi and associates, 62% had a good recovery.[150] Blanc and colleagues reported a significantly better outcome in patients with venous air embolism with a delay in treatment of less than 6 hours (84%), as opposed to more than 6 hours (53%); in contrast, with arterial air embolism, there were no differences between groups with less or more than 6 hours' delay.[4] Ziser and colleagues,[151] studying 17 patients with CAE resulting from extracorporeal circulation, reported a total recovery in 47% compared with 58% in the study by Blanc and associates. However, the time elapsed before $HBO_2$ treatment was 9.6 hours compared with 3.5 hours in the study by Blanc and associates. Although the recovery rates in these very heterogeneous groups of patients vary widely, it

**Table 32-2  Air Embolism in a Clinical or Diving Population Undergoing Hyperbaric Oxygen Therapy**

| Authors | No. of Patients | C/D | Mean Delay/Range | Assessment | Outcome* Fully Recovered | Minor Sequelae | Severe Sequelae | Dead |
|---|---|---|---|---|---|---|---|---|
| Pearson and Goad, 1982[115] | 5 | D | 20 min/5–60 min | Neurologic examination EEG | 80% EEG normal | | | 20% |
| Murphy et al, 1985[149] | 16 | C | 8 hr/0.25–25 hr | Neurologic examination | 50% | 31% | 6% | 12% |
| Leitch and Green, 1986[12] | 89 | D | <10 min[†] | Neurologic examination | 65% | 18% | 16% | 1% |
| Takahashi et al, 1987[150] | 34 | C | 13 hr/0.5–40 hr | Neurologic examination | 62% | 15% | | 24% |
| Neuman and Hallenbeck, 1987[152] | 4 | D | 9 hr/1–15 hr | Neurologic examination CT scan | 75% CT scan normal | 25% CT scan normal | | |
| Bitterman and Melamed, 1988[146] | 6 | C | 24 hr/11–60 hr | Neurologic examination CT scan | 33% CT scan normal | 33% CT scan normal | | 33% |
| Massey et al, 1990[147] | 14 | C | 17.5 hr/1–48 hr | Neurologic examination | 50% | 14% | 14% | 22% |
| Kol et al, 1993[153] | 6 | C | 3 hr/2–20 hr | Neurologic examination | 50% | | 17% | 33% |
| Mushkat et al, 1995[20] | 4 | C | 26 hr/3–48 hr | Neurologic examination CT scan | 75% CT scan normal | | | 25% |
| Ziser et al, 1999[151] | 17 | C | 9.6 hr/1–20 hr | Neurologic examination | 47% | | 35% | 18% |
| Blanc et al, 2002[4] | 86 | C | 3.5 hr/2–8 hr | Neurologic examination | 58% | 24% | 9% | 8% |
| Benson et al, 2003[154] | 19 | C | 8.9 hr/0.5–28 hr | Neurologic examination | 42% | 32% | | 26% |

*The authors used different classifications for the neurologic outcome after completion of the hyperbaric oxygen therapy. In general, minor neurologic sequelae or major improvement means that only sensory deficits remain, whereas severe neurologic sequelae or partially recovered means that motor deficits are still present.
[†]Divers and submariners during free ascent or escape training, where the recompression chamber is on location.
C/D, clinical/diving; CT, computed tomography; EEG, electroencephalogram.

seems that early application of $HBO_2$ therapy plays an important role in the management and treatment of iatrogenic CAE.

## CONCLUSIONS

Air embolism, the entry of gas into the vascular structures, is a mainly iatrogenic clinical problem that can result in serious morbidity and even death. In most cases, gas embolism is actually air embolism, although the medical use of other gases such as carbon dioxide, nitrous oxide, nitrogen, and helium can also result in embolism. Significant amounts of in vivo data demonstrate that cerebral damage is caused by even small volumes of arterial gas. However, the exact relevance of these data for the clinical situation has not yet been fully elucidated. Although data on the morbidity and mortality of air embolism in humans are scarce, many case reports and retrospective studies on small numbers of patients suffering from CAE have shown that $HBO_2$ is the treatment of choice for this complication.

## REFERENCES

1. Murphy BP, Harford FJ, Cramer FS: Cerebral air embolism resulting from invasive medical procedures: Treatment with hyperbaric oxygen. Ann Surg 1985;201:242–245.
2. Muth CM, Shank ES: Gas embolism. N Engl J Med 2000;342:476–482.
3. Heckmann JG, Lang CJG, Kindler K, et al: Neurologic manifestations of cerebral air embolism as a complication of central venous catheterization. Crit Care Med 2000;28:1621–1625.
4. Blanc P, Boussuges A, Henriette K, et al: Iatrogenic cerebral air embolism: Importance of an early hyperbaric oxygenation. Intensive Care Med 2002;28:559–563.
5. Melamed Y, Shupak A, Bitterman H: Medical problems associated with underwater diving. N Engl J Med 1992;326:30–35.
6. Evans DE, Kobrine AI, Weathersby PK, Bradley ME: Cardiovascular effects of cerebral air embolism. Stroke 1981;12:338–344.
7. de la Torre E, Meredith J, Netsky MG: Cerebral air embolism in the dog. Arch Neurol 1062;6:307–316.
8. McGrath BJ, Zimmerman JE, Williams JF, Parmet J: Carbon dioxide embolism treated with hyperbaric oxygen. Can J Anaesth 1989;36:586–589.
9. Mitchell SJ, Benson M, Vadlamudi L, Miller P: Cerebral arterial gas embolism by helium: An unusual case successfully treated with hyperbaric oxygen and lidocaine. Ann Emerg Med 2000;35:300–303.
10. Gomes OM, Pereira SN, Castagña RC, et al: The importance of the different sites of air injection in the tolerance of arterial air embolism. J Thorac Cardiovasc Surg 1973;65:563–568.
11. Walker R: Pulmonary barotrauma in divers. In Edmonds E, Lowry C, Pennefather J (eds): Diving and Subaquatic Medicine, 4th ed. Oxford: Butterworth-Heinemann, 2002, pp 55–71.
12. Leitch DR, Green RD: Pulmonary barotrauma in divers and the treatment of cerebral arterial gas embolism. Aviat Space Environ Med 1986;57:931–938.
13. Schaefer KE, McNulty WP, Carey C, Liebow AA: Mechanisms in development of interstitial emphysema and air embolism on decompression from depth. J Appl Physiol 1958;13:15–29.
14. Malhotra MS, Wright HC: The effects of raised intrapulmonary pressure on the lungs of fresh unchilled cadavers. J Pathol Bacteriol 1961;82:198–202.
15. Halliday P, Anderson DN, Davidson AI: Management of cerebral air embolism secondary to a disconnected central venous catheter. Br J Surg 1994;81:71.
16. Palmon SC, Moore LE, Lundberg J, Toung T: Venous air embolism: A review. J Clin Anesth 1997;9:251–257.
17. Marini JJ, Culver BH: Systemic gas embolism complicating mechanical ventilation in the adult respiratory distress syndrome. Ann Intern Med 1989;110:699–703.
18. Ho AMH, Ling E: Systemic air embolism after lung trauma. Anesthesiology 1999;90:564–575.
19. Bricker MB, Morris WP, Allen SJ, et al: Venous air embolism in patients with pulmonary barotrauma. Crit Care Med 1994;22:1692–1698.
20. Mushkat Y, Luxman D, Nachum Z, et al: Gas embolism complicating obstetric or gynecologic procedures: Case reports and review of the literature. Eur J Obstet Gynecol Reprod Biol 1995;63:97–103.
21. Weissman A, Kol S, Peretz BA: Gas embolism in obstetrics and gynaecology: A review. J Reprod Med 1996;41:103–111.
22. Porter JM, Pidgeon C, Cunningham AJ: The sitting position in neurosurgery: A critical appraisal. Br J Anaesth 1999;82:117–128.
23. Black M, Calvin J, Chan KL, Walley VM: Paradoxic air embolism in the absence of an intracardiac defect. Chest 1999;99:754–755.
24. Fraker TD: Detection and exclusion of interatrial shunts by two-dimensional echo-cardiography and peripheral venous injection. Circulation 1979;59:379–384.
25. Jaffe RA, Pinto FJ, Schnittger I, Brock-Untne JG: Intraoperative ventilator-induced right to left intracardiac shunt. Anesthesiology 1991;75:153–155.
26. Chen WJ, Kuan P, Lien WP, Lin Y: Detection of patent foramen ovale by contrast echocardiography. Chest 1992;101:1515–1520.
27. Dubourg O, Bourdarias JP, Farcot JC: Contrast echocardiographic visualization of cough-induced right-to-left shunt through a patent ovale. J Am Coll Cardiol 1987;4:587–594.
28. Vik A, Jenssen BM, Brubakk AO: Paradoxical air embolism in pigs with a patent foramen ovale. Undersea Biomed Res 1992;19:361–374.
29. Vik A, Jenssen BM, Brubakk AO: Arterial gas bubbles after decompression in pigs with patent foramen ovale. Undersea Hyperbaric Med 1993;20:121–131.
30. Wilmhurst PT, Byrne JC, Webb-Peploe MM: Relation between intracardial shunts and decompression sickness in divers. Lancet 1989;2:1302–1306.
31. Tetzlaf K, Muth CM: Right to left shunts and the risk of decompression illness. Crit Care Med 2003;31:2083.
32. Foster PP, Boriek AM, Butler BD, et al: Patent foramen ovale and paradoxical systemic embolism: A bibliographic review. Aviat Space Environ Med 2003;74:B1–B64.
33. Durant TM, Oppenheimer MJ, Webster MR, Long J: Arterial air embolism. Am Heart J 1949;38:481–500.
34. Blankenstein JH van, Slager CJ, Schuurbiers JCH, et al: Heart function after injection of small air bubbles in coronary artery of pigs. J Appl Physiol 1993;75:1201–1207.
35. Blankenstein JH van, Slager CJ, Soei LK, et al: Effect of arterial blood pressure and ventilation gases on cardiac depression

induced by coronary air embolism. J Appl Physiol 1994;77: 1896–1902.

36. Hossmann KA, Fritz H: Coupling of function, metabolism and blood flow after air embolism of the cat brain. Adv Neurol 1978;20:255–262.

37. Fritz H, Hossmann KA: Arterial air embolism in the cat brain. Stroke 1979;10:581–589.

38. Hossmann KA: Experimental models for the investigation of brain ischemia. Cardiovasc Res 1998;39:106–120.

39. Williams DJ, Doolette DJ, Upton RN: Increased cerebral blood flow and cardiac output following cerebral arterial air embolism in sheep. Clin Exp Pharmacol Physiol 2001;28:868–872.

40. Johansson BB: Cerebral air embolism and the blood-brain barrier in the rat. Acta Neurol Scand 1980;62:201–209.

41. Gorman DF, Browning DM: Cerebral vasoreactivity and arterial gas embolism. Undersea Biomed Res 1986;13:317–335.

42. Dutka AJ, Hallenbeck JM, Kochanek P: A brief episode of severe arterial hypertension induces delayed deterioration of brain function and worsens blood flow after transient multifocal cerebral ischemia. Stroke 1987;18:386–395.

43. Helps SC, Meyer-Witting M, Reilly PL, Gorman DF: Increasing doses of intracarotid air and cerebral blood flow in rabbits. Stroke 1990;21:1340–1345.

44. Meldrum BS, Papy JJ, Vigouroux RA: Intracarotid air embolism in the baboon: Effects on cerebral blood flow and the electroencephalogram. Brain Res 1971;25:301–315.

45. Helps SC, Meyer-Witting M, Reilly PL, Gorman DF: The effect of gas emboli on rabbit cerebral blood flow. Stroke 1990;21: 94–99.

46. Dexter F, Hindman BJ: Recommendations for hyperbaric oxygen therapy of cerebral air embolism based on a mathematical model of bubble absorption. Anesth Analg 1997;84:1203–1207.

47. Hulst van RA, Lameris TW, Hasan D, et al: Effects on cerebral air embolism on brain metabolism in pigs. Acta Neurol Scand 2003;108:118–124.

48. Mitchell SJ, Gorman DF: The pathophysiology of cerebral arterial gas embolism. J Extra Corpor Technol 2002;34:18–23.

49. Hindman BJ, Dexter F, Subieta A, et al: Brain injury after cerebral arterial air embolism in the rabbit as determined by triphenyltetrazolium staining. Anesthesiology 1999;90: 1462–1473.

50. Helps SC, Gorman DF: Air embolism of the brain in rabbits pretreated with mechlorethamine. Stroke 1991;22:351–354.

51. Warren BA, Philip PB, Inwood MJ: The ultrastructural morphology of air embolism: Platelet adhesion to the interface and endothelial damage. Br J Exp Pathol 1973;54:163–172.

52. Ward CA, Koheil A, McCulloch D, et al: Activation of compliment at the plasma-air and serum-air interface of rabbits. J Appl Physiol 1986;60:1651–1658.

53. Ward CA, McCulloch, Yee D, et al: Complement activation involvement in decompression sickness of rabbits. Undersea Biomed Res 1990;18:51–66.

54. Pekna M, Nilsson L, Nilsson-Ekdahl K, et al: Evidence for iC3 generation during cardiopulmonary bypass as the result of blood-gas interaction. Clin Exp Immunol 1993;91:404–409.

55. Francis TJR, Mitchell SJ: Pathophysiology of the decompression sickness. In Brubakk AO, Neuman TS (eds): The Physiology and Medicine of Diving, 5th ed. Philadelphia: WB Saunders, 2003, pp 530–556.

56. Armon C, Deschamps C, Adkinson C, et al: Hyperbaric treatment of cerebral air embolism sustained during an open-heart surgical procedure. Mayo Clin Proc 1991;66:565–571.

57. Stump DA, Rogers AT, Hammon JW, Neuwman SP: Cerebral emboli and cognitive outcome after cardiac surgery. J Cardiothorac Vasc Anesth 1996;10:113–119.

58. Ngai SH, Stinchfield FE, Triner L: Air embolism during total hip arthroplasties. Anesthesiology 1974;40:405–407.

59. Evans RD, Palazzo MG, Ackers JW: Air embolism during total hip replacement: Comparison of two surgical techniques. Br J Anaesth 1989;62:243–247.

60. Giebler R, Kollenberg B, Pohlen G, Peters J: Effect of positive end-expiratory pressure on the incidence of venous air embolism and on the cardiovascular response to the sitting position during neurosurgery. Br J Anaesth 1998;80:30–35.

61. Porter JM, Pidgeon C, Cunningham AJ: The sitting position in neurosurgery: A critical appraisal. Br J Anaesth 1999;82:117–128.

62. Gillen HW: Symptomatology of cerebral gas embolism. Neurology 1968;18:507–512.

63. Peirce EC II: Cerebral gas embolism (arterial) with special reference to iatrogenic accidents. HBO Rev 1980;1:161–184.

64. Mammoto T, Hayashi Y, Ohnishi Y, Kuro Y: Incidence of venous and paradoxical air embolism in neurosurgical patients in sitting position: Detection by transesophageal echocardiography. Acta Anaesthesiol Scand 1998;42:643–647.

65. Boussuges A, Blanc P, Molenat F, et al: Haemoconcentration in neurological decompression illness. Int J Sports Med 1996;17:351–55.

66. Bedford RF, Marshall WK, Butler A, Welsh JE: Cardiac catheters for diagnosis and treatment of venous air embolism: A prospective study in man. J Neurosurg 1981;55:610–614.

67. Annane D, Troché G, Delisle F, et al: Effects of mechanical ventilation with normobaric oxygen therapy on the rate of air removal from cerebral arteries. Crit Care Med 1994;22:851–857.

68. Annane D, Troché G, Delisle F, et al: Kinetics of elimination and acute consequences of cerebral air embolism. J Neuroimaging 1995;5:183–189.

69. Hwang TL, Fremaux R, Sears ES, et al: Confirmation of cerebral air embolism with computerized tomography. Ann Neurol 1983;13:214–215.

70. Hirabuki N, Miura T, Mitomo M, et al: Changes of cerebral air embolism shown by computed tomography. Br J Radiol 1988;61:252–255.

71. Takizawa S, Tokuoka K, Ohnuki Y, et al: Chronological changes in cerebral air embolism that occurred during continuous drainage of infected lung bullae. Cerebrovasc Dis 2000;10:409–412.

72. Hashimoto Y, Yamaki T, Sakakibara T, et al: Cerebral air embolism caused by cardiopulmonary resuscitation after cardiopulmonary arrest on arrival. J Trauma 2000;48:975–977.

73. Inamasu J, Nakamura Y, Saito R, et al: Cerebral air embolism after central venous catheterization. Am J Emerg Med 2001;19:520–521.

74. Sakai N, Nishizawa S: Cerebral air embolism after lung contusion. J Neurosurg 2001;95:909.

75. Söderman M: Cerebral air emboli from angiography in a patient with stroke. Acta Radiol 2001;42:140–143.

76. Hodgson M, Beran RG, Shirtley G: The role of computed tomography in the assessment of neurological sequelae of decompression sickness. Arch Neurol 1988;45:1033–1035.

77. Levin HS, Goldstein FC, Norcross K, et al: Neurobehavioral and magnetic resonance imaging findings in two cases of decompression sickness. Aviat Space Environ Med 1989;60:1204–1210.

78. Francis TJR, Mitchell SJ: Manifestations of decompression disorders. In Brubakk AO, Neuman TS (eds): The Physiology and Medicine of Diving, 5th ed. Philadelphia: WB Saunders, 2003, pp 578–600.

79. Kyttä J, Tanskanen P, Randell T: Comparison of the effects of controlled ventilation with 100% oxygen, 50% oxygen in nitrogen, and 50% oxygen in nitrous oxide on responses to venous air embolism in pigs. Br J Anaesth 1996;77:658–661.

80. Tovar EA, Del Campo C, Borsari A, et al: Postoperative management of cerebral air embolism: Gas physiology for surgeons. Ann Thorac Surg 1995;60:1138–1142.

81. Hulst van RA, Haitsma JJ, Lameris TW, et al: Hyperventilation impairs brain function in acute cerebral air embolism in pigs. Intensive Care Med 2003;30:944–950.

82. Drenthen J, Hulst van RA, Blok JH, et al: Quantitative EEG monitoring during cerebral air embolism and hyperbaric oxygen treatment in a pig model. J Clin Neurophysiol 2003;20:264–272.

83. Bove AA: The basis for drug therapy in decompression sickness. Undersea Biomed Res 1982;2:91–111.

84. Moon RE: Adjuvant therapy in decompression illness: Present and future. S Pacific Undersea Med Soc J 2000;30:99–110.

85. Brunner F, Frick P, Buhlmann A: Post-decompression shock due to extravasation of plasma. Lancet 1964;1:1071–1073.

86. Smith RM, Neuman TS: Elevation of serum creatine kinase in divers with arterial gas embolization. N Engl J Med 1994;330:19–24.

87. Smith RM, Van Hoessen KB, Neuman TS: Arterial gas embolism and hemo-concentration. J Emerg Med 1994;12:147–153.

88. Zhuang J, Shackford SR, Schmoker JD, Pietropaoli JA Jr: Colloid infusion after brain injury: Effect on intracranial pressure, cerebral blood flow and oxygen delivery. Crit Care Med 1995;23:140–148.

89. Dieterich HJ: Crystalloids versus colloid: A never ending story? Anaesthesist 2001;50:367–383.

90. Reasoner DK, Ryu KH, Hindman BJ, et al: Marked hemodilution increases neurological injury after focal cerebral ischemia in rabbits. Anesth Analg 1996;82:61–67.

91. Pulsinelli WA, Levy DE, Sigsbee B, et al: Increased damage after ischemic stroke in patients with hyperglycemia with or without established diabetes mellitus. Am J Med 1983;74:540–544.

92. Lam AM, Winn HR, Cullen BF, Sundling N: Hyperglycaemia and neurological outcome in patients with head injury. J Neurosurg 1991;75:545–551.

93. Lanier WL, Stangland KJ, Scheithauer BW, et al: The effect of dextrose solution and head down position on neurological outcome after complete cerebral ischemia in primates: Examination of a model. Anesthesiology 1987;66:39–48.

94. Leverve XM: Energy metabolism in critically ill patients: Lactate is a major oxidizable substrate. Curr Opin Clin Nutr Metab Care 1999;2:165–169.

95. Leverve XM, Mustafa I: Lactate: A key metabolite in the intercellular metabolic interplay. Crit Care 2002;6:284–285.

96. Mustafa I, Roth H, Hanafiah A, et al: Effect of cardiopulmonary bypass on lactate metabolism. Intensive Care Med 2003;29:1279–1285.

97. Ironside JW, Head MW: Variant Creutzfeldt-Jakob disease: Risk of transmission by blood and blood products. Haemophilia 2004;10(Suppl 4):64–69.

98. Laxenaire MC, Charpentier C, Feldman L: Anaphylactoid reactions to colloid plasma substitutes: Incidence, risk factors, mechanisms. A French multicenter prospective study. Ann Fr Anesth Reanim 1994;13:301–310.

99. Kaplan SS, Park TS, Gonzales ER, Gidday JM: Hydroxyethyl starch reduces leukocyte adherence and vascular injury in the newborn pig cerebral circulation after asphyxia. Stroke 2000;31:2218–2223.

100. Doyle JA, Davis DP, Hoyt DB: The use of hypertonic saline in the treatment of traumatic brain injury. J Trauma 2001;50:367–83.

101. Bhardwaj A, Harukuni I, Murphy SJ, et al: Hypertonic saline worsens infarct volume after transient focal ischemia in rats. Stroke 2000;31:1694–1701.

102. Hartl R, Ghajar J, Hochleuthner H, Mauritz W: Treatment of refractory intracranial hypertension in severe traumatic brain injury with repetitive hypertonic/hyperoncotic infusions. Zentralbl Chir 1997;122:181–185.

103. Schwarz S, Schwab S, Bertram M, et al: Effects of hypertonic saline hydroxyethyl starch solution and mannitol in patients with increased intracranial pressure after stroke. Stroke 1998;29:1550–1555.

104. Linaweaver PG: Dextran in recompression therapy [letter]. Ann Intern Med 1975;82:287.

105. Merton DA, Fife WP, Gross DR: An evaluation of plasma volume expanders in the treatment of decompression sickness. Aviat Space Environ Med 1983;54:218–222.

106. Patel PM, Drummond JC, Cole DJ, et al: Isoflurane and pentobarbital reduce the frequency of transient ischemic depolarizations during focal ischemia in rats. Anesth Analg 1998;86:773–780.

107. Hoffman WE, Charbel FT, Edelman G, Ausman JI: Thiopental and desflurane treatment for brain protection. Neurosurgery 1998;43:1050–1053.

108. Dutka AJ: Therapy for dysbaric central nervous system ischemia: Adjuncts to recompression. In Bennett PB, Moon RE (eds): Diving Accident Management: Proceedings of the Forty-First Undersea and Hyperbaric Medical Society Workshop. Bethesda, MD, 1990, pp 222–235.

109. Butler BD, Hills BA: Transpulmonary passage of venous air emboli. J Appl Physiol 1985;59:543–547.

110. Kindwall EP, Margolis I: Management of severe decompression sickness with treatment ancillary to recompression: A case report. Aviat Space Environ Med 1975;46:1065–1068.

111. Hallenbeck JM, Leitch DR, Dutka AJ, et al: Prostaglandin $I_2$, indomethacin and heparin promote postischemic neuronal recovery in dogs. Ann Neurol 1982;12:145–156.

112. Ryu KH, Hindman BJ, Reasoner DK, Dexter F: Heparin reduces neurological impairment after cerebral arterial air embolism in the rabbit. Stroke 1996;27:303–310.

113. Nishimoto K, Wolman M, Spatz M, Klatzo I: Pathophysiologic correlations in the blood-brain barrier damage due to air embolism. Adv Neurol 1978;20:237–248.

114. Ito U, Ohno K, Suganuma Y, et al: Effects of steroid on ischemic brain edema: Analysis of cytotoxic and vasogenic edema occurring during ischemia and after restoration of blood flow. Stroke 1980;11:166–176.

115. Pearson RR, Goad RF: Delayed cerebral edema complicating cerebral arterial gas embolism: Case histories. Undersea Biomed Res 1982;9:283–296.

116. Kizer KW: Corticosteroids in treatment of serious decompression sickness. Ann Emerg Med 1981;10:485–488.

117. Francis TJR, Dutka AJ: Methylprednisolone in the treatment of acute spinal cord decompression sickness. Undersea Biomed Res 1989;16:165–174.

118. Dutka AJ, Mink RB, Pearson RR, Hallenbeck JM: Effects of treatment with dexamethasone on recovery from experimental cerebral arterial gas embolism. Undersea Biomed Res 1992;19:131–141.

119. McDermott JJ, Dutka AJ, Evans DE, Flynn ET: Treatment of experimental cerebral air embolism with lidocaine and hyperbaric oxygen. Undersea Biomed Res 1990;17:525–534.

120. Shokunbi MT, Gelb AW, Wu XM, Miller DJ: Continuous lidocaine infusion and focal feline cerebral ischemia. Stroke 1990;21:107–111.

121. Nagao S, Murota T, Momma F, et al: The effect of intravenous lidocaine on experimental brain edema and neural activities. J Trauma 1988;28:1650–1655.

122. Rasool N, Faroqui M, Rubenstein EH: Lidocaine accelerates neuroelectrical recovery after incomplete global ischaemia in rabbits. Stroke 1990;21:929–935.

123. Ayad M, Verity MA, Rubenstein EH: Lidocaine delays cortical ischemic depolarization: Relationship to electrophysiologic recovery and neuropathology. J Neurosurg Anesthesiol 1994;6:98–110.

124. Mitchell SJ, Pellett O, Gorman DF: Cerebral protection by lidocaine during cardiac operations. Ann Thorac Surg 1999;67:1117–1124.

125. Spahn DR: Current status of artificial oxygen carriers. Adv Drug Delivery Rev 2000;40:143–151.

126. Lutz J, Hermann G: Perfluorochemicals as a treatment of decompression sickness in rats. Pflugers Arch 1984;401:174–177.

127. Spiess BD, McCarthy RJ, Tuman KJ, et al: Treatment of decompression sickness with a perfluorocarbon emulsion (FC-43). Undersea Biomed Res 1988;15:31–37.

128. Lynch PR, Krasner LJ, Vinciquerrra T, Shaffer TH: Effects of intravenous perfluorocarbon and oxygen breathing on acute decompression sickness in the hamster. Undersea Biomedical Res 1989;16:275–281.

129. Cochran RP, Kunzelman KS, Vocelka CR, et al: Perfluorocarbon emulsion in the cardiopulmonary bypass prime reduces neurological injury. Ann Thorac Surg 1997;63:1326–1332.

130. Tuman KJ, Speiss BD, McCarthy RJ, Ivankovich AD: Cardiorespiratory effects of venous air embolism in dogs receiving a perfluorocarbon emulsion. J Neurosurg 1986;65:238–244.

131. Herren JI, Kunzelman KS, Vocelka C, et al: Angiographic and histological evaluation of porcine retinal vascular damage and protection with perfluorocarbons after massive air embolism. Stroke 1988;29:2396–2403.

132. Peirce EC II: Specific therapy for arterial air embolism. Ann Thorac Surg 1980;29:300–303.

133. Tibbles PM, Edelsberg JS: Hyperbaric oxygen therapy. N Engl J Med 1996;25:1642–1648.

134. Moon RE, Air or Gas Embolism. In Feldmeijer JJ (ed): Hyperbaric oxygen therapy: Committee Report. Kensington, MD: Undersea and Hyperbaric Medical Society, 2003, pp 5–10.

135. Radermacher P, Warninghoff V, Nurnberg JH, et al: Successful treatment with hyperbaric oxygen following severe cerebroarterial gas embolism. Anasthesiol Intensivmed Notfallmed Schmerzther 1994;29:59–61.

136. Leitch DR, Hallenbeck JM: Oxygen in the treatment of spinal cord decompression sickness. Undersea Biomed Res 1985;12:269–289.

137. Shank ES, Muth CM: Decompression illness, iatrogenic gas embolism and carbon monoxide poisoning: The role of hyperbaric oxygen therapy. Int Anesthesiol Clin 2000;38:11–138.

138. Gabb G, Robin ED: Hyperbaric oxygen: A therapy in search for diseases. Chest 1987;92:1074–1082.

139. Layon AJ: Hyperbaric oxygen treatment for cerebral air embolism: Where are the data? Mayo Clin Proc 1991;66:641–646.

140. Leitch DR, Greenbaum LJ, Hallenbeck JM: Cerebral arterial air embolism. I: Is there benefit in beginning HBO treatment at 6 bar? Undersea Biomed Res 1984;11:221–235.

141. Leitch DR, Greenbaum LJ, Hallenbeck JM: Cerebral arterial air embolism. II: Effect of pressure and time on cortical evoked potential recovery. Undersea Biomed Res 1984;11:237–248.

142. Leitch DR, Greenbaum LJ, Hallenbeck JM: Cerebral arterial air embolism. III: Cerebral blood flow after decompression from various pressure treatments. Undersea Biomed Res 1984;11:249–263.

143. Leitch DR, Greenbaum LJ, Hallenbeck JM: Cerebral arterial air embolism. IV: Failure to recover with treatment, and secondary deterioration. Undersea Biomed Res 1984;11:265–274.

144. Sykes JJW, Hallenbeck JM, Leitch DR: Spinal cord decompression sickness: A comparison of recompression therapies in an animal model. Aviat Space Environ Med 1986;57:561–568.

145. Hulst van RA, Drenthen J, Haitsma JJ, et al: Effects of hyperbaric treatment in cerebral air embolism on intracranial pressure, brain oxygenation and brain glucose metabolism in the pig. Crit Care 2005;33:841–846.

146. Bitterman H, Melamed Y: Delayed hyperbaric treatment of cerebral air embolism. In Shields T (ed): Proceedings of the XVth Annual Meeting, European Undersea and Biomedical Society, Aberdeen:1988, pp 1–9.

147. Massey EW, Moon RE, Shelton D, Camporesi EM: Hyperbaric oxygen therapy of iatrogenic air embolism. J Hyperbaric Med 1990;5:15–21.

148. Wherrett CG, Mehran RJ, Beaulieu MA: Cerebral arterial gas embolism following diagnostic bronchoscopy; delayed treatment with hyperbaric oxygen. Can J Anaesth 2002;49:96–99.

149. Murphy BP, Harford FJ, Cramer FS: Cerebral air embolism resulting from invasive medical procedures: Treatment with hyperbaric oxygen. In Cramer FS (ed): Proceedings of the Eighth International Congress on Hyperbaric Medicine. Flagstaff, AZ: Best Publishing, 1985, pp 245–251.

150. Takahashi H, Kobayashi S, Hayase H, Sakakibara K: Iatrogenic air embolism: A review of 34 cases. In Greenbaum L (ed): Ninth International Symposium on Underwater Hyperbaric Physiology. Kensington, MD: Undersea and Hyperbaric Medical Society, 1987, pp 931–948.

151. Ziser A, Adir Y, Lavon H, Shupak A: Hyperbaric oxygen therapy for massive arterial air embolism during cardiac operations. J Thorac Cardiovasc Surg 1999;117:818–821.

152. Neuman TS, Hallenbeck JM: Barotraumatic cerebral air embolism and the mental status examination: A report of four cases. Ann Emerg Med 1987;16:220–223.

153. Kol S, Ammar R, Weisz G, Melamed Y: Hyperbaric oxygenation for arterial air embolism during cardiopulmonary bypass. Ann Thorac Surg 1993;55:401–403.

154. Benson J, Adkinson C, Colliers R: Hyperbaric oxygen therapy of iatrogenic cerebral gas embolism. Undersea Hyperb Med 2003;30:117–127.

# CHAPTER 33

# Blunt Thoracic Trauma

Andreas Reske and Dierk Schreiter

In industrial countries, 75% to 90% of chest injuries are caused by blunt trauma, 80% to 90% are associated with multiple trauma.[1-3] The increasing incidence of chest injuries over the last few decades is the result of the growing numbers of cases of blunt high-velocity traumas. Moreover, advanced prehospital emergency medical services allow critically injured patients to reach the hospital alive, and advances in diagnostic imaging techniques such as computed tomography (CT) have improved the sensitivity for the detection of chest injuries.

Along with chest wall injuries, pulmonary contusion is the most common injury identified in blunt thoracic trauma, and it significantly increases the rate of complications and mortality. The mortality among patients with isolated chest injuries is low and ranges from 0% to 5% in young patients and 10% to 20% in elderly patients,[4-6] whereas the mortality among severely injured patients with accompanying chest injuries and pulmonary contusion is reported to be 15% to 60%, depending on the overall severity of the injury.[3,4,7-14] Although patients with posttraumatic respiratory failure apparently have a low mortality, they are still prone to developing short- and long-term pulmonary dysfunction.[15-17] Therefore, these patients should be routinely screened for risk factors for posttraumatic respiratory failure. Risk factors include an injury severity score greater than 25, pulmonary contusion, age greater than 65 years, hypotension on admission, and a 24-hour transfusion requirement of more than 10 units.[18,19]

## HISTORY

Pulmonary contusion was first described by Morgagni in 1761, when he found it in two autopsies without any evidence of chest wall injuries.[20] After systematic clinical and experimental research, this phenomenon was confirmed by Payne 150 years later. He postulated an increased risk of parenchymal lung injury in blunt thoracic trauma whenever energy-absorbing rib fractures were absent.[21] In 1907, Litten reported that pneumonia and progressive respiratory failure frequently developed after pulmonary contusion. Moreover, he described high mortality and noted that autopsies were significant for infiltration and atelectasis.[22] Further knowledge was gained from examinations of blast injuries during World Wars I and II. The landmark studies of Hooker conducted during 1918 and 1919 showed that pulmonary hemorrhage was actually the predominant pathophysiologic consequence of blast injuries.[23] In 1945, the research of Burford and Burbank was trendsetting. These investigators showed that posttraumatic respiratory failure was caused by an increased amount of interstitial and intraalveolar fluids and described this as "the traumatic wet lung." Applying their newly gained pathophysiologic knowledge, these investigators recommended sufficient pain control, aggressive pulmonary toilet, and positive airway pressure by mask to ensure adequate ventilation.[24] Successful treatment of thoracic trauma by applying mask continuous positive airway pressure (CPAP) was also reported by Jensen.[25] In 1956, Avery and colleagues added controlled mechanical ventilation to the therapeutic approaches to the management of blunt thoracic trauma.[26]

## PATHOPHYSIOLOGY

In nontraumatic subgroups of patients with acute lung injury (ALI) or acute respiratory distress syndrome (ARDS), the precipitating condition can often be identified. In contrast, a variety of factors may contribute to the development of posttraumatic respiratory failure in both isolated blunt thoracic trauma and multiple trauma. Impaired respiratory drive and mechanics originating from cerebral injuries, uncontrolled pain, flail chest, pneumothorax and hemothorax, and intra-abdominal hypertension can affect gas exchange by decreasing alveolar ventilation. In contrast, direct (e.g., pulmonary contusion) and indirect (e.g., shock with massive transfusion) injury to the pulmonary parenchyma may culminate in "real" pulmonary dysfunction (Table 33.1).

Two distinct forms of posttraumatic ALI/ARDS in general populations of trauma patients have been described. Early ALI/ARDS that develops within 48 hours has been attributed to hemorrhagic shock and capillary leak, whereas later-onset ALI/ARDS has been associated with a higher incidence of pneumonia, often occurring in multiple organ failure.[19,27] Moreover, we have observed that many patients present with large bilateral atelectases on admission.[28,29] In our experience, many patients have large bilateral atelectasis already on admission, which can also be a cause of early, and usually reversible, post-traumatic ALI/ARDS. The coexistence of direct mechanical damage to the pulmonary parenchyma and of indirect systemic and pulmonary sequelae of severe trauma increases the likelihood of complications. Although some studies failed to demonstrate a correlation of pulmonary contusion with more severe ALI/ARDS,[27] many authors have reported that the severity of pulmonary contusion correlates with the development of pulmonary infections, respiratory failure, and mortality.[29-31] Moreover, pulmonary contusion is an independent risk factor for ALI/ARDS,[18,32] and the severity of pulmonary contusion has been shown to indicate the need for ventilatory support.[29,31]

The lung is a soft organ capable of large deformation; however, under rapidly applied compressive or concussive loads (i.e., pulmonary contusion), it is highly susceptible to parenchymal laceration and fracture of blood vessels.[30,33] The lung can be mechanically injured by the tearing of tissues when low-density alveolar tissue is stripped from heavier hilar structures because they accelerate at different rates; the lung can also be injured by direct laceration of the lung by displacement of fractured ribs or chest wall compression and by bleeding into uninvolved lung segments. Direct mechanical damage to the lung parenchyma, intraparenchymal hemorrhage, edema formation, and additional indirect injury (originating from trauma-associated triggers of ALI/ARDS such as hemorrhagic shock with massive transfusion), frequently culminate in post-traumatic ALI/ARDS.

Infiltration of the lung by neutrophil granulocytes (polymorphonuclear leukocytes or PMNs) is the hallmark of early post-traumatic ALI/ARDS similar to other causes of ALI/ARDS.[30,34] The influx of PMNs into the pulmonary parenchyma and sequentially into the alveolar

**Table 33-1  Factors Predisposing the Injured Patient to Acute Lung Injury/Acute Respiratory Distress Syndrome**

| Direct Lung Injury | Indirect Lung Injury |
|---|---|
| Pulmonary contusion | Hemorrhagic shock |
| Aspiration of blood or gastric contents | Systemic inflammatory response syndrome |
| Bleeding into uninjured lung segments | Massive transfusion of blood products |
| Reexpansion pulmonary edema | Sepsis |
| Fat embolism | Severe brain injury |
| Pneumonia | Thermal injury |
| Inhalation injury | |

space in ALI/ARDS is a complex process consisting of PMN retention, margination, and endothelial adhesion within the pulmonary microvasculature, followed by migration into the pulmonary interstitium and alveolar space. When the PMNs that migrated into the pulmonary parenchyma are activated, they become capable of releasing numerous cytotoxic products. Among these are reactive oxygen species, elastases, and proteases, whose actions, by damaging the alveolocapillary barrier, result in increased permeability of the barrier and eventually in accumulation of protein-rich interstitial and alveolar edema. Comparable to different forms of ALI/ARDS this high-permeability pulmonary edema not only floods the alveoli and terminal airways, but also destabilizes airspaces by inactivating the surfactant of alveoli and terminal airways whose production and function are already significantly impaired.[36,37] Edema flooding and collapse of airspaces are the mechanisms which gives rise to the clinical phenomena of reduced functional capacity, increased pulmonary elastance, ventilation-perfusion mismatching, raised intrapulmonary shunt, and, finally, hypoxemia.

## INITIAL APPROACH TO DIAGNOSIS AND TREATMENT

The prehospital and emergency room treatment of patients with chest trauma consists of rapid primary evaluation and resuscitation of vital functions and should follow the basic ABCs of major trauma management, which must constantly be reassessed.[38–41] A short and injury-focused medical history helps to identify trauma mechanisms and occult injuries. For all patients, not only patients with chest trauma, the correct diagnosis often results from the combination of a careful history and physical examination and a high degree of suspicion. Accordingly, profound knowledge of trauma mechanisms and typical injury patterns helps to decrease the number of missed thoracic injuries. For example, undamped high-velocity traumas such as traffic accidents or falls from a height are typical causes of severe chest trauma with pulmonary contusion.[42–46] Despite the common misconception, pulmonary contusions frequently occur in the absence of rib fractures.[7,21,30,47] Moreover, the probability of pulmonary contusion also increases with the overall severity of injury.[1,2,42,48] This knowledge has been incorporated into scoring systems that can serve as additional tools to improve the accuracy of the diagnosis of thoracic injuries and of the prediction of complications.[3,49,50] Such scoring systems may be particularly helpful when sophisticated imaging equipment (i.e., CT; see later) is not available because the early and adequate assessment of the thoracic and overall injury severity helps to initiate the appropriate goal-directed management.[3,6]

Besides pulmonary contusion, pneumothorax is the most common injury identified in blunt chest trauma. It accounts for 60% of all chest injuries and occurs in 20% of cases as bilateral pneumothorax.[8,9,51] Therefore, it has to be specifically detected and treated. However, given that the clinical diagnosis of pneumothorax is incorrect in up to 30% of cases,[51] the physical examination should be followed by diagnostic imaging techniques because the absence of visible or palpable injuries does not exclude the presence of visceral injuries.

An initial chest radiograph taken in the emergency room is required by all current guidelines and is obtained in most trauma centers. Although chest radiography can reliably show skeletal injuries, intrathoracic injuries are frequently missed.[47,59–61] This limitation can be overcome in these patients by performing a CT scan. In the past, the time required for CT scanning raised doubts regarding the practicability of the routine use of CT in patients with multiple trauma. Since the introduction of much faster multidetector CT scanners, several groups have incorporated CT scanning into their emergency room procedures for trauma patients.[40,61–65] CT scanning can distinguish chest wall from parenchymal or mediastinal injury early and reliably, whereas this differentiation may not be possible with chest radiography.[65] In addition, significant numbers of pulmonary contusions cannot be identified by initial chest radiographs.[5,7,59–61] In contrast, the sensitivity of CT for detecting pulmonary contusion is 100% immediately after injury.[47,59–61,66] Similar problems exist for the diagnosis of both hemothorax and pneumothorax because plain chest radiographs often miss anterior pneumothoraces.[67] The incidence of pneumothorax identified by CT scans but missed by clinical examination and plain chest radiographs ranges from 5% to 55%; again, CT scanning detects pneumothorax with 100% sensitivity.[68,69]

In addition to qualitative description, the degree of lung injury can be further assessed by quantitative analyses of thoracic CT scans.[16,17,28,29,31,70–73] Miller and colleagues reported that the greater the severity of the parenchymal damage, the greater the incidence of ALI/ARDS and other pulmonary or extrapulmonary complications. These investigators found that patients in whom the volume of the pulmonary contusion measured by CT analysis exceeded 20% of total lung volume were at a significantly higher risk of developing both ALI/ARDS (82% versus 22%) and pneumonia (52% versus 21%) and had a significantly higher mortality (24% versus 3%).[29] The potential of such quantitative parameters to predict the development of posttraumatic ALI/ARDS was also shown by our group.[28,72,74] Unfortunately, this technique is not yet ready for routine clinical use because of the tremendous time requirements involved.

In patients requiring airway management or ventilatory support, published data are conflicting regarding the timing and choice of airway and respiratory support[75–83] (Fig. 33.1). Prehospital intubation performed by untrained medical personnel increases the risk of complications, morbidity, and mortality.[82,83] In contrast, prehospital intubation performed by skilled and properly trained paramedics or physicians using standardized techniques such as rapid-sequence induction for intubation is considered comparable in quality to hospital intubation.[84] Whenever there are indications for intubation, this procedure should be performed at the earliest and safest point in time. Patients with thoracic trauma without manifest respiratory insufficiency and without other indications for immediate intubation should not be intubated in the field. This view is supported by data showing that patients intubated in the field have no benefit with regard to the duration of mechanical ventilation, time to hospital discharge, incidence of sepsis, and mortality; however, their rescue period is significantly prolonged.[85]

## MECHANICAL VENTILATION

Because other supportive treatment modalities for pulmonary contusion such as fluid restriction, diuretics, and corticosteroids have not shown any benefit,[8,30] mechanical ventilation strategies will likely provide the most successful approach to reduce the morbidity and mortality associated with posttraumatic acute respiratory failure.[86] The outstanding importance of mechanical ventilation was already recognized by Ashbaugh and colleagues when they described the beneficial effects of positive end-expiratory pressure (PEEP) in their first description of ARDS. Their results can be translated to posttraumatic ALI/ARDS because 7 of their 12 patients suffered from this condition.[87] Since then, numerous approaches to the mechanical ventilation of critically ill trauma patients have been described, studied, and compared, and the literature is full of respective reports.[26,28,70,80,81,88–95] However, the only approach to mechanical ventilation that was proven beneficial in terms of reduced mortality was ventilation with low tidal volumes and PEEP, as prospectively tested in large numbers of patients.[96,97] Unfortunately, patients with posttraumatic ALI/ARDS were underrepresented in these studies, and concerns regarding practicability and benefits of low–tidal volume ventilation in injured patients have been voiced.[27,98,99] For instance, hypercapnia resulting from ventilation with reduced tidal volumes represents an important drawback, particularly in patients with multiple trauma who have cerebral injuries.[70]

Because of the diversity of this population, it is almost impossible to give universal recommendations for the ventilatory management of traumatized patients[100,101] (Fig. 33.2). In contrast to noninjured patients with ALI/ARDS, whose management is mainly supportive and observant, the intensive care specialist has to be aware of the special challenges and problems faced in the ventilatory management of injured patients. These patients are at high risk of developing ALI/ARDS and ventilator-associated complications.[102,103] Furthermore, they frequently require urgent surgical interventions (i.e., craniotomy or laparotomy), their systemic oxygen delivery may suddenly be impaired by severe hemorrhage, and the usual modes of or adjuncts to mechanical

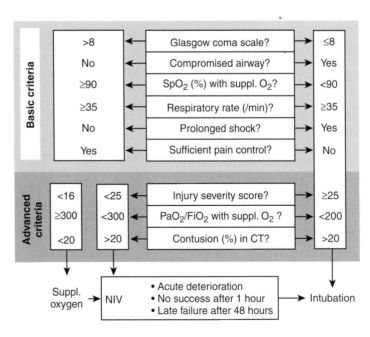

**Figure 33.1** Our approach to the choice of airway and respiratory support is displayed. These criteria are constantly checked throughout prehospital and emergency department treatment, and the level of support is increased when necessary. The decision between NIV and intubation is often not straightforward, in these cases all criteria need to be considered in conjunction with each other. For further information on the "CT V$_{non}$ (%)" criterion, the reader is referred to references 28 and 29. MV, mechanical ventilation; NIV, noninvasive ventilation; SpO2, peripheral oxygen saturation.

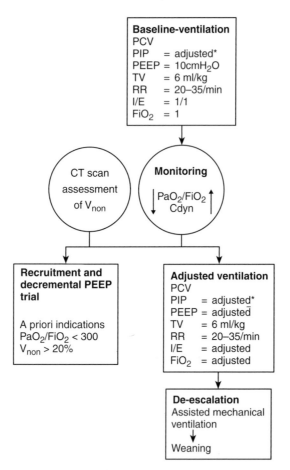

**Figure 33.2** This flow chart illustrates how we adapt the mode of invasive mechanical ventilation in patients with post-traumatic acute lung injury/acute respiratory distress syndrome (ALI/ARDS) in our intensive care unit. We start from baseline ventilation, use changes in oxygenation and dynamic compliance for evaluating the appropriateness of the baseline ventilation, and, if necessary, adjust the ventilator settings. If a patient deteriorates during adjusted ventilation, or whenever a patient meets our a priori criteria, we use recruitment maneuvers and subsequently titrate positive end-expiratory pressure (PEEP) in a decremental fashion. The criterion $V_{non}$ refers to the nonaerated lung volume measured from computed tomography and expressed as percentage of the total lung volume (100%). Using a modification of the method of Miller and colleagues, we measure the nonaerated lung volume instead of the volume of the pulmonary contusion.[29,28] PCV, pressure controlled ventilation; PIP, positive inspiratory pressure; TV, tidal volume; RR, respiratory rate; I/E, inspiratory-to-expiratory ratio; Cdyn, dynamic compliance. * The PIP is adjusted to achieve a TV of 6 ml per kg predicted body weight. We try to keep the PIP <30 cm $H_2O$ and avoid PIPs >35 cm $H_2O$.

ventilation (i.e., low–tidal volume ventilation with permissive hypercapnia or prone positioning) may be precluded by particular injury patterns.

The management of decreased alveolar ventilation is usually straightforward and is less challenging than that of posttraumatic ALI/ARDS. However, improper or delayed management may still precipitate complications. Rapid shallow breathing, for example, promotes the formation of atelectasis, which may remain subclinical until a patient develops complications (e.g., pneumonia). It is important to emphasize the *progressive nature* of post-traumatic pulmonary failure. This term, originally coined to describe the clinical course of patients with pulmonary contusion,[104] also highlights a major threat to multiple trauma patients. Many patients, especially those with isolated blunt thoracic trauma, can be acceptably managed (i.e., oxygenated) with supplemental oxygen during the first few posttraumatic days, but reduced chest excursion and increased intraabdominal pressure carry a high risk of progressive atelectasis formation. Because we routinely subject all patients with multiple trauma to CT scanning of the entire body immediately after initial resuscitation in the emergency department, we have learned that many patients who can be managed with supplemental oxygen have bilateral dorsal atelectasis frequently occupying more than 15% of the total lung volume.[28] On the second or third post-traumatic day, however, many of these patients deteriorate (i.e., desaturate) rapidly, and intubation and mechanical ventilation become necessary to ensure adequate oxygenation. This delayed respiratory decompensation matches descriptions of the later-onset ALI/ARDS in trauma patients.[19,27] It also illustrates how the coexistence of several predisposing factors may culminate in pulmonary failure, which typically occurs on the second or third posttraumatic day.[105] Finally, this progressive and delayed respiratory failure has led several authors to recommend early aggressive mechanical ventilatory support to prevent progressive atelectasis and worsening of arterial oxygenation.[6,100]

One of the most important factors contributing to the development of posttraumatic pulmonary complications is atelectasis. Atelectasis causes ventilation-perfusion-mismatch and hypoxemia refractory to supplemental oxygen, particularly when compensatory mechanisms such as hypoxic pulmonary vasoconstriction become insufficient. It can also inflict additional pulmonary and extra-pulmonary damage potentially leading to increased morbidity and mortality.[106–110] Moreover, atelectasis causes a decrease in clearance of bacteria, particularly *Staphylococcus aureus*, *Klebsiella pneumoniae*, and *Streptococcus pneumoniae*.[108,111,112] This finding is of particular relevance because these bacteria are frequent pathogens in early posttraumatic pneumonia.[113,114] The deleterious interaction between atelectasis and nosocomial pneumonia may, besides other risk factors for pneumonia (e.g., aspiration), help to explain why injured patients who frequently present with substantial atelectasis are so prone to develop early nosocomial pneumonia.[115,116] Moreover, the cyclic recruitment and derecruitment of lung units within atelectatic regions, resulting in the so-called low–lung volume injury, have led to their incorporation into the concept of ventilator-associated lung injury.[117–119]

We agree with other investigators that the approach to mechanical ventilation, not only in injured patients, should be focused on the prevention of lung collapse, the recruitment of collapsed tissue, the minimization of alveolar hyperinflation, and the prevention of additional ventilator-associated lung injury.[7,28,93,97,120–122] Although this concept is based on a sound physiologic basis, it is not yet supported by strong evidence from randomized controlled clinical trials and relies mainly on data from animal experiments[109] and small clinical studies.[93,97] Unfortunately, the ARDS Network studies that provide the greatest contribution to the body of evidence supporting the use of low tidal volumes and PEEP have been repeatedly criticized for their nonphysiologic design.[121,123] Moreover, many authors have argued that the intensive care specialist has to tailor ventilator settings to a single patient instead of a patient population.[121,122] Also under dispute is whether tidal volumes should be set according to the patient's predicted body weight or whether surrogates of the severity of lung injury should govern the choice of ventilator settings. Such surrogates could be morphologic (e.g., the collapsed lung volume or the "potential for recruitment") or mechanical (i.e., dynamic compliance, "stress index," and "lung strain") parameters.[121,124,125] Finally, concerns have been expressed that mechanical ventilation with insufficient PEEP and low tidal volumes does not recruit collapsed alveoli, but rather allows for progressive derecruitment, atelectasis, and hypoxemia that can even occur at moderate to high PEEP levels.[98,126].

We now review some clinically pertinent issues surrounding the ventilatory management of injured patients, discuss approaches to reduce atelectasis, and describe adjuncts to mechanical ventilation. According to the current guidelines of the British Thoracic Society, CPAP is an option in injured patients who remain hypoxic despite adequate pain control and high flow oxygen.[128] This recommendation is supported by a study reporting that CPAP applied by face mask combined with patient-controlled analgesia led to lower mortality and a lower incidence of nosocomial infections.[95] Among the contraindications to non-invasive ventilation in injured patients are impaired consciousness, facial trauma, and undrained pneumothorax. We already discussed the problems surrounding the application of supplemental oxygen by face mask, and we believe that the early institution of noninvasive ventilation in suitable patients represents a valuable means to render more invasive ventilatory support unnecessary. Furthermore, we believe that current protocols that gradually adapt the degree of ventilatory support have already succeeded older recommendations for "prophylactic controlled mechanical

ventilation" in patients with multiple trauma. However, clinicians should frequently reassess whether the method of ventilatory support still meets the demands of the patient's clinical condition. If there are indications that the patient is deteriorating, in terms of oxygenation, ventilation, or lung mechanics, the level of ventilatory support should be appropriately increased without delay. This early change to more invasive mechanical ventilation is supported by the finding that the longer atelectasis is tolerated, the higher the transpulmonary pressures required to reinflate them will be.[129] Moreover, oxygenation goals accepted in some patient populations may not be acceptable in trauma patients. In contrast to the results of the ARDS Network data, hypoxemia on admission is an independent predictor of poor outcome in trauma patients; tolerating borderline arterial oxygen tension values (i.e., 55 mm Hg) can pose a serious threat to patients at risk of significant bleeding or to patients with cerebral injuries and intracranial hypertension.[5,96] Therefore, if a patient deteriorates despite noninvasive ventilatory support, we suggest that invasive ventilation be initiated.

If patients need to be intubated and ventilated invasively, controlled or assisted ventilatory modes can be chosen. Putensen and colleagues presented an interesting approach focused on the maintenance of spontaneous breathing. Their rationale for maintaining spontaneous breathing was that diaphragmatic contractions will recruit dependent atelectatic lung regions and thereby improve both the distribution of ventilation and ventilation-perfusion matching.[93] This goal was achieved by reduced levels of sedation and assisted mechanical ventilation, resulting in beneficial effects such as shorter durations of mechanical ventilation, intubation, and intensive care unit stay. Thus this study confirms the observation that decreasing the level of sedation shortens the time to weaning from mechanical ventilation and to discharge from the intensive care unit.[130]

In clinical practice, however, controlled ventilatory modes are frequently required to treat multiply traumatized patients. Because patients receiving controlled mechanical ventilation are more prone to atelectasis, pneumonia, and other ventilator-associated complications, the ongoing need for controlled mechanical ventilation should be frequently reassessed. During controlled mechanical ventilation, the principles of lung protective ventilation should be followed. Among the evidence-based elements of lung protective ventilation are low tidal volumes and PEEP. However, several other factors also play a role in the concept of lung protective ventilation. We believe that PEEP should not be set according to arbitrarily chosen combinations of PEEP and inspired oxygen fraction values.[96] Instead, we support the suggestion to titrate PEEP decrementally after placing the tidal ventilation on the deflation limb of the pulmonary pressure-volume curve.[28,125,131–133] Placing the ventilatory cycle on the deflation limb (i.e., on top of a higher end-expiratory lung volume) of the pressure-volume curve requires the use of a recruitment maneuver.[28,122,131,132,134,135] Starting from an open lung condition, the decremental PEEP titration aims to identify the pressure at which the lung starts to collapse. Because lung collapse cannot be directly identified at the bedside, surrogate parameters such as oxygenation and dynamic compliance are followed to guide the PEEP titration.[28,131,132,134–136] Nevertheless, recruitment maneuvers and decremental PEEP titration are interdependent (Figs. 33.3 and 33.4). If PEEP is not adequately titrated after a recruitment maneuver, the lung will recollapse; conversely, PEEP cannot be decrementally titrated without a recruitment maneuver.[28,122,136] Although alveolar recruitment maneuvers together with sufficient PEEP are capable of increasing oxygenation and lung aeration, their use relies on data from animal experiments, small clinical studies and physiologic premises.[28,134,136] We believe in the benefits of this concept, but strong evidence is lacking, and considerable controversy and reports of side effects exist.[137,138] A comprehensive discussion of the advantages and disadvantages of alveolar recruitment and high PEEP is beyond the scope of this chapter.

As mentioned earlier, useful adjuncts can be incorporated into the ventilation protocol; these include prone or kinetic positioning and bronchoscopy.[120,139,140] Whenever we have to treat an injured patient with post-traumatic ALI/ARDS with controlled mechanical ventilation, we primarily use kinetic positioning.

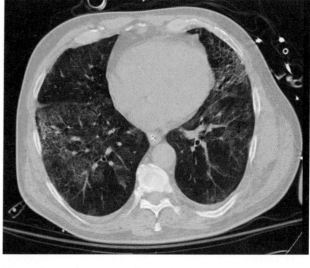

**Figure 33.4** The same patient as in Figure 33.3, 48 hours after a recruitment maneuver (opening pressure 65 cm $H_2O$) and a decremental PEEP trial. The PEEP was 16 cm $H_2O$ at the time of the CT.

Moreover, because many patients with severe chest trauma, and especially those with pulmonary contusion, have some degree of intrapulmonary bleeding, we routinely perform bronchoscopy soon after admission. Bronchoscopy not only aids in the diagnosis and location of intrapulmonary bleeding, but also allows the removal of secretions and mucous plugs.[7,120]

## CONCLUSION

In conclusion, posttraumatic respiratory failure poses a major risk to many patients, and management of this condition is challenging. One of the most important aspects of managing a patient with posttraumatic ALI/ARDS is to identify the precipitating conditions and to treat these problems aggressively. Every step of ventilatory management should be focused on the prevention of complications and the facilitation of early spontaneous breathing and weaning from ventilatory support.

## ACKNOWLEDGMENTS

We thank Hans-Christoph Pape (Professor, Department of orthopedic surgery, University of Pittsburgh Medical Center) for his expert comments and Michael Metze and Harriet Adamson for proofreading the manuscript.

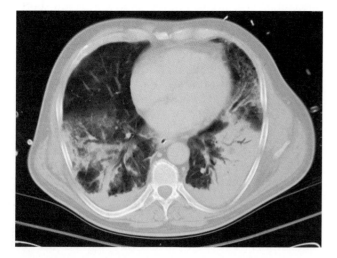

**Figure 33.3** Thoracic CT scan of a patient suffering from multiple trauma with severe pulmonary contusion who developed acute respiratory distress syndrome. The PEEP was 10 cm $H_2O$ at the time of the CT.

# REFERENCES

1. Karmy-Jones R, Jurkovich GJ, Shatz DV, et al: Management of traumatic lung injury: A Western Trauma Association multicenter review. J Trauma 2001;51:1049–1053.

2. Kulshrestha P, Munshi I, Wait R: Profile of chest trauma in a level I trauma center. J Trauma 2004;57:576–581.

3. Pape HC, Remmers D, Rice J, et al: Appraisal of early evaluation of blunt chest trauma: Development of a standardized scoring system of initial clinical decision making. J Trauma 2000;24:496–504.

4. Stellin G: Survival in trauma victims with pulmonary contusion. Am Surg 1991;57:780–784.

5. Hoff SJ, Shotts SD, Eddy VA, et al: Outcome of isolated pulmonary contusion in blunt trauma patients. Am Surg 1994;60:138–142.

6. Nelson LD: Ventilatory support of the trauma patient with pulmonary contusion. Respir Care Clin N Am 1996;2:425–447.

7. Allen GS, Coates NE: Pulmonary contusion: A collective review. Am Surg 1996;62:895–900.

8. Clark GC, Schecter WP, Trunkey DD: Variables affecting outcome in blunt chest trauma: Flail chest vs pulmonary contusion. J Trauma 1988;28:298–304.

9. Gaillard M, Hervé C, Mandin L, et al: Mortality prognostic factors in chest injury. J Trauma 1990;30:93–96.

10. Lewis FR: Thoracic trauma. Surg Clin North Am 1982;62:97–104.

11. LoCicero J, Mattox KL: Epidemiology of chest trauma. Surg Clin North Am 1989;69:15–19.

12. Nast Kolb D, Waydhas C, Gippner-Steppat C, et al: Indicators of the posttraumatic inflammatory response correlate with organ failure in patients with multiple injuries. J Trauma 1997;42:446–451.

13. Pinilla JC: Acute respiratory failure in severe blunt chest trauma. J Trauma 1982;22:221–226.

14. Shorr RM, Crittenden M, Indeck M, et al: Blunt thoracic trauma: Analysis of 515 patients. Ann Surg 1987;206:200–205.

15. Davidson TA, Rubenfeld GD, Caldwell ES, et al: The effect of acute respiratory distress syndrome on long-term survival. Am J Respir Crit Care Med 1999;160:1838–1842.

16. Kishikawa M, Yoshioka T, Shimazu T, et al: Pulmonary contusion causes long-term respiratory dysfunction with decreased functional residual capacity. J Trauma 1991;31:1203–1208; discussion 1208–1210.

17. Kishikawa M, Minami T, Shimazu T, et al: Laterality of air volume in the lungs long after blunt chest trauma. J Trauma 1993;34:908–912; discussion 912–913.

18. Miller PR, Croce MA, Kilgo PD, et al: Acute respiratory distress syndrome in blunt trauma: Identification of independent risk factors. Am Surg 2002;68:845–850; discussion 850–851.

19. Croce MA, Fabian TC, Davis KA, et al: Early and late acute respiratory distress syndrome: Two distinct clinical entities. J Trauma 1999;46:361–366; discussion 366–368.

20. Morgagni GB: De sedibus et causis morborum. Liber IV: De morbis chirurgicis et universalibus. Epist. anatom. medica LIII: De vulneribus et ictibus colli, pectoris et dorsi. Artic. XXXI–XXXIII. Venetiis, 1761.

21. Payne EM, Abert CM: Contusion of the lung without external injuries. BMJ 1909;1:139–142.

22. Litten M: Kontusionspneumonie. Dtsch Med Wochenschr 1907;13:499–502.

23. Hooker DR: Physiological effects of air concussion. Am J Physiol 1924;67:219–274.

24. Burford TH, Burbank B: Traumatic wet lung: Observations on certain physiologic fundamentals of thoracic trauma. J Thorac Surg 1945;14:415–424.

25. Jensen NK: Recovery of pulmonary function after crushing injury to the chest. Chest 1952;22:319–346.

26. Avery EE, Benson DW, Morch ET: Critically crushed chests: A new method of treatment with continuous mechanical hyperventilation to produce alkalotic apnea and internal pneumatic stabilization. J Thorac Surg 1956;32:291–311.

27. Dicker RA, Morabito DJ, Pittet JF, et al: Acute respiratory distress syndrome criteria in trauma patients: Why the definitions do not work. J Trauma 2004;57:522–526; discussion 526–528.

28. Schreiter D, Reske A, Stichert B, et al: Alveolar recruitment in combination with sufficient positive end-expiratory pressure increases oxygenation and lung aeration in patients with severe chest trauma. Crit Care Med 2004;32:968–975.

29. Miller PR, Croce MA, Bee TK, et al: ARDS after pulmonary contusion: Accurate measurement of contusion volume identifies high-risk patients. J Trauma 2001;51:223–228; discussion 229–230.

30. Cohn SM: Pulmonary contusion: Review of a clinical entity. J Trauma 1997;42:5:973–979.

31. Wagner RB, Jamieson PM: Pulmonary contusion: Evaluation and classification by computed tomography. Surg Clin North Am 1989;69:31–40.

32. Pepe PE, Potkin RT, Reus DH, et al: Clinical predictors of the adult respiratory distress syndrome. Am J Surg 1982;144:124–130.

33. Fung YC, Yen RT, Tao ZL, et al: A hypothesis on the mechanism of trauma of lung tissue subjected to impact load. J Biomech Eng 1988;110:50–56.

34. Pallister I, Dent C, Topley N: Increased neutrophil migratory activity after major trauma: A factor in the etiology of acute respiratory distress syndrome? Crit Care Med 2002;30:1717–1721.

35. Doerschuk CM, Mizgerd JP, Kubo H, et al: Adhesion molecules and cellular biomechanical changes in acute lung injury: Giles F. Filley Lecture. Chest 1999;116(Suppl):37S–43S.

36. Gregory TJ, Longmore WJ, Moxley MA, et al: Surfactant chemical composition and biophysical activity in acute respiratory distress syndrome. J Clin Invest 1991;88:1976–1981.

37. Pison U, Seeger W, Buchhorn R, et al: Surfactant abnormalities in patients with respiratory failure after multiple trauma. Am Rev Respir Dis 1989;140:1033–1039.

38. American College of Surgeons: Advanced Trauma Life Support for Doctors, 7th ed. Chicago: American College of Surgeons, 2004.

39. Greenberg M, Rosen C: Evaluation of the patient with blunt chest trauma: An evidence based approach. Emerg Med Clin North Am 1999;17:41–62.

40. Napolitano LM, Genuit T, Rodriguez A: Evaluation of blunt thoracic trauma. In Messick WJ (ed): Initial Management of Injuries: An Evidence-Based Approach. London: BMJ Books, 2001, pp 54–63.

41. Ruchholtz S, Zintl B, Nast-Kolb D, et al: Improvement in the therapy of multiply injured patients by introduction of clinical management guidelines. Injury 1998;29:115–129.

42. Richter M, Krettek C, Otte D, et al: Correlation between crash severity, injury severity, and clinical course in car occupants with thoracic trauma: A technical and medical study. J Trauma 2001;51:10–16.

43. Orzechowski KM, Edgerton EA, Bulas DI, et al: Patterns of injury to restrained children in side impact motor vehicle crashes: The side impact syndrome. J Trauma 2003;54:1094–1101.

44. Viano DC, Lau IV, Andrzejak DV, et al: Biomechanics of injury in lateral impacts. Accid Anal Prev 1989;21:535–551.

45. Viano DC, Lau IV, Asbury C, et al: Biomechanics of the human chest, abdomen, and pelvis in lateral impact. Accid Anal Prev 1989;21:553–574.

46. Pattimore D, Thomas P, Dave S: Torso injury patterns and mechanisms in car crashes: An additional diagnostic tool. Injury 1992;23:123–126.

47. Kunisch-Hoppe M, Bachmann G, Hoppe M, et al: [CT quantification of pleuropulmonary lesions in severe thoracic trauma.] Rofo 1997;167:453–457.

48. Calhoon JH, Trinkle JK: Pathophysiology of chest trauma. Chest Surg Clin N Am 1997;7:199–211.

49. Baker SP, O'Neill B, Haddum W, et al: The injury severity score: A method of describing patients with multiple injuries and evaluating emergency care. J Trauma 1974;14:187–196.

50. Civil ID, Schwab CW: The abbreviated injury scale, 1985 revision: A condensed chart for clinical use. J Trauma 1988;28:87–90.

51. Di Bartolomeo S, Sanson G, Nardi G, et al: A population-based study on pneumothorax in severely traumatized patients. J Trauma 2001;51:677–682.

52. Dunlop MG, Beattie TF, Preston PG, Steedman DJ: Clinical assessment and radiograph following blunt chest trauma. Arch Emerg Med 1989;6:125–127.

53. Bokhari F, Brakenridge S, Nagy K, et al: Prospective evaluation of the sensitivity of physical examination in chest trauma. J Trauma 2002;53:1135–1138.

54. Chen SC, Markmann JF, Kauder DR, et al: Hemopneumothorax missed by auscultation in penetrating chest injury. J Trauma 1997;42:86–89.

55. Hirshberg A, Thomson SR, Huizinga WK: Reliability of physical examination in penetrating chest injuries. Injury 1988;19:407–409.

56. Holmes JF, Sokolove PE, Brant WE, et al: A clinical decision rule for identifying children with thoracic injuries after blunt torso trauma. Ann Emerg Med 2002;39:492–499.

57. Ullman EA, Donley LP, Brady WJ: Pulmonary trauma emergency department evaluation and management. Emerg Med Clin North Am 2003;21:291–313.

58. Di Bartolomeo S: Tension pneumothorax, Achilles, and the turtle. J Trauma 2004;57:926.

59. Schild HH, Strunk H, Weber W, et al: Pulmonary contusion: CT vs plain radiograms. J Comput Assist Tomogr 1989;13:417–420.

60. Trupka A, Waydhas C, Hallfeldt K, et al: Value of thoracic computed tomography in the first assessment of severely injured patients with blunt chest trauma: Results of a prospective study. J Trauma 1997;43:405–411.

61. McGonigal M, Schwab W, Kauder W, et al: Supplemental emergent chest computed tomography in the management of blunt torso trauma. J Trauma 1990;30:1431–1435.

62. Wicky S, Wintermark M, Schnyder P, et al: Imaging of blunt chest trauma. Eur Radiol 2000;10:1524–1538.

63. Kloppel R, Schreiter D, Dietrich J, et al: Early clinical phase of patient's management after polytrauma using 1- and 4-slice helical CT. Radiologe 2002;42:541–546.

64. Navarrete-Navarro P, Vázquez G, Bosch JM, et al: Computed tomography vs clinical and multidisciplinary procedures for early evaluation of severe abdomen and chest trauma: A cost analysis approach. Intensive Care Med 1996;22:208–212.

65. Collins J: Chest wall trauma. J Thorac Imaging 2000;15:112–119.

66. Copes W, Champion H, Sacco W, et al: The injury severity score revisited. J Trauma 1988;23:775–787.

67. Tyburski JG, Collinge JD, Wilson RF, et al: Pulmonary contusions: Quantifying the lesions on chest X-ray films and the factors affecting prognosis. J Trauma 1999;46:833–838.

68. Hill SL, Edmisten T, Holtzman G, et al: The occult pneumothorax: An increasing diagnostic entity in trauma. Am Surg 1999;65:254–258.

69. Neff MA, Monk JS Jr, Peters K, et al: Detection of occult pneumothoraces on abdominal computed tomographic scans in trauma patients. J Trauma 2000;49:281–285.

70. Gentilello LM, Anardi D, Mock Ch, et al: Permissive hypercapnia in trauma patients. J Trauma 1995;39:846–852; discussion 852–853.

71. Voggenreiter G, Majetschak M, Aufmkolk M, et al: Estimation of condensed pulmonary parenchyma from gas exchange parameters in multiple trauma patients with blunt chest trauma. J Trauma 1997;43:8–12.

72. Gattinoni L, Caironi P, Pelosi P, et al: What has computed tomography taught us about the acute respiratory distress syndrome? Am J Respir Crit Care Med 2001;164:1701–1711.

73. Mizushima Y, Hiraide A, Shimazu T, et al: Changes in contused lung volume and oxygenation in patients with pulmonary parenchymal injury after blunt chest trauma. Am J Emerg Med 2000;18:385–389.

74. Malbouisson LM, Muller JC, Constantin JM, et al: Computed tomography assessment of positive end-expiratory pressure-induced alveolar recruitment in patients with acute respiratory distress syndrome. Am J Respir Crit Care Med 2001;163:1444–1450.

75. Spaite DW, Criss EA, Valenzuela TD, et al: Prehospital advanced life support for major trauma: Critical need for clinical trials. Ann Emerg Med 1998;32:480–489.

76. McSwain NE Jr: A plea for uniformity in EMS research. J Trauma 2002;52:1220–1221.

77. Eckstein M, Chan L, Schneir A, et al: Effect of prehospital advanced life support on outcomes of major trauma patients. J Trauma 2000;48:643–648.

78. Liberman M, Mulder D, Sampalis J: Advanced or basic life support for trauma: Meta-analysis and critical review of the literature. J Trauma 2000;49:584–599.

79. Vidhani K, Kause J, Parr M: Should we follow ATLS guidelines for the management of traumatic pulmonary contusion: The role of non-invasive ventilatory support. Resuscitation 2002;52:265–268.

80. Richardson JD, Adams L, Flint LM: Selective management of flail chest and pulmonary contusion. Ann Surg 1982;196:481–487.

81. Goris RJ, Gimbrere JS, van Niekerk JL, et al: Improved survival of multiply injured patients by early internal fixation and prophylactic mechanical ventilation. Injury 1982;14:39–43.

82. Bochicchio GV, Scalea TM: Is field intubation useful? Curr Opin Crit Care 2003;9:524–529.

83. Bochicchio GV, Ilahi O, Joshi M, et al: Endotracheal intubation in the field does not improve outcome in trauma patients who present without an acutely lethal traumatic brain injury. J Trauma 2003;54:307–311.

84. Davis BD, Fowler R, Kupas DF, et al: Role of rapid sequence induction for intubation in the prehospital setting: Helpful or harmful? Curr Opin Crit Care 2002;8:571–577.

85. Ruchholtz S, Waydhas C, Ose C, et al: Prehospital intubation in severe thoracic trauma without respiratory insufficiency: A matched-pair analysis based on the Trauma Registry of the German Trauma Society. J Trauma 2002;52:879–886.

86. O'Keefe GE, Maier RV: New regimens in the management of posttraumatic respiratory failure. Curr Opin Pulm Med 1997;3:227–233.

87. Ashbaugh JD, Bigelow DB, Petty TL, Levine BE: Acute respiratory distress in adults. Lancet 1967;2:319–323.

88. Enderson BL: Inverse ratio ventilation for posttraumatic respiratory failure. J Tenn Med Assoc 1990;83:134–135.

89. Moomey CB Jr, Fabian TC, Croce MA, et al: Cardiopulmonary function after pulmonary contusion and partial liquid ventilation. J Trauma 1998;45:283–290.

90. Gore DC: Hemodynamic and ventilatory effects associated with increasing inverse inspiratory-expiratory ventilation. J Trauma. 1998;45:268–272.

91. Borg UR, Stoklosa JC, Siegel JH, et al: Prospective evaluation of combined high-frequency ventilation in post-traumatic patients with adult respiratory distress syndrome refractory to optimized conventional ventilatory management. Crit Care Med 1989;17:1129–1142.

92. Hurst JM, Branson RD, DeHaven CB: The role of high-frequency ventilation in post-traumatic respiratory insufficiency. J Trauma 1987;27:236–242.

93. Putensen C, Zech S, Wrigge H, et al: Long-term effects of spontaneous breathing during ventilatory support in patients with acute lung injury. Am J Respir Crit Care Med 2001;164:43–49.

94. Sharma S, Mullins RJ, Trunkey DD: Ventilatory management of pulmonary contusion patients. Am J Surg 1996;171:529–532.

95. Gunduz M, Unlugenc H, Ozalevli M, et al: A comparative study of continuous positive airway pressure (CPAP) and intermittent positive pressure ventilation (IPPV) in patients with flail chest. Emerg Med J 2005;22:325–329.

96. Acute Respiratory Distress Syndrome Network: Ventilation with lower tidal volumes as compared with traditional tidal volumes for acute lung injury and the acute respiratory distress syndrome. N Engl J Med 2000;342:1301–1308.

97. Amato MBP, Barbas CS, Medeiros DM, et al: Effect of a protective-ventilation strategy on mortality in the acute respiratory distress syndrome. N Engl J Med 1998;338:347–354.

98. Johannigman JA, Miller SL, Davis BR, et al: Influence of low tidal volumes on gas exchange in acute respiratory distress syndrome and the role of recruitment maneuvers. J Trauma 2003;54:320–325.

99. Wolter TP, Fuchs PC, Horvat N, et al: Is high PEEP low volume ventilation in burn patients beneficial? A retrospective study of 61 patients. Burns 2004;30:368–373.

100. Michaels AJ: Management of post traumatic respiratory failure. Crit Care Clin 2004;20:83–99.

101. Pelosi P, Severgnini P, Chiaranda M: An integrated approach to prevent and treat respiratory failure in brain-injured patients. Curr Opin Crit Care 2005;11:37–42.

102. Hudson LD, Milberg JA, Anardi D, et al: Clinical risks for development of the acute respiratory distress syndrome. Am J Respir Crit Care Med 1995;151:293–301.

103. Gajic O, Frutos-Vivar F, Esteban A, et al: Ventilator settings as a risk factor for acute respiratory distress syndrome in mechanically ventilated patients. Intensive Care Med 2005;31:922–926.

104. Fulton RL, Peter ET: The progressive nature of pulmonary contusion. Surgery 1970;67:499–506.

105. Regel G, Grotz M, Weltner T, et al: Pattern of organ failure following severe trauma. World J Surg 1996;20:422–429.

106. Glasser SA, Domino KB, Lindgren L, et al: Pulmonary blood pressure and flow during atelectasis in the dog. Anesthesiology 1983;58:225–231.

107. Marshall BE: Importance of hypoxic pulmonary vasoconstriction with atelectasis. Adv Shock Res 1982;8:1–12.

108. van Kaam AH, Lachmann RA, Herting E, et al: Reducing atelectasis attenuates bacterial growth and translocation in experimental pneumonia. Am J Respir Crit Care Med 2004;169:1046–1053.

109. Duggan M, McCaul CL, McNamara PJ, et al: Atelectasis causes vascular leak and lethal right ventricular failure in uninjured rat lungs. Am J Respir Crit Care Med 2003;167:1633–1640.

110. Squadrone V, Coha M, Cerutti E, et al: Continuous positive airway pressure for treatment of postoperative hypoxemia: A randomized controlled trial. JAMA 2005;293:589–595.

111. Richardson JD, Woods D, Johanson WG, et al: Lung bacterial clearance following pulmonary contusion. Surgery 1979;86:730–735.

112. Drinkwater DC Jr, Wittnich C, Mulder DS, et al: Mechanical and cellular bacterial clearance in lung atelectasis. Ann Thorac Surg 1981;32:235–243.

113. Singh N, Falestiny MN, Rogers P, et al: Pulmonary infiltrates in the surgical ICU: Prospective assessment of predictors of etiology and mortality. Chest 1998;114:1129–1136.

114. Croce MA, Fabian TC, Mueller EW, et al: The appropriate diagnostic threshold for ventilator-associated pneumonia using quantitative cultures. J Trauma 2004;56:931–934; discussion 934–936.

115. Croce MA, Fabian TC, Waddle-Smith L, et al: Identification of early predictors for post-traumatic pneumonia. Am Surg 2001;67:105–110.

116. Gannon CJ, Pasquale M, Tracy JK, et al: Male gender is associated with increased risk for postinjury pneumonia. Shock 2004;21:410–414.

117. Dos Santos CC, Slutsky AS: Invited review: mechanisms of ventilator-induced lung injury: A perspective. J Appl Physiol 2000;89:1645–1655.

118. Moloney ED, Griffiths MJ: Protective ventilation of patients with acute respiratory distress syndrome. Br J Anaesth 2004;92:261–270.

119. Duggan M, Kavanagh BP: Pulmonary atelectasis: A pathogenic perioperative entity. Anesthesiology 2005;102:838–854.

120. Haenel JB, Moore FA, Moore EE, Read RA: Efficacy of selective intrabronchial air insufflation in acute lobar collapse. Am J Surg 1992;164:501–505.

121. Gattinoni L, Caironi P, Carlesso E: How to ventilate patients with acute lung injury and acute respiratory distress syndrome. Curr Opin Crit Care 2005;11:69–76.

122. Marini JJ, Gattinoni L: Ventilatory management of acute respiratory distress syndrome: A consensus of two. Crit Care Med 2004;32:250–255.

123. Grasso S, Fanelli V, Cafarelli A, et al: Effects of high versus low positive end-expiratory pressures in acute respiratory distress syndrome. Am J Respir Crit Care Med 2005;171:1002–1008.

124. Grasso S, Terragni P, Mascia L, et al: Airway pressure-time curve profile (stress index) detects tidal recruitment/hyperinflation in experimental acute lung injury. Crit Care Med 2004;32:1018–1027.

125. Albaiceta GM, Taboada F, Parra D, et al: Tomographic study of the inflection points of the pressure-volume curve in acute lung injury. Am J Respir Crit Care Med 2004;170:1066–1072.

126. Maggiore SM, Jonson B, Richard JC, et al: Alveolar derecruitment at decremental positive end-expiratory pressure levels in acute lung injury: Comparison with the lower inflection point, oxygenation, and compliance. Am J Respir Crit Care Med 2001;164:795–801.

127. Bendixen HH, Hedley-Whyte J, Laver MB: Impaired oxygenation in surgical patients during general anesthesia with controlled ventilation: A concept of atelectasis. N Engl J Med 1963;269:991–996.

128. British Thoracic Society Standards of Care Committee: Non-invasive ventilation in acute respiratory failure. Thorax 2002;57:192–211.

129. Levine BE, Johnson RP: Effects of atelectasis on pulmonary surfactant and quasi-static lung mechanics. J Appl Physiol 1965;20:859–864.

130. Kress JP, Pohlman AS, O'Connor MF, et al: Daily interruption of sedative infusions in critically ill patients undergoing mechanical ventilation. N Engl J Med 2000;342:1471–1477.

131. Rimensberger PC, Cox PN, Frndova H, et al: The open lung during small tidal volume ventilation: concepts of recruitment and "optimal" positive end-expiratory pressure. Crit Care Med 1999;27:1946–1952.

132. Rimensberger PC, Pristine G, Mullen BM, et al: Lung recruitment during small tidal volume ventilation allows minimal positive end-expiratory pressure without augmenting lung injury. Crit Care Med 1999;27:1940–1945.

133. Hickling KG: Best compliance during a decremental, but not incremental, positive end-expiratory pressure trial is related to open-lung positive end-expiratory pressure: A mathematical model of acute respiratory distress syndrome lungs. Am J Respir Crit Care Med 2001;163:69–78.

134. Lachmann B: Open up the lung and keep the lung open. Intensive Care Med 1992;18:319–321.

135. Hickling KG: Reinterpreting the pressure-volume curve in patients with acute respiratory distress syndrome. Curr Opin Crit Care 2002;8:32–38.

136. Barbas CS, de Matos GF, Pincelli MP, et al: Mechanical ventilation in acute respiratory failure: Recruitment and high positive end-expiratory pressure are necessary. Curr Opin Crit Care 2005;11:18–28.

137. Bein T, Kuhr LP, Bele S, et al: Lung recruitment maneuver in patients with cerebral injury: Effects on intracranial pressure and cerebral metabolism. Intensive Care Med 2002;28:554–558.

138. Rouby JJ: Lung overinflation: The hidden face of alveolar recruitment. Anesthesiology 2003;99:2–4.

139. Voggenreiter G, Neudeck F, Aufmkolk M, et al: Intermittent prone positioning in the treatment of severe and moderate posttraumatic lung injury. Crit Care Med 1999;27:2375–2382.

140. Pape HC, Remmers D, Weinberg A, et al: Is early kinetic positioning beneficial for pulmonary function in multiple trauma patients? Injury 1998;29:219–225.

## SUGGESTED READINGS

Fulton RL, Peter ET, Wilson JN: The pathophysiology and treatment of pulmonary contusions. J Trauma 1970;10:719–730.

Gentilello L, Thompson DA, Tonnesen AS, et al: Effect of a rotating bed on the incidence of pulmonary complications in critically ill patients. Crit Care Med 1988;16:783–786.

Greene R: Lung alterations in thoracic trauma. J Thorac Imaging 1987;2:1–7.

Haenel JB, Moore FA, Moore EE: Pulmonary consequences of severe chest trauma. Respir Care Clin N Am 1996;2:401–424.

Johnson G. Traumatic pneumothorax: Is a chest drain always necessary? J Accid Emerg Med 1996;13:173–174.

Johnson JA, Cogbill TH, Winga ER: Determinants of outcome after pulmonary contusion. J Trauma 1986;26:695–698.

MacLeod J, Lynn M, McKenney MG, et al: Predictors of mortality in trauma patients. Am Surg 2004;70:805–810.

Pape HC, Remmers D, Kleemann W, et al: Posttraumatic multiple organ failure: A report on clinical and autopsy findings. Shock 1994;2:228–234.

Toombs BD, Sandler CM, Lester RG: Computed tomography of chest trauma. Radiology 1981;140:733–738.

Trupka A, Waydhas C, Nast-Kolb D, et al: Early intubation in severely injured patients. Eur J Emerg Med 1994;1:1–8.

Waren LB, Matthay MA: The acute respiratory distress syndrome. N Engl J Med 2000;342:1334–1349.

# SECTION 5

# ADJUNCTS TO VENTILATOR THERAPY

# CHAPTER 34

# Airway Management and Physiologic Control of Ventilation

Denham S. Ward and Jaideep J. Pandit

Mechanical ventilation through an artificial airway replaces the body's own homeostatic control over ventilation and the upper airway. The purpose of this chapter is as follows: (1) to outline the control of ventilation and the upper airway in the normal (physiologic) state, (2) to show how this helps us understand situations in which this control may be impaired, (3) to discuss artificial alternatives to the natural upper airway, (4) to illustrate how these principles may be important for the patient in intensive care (ICU) who is spontaneously breathing, and (5) to show how drugs commonly used in the intensive care setting may interact with this normal control of breathing.

## UPPER AIRWAY: PHYSIOLOGIC CONTROL

The upper airway is the framework of bone, cartilage, and soft tissue beginning at the nose or lips and ending at the larynx. Whenever any part of this structure is not patent, *upper airway obstruction* may result. Commonly, this condition occurs at points that are already naturally narrow or prone to collapse. The nose, the larynx, and the trachea all have bony or cartilaginous support, so the part most prone to collapse is the pharynx. Collapse most readily occurs at the level of the epiglottis, the tongue, and the soft palate. Pathologic abnormalities such as upper airway tumors, foreign bodies, and trauma can also lead to obstruction at any point in the upper airway.[1]

In the supine conscious subject, the genioglossus muscle has high resting tone and phasic activity during the inspiratory part of the respiratory cycle. This keeps the airway patent and allows a gap between the tongue and the posterior pharyngeal wall. However, during sleep, anesthesia, and deep sedation, genioglossus tone is reduced, and the relaxed tongue then collapses against the posterior pharyngeal wall, thus potentially obstructing the airway (Fig. 34.1). Episodic airway obstruction during sleep is quite common, and the incidence increases with age.[2] In natural sleep, this episodic airway obstruction is terminated and then reversed by the process of arousal. During anesthesia and deep sedation, not only are the drives to the pharyngeal dilators diminished,[3] but also the central nervous system arousal that occurs when the airway is obstructed may be diminished or eliminated.[4] Maneuvers that restore airway patency (without the establishment of a surgical airway) include (1) extension of the neck at the atlanto-occipital joint, (2) head extension at the neck (the combination of neck and head extension is known as the "sniffing position"), (3) manual anterior protrusion of the jaw,[5] (4) the use of specific supraglottic airway devices (SADs; the simplest being the Guedel airway), and (5) tracheal intubation. The position of the patient may also improve airway patency in patients prone to obstruction.[6]

Swallowing incorporates a reflex that protects the lower airway from reflux of solid or liquid matter. The larynx is elevated by the constriction of the infrahyoid muscles, and the epiglottis folds backward to occlude the entrance to the larynx. This reflex is impaired by decreased levels of consciousness resulting from sedation or neurologic injury, with the attendant risk of pulmonary aspiration. This risk can be reduced by the use of a cuffed tracheal tube, as described later.

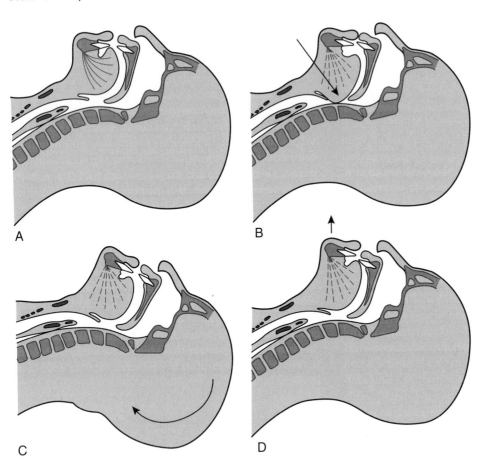

A

B

C

D

**Figure 34.1** Diagrammatic cross section of the upper airway. *A,* Supine subject, awake. *B,* During sleep or anesthesia. The *arrow* points to the tongue, which is falling back to obstruct the airway as a result of loss of genioglossus tone. *C* and *D,* The effects of tilting the head back and thrusting the jaw forward relieve the obstruction.

## IMPAIRED UPPER AIRWAY CONTROL

### Sleep Apnea

*Apnea* is the cessation of airflow, and conventionally it has to exceed 10 seconds' duration to be considered significant. The *respiratory disturbance index* is the number of apneas per hour of sleep. Apnea may be *central,* in which the drive to ventilation ceases and effort is absent, or *obstructive,* in which drive and respiratory effort persist, but upper airway collapse prevents any airflow. Mixed disorders are also common. The *obstructive sleep apnea syndrome* (OSA) occurs when these signs of apnea during sleep are also accompanied by daytime comorbidity such as excessive sleepiness, poor memory and concentration, headache, hypertension, and cardiovascular disorders. The origin of OSA includes many factors that predispose to the airway collapsing during sleep and has been the subject of much research (Box 34.1).[7,8]

Diagnosis of the condition is based on polysomnography (sleep study), which includes electroencephalography, pulse oximetry, transcutaneous carbon dioxide ($CO_2$) determinations, expired minute ventilation (usually using impedance plethysmography), video recording of sleep, and electrocardiography. Other investigations directed to the underlying cause (see Box 34.1) are also undertaken.

Treatment is ideally directed to the underlying cause (see Box 34.1), but it generally involves the use of nocturnal continuous positive airway pressure (CPAP; see later) to prevent nocturnal obstructive episodes. Palatal surgery is also an option in patients with OSA who snore. Tracheostomy is reserved for the treatment

---

**BOX 34-1**

**Factors that Predispose to Obstructive Sleep Apnea**

Obesity
Smoking (from chronic nasal congestion and pharyngeal edema or inflammation)
Nasal obstruction (e.g., septal deviation)
Tonsillar and adenoidal hypertrophy
Craniofacial abnormality (e.g., Down's, Pierre-Robin, Treacher-Collins syndromes)
Laryngeal obstruction (laryngomalacia, tracheomalacia)
Endocrine (e.g., Cushing's disease, hypothyroidism)
Neuromuscular disorders (that also reduce ventilatory drive or control of pharynx)

of life-threatening OSA when invasive forms of respiratory support are not tolerated.

The causes of central sleep apnea include disordered peripheral chemosensitivity, which can occur in cardiac failure or after bilateral carotid body resection, and disordered central ventilatory control (e.g., after stroke, head injury). Central sleep apnea a less common disorder than OSA, although episodes of central apnea are common in patients with sleep apnea and with heart failure.[9,10]

## Obesity

An overlap between obesity and OSA has been recognized, in that many obese patients suffer from OSA, but not all patients with OSA are obese. During anesthesia and sedation, support of the upper airway using the manual maneuvers described earlier can be difficult, and tracheal intubation can also be complicated in obesity. Indeed, even surgical tracheostomy can be difficult in the presence of excess fat or soft tissue in the neck. During spontaneous breathing, the work of breathing is greater in obese persons because the weight and structure of the chest wall contribute to poor compliance, and the shape of the chest wall can sometimes cause the respiratory muscles to work at a mechanical disadvantage. In the supine position, the abdomen may also contribute adversely to all these factors. Finally, obesity often is associated with serious systemic comorbidity such as hypertension, coronary artery disease, and diabetes, all of which further exacerbate the risk of tissue hypoxia.

## SUPPORT OF THE UPPER AIRWAY

In addition to the simple manual maneuvers described earlier, the following additional means are used to provide support to an upper airway that has collapsed or is in danger of collapse: (1) CPAP, (2) SADs, (3) oronasal tracheal intubation, and (4) tracheostomy. These airway devices may be placed for short-term ventilatory support (e.g., during surgery), or they may be necessary for longer-term mechanical ventilation. The method selected for support of the upper airway requires consideration of the patient, the disease, the type of mechanical ventilation, and the anticipated duration of mechanical ventilation.

### Continuous Positive Airway Pressure Ventilation

CPAP and its modifications (e.g., bilevel positive airway pressure [BiPAP] and positive end-expiratory pressure) are discussed in Section 3 of this book. These terms refer to the manner in which airway pressure varies with the respiratory cycle. During normal spontaneous breathing, inspiration is associated with negative airway pressure (relative to atmosphere); during passive expiration, airway pressure is slightly positive. In CPAP, airway pressure is always positive at the same mean level; breathing remains spontaneous, and so airway pressure fluctuates around the positive predetermined set level. In BiPAP, the airway pressure is again always positive, but more so during inspiration than expiration; breathing is spontaneous, and airway pressures fluctuate around the two set levels. Thus, whereas CPAP only opens the upper airway, BiPAP can supply actual ventilatory assistance. In all these modes of pressure application, the continuously positive airway pressure can act as a pneumatic splint against upper airway collapse, can reduce the work of breathing, and can thereby improve oxygenation. These types of airway pressure fluctuations can be applied through an endotracheal tube as part of a strategy of mechanical ventilation. They are most commonly used to assist weaning from a period of prolonged mechanical ventilation to enable the return of spontaneous, unassisted breathing. They can also be used in conjunction with noninvasive ventilation (NIV).

### Noninvasive Ventilation

NIV is discussed in more detail in Chapter 45. It is termed *noninvasive* to distinguish it from methods involving tracheal intubation. Tracheal intubation is termed *invasive* because some degree of anesthesia or sedation is usually needed to site the endotracheal tube properly; NIV does not require these measures. In NIV, the patient's lungs are ventilated through a tight-fitting nasal or face mask. In the ICU, NIV has several potential roles.[11,12] First, it can be used to delay tracheal intubation in patients admitted with worsening lung function. Delaying tracheal intubation may be beneficial; although intubation facilitates positive pressure mechanical ventilation, which the patient needs, it is associated with complications. The act of inducing sedation or anesthesia to facilitate the intubation can itself cause cardiorespiratory collapse; ventilator-associated pneumonia is a serious concern (there is an infection risk of 1% for each day that the patient's lungs are mechanically ventilated), and high inflation pressures can cause barotrauma. Secondly, because NIV is not as sophisticated an intervention as tracheal intubation, it can be introduced at a much earlier stage than one would normally consider intubation; it may therefore "buy time" when expert anesthetic or intensive care support may not be immediately available. Thirdly, it can be used as a means of assisting weaning from endotracheal mechanical ventilation; the patient's lungs can be extubated perhaps earlier than is usual, but then NIV is commenced for a period to provide respiratory support. This approach is often better than extubation directly to spontaneous, unassisted self-ventilation.

However, NIV itself poses problems. Some patients, especially those who are dyspneic, do not tolerate the masks, which can cause pressure sores in up to 2% of patients. There is no evidence that NIV actually decreases tracheal intubation rates in the context of exacerbations of chronic obstructive pulmonary disease, and no controlled trial has compared outcomes using NIV with tracheal intubation to treat exacerbations of this disease. NIV needs specialist nursing, although perhaps to a lesser degree than ventilation using tracheal intubation, and intubation facilities still need to be available. It is not possible to manage the lower airway (e.g., regular suctioning) with NIV, so it is of limited use in patients in whom secretions are a major problem.

## Supraglottic Airway Devices

Perhaps the simplest means of supporting the upper airway is a hand-held face mask. When connected to a suitable supply of oxygen ($O_2$) or anesthetic gas, such a mask may be used to support the airway manually or, if spontaneous ventilation is absent, may allow hand ventilation of the patient's lungs. One problem with the face mask technique is that, during surgery, it does not allow good surgical access to the patient's face, head, or airway. Further, use of the mask requires that one or both of the physician's hands be occupied in airway maintenance, and active ventilation of the patient's lungs can be often inefficient (i.e., not all the tidal volume [$V_T$] administered to the patient enters the lungs, and some is lost as a leak).[13]

SADs were developed to overcome some of these problems. In general, these devices are tubes, often with inflatable distal components to hold the airway in place, that lie in the oropharynx above the level of the glottis. The device most commonly used is the laryngeal mask airway; others include the cuffed oropharyngeal airway and the ProSeal™ laryngeal mask (laryngeal mask company, Henley-on-Thames, UK). SADs allow spontaneous breathing and, like the face mask technique, facilitate active ventilation by hand. However, because SADs lie above the glottic opening and do not seal it, there is a risk that prolonged positive pressure ventilation of the lungs (e.g., if the SAD is connected to a mechanical ventilator) may cause air to enter the esophagus and stomach. If gastric fluid should then regurgitate, SADs will not completely protect the airway from lung soiling. A debate is ongoing concerning the role of some SAD devices in positive pressure ventilation, and some authorities argue that the use of these devices during positive pressure ventilation is justified.[14,15] In particular, it has been argued that the ProSeal™ laryngeal mask airway has certain features that make positive pressure of the lungs more efficient than using the traditional laryngeal mask airway.[15]

SADs have several roles in the ICU. First, they can be used as emergency airway devices to facilitate oxygenation of the lungs when tracheal intubation has failed. Failed intubation is relatively common in the ICU; tracheal tubes often need to be changed (e.g., because of clogging by secretions), and because many patients are edematous secondary to their subacute or chronic underlying disease processes and to repeated endotracheal tube changes, tracheal intubation can be difficult. In this situation, a laryngeal mask may act as a rescue device. Secondly, SADs can be used to facilitate NIV.[16,17] This approach may also aid in weaning from mechanical ventilation. Finally, SADs have found a place in maintaining the airway during percutaneous tracheostomy or formal (open) tracheostomy.[18]

The use of SADs in intensive care has certain limitations. SADs do not easily facilitate suctioning and care of the lower respiratory tract. In addition, sustained cuff pressure can cause erosion or ulceration of surrounding pharyngeal structures, and nerve palsies, especially hypoglossal, have also been reported.[19,20]

## Tracheal Tubes

Endotracheal tubes lie in the trachea and usually have a small cuff at the distal end that protects the airway from soiling (e.g., by blood or regurgitant gastric contents) and improves the efficiency of ventilation by minimizing leaks. Tracheal tubes vary in shape, size, and composition, and these factors are important in relation to their specific use. For example, the RAE (Ring, Aldair, and Elwyn) preformed tube is curved so that, when properly placed, the tip points caudally; this tube is therefore useful in oral and cranial surgery. Ceramic and metallic tubes are laser resistant. Armored (flexible metallic) tubes are more difficult to kink and thus are useful during surgery in which the head position changes or when the patient is prone (Fig. 34.2). However, these tubes can be crushed (e.g., by biting) and must be used cautiously in the ICU setting.

Because tracheal tubes form a sealed conduit into the trachea, they are primarily used when the patient is paralyzed and requires positive pressure ventilation (there is no risk of blowing air into the stomach). It is indeed possible to allow the patient to breathe spontaneously through a tracheal tube, but because the glottis and trachea are richly innervated, deep sedation is usually required to prevent the patient from reflex coughing. The doses of anesthetic agent required to achieve this level of sedation may cause dose-related side effects. Whereas most SAD devices can be used effectively after relatively short periods of training, the techniques used to insert a tracheal tube are more specialized.

Tracheal tubes may be passed either orally or nasally. The distinction between these routes is important, and

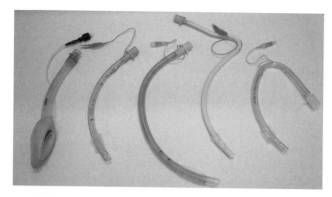

**Figure 34.2** Examples of airways and tracheal tubes. From *left,* Laryngeal mask airway (a supraglottic airway device); "standard" Magill-shaped polyvinyl chloride endotracheal tube; reinforced, flexible metallic endotracheal tube (e.g., for use in head and neck surgery); nasotracheal tube; RAE (Ring, Aldair, and Elwyn) tube.

the route chosen can depend on the type of surgery. For example, a nasotracheal tube facilitates better surgical access for dental surgery, but it is clearly a hindrance during operations on the nose. In intensive care practice, nasal tubes are discouraged because they are a potential source of systemic infection originating from the paranasal sinuses.[21]

## Cuffed versus Uncuffed Tubes

In general, cuffed tubes are used in adult anesthesia, and "plain" or uncuffed tubes are used in prepubertal children. In adults, the narrowest part of the larynx is at the level of the vocal cords. Therefore, if a tube can be passed between the vocal cords, one can be confident that at any point distal to the vocal cords, the tube will be sitting loosely and will not be wedged. A wedged tube can cause epithelial damage. The high-volume, low-pressure cuff can be inflated to provide a loose seal at this level. In children, however, the narrowest part of the larynx is at the level of the cricoid cartilage and not at the vocal cords. It is quite possible therefore to pass a tracheal tube that is small enough to pass through the vocal cords with ease but that may become wedged at the level of the cricoid. Wedging may cause epithelial edema or necrosis at this point. To confirm that the tracheal tube is sitting loosely at all points in the larynx in children, plain tubes are used, and one seeks deliberately to allow a small leak. This leak should be audible on inflation of the chest under positive pressure, and its presence excludes the possibility that the tube is exerting any circumferential pressure on the laryngeal epithelium at its narrowest point. The disadvantages of this small leak are that ventilation may not be as efficient and the lower airway is not definitively secured and protected from soiling from above. For these reasons, if the type of

surgery permits, the laryngeal inlet can be packed with damp ribbon gauze.

It is important to have some notion of the factors in operative surgery that influence the choice of airway support. In general, these factors are either patient-related or surgical.

### Patient-Related Factors Influencing Choice of Airway Device

Certain factors or signs in the patient suggest to most clinicians that a tracheal tube, with the patient consequently artificially ventilated, should be used, rather than an SAD device with the patient breathing spontaneously.

**Gastroesophageal Reflux**   Hiatal hernia, peptic ulcer disease, symptomatic reflux, pregnancy, recent ingestion of solids or particulate liquids, abdominal sepsis, and injury all predispose the patient to regurgitation of gastric contents during induction of anesthesia. Tracheal intubation, as part of rapid-sequence induction of anesthesia, minimizes the risk of lung soiling.

**Obesity**   Obese patients do not always find it easy to breathe when lying supine, even when they are awake. Anesthesia and sedation further increase upper airway resistance and decrease ventilatory efficacy (e.g., through a reduction in functional residual capacity). Thus, many obese patients require positive pressure ventilation through an endotracheal tube.

### Patients with Known or Anticipated Difficult Airway

In any patient whose trachea is known or anticipated to be difficult to intubate, it is reasonable to formulate a plan to intubate the trachea during induction of anesthesia and thereby achieve a definitively secured airway in the patient before the surgical procedure begins. Although it is also acceptable (and sometimes necessary, should tracheal intubation fail) to use an SAD device, the problem is that, should tracheal intubation subsequently be necessary urgently during the course of surgery, this may be difficult or impossible to achieve in a short time. Patients with known difficulty in intubation should be clearly identified if they remain intubated in the postoperative period. A specifically designed warning tag attached to the pilot balloon is an excellent method of identification.

### Surgical Factors Influencing Choice of Airway Device

Certain surgical requirements influence the choice of airway device.

**Factors Related to the Shared Airway**   For certain operations, it is necessary for the surgeon to have an unobstructed view of the relevant anatomy. Because of the large distal cuff, most SAD devices do not permit a good view of structures distal to the oropharynx. Thus, for almost all periglottic, laryngeal, and subglottic operations, a tracheal tube is more suitable or is necessary. SAD devices may, however, be used for operations related to the tonsils, anterior tongue, nose, teeth, and ears without obstructing the surgical field.

**Laser Surgery**  Standard (polyvinyl chloride) tracheal tubes are not laser-resistant and may ignite if struck by a laser beam. Specialized tracheal tubes have been developed that are more laser resistant. The materials used include various metals, Teflon®, and ceramics. Some recent work suggests that the flexible laryngeal mask airway is also suitably laser-resistant, and if used in the presence of laser, its distal cuff should be filled with saline (or methylene blue dye, so rupture can be easily detected).[22]

**Requirement for Neuromuscular Blockade**  For certain operations (e.g., abdominal surgery), it is necessary that the patient's muscles are fully flaccid to facilitate surgery. This is best achieved by use of neuromuscular blocking drugs. Because these drugs also paralyze spontaneous ventilation, artificial mechanical ventilation is required, and a tracheal tube is most commonly used to facilitate this procedure. For some operations, flaccid muscles are not strictly necessary, but it is desirable to minimize risk of the patient's moving, coughing, or swallowing (e.g., base of skull surgery; any ear, nose, and throat operation in combination with neurosurgery; or pharyngeal surgery). This goal is most reliably achieved using neuromuscular blocking drugs.

**Postoperative Plan**  After some major and long operations, it is conventional for the postoperative plan to include admission to an ICU for a period of artificial ventilation, which itself requires the presence of a tracheal tube. This plan may also be necessary if the patient has certain medical conditions (e.g., poor lung function).

In the ICU, important aspects of endotracheal tube management include the following: (1) the tubes are used regularly to suction the lower airway (hence preformed or shaped tubes such as the RAE tubes are generally unsuitable for use in ICU); (2) the tubes are made from a nonirritant, appropriate material (hence the reinforced or metallic endotracheal tubes sometimes used for laser upper airway surgery are not ideal for long-term ventilation); (3) cuff pressure is regularly checked, and cuffs are not overinflated, to prevent trauma and ulceration; and (4) endotracheal tubes may need to be changed (tube exchange) if they are blocked by secretions.

## Tracheostomy

Direct surgical intubation of the trachea percutaneously from the anterior neck is a technique that predated oronasal tracheal intubation by several hundred years. In general, tracheostomy has the following indications.

It can be used in the emergency setting when conventional oronasal tracheal intubation has failed (*failed intubation*) or as an elective procedure during some types of major oral, head, or neck surgeries, in which it facilitates healing of the primary surgical condition. In addition, it is used after laryngectomy (in which case the tracheostomy is permanent), as well as in chronic neuromuscular disorders when long-term tracheal intubation through the oronasal route is impractical. Silver (uncuffed) tracheal tubes are less traumatic and are tolerated for much longer periods than are cuffed polyvinyl chloride plastic tubes. Certain types of tracheostomy tubes also allow speech; the stoma leading to the atmosphere can be blocked digitally, and an opening in the tracheostomy tube forces air through the vocal cords.

In the ICU, for patients undergoing long-term (e.g., >7 to 10 days) ventilation, tracheostomy offers the following advantages. First, it reduces dead-space volume and airway resistance (the dead-space volume and resistance of the short tracheostomy tube lying close to the main bronchi are less than those of the longer endotracheal tube). This facilitates weaning from mechanical ventilation and allows easier suctioning and care of the lower airway. Early tracheostomy has been shown to reduce the length of stay in the ICU, and levels of sedation can be decreased after tracheostomy and can thus also facilitate earlier extubation and recovery. Finally, levels of nosocomial infection are reduced after tracheostomy.

### Methods

*Conventional tracheostomy* is a formal surgical procedure. It can be performed either using local anesthesia (with the patient awake) or using general anesthesia. In the latter situation, the airway has already been secured with either a conventional endotracheal tube or a laryngeal mask airway.

More recently, *percutaneous tracheostomy* performed by anesthesiologists and intensive care specialists, rather than by surgeons, has been used as an alternative to the more formal open surgical tracheostomy.[23] Most methods rely on (1) initial access to the trachea using a large needle (commonly through the second or third tracheal rings), (2) a method of dilation of the access site using serial plastic dilators or forceps, (3) insertion of the definitive tracheostomy tube, and (4) continuous visualization during the procedure using a fiberoptic bronchoscope inserted through the existing endotracheal tube or laryngeal mask airway to ensure that the initial access and dilation are of the trachea and not of the paratracheal structures. Methods currently used include the Ciaglia technique, the "Blue Rhino" method, the Griggs forceps technique, and the Rapitrach method. Percutaneous tracheostomy is essentially a "blind" technique in that no formal surgical dissection is performed to expose the anatomy of the trachea. Therefore, surgical tracheostomy is probably preferable in these circumstances: (1) after previous head and neck surgery, (2) in the presence of goiter and other neck masses, (3) after previous tracheostomy (including previous percutaneous tracheostomy), and (4) in cases of known or established difficult tracheal intubation.

## VENTILATORY CONTROL

It is important to review the control of ventilation in the normal state, to more clearly understand situations in which this control is impaired (or overridden, as in mechanical ventilation). Caruana-Montaldo and associates have provided a clinical overview of the control of breathing.[24]

### Overview of Spontaneous Breathing

Phasic breathing is generated in the respiratory center of the brainstem. A detailed discussion of the interconnections of the respiratory neurons is beyond the scope of this chapter (see the review by Bianchi and colleagues[25]). Briefly, the medulla contains inspiratory and expiratory neurons, which together function to generate the basic respiratory rhythm. The respiratory center neurons receive numerous inputs that further modify and refine the rate and depth of breathing. These inputs may be classified broadly as *feedforward factors* or *feedback factors*. Feedforward factors are those that primarily drive the breathing; they "tell the respiratory system how much work it needs to do."[26,27] Feedback factors are those that feed back to refine the breathing; they "tell the respiratory system how well it is doing."[24] Table 34.1 summarizes some of these factors. An example of a feedforward factor is afferent neural input to the respiratory center from moving joints during muscular exercise. This input carries some information about the degree of exercise performed, and the strength of the signal may indicate to the system how much breathing needs to be done to match breathing to the work performed. Generally, feedback factors are the arterial blood levels of the partial pressure of $O_2$ and $CO_2$ ($PaO_2$ and $PaCO_2$) and hydrogen ions ($H^+$). For example, if breathing is inadequate, then $PaCO_2$ will rise and $PaO_2$ will decline, and these changes are stimuli to the respiratory center for minute ventilation to increase (see later).

**Table 34-1** Feedforward and Feedback Factors*

| Feedforward | Feedback |
|---|---|
| Talking, singing | Arterial $P_{CO_2}$ |
| Other volitional control | Arterial $P_{O_2}$ |
| Muscle spindles | Arterial pH |
| Joint position receptors | Oscillations of above |
| Pain receptors | |
| Flux of $CO_2$ ($\dot{V}_{CO_2}$) back to the lung | |
| Cardiac output (cardiodynamic drive) | |
| Catecholamines | |
| Arterial plasma potassium levels | |
| Arterial oscillations of $P_{CO_2}$, $P_{O_2}$, pH | |

*A full explanation of the mechanisms of these factors is beyond the scope of this chapter, and some factors are still debated (e.g., oscillations).
$CO_2$, carbon dioxide; $P_{CO_2}$, partial pressure of carbon dioxide; $P_{O_2}$, partial pressure of oxygen; $\dot{V}_{CO_2}$, carbon dioxide consumption.

### Output of the Respiratory System

The final output of the respiratory system is the minute ventilation, which is often denoted and measured as expired ventilation in liters per minute ($\dot{V}_M$). In natural, spontaneous breathing, this is the product of $V_T$ (measured in liters) and frequency of breathing (f, measured as $min^{-1}$); however, probably more closely related to the actual neural output is the division into inspiratory flow and inspiratory duty cycle (in the following equation, $T_I$ and $T_B$ are the inspiratory time and breath time, respectively, in seconds; and $V_I$ is the inspiratory $V_T$):

$$\dot{V}_M = f \cdot V_T = \frac{V_I}{T_I} \cdot \frac{T_I}{T_B} \cdot 60$$

### Influence of Changing Alveolar Ventilation on the Alveolar (Arterial) Oxygen and Carbon Dioxide Tension

Changing the alveolar ventilation (the minute ventilation reduced by the dead-space ventilation) alters the alveolar gas composition. For example, in a spontaneously breathing patient, voluntary hyperventilation influences the relative levels of $PO_2$ and $PCO_2$ of gas in contact with the alveoli (the alveolar gas). A similar result is obtained by changing the minute ventilation of the ventilator in a patient being mechanically ventilated. For healthy persons, both the alveolar $PO_2$ ($PAO_2$) and the alveolar $PCO_2$ ($PACO_2$) approximate the arterial levels of these gases ($PaO_2$ and $PaCO_2$). However, in disease, considerable gradients can exist between the alveolar and arterial partial pressures.

Three factors influence the $PaO_2$: (1) the inspired $PO_2$, (2) the alveolar minute ventilation, and (3) $O_2$ consumption ($\dot{V}O_2$, which represents the metabolic uptake of $O_2$). For most subjects at rest, $\dot{V}O_2$ is approximately 200 mL/min, but it can increase with exercise and hyperthermia and decrease with hypothermia, anesthesia, and critical illness. Hyperventilation increases $PaO_2$ toward the inspired level, which is the theoretical absolute maximum level attainable. Hypoventilation decreases $PO_2$. An increase in $\dot{V}O_2$ will tend to reduce $PaO_2$; a decrease in $\dot{V}O_2$ will have the opposite effect.

Only two factors influence the $PaCO_2$ (assuming that there is no rebreathing to increase the inspired $PCO_2$): (1) the alveolar minute ventilation, and (2) $CO_2$ production, which is the metabolic output of $CO_2$. A decline in alveolar ventilation causes alveolar $PCO_2$ to increase; an increase in ventilation will have the opposite effect. An increase in $CO_2$ production (in exercise, hyperthermia) will tend to cause $PaCO_2$ to rise (unless there is a matched increase in alveolar ventilation); a decrease in $CO_2$ production (hypothermia, anesthesia) will have the opposite effect. In terms of Table 34.1, the effect of ventilation on the alveolar (and hence arterial) gas composition can also be considered representative of feedforward mechanisms.

## Influence of Changing Arterial Gas Composition on Alveolar Ventilation

The $PaO_2$ and $PaCO_2$ can be considered as stimuli that act on certain receptors. The activity of these receptors is transmitted to the respiratory neurons in the medulla to influence the minute ventilation. In terms of Table 34.1, these are feedback factors.

### Peripheral Chemoreceptors
The carotid bodies are located at the bifurcation of the carotid arteries bilaterally in the neck and are the main peripheral chemoreceptors. Afferent impulses travel in the carotid sinus branch of the glossopharyngeal nerve to the brainstem respiratory neurons. Aortic bodies are located in the arch of the aorta (afferent nerve branches from the vagus), but their function in humans is thought to be minimal. Histologically, these bodies consist of type I (glomus) cells that are in contact with the afferent nerve endings. The glomus cell is surrounded by type II cells whose function is still obscure. Glomus cells secrete dopamine as well as acetylcholine, norepinephrine, serotonin, adenosine triphosphate, and polypeptides. All these substances may be involved in the process of chemotransduction (see later). There are also efferent nerve endings from the sympathetic superior cervical ganglion. The peripheral chemoreceptors respond by increased afferent impulses to raised $PaCO_2$ (hypercapnia), reduced $PaO_2$ (hypoxia), and raised arterial $H^+$ (low arterial pH; acidosis).

These stimuli *interact* synergistically at the carotid body. The peripheral chemoreceptor responds more to *oscillations* of these stimuli (i.e., rapidly changing absolute levels of stimulus about the same mean value) than it does to a constant mean value of the stimulus (see Table 34.1). Additionally, peripheral chemoreceptors respond to a range of chemicals including arterial plasma potassium levels, catecholamines, and adenosine.

The process by which the hypoxic (or $CO_2$ or acid) signal is converted into an electrical impulse in the nerve is known as *transduction*. Current theories for this complex process are that hypoxia causes membrane depolarization, activation of voltage-sensitive calcium channels in the glomus cell, elevation of cytosolic calcium, and release of neurotransmitter, which then acts on the afferent nerve ending. The details of each of these steps are still under investigation.

### Central Chemoreceptors
Animal studies have revealed chemosensitive areas in the brainstem. Local application of acid solutions and solutions rich in $CO_2$ to superficial areas of the ventral medulla can give rise to an increase in ventilation or phrenic nerve output in experimental animals. The observation that humans deprived of their carotid bodies (after surgery for carotid body tumors) remain responsive to $PCO_2$, but not to hypoxia or to acute metabolic acidosis, suggests that the central chemosensitive areas are stimulated by $PCO_2$ (which crosses the blood-brain barrier), but not by hypoxia or by $H^+$ ions (because $H^+$ ions do not cross the blood-brain barrier).

A discrete chemoreceptor has not been identified; rather, collections of neurons that respond appropriately to the applied $CO_2/H^+$ stimulus have been identified. These neurons appear to respond to changes in extracellular fluid composition, rather than to cerebrospinal fluid composition.

## Ventilatory Response to Changes in Arterial Carbon Dioxide and Oxygen and pH

The integration of chemoreceptor outputs with other factors affecting ventilation results in an overall ventilatory response. In quantitative or mathematical terms, minute ventilation is directly proportional to the prevailing value of $PaCO_2$, a relationship potentiated by concomitant hypoxia. Minute ventilation is quantitatively inversely proportional to the prevailing value of $PaO_2$, a relationship potentiated by concomitant hypercapnia. Changes in pH mirror the expected extracellular change in $CO_2$. These relationships are discussed further in the literature.[24,28]

## PHARMACOLOGY

During mechanical ventilation, drug effects on the control of breathing are of little importance, but during and after the weaning process, any depression of ventilatory control may require the reinstitution of mechanical ventilation. These drug effects on the control of breathing are complex and can affect breathing by alterations in (1) the chemoreflexes (both hypoxic and hypercapnic), (2) upper airway tone, or (3) the nonchemoreflex or wakefulness drive. Because the control of ventilation is under both feedback and feedforward control, the effects of specific drugs can vary greatly, depending on the patient's physiologic state. During sleep, adequate ventilation may depend solely on the chemoreflexes; when the patient is awake, feedforward influences from the higher centers may predominate. Thus, ventilation may be adequate when the patient is awake and aroused but may become inadequate during sleep. The interaction of drugs and the sleep state may be particularly important because sleep-deprived patients in ICUs may have *rapid eye movement (REM) rebound* as their status improves.[29] This REM rebound may make them at risk for upper airway obstruction, although postoperative patients may be at risk for airway obstruction even when they are awake.[30,31] It has long been appreciated that sleep and opioids have a marked interaction with the hypercapnic chemoreflex.[29,32]

Mechanical ventilation is facilitated by many drugs that can impede the physiologic control of breathing after the weaning process. Foremost are the opioids, sedatives, and neuromuscular blocking agents. When mechanical ventilation is terminated rapidly, as at the end of surgery, it is particularly important that residual effects of anesthetic agents be adequately dissipated or reversed. Adequate spontaneous ventilation is readily possible during surgical levels of anesthesia so long as the airway is maintained, but (almost paradoxically) a picture resembling sleep apnea may be induced at lighter planes of anesthesia that requires control of the airway.[33] Thus, many of the problems noted on termination of mechanical ventilation are related to the simultaneous termination of mechanical support of the upper airway.

Many good reviews and monographs on the pharmacology of the control of breathing have been published,[27,28,34] as well as reports of the respiratory effects seen during recovery from anesthesia and mechanical ventilation.[35] This brief section covers some issues that may be important to patients who have recently been weaned from mechanical ventilation.

## Opioids and Sedatives

Opioids are the mainstays in the treatment of severe pain, and thus they are frequently used in patients in the ICU. Bailey and Thakur have reviewed the respiratory effects of pain management techniques, including opioid use.[36] Opioids are, of course, the classic respiratory depressants and have a dose-related depression of total ventilation through a decrease in both VT and respiratory frequency. The hypoxic chemoreflex sensitivity is decreased,[37] whereas at lower doses there is no decrease in the hypercapnic sensitivity (but there is a parallel shift to a lower ventilation at the same $CO_2$ level[38]). Higher opioid doses decrease the hypercapnic sensitivity, but this effect may also be related to the sedation induced at the higher doses, rather than to direct opioid action on the chemoreflex. The respiratory depressant effect is a central μ receptor action of the opioid.[39] As far as respiratory depression is concerned, there is little to recommend one opioid over another. However, the pharmacokinetic characteristics of the different opioids may have a profound impact, and opioids that are short acting after a single dose may produce extended respiratory depression after prolonged infusion.[40] When an opioid is given, the increase in $CO_2$ secondary to the reduction in spontaneous minute ventilation will tend to counter the ventilatory depression if the onset of the opioid is slow. However, a bolus of a rapid-onset opioid may induce apnea before the $CO_2$ can increase sufficiently to stimulate ventilation.[41]

The route by which the opioid reaches the brainstem seems not to be important, and neuraxially given opioids (e.g., epidural or intrathecal) depress both the hypoxic and hypercapnic responses even though the plasma levels are not significant.[42,43] However, with neuraxial administration, delayed depression must be considered, particularly if lipophilic opioids are used. Postoperatively, opioid administration is associated with upper airway obstruction and desaturation.[44]

Midazolam and propofol are commonly used in ventilated and ICU patients for sedation, and both drugs may have respiratory depressant effects. Because propofol is the more shorter-acting drug, its effects are usually not problematic once the infusion is terminated. Neither drug has pronounced respiratory effects at usual levels of sedation, but again, their effects on the upper airway may be more important than their effects on decreasing respiratory drive.[45] Both drugs reduce the hypercapnic and hypoxic chemoreflexes, but the loss of the wakefulness drive may account for most of the observed mild reduction in hypercapnic sensitivity.[46-49] There is no specific reversal agent for propofol, but flumazenil reverses both the sedative and respiratory depressant effects of midazolam (sedation reversal may outlast reversal of the respiratory depression).[50]

Dexmedetomidine is a centrally acting $\alpha_2$-agonist used in the ICU for sedation. This drug may be continued after mechanical ventilation and upper airway support have been removed. The respiratory effects of this drug seem to be relatively modest,[51] but it has probably not been completely studied, particularly in drug combinations. However, the combination of clonidine (another $\alpha_2$-agonist) with morphine did not result in pronounced ventilatory depression.[52] In addition, clonidine, given intravenously, orally, and epidurally, has been shown to cause apnea.[53,54] Although even high-dose dexmedetomidine does not seem to induce clinically significant apnea,[55] it seems prudent to use this drug cautiously, especially in patients with risk factors for OSA.

## Drug Combinations

The combination of opioids and sedatives can be synergistic in the amount of respiratory depression produced.[56] This synergism may result from the effect of the sedative on the wakefulness drive and the effect of the opioid on the chemoreflex. Bailey and colleagues noticed that the combination of fentanyl and midazolam caused frequent apneic episodes and observed that such episodes were not seen with either drug alone.[57]

## Neuromuscular Blocking Drugs

Neuromuscular blocking drugs are frequently used to facilitate mechanical ventilation, both short term in the operating room and for longer periods in the ICU. It is essential to ensure that recovery or reversal from neuromuscular blockade is achieved before either airway support or mechanical ventilation is removed. In addition to their predictable effects on the phrenic nerve-diaphragm neuromuscular junction, neuromuscular blocking drugs also have deleterious effects on both chemoreception and upper airway patency. The reader is referred to the recent review by Eriksson.[58]

It is currently generally accepted that the neuromuscular blocking drugs act to block the *neuromuscular junction* nicotinic receptors, but they have little effect on *neuronal* nicotinic receptors. Although the exact role of acetylcholine and acetylcholine receptors in the signal transduction cascade in the carotid body is controversial,[59] low doses of vecuronium do, however, appear to depress hypoxic ventilatory drive through depression of carotid body chemosensitivity in both rats[60] and humans.[61] These observations raise the possibility that these drugs may also act on some neuronal nicotinic receptors.

## Cardiovascular Drugs

Patients undergoing mechanical ventilation frequently need medications to support cardiovascular functions. These drugs can have significant respiratory effects, but fortunately, most of them do not cause major clinical problems. Ward and Karan have reviewed this topic.[62]

Dopamine has the most pronounced ventilatory effects, because even low doses significantly blunt the hypoxic ventilatory response.[63] Studies have demonstrated that a low-dose dopamine infusion, given during hypoxia or during states with compromised $O_2$ delivery to tissues (e.g., congestive heart failure), has depressant effects on minute ventilation.[64,65] Other cardiovascular drugs, including adrenergic agents, adenosine, and digoxin, have ventilatory effects that can be readily measured, but there is no evidence that any of these effects is clinically significant.[62]

## REFERENCES

1. Pandit JJ, Popat M: Difficult airway management in maxillofacial trauma. In Katz RL, Patel, RV (eds): Seminars in Anesthesia, Perioperative Medicine and Pain, vol 20: The Difficult Airway. Philadelphia: WB Saunders Company, 2001, pp 144–153.
2. Young T, Paeta M, Dempsey J, et al: The occurrence of sleep-disordered breathing among middle-aged adults. N Engl J Med 1993;328:1230–1273.
3. Eastwood PR, Szollosi I, Platt PR, Hillman DR: Collapsibility of the upper airway during anesthesia with isoflurane. Anesthesiology 2002;97:786–793.
4. Drummond GB: Keep a clear airway [editorial]. Br J Anaesth 1991;66:153–156.
5. Isono S, Tanaka A, Tagaito Y, et al: Pharyngeal patency in response to advancement of the mandible in obese anesthetized persons. Anesthesiology 1997;87:1055–1062.
6. Isono S, Tanaka A, Nishino T: Lateral position decreases collapsibility of the passive pharynx in patients with obstructive sleep apnea. Anesthesiology 2002;97:780–785.
7. Cherniack N: Apnea and periodic breathing during sleep. N Engl J Med 1999;341:985–987.
8. Younes M: Contributions of upper airway mechanics and control mechanisms to severity of obstructive apnea. Am J Respir Crit Care Med 2003;168:645–658.
9. Young T, Peppard PE, Gottlieb DJ: Epidemiology of obstructive sleep apnea: A population health perspective. Am J Respir Crit Care Med 2002;165:1217–1239.
10. Javaheri S: A mechanism of central sleep apnea in patients with heart failure. N Engl J Med 1999;341:949–954.
11. Brochard L: Noninvasive ventilation for acute respiratory failure. JAMA 2002;288:932–935.
12. Evans TW: International Consensus Conferences in Intensive Care Medicine: Non-invasive positive pressure ventilation in acute respiratory failure. Intensive Care Med 2001;27:166–178.
13. Goodwin M, Pandit JJ, Hames K, et al: The effect of neuromuscular blockade on the efficiency of mask ventilation of the lungs. Anaesthesia 2002;58:60–63.
14. Sidaras G, Hunter JM: Laryngeal mask airway and positive pressure ventilation. Br J Anaesth 2001;86:749–753.

15. Verghese C, Jago R: Is it safe to artificially ventilate paralysed patients through a laryngeal mask? Br J Anaesth 2002;88:149–150.

16. Arosio EM, Conci F: Use of the laryngeal mask airway for respiratory distress in the intensive care unit. Anaesthesia 1995;50:635–636.

17. Glaisyer HR, Parry M, Lee J, Bailey PM: The laryngeal mask airway as an adjunct to extubation on the intensive care unit. Anaesthesia 1996;51:1187–1188.

18. Cook TM, Taylor M, McKinstry C, et al: Use of the ProSeal™ laryngeal mask airway to initiate ventilation during intensive care and subsequent percutaneous tracheostomy. Anesth Analg 2003;97:848–850.

19. Keller C, Brimacombe J: Mucosal pressures from the cuffed oropharyngeal airway vs the laryngeal mask airway. Br J Anaesth 1999;82:922–924.

20. Umapathy N, Eliathamby TG, Timms MS: Paralysis of the hypoglossal and pharyngeal branches of the vagus nerve after use of a LMA and ETT. Br J Anaesth 2001;87:322.

21. Fassoulaki A, Pamouktsoglou P: Prolonged nasotracheal intubation and its association with inflammation of paranasal sinuses. Anesth Analg 1989;69:50–52.

22. Pandit JJ, O'Malley S, Chambers P: KTP laser-resistant properties of the reinforced laryngeal mask airway. Br J Anaesth 1997;78:594–600.

23. Ambesh SP, Pandey CK, Srivastava S, et al: Percutaneous tracheostomy with single dilatation technique: A prospective, randomized comparison of Ciaglia blue rhino versus Griggs' guidewire dilating forceps. Anesth Analg 2002;95:1739–1745.

24. Caruana-Montaldo B, Gleeson K, Zwillich CW: The control of breathing in clinical practice. Chest 2000;117:205–225.

25. Bianchi AL, Denavit-Saubié M, Champagnat J: Central control of breathing in mammals: Neuronal circuitry, membrane properties, and neurotransmitters. Physiol Rev 1995;75:1–45.

26. Guz A: Brain, breathing and breathlessness. Respir Physiol 1997;109:197–204.

27. Ward DS, Karan S: Effects of pain and arousal on the control of breathing. J Anesth 2002;16:216–221.

28. Ward DS, Temp JA: Neuropharmacology of the control of ventilation. In Biebuyck J, Lynch C, Maze M, et al (eds): Anesthesia: Biologic Foundations. Philadelphia: Lippincott-Raven, 1997, pp 1367–1394.

29. Knill RL, Moote CA, Skinner MI, et al: Anesthesia with abdominal surgery leads to intense REM sleep during the first postoperative week. Anesthesiology 1990;73:52–61.

30. Rahman MQ, Kingshott RN, Wraith P, et al: Association of airway obstruction, sleep, and phasic abdominal muscle activity after upper abdominal surgery. Br J Anaesth 2001;87:198–203.

31. Wu A, Drummond GB: Sleep arousal after lower abdominal surgery and relation to recovery from respiratory obstruction. Anesthesiology 2003;99:1295–1302.

32. Forrest WH Jr, Bellville JW: The effect of sleep plus morphine on the respiratory response to carbon dioxide. Anesthesiology 1964;25:137–141.

33. Eastwood PR, Szollosi I, Platt PR, Hillman DR: Comparison of upper airway collapse during general anaesthesia and sleep. Lancet 2002;359:1207–1209.

34. Dahan A, Teppema LJ: Influence of anaesthesia and analgesia on the control of breathing. Br J Anaesth 2003;91:40–49.

35. Isono S, Rosenberg J: Recovery from anesthesia. In Ward DS, Dahan A, Teppema LJ (eds): Pharmacology and Pathophysiology of the Control of Breathing. New York: Marcel Dekker, 2005.

36. Bailey PL, Thakur RBB: Pain management and regional anesthesia. In Ward DS, Dahan A, Teppema LJ (eds): Pharmacology and Pathophysiology of the Control of Breathing. New York: Marcel Dekker, 2005.

37. Santiago TV, Johnson J, Riley DJ, Edelman NH: Effects of morphine on ventilatory response to exercise. J Appl Physiol 1979;47:112–118.

38. Bourke DL, Warley A: The steady-state and rebreathing methods compared during morphine administration in humans. J Physiol (Lond) 1989;419:509–517.

39. Sarton E, Teppema L, Nieuwenhuijs D, et al: Opioid effect on breathing frequency and thermogenesis in mice lacking exon 2 of the mu-opioid receptor gene. Adv Exp Med Biol 2001;499:399–404.

40. Shafer SL, Varvel JR: Pharmacokinetics, pharmacodynamics, and rational opioid selection. Anesthesiology 1991;74:53–63.

41. Bouillon T, Schmidt C, Garstka G, et al: Pharmacokinetic-pharmacodynamic modeling of the respiratory depressant effect of alfentanil. Anesthesiology 1999;91:144–155.

42. Bailey PL, Lu JK, Pace NL, et al: Effects of intrathecal morphine on the ventilatory response to hypoxia. N Engl J Med 2000;343:1228–1234.

43. Bailey PL, Rhondeau S, Schafer PG, et al: Dose-response pharmacology of intrathecal morphine in human volunteers. Anesthesiology 1993;79:49–59.

44. Catley DM, Thorton M, Jordan C, et al: Pronounced, episodic oxygen desaturation in the postoperative period: Its association with ventilatory pattern and analgesic regimen. Anesthesiology 1985;63:20–28.

45. Gross JB, Cerza DA: Ventilatory effects of medications used for moderate and deep sedation. In Ward DS, Dahan A, Teppema LJ (eds): Pharmacology and Pathophysiology of the Control of Breathing. New York: Marcel Dekker, 2005.

46. Alexander CM, Gross JB: Sedative doses of midazolam depress hypoxic ventilatory responses in humans. Anesth Analg 1988;67:377–382.

47. Blouin RT, Conrad PF, Gross JB: Time course of ventilatory depression following induction doses of propofol and thiopental. Anesthesiology 1991;75:940–944.

48. Blouin RT, Seifert HA, Babenco D, et al: Propofol depresses the hypoxic ventilatory response during conscious sedation and isohypercapnia. Anesthesiology 1993;79:1177–1182.

49. Power SJ, Morgan M, Charkrabarti MK: Carbon dioxide response curves following midazolam and diazepam. Br J Anaesth 1983;55:837–841.

50. Flogel CM, Ward DS, Wada DR, Ritter JW: The effects of large-dose flumazenil on midazolam-induced ventilatory depression. Anesth Analg 1993;77:1207–1214.

51. Belleville JP, Ward DS, Bloor BC, Maze M: Effects of intravenous dexmedetomidine in humans. I. Sedation, ventilation and metabolic rate. Anesthesiology 1992;77:1125–1133.

52. Bailey PL, Sperry RJ, Johnson GK, et al: Respiratory effects of clonidine alone and combined with morphine, in humans. Anesthesiology 1991;74:43–48.

53. Benhamou D, Veillette Y, Narchi P, Ecoffey C: Ventilatory effects of premedication with clonidine. Anesth Analg 1991;73:799–803.

54. Narchi P, Benhamou D, Hamza J, Bouaziz H: Ventilatory effects of epidural clonidine during the first 3 hours after caesarean section. Acta Anaesthesiol Scand 1992;36:791–795.

55. Zornow MH: Ventilatory, hemodynamic and sedative effects of the $\alpha_2$ adrenergic agonist, dexmedetomidine. Neuropharmacology 1991;30:1065–1071.

56. Nieuwenhuijs DJ, Olofsen E, Romberg RR, et al: Response surface modeling of remifentanil-propofol interaction on cardiorespiratory control and bispectral index. Anesthesiology 2003;98:312–322.

57. Bailey PL, Pace NL, Ashburn MA, et al: Frequent hypoxemia and apnea after sedation with midazolam and fentanyl. Anesthesiology 1990;73:826–830.

58. Eriksson LI: Neuromuscular blocking agents and ventilation. In Ward DS, Dahan A, Teppema LJ (eds): Pharmacology and Pathophysiology of the Control of Breathing. New York: Marcel Dekker, 2005.

59. Fitzgerald RS: Oxygen and carotid body chemotransduction: The cholinergic hypothesis. A brief history and new evaluation. Respir Physiol 2000;120:89–104.

60. Igarashi A, Amagasa S, Horikawa H, Shirahata M: Vecuronium directly inhibits hypoxic neurotransmission of the rat carotid body. Anesth Analg 2002;94:117–122.

61. Eriksson LI, Sato M, Severinghaus JW: Effect of a vecuronium-induced partial neuromuscular block on hypoxic ventilatory response. Anesthesiology 1993;78:693–699.

62. Ward D, Karan S: Cardiovascular drugs and the control of breathing. In Ward DS, Dahan A, Teppema LJ (eds): Pharmacology and Pathophysiology of the Control of Breathing. New York: Marcel Dekker, 2005.

63. Dahan A, Ward DS, van den Elsen M, et al: Influence of reduced carotid body drive during sustained hypoxia on hypoxic depression of ventilation in humans. J Appl Physiol 1996;81:565–572.

64. Huckauf H, Ramdohr B, Schroder R: Dopamine induced hypoxemia in patients with left heart failure. Int J Clin Pharmacol Biopharm 1976;14:217–224.

65. van de Borne P, Oren R, Somers VK: Dopamine depresses minute ventilation in patients with heart failure. Circulation 1998;98:126–131.

# CHAPTER 35

# Current Sedation Practices in the Intensive Care Unit

Jayashree Raikhelkar and Peter J. Papadakos

Sedation in the intensive care unit (ICU) has changed dramatically over the past decade. An understanding of newer sedative and analgesics has enabled critical care practitioners to titrate agents for specific patient populations. The advent of shorter-acting agents for sedation has meant that clinicians no longer must resort to using very long-acting compounds, which have undesirable side effects. This advance allows patients to be comfortable while intubated and mechanically ventilated and also permits caregivers in the ICU to assess patients frequently for weaning from mechanical ventilation. The results are a reduction in overall days on the ventilator and a shorter ICU stay.

## AGITATION AND ANXIETY

Almost 75% patients in ICUs develop some form of agitation or anxiety during the course of their stay. The optimum level of sedation varies among patients. Sedation should be titrated to an individual's comorbidities and safety. Because the origin of agitation is multifactorial, a stepwise approach must be sought to find its underlying cause. Both agitation and anxiety are common in all age groups. The causes of agitation include extreme anxiety, delirium, adverse drug effects (Table 35.1), and pain. Inadequate pain control is especially common in postoperative patients. Because of fears of respiratory depression and dependence potential, opioids are often administered at subtherapeutic doses, and the result is inadequate pain control.

Hypoxemia has long been associated with agitation. This association has led to monitoring of oxygen saturation by pulse oximetry or arterial partial pressure of oxygen in all patients. A partial pressure of oxygen lower than 60 mm Hg or oxygen saturation less than 90% can be reflective of agitation. Hypotension and its resulting reduction in cerebral perfusion can also lead to agitation. Abnormalities in blood glucose, especially hypoglycemia, must be excluded. Sepsis can also manifest as agitation.

Patients with head injury can present with minor to severe degrees of agitation. Intracranial hemorrhages, thrombotic strokes, brain neoplasms, and infections all may be associated with some degrees of agitation.

One of the most common problems confronting critical care physicians is withdrawal of patients from alcohol or other agents such as cocaine, opioids, and benzodiazepines. Another commonly overlooked agent that affects agitation in the ICU is nicotine.

In the ICU, a common cause of agitation is ventilator dyssynchrony in mechanically ventilated patients. This is usually the result of poor ventilator settings that delay responses to a patient's own spontaneous breathing. However, this situation has become less common since the advent of computer-controlled ventilators. Intubated and alert patients may develop agitation from the endotracheal tube itself or from an inability to communicate with their caregivers and family. The ICU environment, with its sounds, monitors, and lack of natural light, is a significant contributor to further agitation.

In current ICU practice, patients receive multiple-drug regimens. As a consequence of numerous drug interventions and interactions, the incidence of agitation

**Table 35-1    Medications Associated with Agitation in the Intensive Care Unit**

| | |
|---|---|
| Antibiotics | Acyclovir, amphotericin B, cephalosporins, ciprofloxacin, ketoconazole, penicillin, rifampin |
| Anticonvulsants | Phenobarbital, phenytoin |
| Cardiac drugs | Captopril, clonidine, digoxin, dopamine, labetalol, nifedipine, quinidine |
| Corticosteroids | Dexamethasone, methylprednisolone |
| Narcotic analgesics | Codeine, meperidine, morphine sulfate |
| Miscellaneous | Theophylline, hydroxyzine, ketamine, nonsteroidal anti-inflammatory drugs |

dramatically increases. A brief list of medications associated with agitation is given in Table 35.1. When a drug is suspected of increasing agitation, one may have to wait for several days after withdrawal of the drug and of its metabolites to see a response in the patient.

Because of the complexity of disease states and the dynamic nature of hemodynamics in patients in the ICU, the requirements and priority to treat agitation fluctuate with time. The clinician must frequently reassess and redefine the goals of therapy. Ideally, scales for monitoring sedation and agitation should be simple to apply and easy to understand, to allow for quick recognition of changes in sedation level and titration of pharmacologic and nonpharmacologic interventions.

Numerous sedation scales for the ICU have been published, although no single "gold standard" exists. Most ICUs follow modifications of scales described in the literature. The development of unit-based scales and protocols is important for easy acceptance by all the members of the health care team.

## SEDATION SCALES

One of the most commonly used measures of sedation is the *Ramsay Sedation Scale*. It divides a patient's level of sedation into six categories ranging from severe agitation to deep coma. Despite its frequent use, the Ramsay Sedation Scale has shortcomings in patients with complex cases. When the scale is applied at the bedside, many patients appear to conform to more than one level of sedation. For example, patient may appear to be asleep, with a sluggish response to the glabellar tap, and at the same time may be restless and anxious.

Because of the scale's simplicity, however, it is widely used in the ICU.

The *Riker Sedation-Agitation Scale* (SAS) was the first scale tested and developed for the ICU. The SAS identifies seven levels of sedation and agitation, which range from dangerous agitation to deep sedation, with a thorough description of patient behavior. This scale allows the clinician to distinguish easily between each level (Table 35.2).

The *Motor Activity Assessment Scale* (MAAS) is similar in structure to the SAS because it uses patients' behavior to describe different levels of agitation. Like the SAS, the MAAS has seven levels of agitation that range from unresponsive to dangerously agitated (see Table 35.2).

One of the newest assessment tools for the ICU is the *Confusion Assessment Method for the ICU* (CAM-ICU). It was described by Ely and colleagues and has been validated in critically ill patients with delirium. It is used in combination with the Glasgow Coma Scale for highly complex, agitated patients. The CAM-ICU is simple to apply at the bedside and has been found to be highly reliable, sensitive, and specific.

All the aforementioned scales rely on the clinician's interpretation for evaluation of a patient's agitation. There is hope that one day a computer-based, real-time monitor of brain function will be developed that will remove human variability in ICU assessments of agitation and sedation. One such monitor does exist and is popular in the operating room. Called the *Bispectral Index* (BIS), this monitor provides discrete values ranging from 100 (completely awake) to less than 60 (deep sedation), to less than 40 (coma) by incorporating several frontal electroencephalogram components. Although valid in the operating room, it has not been widely studied in the ICU.

**Table 35-2    Sedation Scales**

| | | **Riker Sedation-Agitation Scale*** |
|---|---|---|
| 7 | Dangerously agitated | Pulling at endotracheal tube, trying to remove catheters, climbing over bed rail, striking at staff, thrashing from side to side |
| 6 | Very agitated | Not calm despite frequent verbal reminding of limits, requiring physical restraints, biting endotracheal tube |
| 5 | Agitated | Anxious or mildly agitated, attempting to sit up, calming down to verbal instructions |
| 4 | Calm and cooperative | Calm, awakening easily, following commands |
| 3 | Sedated | Difficult to arouse, awakening to verbal stimuli or gentle shaking but drifting off again, following simple commands |
| 2 | Very sedated | Arousing to physical stimuli but not communicating or following commands, possibly moving spontaneously |
| 1 | Unarousable | Minimal or no response to noxious stimuli, not communicating or following commands |
| | | **Motor Activity Assessment Scale†** |
| 6 | Dangerously agitated | No external stimulus required to elicit movement; patient uncooperative, pulling at tubes or catheters, thrashing from side to side, striking at staff, or trying to climb out of bed; does not calm down when asked |
| 5 | Agitated | No external stimulus required to elicit movement; patient attempts to sit up or moves limbs out of bed and does not consistently follow commands (e.g., will lie down when asked but soon reverts back to attempts to sit up or move limbs out of bed) |
| 4 | Restless and cooperative | No external stimulus required to elicit movement; patient picking at sheets or tubes or uncovering self and following commands |
| 3 | Calm and cooperative | No external stimulus required to elicit movement; patient adjusting sheets or clothes purposefully and following commands |
| 2 | Responsive to touch or name | Opens eyes or raises eyebrows or turns head toward stimulus or moves limbs when touched or name is loudly spoken |
| 1 | Responsive only to noxious stimulus | Opens eyes or raises eyebrows or turns head toward stimulus or moves limbs with noxious stimulus |
| 0 | Unresponsive | Does not move with noxious stimulus |
| | | **Ramsay Scale††** |
| 1 | Awake | Patient anxious and agitated or restless or both |
| 2 | | Patient cooperative, oriented, and tranquil |
| 3 | | Patient responds to commands only |
| 4 | Asleep | Brisk response to light glabellar tap or loud auditory stimulus |
| 5 | | Sluggish response to light glabellar tap or loud auditory stimulus |
| 6 | | No response to light glabellar tap or loud auditory stimulus |

*Data from Riker RR, Fraser GL: Monitoring sedation, agitation, analgesia, neuromuscular blockade, and delirium in adult ICU patients. Semin Respir Crit Care Med 2001;22:189–198.

†Data from Devlin JW, Boleski G, Mlynarek M, et al: Motor Activity Assessment Scale: A valid and reliable sedation scale for use with mechanically ventilated patients in an adult surgical intensive care unit. Crit Care Med 1999;27:1271–1275.

††Ramsay MAE, Savage TM, Simpson BRJ, et al: Controlled sedation with alphaxalone. BMJ 1774;2:656-650.

## REVIEW OF COMMON SEDATIVE AND ANALGESIC AGENTS USED IN THE INTENSIVE CARE UNIT

The mainstays of supportive care in the ICU are sedatives and analgesics. Many novel, easily titratable agents have been introduced that have greatly enhanced patient care. The pharmacology of these agents, as well as that of more classic agents, is reviewed (Table 35.3).

### Opioids

The primary agents used for analgesia are opioids. Most are lipid soluble, and they mediate their effect largely through the μ receptor at central, spinal, and peripheral sites. All the opioids share common therapeutic properties but vary in potency and pharmacokinetics.

Although opioids can be given by multiple routes of administration, the intravenous route is commonly used because of its convenience. More recently, epidural, intrathecal, transdermal, and transmucosal delivery systems have been developed. The advice of an anesthesiologist is warranted when implementing and standardizing pathways for such delivery systems. At therapeutic doses, opioids may cloud the sensorium, but they do not possess amnestic properties.

The control of pain is of paramount importance in the ICU. If left unchecked, unrelieved pain can evoke a powerful stress response resulting in tachycardia, hypertension, increased myocardial consumption, hypercoagulability, immunosuppression, and persistent catabolism. Adequate pain relief may also reduce pulmonary complications in postoperative patients.

When administrating a selective agent in the ICU, the clinician must be thoroughly knowledgeable about its pharmacology and side effect profile. The ideal opioid should have a rapid onset, be easily titratable, lack accumulation of metabolites, and be inexpensive.

*Morphine sulfate* remains the most common and most frequently administered opioid in the ICU. Its popularity stems from its familiarity and low cost. Morphine has lower lipid solubility than most narcotics, and this property may result in a delayed onset of action. Morphine induces histamine release in some individuals that may lead to a profound drop in arterial blood pressure and systemic vascular resistance. Thus, morphine should be used with caution in patients with unstable hemodynamics and reactive airway disease. The effect of histamine release can be minimized by slow infusions and adequate volume pretreatment. Morphine is primarily metabolized in the liver; however, the kidneys excrete more than 40% of the drug. The major metabolite of morphine (morphine-6-glucuronide) is excreted in the urine. This metabolite is thought to be responsible for the increased sensitivity to morphine observed in patients with renal failure.

*Fentanyl* is a synthetic opioid with 50 to 100 times the potency of morphine. It is highly lipid soluble with a rapid onset of action and no active metabolites. It is a selective μ agonist producing profound dose-dependent analgesia. Hemodynamically, fentanyl can rarely cause hypotension by producing bradycardia and decreased sympathetic tone. Because of its short duration of action, fentanyl should be administered as a continuous infusion. At high doses, it can cause loss of consciousness and muscle rigidity. Because fentanyl causes no histamine release and its pharmacokinetic profile not altered by renal failure, it is the analgesic of choice for critically ill and unstable patients. During prolonged infusions, saturation of redistribution sites and drug accumulation occur. In these situations, the terminal half-life of the drug can be as long as 16 hours.

*Remifentanil* (Ultiva) is an ultrashort-acting narcotic with a rapid onset and very short context-sensitive (half-life). Although not well studied in patients in ICUs, this drug is best indicated for patients who require serial neurologic evaluations. Remifentanil is rapidly hydrolyzed by circulating and tissue nonspecific esterases; therefore, it must be given as a continuous infusion. There appears to be no cumulative effect during long infusions, and organ dysfunction does not appear to alter drug metabolism. The side effects of this drug include respiratory depression, skeletal muscle rigidity, hypotension, and bradycardia. Prior administration of an induction agent or a paralytic can attenuate the rigidity seen with this drug.

*Meperidine* was once commonly used for pain relief, but it is no longer recommended for repetitive use. It has a rapid onset, binding to both μ and κ receptors. Through κ-receptor activation, meperidine can suppress shivering and can prevent associated metabolic and cardiac demands. Meperidine's active metabolite, normeperidine, may accumulate in patients with renal failure and has neurotoxic properties (tremors, delirium, and seizures). At higher doses, meperidine can act as a myocardial depressant. It may also interact with antidepressants (*contraindicated with monoamine oxidase inhibitors and should be used with caution with selective serotonin reuptake inhibitors*). Because of its multiple drug interactions, meperidine is infrequently used in critically ill patients.

Most of the opioid analgesics have a common adverse effect profile. Ventilatory depression and hypoxemia are of particular concern in spontaneously breathing patients or in those with partial ventilatory support. Weaning from the ventilator may be prolonged. Hypotension, pruritus, and increases in common bile duct pressures and urinary retention are also frequent. Opioids may increase intracranial pressure in patients with traumatic brain injury, although those data are inconsistent.

**Table 35-3   Analgesics Used in Intensive Care**

| Agent | Analgesic Dose (IV) | Half-Life | Metabolic Pathway | Active Metabolites (Effect) | Adverse Effects | Intermittent Dose* | Infusion Dose Range (Usual) | Infusion Cost/Day (70 kg) |
|---|---|---|---|---|---|---|---|---|
| Fentanyl | 200 μg | 1.5–6 hr | Oxidation | No metabolite, parent accumulates | Rigidity with high doses | 0.35–1.5 μg/kg IV q0.5–1h | 0.7–10 μg/kg/hr | 100 μg/hr: $26.00 |
| Hydromorphone | 1.5 mg | 2–3 hr | Glucuronidation | None | — | 10–30 μg/kg IV q1–2h | 7–15 μg/kg/hr | 0.75 mg/hr: $5.00–$11.00 |
| Morphine | 10 mg | 3–7 hr | Glucuronidation | Yes (sedation, especially in renal insufficiency) | Histamine release | 0.01–0.15 mg/kg IV q1–2h | 0.07–0.5 mg/kg/hr | 5 mg/hr: $3.50–$12.00 |
| Meperidine | 75–100 mg | 3–4 hr | Demethylation and hydroxylation | Yes (neuroexcitation, especially in renal insufficiency or high doses) | Avoid with MAOIs and SSRIs | Not recommended | Not recommended | — |
| Codeine | 120 mg | 3 hr | Demethylation and glucuronidation | Yes (analgesia, sedation) | Lacks potency, histamine release | Not recommended | Not recommended | — |
| Remifentanil | — | 3–10 min | Plasma esterase | None | — | — | 0.6–15 μg/kg/hr | 10 μg/kg/hr: $170.00 |
| Ketorolac | — | 2.4–8.6 hr | Renal | None | Risk of bleeding, GI and renal adverse effects | 15–30 mg IV q6h, decrease if age >65 yr or weight <50 kg or renal impairment, avoid >5 days use | | — |
| Ibuprofen | — | 1.8–2.5 hr | Oxidation | None | Risk of bleeding, GI and renal adverse effects | 400 mg PO q4–6h | — | — |
| Acetaminophen | — | 2 hr | Conjugation | — | — | 325–650 mg PO q4–6h, avoid >4 g/day | — | — |

*More frequent doses may be needed for acute pain management in mechanically ventilated patients.

GI, gastrointestinal; IV, intravenously; MAOI, monoamine oxidase inhibitor; PO, orally; SSRI, selective serotonin reuptake inhibitor.

## Nonopioid Analgesics

Nonopioid agents are used with increasing frequency in the ICU. They include salicylates, acetaminophen, and nonsteroidal anti-inflammatory drugs (NSAIDS). The primary mode of action of NSAIDS is nonselective competitive inhibition of cyclooxygenase, a critical enzyme required for prostaglandin-mediated amplification of pain pathways. When given with an opioid, nonopioids tend to reduce opioid requirements. They are not respiratory depressants and are less likely to cause nausea and vomiting. Ketorolac tromethamine is available in intravenous form, which is convenient in the ICU setting. Of course, NSAIDs are not without side effects. Their antiplatelet action may precipitate gastrointestinal bleeding and can impair renal blood flow autoregulation. Because of increased cardiovascular risks, some cyclooxygenase 2 agents have been withdrawn from the market.

## Benzodiazepines

Benzodiazepines are the most widely used sedatives and hypnotics today. In the ICU setting, these drugs are commonly used for sedation and for the treatment of anxiety, agitation, and alcohol withdrawal. They have no analgesic properties alone. They enhance the inhibitory effects of γ-aminobutyric acid (GABA) on neuronal transmission primarily in the limbic system, the thalamus, the hypothalamus, and the spinal level.

Benzodiazepines are metabolized in the liver. Because of decreased metabolism, these drugs may accumulate with prolonged and continuous infusions in critically ill patients or in patients with liver disease. Prolonged oversedation and somnolence have been seen in elderly patients after they stop the drug; these effects are the result of accumulation and long half-lives of the parent drug or active metabolites. Therefore, these drugs should be carefully titrated.

To avoid these complications, benzodiazepines should be titrated to a predefined end point with serial bolus loading. Sedation is maintained with intermittent or as-needed (PRN) doses of midazolam, lorazepam, or diazepam.

The Society of Critical Care Medicine's (SCCM's) current clinical practice guidelines recommend lorazepam as the sedative of choice. It can be given in either intermittent intravenous doses or as a continuous infusion. Lorazepam is an intermediate-acting benzodiazepine with fewer lipophilic properties than diazepam and therefore less potential for accumulation. Unlike midazolam, lorazepam has no active metabolite; its metabolism is less affected in elderly patients and in liver failure. Lorazepam should be use with caution. Prolonged use has been associated with *propylene glycol toxicity*, and propylene glycol accumulation has led to acidosis and renal failure.

Another commonly used benzodiazepine is midazolam. Initially only used in the operating room, midazolam is now used in the ICU. It is a short-acting, water-soluble benzodiazepine whose structure undergoes transformation to more lipophilic compounds in the bloodstream. Midazolam exhibits dose-related respiratory depression, and at larger doses it may cause vasodilation and hypotension. It is metabolized in the liver to a less potent but active compound. The new SCCM guidelines recommend midazolam for short-term use and rapid sedation of actively agitated patients. Midazolam produces unpredictable awakening and prolonged extubated times when infusions continue for longer than 48 to 72 hours.

One of the side effects of benzodiazepines is paradoxical agitation. This effect is most commonly seen in elderly patients and may result from drug-induced amnesia or disorientation. The benzodiazepine receptor antagonist, flumazenil (Romazicon), can reverse the effects of these drugs. Doses of 0.1 to 0.2 mg produce partial antagonism, and 0.4 to 1 mg causes complete reversal. The use of flumazenil has been associated with seizures and with increased oxygen consumption. Moreover, flumazenil may precipitate withdrawal in patients with a history of long-term benzodiazepine consumption. Therefore, flumazenil should be carefully titrated, and the dose should be individualized.

## Propofol

Propofol has now become a popular sedative agent in the ICU. It is structurally 2,6-diisopropylphenol, which is manufactured as a 1% aqueous emulsion containing soybean oil, glycerol, and egg phosphatide. Propofol's mechanism of action is not fully understood. It involves the activation of GABA receptors in the central nervous system. Its onset is rapid, within 1 to 2 minutes of injection. Its duration is short, resulting in awakening only 10 to 15 minutes after discontinuation, because of its rapid redistribution from the central nervous system. Therefore, propofol is an ideal agent in patients requiring intermittent awakening. Used alone, this drug is an incomplete anesthetic because it lacks analgesic properties. Propofol is cleared primarily by the liver, but it appears to have extrahepatic sites of elimination. Long-term infusions have resulted in accumulation in lipid stores and prolonged sedation.

Because of its short contact-specific half-life, propofol can be used for anything from light sedation to general anesthesia. It has a marked respiratory and cardiac depressant effect. Therefore, it should be used with caution in patients with difficult airways or hypovolemia. When given as a bolus, propofol invariably causes hypotension by reducing systemic vascular resistance. Propofol is safe to use in patients with increased intracranial pressure because it reduces the cerebral metabolic rate and blood flow. Other advantageous effects include bronchodilation and antiemesis. Because propofol can cause hypertriglyceridemia, it should be used with caution in patients with pancreatitis and hyperlipidemia.

Propofol is a highly cost-effective agent, especially in the ICU. Using propofol as a sedative during the weaning process has resulted in a reduction in days spent weaning and on mechanical ventilation. The results of a large Spanish study concluded that sedation with propofol in critically ill patients resulted in reduced weaning times and fewer ventilator-dependent days than did sedation with equivalent doses of midazolam. Because of its favorable economic profile and rapid awakening, it is also the drug of choice for many fast-track surgical procedures.

After the introduction of propofol in the United States, numerous infections were reported in surgical patients treated with this drug. Most of these infections were thought to be the result of poor aseptic technique by health care providers. This finding led to the addition of the preservative ethylenediaminetetraacetic acid (EDTA) to the original formulation to help retard the growth of microorganisms. Since then, infection rates have dropped substantially. EDTA is a known chelator of cations including calcium and magnesium. The safety and efficacy of propofol with EDTA have been studied. Investigators found that EDTA-containing formulations did not affect calcium or magnesium homeostasis.

Propofol formulations with EDTA have been proven to modulate the systemic inflammatory response. This subject was studied by Herr and colleagues in surgical ICU patients. Patients receiving propofol with EDTA had significantly lower mortality rates at 7 and 28 days than did those receiving propofol alone. This effect of propofol with EDTA may be related to the ability of EDTA to bind to and excrete the mineral zinc. This property is speculated to prevent the release of cytokines and generation of free radicals and other oxidases in the inflammatory stress response.

Two generic formulations of propofol are available in the United States. One contains the preservative sodium metabisulfite (0.025%). It currently carries a warning by the Food and Drug Administration regarding use in patients who are sensitive to sulfite compounds, and use of this formulation in these patients is discouraged. The other contains benzyl alcohol and may cause several metabolic problems. It is therefore imperative that clinicians be aware of which formulation is used in their facility.

The use of propofol *in pediatric patients in the ICU is currently not recommended*. Cases of bradyarrhythmias, metabolic acidosis, and fatal myocardial depression have been reported in association with continuous infusions and high doses in critically ill children. However, these were highly complex cases with high mortality indices.

The SCCM recommends propofol as the agent of choice when rapid awakening and early extubation are required. Because the drug is a lipid emulsion, triglyceride levels should be monitored routinely when propofol infusions are used. Consequently, the addition of this extra lipid must be kept in mind when calculating the total caloric intake of patients.

## Haloperidol

The butyrophenone haloperidol is the neuroleptic of choice in the treatment of delirium in critically ill patients. Because it is not a respiratory depressant, haloperidol can be used in patients with agitation and compromised pulmonary function. Patients are generally calmer and are able to respond appropriately to commands. Because it has no amnesic and analgesic activity, haloperidol should not be used as the sole agent in intubated patients.

The adverse effect profile of haloperidol includes occasional hypotension from the α-blocking properties of the drug. Rarely, with intravenous use, haloperidol may cause extrapyramidal effects such as drowsiness, lethargy, rigidity, and akathisia. A highly dangerous side effect is neuroleptic malignant syndrome. This syndrome continues to have a mortality rate of 20% to 30%. It has an insidious onset, developing over 24 to 72 hours after drug administration and lasting up to 10 days after discontinuation. Cardiac arrhythmias can also occur. Well-documented reports of torsade de pointes have occurred after administration. Routine monitoring of the electrocardiographic QT interval is recommended. If a patient has a corrected QT interval exceeding 480 milliseconds, the drug should be stopped.

## Etomidate

Etomidate is a well-known hypnotic agent commonly used in rapid-sequence endotracheal intubations. Structurally, it is a nonbarbiturate, carboxylated imidazole-containing compound. For the induction of anesthesia, a bolus dose of 0.2 to 0.6 mg/kg is used. The advantage of etomidate is that is has few cardiovascular side effects. Adverse effects include transient myoclonus (33%) and inhibition of 11-β-hydroxylase, an enzyme important in adrenal steroid production. A single dose can block stress-induced cortisol production. Therefore, infusions of etomidate are not recommended.

## Dexmedetomidine

Dexmedetomidine (Precedex) is a relatively new $\alpha_2$-adrenergic agent approved for short-term ICU use. Eight times as potent as its counterpart, clonidine, dexmedetomidine has excellent sympatholytic sedative and analgesic effects.

Dexmedetomidine has two sites of action. It stimulates presynaptic $\alpha_2$-adrenoceptors, thus inhibiting the release of norepinephrine and hence the propagation of pain signals. It also works postsynaptically to produce a decrease in blood pressure and heart rate.

Dexmedetomidine has many advantages that make it a valuable agent in the ICU setting. Because the drug lacks respiratory depressant effects, patients can be weaned from other sedatives and mechanical ventilation faster and can be extubated without discontinuing the drug. When added to a preexisting opioid pain regimen, dexmedetomidine decreases opioid requirements and side effects. This is particularly helpful in weaning patients with alcohol and other drug dependencies.

Dexmedetomidine is primarily metabolized in the liver, so doses should be adjusted for hepatic failure. Dexmedetomidine should be used with caution in patients with preexisting cardiac conduction defects, bradycardia, or hypovolemia.

Dexmedetomidine is a multifaceted drug with great promise in the ICU setting. More study and research are still necessary to identify the long- and short-term indications of this drug.

## CONCLUSION

The most important aspect of ICU sedation is an understanding of each drug, including its advantages and disadvantages. The clinician must learn to identify the best drugs for each individual patient. It is crucial for the clinician to develop guidelines and protocols for the use of each drug, to enable patients to be comfortable and anxiety free in the ICU. Inadequate levels of sedation should no longer exist. New drugs and their immunomodulatory properties must be explored. This research will lead to greater understanding of sedative drugs and will ultimately result in better patient care.

## SUGGESTED READINGS

Jacobi J, Fraser GL, Coursin DB, et al: Clinical practice guidelines for the sustained use of sedatives and analgesics in the critically ill adult. Crit Care Med 2002;30:119–141.

Cohen IL, Abraham E, Dasta JF, et al: Management of the agitated intensive care unit patient. Crit Care Med 2002;30(Suppl): S97–S123.

Fraser GL, Prato BS, Riker RR, et al: Frequency, severity, and treatment of agitation in young versus elderly patients in the ICU. Pharmacotherapy 2000;20:75–82.

Hassan E, Fontaine DK, Nearman HS: Therapeutic considerations in the management of agitated or delirious critically ill patients. Pharmacotherapy 1998;18:113–129.

Hansen-Flaschen J, Cowen J, Polomano RC: Beyond the Ramsay scale: Need for a validated measure of sedating drug efficacy in the intensive care unit. Crit Care Med 1994;22:732–733.

Riker RR, Picard JT, Fraser GL: Prospective evaluation of the Sedation-Agitation Scale for adult critically ill patients. Crit Care Med 1999;27:1271–1275.

Devlin JW, Boleski G, Mlynarek M, et al: Motor Activity Assessment Scale: A valid and reliable sedation scale for use with mechanically ventilated patients in an adult surgical intensive care unit. Crit Care Med 1999;27:1271–1275.

Ely EW, Margolin R, Francis J, et al: Evaluation of delirium in critically ill patients: Validation of the Confusion Assessment Method for the Intensive Care Unit (CAM-ICU). Crit Care Med 2001;29:1370–1379.

Riker RR, Fraser GL: Monitoring sedation, agitation, analgesia, neuromuscular blockade, and delirium in adult ICU patients. Semin Respir Crit Care Med 2001;22:189–198.

Brook AD, Ahrens TS, Schaiff R, et al: Effect of a nursing-implemented sedation protocol on the duration of mechanical ventilation. Crit Care Med 1999;27:2609–2615.

Kress JP, Pohlman AS, O'Connor MF, Hall JB: Daily interruption of sedation infusions in critically ill patients undergoing mechanical ventilation. N Engl J Med 2000;342:1471–1477.

Lund N, Papadakos PJ: Barbiturates, neuroleptics, and propofol for sedation. Crit Care Clin 1995;11:875–886.

Levine RL: Pharmacology of intervenous sedatives and opioids in the critically ill patients. Crit Care Clin 1994;51:1539–1554.

Lewis KS, Whipple JK, Micheal KA, Quebbeman EJ: Effect of analgesic treatment on the physiological consequences of acute pain. Am J Hosp Pharm 1999;51:1539–1554.

Shapiro BA, Warren J, Egol AB, et al: Practice parameters for intervenous analgesia and sedation for adult patients in the intensive care unit: An executive summary. Society of Critical Care Medicine. Crit Care Med 1995;23:1596–1600.

Tipps LB, Coplin WM, Murry KR, Rhoney DH: Safety and feasibility of continuous infusion of remifentanil in the neurosurgical intensive care unit. Neurosurgery 2000;46:596–602.

Albanese J, Viviand X, Potie F, et al: Sufentanil, fentanyl, and alfentanil in head trauma patients: A study on cerebral hemodynamics. Crit Care Med 1999;27:407–411.

Watling SM, Dasta JF, Seidl EC: Sedatives, analgesics and paralytics in the ICU. Ann Pharmcother 1997;31:148–153.

Gilliland HE, Prasad BK, Mirakhur RK, Fee JP: An investigation of the potential morphine-sparing effect of midazolam. Anaesthesia 1996;51:808–811.

Watling SM, Johnson M, Yanos J: A method to produce sedation in critically ill patients. Ann Pharmacother 1996;30:1227–1231.

Shafer A: Complications of sedation with midazolam in the intensive care unit and a comparison with other sedative regimes. Crit Care Med 1998;26:947–956.

Young C, Knudsen N, Hilton A, Reves JG: Sedation in the intensive care unit. Crit Care Med 2000;28:854–866.

Kamijo Y, Masuda T, Nishikawa T, et al: Cardiovascular response and stress reaction to flumazenil injection in patients under infusion with midazolam. Crit Care Med 2000;28:318–323.

Bailie GR, Cockshott ID, Douglas EJ, Bowles BJ: Pharmacokinetics of propofol during and after long term continuous infusion for maintenance of sedation in ICU patients. Br J Anaesth 1992;68:486–491.

Barrientos-Vega R, Mar Sanchez-Soria M, Morales-Garcia C, Robas-Gomaz A, et al: Prolonged sedation of critically ill patients with midazolam or propofol: Impact on weaning and costs. Crit Care Med 1997;25:33–40.

Bennett SN, McNeil MM, Bland LA, et al: Postoperative infections traced to contamination of an intervenous anaesthetic, propofol. N Engl J Med 1995;333:147–154.

Abraham E, Papadakos PJ, Tharratt RS, et al: Effects of propofol containing EDTA on mineral metabolism in medical ICU patients with pulmonary dysfunction. Intensive Care Med 2000;26(Suppl 4):S422–S432.

Herr DL, Kelly K, Hall JB, et al: Safety and efficacy of propofol with EDTA when used for sedation of surgical intensive care unit patients. Intensive Care Med 2000;26(Suppl 4):S452–S462.

Mirenda J, Broyles G: Propofol as used for sedation in the ICU. Chest 1995;198:539–548.

Cremer OL, Moons KG, Bouman EA, et al: Long-term propofol infusion and cardiac failure in adult head-injured patients. Lancet 2001;357:117–118.

Padegal V, Venkata B, Papadakos PJ: Neuroleptic malignant syndrome and malignant hyperthermia. In Kruse JA, Fink MP,

Carlson RW (eds): Saunders Manual of Critical Care. Philadelphia: WB Saunders, 2002, pp 301–303.

Gertler R, Brown C, Mitchell DH, Silvius EN: Dexmedetomidine: A novel sedative-analgesic agent. Proc (Bayl Univ Med Cent) 2001;14:13–21.

Chhangani SV, Papadakos PJ: The use of dexmedetomidine for sedation in patients with traumatic brain injury. Am Soc Crit Care Anesthesiol 2002;97:B20.

Barreiro TJ, Papadakos PJ: Current practices in intensive care unit sedation. In Papadakos PJ, Szalados JE (eds): Critical Care: The Requisites in Anesthesiology. Philadelphia: Elsevier Mosby, 2005.

Papadakos PJ: Current practices in ICU sedation. Anesthesiol News 2005;Spec Ed:1–7.

# CHAPTER 36

# Use of Special Beds

Davide Chiumello, Milena Milena Racagni, and Paolo Pelosi

Because of the high incidence in critically ill patients of nosocomial infections that significantly increase morbidity, mortality, and health care costs, it is imperative to apply every effective pharmacologic and nonpharmacologic strategy to reduce the risk of infection.[1-3] *Ventilator-associated pneumonia,* which is defined as a type of nosocomial bacterial pneumonia occurring in patients who are receiving invasive mechanical ventilation, is associated with a significant increase in morbidity and mortality.[4] Among the nonpharmacologic strategies suggested to reduce the risk of infection, body positioning in critically ill patients is particularly important. Body position strategies used to prevent ventilator-associated pneumonia include the semirecumbent position, turning of the patient, kinetic bed therapy, and prone positioning.[5,6] In this chapter, we discuss the rationale for, clinical data concerning, and major benefits seen in randomized clinical trials of body position in preventing ventilator-associated pneumonia.

The development of nosocomial pneumonia in critically ill patients is associated with a mortality of approximately 30%. Ventilator-associated pneumonia complicates recovery in 10% to 30% of critically ill patients.[7,8]

Craig and Connelly, who studied a large group of critically ill patients who presented with ventilator-associated pneumonia and matched them with a group of patients who did not develop pneumonia, found that patients with ventilator-associated pneumonia stayed three times longer in the intensive care unit (12 days versus 3 days) and had a fourfold greater mortality than controls (20.3% versus 5.6%).[9] Similarly, Heyland and colleagues found crude mortality rates for patients with ventilator-associated pneumonia and for patients without pneumonia of 23.7% and 17.9%, respectively, with a

relative risk attributable to ventilator-associated pneumonia of 32%.[10] In addition, medical patients had a much longer stay in the intensive care unit than did surgical patients: 6.5 versus 0.7 days, with a mortality of 65% versus 27%, respectively.

Ventilator-associated pneumonia is usually defined as *early-onset type* when it occurs within 48 to 72 hours of intubation and as *late-onset type* when it develops later.[4,7] Invasive mechanical ventilation is one of the strongest risk factors for nosocomial pneumonia. A prospective multicenter study showed that the frequency of ventilator-associated pneumonia rose from 5% for patients receiving mechanical ventilation for 1 day to 69% for patients ventilated for more than 30 days.[11,12] In addition, several other risk factors have been found to increase the incidence of ventilator-associated pneumonia, in particular recovery from thoracic or upper abdominal surgery, the severity of underlying disease, use of antibiotics, use of an endotracheal tube, leakage of secretions around the cuffs, the need for reintubation, and use of paralytic agents.[7]

Although the pathogenesis of ventilator-associated pneumonia is multifactorial and can be favored by intrinsic and extrinsic factors (Box 36.1), two important processes must be present: (1) colonization of the aerodigestive tract by bacteria and (2) aspiration of contaminated secretions into the lower airway. Infectious organisms implicated in ventilator-associated pneumonia are generally different from those associated with community-acquired pneumonia. Gram-negative aerobes, in particular *Pseudomonas aeruginosa, Enterobacter* species, *Klebsiella pneumoniae, Acinetobacter,* and methicillin-resistant *Staphylococcus aureus* are present, whereas anaerobic bacteria have a very limited role in the

**Independent Risk Factors for Ventilator-Associated Pneumonia**

Age >60 years
Chronic obstructive pulmonary disease
Coma
Head trauma
Large volume of gastric aspiration
Upper respiratory tract colonization
Gastric colonization
Sinusitis
Previous antimicrobial agents
Stress ulcer prophylaxis
Enteral feeding
Supine head position
Respiratory equipment
Reintubation

pathogenesis of this disorder.[13] Efforts to reduce ventilator-associated pneumonia should be aimed at decreasing bacterial colonization of the aerodigestive tract and the risk of aspiration of secretions into the airway.

Guidelines for preventing ventilator-associated pneumonia suggest several disinfections, periodic maintenance of equipment, and the use of devices to prevent the transmission of microorganisms.[14] These guidelines advise against routine sterilization or disinfection of the internal machinery of mechanical ventilators and recommend periodic drainage and discarding of any condensate that collects in the ventilator tubing. There is no clear evidence in favor of heat moisture exchange or heated humidifiers in patients receiving mechanical ventilation for conditioning medical gases. Regarding the prevention of aspiration of secretions, it seems safe to remove the endotracheal or tracheotomy and enteral tube as soon as the clinical indications for tube placement are no longer applicable. Noninvasive positive pressure ventilation should always be used, when clinically indicated, as a first-line method of ventilation, before invasive mechanical ventilation is considered. No recommendations exist for using sucralfate, histamine ($H_2$) antagonists, or antacids for stress bleeding prophylaxis and selective decontamination.

## SEMIRECUMBENT POSITION

Bacterial colonization of gastric contents and oropharyngeal secretions, with subsequent tracheal aspiration, is a common risk factor for the development of ventilator-associated pneumonia. The presence of gastroesophageal reflux with bacterial colonization may also increase the risk of ventilator-associated pneumonia. To determine the possible role of gastric aspiration, several studies showed that, when gastric contents were radioactively labeled with technetium, radioactivity in endobronchial secretions was higher in samples obtained when patients were supine than when patients were semirecumbent.[15,16]

In critically ill patients, impairment of the physiologic swallowing dynamics as a result of the use of sedative agents or the presence of an endotracheal tube or of a nasogastric tube for enteral feeding may promote gastroesophageal reflux. Investigators have hypothesized that gastroesophageal reflux may additionally increase the risk of bacterial colonization of the lower airways.

Orozco-Levi and colleagues evaluated gastroesophageal reflux in a group of 15 patients, both supine and semirecumbent (45-degree angle), who were mechanically ventilated and had a nasogastric tube in place; these investigators measured the level of radioactivity in samples of gastric, pharyngeal, and bronchial secretions and blood.[17] Although the level of radioactivity was higher in the pharyngeal secretions, it was similar in the bronchial secretions in the supine and the semirecumbent positions. Thus, the semirecumbent position may protect from oropharyngeal colonization of gastric contents but not from pulmonary aspiration of gastric contents. In a study of nosocomial infection, Kollef demonstrated a threefold risk increase of pneumonia in patients who were lying in the supine head position during the first day of mechanical ventilation.[18]

Based on the foregoing data, a subsequent clinical trial evaluated the frequency of pneumonia in patients in semirecumbent and supine positions.[19] Patients were subjected to standard measures of general critical care, with local and systemic stress ulcer prophylaxis in addition to parenteral or enteral nutrition. Eighty-six patients were enrolled in the clinical trial; pneumonia was suspected in 16 of 47 patients (34%) in the supine group and in 3 of 39 patients (8%) in the semirecumbent group, with a risk reduction of 76%. Most of the cases of suspected pneumonia were of the late-onset type. However, there was only a trend in the reduction of days of mechanical ventilation until pneumonia occurred in patients in the semirecumbent body position. Multivariate analysis revealed that enteral nutrition (adjusted odds ratio, 11.8 [1.4 to 98.5]; $P = .022$) and supine body position (adjusted odds ratio, 6.1 [1.2 to 30.8]; $P = .038$) were independent risk factors. In addition, enteral feeding and body position were significantly interrelated (i.e., the frequency of pneumonia was higher when enteral feeding was given in patients in the supine position). However, this study was not able to show any difference in clinical outcome between the semirecumbent position and the supine position. In a previous study, the supine position during the first 24 hours of mechanical ventilation was an independent risk factor of a poor prognosis in patients with nosocomial pneumonia.[18]

To prevent aspiration associated with enteral feeding, investigators have proposed that the patient's head should always be elevated at an angle of 30 to 45 degrees, in the absence of mechanical contraindications, during invasive mechanical ventilation with an enteral tube in place. This maneuver was suggested in the published guidelines for preventing ventilator-associated pneumonia and is supported by clinical epidemiologic studies and strong theoretical rationale.[14] Clinically, however, use of the semirecumbent position is not standard practice. One survey of French physicians showed that only 58% of their patients were semirecumbent.[2]

A prospective, cross-sectional, observational study of Canadian intensive care units with at least eight beds evaluated protocols with respect to pneumonia prevention; the investigators asked medical or nursing directors about their current practices and also observed patient care directly.[20] For all patients who had an elevation of the head of the bed measured, the average elevation was 29.9 degrees (range, 0 to 90 degrees).[21] More important, of all the intensive care units that reported elevation of the head of the bed, 34 of 63 (54%) had an average bed elevation of less than 30 degrees.

Another study investigated the accuracy of clinical estimation of trunk flexion and agreement among intensive care specialists and nurses.[22] Nurses estimated trunk flexion at 24±12 degrees, and intensive care specialists estimated 21±13 degrees, whereas the standard measurement by goniometry was 16±90 degrees.

Both pulmonary and nonpulmonary factors have been advocated as determinants of patient position. Investigators have shown that the process of weaning from mechanical ventilation and the presence of pulmonary secretions increased the use of the semirecumbent position, whereas lateral placement for postural drainage, low cerebral perfusion pressure, and cervical spinal instability decreased the use of this position.[20] When clinicians were asked about current knowledge on optimal body positions for patients who were mechanically ventilated, numerous positions were suggested, including the following: simple supine position; elevation of the head by 10 to 20 degrees, 20 to 30 degrees, or 45 degrees; reverse Trendelenburg position, and various lateral positions. The potential risk of harm, low safety, lack of resources, hemodynamic instability, and the availability of alternative positions were identified as the principal barriers to semirecumbency.

Education can be helpful in promoting the use of the semirecumbent position. Investigators showed that, before an active educational program was instituted, only 31% of nursing staff members agreed that a 45-degree head elevation was the optimal body position.[23] The presence of an order specifically addressing the head of bed position, such as: "Head of bed at 45 degrees continuously in mechanically ventilated patients," in addition to each of the standard orders used by physicians, was able to increase the percentage of semirecumbent position use from 26% to 85% for a position angle greater than 30 degrees and from 3% to 16% for a position angle greater than 45 degrees. Six months after completion of an educational program, the semirecumbent position was still applied in the same percentage of patients.

Use of the semirecumbent position should be recommended in every patient who has no clinical contraindications. It is easily performed and inexpensive, and it may reduce the incidence of ventilator-associated pneumonia. Whether it reduces mortality remains to be determined, however.

## TURNING THE PATIENT

Because of the severity of their underlying disease (e.g., septic shock, acute respiratory failure, cardiogenic shock, coma), critically ill patients are relegated to strict bed rest, they are usually sedated, and they are sometimes paralyzed for better adaptation to mechanical ventilation. However, prolonged immobilization in these patients may promote several complications, including loss of muscle strength and tone, muscle atrophy, pulmonary dysfunction, and pressure sores.[24,25]

The most obvious complication is loss of muscle strength. A muscle may lose up to 10% to 15% of its original strength each week when it is at complete rest, and after 3 to 5 weeks of immobilization, nearly half its normal strength is lost. The antigravity muscles are the most dramatically affected.

Unfortunately, because of the low rate of recovery, the complications of immobilization are much easier to prevent than to treat. Investigators have reported that disuse weakness is reversed at a rate of only 6% per week, whereas muscle strength can be maintained without loss or gain with daily muscle contractions of just 20% of maximal tension for several seconds each day. Besides the loss of muscle strength, a reduction in muscle mass occurs. Half a muscle's bulk can be lost after only 2 months of resting.

The loss of strength usually affects the respiratory muscles, with a consequent reduction in tidal volume and minute ventilation and a compensatory (sometimes partial) increase in respiratory rate. Immobilized patients have difficulty in contracting respiratory muscles and in fully expanding the chest wall. They also have a reduced capability to clear secretions, which then accumulate in the lower airways, promote atelectasis, and increase the risk for pulmonary infections.

Because of the weight of the lung, the alveoli in the most dependent lung zone (i.e., near the spine) are collapsed, and alveolar ventilation is reduced. If this zone remains perfused, a ventilation-perfusion mismatch will develop, with consequent arterial hypoxemia.

*Pressure sores* are defined as localized areas of cellular necrosis that develop when the external pressure is greater than the capillary pressure. These sores are usually localized over bony prominences, and the risk of necrosis increases with the degree of external pressure and the extent of distortion.

Alveolar collapse is favored by impairment of mucociliary clearance. In studies of intubated patients who were receiving prolonged mechanical ventilation, mucociliary clearance, as measured by the motion of a radioactive bolus in the trachea, was found to be deeply reduced compared with healthy subjects (0.8 to 1.4 mm/minute versus 10 mm/minute).[26,27] Patients who developed pulmonary complications had significantly lower velocities of mucus transport compared with patients without pulmonary complications. Conversely, patients receiving general anesthesia for abdominal or thoracic surgery, but without prolonged mechanical ventilation (i.e., temporary mechanical ventilation), did not have reductions in bronchial transport velocity. Intubated patients who had lower velocities of mucus transport had reductions in surface of the ciliated area.[28] This reduction of mucus transport was correlated with the ciliated area on the luminal surface. The use of mechanical ventilation, with its high oxygen fraction, colonization of the trachea by bacteria, tracheal suctioning, pulmonary inflammatory responses, and administration of several drugs, may favor impairment of the mechanism of mucociliary clearance.

To prevent pulmonary complications, investigators have suggested that critically ill patients be turned from the supine position every 2 hours.[27] Previous studies showed that, when atelectatic lung regions were reopened by applying mechanical ventilation with an adequate positive end-expiratory pressure level, the rates of bacterial growth in the lung and translocation from the lung to the bloodstream were lower.[29–31] Pulmonary surfactant is able to lower alveolar surface tension and may prevent alveolar collapse and edema. In an experimental model of pneumonia with surfactant deficiency, instillation of exogenous surfactant significantly reduced bacterial proliferation in the lung and bloodstream.[32]

Radiographically demonstrated atelectasis can be present in 50% to 90% of postsurgical patients,[33] and after cardiac surgery, the percentage is as high as 84%.[34] Consequently, in an attempt to decrease the incidence of atelectasis, investigators have suggested turning patients postoperatively, starting on the first day of recovery. Chulay and colleagues evaluated whether immobility or systematic turning in the first 72 hours postoperatively had a clinical physiologic impact after coronary artery bypass surgery; 35 patients were studied, 18 in the control group and 17 in the turning treatment group.[34] This latter group received the same medical and nursing care as the control group, except for the first 24 hours after surgery, body position was systematically changed every 2 hours between a supine position and a left or right lateral posture at a 45-degree angle. These investigators found a marked difference between the two groups in the duration of postoperative fever; the turned patients spent 32% less time in the intensive care unit. Control patients had temperatures higher than 38°C for 44±11 hours, whereas the turned patients had only 26±14 hours of fever. There were no differences in the length of endotracheal intubation, radiographic abnormalities, and arterial oxygenation. Although this study did not elucidate the mechanisms of fever reduction, a possible reason could be the prevention of dependent pulmonary congestion with less small airway obstruction, which may increase the inflammatory response and distal atelectasis.

To assess the attitudes of physicians toward turning of critically ill patients, Krishnagopalan and associates conducted an electronic mail survey of intensive care specialists; 83% of the physicians agreed that the standard of their intensive care unit was to turn the patient every 2 hours, and 90% affirmed that this standard prevented complications.[27] However, only 57% answered that this standard was achieved in intensive care. These data suggest that although turning of the patient can decrease pulmonary complications, most critically ill patients do not receive the standard of care and thus are at increased risk for the complications of immobilization.

## KINETIC BED THERAPY

Prolonged immobilization increases the risk of pulmonary complications after major surgery. Thus, prompt postoperative mobilization is now standard practice. In patients whose underlying disease requires a regimen of bed rest, kinetic bed therapy, by turning the patient, can be a useful tool to prevent atelectasis and ventilator-associated pneumonia. In kinetic bed therapy, the bed rotates at least 40 degrees from side to side, whereas for continuous lateral rotation therapy, the bed rotates less than 40 degrees from side to side.[35]

Although the concept of kinetic bed therapy is long established, kinetic beds became available in intensive care in the 1970s with the introduction of the RotoRest Bed.[36] The RotoRest system allowed continuous turning up to 62 degrees (i.e., an arc of 124 degrees).

The rationale for kinetic bed therapy arises from the physiologic mobility of healthy persons.[37] Both day and night, healthy persons move their bodies to varying degrees.

Investigators have reported that sleeping persons usually moves their bodies about every 15 minutes. Consequently, it was hypothesized that frequent rotation of the patient would resemble physiologic mobility and would thus increase secretion removal and decrease the risk of infections.

## Ventilator-Induced Lung Injury

Acute lung injury and acute respiratory distress syndrome (ARDS) are characterized by noncardiogenic pulmonary edema with an increase in lung weight. The edema is responsible for lung compressive atelectasis and impairment of gas exchange. Although mechanical ventilation is an invaluable tool for guaranteeing adequate gas exchange, positive pressure ventilation may activate or increase the inflammatory response, with the release of several mediators that could induce local or systemic damage known as *ventilator-induced lung injury*.[38] A lung protective ventilator approach that minimizes lung stress was found to reduce ventilator-induced lung injury.[39]

By achieving more homogeneous distribution of transpulmonary pressure (the opening pressure that causes lung stress), kinetic bed therapy was hypothesized to decrease the risk of ventilator-induced lung injury. To verify this hypothesis, a group of healthy baboons, which were sedated, paralyzed, and mechanically ventilated for 11 days, received continuous bed rotation to 45 degrees compared with a control group.[40] The standard care group was turned from the supine position to a 90-degree angle every 2 hours. Lung injury was estimated by evaluating the composition of bronchoalveolar lavage and by lung histopathologic examination. The percentage of neutrophils in the bronchoalveolar lavage fluid at day 7 and day 11 was significantly lower in the continuous rotation group compared with the control group. Similarly, the lung histopathologic evaluation showed only one animal with mild focal pneumonia and a rare mucus plug. The degree of consolidation was 0.6%, as opposed to 11% in the control group. These data suggest that continuous rotation may induce protective effects.

## Mucus Transport

To determine the effect of continuous rotational therapy on pulmonary mucus transport, an inhaled tracer aerosol of 99m-technetium sulfur colloid was used. These patients were studied in the supine position on a stationary bed, during a rotation of 30 degrees to each side, and then again in the supine position.[41] The investigators found no improvement in mucus clearance during the rotational period. A possible explanation for these negative results could be the low degree of rotation attained in this study, approximately 30 degrees, less than the 45 degrees commonly suggested. Another factor could be the relatively brief duration of rotation (only 90 minutes), which may have been insufficient to increase mucus clearance.

## Atelectasis and Arterial Oxygenation

As stated earlier, critically ill patients who are mechanically ventilated are at high risk for ventilator-associated pneumonia. Investigators have hypothesized that lung atelectasis may predispose patients to pneumonia. *Atelectasis* is defined as a loss of aeration and can be segmental, lobar, or of an entire lung, depending on the chest radiograph extension. In the supine position, the cephalic displacement of the diaphragm resulting from the reduction or loss of muscular tone and lung edema may favor the development of compressive atelectasis. Compressive atelectasis is usually located in dependent lung zones, near the spine and the juxtadiaphragmatic portion. The pooled and stagnant secretions in these atelectatic regions may promote bacterial proliferation and increase the risk of infection.

Unlike in critically ill patients, who are restricted to the supine position, healthy subjects usually change their position during sleep every 11 minutes. This phenomenon was described by Keane as "the minimum physiologic mobility requirement."[42] Kinetic therapy mimics physiologic mobility and thus avoids the risk of compressive atelectasis. In one study, critically ill patients with respiratory failure and evidence of atelectasis on chest radiographs were managed with kinetic therapy and percussion therapy or with manual repositioning.[43] Kinetic therapy was applied using an angle of rotation of 45 degrees on each side, with a minimum duration of rotation of 18 hours out of every 24 hours. Kinetic therapy caused complete or partial resolution of atelectasis in 14 of 17 patients (82%), whereas only 1 of 7 control patients (14%) demonstrated this improvement. In addition, none of the patients treated with kinetic therapy required bronchoscopy for resolution of atelectasis.

Similarly, in patients with orthopedic injuries or with head or spinal injuries, kinetic therapy (rotation at 62 degrees for each side) significantly reduced atelectasis (42% versus 18%) compared with a conventional regimen of turning every 2 hours.[44] However, patients receiving kinetic therapy were rotated for only 13 hours every day.

Ahrens and colleagues evaluated kinetic therapy in comatose patients with a Glasgow coma scale score less than 11.[35] Kinetic therapy was delivered at an angle of 40 degrees of rotation and was able to reduce the incidence of lobar atelectasis compared with the standard of care.

During kinetic therapy, it is essential for the patient to be comfortable, to allow a long duration of treatment. Neurologically depressed patients or deeply sedated patients do not present particular problems; conversely, alert patients require some form of sedation to improve comfort.

The areas of lung atelectasis that remain perfused are responsible for arterial hypoxemia. Kinetic therapy was found to improve arterial oxygenation compared with the standard of care. In addition, in a group of patients with acute lung injury, the ventilation-perfusion ratio was assessed during continuous rotation therapy.[45] The ventilation-perfusion ratio was determined by the multiple inert gas elimination technique. Briefly, a mixture of six inert gas was infused, and arterial, mixed venous, and mixed expired gas samples were taken simultaneously. Arterial oxygenation was significantly improved during continuous rotation compared with the supine position. The shunt, defined as a ventilation-perfusion ratio of less than 0.005, decreased from 23% to 19%, and area of normal ventilation and perfusion, defined as a ventilation-perfusion ratio between 0.1 and 10, increased from 73% to 78%. Because the tidal volume did not change, the reduction in shunt was the result of redistribution of pulmonary blood flow from poorly ventilated to well-ventilated lung units during continuous rotation therapy.

## Nosocomial Pneumonia and Outcome

With regard to lower respiratory tract infections, several randomized controlled studies showed that kinetic therapy significantly reduced the incidence of tracheobronchitis and pneumonia[46–48] (Table 36.1). De Boisblanc and associates evaluated the occurrence of pneumonia during the first 5 days of intensive care stay.[49] The incidence of early-onset pneumonia was significantly lower in patients receiving kinetic therapy (9%) compared with patients receiving the standard of care (22%). Moreover, the lowest reduction was obtained in patients with sepsis, as compared with patients with obstructive pulmonary disease.

Fink and colleagues reported a reduction in intensive care and hospital length of stay from 8 to 5 days and from 44.5 to 20 days with kinetic therapy.[46] Among patients with sepsis and pneumonia, kinetic therapy decreased intensive care stay by an average of 3 days, whereas patients with obstructive pulmonary disease obtained the highest reduction, an average of 6 days.[25]

Unfortunately these encouraging data on the reduction of pulmonary infections and on the length of stay are not mirrored by significant differences in outcome. Possible explanations for the discrepancy between the lowered incidence of pneumonia and the lack of change in outcome could include the following: (1) these randomized studies were underpowered to demonstrate a difference in mortality because of the relatively small number of patients studied, (2) patients spent few hours in kinetic therapy, and (3) the clinical incidence of pneumonia could have been overestimated as a result of the erroneous classification of parenchymal congestion and atelectasis as pneumonia. Thus, it is possible that kinetic therapy also decreased noninfectious causes of parenchymal infiltration without affecting survival.

## PRONE POSITIONING

In patients with acute lung injury and ARDS, the prone position is often used to improve gas exchange, to reduce barotrauma, and to remove secretions. However in certain conditions or when therapeutic or nursing maneuvers are necessary, the prone position may be inadvisable, and continuous rotational therapy could be a useful tool to improve gas exchange.

The mechanisms in the improvement in gas exchange in prone positioning are different from those in continuous rotational therapy. In the prone position, reduction of chest wall compliance, blood flow redistribution, change in diaphragmatic motion, improved ventilation-perfusion ratio, and recruitment of previously collapsed zones have been implicated. In continuous rotational therapy, mobilization of secretions, recruitment of collapsed lung regions, and prevention of atelectasis may contribute to

| Table 36-1 | Randomized Clinical Studies of Kinetic Therapy: Pneumonia Rates and Length of Stay | | |
|---|---|---|---|
| **Authors** | **Population** | **Pneumonia Rates** | **Length of Stay** |
| Gentilello et al.[45] | Trauma patients | 21% versus 15% | No difference |
| Summer et al.[49] | Medical patients | 22% versus 9% | Decreased |
| Fink et al.[47] | Trauma patients | 40% versus 14% | No difference |
| De Boisblanc et al.[50] | Medical patients | 22% versus 9% | No difference |

the effects on gas exchange. In patients in whom prone positioning seems unsafe, continuous rotational therapy could be an alternative in the management of patients with ARDS.

Staudinger and colleagues compared the use of the prone position and continuous rotational therapy in patients suffering from ARDS. Patients randomized to be prone were turned supine each day for as short as possible to permit therapeutic or nursing maneuvers, whereas patients in the kinetic therapy group had a dedicated therapeutic bed allowing continuous axial rotation from one lateral position to the other with a maximum angle of 124 degrees.[50] Arterial oxygenation and the intrapulmonary shunt fraction improved in both groups. Arterial oxygenation improved in 10 of 12 patients in the prone position compared with 7 of 14 patients in the kinetic therapy group. Similarly, the intrapulmonary shunt fraction decreased in both groups. Comparing the areas under the curves during the first 72 hours, there were no differences with respect to arterial oxygenation and intrapulmonary shunt. The prone position was well tolerated without any hemodynamic changes, whereas kinetic therapy caused relative hemodynamic instability in three patients. Besides improving gas exchange, the prone position could favor the drainage of secretions, with a possible reduction of bacterial colonization and infection of the lower airway.

In a small, randomized study enrolling mechanically ventilated patients who had a Glasgow coma scale score of 9 or less, the prone position was compared with the supine position in terms of the incidence of ventilator-associated pneumonia.[51] Patients were randomized during the first 24 hours after intubation and were prone for 4 hours once daily. The incidence of microbiologically confirmed ventilator-associated pneumonia was lower in the prone position compared with the supine, although results were not significant: 38% versus 20%, without any difference in the duration of mechanical ventilation before the development of pulmonary infection. In a subsequent, larger, randomized controlled trial, the prone position significantly reduced ventilator-associated pneumonia (91 versus 85 episodes).[52] Therefore, prone position may be considered a means of preventing ventilator-associated pneumonia along with postural changes and the semirecumbent position.

## CONCLUSION

Current data clearly demonstrate the importance of an appropriate policy of body positioning to reduce the incidence of ventilator-associated pneumonia in critically ill patients. However, further studies will be necessary to evaluate more fully the effect of this strategy on clinical outcome.

## REFERENCES

1. Bueno-Cavanillas A, Delgado-Rodriguez M, Lopez-Luque A, et al: Influence of nosocomial infection on mortality rate in an intensive care. Crit Care Med 1994;22:55–60.
2. Cook D, Ricard JD, Reeve B, et al: Ventilator circuit and secretion management strategies: A Franco-Canadian survey. Crit Care Med 2000;28:3547–3554.
3. Giron E, Stephan F, Novara A: Risk factors and outcome of nosocomial infections: Results of a matched case control study of ICU patients. Am J Respir Crit Care Med 1998;157:1151–1158.
4. Kollef MH: The prevention of ventilator-associated pneumonia. N Engl J Med 1999;340:627–634.
5. Cook D, De Jonghe B, Brochard L, et al: Influence of airway management on ventilator-associated pneumonia. JAMA 1998;279:781–787.
6. Dodek P, Keenan S, Cook D, et al: Evidence-based clinical practice guideline for the prevention of ventilator-associated pneumonia. Ann Intern Med 2004;141:305–313.
7. Chastre J, Fagon JY: Ventilator-associated pneumonia. Am J Respir Crit Care Med 2002;165:867–903.
8. Kollef MH: Prevention of hospital-associated pneumonia and ventilator-associated pneumonia. Crit Care Med 2004;32:1396–1405.
9. Craig CP, Connelly S: Effect of intensive care unit nosocomial on duration: Stay and mortality. Am J Infect Control 1984;12:233–238.
10. Heyland DK, Cook DJ, Griffith L, et al: The attributable morbidity and mortality of ventilator-associated pneumonia in the critically ill patient. Am J Respir Crit Care Med 1999;159:1249–1256.
11. Chevret S, Hemmer M, Carlet J, et al: Incidence and risk factors of pneumonia acquired in intensive units: Results from a multicenter prospective study on 996 patients. European Cooperative Group on Nosocomial Pneumonia. Intensive Care Med 1993;19:256–264.
12. Mosconi P, Langer M, Cigada M, et al: Epidemiology and risk factors of pneumonia in critically ill patients: Intensive Care Unit Group for Infection Control. Eur J Epidemiol 1991;7:320–327.
13. Shorr AF, Sherner JH, Jackson WL, et al: Invasive approaches to the diagnosis of ventilator-associated pneumonia: A meta-analysis. Crit Care Med 2005;33:46–53.
14. Tablan OC, Anderson LJ, Besser R, et al: Guidelines for preventing health-care–associated pneumonia, 2003: Recommendations of CDC and the Healthcare Infection Control Practices Advisory Committee. MMWR Recomm Rep 2004;53:1–36.
15. Ibanez J, Perrafiel A, Raurich JM, et al: Gastroesophageal reflux in intubated patients receiving enteral nutrition: Effect of supine and semirecumbent positions. JPEN J Parenter Enteral Nutr 1992;16:419–422.
16. Torres A, Serra-Batlles J, Ros E, et al: Pulmonary aspiration of gastric contents in patients receiving mechanical ventilation: The effect of body position. Ann Intern Med 1992;116:540–543.
17. Orozco-Levi M, Torres A, Ferrer M, et al: Semirecumbent position protects from pulmonary aspiration but not completely from gastroesophageal reflux in mechanically ventilated patients. Am J Respir Crit Care Med 1995;152:1387–1390.
18. Kollef MH: Ventilator-associated pneumonia: A multivariate analysis. JAMA 1993;270:1965–1970.
19. Drakulovic MB, Torres A, Bauer TT, et al: Supine body position as a risk factor for nosocomial pneumonia in mechanically ventilated patients: A randomised trial. Lancet 1999;354:1851–1858.

20. Cook DJ, Meade MO, Hand LE, et al: Toward understanding evidence uptake: Semirecumbency for pneumonia prevention. Crit Care Med 2002;30:1472–1477.

21. Heyland DK, Cook DJ, Dodek PM: Prevention of ventilator-associated pneumonia: Current practice in Canadian intensive care units. J Crit Care 2002;17:161–167.

22. McMullin JP, Cook DJ, Meade MO, et al: Clinical estimation of trunk position among mechanically ventilated patients. Intensive Care Med 2002;28:304–309.

23. Helman DL Jr, Sherner JH III, Fitzpatrick TM, et al: Effect of standardized orders and provider education on head-of-bed positioning in mechanically ventilated patients. Crit Care Med 2003;31:2285–2290.

24. Dittmer DK, Teaselli R: Complications of immobilization and bed rest. Part 1. Can Fam Physician 1993;39:1428–1437.

25. Teaselli R, Dittmer DK: Complications of immobilization and bed rest. Part 2. Can Fam Physician 1993;39:1440–1446.

26. Konrad F, Schreiber T, Brecht-Kraus D, et al: Mucociliary transport in ICU patients. Chest 1994;105:237–241.

27. Krishnagopalan S, Johnson EW, Low LL, et al: Body positioning of intensive care patients: Clinical practice versus standards. Crit Care Med 2002;30:2588–2592.

28. Konrad F, Schiener R, Marx T, et al: Ultrastructure and mucociliary transport of bronchial respiratory epithelium in intubated patients. Intensive Care Med 1995;21:482–489.

29. Pison U, Max M, Neuendank A, et al: Host defence capacities of pulmonary surfactant: Evidence for nonsurfactant functions of the surfactant system. Eur J Clin Invest 1994;24:586–599.

30. Steinberg JM, Schiller HJ, Halter JM, et al: Alveolar instability causes early ventilator induced lung injury independent of neutrophils. Am J Respir Crit Care Med 2003;169:57–63.

31. Verbrugge SJ, Sorm V, van't Veen A, et al: Lung overinflation without positive end expiratory pressure promotes bacteremia after experimental *Klebsiella pneumoniae* inoculation. Intensive Care Med 1998;24:172–177.

32. Van Kaam AH, Lachman RA, Herting E, et al: Reducing atelectasis attenuates bacterial growth and translocation in experimental pneumonia. Am J Respir Crit Care Med 2004;169:1046–1053.

33. Bernheim HA, Block LH, Atkins E: Fever: Pathogenesis, pathophysiology and purpose. Ann Intern Med 1979;91:261–270.

34. Chulay M, Brown J, Summer W: Effect of postoperative immobilization after coronory artery bypass surgery. Crit Care Med 1982;10:176–179.

35. Ahrens T, Kollef M, Stewart J, et al: Effect of kinetic therapy on pulmonary complications. Am J Crit Care 2004;13:376–382.

36. Keane FX: Roto rest. BMJ 1967;3:731–733.

37. Sahn SA: Continuous lateral rotational therapy and nosocomial pneumonia. Chest 1991;99:1236–1267.

38. Dos Santos CC, Zhang H, Slutsky AS: From bench to bedside: Bacterial growth and cytokines. Crit Care 2002;6:4–6.

39. Ranieri VM, Suter PM, Tortorella C, et al: Effect of mechanical ventilation on inflammatory mediators in patients with acute respiratory distress syndrome: A randomized controlled trial. JAMA 1999;282:54–61.

40. Anzueto A, Peters JI, Seidner SR, et al: Effects of continuous bed rotation and prolonged mechanical ventilation on healthy, adult baboons. Crit Care Med 1997;25:1560–1564.

41. Dolovich M, Rushbrook J, Churchill, et al: Effect of continuous lateral rotational therapy on lung mucus transport in mechanically ventilated patients. J Crit Care 1998;13:119–125.

42. Keane FX: The minimum physiological mobility requirement for man supported on a soft surface. Paraplegia 1978;16:383–389.

43. Raoof S, Chowdhrey N, Raoof S, et al: Effect of combined kinetic therapy and percussion therapy on the resolution of atelectasis in critically ill patients. Chest 1999;115:1658–1666.

44. Gentilello L, Thompson DA, Tonnesen AS, et al: Effect of a rotating bed on the incidence of pulmonary complications in critically ill patients. Crit Care Med 1988;16:783–786.

45. Bein T, Reber A, Metz C, et al: Acute effects of continuous rotational therapy on ventilation-perfusion inequality in lung injury. Intensive Care Med 1998;24:132–137.

46. Fink M, Helsmoortel CM, Stein KL, et al: The efficacy of an oscillating bed in the prevention of lower respiratory tract infection in critically ill victims of blunt trauma. Chest 1990;97:133–137.

47. Kirschenbaum L, Azzi E, Sfeir T, et al: Effect of continuous lateral rotational therapy on the prevalence of ventilator-associated pneumonia in patients requiring long-term ventilatory care. Crit Care Med 2002;30:1983–1986.

48. Summer WR, Curry P, Haponik EF, et al: Continuous mechanical turning of intensive care unit patients shortens length of stay in some diagnostic-related groups. J Crit Care 1989;4:45–53.

49. De Boisblanc BP, Castro M, Everret B, et al: Effect of air-supported, continuous, postural oscillation on the risk of early ICU pneumonia in nontraumatic critical illness. Chest 1993;103:1543–1547.

50. Staudinger T, Kofler J, Mullner M, et al: Comparison of prone positioning and continuous rotation of patients with adult respiratory distress syndrome: Results of a pilot study. Crit Care Med 2001;29:51–56.

51. Beuret P, Carton MJ, Nourdine K, et al: Prone position as prevention of lung injury in comatose patients: A prospective, randomised, controlled study. Intensive Care Med 2002;28:564–569.

52. Guerin C, Gaillard S, Lemasson S, et al: Effects of systematic prone positioning in hypoxemic acute respiratory failure. JAMA 2004;292:2379–2387.

## SUGGESTED READINGS

Clemmer TP, Green S, Ziegler B, et al: Effectiveness of the kinetic treatment table for preventing and treating pulmonary complications in severely head-injured patients. Crit Care Med 1990;18:614–617.

De Clercq H, De Decker G, Alexander JP, et al: Cost evaluation of infections in intensive care. Acta Anaesthesiol Belg 1983;34:179–189.

# CHAPTER 37

# Oxygen Therapy in Acutely Ill Patients

George E. Karras, Jr.

The addition of supplemental oxygen ($O_2$) to improve tissue $O_2$ delivery ($DO_2$) can often play a pivotal role in acutely ill patients. In some circumstances, the indications and concentrations provided can be somewhat controversial. This chapter discusses the concepts of $DO_2$ and $O_2$ consumption ($VO_2$) and arterial hypoxemia in the context of $O_2$ therapy, its indications, and its potential complications. It also reviews delivery systems for $O_2$ therapy and then briefly surveys the issue of lung injury associated with hyperoxia.

## OXYGEN DELIVERY AND CONSUMPTION

To appreciate fully the role of $O_2$ therapy in an acutely ill patient, it is helpful to review the process of tissue oxygenation. Adequacy of $DO_2$ is essential to the normal aerobic metabolism that occurs in all human cells. *Shock* is defined as inadequate tissue perfusion, leading to tissue hypoxia ($O_2$ debt), anaerobic metabolism, lactate production, and, ultimately, cell death. In this context, lactic acidosis is the hallmark of $O_2$ debt. During times of poor tissue perfusion, acute $O_2$ therapy can play an integral role in the treatment of tissue hypoxia.

### Physiology of Oxygen Delivery and Consumption

Under normal circumstances, $VO_2$, defined as CI × ($CaO_2$ − $CvO_2$), where CI is cardiac index and $CaO_2$ and $CvO_2$ are arterial and venous $O_2$ content respectively, is independent of $DO_2$. As $DO_2$ decreases, this independence is preserved by the tissue's ability to increase $O_2$ extraction

proportionally to the decrease in $DO_2$.[1] This is expressed as the $O_2$ extraction ratio, calculated as follows:

$$O_2 \text{ ext} = CaO_2 - CvO_2/CaO_2$$

This ability to preserve increases in $O_2$ extraction continues to a critical decrease in $DO_2$, below which $O_2$ extraction is no longer able to compensate for the decrease in $DO_2$. At this point, termed *critical* $DO_2$, $VO_2$ decreases proportionally to $DO_2$; that is, $VO_2$ is now dependent on $DO_2$ (Fig. 37.1). Blood lactate increases as $DO_2$ falls below this critical level, a finding indicating that metabolic demands of the cell are no longer being met.

### Pathophysiology of Oxygen Delivery and Consumption

Multiple clinical studies of critically ill patients with severe sepsis, septic shock, acute respiratory distress syndrome (ARDS), and multisystem organ failure demonstrated a pathologic dependence of $VO_2$ on $DO_2$[2-5] (Fig. 37.2). The reason for this dependence appears to be that the $O_2$ extraction ratio is lower in critically ill patients secondary to altered distribution of blood flow and/or impaired $O_2$ extraction at the cellular level.[6] Nevertheless, demonstration of this abnormal relationship fostered a decade-long controversy regarding the clinical efficacy of increasing $DO_2$ to supranormal levels in critically ill adult patients and thus decreasing the incidence of multiple-system organ failure and mortality.[7-11] More recent evidence indicates that targeting specific end points such as blood lactate and mixed venous $O_2$ saturation ($SvO_2$) by increasing $DO_2$ may improve outcome.[12]

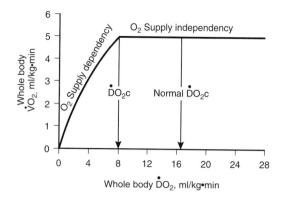

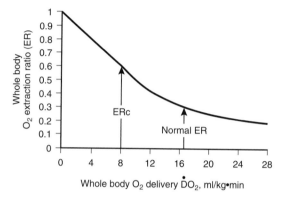

**Figure 37.1**  The biphasic $\dot{V}O_2$-$\dot{D}O_2$ model. The top panel shows the relationship between $\dot{V}O_2$ and $\dot{D}O_2$. The bottom panel reveals the parallel relationship between oxygen extraction ratio (ER) and $\dot{D}O_2$. Note the critical ER (ERC) is normally about 30% and corresponds to the critical $\dot{D}O_2$ ($\dot{D}O_2C$). (From Schlichtig R: $O_2$ uptake, critical $O_2$ delivery, and tissue wellness. In Pinsky M, Dhainaut JF [eds]: *Pathologic Foundations of Critical Care*. Baltimore: Williams & Wilkins, 1993, p 121.)

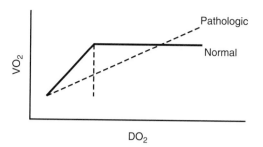

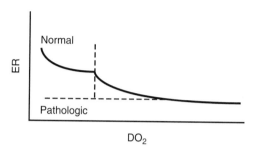

**Figure 37.2**  The normal and pathologic relationship between oxygen delivery and oxygen consumption. The normal critical $DO_2$ is seen at the point where the shape of the curve changes, separating the independent from dependent portions of the normal $DO_2$–$VO_2$ relationship. The pathologic relationship is defined by a greater critical $DO_2$ compared to normal. Clinical studies have not demonstrated a plateau of $VO_2$ in patients with a pathologic dependency on $VO_2$ or $DO_2$. In the pathology relationship, the oxygen extraction ratio remains relatively constant and therefore $VO_2$ is dependent on $DO_2$. (From Russell JA, Phang PT: The oxygen delivery/consumption controversy: Approaches to management of the critically ill. Am J Respir Crit Care 1994;149:534.)

## CAUSES OF INADEQUATE TISSUE PERFUSION AND TISSUE HYPOXEMIA

$$\text{Oxygen delivery} = \text{Cardiac output} \times \text{CaO}_2$$
$$\text{CaO}_2 = (\text{Hgb} \times 1.34 \times \text{SaO}_2) + (\text{PaO}_2 \times 0.00031)$$

where Hgb is hemoglobin, $SaO_2$ is arterial $O_2$ saturation, and $PaO_2$ is arterial oxygen tension. Therefore, it is possible to describe alterations in flow, Hgb, and $O_2$ tension that will contribute to tissue hypoxemia. Further, abnormalities in $VO_2$ and $O_2$ extraction can also lead to $O_2$ debt.

### Abnormalities in Circulation

There are four basic causes of shock:

1. *Cardiogenic shock* implies that the heart can no longer effectively provide forward flow. This can happen when a critical amount of myocardial tissue has been injured or destroyed, as in myocardial ischemia or infarction. This condition can also be seen during a hemodynamically significant arrhythmia or in patients with significant valvular dysfunction or septal defects.

2. *Hypovolemic shock* occurs because of a critical decrease in effective circulating blood volume causing an underfilled heart and consequent decreased blood flow.

3. *Obstructive shock* can result from pericardial tamponade or large pulmonary embolus, thus limiting cardiac output.

4. *Distributive shock* or *vasodilatory shock* can cause tissue hypoxemia from maldistribution of blood flow, precapillary shunting, abnormalities in $O_2$ extraction, and relative hypovolemia from changes in venous capacitance.

### Abnormalities in Arterial Oxygen Content and Oxygen Extraction

Blood $O_2$ content is a reflection of Hgb, $O_2$ saturation, and dissolved $O_2$. The process of $O_2$ extraction involves the diffusion of $O_2$ from the Hgb molecule to the tissues and the utilization of that $O_2$ by the cell mitochondria.

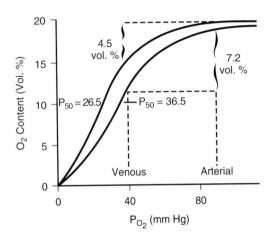

**Figure 37.3** The oxygen-hemoglobin dissocation curve (ODC). The shape of the ODC results in 90% hemoglobin saturation at a PaO$_2$ of 60 mmHg. The P$_{50}$ is the PaO$_2$ at which hemoglobin is 50% saturated. Notice the right-ward shifted curve is able to release 60% more O$_2$, which is available to the tissues, compared to the left-ward shifted curve. (From Bone RC: Monitoring respiratory and hemodynamic function in the patient with respiratory failure. In Kirby RR, Smith RA, Desautels DA [eds]: *Mechanical Ventilation*. New York: Churchill Livingstone, 1985, p 146.)

Therefore, O$_2$ extraction can be compromised by alterations in the amount of Hgb and O$_2$-Hgb affinity.

The O$_2$-Hgb dissociation curve (ODC) (Fig. 37.3) defines the relationship between O$_2$ dissolved in blood and the amount of O$_2$ carried by Hgb. The position of the curve is expressed as P$_{50}$, the PaO$_2$ at which Hgb is 50% saturated. In states in which total Hgb is decreased (anemia), DO$_2$ is decreased, and O$_2$ extraction will increase until a critical DO$_2$ is reached, thereby causing tissue hypoxia. Under these circumstances, the ODC is shifted to the right (P$_{50}$ is higher), and O$_2$ unloading from Hgb is enhanced.[13]

Altered O$_2$-Hgb affinity is manifested either by a reduced ability to release O$_2$ from Hgb or an inability to bind O$_2$ to Hgb.[13] Examples of the former include hemoglobinopathies and decreased levels of red cell 2,3-diphosphoglycerate. Methemoglobinemia and carbon monoxide poisoning severely limit the affinity of O$_2$ for Hgb; the results are decreased SaO$_2$ and tissue hypoxia, but often normal dissolved arterial O$_2$ levels. Under these conditions, the ODC is shifted to the left (P$_{50}$ is decreased).[13-16]

The vasodilatory defects associated with sepsis and the systemic inflammatory response syndrome contribute to the maldistribution of blood flow and precapillary shunting referenced earlier.[17] An abnormally low O$_2$ extraction ratio is one of the consequences of this process and is often a contributing factor to tissue hypoxia and lactic acidosis seen in these syndromes.[17-20] Tissue hypoxia resulting from defects in O$_2$ utilization at the cellular level can contribute

to the formation of O$_2$ debt. The classic example of cyanide toxicity with its inhibition of oxidative phosphorylation is well known. This process impedes the formation of adenosine triphosphate through oxidative phosphorylation.[14] It results in the formation of lactic acidosis in the context of a normal SaO$_2$, decreased VO$_2$, and normal or elevated SvO$_2$. Endotoxin has also been linked to the inhibition and uncoupling of mitochondrial respiration, a finding suggesting that cellular defects of O$_2$ utilization are independent of tissue perfusion in septic shock.[18]

## Causes of Arterial Hypoxemia (Decreased Oxygen Tension of Arterial Blood)

Arterial blood gas tension is determined by the composition of alveolar gas and the efficiency of gas transfer between the alveoli and the pulmonary capillary blood. Alveolar gas tension is a function of the mixture of inspired gas, the matching of ventilation and blood flow in the lungs, and the composition of mixed venous blood.[13] The causes of arterial hypoxemia include hypoventilation, shunt, ventilation-perfusion (V/Q) mismatch, diffusion block, and increased O$_2$ extraction with decreased SvO$_2$.

### Hypoventilation or Hypercapnic Respiratory Failure

The hallmark of hypoventilation is carbon dioxide (CO$_2$) retention, which is *always* present. The simplified alveolar gas equation is expressed as follows:[13,21]

$$PaCO_2 = PiO_2 - PaCO_2/R$$

where PaCO$_2$ is alveolar CO$_2$ tension, PiO$_2$ is inspired PaO$_2$, PaCO$_2$ is arterial CO$_2$ tension, and R is the respiratory quotient of 0.8.

This equation tells us two things. First, PaO$_2$ is directly and inversely proportional to alveolar ventilation; that is, when patients breathe ambient air while hypoventilating, hypoxia results secondary to an increase in alveolar CO$_2$. Second, hypoxemia of pure hypoventilation can be readily ameliorated by increasing the fraction of inspired O$_2$ (FiO$_2$).

These two points become particularly important when monitoring patients for airway or ventilatory adequacy in the intensive care unit (ICU), as well as when monitoring patients during opiate therapy or procedural intravenous sedation. As Stemp and Ramsay noted in patients breathing room air,[22] a fall in SpO$_2$ on pulse oximetry would be indicative of alveolar hypoventilation or possible airway obstruction. Early detection of this phenomenon would allow for early intervention. The use of supplemental O$_2$ in these settings, however, can mask the progression of bradypnea to apnea, can prevent the onset of hypoxemia as evidenced by pulse oximetry, and can lead to unrecognized severe hypoventilation with potentially disastrous results.[22] The pulse oximeter therefore becomes a tool for monitoring not only oxygenation but also, and more importantly, the adequacy of ventilation when supplemental $O_2$ is not in use.[23]

The causes of hypoventilation are myriad and include the following: ventilatory muscle dysfunction, depressed central drive, increased minute ventilation, V/Q inequality, and injudicious use of $O_2$.[21,24] The muscles and bones of the thorax are vulnerable to disease and injury that can lead to high $PaCO_2$ and low alveolar oxygen tension ($PaO_2$). Diseases of the central nervous system can affect the respiratory muscles and the level of consciousness. Examples include Guillain-Barré syndrome, myasthenia gravis, diphtheria, poliomyelitis, hemorrhage and trauma to the cervical spine and brain. Chest wall abnormalities, such as severe kyphoscoliosis, or injuries, such as rib fractures or flail chest, or postoperative thoracotomy pain can lead to ventilatory failure. Upper airway obstruction secondary to hematoma formation or severe inflammation or infection can significantly increase the inspiratory work of breathing and respiratory muscle fatigue. Another example of increasing inspiratory load on breathing is morbid obesity leading to hypoventilation.[24] Indeed, severe cases of obstructive airways disease or pulmonary edema can cause respiratory muscle fatigue and hypercapnia.

Depressed central drive is commonly caused by drug overdoses, especially sedative-hypnotics and narcotics. However, this condition is also seen in diseases affecting the medulla of the brain such as encephalitis and hemorrhage. Metabolic derangements can also suppress central drive. Severe hypothyroidism and metabolic alkalosis[24] can, at times, lead to significant $CO_2$ retention.

In circumstances of borderline ventilatory reserve, nonpulmonary causes of elevated minute ventilation can overwhelm a patient's ability to excrete excess $CO_2$. When nutritional support with a high percentage of carbohydrate calories is provided, the respiratory quotient increases, thus producing more $CO_2$, increasing minute ventilation, and subsequently exacerbating hypercapnic respiratory failure.[25] Other causes of increased minute ventilation include metabolic acidosis (common in patients receiving crystalloid resuscitation), sepsis, anxiety, and agitation.

V/Q inequalities contribute to hypercapnia in patients with chronic obstructive pulmonary disease (COPD),[26] and the associated hypoxemia is more severe in relation to hypercapnia than in other forms of hypoventilation.

Injudicious use of $O_2$ therapy in patients with COPD can worsen hypercarbia and ventilatory failure. This effect is often attributed to a decrease in hypoxic ventilatory drive associated with this group of patients, although this concept is controversial.[27] Hanson and colleagues[28] described the development of Haldane dead space, secondary to loss of hypoxic vasoconstriction, sufficient to account for the development of hypercarbia seen in these patients. More recently, investigators suggested that an overall reduction in ventilation occurred when high concentrations of $O_2$ were given to patients believed to be $CO_2$ retainers, as opposed to nonretainers, during acute exacerbation of COPD.[29] Significant release of hypoxic vasoconstriction was also noticed, but to a similar degree in both groups. Another study concluded that supplemental $O_2$ could be safely given to patients with COPD following a period of mechanical ventilation, because new V/Q relationships had been established during normoxic ventilation.[30] In most patients with hypoventilation, hypoxemia is easily reversed with supplemental $O_2$ therapy. The main thrust of management is treating the cause of hypoventilation.

**Shunt** Hypoxemia caused by shunt is defined by a decrease in arterial $O_2$ content in the context of constant alveolar ventilation. Venous blood passes through areas of unventilated lung to the arterial system. The shape of the ODC dictates an important diagnostic element of shunt.[24] The addition of supplemental $O_2$ cannot ameliorate the hypoxemia. Because the saturation of nonshunted blood is on the flat portion of the ODC, additional $O_2$ has little impact in raising $PaO_2$. When this blood mixes with poorly oxygenated shunted blood, the $PaO_2$ drops precipitously. In contrast, in hypoventilation, diffusion abnormality, and V/Q inequality, arterial hypoxemia is easily resolved with $O_2$ therapy.[21]

Extrapulmonary causes of shunt include cardiac defects such as atrial septal defect, patent ductus arteriosus, and ventricular septal defect associated with increased right heart pressures. Pulmonary disorders such as pneumonia, ARDS, and cardiogenic pulmonary edema represent causes of shunt commonly seen in the ICU. Moreover, treatment with 100% $O_2$, which causes nitrogen washout, can result in alveolar collapse. The consequent area of low V/Q ratio can worsen the hypoxemia seen in patients with V/Q abnormalities.

**Ventilation-Perfusion Mismatch** V/Q mismatch is the most common cause of arterial hypoxia.[26] Various lung units or regions receive variable proportions of ventilation and flow. Some receive high flow relative to ventilation (low V/Q), and others receive high ventilation relative to flow (high V/Q). Therefore, total gas exchange is inefficient. In areas of low V/Q, mixed venous blood picks up alveolar $O_2$ at a faster rate than alveolar ventilation can replace it.[31] Alveolar $O_2$ remains low. Arterial hypoxemia persists because the well-oxygenated blood from areas of high V/Q cannot compensate for the poorly oxygenated mixed venous blood from areas of low V/Q.[24,32] Again, the shape of the ODC is responsible for this limitation just as seen with $O_2$ supplementation and right-to-left shunt noted earlier.[24] In contrast to shuntlike hypoxia, however, $O_2$ therapy ameliorates the hypoxia of V/Q mismatch by increasing the rate of delivery of oxygen to areas of low V/Q. Because the rate of $O_2$ uptake does not change, alveolar $O_2$ increases, and arterial oxygenation improves.[24] V/Q mismatch causes hypoxemia in multiple disease processes including acute lung injury, COPD, asthma, interstitial lung disease, pulmonary edema, and pulmonary embolus. $O_2$ therapy usually easily improves $PaO_2$ in patients with V/Q abnormalities.

**Diffusion Impairment** The term *diffusion impairment* describes the lack of equilibrium between $PaO_2$ in pulmonary capillary blood and alveolar gas. This can occur when the alveolar capillary membrane is thickened, thereby limiting the rate of diffusion of $O_2$ between the alveoli and the capillary.[21] Interstitial fibrosis from multiple causes serves as a classic example.

Damage or loss of whole lung units reduces capillary volumes and alveolar capillary surface area. This process results in decreased red cell transit time through alveolar capillaries and lack of equilibrium. Increases in cardiac output such as those observed in severe sepsis or septic shock could decrease transit time through alveolar capillaries, thus worsening arterial hypoxemia in the context of an already diseased lung.

**Increased Oxygen Extraction (Decreased Mixed Venous Oxygen)** Decreases in $DO_2$ because of poor cardiac output or low arterial $O_2$ content can cause a reduction in $SvO_2$. Shunting of this blood can cause significant arterial hypoxemia. It can also worsen existing hypoxemia associated with pulmonary shunt or V/Q mismatch.

## ASSESSMENT OF TISSUE HYPOXIA

The signs and symptoms associated with tissue hypoxia include tachycardia, tachypnea with increased minute ventilation, dyspnea, and altered mental status. In acutely ill elderly patients, new-onset delirium or agitation secondary to acute hypoxemia can be confused with ICU psychosis or "sundowning." As hypoxemia worsens or its duration increases, respiratory distress, respiratory muscle paradox, and arrhythmias ensue, with elevations in myocardial $VO_2$. Ultimately, respiratory muscle fatigue, coma, and respiratory and cardiac arrest may occur. In fact, hypoxia is a potentially reversible cause of pulseless electrical activity. Cyanosis is often a late and unreliable indicator of hypoxemia.[31]

Direct measurement of $PaO_2$ or $SaO_2$ is easily obtained at the patient's bedside, and it remains the most practical laboratory assessment for arterial hypoxemia. This measurement can be done either invasively through arterial blood gas determination or noninvasively by pulse oximetry. Arterial blood gas samples allow assessment of $PaO_2$ and $SaO_2$, as well as alveolar-arterial $O_2$ tension difference ($PA$-$aO_2$), venous admixture, and estimated shunt.[33] Limitations of arterial blood gas analysis include the following: the technique is invasive, measurements are intermittent and may potentially miss sudden changes in patient status, and inaccuracies may occur related to sampling. Pulse oximetry is frequently used as a measurement of blood oxygenation. It is done continuously and noninvasively and reduces the need for invasive blood gas analysis.[33]

Neither arterial blood gas analysis nor pulse oximetry is helpful when tissue hypoxia exists but $PaO_2$ and $SaO_2$ values are normal. Such situations can occur during states of low cardiac output, decreased Hgb, or increased $VO_2$. Within these contexts, assessment of $SvO_2$ or blood lactate provides a better index of tissue perfusion.[12,18,19,34] Either a central venous catheter with the tip in the superior vena cava[12] or a pulmonary artery catheter is required for sampling mixed venous blood.

## INDICATIONS FOR OXYGEN THERAPY

Increasing $O_2$ transport is the main goal in treating tissue hypoxia. $O_2$ therapy often plays a key role in this endeavor, particularly when $CaO_2$ is decreased secondary to arterial hypoxia.

### Treating the Causes of Arterial Hypoxemia

As previously mentioned, the $O_2$ dissociation curve defines the relationship between $PaO_2$ and $SaO_2$. Because a $PaO_2$ of 60 mm Hg results in an $SaO_2$ of approximately 90%, the aim is to maintain a $PaO_2$ greater than or equal to 60 mm Hg with supplemental $O_2$.[35] The ODC becomes steep at this point, and any further decrease in $PaO_2$ would result in a marked drop in $SaO_2$.

### Hypoventilation or Hypercapnic Respiratory Failure

The alveolar gas equation allows us to predict a parallel rise in $PaO_2$ with supplemental $O_2$ use, assuming ventilation and metabolic rates are unchanged.[21] The level of hypoxemia is usually not severe and is easily reversed by the use of $O_2$. For example, patients with drug overdose or acute neuromuscular disease often have normal lungs. The primary goals of management are therefore recognition and treatment of the underlying cause of hypoventilation.

COPD is also a major cause of hypercapnic respiratory failure. V/Q mismatch plays a major role in the pathophysiology of increased $PCO_2$ in these patients.[26,32] $O_2$ is titrated carefully in patients with chronic COPD because too high an $FiO_2$ can either abolish hypoxic ventilatory drive or reduce hypoxic vasoconstriction, thereby leading to an increase in dead space.[28] Both mechanisms can contribute to dangerously high levels of

$P_{CO_2}$ and ventilatory failure. Despite this concern, adequacy of tissue perfusion is the primary goal in these critically ill patients. Sacrificing adequate arterial $O_2$ levels and $D_{O_2}$ to improve hypercarbia is not recommended. If after careful titration of $O_2$, $P_{CO_2}$ is still dangerously high (as indicated by a patient's clinical status and arterial pH) and $Sa_{O_2}$ is too low (decreased $Sv_{O_2}$ or increased blood lactate), then options such as bilevel noninvasive positive pressure ventilation or intubation and mechanical ventilation can be utilized.

## Ventilation-Perfusion Mismatch

V/Q abnormalities are ubiquitous in almost all forms of lung disease.[26] Supplemental $O_2$ increases $Pa_{O_2}$, but the extent of increase depends on the predominant pattern of inequality. Therefore, the response may be unpredictable and could take many minutes.[36] Treatment with 100% $O_2$ can increase $Pa_{O_2}$ to very high levels; however, nitrogen washout can cause alveolar collapse that can turn areas of low V/Q to true shunt.

The rise in $Pa_{O_2}$ with the use of intermediate levels of $O_2$ depends on the pattern of V/Q mismatch. Further, with $O_2$ therapy, hypoxic vasoconstriction may be eliminated. Nitrogen washout and elimination of hypoxic vasoconstriction may limit any potential improvement in arterial hypoxemia.[21,26] In addition to $O_2$ therapy, treatment is aimed at improving the V/Q abnormality. This includes the use of bronchodilators for patients with asthma and COPD, antibiotics for patients with pneumonia, and positive end-expiratory pressure for patients with acute lung injury and pulmonary edema.

## Diffusion Impairment

Hypoxemia-associated diffusion block is easily overcome by supplemental $O_2$. The rate of movement of $O_2$ across the alveolar-capillary membrane depends on the pressure difference between the capillary and the alveolus. Increasing $Pa_{O_2}$ raises driving pressure and thus improves $Pa_{O_2}$.

## Shunt

Hypoxia caused by shunt is less responsive to supplemental $O_2$. However, meaningful increases in $Pa_{O_2}$ can occur with use of high concentrations of $O_2$ in these patients. At high $Pa_{O_2}$, there is significant additional dissolved $O_2$.[21] By increasing $Pa_{O_2}$ from 100 to 600 mm Hg with 100% $Fi_{O_2}$, the dissolved $O_2$ in capillary blood increases from 0.3 to 1.8 mL $O_2$/100 mL of blood. Assuming a cardiac output of 6 L/minute and an $O_2$ uptake of 300 mL/minute, a graph created by West (Fig. 37.4) demonstrates increases in $Pa_{O_2}$ at different $Fi_{O_2}$ concentrations relative to changing shunt fractions. Important increases in $Ca_{O_2}$ and $O_2$ saturations can occur as $Fi_{O_2}$ is increased. However, with shunt fractions of 50% or greater, little benefit to high concentrations of supplemental $O_2$ is seen.

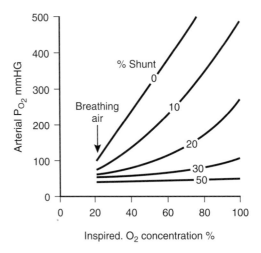

**Figure 37.4** Arterial oxygen tension in response to increases in inspired oxygen concentrations in lung with various amounts of shunt. Useful gains in oxygenation occur even with severe shunting. (From West JB: *Pulmonary Pathophysiology: The Essentials*. Baltimore: Williams & Wilkins, 1977, p 174.)

## Oxygen Therapy in States of Decreased Flow, Arterial Oxygen Content, and Altered Oxygen Extraction

Acute anemia often appears within the context of normal arterial oxygenation. In this situation, it seems prudent to utilize supplemental $O_2$ to maintain an $Sa_{O_2}$ greater than 90% while definitive treatment with blood product transfusion is undertaken.[35] When inhaled, carbon monoxide diffuses rapidly across the alveolar capillary membrane and binds tightly (but reversibly) to Hgb with an affinity at least 200 times that of $O_2$.[35] A reduced amount of $O_2$ is available for delivery to the tissues as the ODC is shifted to the left. Consequently, significant tissue hypoxia occurs with decreased $Sv_{O_2}$ and $Sa_{O_2}$ and increased lactate[14,37,38] but normal $Pa_{O_2}$. Administration of 100% $O_2$ reduces the half-life of carboxyhemoglobin from approximately 320 minutes to 60 to 80 minutes. The high volume of $O_2$ in solution causes detachment of carbon monoxide from Hgb and allows for pulmonary elimination.[35] Treatment with hyperbaric $O_2$ reduces the half-life even further and is indicated in patients with evidence of end-organ damage or tissue hypoxia.[35,37,38]

Supplemental $O_2$ is recommended during low flow in so far as the ability exists to increase dissolved $O_2$ in the blood with use of high $Fi_{O_2}$ and to assist with improving $D_{O_2}$. Assessing and treating the underlying cause of decreased tissue perfusion with fluids, blood, inotropes, vasopressors, and antibiotics are critical interventions. As previously mentioned, as $D_{O_2}$ decreases, $O_2$ extraction increases (with the possible exception of distributive shock), and $Sv_{O_2}$ falls. This situation can contribute to arterial hypoxemia, especially because many of the disease processes causing inadequate tissue perfusion are often associated with V/Q abnormalities of the lung. Several studies have demonstrated a rightward shift of the ODC in critically ill patients[39] and in patients with ARDS.[40]

## Supplemental Oxygen Use in Acute Myocardial Infarction

Although supplemental $O_2$ is commonly prescribed to patients with uncomplicated myocardial infarction, the one controlled study conducted to evaluate this practice failed to demonstrate benefit.[41] However, acute myocardial infarction is often complicated by left ventricular dysfunction and pulmonary edema, as well as atelectasis or pneumonia. The resultant V/Q abnormality and shunt often cause arterial hypoxemia.[32] $O_2$ therapy is indicated to improve $PaO_2$ and $DO_2$.

## Perioperative Use of Oxygen

Two randomized controlled trials that examined the use of perioperative hyperoxia to reduce the incidence of surgical wound infections yielded conflicting results.[42,43] Because of important differences in study populations and in management paradigms, further study is needed to identify those groups of patients who will benefit from higher concentrations of supplemental perioperative $O_2$. For now, therapy should be aimed at maintaining adequate tissue $DO_2$.

## OXYGEN DELIVERY SYSTEMS

$O_2$ delivery systems vary in complexity and precision. Outside of operating room settings, all systems are nonrebreathing. Because exhaled gas is sequestered by one-way valves to avoid rebreathing, no inspiratory gas is made up of exhaled tidal volume.[9] The only $CO_2$ inhaled is that of entrained ambient room air. These systems are designed to provide inspired gases in sufficient volume and flow to allow for variable respiratory patterns common in critically ill patients. $O_2$ delivery systems are divided into low-flow and high-flow systems.

## Low-Flow Systems

Low-flow systems supply $O_2$ at flow rates less than inspiratory demand and therefore depend on entrained room air to meet the inspiratory flow and volume needs of the patient. The $FiO_2$ may be either high or low. Flow is low, generally less than or equal to 6 L/minute. The $FiO_2$ delivered to the patient depends on the amount of room air entrained.[29] Therefore, in patients with variable respiratory patterns, frequencies, or volumes, the delivered

$FiO_2$ is also highly variable. The greater the minute ventilation, the lower the $FiO_2$ will be for a given $O_2$ flow rate.[36] Because of these variabilities, when delivery of fixed or constant $FiO_2$ is required, as in patients with COPD, low-flow systems should not be used.

## Nasal Cannulas

Nasal cannulas are the most commonly used devices for delivering low-flow $O_2$. Provided $FiO_2$ values to the nasopharynx range from 0.24 to 0.44, with flows of 1 to 6 L/minute. Flows greater than 6 L/minute provide no significant increase in delivered $FiO_2$. Nasal cannulas are usually very well tolerated, but complications can occur and include drying of mucous membranes, nasal trauma, and epistaxis. In addition, because $O_2$ is an important part of combustion, fire hazard exists with any type of $O_2$ therapy.

## Simple Oxygen Masks

Simple $O_2$ masks cover the nose and mouth with a reservoir of 100 to 200 mL. This design allows for increases in $FiO_2$ to 50% to 60% with $O_2$ flow rates of 5 to 6 L/minute. Holes on the side of the mask exhaust exhaled gas and entrain room air. The somewhat higher flow rates avoid $CO_2$ rebreathing.[31,35] Increasing flow to greater than 8 L/minute offers little advantage in terms of increased $FiO_2$. Use of the face mask permits humidification of gas and thereby reduces mucous membrane drying. Disadvantages of these masks include an increased risk of gastric aspiration in somnolent or lethargic patients. In addition, the mask requires removal when eating or drinking and for pulmonary toilette.

## Masks with Reservoir Bags

Attachment of a 600- to 1000-mL reservoir bag to a simple face mask allows the delivery of $FiO_2$ of 50% to 80 %. Flow rates of 5 to 8 L/minute are required to keep the bag inflated, to flush out $CO_2$ from the mask, and to prevent entrainment of room air. Partial rebreathing masks can provide an $FiO_2$ of 60%. Partial nonrebreathing masks can provide an $FiO_2$ of 80% to 85% by applying a one-way valve between the mask and the reservoir bag. Thus, the patient only inhales through the reservoir bag and exhales through the separate valves on either side of the mask.[14] As a low-flow system, $FiO_2$ can vary with changes in minute ventilation. Moreover, the use of high $FiO_2$ carries a risk of absorption atelectasis and worsening shunt.

## High-Flow Oxygen Systems

Gas flow through the mask of high-flow systems is able to meet patients' total inspiratory demand and ensures that breathing pattern or minute ventilation will not adversely affect $FiO_2$. This objective is met by the presence of a reservoir that is greater than anatomic dead space and with very high flow rates. Gas flow rates of 30 to

40 L/minute are adequate to meet peak inspiratory flow rates of critically ill patients.[36] In addition, the use of high flow systems is important in patients at risk for losing their hypoxic drive to breathe because, in this setting, delivery of controlled amounts of $FiO_2$ is essential.

### Venturi Mask

This mask operates on the Bernoulli principle of jet mixing of gas. Pure $O_2$ flows through a narrow orifice. This high-velocity stream entrains a constant proportion of room air through side ports at the base of the mask.[36] This occurs because as the velocity of flow of $O_2$ increases, pressure at the side of the stream of flow decreases, thereby entraining more room air and determining $FiO_2$. Because air entrainment depends on the velocity of flow of gas and the size of the ports, $FiO_2$ can be well controlled and accurate between 24% and 50%.[36] With the use of Venturi masks, reliability of inspiratory $O_2$ tension is afforded to patients with COPD. This technique minimizes the risk of abolishing hypoxic respiratory drive or hypoxic vasoconstriction and is unaffected by the patient's respiratory pattern.

### Oxygen Nebulizers

Air entrainment of reservoir nebulizers provides patients with high gas flows and predictable $FiO_2$ in an aerosolized mist.[31] An $FiO_2$ of 35% to 100% can be delivered. Ascertaining whether patient flow demands are being met can be done by observing that the mist of the system is not flowing out of the mask side ports during inspiration. This finding implies that room air is being entrained and that the $FiO_2$ is lower than the set $FiO_2$.[31]

### High-Flow Nasal Cannula Systems

Humidifier and heater designs allow these relatively new systems to deliver gas at flow rates of 1 to 50 L/minute through a nasal cannula. The relative humidity has been shown to be 99% to 100% throughout all flow settings with mean temperatures of 36°C to 37°C.[44] Both humidity and temperature levels provide for surprisingly good patient tolerance and comfort. Although no large-scale clinical trials using these systems have been conducted, abstracts have demonstrated efficacy in delivery of increased concentrations of $O_2$ equal to or greater than concentrations with nonrebreathing masks.[45] There is also some evidence in abstract form and much anecdotal evidence that the high-flow nasal cannula systems improve ventilation in patients with COPD and may help to decrease the work of breathing in patients with pneumonia and acute lung injury and in states of elevated minute ventilation.[46,47] Clearly, however, controlled, randomized trials are needed to determine the effectiveness of these systems in reducing the work of breathing and even assessing their ability to forgo intubation and mechanical ventilation in selected patients.

## COMPLICATIONS ASSOCIATED WITH HYPEROXIA

The use of supplemental $O_2$ increases tissue concentration of molecular $O_2$, an increase that in and of itself poses no risk. Most molecular $O_2$ is reduced by mitochondrial cytochrome oxidase, and water is the final end product. However, other enzymatic auto-oxidation reactions produce $O_2$-derived free radicals, including hydrogen peroxide, superoxide radical, and hydroxyl radical. The high capacity of these free radicals to capture electrons results in oxidative injury of lipid and protein structures. Consequently, cell membrane and DNA destruction causes cell death.[48,49] Naturally occurring antioxidant defense mechanisms scavenge these $O_2$-derived free radicals and protect the cell from destruction. Superoxide dismutase, catalase, and glutathione peroxidase are examples of enzymatic responses. Vitamins C and E are nonenzymatic substances with antioxidant activity.[48,49]

Tolerance to hyperoxia appears to depend on the balance between the formation of $O_2$-derived free radicals and the organism's capacity to produce an adequate antioxidant defense. If this balance is upset, $O_2$ radicals increase within the cell, and cell death ensues.[48] Although it is likely that long-term exposure of normal lungs to high $FiO_2$ will lead to lung injury secondary to the formation of free radicals, there is little clinical evidence that short-term exposure has worrisome consequences. Several studies revealed that volunteers with normal lungs could be exposed to 100% $O_2$ at sea level for between 6 and 44 hours without detectable pulmonary physiologic changes.[49,50] Another study detected indirect evidence of alveolar capillary injury by assessing bronchoalveolar lavage fluid in normal volunteers exposed to an $FiO_2$ of 0.95 for 17 hours.[51] However, an earlier prospective study, by Barber and colleagues,[52] demonstrated a lower P/F ratio and an increase in radiographic abnormalities in brain-dead patients exposed to 100% $O_2$ for 40 hours compared with those exposed to room air. No difference in lung histology was reported between the two groups. This finding suggested that atelectasis was the major hypoxic effect during positive pressure ventilation. Finally, tracheitis and decreased tracheal mucus velocity were noted in physiologically normal persons breathing 90% to 95% $O_2$ for 6 hours.[53]

It appears likely that, except for some cases of early tracheitis, supplemental $O_2$ in concentrations between 0.5 and 1.0 can be administered to patients for 24 to 48 hours with relative impunity. In fact, absorption atelectasis, caused by nitrogen washout, is the earliest and most common pulmonary pathophysiologic change when using high concentrations of inspired $O_2$ (near 100%).[48] This condition likely accounts for early decreases in vital capacity and diffusing capacity seen in this setting,[50] and it has been noted as an important cause of impaired gas exchange during and after general anesthesia. Investigators have therefore suggested that using lower $O_2$ concentrations during general anesthesia may be beneficial.[54]

Practically speaking, high levels of inspired $O_2$ are most often administered for longer than 48 hours to patients with significant lung injury (e.g., patients with ARDS, sepsis, or pneumonia). In these patients, it is extremely difficult to distinguish pulmonary effects caused by the underlying disease process from those caused by $O_2$ toxicity or the use of mechanical ventilation.[48] Some experimental models demonstrated that cytokines increase the level of enzymes related to cellular antioxidant defense.[55] This finding raises the possibility that sepsis and acute lung injury induce tolerance to hyperoxia.[48]

Accumulating evidence has demonstrated that cyclic mechanical stretching of the diseased lung is detrimental during mechanical ventilation with high tidal volumes or high peak and plateau pressures. This stretching, associated with the release of proinflammatory mediators, contributes to the formation of ventilator-induced lung injury. Indeed, several studies showed improved mortality when lung protective strategies were utilized during mechanical ventilation.[56,57] It is therefore compelling to consider that ventilator-induced lung injury may be more deleterious than the effects of hyperoxia in patients with acute lung injury.[48]

## CONCLUSION

Provision of $O_2$ therapy can be a lifesaving maneuver in acutely hypoxemic patients. Keeping the ODC in mind can provide a conceptual reference regarding delivery of $O_2$ to the tissues. Careful consideration of the cause of hypoxemia allows for titration of $O_2$ at the patient's bedside, to avoid some of the untoward effects of this therapy.

In those patients with decreased tissue perfusion who are not hypoxemic, therapy is primarily directed at treating the cause of shock, although it is likely that supplemental $O_2$ is also beneficial. High concentrations of $O_2$ are usually well tolerated in most patients for up to 48 hours. In patients with significant lung injury, hyperoxia may be less deleterious than previously thought.

## ACKNOWLEDGMENTS

I gratefully acknowledge the research assistance provided by Roger S. Manahan, M.L.S., and the editorial assistance of Jeanne C. Esposito, Ph.D., and Christine M. Hall, A.S.

## REFERENCES

1. Russell JA, Phang PT: The oxygen delivery/consumption controversy: Approaches to management of the critically ill. Am J Respir Crit Care Med 1994;149:533–537.
2. Danek SJ, Lynch JP, Weg JG, Dantzker DR: The dependence of oxygen uptake on oxygen delivery in the adult respiratory distress syndrome. Am Rev Respir Dis 1980;122:387–395.
3. Mohsenifar Z, Goldbach P, Tashkin DP, Campisi DJ: Relationship between $O_2$ delivery and $O_2$ consumption in the adult respiratory distress syndrome. Chest 1983;84: 257–270.
4. Guitierrez G, Pohil J: Oxygen consumption is linearly related to $O_2$ supply in critically ill patients. J Crit Care 1986;1:45–53.
5. Kaufman BS, Rackow EC, Falk JL: The relationship between oxygen delivery and consumption during fluid resuscitation of hypovolemic and septic shock. Chest 1984;85:336–340.
6. Hayes MA, Yau EH, Timmins AC, et al: Response of critically ill patients to treatment aimed at achieving supranormal oxygen delivery and consumption. Chest 1993;103:886–895.
7. Tuchschmidt J, Fried J, Astiz M, Rackow E: Elevation of cardiac output and oxygen delivery improves outcome in septic shock. Chest 1992;102:216–220.
8. Gutierrez G, Palieas F, Doglio G, et al: Gastric intramucosal pH as therapeutic index of tissue oxygenation in critically ill patients. Lancet 1992;339:195–199.
9. Yu M, Levy MM, Smith P, et al: Effect of maximizing oxygen delivery on morbidity and mortality rates in critically ill patients: A prospective, randomized, controlled study. Crit Care Med 1993;21:830–837.
10. Ronco JJ, Fenwick JC, Tweeddale MG, et al: Identification of the critical oxygen delivery for anaerobic metabolism in critically ill septic and nonseptic humans. JAMA 1993;270:1724–1730.
11. Hayes MA, Timmius AC, Yau EHS, et al: Elevation of systemic oxygen delivery in the treatment of critically ill patients. N Engl J Med 1994;330:1717–1722.
12. Rivers E, Nguyen B, Haustad S, et al: Early goal-directed therapy in the treatment of severe sepsis and septic shock. N Engl J Med 2001;345:1368–1377.
13. Bone RC: Monitoring respiratory and hemodynamic function in the patient with respiratory failure. In Kirby RR, Smith RA, Desautels DA (eds): *Mechanical Ventilation.* New York: Churchill Livingstone, 1985, pp 137–170.
14. Beer MF: Oxygen therapy and pulmonary oxygen toxicity. In Fishman AP (ed): *Fishman's Pulmonary Diseases and Disorders,* 3rd ed. New York: McGraw-Hill, 1998, pp 2627–2642.
15. Zwart A, Kwant G, Oeseburg B, Zijlstra WG: Human whole-blood oxygen affinity: Effect of carbon monoxide. J Appl Physiol 1984;57:14–20.
16. Curry SC, Arnold-Capell P: Nitroprusside, nitroglycerin, and angiotensin-converting enzyme inhibitors. Crit Care Clin 1991;7:555–581.
17. Seigel JH, Greenspan M, Del Guercio LPM: Abnormal vascular tone, defective oxygen transport and myocardial failure in human septic shock. Ann Surg 1973;165:504–517.
18. Rackow EC, Astiz ME, Weil MH: Cellular oxygen metabolism during sepsis and shock: The relationship of oxygen consumption to oxygen delivery. JAMA 1988;259: 1989–1993.
19. Gilbert EM, Haupt MT, Mandanas RY, et al: The effect of fluid loading, blood transfusion, and catecholamine infusion on oxygen delivery and consumption in patients with sepsis. Am Rev Respir Dis 1986;134:873–878.

20. Vincent JL, Roman A, DeBacker D, Kahn RJ: Oxygen uptake/supply dependency: Effects of short-term dobutamine infusion. Am Rev Respir Dis 1990;142:2–7.

21. West JB: *Pulmonary Pathophysiology: The Essentials.* Baltimore: Williams & Wilkins, 1982.

22. Stemp LS, Ramsay MA: Oxygen may mask hypoventilation: Patient breathing must be ensured. APSF Newslett 2004;20:80.

23. Fu ES, Downs JB, Schweiger JW: Supplemental oxygen impairs detection of hypoventilation by pulse oximetry. Chest 2004;126:1552–1558.

24. Aldrich TK, Prezant DJ: Indications for mechanical ventilation. In Tobin MJ (ed): *Principles and Practice of Mechanical Ventilation.* New York: McGraw-Hill, 1994, pp 155–189.

25. Askanazi J, Wordenstrom J, Rosenbaum SH, et al: Nutrition for the patient with respiratory failure: Glucose vs fat. Anesthesiology 1981;54:373–377.

26. West JB: Assessing pulmonary gas exchange. N Engl J Med 1987;316:1336–1338.

27. Hoyt JW: Debunking myths of chronic obstructive pulmonary disease. Crit Care Med 1997;25:1450–1451.

28. Hanson CW 3rd, Marshall BE, Frasch HF, Marshall C: Causes of hypercarbia with oxygen therapy in patients with chronic obstructive pulmonary disease. Crit Care Med 1996;24:23–28.

29. Robinson T, Freiberg D, Regnis JA, Young IH: The role of hypoventilation and ventilation-perfusion redistribution in oxygen-induced hypercapnia during acute exacerbations of chronic obstructive pulmonary disease. Am J Respir Crit Care Med 2002;161:1524–1529.

30. Crossley DJ, McGuire GP, Barrow PM, Houston PL: Influence of inspired oxygen concentration on dead space, respiratory drive, and $PaCO_2$ in intubated patients with chronic obstructive pulmonary disease. Crit Care Med 1997;25:1522–1526.

31. O'Connor BS, Vender JS: Oxygen therapy. Crit Care Clin 1995;11:67–78.

32. West JB: Ventilation-perfusion relationships. Am Rev Respir Dis 1977;116:919–943.

33. Jubray A, Tobin MJ: Monitoring gas exchange during mechanical ventilation. In Tobin MJ (ed): *Principles and Practice of Mechanical Ventilation.* New York: McGraw-Hill, 1994, pp 919–943.

34. Bakker J, Coffernils M, Leon M, et al: Blood lactate levels are superior to oxygen-derived variables in predicting outcome in human septic shock. Chest 1991;99:956–962.

35. Fulmer JD, Snider GL: ACCP-NHLBI national conference of oxygen therapy. Chest 1984;86:234–247.

36. Leach RM, Bateman NT: Acute oxygen therapy. Br J Hosp Med 1993;49:637–644.

37. Youngberg T, Myers RAM, Piantadosi CA: Use of hyperbaric oxygen in carbon monoxide, cyanide, and sulfide intoxication. In: Camparesi EM and Barker AC (eds): Hyperbaric Oxygen Therapy: A critical review. Bethesda: Undersea and Hyperbaric Medical Society, 1991, pp 23–53.

38. Snider GL, Rinaldo JE: Oxygen therapy in medical patients hospitalized outside of the intensive care unit. Am Rev Respir Dis 1980;122:29–36.

39. Tulli, G, Vignali G, Guadagnucci A, Mondello V: The oxygen status of the arterial blood in the critically ill. Scand J Clin Lab Invest 1990;203(Suppl):107–118.

40. Clerbaux T, Detry B, Reynaert M, Frans A: Right shift of the oxyhemoglobin dissociation curve in acute respiratory distress syndrome. Pathol Biol (Paris) 1997;45:269–273.

41. Rawles JM, Kenmore ACE: Controlled trial of oxygen in uncomplicated myocardial infarction. BMJ 1976;1:10121–10123.

42. Greif R, Ozan A, Horn EP, et al: Supplemental perioperative oxygen to reduce the incidence of surgical-wound infection. N Engl J Med 2000;342:161–167.

43. Pryor KO, Fahey TJ, Lien CA, Goldstein PA: Surgical site infection and the routine use of perioperative hypoxia in a general surgical population. JAMA 2004;291:79–87.

44. Voss C, Johnson S, Haile Z, et al: Can the Vapotherm high flow nasal cannula system substitute for non-rebreathing mask in select patients. Respir Care 2003;48:A1083.

45. Malinowski T, Lambert J: Oxygen concentrations via nasal cannula at high flow rates. Respir Care 2002;47:A1039.

46. Patel NB, Criner GJ, Chatila W: Effect of Vapotherm in patients hospitalized for acute exacerbation of COPD. Am J Respir Crit Care Med 2003;167:A232.

47. Manning C, Dominy L, Nguyen V: High flow oxygen via nasal cannula during respiratory insufficiency following pneumonectomy. Respir Care 2004;49:A1368.

48. Caralho CRR, de Paula Pinto Schettino G, Maranhao B, Bethlem EP: Hyperoxia and lung disease. Curr Opin Pulm Med 1998;4:300–304.

49. Deneke SM, Fanburg BL: Normobaric oxygen toxicity of the lung. N Engl J Med 1980;303:76–86.

50. Van De Water JM, Kagey KS, Miller IT, et al: Response of the lung to six to 12 hours of 100 percent oxygen inhalation in normal man. N Engl J Med 1970;285:621–626.

51. Davis WB, Rennard SI, Bitterman PB, Crystal RG: Pulmonary oxygen toxicity: Early reversible changes in human alveolar structures induced by hyperoxia. N Engl J Med 1983;309:878–883.

52. Barber RE, Lee J, Hamilton WK: Oxygen toxicity in man: A prospective study in patients with reversible brain damage. N Engl J Med 1970;283:1478–1484.

53. Sackner MA, Lauda J, Hirsch J, Zapata A: Pulmonary effects of oxygen breathing: A 6-hour study in normal men. Ann Intern Med 1975;82:368–374.

54. Rothen HU, Sporre B, Engberg G, et al: Prevention of atelectasis during general anesthesia. Lancet 1995;345:1387–1391.

55. Heffner JE, Repine JE: Pulmonary strategies of antioxidant defense. Am Rev Respir Dis 1989;140:531–554.

56. Amato MBP, Barbas CSU, Medeiros DM, et al: Effect of a protective ventilation strategy on mortality in the acute respiratory distress syndrome. N Engl J Med 1998;338:355–361.

57. Acute Respiratory Distress Syndrome Network: Ventilation with lower tidal volumes as compared with traditional tidal volumes for acute lung injury and the acute respiratory distress syndrome. N Engl J Med 2000;342:1301–1313.

# CHAPTER 38

# Respiratory Pharmacology and Aerosol Therapy

Peter J. Papadakos and Younsuck Koh

Many patients who are undergoing mechanical ventilation receive medications that modulate their lung function. The lung contains a large surface area for both absorption and function of medications and gases. Over the last 10 years, there has been an explosion in the development of pharmacologic agents that not only modulate bronchodilation and bronchoconstriction but also affect lung function and gas exchange in respiratory failure. These therapeutic agents and advances have greatly added to our understanding of how the lung functions during normal and pathologic states.

We are challenged each day by patients with complex lung diseases who present for many levels of ventilatory support, both invasive and noninvasive. The importance of a rapid, comprehensive workup, with a complete history and physical examination and specific tests including an arterial blood gas analysis, cannot be overemphasized. All too often, patients are cared for without collection of proper information. The preoperative and postoperative course in patients with pulmonary diseases will be facilitated if the pulmonary diagnosis and severity of pulmonary dysfunction are established before the start of surgery. It is wise at least to record preoperative blood gas determinations and to collect measurements of lung volumes and flow rates, to ascertain the degree of functional impairment and baseline pulmonary function. However, any preoperative laboratory data can reliably predict postoperative lung complications. For optimal lung care, we must become expert in the function of many drugs and treatment modalities that act on the physiology of the lung. With proper utilization and early intervention, we can improve outcome in the care of patients with baseline disease states as well as those with acute lung diseases.

## AIRWAY STRUCTURE AND FUNCTION

A basic understanding of pulmonary anatomy and function will help us to understand the pharmacologic actions of treatment modalities. Gas enters the thorax, through the mouth, nose, or artificial airway, into the trachea, which divides into the right and left mainstem bronchi. The airways continue to branch, and each division results in two daughter branches that are unequal in diameter, length, and takeoff.[1] The primary function of these airways is to conduct gas through the airway to the gas exchange zones. The increasing cross-sectional area of the airway leads to a reduction in airflow resistance as gas moves to the periphery, thus facilitating mass flow of gas. In respiratory bronchioles and alveolar ducts, gas diffusion is more important than mass gas flow and is facilitated by the large cross-referenced area present.

The airway wall consists of layers of mucosa and smooth muscle and, finally, a connective tissue sleeve. Bronchi and small bronchi contain cartilage within the wall, whereas bronchioles contain no cartilage. Respiratory bronchioles contain alveoli that increase in number with each branching such that only alveoli line the alveolar ducts and sacs. In the bronchi, the mucosal layer contains tall, ciliated epithelial cells, as well as mucus-producing glands, goblet cells, and Clara cells.[2] In the periphery, the mucosal layer thins, and ciliated cells become more cuboidal. In the bronchioles, glands disappear, and goblet cells decrease in number and finally disappear as the number of Clara cells increases. The Clara cells decrease and also finally disappear within respiratory bronchioles and alveolar ducts, which are lined with epithelial cells.[3]

The smooth muscle layer is continuous from the trachea to the alveolar ducts. The smooth muscle bundles encircle the airways in an oblique course. Contraction results in airway narrowing as well as shortening.[1] In the alveolar ducts, the muscle bundles are found in the alveolar entrance rings.[1]

The pulmonary blood supply from the right and left arteries follows the mainstem bronchi into the lung parenchyma. Both the arteries and the bronchi then follow the branching pattern to the level of the respiratory bronchiole about 17 to 23 orders or generations. The arteries give rise to arteriolar and capillary networks within the walls of the alveolar ducts and alveoli.[4] These vessels produce a massive surface area; the pulmonary arteries and arterioles have a surface area of about 2.5 $m^2$, and the capillary surface area is estimated at 50 to 150 $m^2$. From this large surface area, drugs can be absorbed into the circulation.

Airway caliber and tone are regulated by the parasympathetic and sympathetic divisions of the autonomic nervous system.[5,6] The vagally mediated mechanisms of the parasympathetic nervous system are the primary determinants of normal bronchomotor tone and bronchial submucosal gland secretion.[5,7] On stimulation of the vagal efferent nerves, the neurotransmitter acetylcholine is released from the presynaptic nerve terminal. Acetylcholine then diffuses through the synaptic cleft and binds to muscarinic cholinergic receptors found throughout the respiratory tree. Stimulation of the cholinergic receptors results in an increase in the intracellular levels of cyclic 3',5'-guanosine monophosphate (cGMP) in the cytoplasm.[7] These acetylcholine receptors are located in or are adjacent to the respiratory epithelium submucosal glands, mast cells, and smooth muscle.[5,6,8] Stimulation of these acetylcholine receptors in the lung triggers bronchoconstriction and a decrease in airway caliber, as well as activation of mast cell degranulation and an increase in glandular secretion.[9]

The direct sympathetic nervous system innervation of the respiratory tree is sparse. Nevertheless, the bronchial smooth muscle cells, especially those located in the small airways, are well populated with noninnervated $\beta_2$-adrenergic receptors.[10] $\beta_1$-Adrenergic receptors are also present but have only a minimal role in lung physiology. $\beta_2$-Adrenergic receptors are stimulated by adrenergic agonists, both endogenous (the presynaptic neurotransmitter norepinephrine, or epinephrine released by the adrenal medulla) and exogenous (pharmacologic agents). This stimulation results in activation of membrane-bound adenylate cyclase to catalyze the conversion of adenosine triphosphate (ATP) to cyclic 3',5'-adenosine monophosphate (cAMP).[11] Activation of an enzymatic cascade then occurs, resulting in bronchodilation and possibly increased secretion of mucus.

$\alpha$-Adrenergic receptors are also found in the lung.[8] Stimulation of these receptors, located predominantly in the bronchial and vascular smooth muscle and submucosal glands, causes bronchoconstriction and increased mucus secretion. In the lung, $\alpha_2$-receptors are located on the postsynaptic nerve terminal, although they are also found presynaptically elsewhere in the body. Presynaptic $\alpha_2$-receptors regulate the release of norepinephrine from the presynaptic nerve terminal.[12]

A third nonadrenergic, noncholinergic (NANC) system of the lung has been demonstrated in the airways all the way to the small bronchi.[13] A major component of this system appears to be the principal inhibitor system in human airways, and it causes bronchodilation when stimulated. The neurotransmitter involved is a vasoactive intestinal polypeptide, which is more potent than isoproterenol. The NANC also has an excitatory component, probably mediated by a peptide, substance P, that causes bronchoconstriction when it is stimulated. The exact function of the NANC system continues to be an active avenue of investigation. Various endogenous substances, such as histamine, prostaglandins, platelet-activating factor, bradykinin, and various leukotrienes, also have documented inflammatory effects on smooth muscle tone that have been demonstrated to cause bronchoconstriction.[14,15]

The alveolar macrophages, when stimulated by a systemic inflammatory response, also modulate a cascade that releases various leukotrienes and cytokines that act both locally and in the systemic circulation.[16] We have also discovered that the alveolar surfactant system may be involved in protecting the lung against its own mediators (e.g., angiotensin II) and in protecting the cardiocirculatory system against mediators and cytokines produced by the lung.[17]

# BRONCHODILATORS AND BRONCHOACTIVE DRUGS

The basic way to think of bronchodilator drugs is based on their action: (1) direct respiratory smooth muscle relaxants—theophylline and related salts; (2) $\beta$-adrenergic agonists—isoetharine isoproterenol, epinephrine, metaproterenol, albuterol, terbutaline, bitolterol, and pirbuterol; and (3) anticholinergics—atropine, glycopyrrolate, and ipratropium. Their sites of action are depicted in Figure 38.1, as summarized by Kelly.[18]

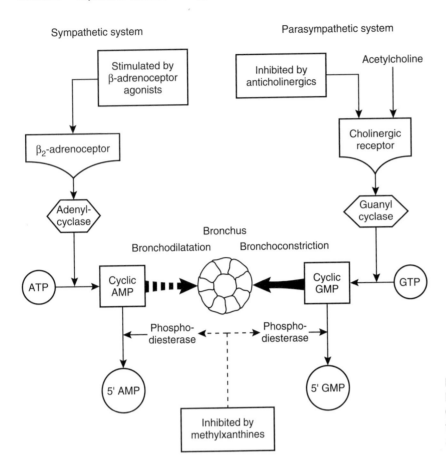

**Figure 38.1** Mechanism of action of bronchodilator drugs. (From Kelly HW: Controversies in asthma therapy with theophylline and the beta 2-adrenergic agents. Clin Pharm 1984;3:386–395.)

## Theophylline

Theophylline, a naturally occurring methylxanthine closely related to caffeine and found in tea, has been used to treat bronchospasm for more than 100 years.[19] At one time, it was the most widely used drug in the treatment of reactive airway disease, but because of conflicting reports of efficacy and safety, use of theophylline in the treatment of acute bronchospasm remains controversial.[20] Nonetheless, theophylline has become one of the most extensively prescribed drugs in the world for the treatment of reversible airway obstruction. The development of methods to monitor serum theophylline concentrations in patients has contributed to the safe and effective clinical use of this drug in this era.

### Pharmacology

The exact mechanism by which theophylline exerts its pharmacologic effect is not completely known.[21] It is well established that theophylline competitively inhibits the activity of cytoplasmic phosphodiesterase, the enzyme that catalyzes the degradation of cAMP and cGMP to their inactive 5′-mononucleotides, 5′-AMP and 5′-GMP.[22] Previously, this was thought to be the mechanism of action; however, the in vitro doses used to achieve phosphodiesterase inhibition appear to be too high to achieve clinically.[23]

In guinea pig and dog trachea muscle preparations, theophylline levels achievable in humans had no effect on cAMP or cGMP, but they did increase calcium ion uptake and redistribution, consistent with a decrease of myoplasmic calcium ion and calcium sequestration in the mitochondrion.[23] Other postulated mechanisms of action include prostaglandin inhibition,[24] indirect β-adrenergic stimulation through release of catecholamines,[25] and increased binding of cAMP to cAMP-binding protein.[26] Adenosine receptor antagonism has been proposed as the primary mediator of the pharmacologic and therapeutic actions of methylxanthines; however, the exact cellular mechanisms underlying bronchial smooth muscle relaxation remain to be clarified.

Regardless of its mechanism of action, theophylline is a direct bronchial smooth muscle relaxant. If bronchospasm is not present, the effects of this agent on air flow and respiratory mechanics are minimal. The drug also acts by decreasing mucosal edema and reducing the production of excessive secretions.[27] Theophylline seems to have anti-inflammatory and immunomodulatory actions,[28] in addition to stimulating respiratory drive.[29] Other effects of theophylline include the following: direct augmentation of myocardial inotropy and chronotropy; stimulation of respiratory muscle contractility; dilation of coronary, pulmonary, renal, and systemic arterioles and veins; diuresis; stimulation of epinephrine and norepinephrine synthesis and release by the adrenal medulla; stimulation of the medullary respiratory center; and decreased cerebral blood flow. In physiologically normal patients, theophylline causes a chronotropic effect, a decrease in coronary artery blood flow, an increase in myocardial oxygen extraction, and a decrease in left ventricular ejection time.[30] In patients with chronic obstructive pulmonary disease (COPD) and cor pulmonale, increase in heart rate, stroke volume, and cardiac output and decreases in right ventricular end-diastolic pressure, left ventricular end-diastolic pressure, wedge pressure, and systemic vascular resistance can occur.[30]

## Side Effects

The use of theophylline has declined, especially in patients with bronchial asthma, because of concerns related to its narrow therapeutic window and as a result of the introduction of newer potent bronchodilators. The most common side effects of theophylline are gastrointestinal and include nausea, vomiting, and anorexia.[31] Gastrointestinal adverse affects associated with oral use can be minimized by administering the drug with food. Central nervous system effects include headache, irritability, restlessness, nervousness, dizziness, and seizures.[20] Theophylline-induced seizures are often unresponsive to standard anticonvulsive therapy, and the mortality rate is very high, in the range of 50%.[32] Theophylline may cause cardiovascular side effects that are often poorly tolerated by critically ill patients. These side effects include the following: palpitations; arrhythmias such as tachycardia, including multifocal atrial tachycardia, extrasystoles, profound bradycardia, and ventricular arrhythmias; hypotension; and circulatory collapse. The rapid intravenous injection of aminophylline and theophylline may increase the incidence of side effects; therefore, slow intravenous titration or the use of an infusion pump is suggested. Cardiac arrest may follow the rapid administration of a bolus dose of aminophylline. Other side effects may include dizziness and flushing.

An important consideration is the pharmacologic preparation of theophylline. Before 1983, the only parenteral form of theophylline was aminophylline. Aminophylline is theophylline compounded with ethylenediamine, which confers water solubility to the insoluble theophylline molecule. This ethylenediamine contributes to the respiratory and cardiac stimulant effects of theophylline. Also of great importance is that ethylenediamine can induce hypersensitivity reactions characterized by urticaria, generalized pruritus, angioedema, and bronchospasm.[31]

## Pharmacokinetics

Theophylline is manufactured as a variety of salts for oral, rectal, and parenteral administration. Rectal use of theophylline mixtures is no longer recommended because of its erratic absorption. Liquid and plain tablet forms of theophylline are rapidly and completely absorbed.[33] Slow-release preparations now dominate the market. The intravenous forms of theophylline are limited primarily to hospitalized patients and emergency use.

The pharmacokinetic properties of theophylline are well described. Once absorbed, the drug is distributed rapidly throughout the body water, more prominently in the extracellular than the intracellular body water.[31] Theophylline binding to serum proteins, principally albumin, varies from 50% to 60%, a percentage that increases as serum pH increases. Theophylline can freely pass into breast milk and crosses the placenta. Theophylline achieves a volume of distribution of 0.3 to 0.7 L/kg in children and adults.[31] Oral standard, non–time release preparations give a peak serum level within 1 to 2 hours after administration. In contrast, extended-release and slow-release tablets release theophylline over a longer period of time, and peak levels are reached approximately 4 hours after administration. Administration of theophylline by intravenous infusion produces the highest and most rapidly achieved peak serum concentration. In healthy, nonsmoking adults, a standard 5 mg/kg infusion over 30 minutes produces an average peak serum concentration of 10 μg/mL.[31]

Hepatic metabolism of theophylline is through the cytochrome P-450 system, which is also its principal method of elimination. Approximately 10% of the drug is eliminated unchanged through the kidney. Metabolism can be affected by the ingestion of other drugs. The half-life is increased in patients using cimetidine, ranitidine, erythromycin, allopurinol, propranolol, mexiletine, oral contraceptives, quinolones, verapamil, and diltiazem. Disease states, especially liver disease, can also affect and lengthen the half-life of theophylline. In patients who smoke either cigarettes or marijuana, the average elimination half-life is much shorter, in the range of 4 to 5 hours. In contrast, in patients with congestive heart failure, cor pulmonale, COPD, or liver disease, the drug has a markedly prolonged elimination half-life, in some cases longer than 12 hours.[31]

Great care must be taken in the administration of theophylline because of its low therapeutic ratio. With close monitoring of levels, however, the drug can be given safely. If caution is used, there should be few cardiovascular side affects and no convulsions or deaths. Theophylline had a bad reputation in the 1970s and 1980s, before the institution of rational dosage schedules and widespread monitoring. The therapeutic range for theophylline is frequently reported to be between 10 and 20 µg/mL in plasma. Marked interpatient and intrapatient variability exists for dose-response curves. Therefore, the ideal way to use the drug is to titrate serum levels to the optimal drug level to maximal bronchodilation within the therapeutic range.

The clinical use of theophylline is for the prevention of bronchospasm in patients with hyperactive airway disease. No theophylline products are currently used for the initial treatment of acute bronchospasm. Rather, they are second-line drugs only if an inhaled β-adrenergic agonist gives a suboptimal effect. In these patients, 5 mg/kg is administered as a loading dose over 30 minutes, if they have not received the drug within 24 hours. In patients taking theophylline, the dose is lowered to one half. Subsequent intravenous infusions are administered to clinical effect with very close monitoring. Most patients now taking theophylline are using it for prophylaxis of chronic bronchospasm.

## β-Adrenergic Receptor Agonists

The introduction of inhaled $β_2$-agonists greatly improved the care of patients with pulmonary diseases. The $β_2$-agonists are the most effective bronchodilators available. They have now gained widespread use both in maintenance therapy and in the acute care of patients.

$β_2$-adrenergic receptor stimulation activates adenyl cyclase, which produces an increase in intracellular cAMP. cAMP induces airway relaxation through phosphorylation of muscle regulatory proteins and decreases unbound intracellular calcium concentration.[34] Selective $β_2$-adrenergic receptor agonists have antiallergic activity by suppressing immunoglobulin E (IgE)–mediated release of mediators from lung mast cells and basophils. These agents increase mucociliary clearance and inhibit pulmonary vascular leakage.[35] $β_2$-Adrenergic stimulation also activates sodium/potassium-ATPase, produces gluconeogenesis, enhances insulin secretion, and produces a mild to moderate decrease in serum potassium concentration by driving potassium intracellularly. All β-adrenergic receptor agonists act by binding $β_1$ and $β_2$ cell membrane receptors. This action induces relaxation of bronchial and vascular smooth muscle. These agents may also induce increased mucociliary transport of respiratory secretions. Stimulation of these receptors affects mast cells and inhibits the release of the mediators of bronchospasm, such as histamine and the slow-reacting substance of anaphylaxis.

These sympathomimetic bronchodilators have been used widely for many years to induce bronchodilation. Figure 38.2 displays the structures of the sympathomimetic drugs. Inhalational use of $β_2$-adrenergic receptor stimulators is more advantageous than oral administration in terms of efficacy and side effects. Regular use of these drugs raised concern about increased asthma-related morbidity and mortality; therefore, these agents are recommended on an as-needed basis for symptomatic relief.

### Epinephrine

Epinephrine (adrenaline) is a naturally occurring catecholamine that is synthesized, stored, and released from the adrenal medulla and certain adrenergic nerve terminals. Because of its broad stimulation of adrenergic receptors, epinephrine is the drug of choice in systemic hypersensitivity reactions, for which it is usually given in a subcutaneous dose of 0.3 to 1.0 mL of a 1:1000 aqueous solution. Similar doses can be used to treat acute bronchospasm. Subcutaneous epinephrine, 0.3 to 0.5 mL of a 1:1000 aqueous solution, can be used for acute wheezing. Epinephrine is an excellent drug and appears to have no more cardiovascular side effects than subcutaneous terbutaline, but it has a shorter (1 to 2 hours versus 2 to 4 hours) duration of action than terbutaline.[36] The usual way to deliver epinephrine in its racemic form is by metered dose inhaler (MDI) or in solution delivered by a nebulizer. In many cases, epinephrine is still used to break highly resistant bronchospasm. Norepinephrine, a weak $β_2$-agonist, has little utility in the treatment of airway and lung disease.

### Isoproterenol and Isoetharine

Isoproterenol is the most potent $β_1$- and $β_2$-agonist. It is currently available either in an MDI or in solution for use in a hand-held or gas-powered nebulizer. Because of its cardiovascular effects, however, isoproterenol has been largely replaced by more selective agents.

Isoetharine has one tenth the potency of isoproterenol and has a duration of action of up to 3 hours. It is available as an MDI and in solution for use in a nebulizer. The aerosolized dose is 0.25 to 0.5 mL diluted in 1 mL of sterile water or saline or 0.68 mg (two puffs) from an MDI. Like isoproterenol, isoetharine has been replaced by more selective $β_2$-agonists.

### Terbutaline

Terbutaline is a slightly less potent bronchodilator than isoproterenol, but with far fewer cardiovascular side effects, and it has a duration of action up to 6 or 7 hours orally or by aerosol. When terbutaline is given subcutaneously, the incidence of cardiovascular side effects is similar to that of epinephrine even though the duration of bronchodilation is longer. The oral dose range is from 1.25 to 5.0 mg every 6 hours.

The MDI dose of terbutaline is 200 µg/puff, and the usual dosage is two puffs every 4 to 6 hours. The injectable form of terbutaline can be nebulized by being diluted to a total volume of 2 to 3 mL with sterile water

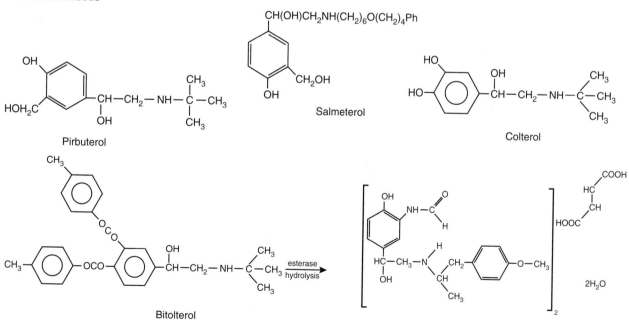

**Figure 38.2** The structures of sympathomimetic drugs.

or saline. The usual dose is 1 mg every 4 to 6 hours. It is a very popular drug.

## Albuterol (Salbutamol)

Albuterol is the most commonly used agent. It has the fewest cardiovascular side effects of the sympathomimetic bronchodilators. Orally or by aerosol, its peak action occurs within 2 hours, and its duration of action is up to 6 hours.[35]

Oral doses range from 1 to 8 mg every 6 hours for the standard, short-acting preparation to 4 to 8 mg every 12 hours for the sustained-release preparation. Clinical studies have shown similar improvements in pulmonary function with the sustained-release preparations given every 12 hours as compared with the standard product given four times daily.

The MDI dose is 0.18 mg (two puffs) every 4 hours. The nebulizer dose is up to 3.0 mg. The frequency of administration depends on the severity of bronchospasm and wheezing: every half-hour to 1 hour for acute, severe asthma, to every 4 to 6 hours for stable airway disease.

## Pirbuterol

Pirbuterol is a relatively selective β-agonist, but does have both bronchodilatory and cardiovascular effects.[37–40] Pirbuterol is 9 times more selective for pulmonary tissue than albuterol and 1520 times more selective than isoproterenol.

The onset of pirbuterol activity occurs 5 minutes after aerosol administration and within 1 hour after oral administration. The peak activity is 30 minutes for aerosol use and 1 hour for oral use. The activity of pirbuterol is equipotent to that of albuterol. The lowest doses that apparently produce maximum bronchodilation are 0.4 mg by aerosol and 15 mg of the oral preparation.[41]

The usual MDI dose is two inhalations (200 μg/puff) up to every 4 hours. The recommended oral dose of pirbuterol is 10 to 15 mg three to four times per day. The complication profile is similar to other β$_2$-agonists in which the neuromuscular side effects are more marked than the cardiovascular side effects.

## Metaproterenol

Metaproterenol was the first synthetic noncatecholamine bronchodilator introduced into clinical practice in the United States. It has a duration of action up to 4 hours. It was also the first oral agent introduced. It has fewer cardiovascular effects than isoproterenol but is a weak bronchodilator. Oral doses of 5 to 20 mg can be used every 4 to 6 hours. The major side effects are neuromuscular (shakiness, tremor, cramps) or cardiovascular (tachycardia). The peak effect usually occurs within 1 to 2 hours.

Metaproterenol is also delivered by MDI and in solution for nebulization. The usual MDI dose is 1.3 mg (two puffs) given as needed up to every 3 to 4 hours for the onset of wheezing. The usual aerosolized dose is 10 to 15 mg (0.2 to 0.3 mL) diluted to 2 to 3 mL with sterile water or saline and given every 3 to 4 hours.

## Long-Acting Agents

The introduction of long-acting, inhaled β$_2$-agonists was a major therapeutic development and led to a fundamental reappraisal of β-agonist use in asthma management.[37] However, the long-acting agents are significantly slower than short-acting β$_2$-adrenergic receptor stimulators in reversing bronchoconstriction. Therefore, the long-acting agents should not be used as rescue medication in acute asthmatic attacks. Salmeterol and formoterol are highly selective β$_2$-agonists with a bronchodilating effect lasting for at least 12 hours after a single inhalation.[38,39]

Salmeterol is the result of a specific program to achieve prolonged duration of action by molecular modification of the short-acting β$_2$-agonist salbutamol (albuterol). Formoterol, a formanilide-substituted phenoethanolamine, was serendipitously found to be long acting when given by inhalation.[37] Sufficient drug remains available in the aqueous biophase to allow immediate interaction with the active side of the receptor, thus accounting for the rapid onset of action. Formation of a depot within the plasmalemma seems to require high topical concentrations of formoterol in the bronchi. This finding may explain why inhaled formoterol has a longer duration of action than when given orally because the inhaled route achieves higher topical concentrations in the periciliary fluid of the bronchi.[42]

In addition to their difference in molecular structure, formoterol and salmeterol also have distinct pharmacologic features. As reflected in the routinely advocated dose for human use, formoterol has a higher potency than salmeterol.[43] Comparative studies in healthy volunteers indicated that formoterol and salmeterol dose dependently cause side effects with a potency ratio of approximately 5:1.[44] This is very similar to the difference in bronchodilator potency between these drugs in asthmatic patients. A few published case reports showed a significantly stronger bronchodilating effect with formoterol than with salmeterol in severe asthma.[45,46] However, in a larger comparative study with patients with persistent severe asthma, no differences were observed in the bronchodilating effects of these agents.[45] Moreover, long-term treatment with salmeterol does not hamper the bronchodilating effects of salbutamol in the acute phase in the emergency room.

Over the past few years, long-acting inhaled β$_2$-agonists have gained acceptance as the preferred form of "add-on" treatment in persistent asthma. Combining these agents with inhaled glucocorticosteroids is the present standard formula of asthma care. In the majority of patients, the addition of these long-acting agents improves both lung function and symptoms.

## Anticholinergics

Anticholinergic agents have been used in the treatment of asthma for several hundred years in the form of stramonium herbal preparations.[47] Anticholinergic bronchodilators are competitive inhibitors of muscarinic receptors. Unlike $\beta_2$-agonists and theophylline, anticholinergics are not functional antagonists; they produce bronchodilation only in cholinergically mediated bronchoconstriction. Normal bronchial tone is maintained through parasympathetic innervation of the airways by the vagus nerve. Certain well-known triggers of asthma and bronchospasm (histamine, prostaglandins, sulfur dioxide, allergens) produce bronchoconstriction.[47] Studies of asthmatic patients consistently demonstrate that anticholinergics are effective bronchodilators, although they are not as potent as $\beta_2$-agonists.

The most commonly used agent is ipratropium bromide, a quaternary ammonium derivative. Ipratropium bromide consistently produces a 10% to 20% improvement in forced expiratory volume in 1 second ($FEV_1$) over $\beta_2$-agonists alone in acute, severe bronchospasm.[48] However, significant interpatient variability is notable; some patients obtain significantly greater (40% to 80%) improvement, and others have little or no improvement. This agent has also been shown not to improve outcome in chronic asthma over $\beta_2$-agonists alone.[49]

The currently available anticholinergics are nonselective muscarinic receptor blockers. Blockade of inhibitory muscarinic receptors could theoretically result in increased release of acetylcholine that could overcome the block on smooth muscle receptors. This important mechanism may explain why some patients have experienced paradoxical bronchoconstriction from nebulized anticholinergics. Only the quaternary ammonium derivative ipratropium bromide should be used because these agents have the advantage of poor absorption across mucosae and the blood-brain barrier as a result of the charge associated with the five-valent tropane nitrogen atom. These agents have only negligible systemic effects and a prolonged, desired local effect (i.e., bronchodilation). They also have no effect on affect mucociliary clearance.[47] These agents have a duration of action of 4 to 8 hours, and both intensity and duration of action are dose dependent. The optimal dose of ipratropium in adults is 500 µg by nebulizer and 40 to 80 µg by MDI in younger adults with asthma. The optimal MDI dose in older adults with severe airflow limitation is two to four times higher. High doses of ipratropium should be used with caution in older patients with prostatic hypertrophy. The time to maximal bronchodilation is considerably slower than with aerosolized short-acting $\beta_2$-agonists

(2 hours versus 30 minutes). This factor, however, is of little clinical consequence because some bronchodilation is seen within 30 seconds, 50% of maximum response occurs within 3 minutes, and 80% of maximum is reached within 30 minutes.[47]

In summary, the role of anticholinergics in the treatment of bronchospasm and asthma is limited. These agents are not currently recommended for the long-term control of these disease processes.[49] However, most studies show that anticholinergic agents provide at least as great and prolonged an improvement in airflow in COPD as other agents, including long acting $\beta_2$-agonists.[50] Therefore, the use of inhaled anticholinergics on a scheduled basis is recommended as a first-line of therapy in patients with COPD.[51]

## Cromolyn Sodium and Nedocromil Sodium

Cromolyn sodium has been used for the prophylactic treatment of asthma for more than 20 years. A newer, related agent, nedocromil sodium, which is a pyranoquinoline dicarboxylic acid, was released in the United States in the 1990s.[49] The exact mechanism of action for these agents is still unknown. Although these agents have minor differences in activity, their principal differences appear to be in potency; 4 mg of nedocromil by MDI is equivalent to 20 mg of cromolyn sodium by Spinhaler.[52] These drugs produce mast cell membrane stabilization. Both agents inhibit in vitro activation of human neutrophils, macrophages, and eosinophils.[47,52] These drugs also inhibit neurally mediated bronchoconstriction through C-fiber sensory nerve stimulation in the airways.[52] These drugs do not have any bronchodilatory effects, however.

Both agents are effective by inhalation only and are available as MDIs, whereas cromolyn also comes as a nebulizer solution. These drugs are not bioavailable orally, but the portion of the drug that reaches the lung is completely absorbed.[47] Absorption from the airway is slower than elimination (hours versus minutes). Both the intensity and the duration of protection against various challenges are dose dependent.[52]

These drugs have a highly nontoxic profile. The common side effects, cough and wheezing, have been reported following inhalation of each agent, and bad taste and headache have been associated more strongly with nedocromil. The taste of nedocromil is so unpleasant that some patients (~20%) are unable to take the drug. Cromolyn has the best nontoxic profile of any compound to treat bronchospasm and asthma; adverse effects occur in less than 1 in 10,000 patients.[53]

Cromolyn and nedocromil are indicated for the prophylaxis of mild asthma in both children and adults, regardless of the cause. These drugs are particularly effective for patients with allergic asthma on a seasonal basis or just before an acute exposure such as entering a home with a pet. These drugs can be used in combination with $\beta_2$-agonists in patients with severe symptoms. The efficacy of these drugs is directly related to their degree of deposition in the lung. These compounds therefore do not work during active bronchospasm. Patients should initially receive cromolyn or nedocromil four times daily; after stabilization, the frequency may be reduced to twice daily.

## Leukotriene Modifiers

The newest treatment agents, approved since 1996, address a novel therapeutic pathway. They act by inhibiting the action of cysteinyl leukotrienes ($LTC_4$, $LTD_4$, and $LTE_4$).[54] These medications, zafirlukast (Accolate), montelukast (Singulair), and zileuton (Zylfo), all work by blocking the leukotriene receptor. Leukotrienes are proinflammatory modulators that increase microvascular permeability and airway edema and thus produce bronchoconstriction.

Zafirlukast has been shown to improve pulmonary function, by increasing $FEV_1$ and reducing symptoms and bronchodilator medication requirements in patients.[55] At doses of 20 mg twice daily, zafirlukast has reduced airway responses to inhaled allergen, platelet-activating factor, and exercise. Adverse effects are minimal, although experience with this medication is limited. Rare cases of hepatotoxicity and eosinophilic vasculitis have been reported. Food may impair absorption, and zafirlukast interacts with warfarin, resulting in prolonged prothrombin time.

Zileuton directly inhibits 5-lipozygenase, whereas other drugs in development bind to and prevent translocation of 5-lipoxygenase–activating protein.[54] Zileuton reduces bronchoconstriction caused by allergens, exercise, aspirin, and cold, dry air.[54] Doses of 600 mg four times daily reduce symptoms and bronchodilator requirements and improve pulmonary function. Zileuton may produce elevated liver enzymes, and patients need to be monitored closely. This drug also affects hepatic isozymes and therefore increases concentrations of warfarin and theophylline.[49]

Neither zafirlukast nor zileuton completely attenuated induced bronchospasm in several challenge models.[54] These newer agents show great promise, but their place in the scheme of asthma management is still in evolution. National Asthma Education and Prevention Program guidelines suggest that these compounds may be used as alternatives to low-dose inhaled steroids in mild persistent asthma. They also have the advantage that they are oral medications, and compliance may be improved over inhaled medications.

## Magnesium Sulfate

Intravenous magnesium sulfate, as a smooth muscle relaxant, had been advocated for patients with severe asthma who exhibited a suboptimal response. However, these initial trials did not use adequate doses of inhaled $\beta_2$-agonists, and bronchodilation from magnesium sulfate was only modest and did not exceed the $\beta_2$-agonist response.[49]

## Glucocorticoid Therapy

The most important therapeutic agents for bronchospasm and asthma are the inhaled corticosteroids. Actions of this class of compounds include (1) increasing the number of $\beta_2$-adrenergic receptors and improving the receptor responsiveness to $\beta_2$-adrenergic receptors to $\beta_2$-adrenergic stimulation, (2) reducing mucus production and hypersecretion, and (3) inhibiting the inflammatory response.[56] The anti-inflammatory effects of possible benefit in asthma include the following: decreases in the synthesis and release of several proinflammatory cytokines such as interleukin-1 (IL-1), IL-3, IL-4, IL-5, IL-6, IL-8, and granulocyte-macrophage colony-stimulating factor; reduction in inflammatory cell activation, recruitment, and infiltration; and decreases in vascular permeability.[56] Regular use of a steroid inhaler in combination with long-acting inhaled $\beta_2$-agonists was reported to improve lung function and to reduce the severity of dyspnea compared with individual drugs in patients with COPD.[57]

### Systemic Glucocorticoid Therapy

In severe acute asthma, status asthmaticus, the standard of care is treatment with systemic glucocorticoids combined with frequent administration of inhaled $\beta_2$-agonists.[49] Glucocorticoids can be administered by the parenteral route (methylprednisolone sodium succinate, hydrocortisone sodium succinate) or alternatively by the oral route (prednisone, methylprednisolone), either of which provides rapid onset of action and systemic effects.[58]

The glucocorticoids used in asthma are compared in Table 38.1. Recommended doses for acute asthma are listed in Table 38.2. There is no difference in response between intravenous and oral administration of steroids.[58] Evidence suggests that divided doses should be used initially. Following resolution of symptoms (decrease in obstruction achievement of >50% of predicted normal $FEV_1$, generally occurring in the first 48 hours), the steroid dose is reduced to one or two doses orally.[58] The duration of treatment depends on the response of individual patients and their response to these agents in the past. Tapering the dose after treatment is recommended, as with all steroids, to prevent adrenal insufficiency.

Systemic glucocorticoids are also recommended for the treatment of impending episodes of severe bronchospasm unresponsive to bronchodilator therapy.[49] Prednisone, at 1 to 2 mg/kg/day (≤40 to 60 mg/day),

**Table 38-1  Glucocorticoid Comparison Chart**

| Systemic | Relative Anti-Inflammatory Potency | Relative Sodium-Retaining Potency | Duration Biologic Activity (hr) | Plasma Elimination Half-Life (hr) |
|---|---|---|---|---|
| Hydrocortisone | 1 | 1.0 | 8–12 | 1.5–2.0 |
| Prednisone | 4 | 0.8 | 12–36 | 2.5–3.5 |
| Methylprednisolone | 5 | 0.5 | 12–36 | 3.3 |
| Dexamethasone | 25 | 0 | 36–54 | 3.4–4.0 |
| **Aerosol** | **Topical Potency** | **Receptor-Binding** | **Receptor Complex** | **Oral Bioavailability** |
| Flunisolide (FLU) | 330 | 1.8 | 3.5 | 21 |
| Triamcinolone acetonide (TAA) | 330 | 3.6 | 3.9 | 10.6 |
| Beclomethasone dipropionate (BDP) | 600 | 13.5 | 7.5 | 20 |
| Budesonide (BUD) | 980 | 9.4 | 5.1 | 11 |
| Fluticasone propionate (FP) | 1200 | 18 | 10.5 | <1 |

is administered orally in two divided doses for 3 to 10 days.[49] If an adequate response is not achieved, administration of prednisone three times daily may be worthwhile.

The balance between the control of symptoms and the occurrence of drug-related toxicity is always in the forefront. Because short-term (1 to 2 weeks) high-dose steroids (1 to 2 mg/kg/day prednisone) do not produce serious toxicity, it is unnecessary to taper following this course.[49]

Extended use may affect adrenal cortisol release. However, hypothalamic-pituitary-adrenal axis suppression

is short-lived (1 to 3 days) and readily reversible following short bursts (10 days or less) of pharmacologic doses.[58] Therefore, in patients who require long-term systemic glucocorticoids, the lowest possible dose required to control symptoms should be used. An accepted method to decrease toxicity is alternate-day therapy or use of inhaled glucocorticoids.

## Inhaled Glucocorticoids

The largest breakthrough in the treatment of bronchoconstriction was the development of inhaled steroids. These agents are now considered first-line

**Table 38-2  Corticosteroids**

| Medications | Adult Dosage | Comments |
|---|---|---|
| Prednisone Methylprednisolone Prednisolone | 120–180 mg in three or four divided doses for 48 hr, then 60–80 mg/day until peak expiratory flow reaches 70% of personal best | For outpatient "burst," use 1–2 mg/kg/day (maximum, 60 mg for 3–7 days); it is unnecessary to taper following the course |

steroid therapy. As with all steroids used in low to moderate doses, the risk of systemic complications is low. The inhaled glucocorticoids demonstrate a favorable topical systemic potency ratio, but they are far from benign. If an "ideal" glucocorticoid were developed, it would have a high degree of topical potency, minimal systemic absorption of active drug, and minimal local or systemic side effects. No such agent is available.

The inhaled glucocorticoids have high topical anti-inflammatory effects and are either poorly absorbed or metabolized to less active substances after absorption.[59] The systemic affects vary from agent to agent. Aerosol delivery of the preparations varies from 10% to 30%, and this can make a difference in both topical potency and systemic activity.[60] The delivery system can therefore make a significant difference in relative comparable dose.[49]

Optimal dosages of inhaled steroids have not been thoroughly studied, but most patients may control their disease with twice-daily doses. However, investigations demonstrated an improved asthma response with decreased systemic effects by giving the same total daily dose four times daily as opposed to twice daily.[49]

There is an apparent additive effect of long-acting β-agonists and inhaled glucocorticoids in current patient management. A possible explanation is that steroids are anti-inflammatory, whereas the smooth muscle relaxing effect of long-acting β-agonists results in prolonged bronchodilation and bronchoprotection. It can be assumed that the combination of both pharmacologic activities is particularly clinically beneficial.

## Experimental Drugs

### Potassium Channel Openers

The plasma membrane of airway smooth muscle has a high density of potassium channels. The opening of potassium ion channels in the cell membrane would allow potassium ions to move out from cells, an action normally maintained by the ion transporter potassium/sodium-ATPase. The opening of potassium channels in cell membranes results in membrane hyperpolarization, which inhibits the cellular influx of calcium through voltage-dependent channels and leads to relaxation of airway smooth muscle cells.[61] Few clinical trials have addressed the bronchodilatory effect of potassium channel openers (KCOs). Cromakalim, a benzopyran prototype, given orally significantly reduced the fall in early morning lung function of asthmatic patients.[62] However, levcromakalim, another KCO, did not cause significant bronchodilation or changes in airway responsiveness in other studies.[63,64] Therefore, it remains to be determined whether KCOs will be useful bronchodilators.

## Tachykinin and Kinin Receptor Antagonists

The tachykinins, substance P, neurokinin A, and neurokinin B, belong to a structural family of peptides. Bradykinin belongs to a family of short peptide. Tachykinins and bradykinin seem to be involved in exaggerated neurogenic airway inflammation such as bronchoconstriction and plasma extravasation.[65,66] Cold air–induced bronchoconstriction seems to be mediated by kinin and tachykinins.[67] The biologic actions of tachykinin and kinin are mediated by receptors: neurokinin $(NK)_1$, $NK_2$, and $NK_3$ receptors versus $B_1$ and $B_2$ receptors, respectively. Clinical studies with tachykinin and kinin receptor antagonists in human airways are scarce. In a double-blind, placebo-controlled, crossover trial with nine patients with stable asthma, a selective $NK_1$ receptor antagonist, FK-888, did not attenuate the maximal fall by exercise in specific airway conductance.[68] However, recovery from exercise-induced airway narrowing was significantly faster after inhalation of FK-888.[68] Inhalation of a bradykinin receptor antagonist, Hoe 140, had some protective effect in moderate asthma in a 4-week study.[69] Although tachykinin and bradykinin receptor antagonists are unlikely to play a major role in patients with asthma, they may possibly be useful in selected types of asthma such as nocturnal asthma induced by gastroesophageal reflux[70] or hyperpnea-induced bronchoconstriction.[71]

## Antiallergic Drugs

Selective $\beta_2$-receptor agonists, glucocorticoids, disodium cromoglycate, and nedocromil are traditional antiallergic agents to block allergic response in several ways. As a new antiallergic drug, suplatast tosilate (IPD-1151T) modulates T-helper type 2 cell cytokine production.[72] Oral administration of suplatast tosilate suppressed airway hyperresponsiveness in patients with asthma by reducing eosinophilic inflammation in the airways.[73] A recombinant humanized monoclonal anti-IgE antibody (omalizumab), which forms complexes with free IgE, blocks its interaction with mast cells and basophils, and lowers free IgE levels in the circulation, provided clinical benefit in a dose-dependent fashion in patients with seasonal allergic rhinitis.[74] Other antiallergic agents are under investigation.

## Drugs Targeting Cell Signaling Pathways

Cellular inflammation is regulated by intracellular signaling pathways to control specific cell response. The overexpression of multiple gene-encoding inflammatory agents leads to diverse diseases. For example, the intracellular protein kinase C, which is a serine-threonine protein kinase enzyme, has an important role in the genesis of pulmonary edema.[75] Targeting key signaling components of intracellular transduction as a therapeutic measure would correct the underlying cause of disease, not simply modify the associated symptoms. Although many substances to block signaling pathways are under investigation, no clinically proven multiple kinase inhibitor for lung disorders is currently on the market.

## Nitric Oxide

Nitric oxide (NO), in it role as an endothelial-derived relaxing factor, has been recognized as an important endogenous mediator for smooth muscle relaxation.[76,77] Therefore, exogenously administered, inhaled NO could be expected to cause vasodilation in well-aerated areas of the lung with no systemic hemodynamic effects. Inhaled NO-induced vasodilation of pulmonary vessels should increase blood flow to well-ventilated areas of the lung and preferentially shunt blood away from poorly venti-lated areas.

In the 1990s, there was interest in the use of NO in the treatment of acute respiratory distress syndrome (ARDS). Early studies showed some promise.[78] In a large multi-centered study,[76] however, no change in mortality was noted. Nonetheless, the study did show that NO was well tolerated, and it improved oxygenation compared with placebo over the first 4 hours of treat-ment. The complex nature of ARDS and cytokine mod-ulation may have led to the failure to affect mortality. NO is still used in several centers as bridge therapy when traditional support therapy for ARDS is failing.

NO has a place in some neonatal centers. It lowers the need for extracorporeal membrane oxygenation in respiratory failure of the newborn.[79] The drug also plays a role in the treatment of pulmonary hypertension of the newborn.[79,80] In this disorder, NO can increase oxygena-tion and decrease pulmonary arterial pressure. These studies, however, typically involved few patients, examined only the acute physiologic changes associated with administration of inhaled NO, and lacked concurrent placebo groups.

Further examination of NO along with more advanced modes of mechanical ventilation that do not add to cytokine load may lead to better outcomes in long-term survival. We must design more controlled trials that study only one aspect of the acute process and the way in which specific tissues react to NO.

## Surfactant

The presence of this substance has been known since 1959, when Avery and Mead published direct evidence linking the absence of a surface-active material in the lung to that of a substance that actively changed the sur-face tension of the alveoli of the lung.[81] This material was later named pulmonary surfactant. Pulmonary surfactant is a complex of phospholipids (80% to 90%), neutral lipids (5% to 10%), and at least four specific surfactant proteins (5% to 10%; SP-A, SP-B, SP-C, and SP-D) that lie as a layer at the air-liquid interface in the alveoli[82,83] and small airways, thus lowering surface tension. Surfactant is synthesized by the alveolar type II cells and is secreted into alveolar spaces.[83]

A further possible function of bronchial surfactant, which to date has not been studied, is its masking of receptors on smooth muscle with respect to substances that induce contraction and lead to airway obstruction. This means that surfactant could also possibly be involved in asthma.[84] Moreover, investigators have demonstrated that surfactant plays a role in the lung's defense against infection.[85] Surfactant, and in particular SP-A, enhances the antibacterial and antiviral defense of alveolar macrophages. Surfactant may also be important in protecting the lung from lung-released mediators (e.g., angiotensin II) and in protecting the cardiopulmonary system against mediators produced by the lung.[17,87]

Disturbances of the surfactant system can result from different factors. The most common is damage to the alveolar-capillary membrane, which leads to high-permeability edema with washout dilution of the surfactant or inactivation of the surfactant by plasma components, such as fibrinogen, albumin, globulin, and transferred hemoglobin and cell membrane lipids. In addition, surfactant can be easily depleted by the cyclic opening and closing of alveoli during mechanical ventilation; this disturbed synthesis, storage, or release of surfactant is secondary to direct injury of type II cells.[86,87] The dimin-ished surfactant in mechanical ventilation may play an important role in respiratory failure in ARDS.

Diminished pulmonary surfactant has far-reaching consequences for lung function. Independent of cause, decreased surfactant function leads directly or indirectly to (1) decreased pulmonary compliance, (2) decreased functional residual capacity, (3) atelectasis and enlarge-ment of the functional right-to-left shunt, (4) decreased gas exchange and respiratory acidosis, (5) hypoxemia with anaerobic metabolism and metabolic acidosis, and (6) pulmonary edema with further inactivation of surfac-tant by plasma constituents.

## Treatment

Surfactant replacement therapy has been used in preterm infants for the last 20 years with great success.[88] The rate of mortality has fallen because we are better able to deliver surfactant to these preterm infants. After preterm infants are born, respiratory distress can be prevented or its severity can be reduced by the intratracheal adminis-tration of synthetic or natural surfactants. Synthetic (lecithin, tyloxapol, hexadecanol) or natural (fortified extract of cow lungs) surfactant has also been adminis-tered repeatedly during the course of this disease process.

Ongoing research in surfactant replacement therapy in adults has not yet led to a decrease in mortality. Several formulations are under investigation, along with systems to deliver the agent into the adult lung. Multiple technical problems in the delivery of surfactant into the adult lung in ARDS have yet to be overcome. In addition, the maturity of the immune system may also play a role in the lack of positive outcomes in adult studies. New formulations are currently under development and may lead to more positive results in the adult population.

## CONCLUSION

Many agents are now available to maximize pulmonary function in multiple disease states. The physician who cares for these patients should be expert in the pharmacology of these drugs, from the older agents such as theophylline and atropine to the newer, long-acting $\beta_2$-agonists and leukotriene modulators. Most patients with severe airflow limitation need combination therapy, consisting of glucocorticoids and $\beta_2$-agonists with or without theophylline or anticholinergics.

We should also be familiar with the newer aerosol delivery systems. Aerosol delivery of drugs for asthma has the advantage of being site specific. For example, inhalation of short-acting $\beta_2$-agonist provides faster bronchodilation than administration of oral agents. The various devices used to generate therapeutic aerosols include MDIs, jet nebulizers, ultrasonic nebulizers, and dry powder inhalers. The single most important device factor determining the site of aerosol deposition is particle size. As anesthesiologists and intensive care specialists, we should also review our ability to deliver these drugs down an endotracheal tube. Important determinants of aerosol deposition in ventilator-supported patients include the delivery system, particle size, number of puffs or amount of nebulization, characteristics of the ventilator circuit, ventilator mode, and patient-related factors. These factors should make us develop a treatment plan for each of our high-risk patients before bronchospasm occurs.

## REFERENCES

1. Weibel ER, Taylor CR: Design and structure of the human lung. In Fishman AP (ed): Pulmonary Diseases and Disorders, 2nd ed. New York: McGraw-Hill, 1988, pp 11–20.
2. Breeze RG, Wheeldon EB: The cells of the pulmonary airways. Am Rev Respir Dis 1977;116:705–777.
3. Cauldwell FW, Siebert RG, Lininger RE, et al: Anatomic study of 150 human cadavers. Surg Gynecol Obstet 1948;86: 395–412.
4. Jerome EH: Pulmonary circulation. In Hemmings H, Hopkins P (eds): Foundations of Anesthesia: Basic and Clinical Sciences. London: Mosby, 2000, pp 465–481.
5. Barnes PJ: State of the art: Neural control of the human airways in health and disease. Am Rev Respir Dis 1986;134:1289–1314.
6. Barnes PJ: New concepts in the pathogenesis of bronchial hyperresponsiveness and asthma. J Allergy Clin Immunol 1989;83:1013–1026.
7. Gross NJ, Skorodin MS: The place of anticholinergic agents in the treatment of airway obstruction. Immunol Allergy Pact 1986;7:224–231.
8. Richardson JB, Farguson CC: Neuromuscular structure and function in the airways. Fed Proc 1979;38:202–208.
9. Boushey HA, Holtzman MJ, Shellar JR, et al: State of the art: Bronchial hyperactivity. Am Rev Respir Dis 1980;121: 389–413.
10. Theodore AL, Beer DJ: Pharmacotherapy of chronic obstructive pulmonary disease. Clin Chest Med 1986;7:657–671.
11. Lefkowitz RJ: Clinical physics of adrenoreceptor regulation. Am J Physiol 1982;243:E43–E47.
12. Seligman M, Chernow B: Use of adrenergic agents in the critically ill patient. Hosp Formul 1987;223:348–360.
13. Richardson JO: Non-adrenergic inhibitory innervation of the lung. Lung 1982;159:315–322.
14. Barnes PJ: Neural control of human airways in health and disease. Am Rev Respir Dis 1986;134:1286–1314.
15. Burgess C, Crane J, Pearce N, Beasley R: $\beta_2$-Agonists and New Zealand asthma mortality. Lancet 1991;337:982–983.
16. Villar J, Petty TL, Slutsky AS: ARDS in its middle age: What have we learned. Appl Cardiopulm Pathophysiol 1998;7:167–172.
17. So KL, Gommers D, Lachmann B: Bronchoalveolar surfactant system and intratracheal adrenaline. Lancet 1993;341:120–121.
18. Kelly HW: Controversies in asthma therapy with theophylline and the beta 2-adrenergic agents. Clin Pharm 1984;3:386–395.
19. McFadden ER: Clinical use of $\beta$-adrenergic agonists. J Allergy Clin Immunol 1985;76:352–356.
20. McFadden ER Jr: Methylxanthines in the treatment of asthma: The rise, the fall, and the possible rise again [editorial]. Ann Intern Med 1991;115:323–324.
21. Gora-Harper ML: The Injectable Drug Reference. Princeton, NJ: Society of Critical Care Medicine, Bioscientific Resources, 1998.
22. Weinberger M, Hendeles L: Slow-release theophylline: Rationale and basis for product selection. N Engl J Med 1983;308:76–64.
23. Persson CGA: Overview of effects of theophylline. J Allergy Clin Immunol 1986;78:780–787.
24. Horrobin DF, Manku MS, Franks DJ, et al: Methylxanthine phosphodiesterase inhibitors behave as prostaglandin antagonists in a perfuse rat mesenteric artery preparation. Prostaglandins 1977;13:33–40.
25. Murphy CM, Coonce SL, Simon PA: Treatment of asthma in children. Clin Pharm 1992;10:685–703.
26. Miech RP, Niedzwicki JG, Smith TR: Effect of theophylline on the binding of c-AMP to soluble protein from tracheal smooth muscle. Biochem Pharmacol 1979;28:3687–3688.
27. Hendeles L, Weinberger M: Theophylline: A state of the art review. Pharmacotherapy 1983;3:2–44.
28. Kidney J, Dominguez M, Taylor PM, et al: Immunomodulation by theophylline in asthma: Demonstration by withdrawal of therapy. Am J Respir Crit Care Med 1995;151:1907–1914.
29. Ashutosh K, Sedat M, Fragale-Jackson J: Effects of theophylline on respiratory drive in patients with chronic obstructive pulmonary disease. J Clin Pharmacol 1997;37:1100–1107.
30. Parker JO, Kelkar K, West RS: Hemodynamic effects of aminophylline in cor pulmonale. Circulation 1966;38:17–25.

31. McEvoy GK: Theophylline. In McEvoy GK (ed): *AHFS Drug Information 1993.* Bethesda, MD: American Society of Hospital Pharmacists, 1993, pp 2278–2285.

32. Bergstrand H: Phosphodiesterase inhibition and theophylline. Eur J Respir Dis 1980;61(Suppl 109):37–44.

33. Weinberger M, Hendeles L, Bighley L: Relationships of product formulation to absorption of oral theophylline. N Engl J Med 1978;299:852–857.

34. Johnson M: The beta-adrenoceptor. Am J Respir Crit Care Med 1998;158:S146–S153.

35. Nelson HS: Beta-adrenergic bronchodilators. N Engl J Med 1995;333:499–506.

36. Amory DW, Burnham SC, Cheney FW Jr: Comparison of the cardiopulmonary effects of subcutaneously administered epinephrine and terbutaline in patients with reversible airway obstruction. Chest 1975;67:279.

37. Kips JC, Pauwels RA: Long-acting inhaled $\beta_2$-agonist therapy in asthma. Am J Respir Crit Care Med 2001;164:923–932.

38. Ullman A, Suedmyr N: Salmeterol, a new long-acting inhaled $\beta_2$-adrenoceptor agonist: Comparison with salbutamol in adult asthmatic patients. Thorax 1988;43:674–678.

39. Lofdahl CG, Suedmyr N: Formoterol fumarate, a new $\beta_2$-adrenoceptor agonist: Acute studies of selectivity and duration of effect after inhaled and oral administration. Allergy 1989;44:264–271.

40. Moore PF, Constantine JW, Barth WE: Pirbuterol selective $\beta_2$-adrenergic bronchodilator. J Pharmacol Exp Ther 1978;207:410–418.

41. Littner MR, Tashkin DP, Culvarese B, Raotista M: Bronchial and cardiovascular effects of increasing doses of pirbuterol acetate aerosol in asthma. Ann Allergy 1982;48:141–144.

42. Anderson GP, Linden A, Rabe KF: Why are long-acting $\beta$-adrenoceptor agonists long-acting? Eur Respir J 1994;7:569–578.

43. Kallstrom BL, Sjoberg J, Waldeck B: The interaction between salmeterol and $\beta_2$-adrenoceptor agonists with higher efficacy on guinea pig trachea and human bronchus in vitro. Br J Pharmacol 1994;113:687–692.

44. Guhan AR, Cooper S, Oborne J, et al: Systemic effects of formoterol and salmeterol: A dose-response comparison in healthy subjects. Thorax 2000;55:650–656.

45. Nightingale JA, Rogers DF, Barnes PJ: Comparison of the effects of salmeterol and formoterol in patients with severe asthma. Am J Respir Crit Care Med 2000;161:A190.

46. Noppen M, Vincken W: Bronchodilating effect of formoterol but not of salmeterol in two asthmatic patients [letter]. Respiration 2000;67:112–113.

47. Weiss EB, Stein M (eds): *Bronchial Asthma: Mechanisms and Therapeutics,* 3rd ed. Boston: Little, Brown, 1993.

48. Kelly HW, Murphy S: Should anticholinergics be used in acute severe asthma? Ann Pharmacother 1990;24:409–416.

49. National Heart, Lung and Blood Institute: National Asthma Education and Prevention Program, expert panel report 2. Guidelines for Diagnosis and management of Asthma. NIH publication no. 97–4051. Bethesda, MD: National Institutes of Health, National Heart, Lung and Blood Institute, 1997.

50. Beeh KM, Welte T, Buhl R: Anticholinergics in the treatment of chronic obstructive pulmonary disease. Respiration 2002;69:372–379.

51. National Heart, Lung and Blood Institute, World Health Organization: Global Strategy for the Diagnosis, Management, and Prevention of Chronic Obstructive Pulmonary Disease. NHLBI/WHO workshop report, publication no. 2701. Bethesda, MD: National Institutes of Health, National Heart, Lung and Blood Institute, 2001.

52. Wasserman SI (ed): Nedocromil sodium: A pyranoquinoline anti-inflammatory agent for the treatment of asthma. J Allergy Clin Immunol 1993;92(Suppl):143–216.

53. Murphy S, Kelly HW: Cromolyn sodium: A review of mechanisms and clinical use in asthma. Drug Intell Clin Pharm 1987;21:22–35.

54. Hendeles L, Scheife RT (eds): New frontiers in asthma therapy: Leukotriene receptor antagonists and 5-lipoxygenase inhibitors. Pharmacotherapy 1997;17(Suppl):1S–54S.

55. Spector SL, Smith LJ, Glass M: Effects of six weeks of therapy with oral doses of ICI 204, 219, a leukotriene $D_4$ receptor antagonist. Crit Care Med 1994;150:618–623.

56. Baraniuk JN (ed): Steroids in asthma: Molecular mechanisms of glucocorticoid actions. J Allergy Clin Immunol 1996;97(Suppl):141–182.

57. Mahler DA, Wire P, Horstman D, et al: Effectiveness of fluticasone propionate and salmeterol combination delivered via Diskus device in the treatment of chronic obstructive pulmonary disease. Am J Respir Crit Care Med 2002;166:1084–1091.

58. Kelly HW, Murphy S: Corticosteroids for acute severe asthma. Ann Pharmacother 1991;25:72–79.

59. Barnes PJ: Inhaled glucocorticoids for asthma. N Engl J Med 1995;332:868–875.

60. Kelly HW: Comparison of inhaled corticosteroids. Ann Pharmacother 1998;32:220–232.

61. Small RC, Berry JL, Burka JF, et al: Potassium channel activators and bronchial asthma. Clin Exp Allergy 1992;22:11–18.

62. Williams AJ, Lee TH, Cochrane GM, et al: Attenuation of nocturnal asthma by cromakalim. Lancet 1990;336:334–336.

63. Kidney JC, Fuller RW, Worsdell YM, et al: Effect of an oral potassium channel activator, BRL 38227, on airway function and responsiveness in asthmatic patients: Comparison with oral salbutamol. Thorax 1993;48:130–133.

64. Faurschou P, Mikkelsen KL, Steffensen I, Franke B: The lack of bronchodilator effect and the short-term safety of cumulative single doses of an inhaled potassium channel opener (bimakalim) in adult patients with mild to moderate bronchial asthma. Pulm Pharmacol 1994;7:293–297.

65. Joos G, Kips J, Pauwels R, Van der Straeten M: The respiratory effects of neuropeptides. Eur J Respir Dis 1986;144:107–136.

66. Frossard N, Advenier C: Tachykinin receptors and the airways. Life Sci 1991;49:1941–1953.

67. Yoshihara S, Nadel JA, Figini M, et al: Endogenous nitric oxide inhibits bronchoconstriction induced by cold-air inhalation in guinea pigs: Role of kinins. Am J Respir Crit Care Med 1998;157:547–552.

68. Ichinose M, Miura M, Yamauchi H, et al: A neurokinin 1-receptor antagonist improves exercise-induced airway narrowing in asthmatic patients. Am J Respir Crit Care Med 1996;153:936–941.

69. Akbary AM, Wirth KJ, Scholkens BA: Efficacy and tolerability of Icatibant (Hoe 140) in patients with moderately severe chronic bronchial asthma. Immunopharmacology 1996;33:238–242.

70. Ricciardolo FLM, Rado V, Fabbri LM, et al: Bronchoconstriction induced by citric acid inhalation in guinea pigs: Role of tachykinin, bradykinin, and nitric oxide. Am J Respir Crit Care Med 1999;159:557–562.

71. Solway J, Kao BM, Jordan JE, et al: Tachykinin receptor antagonists inhibit hyperpnea-induced bronchoconstriction in guinea pigs. J Clin Invest 1993;92:315–323.

72. Furukido K, Takeno S, Ueda T, et al: Suppression of the Th 2 pathway by suplatast tosilate in patients with perennial nasal allergies. Am J Rhinol 2002;16:329–336.

441

73. Yoshida M, Aizawa H, Inoue H, et al: Effect of suplatast tosilate on airway hyperresponsiveness and inflammation in asthma patients. J Asthma 2002;39:545–552.

74. Casale TB, Condemi J, LaForce C, et al: Effect of omalizumab on symptoms of seasonal allergic rhinitis: A randomized controlled trial. JAMA 2001;286:2956–2967.

75. Siflinger-Birnboim A, Johnson A: Protein kinase C modulates pulmonary endothelial permeability: A paradigm for acute lung injury. Am J Physiol 2003;284:L435–L451.

76. Dellinger RP, Zimmerman JL, Taylor RW, et al: Inhaled nitric oxide in patients with acute respiratory distress syndrome: Results of a randomized phase II trial. Crit Care Med 1998;26:15–23.

77. Moncada S, Palmer RMJ, Higgs HA: Nitric oxide: Physiology, pathophysiology and pharmacology. Pharmacol Rev 1991;43:109–142.

78. Rossaint R, Falke KJ, López F, et al: Inhaled nitric oxide for the adult respiratory distress syndrome. N Engl J Med 1993;328:399–405.

79. Neonatal Inhaled Nitric Oxide Study Group: Inhaled nitric oxide in full-term and nearly full-term infants with hypoxic respiratory failure. N Engl J Med 1997;336:597–604.

80. Roberts JD, Polaner DM, Lang P, et al: Inhaled nitric oxide in persistent pulmonary hypertension of the newborn. Lancet 1992;340:818–819.

81. Avery MA, Mead J: Surface properties in relation to atelectasis and hyaline membrane disease. Am J Dis Child 1959;97:517–523.

82. Lachmann B, Winsel K, Reutgen H: Der Anti-Atelektase-Faktor der Lunge. Z Erkr Atmungsorgane Folia Bronchol 1972;137:267–287.

83. van Golde LMG, Batenburg JJ, Robertson B: The pulmonary surfactant system: Biochemical aspects and functional significance. Physiol Rev 1988;68:374–455.

84. Lachmann B, Becher G: Protective effect of lung surfactant on allergic bronchial constriction in guinea pigs. Am Rev Respir Dis 1986;133:A118.

85. Van Iwaarden F: Surfactant and pulmonary defense system. In Robertson B, Van Golde LMG, Battenburg JJ (ed): *Pulmonary Surfactant*. Amsterdam: Elsevier, 1992, pp 215–253.

86. Verbrugge SJC, Lachmann B: Mechanisms of ventilation-induced lung injury and its prevention role of surfactant. Appl Cardiopulm Pathophysiol 1998;7:173–198.

87. Papadakos PJ: Artificial ventilation. In Hemmings H, Hopkins P (eds): *Foundations of Anesthesia: Basic Clinical Sciences*. London: Mosby, 2000, pp 507–514.

88. Tobin N: Asthma, airway biology and nasal disorders in AJRCCM, 2001. Am J Respir Crit Care Med 2002;165:598–618.

442

# CHAPTER 39

# Antibiotic Use in the Mechanically Ventilated Patient

Michael S. Niederman

Antibiotics are the foundation of therapy for respiratory tract infections in mechanically ventilated patients. The infections treated in this patient population include severe community-acquired pneumonia (CAP), ventilator-associated pneumonia (VAP), severe nosocomial and health care–associated pneumonia (HCAP), and nosocomial tracheobronchitis. Most of these infections are treated with systemic antibiotics, but there may also be a role for aerosolized antibiotic therapy as an adjunct to systemic therapy in some patients and as sole therapy for selected patients with nosocomial tracheobronchitis. In the mechanically ventilated patient, nosocomial pneumonia may arise after at least 48 hours of ventilatory support, and this type of pneumonia is termed VAP.[1] Alternatively, patients with CAP, HCAP, or nosocomial pneumonia may be so severely ill that management requires ventilatory support, although by definition, these patients do not have VAP if the reason for initial ventilation is the severe pneumonia itself. HCAP is a more recently defined entity that includes patients coming from nursing homes, those in the hospital for more than 2 out of the past 90 days, those from dialysis centers, or those receiving home wound care.[1,2] When pneumonia makes these patients severely ill, they require therapy with mechanical ventilation. Because of their exposure to the health care environment, patients with HCAP are at risk for infection with drug-resistant pathogens and are managed similarly to patients with nosocomial pneumonia and not CAP.

The longer a patient is ventilated, the greater is the risk of respiratory infection, although the daily risk of infection drops over time in patients who are managed with short-term ventilation. The risk of VAP is 3% per day for the first 5 days of ventilation, 2% per day for days 6 to 10, and 1% per day for the next 5 days.[3] Although most chronically tracheostomized and ventilated patients develop respiratory infection, the risk is greater for developing tracheobronchitis than for pneumonia, and patients who survive to the point of long-term ventilation have a relatively low daily risk of developing pneumonia, although the cumulative risk is high.[4,5]

When antibiotics are used for most patients, initial therapy is aimed at a broad spectrum of likely pathogens and is thus empiric because the infecting pathogen is often not known. Therapy can be more specifically focused later, on the basis of the results of diagnostic tests. In some cases, initial empiric therapy must be continued because no etiologic pathogen is identified. When a pathogen is recovered, the term *appropriate* refers to the use of at least one antimicrobial agent that is active in vitro against the etiologic pathogen.[1] The term *adequate* includes not only appropriate therapy, but also the use of that agent in the correct dose, by the right route, given in a timely fashion, and with penetration to the site of infection. Timely and appropriate antibiotic therapy can improve survival in patients with severe CAP and nosocomial pneumonia, and the benefits are most evident in patients who are not otherwise terminally ill.[1,6–10] However, even with the use of the correct agents, not all patients recover. That some ventilated patients die in spite of microbiologically appropriate therapy is a reflection of the degree of antibiotic efficacy, as well as a reflection of host response capability (which may, in part, have a genetic determination) and the fact that not all deaths are the direct result of infection. In some patients, death is the result of underlying serious illness; the percentage of deaths that result from infection is termed the *attributable mortality*. In patients with VAP, this rate has been estimated to be as high as 50% to 60%.[10] However, the use of timely and appropriate antimicrobial therapy can reduce attributable mortality to as low as 20%.

The need for initial therapy to be accurate has led to the frequent and prolonged use of multiple antibiotics in critically ill patients; this approach, in turn, has promoted the development of multidrug-resistant (MDR) pathogens, which are common in many infections.[11] Modern management of these patients requires initial broad-spectrum therapy, followed by a narrowing and focusing of therapy as clinical and culture data become available. This "de-escalation" approach is often accompanied by efforts to use short-duration therapy.[12]

Numerous guidelines for empiric therapy for both CAP and nosocomial pneumonia have been developed, but several caveats should be remembered.[1,6] First, although current guidelines for empiric therapy are evidence based, very few outcome studies have been conducted to demonstrate the utility of these guidelines in improving mortality and other outcomes. Second, guidelines must be reevaluated relative to local patterns of antibiotic susceptibility. In the case of CAP, the emergence of penicillin-resistant pneumococcus, community-acquired methicillin-resistant *Staphylococcus aureus* (MRSA), and epidemic viral illness (influenza, severe acute respiratory syndrome [SARS]) may affect the selection of initial therapy, particularly if resistance is prevalent in a specific community. In the setting of VAP, each hospital has its own unique flora and antibiotic susceptibility patterns; knowledge of such patterns is essential.[1,13]

## PRINCIPLES OF ANTIBIOTIC USE

### Mechanisms of Action

When an antibiotic interferes with the growth of bacteria, it does so by undermining the integrity of the cell wall or by interfering with bacterial protein synthesis or common metabolic pathways. The effect is termed either *bactericidal* or *bacteriostatic*. These broad categorizations may not apply for a given agent against all organisms, however.[14] Bactericidal antibiotics kill bacteria, generally by inhibiting cell wall synthesis or by interrupting a key metabolic function of the organism. Agents of this type include the penicillins, cephalosporins, aminoglycosides, fluoroquinolones, vancomycin, daptomycin, rifampin,

and metronidazole. Bacteriostatic agents inhibit bacterial growth, do not interfere with cell wall synthesis, and rely on host defenses to eliminate bacteria. Agents of this type include the macrolides, tetracyclines, sulfa drugs, chloramphenicol, linezolid, and clindamycin. The use of specific agents is dictated by the susceptibility of the causative organism, at a given location, to individual antibiotics. However, when neutropenia is present, or if there is accompanying endocarditis or meningitis, the use of a bactericidal agent is preferred. Thus, for most patients with pneumonia, it is not essential to choose a bactericidal agent. One additional consideration is that certain organisms can produce toxins, and antibiotics that inhibit protein synthesis (linezolid, clindamycin) may have an advantage in toxin-mediated illnesses, such as those caused by certain strains of *S. aureus*, when compared with cell wall–active bactericidal antibiotics.[15]

The antimicrobial activity of a specific agent is often described by the terms *minimum inhibitory concentration* (MIC) and *minimum bactericidal concentration* (MBC). MIC refers to the minimum concentration of an antibiotic that inhibits the growth of 90% of a standard sized inoculum, leading to no visible growth in a broth culture. At this concentration, not all the bacteria have necessarily been killed. MBC refers to the minimum concentration needed to cause a 3-logarithmic decrease (99.9% killing) in the size of the standard inoculum; generally, all pathogenic bacteria are killed at this concentration. The MIC is used to define the *sensitivity* of a pathogen to a specific antibiotic, under the assumption that the concentration required for killing (the MIC) can be reached in the serum in vivo. However, these terms must be interpreted cautiously in patients with pneumonia because the MIC data do not consider the penetration of an agent into lung tissues and sites of infection. Thus, if an agent achieves infection site concentrations that exceed serum concentrations, the efficacy may be better than predicted by the MIC data. Concerns about antimicrobial resistance have led to the emergence of a newer term, the *mutant prevention concentration* (MPC).[16] The MPC is defined as the lowest concentration of an antimicrobial that prevents bacterial colony formation from a culture containing greater than $10^{10}$ bacteria. At lower than MPC concentrations, spontaneous mutants can persist and be enriched among the organisms that remain during therapy. The clinical relevance of this concept is still uncertain.

### Penetration into the Lung

The concentration of an antibiotic in the lung depends on the permeability of the capillary bed at the site of infection (the bronchial circulation), the degree of protein binding of the drug, and the presence or absence of an active transport site for the antibiotic in the lung.[17]

In the lung, the relevant site to consider for antibiotic penetration is controversial, but concentrations in lung parenchyma, epithelial lining fluid, and cells such as macrophages and neutrophils are probably important in pneumonia, whereas bronchial concentrations may be more important in tracheobronchitis. In addition, certain organisms are intracellular, such as *Legionella pneumophila* and *Chlamydophila pneumoniae;* for these organisms, macrophage concentrations may be important. Conditions at the site of infection may also be important, and some agents can be inactivated by certain local conditions. Aminoglycosides have reduced activity at acidic pH, which may be present in infected lung tissues. In addition, certain bacteria develop resistance by producing destructive enzymes (such as β-lactamases), by altering the permeability of the outer cell wall, by changing the target site of antimicrobial action, or by pumping (efflux) of the antimicrobial from the interior of the cell. In all these conditions, a high local concentration of antimicrobial agent may help offset the bacterial resistance mechanisms.

The concentration of an antibiotic in lung parenchyma depends on its penetration through the bronchial circulation capillaries. The bronchial circulation has a fenestrated endothelium, so antibiotics penetrate in proportion to their molecular size and protein binding. Small molecules that are not highly protein bound pass readily into the lung parenchyma. Penetration through the bronchial circulation is inflammation dependent, whereas the pulmonary vascular bed has a nonfenestrated epithelium, which is inflammation independent; penetration is best for lipophilic agents.[17] These lipophilic drugs include chloramphenicol, the macrolides (including the azalides and ketolides), linezolid, clindamycin, the tetracyclines, the quinolones, and trimethoprim-sulfamethoxazole. Agents that are poorly lipid soluble are inflammation dependent for their entry into the epithelial lining fluid and include the penicillins, cephalosporins, aminoglycosides, vancomycin, carbapenems, and monobactams.[18]

If the volume of distribution exceeds 3 L, this finding implies distribution outside the plasma.[16] Some lipophilic agents, such as the macrolides and quinolones, are distributed extensively to body tissues, and the serum levels underestimate their effect at sites of infection, especially for drugs that achieve a high intracellular concentrations in phagocytes. The volume of distribution can also be increased by obesity. Therefore, dosing based on ideal body weight may lead to underdosage, but basing doses of hydrophilic antibiotics on total body weight may result in overdosage.[16]

## Aerosol Antibiotic Therapy

For some drugs, such as the aminoglycosides, penetration into the epithelial lining fluid and lung secretions is not optimal, and systemic therapy of pneumonia is often less effective than treatment of bacteremia. For this reason, these agents have been studied for delivery through the aerosol route. Local administration of antimicrobials has been used in the therapy of bronchiectasis, especially in the setting of cystic fibrosis, and in the treatment of VAP. Direct delivery of antibiotics is usually achieved by nebulization. This approach achieves high intrapulmonary concentrations, and it may do so without substantial systemic absorption. Thus, the risk of systemic toxicity is reduced. The use of this approach in mechanically ventilated patients is somewhat anecdotal, and not carefully studied, but it has been proposed for patients with either infectious tracheobronchitis or VAP.[19,20] Both infections can involve highly resistant gram-negative bacteria, and the local delivery of antibiotics may effectively treat some pathogens that cannot be eradicated by systemic therapy.

In mechanically ventilated patients, local antibiotic administration, by instillation or nebulization, has been used to prevent pneumonia. In general, this approach is not recommended, because even when it has been successful, there has been concern about the emergence of MDR gram-negative bacteria in patients who subsequently do develop infection, and these organisms may be difficult to treat. Only one prospective randomized trial has examined the impact of the adjunctive use of locally instilled tobramycin with intravenous agents in the management of VAP.[21] Although the addition of endotracheal tobramycin did not improve clinical outcome compared with placebo, microbiologic eradication was significantly greater in the patients receiving aerosolized antibiotics.

In spite of these data, uncontrolled case series have shown that when patients have VAP caused by MDR *Pseudomonas aeruginosa* or *Acinetobacter* species, aerosolized aminoglycosides, polymyxin, or colistin may be helpful as adjuncts to systemic antibiotics.[1,19,20] One side effect of aerosolized antibiotics has been bronchospasm, which can be induced by the antibiotic or the associated diluents present in certain preparations. A specially formulated preparation of tobramycin for aerosol administration is available and may avoid this complication.

Although the optimal method of administration of aerosol therapy is unknown, most studies have shown that nebulization can be effective and can achieve more uniform distribution than direct instillation. When aerosol therapy is used in mechanically ventilated patients, it must be carefully synchronized with the ventilator cycle, and the optimal delivery device is not yet defined. In an animal model, investigators found that by using an ultrasonic nebulizer placed in the inspiratory limb of the ventilator circuit, proximal to the Y-connector, up to 40% of the administered dose could be retained in the lung; the tissue concentrations achieved were

10 times higher than possible with comparable doses given systemically, and systemic absorption was minimal.[22,23] To optimize delivery, inspiratory time may need to be as high as 50% of the ventilatory cycle, and routine humidification should be stopped during antibiotic administration. In ventilated patients, the ventilator may need to be set with a tidal volume of 8 to 10 mL/kg, with no humidification system in use during the use of the ultrasonic nebulizer, which should be set to deliver 8 L/minute.

## Pharmacokinetics and Pharmacodynamics

*Pharmacokinetics* is the study of the absorption, distribution, and elimination of a drug in the body. This information can be used to describe the concentration in serum. Pharmacokinetics also includes the study of the concentration at other sites of the body, including the site of infection and the relationship between drug concentrations and their pharmacologic or toxic effect.[16] For antibiotics, this means the relationship of antibiotic concentrations at the site of infection, compared with the MIC of the target organism. *Pharmacodynamics* refers to the action of a drug on the body, including its therapeutic effect.

Some antibiotics kill bacteria in relation to how long their concentration stays at levels higher than the MIC of the target organism (time-dependent killing), whereas other agents are effective in relation to the peak concentration achieved (concentration-dependent killing).[16] If antibiotic killing is time dependent, dosing schedules should be chosen to achieve the maximal time greater than the MIC of the target organism. However, for many organisms, the concentration of the antibiotic needs to be greater than the MIC for only 40% to 50% of the dosing interval, and possibly for as little as 20% to 30% of the interval in the case of carbapenems. Antibiotics of this type include the β-lactams (penicillins and cephalosporins), carbapenems, aztreonam, macrolides, and clindamycin. The rate of killing is saturated once the antibiotic concentration exceeds four times the MIC of the target organism. Continuous infusion of β-lactams is under study to optimize time-dependent killing with these agents.

When bacterial killing is concentration dependent, activity is determined by the degree of concentration achieved at the site of infection and the size of the *area under the curve* (AUC; of drug concentration plotted versus time) in relation to the MIC of the target organism. Alternatively, the action of these agents can be described by how high the peak serum concentration (Cmax) is in relation to the organism MIC. Classic agents of this type include the aminoglycosides and the fluoroquinolones, but the ketolides are also concentration-dependent antibiotics.[16] For these types of agents, the optimal killing of bacteria is defined by the ratio of AUC to MIC,

often referred to as the *area under the inhibition curve* (AUIC). The target AUIC for gram-negative bacteria is 125 or greater.[24]

For both the aminoglycosides and quinolones, some studies have shown that efficacy can also be defined by the Cmax/MIC ratio, aiming for a target of 12 for quinolones against pneumococcus.[25] Optimal use of these agents would entail infrequent administration but with high doses, the underlying principle behind the once-daily administration of aminoglycosides. With once-daily aminoglycoside dosing, the patient achieves a high peak concentration (maximal killing) and a low trough concentration (minimal nephrotoxicity); this regimen relies on the *postantibiotic effect* (PAE) to maintain the efficacy of the antibiotic after the serum (or lung) concentrations fall to less than the MIC of the target organism. If an antibiotic has a PAE, it is capable of suppressing bacterial growth even after its concentration falls to less than the MIC of the target organism. In clinical practice, the use of once-daily aminoglycoside dosing has had variable benefits in both efficacy and toxicity.[26] Most of the agents that kill in a concentration-dependent fashion have a prolonged PAE, whereas agents with little or no PAE against gram-negative bacteria are generally also agents that kill in a time-dependent fashion, hence they are given several times daily.

## ANTIBIOTIC THERAPY OF RESPIRATORY INFECTION IN THE MECHANICALLY VENTILATED PATIENT

Although it is necessary to initiate prompt and accurate antibiotic therapy for the patient with severe pneumonia, initial therapy is usually empiric because it is often impossible to identify a specific etiologic agent when the pneumonia is first diagnosed. The choice of empiric therapy is based on knowledge of the likely etiologic pathogen for each clinical setting, modified by knowledge of local patterns of bacteriology and the prevalence of specific types of antimicrobial resistance in a given region or a specific hospital setting. The American Thoracic Society and the Infectious Diseases Society of America have developed algorithms for initial empiric therapy of severe pneumonia arising in both the community and the hospital.[1,6,27]

### Severe Community-Acquired Pneumonia

The primary etiologic pathogen for severe CAP is pneumococcus, and patients requiring mechanical ventilation to treat CAP should be treated for possible drug-resistant *Streptococcus pneumoniae* (DRSP), along with other likely pathogens including *L. pneumophila*. Other organisms to be treated include *Haemophilus influenzae, Mycoplasma pneumoniae, C. pneumoniae*, aspiration organisms (which usually are enteric gram-negative organisms more than anaerobes), and aerobic gram-negative bacilli (including *P. aeruginosa*).[6,27] There has been some controversy about whether enteric gram-negative bacteria are common in CAP, and the identified risk factors have included features that would reclassify some affected patients as having HCAP and not CAP. Thus, patients admitted from a nursing home or dialysis center, or those who have been hospitalized in the previous 90 days, should be treated by the HCAP algorithm. Risk factors for gram-negative organisms include aspiration, pulmonary comorbidity, and recent antibiotic therapy (>7 days in the past month). Concern for *P. aeruginosa* infection is increased in patients with bronchiectasis, malnutrition, human immunodeficiency virus infection, or corticosteroid therapy (>10 mg/day).[6,27,28] In the patient with severe CAP following influenza, another consideration is *S. aureus*, and there has been some concern with severe CAP in this setting caused by community-acquired MRSA.[15,29]

Patients with CAP who are admitted to intensive care units (ICUs) are divided into those at risk for *P. aeruginosa* and those who are not. All patients require combination therapy. Monotherapy is not recommended for any ICU-admitted CAP patient because of the absence of efficacy data for any single agent in this setting. For patients not at risk for *P. aeruginosa*, therapy should be with a selected β-lactam combined with either a macrolide or a quinolone.[6,27] Recommended β-lactams include ceftriaxone, cefotaxime, and ampicillin-sulbactam. Ceftriaxone can be given from 1 g daily to 2 mg twice daily; the latter is recommended for severe pneumococcal infection, especially with associated meningitis. All patients require the addition of either a macrolide or a quinolone for possible atypical pathogen (*Legionella* spp., *M. pneumoniae*, or *C. pneumoniae*) infection, either as the sole cause or as part of a mixed infection. Some studies, including those involving severe CAP, have shown that the addition of this type of coverage is associated with a lower mortality rate than when other regimens are used.[30-32] The recommended macrolide is intravenous azithromycin (500 mg/day for 7 to 10 days) because it is better tolerated than erythromycin. The recommended quinolone is moxifloxacin (400 mg/day), regardless of renal function or levofloxacin (750 mg/day), for patients with normal renal function. In patients with abnormal renal function, levofloxacin doses should be adjusted, after using the same initial starting dose for all patients. In addition, several retrospective studies of patients with bacteremic pneumococcal pneumonia demonstrated that dual therapy including a β-lactam combined with a macrolide or a quinolone is associated with improved outcome, compared with single-agent β-lactam therapy.[33,34]

For the penicillin-allergic patient, therapy should be with an antipneumococcal quinolone (levofloxacin or moxifloxacin) in addition to aztreonam.

When risk factors for *P. aeruginosa* are present, the patient should be treated with two antipseudomonal agents in addition to coverage for DRSP and *Legionella*. Effective antimicrobials that can be used for this type of patient with severe CAP are selected β-lactams (cefepime, piperacillin-tazobactam, imipenem, meropenem), in combination with an antipseudomonal quinolone (ciprofloxacin, high-dose levofloxacin: at 750 mg/day). Alternatively, the foregoing β-lactams can be combined with an aminoglycoside and either azithromycin or a non-pseudomonal quinolone (moxifloxacin). In the penicillin-allergic patient, aztreonam can be combined with an aminoglycoside and an antipneumococcal fluoroquinolone (Box 39.1).

Monotherapy with an antipneumococcal fluoroquinolone for severe CAP has not yet been proven safe and effective. Moxifloxacin is efficacious for CAP, even in elderly patients, but few patients with severe CAP have been studied. Although in the Community-Acquired Pneumonia Recovery in the Elderly (CAPRIE) study, which compared moxifloxacin with levofloxacin for CAP in elderly patients, the cure rate for moxifloxacin (94.7%) was greater than that for levofloxacin (84.6%), few patients in this study were mechanically ventilated.[35] In a recent study of severe CAP that compared levofloxacin with combination ceftriaxone-ofloxacin therapy, equivalent clinical responses were observed in both treatment groups (79.1% with levofloxacin compared with 79.5% with combination therapy).[36] However, patients with shock were excluded from the study, and in patients with mechanical ventilation, treatment with levofloxacin resulted in a lower clinical cure rate (63% compared with 72% with combination therapy).[36] Current guidelines recommend that if quinolones are used for severe CAP, they should be used as a replacement for a macrolide and should be part of a combination regimen, usually with a β-lactam.[6,27] However, in a recent report, the use of initial empiric therapy with a β-lactam with a fluoroquinolone for severe CAP was associated with increased short-term mortality (odds ratio, 2.71; 95% confidence interval, 1.2 to 6.1), in comparison with other guideline-recommended antimicrobial regimens.[37]

If a specific organism is later recovered from culture, then therapy can be modified and focused, with the previous caveat about bacteremic pneumococcal pneumonia kept in mind. In addition, if the patient's history contains certain epidemiologic clues (travel, comorbid illness, animal exposure), therapy should be modified to cover the suspected organism. For example, those patients with chronic obstructive pulmonary disease should be treated for *H. influenzae* and *Moraxella catarrhalis*. In addition, if a sputum

---

**BOX 39-1**

**Principles of Antibiotic Therapy for the Mechanically Ventilated Patient with Community-Acquired Pneumonia**

- Administer the first dose of antibiotic therapy within 4–6 hours of arrival to the hospital.
- Treat all patients for pneumococcus (including DRSP) and *Legionella*, and consider coverage of *Haemophilus influenzae*, enteric gram-negative bacteria (including *Pseudomonas aeruginosa*), *Staphylococcus aureus* (including MRSA), and atypical pathogens (*Mycoplasma pneumoniae*, *Chlamydophila pneumoniae*).
- Limit macrolide monotherapy to outpatients or inpatients with no risk factors for DRSP, enteric gram-negative bacteria, or aspiration, who do not have severe illness.
- Use EITHER a selected β-lactam with a macrolide (azithromycin) OR quinolone (levofloxacin or moxifloxacin) for patients not at risk for *P. aeruginosa* infection.
  - If penicillin allergic, use an antipneumococcal quinolone PLUS aztreonam.
- For those at risk for *P. aeruginosa* infection, use an antipseudomonal β-lactam PLUS either ciprofloxacin or levofloxacin OR combine with an aminoglycoside AND either a macrolide or an antipneumococcal quinolone (levofloxacin or moxifloxacin).
  - If penicillin allergic, use aztreonam PLUS an aminoglycoside PLUS an antipneumococcal quinolone.
- To cover DRSP, the selected acceptable intravenous β-lactams include ceftriaxone, cefotaxime, ertapenem, and ampicillin/sulbactam.
- Antipseudomonal β-lactams include cefepime, imipenem, meropenem, and piperacillin/tazobactam.
- Do not administer quinolone monotherapy to any patient with intensive care unit–admitted CAP.
- The newer antipneumococcal quinolones, in order of decreasing antipneumococcal activity, are gemifloxacin (oral only), moxifloxacin (oral and intravenous), and levofloxacin (oral and intravenous).
- Vancomycin and linezolid should be used rarely and only in patients with severe CAP and either meningitis (vancomycin) or severe necrotizing pneumonia after influenza.
  - If community-acquired, toxin-producing, MRSA is suspected, use EITHER linezolid alone OR consider adding clindamycin to vancomycin.

*CAP, community-acquired pneumonia; DRSP, drug-resistant* Streptococcus pneumoniae; *MRSA, methicillin-resistant* Staphylococcus aureus.

---

Gram stain is obtained and shows gram-positive cocci in clusters, particularly in a patient with severe pneumonia following a recent viral or influenza infection, therapy for *S. aureus* should be added.

Although community-acquired MRSA is not common in CAP, it has been reported following influenza or viral infection in otherwise healthy patients with severe, bilateral, necrotizing pneumonia.[15,29] This organism is different from nosocomial MRSA because it occurs in previously healthy people, produces the Panton-Valentine leukocidin (a virulence factor that causes tissue necrosis), and is usually of the USA 300 clonal type.[29] Treatment for this type of pneumonia is uncertain, but vancomycin alone may not be effective. One case series suggested that therapy include an antibiotic that inhibits toxin, such as clindamycin (added to vancomycin) or linezolid (used alone).[15]

All the foregoing recommended therapies are effective for DRSP, which is now common in the United States. Pneumococcus resistant to penicillin (>0.1 mg/L) may account for up to 40% of clinical isolates in the United States, and it is more common in patients who are immunocompromised and in those who have received β-lactam antibiotics in the past 3 months.[6,38] Most of the penicillin resistance seen in patients with pneumonia is of the intermediate type and is not high level (minimal inhibitory concentration ≥2.0 mg/L). This observation may explain the findings that outcome in CAP is generally not worsened by the presence of penicillin-resistant organisms, compared with penicillin-sensitive organisms. Effective therapy has been achieved with ceftriaxone and with cefotaxime, which are probably more likely to be effective than cefuroxime.[39,40] The antipneumococcal quinolones moxifloxacin and levofloxacin (at the 750-mg dose) are also effective. If *Legionella* infection is documented, a quinolone may be the most reliable therapy.[41]

In mechanically ventilated patients with severe CAP, consideration should be given to adjunctive therapy with corticosteroids. Three clinical situations may necessitate this approach. First, if a patient has pneumococcal pneumonia with meningitis, therapy with corticosteroids, started before antibiotics, has improved the likelihood of a good neurologic outcome.[42] Second, when a patient with severe CAP is hypotensive, relative adrenal insufficiency is common, and physiologic replacement doses of corticosteroids may be helpful.[43] Finally, one prospective, randomized trial of severe CAP showed improved outcomes, including mortality, when patients received a continuous infusion of low- to moderate-dose corticosteroids.[44] In addition to corticosteroids, the use of activated protein C may be helpful for severe CAP, although the documented benefit was minimal in patients who received accurate and appropriate antibiotic therapy, compared with those who did not.[45]

## Hospital-Acquired Pneumonia

The hospital-acquired pneumonia (HAP) group includes patients with VAP and those with severe nosocomial pneumonia who require mechanical ventilation to support them at a time of severe infection. All these patients are at risk for infection with a group of core pathogens, but some are also at risk for infection by additional organisms, particularly MDR pathogens, based on the presence of risk factors.[1] The core pathogens include pneumococcus, *H. influenzae*, MRSA, and nonresistant enteric gram-negative organisms (*Escherichia coli*, *Klebsiella* species, *Enterobacter* species, *Proteus* species, and *Serratia marcescens*). Patients who have risk factors for MDR pathogens are at risk for infection with the core pathogens as well as for infection with *P. aeruginosa*, *Acinetobacter* species, and methicillin-sensitive S. aureus (MSSA). Risk factors for infection with MDR organisms include the presence of HCAP, current hospitalization for at least 5 days, antibiotic therapy within the previous 90 days, immunosuppressive illness or therapy (corticosteroids or chemotherapy), and admission to a unit with a high rate of MDR organisms. Depending on the time of onset of infection, patients with VAP may not always be at risk for infection with MDR pathogens, but patients with HCAP are, by definition, at risk for infection with these organisms.

Although these general patterns apply to most patients, bacteriologic features vary from one hospital to another, from one ICU to another, and from one time period to another. Therefore, it is necessary to have a knowledge of local microbiologic data when adapting treatment recommendations to a specific clinical setting.[13] Some patients, particularly those with acute respiratory distress syndrome, can have polymicrobial infection, in which multiple bacterial pathogens act synergistically. Pure anaerobic pneumonia is uncommon in patients with HAP, including those with aspiration risk factors, and in this latter population, enteric gram-negative organisms are still the dominant concern.[28,46] Although fungal and viral pathogens can cause HAP, this situation is relatively uncommon, based on current data. *Candida* is generally an uncommon pathogen, but a common colonizer, and it rarely causes pneumonia. Conversely, *Aspergillus* can be an important cause of HAP, particularly in patients who have had a prolonged hospital stay with antibiotic and corticosteroid therapy.

Once there is a clinical suspicion of HAP in a mechanically ventilated patient, the patient should be treated with antibiotics, unless the suspicion of infection is low and a Gram stain of an endotracheal suction aspirate is negative. The antibiotic choice is either a narrow-spectrum regimen or a broad-spectrum regimen, the latter directed at MDR pathogens. The narrow-spectrum approach is used if the patient has pneumonia that started in the first 4 days of hospitalization, if no other risk factors for MDR pathogens are present, and if the patient does not have HCAP. All other patients, including those with HCAP, receive broad-spectrum therapy.[1]

Narrow-spectrum therapy is directed at the core pathogens and is generally achieved with a single agent. Options are ceftriaxone, ampicillin-sulbactam, ertapenem, levofloxacin, moxifloxacin, and ciprofloxacin. If the patient is allergic to penicillin, a quinolone can be used, or the patient can be given the combination of clindamycin and aztreonam.[1] When the patient has risk factors for MDR pathogens, therapy is directed not only at core pathogens, but also at *P. aeruginosa*, *Acinetobacter* species, and, in many instances, MRSA. To provide this spectrum of coverage, therapy includes at least two and often three antibiotics. The recommended therapy is to use either an aminoglycoside or an antipseudomonal quinolone (ciprofloxacin or levofloxacin) in combination with an antipseudomonal β-lactam. The choices of β-lactams are cefepime, ceftazidime, imipenem, meropenem, and piperacillin-tazobactam. In choosing among these options, it is important to use a different agent from any the patient received in the previous 14 days, because repeated use of the same agent may lead to clinical failure related to selection of resistance as a result of recent exposure[47] (Box 39.2).

If there are concerns about MRSA because of risk factors, a high local prevalence, or the presence of clusters of gram-positive organisms on a Gram stain of a tracheal aspirate sample, then a third agent, either linezolid or vancomycin, should be added. If culture data from tracheal aspirates become available, then therapy can sometimes be more specific. For example, if MRSA is documented in the ventilated patient, some data suggest an advantage of linezolid over vancomycin.[48] For *Acinetobacter* species, the drug of choice is a carbapenem, but if resistance to this class of antibiotics is present, the recommended therapy is colistin, although tigecycline may become an option in the future, once more clinical data in this setting are available.

The value of combination therapy is controversial. In general, no strong data show that the use of an aminoglycoside with a β-lactam is more effective than β-lactam monotherapy, unless the patient is neutropenic or has pseudomonal bacteremia.[1,49] Thus, when the mechanically ventilated patient is given combination therapy, the major justification is to provide a broad enough spectrum of therapy to treat MDR pathogens effectively in a patient with risk factors. It is important to use the correct dose of antibiotics in critically ill ventilated patients

**BOX 39-2**

---

Principles of Antibiotic Use in the Therapy of the Mechanically Ventilated Patient with Nosocomial Pneumonia

---

- Initiate therapy as soon as there is a clinical suspicion of infection.
- Obtain a lower respiratory tract culture (tracheal aspirate, protected brush, bronchoalveolar lavage) before initiation of antibiotic therapy. Samples can be obtained bronchoscopically or otherwise and cultured quantitatively or semiquantitatively. Do not delay therapy for the purpose of collecting a culture.
- Choose a narrow-spectrum agent for patients with no risk factors for MDR pathogens and no HCAP.
  - Options include ceftriaxone, ampicillin/sulbactam, ertapenem, levofloxacin, moxifloxacin and ciprofloxacin.
  - For penicillin allergy, use a quinolone OR the combination of clindamycin and aztreonam.
- Choose a broad-spectrum regimen with at least two drugs for patients with risk factors for MDR pathogens. Use a knowledge of local microbiology to guide choices.
  - Use an aminoglycoside or an antipneumococcal quinolone (ciprofloxacin or high-dose levofloxacin) PLUS an antipseudomonal β-lactam such as cefepime, ceftazidime, imipenem, meropenem, or piperacillin-tazobactam. If there is concern about MRSA, add EITHER linezolid OR vancomycin.
- Use the correct therapy in recommended doses.
  - Recommended doses for patients with normal renal function are: cefepime, 1–2 g every 8–12 hours; imipenem, 500 mg every 6 hours or 1 g every 8 hours; meropenem, 1 g every 8 hours; piperacillin-tazobactam, 4.5 g every 6 hours; levofloxacin, 750 mg/day, or ciprofloxacin, 400 mg every 8 hours; vancomycin, 15 mg/kg every 12 hours leading to a trough level of 15–20 mg/L; linezolid, 600 mg every 12 hours; and aminoglycosides of 7 mg/kg per day of gentamicin or tobramycin and 20 mg/kg of amikacin.
- Choose an empiric therapy that uses agents from a class of antibiotics different from those the patient has received in the past 2 weeks.
- The drug of choice for *Acinetobacter* infection is a carbapenem, but colistin should be considered if there is carbapenem resistance. In the future, tigecycline may be an appropriate choice.
- Consider linezolid as an alternative to vancomycin, especially in patients with renal insufficiency, those receiving other nephrotoxic medications, and those with proven MRSA ventilator-associated pneumonia.
- Adjunctive aerosolized aminoglycosides can be used for patients with highly resistant gram-negative pathogens, but systemic therapy should be continued.

---

*HCAP, health care–associated pneumonia; MDR, multidrug resistant; MRSA, methicillin-resistant* Staphylococcus aureus.

with pneumonia. Based on clinical trial data, the correct doses for patients with normal renal function include the following: cefepime, 1 to 2 g every 8 to 12 hours; imipenem, 500 mg every 6 hours or 1 g every 8 hours; meropenem, 1 g every 8 hours; piperacillin-tazobactam, 4.5 g every 6 hours; levofloxacin, 750 mg/day, or ciprofloxacin, 400 mg every 8 hours; vancomycin, 15 mg/kg every 12 hours leading to a trough level of 15 to 20 mg/L; linezolid, 600 mg every 12 hours; and aminoglycosides of 7 mg/kg/day of gentamicin or tobramycin and 20 mg/kg of amikacin.[1]

To use antibiotics effectively and responsibly for these patients, it is necessary to implement a de-escalation strategy, which implies the prompt use of broad-spectrum empiric therapy whenever there is a clinical suspicion of infection with MDR pathogens. The reasons for this approach are to avoid delaying therapy and to use a broad-enough spectrum regimen to cover the likely pathogens.[1,12] However, to avoid overuse of antibiotics, a key decision point comes on day 2 to 3, when culture and clinical response data become available. It then becomes possible to narrow and focus therapy or, in some cases, to stop therapy altogether or aim for a short duration of treatment. Based on culture data, de-escalation

is often possible. Therefore, if an aminoglycoside was used with a β-lactam, the maximal benefit may have been achieved after 5 days of dual therapy, and the aminoglycoside can usually be stopped at that point.[1,50] If a non-resistant gram-negative organism is identified, therapy can immediately be de-escalated to a single agent. Drugs shown effective for critically ill mechanically ventilated patients are ciprofloxacin, levofloxacin, imipenem, meropenem, piperacillin-tazobactam, and cefepime. De-escalation can be done as soon as culture data are available. It can also be done in patients who have negative cultures, and even in those with MDR pathogens, provided an effective single agent is identified from sensitivity testing results.[12] This approach has led to less total antibiotic use, and in some instances, reduced mortality.[51] Another way to use less antibiotic is to shorten the duration of therapy. Several studies have shown that it is possible to treat VAP effectively with 6 to 8 days of therapy, provided the initial therapy was appropriate.[51,52] The optimal duration of therapy for infections caused by *P. aeruginosa* and MRSA is still uncertain, but prolonged therapy may be no better than short-duration therapy, in the absence of bacteremia.

## Nosocomial Tracheobronchitis

There are no well-controlled studies of the need for antibiotic therapy of nosocomial tracheobronchitis in mechanically ventilated patients. *Nosocomial tracheobronchitis* is usually defined as a condition in which the patient has fever, increased (usually purulent) sputum, and a positive endotracheal aspirate culture during mechanical ventilation, but in the absence of radiographic pneumonia.[4] These patients usually have infection with *P. aeruginosa*, and their mortality and length of stay may be higher than in ventilated patients without this complication. In spite of adverse outcomes, it remains uncertain whether specific antimicrobial therapy is needed. Anecdotal experience has shown that in some patients who do not have signs of systemic sepsis, therapy with only aerosolized antibiotics (usually aminoglycosides or colistin) may be effective.[19,20]

## Duration of Therapy and Expected Response

In severely ill patients with CAP or nosocomial pneumonia, patients should rapidly improve with effective therapy. Patients who do improve can be treated with antibiotics for 7 to 10 days, whereas those who do not need careful reevaluation. In patients with severe pneumonia, some improvement usually occurs by day 3, and thus this becomes the time point for deciding whether the patient has made an appropriate response to therapy.[6,27]

Treatment failure in severe CAP can occur in up to 15% of all patients and is present either early or late.[53] Most studies of clinical response in CAP examined patients who were not mechanically ventilated. These studies focused on improvements in symptoms of cough, sputum production, and dyspnea, along with the ability to take medications by mouth, and an afebrile status for at least two occasions 8 hours apart. In a ventilated patient, serial measurements of oxygenation are a good indicator of response, and radiographic improvement usually lags behind clinical improvement.

When a patient with severe CAP fails to respond to therapy in the expected time interval, it is necessary to consider infection with a drug-resistant or unusual pathogen (*Mycobacterium tuberculosis*, *Bacillus anthracis* [anthrax], *Coxiella burnetii*, *Burkholderia pseudomallei*, *Pasteurella multocida*, endemic fungi, or hantavirus), a pneumonic complication (lung abscess, endocarditis, empyema), or a noninfectious process that mimics pneumonia (bronchiolitis obliterans with organizing pneumonia, hypersensitivity pneumonitis, pulmonary vasculitis, bronchoalveolar cell carcinoma, lymphoma, pulmonary embolus). The evaluation of the nonresponding patient should be individualized, but it may include computed tomography of the chest, pulmonary angiography, bronchoscopy, and occasionally open lung biopsy.

If the patient has VAP or nosocomial pneumonia, clinical improvement should also occur by day 2 to 3, and serial measurement of the Clinical Pulmonary Infection Score may be the best way to evaluate clinical response.[54] Of all clinical parameters, serial improvement in oxygenation is the best measure of a good response to therapy, and usually this occurs by day 3 in patients who are likely to survive.[54] For the patient who is not responding, the first step is to check respiratory tract cultures, just to be sure that the therapy is active against the pathogen isolated. In addition, more cultures and diagnostic testing are needed to rule out infection with an unusual pathogen (fungus), another diagnosis (inflammatory lung disease), or another site of infection or pneumonia complication (central line infection, empyema, antibiotic-induced colitis). When a patient is not responding to initial therapy, a change in antibiotics, combined with an aggressive diagnostic reevaluation, should be carried out no later than day 3.

## REFERENCES

1. Niederman MS, Craven DE, Bonten MJ, et al: Guidelines for the management of adults with hospital-acquired, ventilator-associated, and healthcare-associated pneumonia. Am J Respir Crit Care Med 2005;171:388–416.
2. Kollef MH, Shorr A, Tabak YP, et al: Epidemiology and outcomes of health-care–associated pneumonia: Results from a large US database of culture positive patients. Chest 2005;128:3854–3862.
3. Cook DJ, Walter SD, Cook RJ: Incidence of and risk factors for ventilator-associated pneumonia in critically ill patients. Ann Intern Med 1998;129:433–440.
4. Nseir S, Di Pompeo C, Soubrier S, et al: Effect of ventilator-associated tracheobronchitis on outcome in patients without chronic respiratory failure: A case-control study. Crit Care 2005;3:R238–R245.
5. Harlid R, Andersson G, Frostell CG, et al: Respiratory tract colonization and infection in patients with chronic tracheostomy: A one-year study in patients living at home. Am J Respir Crit Care Med 1996;154:124–129.
6. Niederman MS, Mandell LA, Anzueto A, et al: Guidelines for the management of adults with community-acquired lower respiratory tract infections: Diagnosis, assessment of severity, antimicrobial therapy and prevention. Am J Respir Crit Care Med 2001;163:1730–1754.
7. Houck PM, Bratzler DW, Nsa W, et al: Timing of antibiotic administration and outcomes for Medicare patients hospitalized with community-acquired pneumonia. Arch Intern Med 2004;164:637–644.
8. Luna CM, Vujacich P, Niederman MS, et al: Impact of BAL data on the therapy and outcome of ventilator-associated pneumonia. Chest 1997;111:676–685.
9. Leroy O, Santré C, Beuscart C, et al: A five-year study of severe community-acquired pneumonia with emphasis on prognosis in patients admitted to an intensive care unit. Intensive Care Med 1995;21:24–31.
10. Heyland DK, Cook DJ, Griffith L, et al: The attributable morbidity and mortality of ventilator-associated pneumonia in

the critically ill patient: The Canadian Critical Trials Group. Am J Respir Crit Care Med 1999;159:1249–1256.

11. Gaynes R, Edwards JR, National Nosocomial Infections Surveillance System: Overview of infections caused by gram-negative bacilli. Clin Infect Dis 2005;41:848–854.

12. Hoffken G, Niederman MS: Nosocomial pneumonia: The importance of a de-escalating strategy for antibiotic treatment of pneumonia in the ICU. Chest 2002;122:2183–2196.

13. Rello J, Sa-Borges M, Correa H, et al: Variations in etiology of ventilator-associated pneumonia across four treatment sites: Implications for antimicrobial prescribing practices. Am J Respir Crit Care Med 1999;160:608–613.

14. Finberg RW, Moellering RC, Tally FP, et al: The importance of bactericidal drugs: Future directions in infectious disease. Clin Infect Dis 2004;39:1314–1320.

15. Micek ST, Dunne M, Kollef MH: Pleuropulmonary complications of Panton-Valentine leukocidin-positive community-acquired methicillin-resistant *Staphylococcus aureus*: Importance of treatment with antimicrobials inhibiting exotoxin production. Chest 2005;128:2732–2738.

16. Andes D, Anon J, Jacobs MR, Craig WA: Application of pharmacokinetics and pharmacodynamics to antimicrobial therapy of respiratory tract infections. Clin Lab Med 2004;24:477–502.

17. Honeybourne D: Antibiotic penetration into lung tissues. Thorax 1994;49:104–106.

18. Panidis D, Markantonis SL, Boutzouka E, et al: Penetration of gentamicin into alveolar lining fluid of critically ill patients with ventilator-associated pneumonia. Chest 2005;128:545–552.

19. Badia JR, Soy D, Adrover M, et al: Deposition of instilled versus nebulized tobramycin and imipenem in ventilated intensive care unit patients. J Antimicrob Chemother 2004;54:508–514.

20. Michalopoulos A, Kasiakou SK, Mastora Z, et al: Aerosolized colistin for the treatment of nosocomial pneumonia due to multidrug-resistant gram-negative bacteria in patients without cystic fibrosis. Crit Care 2005;9:R53–R59.

21. Brown RB, Kruse JA, Counts GW, et al: Double-blind study of endotracheal tobramycin in the treatment of gram-negative bacterial pneumonia: The Endotracheal Tobramycin Study Group. Antimicrob Agents Chemother 1990;34:269–272.

22. Goldstein I, Wallet F, Robin AN, et al: Lung deposition and efficiency of nebulized amikacin during *Escherichia coli* pneumonia in ventilated piglets. Am J Respir Crit Care Med 2002;166:1375–1381.

23. Goldstein I, Wallet F, Robert J, et al: Lung tissue concentrations of nebulized amikacin during mechanical ventilation in piglets with healthy lungs. Am J Respir Crit Care Med 2002;165:171–175.

24. Forrest A, Nix DE, Ballow CH, et al: Pharmacodynamics of intravenous ciprofloxacin in seriously ill patients. Antimicrob Agents Chemother 1993;37:1073–1081.

25. Preston SL, Drusano GL, Berman AL, et al: Pharmacodynamics of levofloxacin: A new paradigm for early clinical trials. JAMA 1998;279:125–129.

26. Hatala R, Dinh T, Cook DJ: Once-daily aminoglycoside dosing in immunocompetent adults: A meta analysis. Ann Intern Med 1996;124:717–725.

27. File TM, Niederman MS: Antimicrobial therapy of community-acquired pneumonia. Infect Dis Clin North Am 2004;18:993–1016.

28. Arancibia F, Bauer TT, Ewig S, et al: Community-acquired pneumonia due to gram-negative bacteria and *Pseudomonas aeruginosa*: Incidence, risk and prognosis. Arch Intern Med 2002;162:1849–1858.

29. Francis JS, Doherty MC, Lopatin U, Johnston CP, et al: Severe community-onset pneumonia in healthy adults caused by methicillin-resistant *Staphylococcus aureus* carrying the Panton-Valentine leukocidin genes. Clin Infect Dis 2005 40:100–107.

30. Gleason PP, Meehan TP, Fine JM, et al: Associations between initial antimicrobial therapy and medical outcomes for hospitalized elderly patients with pneumonia. Arch Intern Med 1999;159:2562–2572.

31. Houck PM, MacLehose RF, Niederman MS, Lowery JK: Empiric antibiotic therapy and mortality among Medicare pneumonia inpatients in 10 Western states: 1993, 1995, 1997. Chest 2001;119:1420–1426.

32. Brown RB, Iannini P, Gross P, Kunkel M: Impact of initial antibiotic choice on clinical outcomes in community-acquired pneumonia: Analysis of a hospital claims-made database. Chest 2003;123:1503–1511.

33. Wunderink RG, Rello J, Cammarata SK, et al: Linezolid vs vancomycin: Analysis of two double-blind studies of patients with methicillin-resistant *Staphylococcus aureus* nosocomial pneumonia. Chest 2003;124:1789–1797.

34. Martinez JA, Horcajada JP, Almela M, et al: Addition of a macrolide to a B-lactam–based empirical antibiotic regimen is associated with lower in-patient mortality for patients with bacteremic pneumococcal pneumonia. Clin Infect Dis 2003;36:389–395.

35. Anzueto A, Niederman MS, Pearle J, et al: Community-acquired pneumonia recovery in the elderly (CAPRIE): Efficacy and safety of moxifloxacin therapy versus that of levofloxacin therapy. Clin Infect Dis 2006;42:73–81.

36. Leroy O, Saux P, Bedos JP, Caulin E: Comparison of levofloxacin and cefotaxime combined with ofloxacin for ICU patients with community-acquired pneumonia who do not require vasopressors. Chest 2005;128: 172–183.

37. Mortensen EM, Restrepo MI, Anzueto A: The impact of empiric antimicrobial therapy with a beta-lactam and fluoroquinolone on mortality for patients hospitalized with severe pneumonia. Crit Care 2005;10:R8.

38. Vanderkooi OG, Low DE, Green K, et al: Predicting antimicrobial resistance in invasive pneumococcal infections. Clin Infect Dis 2005;40:1288–1297.

39. Lujan ML, Gallego M, Fontanals D, et al: Prospective observational study of bacteremic pneumococcal pneumonia: Effect of discordant therapy on mortality. Crit Care Med 2004;32:625–631.

40. Yu VL, Chiou CC, Feldman C, et al: An international prospective study of pneumococcal bacteremia: Correlation with in vitro resistance, antibiotics administered, and clinical outcome. Clin Infect Dis 2003;37:230–237.

41. Mykietiuk A, Carratala J, Fernandez-Sabe N, et al: Clinical outcomes for hospitalized patients with *Legionella* pneumonia in the antigenuria era: The influence of levofloxacin therapy. Clin Infect Dis 2005;40:794–799.

42. de Gans J, van de Beek D, European Dexamethasone in Adulthood Bacterial Meningitis Study Investigators: Dexamethasone in adults with bacterial meningitis. N Engl J Med 2002;347:1549–1456.

43. Salluh JI, Verdeal JC, Mello GW, et al: Cortisol levels in patients with severe community-acquired pneumonia. Intensive Care Med 2006;32:595–598.

44. Confalonieri M, Urbino R, Potena A, et al: Hydrocortisone infusion for severe community-acquired pneumonia: A preliminary randomized study. Am J Respir Crit Care Med 2005;171:242–248.

45. Laterre PF, Garber G, Levy H, et al: Severe community-acquired pneumonia as a cause of severe sepsis: Data from the PROWESS study. Crit Care Med 2005;33:952–961.

46. El Solh AA, Pietrantoni C, Bhat A, et al: Microbiology of severe aspiration pneumonia in institutionalized elderly. Am J Respir Crit Care Med 2003;167:1650–1654.

47. Trouillet JL, Vuagnat A, Combes A, et al: *Pseudomonas aeruginosa* ventilator-associated pneumonia: Comparison of episodes due to piperacillin-resistant versus piperacillin-susceptible organisms. Clin Infect Dis 2002;34:1047–1054.

48. Wunderink RG, Rello J, Cammarata SK, et al: Linezolid vs vancomycin: Analysis of two double-blind studies of patients with methicillin-resistant *Staphylococcus aureus* nosocomial pneumonia. Chest 2003;124:1789–1797.

49. Paul M, Benuri-Silbiger I, Soares-Weiser K, Liebovici L: Beta-lactam monotherapy versus beta-lactam–aminoglycoside combination therapy for sepsis in immunocompetent patients: Systematic review and meta-analysis of randomised trials. BMJ 2004;328:668.

50. Gruson D, Hilbert G, Vargas F, et al: Strategy of antibiotic rotation: Long-term effect on incidence and susceptibilities of gram-negative bacilli responsible for ventilator-associated pneumonia. Crit Care Med 2003;31:1908–1914.

51. Kollef MH, Morrow LE, Niederman MS, et al: Clinical characteristics and treatment patterns among patients with ventilator-associated pneumonia. Chest 2006;129:1210–1218.

52. Soo Hoo GW, Wen E, Nguyen TV, Goetz MD: Impact of clinical guidelines in the management of severe hospital-acquired pneumonia. Chest 2005;128:2778–2787.

53. Menendez R, Torres A, Zalacain R, et al: Risk factors for treatment failure in community acquired pneumonia: Implications for disease outcome. Thorax 2004;59:960–965.

54. Luna CM, Blanzaco D, Niederman MS, et al: Resolution of ventilator-associated pneumonia: Prospective evaluation of the clinical pulmonary infection score as an early clinical predictor of outcome. Crit Care Med 2003;31:676–682.

# SECTION 6

## MONITORING MECHANICAL VENTILATION

# CHAPTER 40

# Blood Gas Analysis

Per A. J. Thorborg

## HISTORY OF BLOOD GAS ANALYSIS: TECHNOLOGY AND CONCEPT DEVELOPMENT

From a historical perspective, our current understanding of human physiology has developed only fairly recently. Anatomists of antiquity and later, in the 16th and 17th centuries, had described the structure of airways, lungs, heart, and vasculature. However, functional relationships, particularly with respect to metabolic activities, became slowly and gradually understood after the discovery of the constituents of air in the 18th century. The technical and conceptual advances that led to the first automated blood gas machine are detailed later in this chapter.[1,2] Table 40.1 gives an overview of the history of blood gas analysis.

Antoine L. Lavoisier (1743–1794), after careful quantitative measurements of the oxidation process, described the nature of respiration. In 1776 and 1777, he realized that the composition of air was a mixture of gases, and the "fixed air" of Joseph Black must contain coal. In 1779, Lavoisier coined the term *oxygen* from the Greek "to form acid." In careful studies, Pierre Simon de Laplace (1749–1827) and Lavoisier showed that consumption of oxygen ($Vo_2$) by animals generated heat, as if the animal had been burning coal, resulting in carbon dioxide ($CO_2$) and water. In his *Traité élémentaire de chimie*, published in 1789, Lavoisier rejected the phlogiston theory and started a new era in chemistry and physiology. At the time, $Vo_2$ was believed to take place in the lung itself. It was not then known where the "furnace" of the body was located. Lazarro Spallanzani (1729–1799) was perhaps the first physiologist to suggest that the furnace consisted of the muscles and other organs of the body, not the heart, blood, or lungs. Using a vacuum technique, Humphry Davy (1778–1829) was the first to show the presence of $CO_2$ and $O_2$ in the blood, and he also showed that venous blood was capable of taking up $O_2$. The first report of arterial puncture in humans was published by Hürter in 1912,[3] who described arterial $O_2$ saturation ($Sao_2$) at 93% to 100% in four subjects.

The first attempt at quantitative blood gas analysis by Heinrich Gustav Magnus (1802–1870) in 1837 showed higher $O_2$ content in the arterial blood and higher $CO_2$ in the venous blood, so Magnus believed that $CO_2$ had to be formed in the circulation. The amount of gases dissolved varied by gas.[4] It was not until 20 years later that Lothar Meyer (1830–1895), in *Die Gase des Blutes*, determined that $O_2$ binds chemically to some component of the blood and thereby maintains high $O_2$ content over a broad range of partial pressures. Carl Ludwig and J. M. Setchenow (1829–1905) had developed a vacuum-based blood gas analyzing setup requiring 100 mL of blood; the analysis took all day to perform.

Technical improvements by Alexander Schmidt (1831–1894) established that $O_2$ was bound to the red cells, whereas $CO_2$ occurred mainly in the plasma. Felix Hoppe-Seyler (1825–1895) was the first to produce the red blood pigment, which he called *hemoglobin*, and he believed that it was this compound that bound $O_2$ (oxyhemoglobin) in the blood. Eduard Pfluger (1828–1910) was the first to show that $Vo_2$ took place in the cells, not in the blood or the lungs. The blood $O_2$ tensions ($Po_2$) measured at the time were very low (20 to 30 torr [mm Hg]), but values close to 80 mm Hg were produced after methodologic improvements in 1880.

**Table 40-1   History of Blood Gas Analysis**

| Author | Chemistry | Physiology | Author |
|---|---|---|---|
| Black, 1755 | Fixed air $CO_2$ | | |
| Priestley, 1774 | Dephlogisticated air ($O_2$) | | |
| Scheele, 1777 | Fire air ($O_2$) | Respiration | Lavoisier and Laplace, 1777 |
| Davy, 1797 | $O_2$ and $CO_2$ present in blood | $O_2$ | *Traité elementaire de chimie* |
| Henry, 1802 | Gas solubility in water | | |
| | Gas partial pressures | | |
| Dalton, 1803 | Water vapor pressure | | |
| | Atomic theory | Animal chemistry lectures | Berzelius, 1806–1808 |
| | | Atomic weights | Berzelius, 1810–1818 |
| Graham, 1829 | Law of diffusion | Quantitative chemistry | |
| Magnus, 1837 | First quantified ABG: $Pao_2 > Pvo_2$ and $Pvco_2 > Paco_2$ | CO to liberate $O_2$ from blood | Bernard, 1858 |
| Meyer, 1857 | $O_2$ binds chemically to something in the blood | Blood gas vacuum pump | Ludwig and Setschenow, 1859 |
| Hoppe-Seyler, 1862 | Hemoglobin | | |
| | | Improved blood gas pump | Schmidt, 1867 |
| | | $O_2$, RBC, $CO_2$, plasma | |
| | | Aerotonometer/gas tension | Pfluger, 1872 |
| | | $O_2$ consumption by cells drives $O_2$ uptake by lungs | Pfluger, 1875 |
| Von Hufner, 1894 | Hemoglobin $O_2$–binding capacity | Relation between $Cao_2$ and $Pao_2$ | Bert, 1878 |
| | | Hemataerometer | Bohr, 1885 |
| | | Ferricyanide method for $Cao_2$: 20 mL required | Haldane and Barcroft, 1900 |
| | | S-shaped oxyhemoglobin DC | Bohr, 1903 |
| | | Oxyhemoglobin DC possibly dependent on $CO_2$ tension | Bohr, Krogh, and Hasselbalch, 1904 |
| | | Alveolar $CO_2$ stable, affects ventilation | Haldane and Priestley, 1905 |

**Table 40-1** History of Blood Gas Analysis—cont'd

| Author | Chemistry | Physiology | Author |
|---|---|---|---|
| | | Microtonometer: $O_2$ diffusion in lungs, not active secretion; capillary blood flow | Krogh, 1910 NP |
| | | Acid displaces oxyhemoglobin DC, effect of temperature | Barcroft, 1910 |
| | | Mathematical description of oxyhemoglobin DC | Hill, 1910 |
| Fisher, 1927 NP | Synthesized hemoglobin | Fetal oxyhemoglobin DC left shifted | Barcroft, 1933 |
| Pauling, 1954 NP | Secondary structure of hemoglobin | | |
| | | Slide ruler: $Cao_2$, $Sao_2$ at different pH and temperature | Severinghaus, 1966 |
| | | pH effect mediated by 2,3-DPG in RBC | Benesch and Chanutin, 1967 |

ABG, arterial blood gas; $Cao_2$, arterial oxygen content; DC, dissociation curve; 2,3-DPG, 2,3-diphosphoglycerate; NP, not published; $Paco_2$, arterial carbon dioxide tension; $Pao_2$, arterial oxygen tension; $Pvco_2$, venous carbon dioxide tension; $Pvo_2$, venous oxygen tension; RBC, red blood cell; $Sao_2$, arterial oxygen saturation.

Christian Bohr (1855–1911), with Haldane and Lorraine Smith, improved the tonometer and called it a *hemataerometer*, which served for measurements at high altitude. However, Bohr strongly believed that $O_2$ was actively secreted into the blood by the lungs. August Krogh and his wife and collaborator Marie Krogh finally dispelled this notion through their studies with an improved hemataerometer, which they called a *microtonometer*.[5] According to John Peters (1887–1955), the accuracy of this new tonometer was 4 to 5 mm Hg, double the accuracy of Haldane's device. In 1894, Carl Gustav von Hüfner (1840–1908) established that 1 g hemoglobin bound 1.34 mL of $O_2$ under standardized conditions and using two different methods. Hans Fisher synthesized hemoglobin in 1927, and Linus Pauling later discovered the secondary structure of hemoglobin and the helices of the peptide chains.

In his 1878 book, *La Pression Barometrique*, Paul Bert (1833–1886) showed convincing results from his studies in barometric chambers that high-altitude hypoxia was not the result of low barometric pressure but rather was caused by lack of $O_2$. Bert's curves were the first to show the relationship between $Po_2$ and $O_2$ content. Seven years later, Bohr reproduced this finding; he used dilute hemoglobin solutions and produced hyperbolic curves.

In 1903, Bohr demonstrated that the whole blood dissociation curve was S shaped, and in 1904 Bohr, Krogh, and K. A. Hasselbalch showed that the position of the curve was influenced by the amount of $CO_2$ in the solution.

Haldane later called this dependence the *Bohr effect*. Haldane's best-known publication, written in 1905 with John G. Priestley, showed the stability of alveolar $CO_2$ and its ability to influence ventilation. Barcroft and Haldane's ferrocyanide method to release respiratory gases from blood allowed for greater precision than previous (0.2%) measurements, and in 1910 these investigators showed that pH and temperature influenced the position of the curve. Archibald Hill described the curve mathematically in 1910. Haldane's equation describes the effect of carbon monoxide on the position of the hemoglobin dissociation curve. Barcroft's studies in the early 1930s yielded a left shifted curve for fetal hemoglobin. Several groups of researchers worked on the shape of the standard hemoglobin dissociation curve in the 1950s and 1960s. John W. Severinghaus, in 1966, presented a slide rule "blood gas calculator" that allowed for $O_2$ saturation and content calculation at different temperatures and pH using a standard hemoglobin dissociation curve.

$CO_2$ transport proved more difficult to understand because of the later discovery of essential knowledge.

Svante Arrhenius' concept of ionization came in 1887, but Henderson's equation describing the equilibrium among hydrogen ion, carbonic acid ($H_2CO_3$) or dissolved $CO_2$, and bicarbonate ($HCO_3^-$) was not published until 1908. Hartog Hamburger first showed the presence of chloride ions in the red blood cell, and in 1924, D. D. Van Slyke, H. Wu, and F. C. McLean showed that a chloride shift across the red blood cell membrane occurred at increasing $CO_2$ tensions ($PCO_2$). The existence of carbonic anhydrase was demonstrated in 1932 by N. U. Meldrum and F. J. W. Roughton. This explained the rapid catalysis of $H_2CO_3$ to water and $CO_2$ in the lungs, an unsolved problem at the time, because Carl Faurholt had shown in 1924 that this catalysis was a slow process in plasma. According to Roughton, carbonic anhydrase speeds up the release of $CO_2$ in the lungs some 13,000 times.

In the work eventually leading up to actual pH measurements, Sören P. L. Sörensen introduced the pH concept in 1909, as well as the buffer concept. In 1917, K. A. Hasselbalch converted the Henderson equation to the logarithmic scale (and also converted the dissociation constant by its negative logarithm according to Bjerrum). The result is known as the *Henderson-Hasselbalch equation*. Hasselbalch also used a hydrogen electrode to measure pH and to classify acid-base disorders as either "compensated" or "noncompensated."

Electrochemical measurement of hydrogen ions in a solution was first described in 1823 by A. C. Becquerel. $O_2$ and hydrogen gases were produced, respectively, at the two poles. W. Ostwald realized that the decisive factor was the hydrogen and hydroxide ion concentrations, respectively, and so was able to determine the dissociation constant of water. The *Nernst equation*, based on van't Hoff's and Boyle-Mariotte's laws, permitted calculation of the electromotive force, the driving energy in both gas and liquid cells, according to Ostwald. W. C. Bottger used a hydrogen liquid cell in 1897 to measure changes in acidity for titrations, and in 1900 R. Hober used it in blood for the first time, with erroneous results. Although this setup became feasible after later methodologic modifications were made by Hasselbalch, it remained too difficult for hospitals at the time. The hydrogen gas pH electrode had its problems, particularly for blood; the solution had to be free of $O_2$, it had to be calibrated to a known hydrogen and $CO_2$ pressure, the process was slow, and both oxidizing and reducing agents were able to interfere with the measurement. Fritz Haber constructed a glass pH electrode in 1909, termed the *Haber electrode*. An indirect method for calculation of blood pH, based on measurement of blood $PCO_2$, was suggested by Hasselbalch in 1916, and this yielded more accurate values than direct pH determination. The only trouble was the $PCO_2$ determination was not that easily performed until the advent of Donald Van

Slyke's manometric method,[6] which was based on Pfluger's aerotonometer method. In this method, blood $O_2$ was first purged with ferrocyanide, and acid was added to release the $CO_2$, which then could be measured tonometrically. In the hospital, it was the resident's duty to perform this time-consuming blood gas titration for $CO_2$ when needed.

The Copenhagen poliomyelitis epidemic of 1952 to 1953 produced several thousand victims and an unusually high incidence of bulbar paralysis leading to respiratory failure. The few existing negative pressure (cuirasse) ventilators were not very effective at ventilating patients, and many well-oxygenated patients died of mysterious alkalosis. The anesthesiologist Bjorn Ibsen, however, considered the alkalosis interpretation erroneous and believed that the condition was the result of $CO_2$ retention with high $HCO_3^-$ levels. After a pH determination and repeat $PCO_2$ measurement after adequate ventilation, Ibsen showed his interpretation to be correct, and thereafter patients who showed signs of respiratory paresis were tracheotomized and ventilated with a bag and $CO_2$ lime absorber. Hundreds of medical and dental students from Copenhagen were recruited to hand ventilate the approximately 100 patients who required assisted ventilation around the clock for several weeks. It became clear that respiratory acidosis had been confused with metabolic alkalosis and that $HCO_3^-$ could not be used as the sole parameter to (indirectly) measure pH. Further clarification was thus obtained by Astrup, who measured both pH (using a glass electrode) and $CO_2$ content (using the Van Slyke apparatus) and used the Henderson-Hasselbalch equation to demonstrate the linear relationship between pH and log $PCO_2$. With this method, $PCO_2$ as a guide to ventilation efforts could be deduced from pH measurement using the nomogram. In 3 months, mortality in patients with bulbar paralysis had gone from 90% to 10% as a result of assisted ventilation.

Baird and Hastings introduced the concept of *buffer base* to describe the total amount of base bound to the buffer systems in the blood. The difference between the normal buffer base and measured buffer base (at two different $PCO_2$ values) was later was called the *base excess* (BE). Zero was normal, a negative value was base deficit (excess acid), and a positive value was BE. Based on three pH measurements, one before and two after calibrations, BE could be calculated. Ole Siggaard-Andersen published a nomogram for calculation of BE in 1963.

With the establishment of an "observation room" in the Municipal Hospital in Copenhagen in 1953, Bjorn Ibsen was the first to establish an around-the-clock general intensive care unit.[7] At the time, Ibsen did not perceive this as an important event, and the first publication with data from this unit was not published until 5 years later.[8]

## DEVELOPMENT OF THE PH, Pco₂, AND Po₂ ELECTRODES

After Arrhenius discovered ionization (thus linking chemistry to physics), and Ostwald was able to measure the hydrogen ion concentration using the hydrogen electrode, van't Hoff showed that ions behave osmotically. This discovery enabled Nernst to link the potential to ion activity, which became the basis for the development of the pH, $Pco_2$, and $Po_2$ electrodes.

Not until Hasselbalch improved the hydrogen electrode in 1913, by trapping the $CO_2$ first, could it be used to measure pH in blood or plasma. Practical glass electrodes for pH determination came in the early 1930s, and pH was measured in a room heated to 37°C. What previously had been an exercise in physiologic chemistry became a clinical necessity during the Copenhagen polio epidemic in which the $CO_2$ content was measured using the van Slyke method for calculation of $Pco_2$ to give feedback to the medical students who were hand ventilating hundreds of polio patients. Astrup developed a simpler method by using the pH electrode. After equilibration to $Pco_2$ at 40 mm Hg and to two other $CO_2$ gas mixtures, pH was plotted as a linear function against log $Pco_2$. The three pH points described a line that also gave both $HCO_3^-$ and $Pco_2$. In 1956, Astrup had developed a thermostatically controlled pH glass electrode containing a reference electrode and Van Slyke's method of using mercury to pull blood down past the electrode. Jorgensen and Astrup introduced the term *standard $HCO_3^-$* to describe the $HCO_3^-$ at $Pco_2$ of 40 in oxygenated blood at 38°C, as a measure of the nonrespiratory component of the acid-base state. In 1958, Astrup presented a method to measure blood pH in only 25 μL (one drop of blood), based on the Sanz microtonometer. In 1960, using this apparatus, Siggaard-Andersen presented a pH/log $Pco_2$ diagram at three different hemoglobin levels titrated with nonvolatile acid or base to define what he called the BE, the metabolic component of an acid-base imbalance.[9] He went on to present the *alignment nomogram* for calculating BE and $HCO_3^-$ from pH and $Pco_2$ in 1963. In an attempt to resolve terminology conflicts with some researchers in the United States, Siggaard-Andersen in 1971 published the *acid-base chart*, which was a pH/log $Pco_2$ chart showing expected responses to primary and compensatory acid-base abnormalities.

In 1954, Richard Stow described a $Pco_2$ electrode based on a membrane-covered pH electrode that was sensitive to $Pco_2$ but not to acids or bases. Severinghaus improved this concept by adding an $HCO_3^-$ buffer between the pH electrode and the outside membrane to make the device more stable and sensitive to $Pco_2$. This polarographic electrode became predominant in the automatic blood gas machines developed later. The term *polarography*, coined by Heyrovsky, describes a relationship between applied voltage and the resulting current. Thus, at a constant voltage, the current will vary with the quantity of substance measured or, in the case of gases, its partial pressure.

Early polarographic $O_2$ microelectrodes were described in 1942 by Phillip Davies and Frank Brink at the University of Pennsylvania in Philadelphia. These investigators used platinum, but although tissue $Po_2$ measurements were successful, the electrode quickly became occluded ("poisoned") by protein deposits when it was submerged in blood. In 1953, Leland C. Clark and colleagues solved this problem in their work on extracorporeal oxygenation by covering a platinum electrode with a semipermeable (cellophane) membrane.[10] The first automatic blood gas machine containing a Clark $Po_2$ electrode and a Stow/Severinghaus $Pco_2$ electrode was presented in 1958 by Severinghaus and Bradley.[11] Eventually, a three-electrode machine (pH, $Po_2$, $Pco_2$) was produced by the same team. Work to improve sensitivity and speed and to reduce the need for stirring of blood around the $O_2$ electrode was achieved by reducing the size of the electrode down to 12 to 25 μm. $O_2$ content was measured by a large platinum electrode that consumed all $O_2$ in solution, as described by Hersch in 1952. The first automated three-electrode blood gas machine, the ABL-1 (Radiometer, Copenhagen), came on the market in 1973.

Based on optode technology known since the mid-1970s, blood gas monitors that measure $Po_2$, $Pco_2$, and pH optically have been developed and marketed since the 1990s but are not widely used in the United States. The optode is introduced through a radial artery catheter and performs intermittent samples without removing the patient's blood. This approach also introduces potential problems.[12] With the development of relatively inexpensive point-of-care traditional blood gas machines, turnaround time for a blood gas in the operating room or the intensive care unit is now a few minutes. This obviates some of the apparent advantages of indwelling blood gas monitor catheters.

Optical spectrophotometry in tissues analyzing the hemoglobin $O_2$ saturation was first introduced by L. Nicolai in 1932. The use of two wavelengths of light, one sensitive to saturated hemoglobin and one sensitive to desaturated hemoglobin, was described by K. Matthes in 1935. Glen Millikan suggested the term *oximetry*, which is used to this day. The oximetric earpiece was used for high-altitude unpressurized airplanes, but it was cumbersome and fragile.[2] Fiberoptic oximetry was introduced in the early 1970s in cardiac catheters. The pulse oximeter was developed by Takuo Aoyagi in 1972 for use on the finger, and it remains the standard of care in critical care medicine and many other clinical situations.[13]

Normal ranges for the arterial blood gas (sea level, inspired $O_2$ fraction [$FiO_2$] of 0.21) are as follows:

pH: 7.35 to 7.45
Arterial partial pressure of $CO_2$ ($PaCO_2$): 35 to 45 mm Hg
Arterial partial pressure of $O_2$ ($PaO_2$): 70 to 100 mm Hg
$SaO_2$: 93% to 98%
$HCO_3^-$: 22 to 26 mmol/L
Base deficit: +2.0 to −2.0

## ASSESSMENT OF OXYGENATION

### Arterial Oxygenation: Air to Pulmonary Capillary

In *dry air* at sea level, the $PO_2$ is 20.93% of 760 mm Hg, or 159 mm Hg. Before the $O_2$ reaches the alveoli, it is diluted by airway *water vapor pressure*:

$$(P_{H_2O}\ 47\ \text{mm Hg at } 37°C) \text{ to } [760 - 47] \times 20.93\% = 149\ \text{mm Hg}$$

At increasing altitude, the barometric pressure drops in a linear fashion, finally to equal that of water vapor pressure at 63,000 ft (19 km). The alveolar $PO_2$ and $PCO_2$ at this altitude are then zero. For a glimpse of the physiology of high altitude, see the later discussion of extreme exposure; for a more in-depth view, see Hultgren's text.[14] Hyperbaric exposure is complicated by physical changes of gases, gas toxicity, and tissue solubility, as well as physiologic changes. These topics are comprehensively dealt with in Brubakk and Neuman's text of hyperbaric medicine for physicians.[15]

Factors that influence alveolar $O_2$ tension ($PaO_2$) include $FiO_2$, barometric pressure ($PB$), alveolar ventilation, and $O_2$ uptake. The simplified formula for the *alveolar gas equation* is as follows:

$$PaO_2 = FiO_2\ [PB - P_{H_2O}] - PaCO_2/R$$

The R in this equation is the respiratory exchange ratio, which is $CO_2$ production (200 mL) divided by $VO_2$ (250 mL). This ratio is usually close to 0.8 for most clinical purposes, although it may vary slightly with nutritional content. Just like water vapor pressure, the addition of a third gas (e.g., an inert anesthetic gas) will have a dilutional effect on the alveolar $O_2$ pressure during gas off-loading. In essence, during air breathing, the $PaO_2$ in a normal lung is 100 mm Hg, and this results in a $PaO_2$ of approximately 95 mm Hg.

$O_2$ diffuses into the lung capillary, where the red blood cell is rapidly loaded with $O_2$ already one third way of the pulmonary capillary. The normal alveolar-arterial $PO_2$ difference ($PA\text{-}aO_2$) is usually less than 15 mm Hg, it but can rise with age to 35 to 40 mm Hg even in apparently healthy adults secondary to the combined effects of age-related changes in diffusion and ventilation-perfusion (V/Q) inequalities within the normal lung. In theory, in the normal lung, there is a range of V/Q ratios dependent on gravity and lung compliance such that the upper lung portions are relatively overventilated and underperfused, whereas the opposite is true for the dependent lung portions.

Diffusing capacity of the lung was first studied by Marie Krogh, who used carbon monoxide, and it became more widely known in 1955 with the publication of an article by Bates.[16] A simplified law for this diffusion is *Fick's law of diffusion*, which describes the diffusion rate as a product of diffusion gradient, surface area, and temperature divided by distance and the square root of the gas molecular weight. Diseases in which diffusion becomes limiting are uncommon, but they can be exemplified by alveolar fibrosis. Early work on V/Q mismatch was done during World War II by the physiologists W. Fenn, H. Rahn, A. Otis, and R. Riley. Riley's three-compartment model of the lung became the gold standard in patient assessment. It was not until 1974 that the multiple inert gas elimination technique was presented, known today as the *Wagner West method*,[17] and it remains the standard in research of V/Q inequality. A meta-analysis of 12 studies noted that $PaO_2$ decreases linearly with age according to the following formula:

$$102 - 0.33 \times \text{age in years}$$

with 95% confidence limits of ±10 mm Hg.[18]

Hypoxic pulmonary vasoconstriction helps to minimize the effect of V/Q mismatching. Many anesthetic gases reduce this protective reflex and produce increased shunting. Shunting greater than 20% to 25% has a devastating effect on arterial oxygenation because additional $O_2$ has little effect on $PaO_2$.

An alternate descriptor is the $PaO_2/PaO_2$ *ratio*, which is less dependent on V/Q matching and $FiO_2$ than the $PA\text{-}aO_2$. It may be thus be preferable as an index of gas exchange to predict a $PaO_2$ response to a change in $FiO_2$.[19] The $PaO_2/FiO_2$ *ratio* is easier to calculate but does not include the $PaCO_2$ factor. When this ratio is less than 200, it has been reported to correlate with shunt greater than 20%.[20] The *respiratory index* $PA\text{-}aO_2/PaO_2$ was developed in an attempt to minimize the problems associated with $PA\text{-}aO_2$.[21]

### Oxygen Content

The formula for calculating *arterial $O_2$ content* ($CaO_2$) describes $O_2$ transport in blood as both bound to hemoglobin and dissolved in plasma. This latter fraction is very small in normobaric and hypobaric conditions and depends on the $P_{O_2}$:

$$CaO_2 \text{ [mL/100 mL blood]} = \text{Hemoglobin} \\ \text{[g/100 mL]} \times 1.306 \times SaO_2 + 0.003 \times \\ PaO_2 \text{ [mm Hg] at } 37°C$$

When one is breathing air at sea level, the plasma-carried $O_2$ part is 0.25 to 0.30 mL/100 mL blood, whereas it increases to 2 mL/100 mL when one breathes 100% $O_2$ at sea level and to 6 mL/100 mL at 3 atmospheres of $O_2$ breathing. The hemoglobin-carried part of $O_2$ in a physiologically normal person who is breathing air is closer to 20 mL/100 mL blood, which resembles the $O_2$ content in air. In hyperbaric conditions, the plasma part alone may then become sufficient for normal arteriovenous $O_2$ extraction, at least in resting conditions. $O_2$ solubility increases with decreasing temperature. All $O_2$ in transit will be in the plasma phase at one point, but $O_2$ has low plasma solubility and will transit faster through the lipid phase of cell membranes than through plasma. *Venous $O_2$ content* is calculated using the same formula and data from a venous sample.

The major portion of $O_2$ content is described by the first part of the formula, with each gram of hemoglobin carrying a (theoretical) maximal 1.39 mL of $O_2$. Until 1963, this value was believed to be 1.34, Hüfner's number based on his measurements in 1894. In 1974, it was suggested that the true numbers are 1.306 for adults and 1.312 for fetal blood.[22] Today, 1.306 is usually used for adults. A few hemoglobin molecules do not carry $O_2$ for various reasons, such as those in which the iron molecule ($Fe^{2+}$) has become oxidized ($Fe^{3+}$) to methemoglobin or binds with carbon monoxide to form carboxyhemoglobin.

It was Christian Bohr who first discovered the sigmoidal shape of the hemoglobin-$O_2$ dissociation curve and, also in 1904, in collaboration with K. A. Hasselbalch and A. Krogh, observed the influence of $CO_2$ on the position of the curve. The influence of $CO_2$ on the position of the curve was shown by Sir J. Barcroft in 1914 to be essentially a pH effect.[23] Hasselbalch reported in 1967 that 2,3-diphosphoglycerate (2,3-DPG) was the mediator of the pH effect in the red blood cell. Barcroft started using the $O_2$ half-saturation pressure of hemoglobin ($P_{50}$) to describe the position of the curve as reproducibility improved in his laboratory. The 1910 *Hill plot* described the middle portion of the rectilinear curve (between 10% and 95% saturation) of $O_2$ saturation versus $O_2$ content. The normal human hemoglobin at standard conditions has a $P_{50}$ of 26 mm Hg. Various abnormal hemoglobins with either higher or lower than normal $P_{50}$ have been described. For example, thalassemia carriers have a left-shifted hemoglobin-$O_2$ dissociation

curve caused by the abnormal presence of fetal hemoglobin in adults.

$O_2$ saturation varies with hemoglobin affinity for $O_2$,[24] owing to the interaction of the following factors: 2,3-DPG, pH (Bohr effect), $P_{CO_2}$ (Haldane effect[25]), and temperature. In the tissues, increasing $P_{CO_2}$, decreasing pH, and increasing temperature facilitate $O_2$ off-loading, as does increased 2,3-DPG. In the lung, the opposite conditions facilitate $O_2$ loading onto hemoglobin. Although 2,3-DPG has been known as a powerful allosteric modifier of hemoglobin $O_2$ affinity (and thus $P_{50}$),[26,27] situations in which this may be clinically important are still elusive,[28,29] with the exception of blood banking. In old bank blood, in which 2,3-DPG levels after 2 weeks are effectively zero, it takes the transfused cells 7 hours to reach 50% and 48 hours to reach normal 2,3-DPG levels (12 µmol/g hemoglobin).[30] This situation should not cause tissue hypoxia, except perhaps in patients with massive transfusion. In chronic anemia, increased 2,3-DPG levels help to off-load $O_2$ at the tissue level.

The question whether these lateral displacements of the hemoglobin-$O_2$ dissociation curve are large enough to matter clinically was addressed by Kelman and Nunn.[31] It appears that the clinically most significant lateral displacement is by $P_{CO_2}$, the Bohr effect. Temperature and 2,3-DPG changes usually result in $P_{50}$ changes of smaller magnitude. Today, automated blood gas machines calculate the $SaO_2$ from a measured $P_{O_2}$ using correction factors for temperature, pH, and BE, as opposed to the co-oximeter, which measures it directly in a blood sample.

## Global Oxygen Delivery and Oxygen Consumption

Global $O_2$ delivery ($DO_2$) can be calculated using the following formula:

$$DO_2 = CaO_2 \times CO$$

where cardiac output (CO) commonly is measured using a pulmonary artery catheter. Cardiac index is calculated by dividing CO with the body surface area. To increase $DO_2$, manipulation of CO usually has the highest impact. If hemoglobin drops from 15 to 14, $DO_2$ will decrease 69 mL/L. A 1% decrease in $SaO_2$ changes $DO_2$ 10 mL/L, whereas a 1-L decrease in CO decreases $DO_2$ 200 mL/L, other factors being constant (hemoglobin, 15; $SaO_2$, 100%; CO, 5 L). Normal $DO_2$ (550 to 720 mL/minute/$m^2$) does not imply that all cells are free to extract this $O_2$. That depends on the local flow regulation in the tissues, influenced by tissue perfusion pressure and baroreceptor reflex activity (in hypotensive situations), as well as local factors such as the balance between vasodilators (e.g., prostacyclin and nitric oxide) and vasoconstrictors (e.g., endothelin-1). Organs with high metabolic activity (e.g., heart, brain, liver) thus regulate perfusion to meet their metabolic demands, whereas organs with low metabolic activity (e.g., resting skeletal muscle) have only intermittent perfusion.

Global $Vo_2$ can be calculated by using the following formula:

$$Vo_2 = CO \times C(a\text{-}v)o_2$$

where $C(a\text{-}v)o_2$ is the arteriovenous $O_2$ content difference (according to Fick). Global $Vo_2$ can also be calculated using a metabolic cart (indirect calorimetry) in which inspired and expired $O_2$ content are measured. In the Fick type of analysis, the $Vo_2$ of the lungs is not included in the calculations because mixed venous blood is drawn from the pulmonary artery catheter before it passes through the lungs. In contrast, indirect calorimetry includes lung $Vo_2$. Theoretically, the difference between these two methods could be used to calculate lung $Vo_2$, but in reality, this approach is technically demanding and problematic because of high variability. Global $Vo_2$ is just that, a single number that does not consider individual organ differences in flow and $O_2$ extraction or their relative contribution. Thus, $Vo_2$ cannot be used to assess individual organ function. Normal $Vo_2$ is 100 to 180 mL/minute/m$^2$. The $O_2$ extraction ratio is calculated by using the following formula:

$$O_2 \text{ extraction} = Vo_2/Do_2$$

The normal value is 22% to 30%.

$O_2$ stores in the body during air breathing have been calculated to be approximately 1550 mL: 450 mL in the lung, 850 mL in the blood, and 250 mL dissolved or bound in tissues. Although breathing 100% $O_2$ increases these stores to 4250 mL, most of the increase results from filling the functional residual capacity with $O_2$. This process increases the lung stores to 3000 mL, the blood stores to 950 mL, and the tissue stores to 300 mL. Preoxygenation before induction of anesthesia, or before planned endotracheal intubation in the intensive care unit, therefore significantly increases the time before desaturation in the event of intubation or ventilation problems.

## Oxygen Extraction

Theoretically, by comparing arterial and venous $O_2$ content for a particular organ, it becomes clear that the organ in question has extracted the difference between the two. To calculate the organ's $Vo_2$, organ $O_2$ content as well as blood flow must be known. By extension, if the extraction is within the normal range, the $Vo_2$ is normal, and presumably organ oxygenation should be normal. This concept may hold true for a single organ, but is it true for the whole body? It is often assumed to be, but although the numbers may be within the normal range, the patient may still exhibit signs of organ failure resulting from poor organ blood flow in a particular organ. Whole body numbers of oxygenation therefore cannot be used to predict the oxygenation state of individual organs reliably. A better measure of organ oxygenation is tissue oxygenation, which is unfortunately rarely available in the clinical setting.

Mixed venous saturation ($Svo_2$) is often used as an indicator of whole body $O_2$ extraction. When $Svo_2$ is low, this finding is interpreted as representative of high $O_2$ extraction. A decrease in $Svo_2$ from the normal 65% to 75% (in patients without anemia) to less than 55% is used as a clinical sign of increased $O_2$ extraction, a sign of too little $Do_2$ in relation to metabolic demands. The clinical availability of pulmonary artery catheters with continuous $Svo_2$ monitoring has also been shown to be valuable for monitoring early resuscitation in septic patients.[32] Increased cerebral blood flow is known to counteract cerebral hypoxia, and similarly, a jugular bulb $Svo_2$ catheter is sometimes used to monitor brain $O_2$ extraction.

An additional interesting use of $Svo_2$ monitoring is to follow the perioperative liver transplant recipient. At the beginning of the operation, the function of the old liver is usually so poor that $Svo_2$ is approximately 90%, significantly higher than normal, a finding indicating that the liver normally contributes significantly to total body $Vo_2$. Once the new donor liver is in place and is working, the $O_2$ extraction increases, and $Svo_2$ decreases toward the normal range. Therefore, in that situation, $Svo_2$ can be used as an indicator of good function of the donor liver.

## Hypoxemia and Oxygen Deficit

In hypoxemic patients, the most common pulmonary (or central) causes of hypoxemia include hypoventilation, V/Q mismatch, and diffusion problems. Hypoxemia reduces $Sao_2$ as calculated in the $Do_2$ formula above. Severe anemia reduces $Cao_2$ but not $Sao_2$. Cardiac causes of hypoxemia include those resulting in low CO. On the $Vo_2$ side is the metabolic rate, which is not only organ specific but also temperature dependent. Respiratory failure may lead to high energy expenditure that is out of proportion for ventilation. Sepsis and the systemic inflammatory response may lead to cellular metabolic abnormalities related to higher than normal $Do_2$ requirements and may thus be associated with relative tissue hypoxia without pronounced hypoxemia. The exact events behind these findings remain to be elucidated.

Hypoxemia is frequently *defined* as a $Pao_2$ of less than 80 mm Hg, but more serious hypoxemia is seen with a

$PaO_2$ of less than 60 mm Hg. $SaO_2$ has then dropped to 90%. A further drop in $PaO_2$ to 40 mm Hg can be called severe because a concomitant tissue oxygenation deficit appears focally, at least in high-extraction tissues such as heart, liver, and brain. Loss of consciousness can be expected as $PO_2$ decreases acutely to less than 30 mm Hg. At the cellular level, the $O_2$ deficit will, if severe enough, lead to depletion of high-energy compounds (adenosine triphosphate [ATP]) with accumulation of adenosine diphosphate, accumulation of reduced nicotinamide adenine dinucleotide (NADH), and lactic acid (owing to activation of 6-phosphofructokinase–associated glycolysis). ATP-dependent membrane pumps become unable to maintain intracellular potassium levels, and this situation leads to membrane depolarization. This condition allows extracellular calcium to enter the cell, thus leading to activation of several enzymatic systems (e.g., phospholipase A), with further amplification of cellular injury and production of cytokines.

Hypoxemia can be acute or chronic and can have a variety of causes. A common sign of hypoxemia is cyanosis of the lips and fingers. Cyanosis appears in patients who have more than 5 g of reduced hemoglobin/100 mL of capillary blood.[33] Therefore, in severe anemia, cyanosis may be difficult to detect visually. In the absence of anemia, cyanosis is usually detected in 50% of patients with an $SaO_2$ of 93%; in 95% of patients with an $SaO_2$ of 89%,[34] the diagnosis of cyanosis is missed in 5%. Pulse oximetry ($SpO_2$) is therefore a valuable clinical monitor of $SaO_2$. Confounding situations occur when methemoglobinemia is higher than 1.5g/100 mL; in these patients, the skin may appear bluish gray.

Acute hypoxemia elicits *compensatory responses* for protection of tissue function. The most common response consists of increased capillary perfusion and $O_2$ extraction. Hyperventilation, by stimulation of the respiratory center in the medulla, is a relatively late response when $PaO_2$ is lower than 52 mm Hg. Hyperventilation increases on further $PaO_2$ reduction. Improved matching of perfusion to ventilated areas of the lung is a result of increased pulmonary arterial pressure. Increased CO improves organ perfusion. Catecholamine release is increased, initially by a reflex response and then followed by the release of circulating catecholamines. Hemoglobin concentration increases only in long-term exposure to hypoxia, such as at high altitude, in chronic respiratory disease, or in breath-holding free divers. A right-shifted hemoglobin-$O_2$ dissociation curve caused by increased 2,3-DPG production and acidosis may also be present.

## When $PaO_2$ and $SaO_2$ Do Not Appear to Correlate

In the blood gas machine, $SaO_2$ is calculated from the measured $PaO_2$. Situations in which calculated $SaO_2$ does not adequately reflect the $PaO_2$ occur when the $CaO_2$ is low.

In contrast, the co-oximeter uses four wavelengths to measure and distinguish among the $SaO_2$, carboxyhemoglobin, methemoglobin, and hemoglobin content. In severe anemia, in carbon monoxide poisoning, or in severe methemoglobinemia, the amount of $O_2$ ($CaO_2$) carried on the available $O_2$-binding hemoglobin decreases dramatically. Thus, although the saturation of hemoglobin may appear high, less than normal $O_2$ is actually transported on hemoglobin to the tissues, and the patient may develop signs of tissue hypoxia. Endogenous nitric oxide and certain drugs (e.g., prilocaine, benzocaine, nitrates, dapsone) are well known to cause methemoglobin transformation. Although endogenous reductase systems slowly reconvert methemoglobin to hemoglobin, elevated methemoglobin levels (>15%) can, in an emergency, be treated with methylene blue (1 to 2 mg/kg). The diagnosis is established by co-oximeter. The pulse oximeter shows falsely high values.

Hemoglobin's affinity for carbon monoxide is 230 times greater than that for $O_2$. Nonsmokers usually have a carboxyhemoglobin content of less than 1.5% as a result of air pollution and passive smoking. Carboxyhemoglobin can increase after accidental smoke inhalation or, to a lesser degree, in heavy smokers (2% to 12%). The available hemoglobin for $O_2$ transport is then reduced, and worse, reduced 2,3-DPG levels cause a left shift of the hemoglobin-$O_2$ dissociation curve. Carboxyhemoglobin levels higher than 3% may impair patients with coronary artery disease, and those levels greater than 5% limit exercise tolerance and vigilance in healthy persons. Values higher than 50% have been associated with coma and death. Because the pulse oximeter cannot distinguish clearly between oxyhemoglobin and carboxyhemoglobin, the $SpO_2$ shows falsely high values. The diagnosis is made by co-oximeter. Treatment is with 100% $O_2$ or hyperbaric $O_2$ if available. In cyanide poisoning, cellular energy metabolism is blocked, so tissue hypoxia may be seen in association with high $PaO_2$ and $SaO_2$ values.

## Venous Blood Gases

The normal mixed venous blood gas values (sea level, $FiO_2$ 0.21, at rest) are as follows:

pH: 7.32 to 7.41
$PCO_2$: 42 to 52 mm Hg
$PO_2$: 35 to 40 mm Hg
$SvO_2$: 65% to 75%
$HCO_3^-$: 24 to 28 mmol/L

Venous $PO_2$ ($PvO_2$) cannot be used to predict $PaO_2$ because $O_2$ extraction is variable. Conversely, mixed venous gases can be used together with the arterial value to calculate the arteriovenous $CaO_2$ difference, $C(a-v)O_2$, describing tissue $O_2$ extraction. Even though the other parameters in the venous blood gas have a predictable statistical correlation with the arterial blood gas, limits of agreements are generally too wide to be used clinically as a substitute for an arterial blood gas determination.

## The Elusive Tissue Oxygenation

The gradual drop in $O_2$ pressure from that in ambient air down to that in cellular mitochondria (close to 0 mm Hg) is sometimes referred to as the $O_2$ cascade. The high $O_2$ gradient required for adequate $DO_2$ to sustain $VO_2$, and ultimately tissue function, is in contrast to that of $CO_2$, and it reflects the low plasma solubility and hemoglobin transport of $O_2$. Therefore, what the clinician would really like to know is the patient's tissue or cellular oxygenation, but it usually has to be inferred based on blood gases and other indirect indices relating to tissue function. Such indices include mixed $PvO_2$, $O_2$ extraction, neurologic signs of intact cerebral function, urine output, and intact cardiac and liver function.

Newer methods to measure tissue oxygenation in the laboratory setting have potential, however, and technologies used for this purpose are briefly compared later.[35] These methods may involve measurement of $PO_2$ or of the local concentration of $O_2$. They may also entail determinations of indirect events believed to be related to the local availability of $O_2$. The local $PO_2$ may be more closely related to $O_2$ diffusion (and therefore local $O_2$ solubility), whereas the local $O_2$ concentration may be more closely related to local $VO_2$ by chemical reactions. All these technologies have underlying assumptions that can influence the validity of the measurements.

Although tissue oxygenation varies from point to point in a particular tissue (basically describing the pathway of $O_2$ diffusion from arterioles and capillaries to the mitochondria), a range or distribution of tissue $O_2$ pressures will best describe the state of tissue oxygenation at a given time. Because of variable metabolic state and blood flow rates, different organs have different normal ranges or $O_2$ pressure distributions, as measured by tissue $O_2$ probes. Exact determination of the presence of tissue hypoxia has been problematic and requires other simultaneous measurements of tissue or cellular function.

The *polarographic* probes require invasive techniques and are not suitable for routine clinical measurements. Both single-point needle-type electrodes and surface-type multielectrodes have been used for this purpose. These probes remain the gold standard for tissue $O_2$ measurement, and they also have the highest resolution, depending on their size.

*Near-infrared spectroscopy* can be used noninvasively to determine the state of oxygenation of hemoglobin and cytochrome $a_3$ (e.g., brain), but this technique has suffered from interference from blood flow in other tissues (scalp), as well as from issues with calibration and defining normal range. Resolution is $10^2$ to $10^3$ lower than with polarography.

*Phosphorescence and fluorescence* methods based on redox states or $O_2$ quenching have fairly high resolution and can give information on intracellular oxygenation. However, they require optode placement in or on tissues. Resolution is 10 times lower than with polarography. *Electron paramagnetic resonance oximetry*, which is based on solid particles or soluble materials, requires administration of materials but has much lower resolution than polarography. Electron paramagnetic resonance oximetry can cause minimal heating of tissues and has limited penetration. *Nuclear magnetic resonance (NMR) spectroscopy* is a more indirect technique for monitoring $O_2$-related events. It has more limited sensitivity, but measurements do not disturb the events measured. The equipment is widely available. NMR use for perfluorocarbon relaxation, proton NMR spectra of myoglobin, NMR Overhauser effect, and NMR Bold effect are other methods with lower resolution that are under investigation. Problems with these complex methods include the difficulty of defining the exact resolution of the technique (what is being measured), as well as penetration and calibration issues.

To define cellular hypoxia based on measurements of tissue oxygenation presents considerable difficulty because most of these data come from research laboratories under specific conditions (e.g., anesthetized animals). Muscle is very resistant to hypoxemia, and critical $PO_2$ values in intact muscle cells are probably in the range of 3 to 10 mm Hg (close to end-capillary values), whereas isolated mitochondria can function at levels as low as 0.1 mm Hg.[36] This number appears to be higher for the brain, because unconsciousness usually appears when jugular vein $PO_2$ drops to less than 20 mm Hg. Significant additional research is required to understand the pathophysiology of cellular and tissue function adequately as related to $O_2$ as well as to the development of noninvasive monitoring for the clinical setting.

## Assessment of Ventilation

### Carbon Dioxide Transport in Blood

As the end product of aerobic metabolism, $PcO_2$ is highest in the mitochondria; it diffuses in venous blood and is transported to the pulmonary capillaries, where normal $PcO_2$ is 46 mm Hg. The diffusion gradient out to the alveoli is determined by the equilibrium between $CO_2$ production and alveolar ventilation. $PaCO_2$ has essentially the same $PcO_2$ as the alveolar gas, 40 mm Hg in physiologically normal persons. In water solution, $CO_2$ hydrates to form $H_2CO_3$, facilitated by carbonic anhydrase present in the red blood cells and in the pulmonary endothelium (but not in plasma).

$H_2CO_3$ dissociates rapidly to $HCO_3^-$ and hydrogen ion. Carried in part by hemoglobin as carbaminohemoglobin, $HCO_3$ contributes to the Haldane effect. $CO_2$ is transported in three forms: as physically dissolved (8.3%), as $HCO_3^-$ (62.6%), or as bound to predominantly reduced hemoglobin (carbaminohemoglobin) (29.1%). $HCO_3^-$ formed within the red blood cell is then rapidly exchanged for chloride by an enzyme known as Band 3, thus allowing the dissociation of $H_2CO_3$ to continue.

The relationships between pH and $P_{CO_2}$, as described by Astrup and later by Siggaard-Andersen, are discussed earlier. Changes in $PaCO_2$ result in a new steady-state pH. The plasma level of $CO_2$ depends on the balance between its production and its elimination. Because metabolic activities are tissue specific, venous $P_{CO_2}$ ($PvCO_2$) from a specific organ will vary depending on the metabolic rate of that tissue, as will its perfusion. The mixed $PvCO_2$ is therefore a flow-weighted average of all perfused tissues. Normally, the resulting $CO_2$ output through the lungs is approximately 200 mL/minute. Factors that may alter $CO_2$ production include changes in temperature (10% per degree), muscular activity (three to five times), stress, systemic inflammatory response syndrome, and overfeeding (of glucose).

## $PaCO_2$ and Alveolar Ventilation

Alveolar $CO_2$ is determined by the $CO_2$ output and alveolar ventilation, assuming that inspired $CO_2$ is close to zero. If dead space increases, inspired $CO_2$ may not be close to zero. When $CO_2$ output is stable, alveolar ventilation becomes the main determinant of alveolar $CO_2$. Alveolar ventilation itself is determined by dead space, tidal volume, and respiratory frequency. Total ventilation is the sum of dead space and alveolar ventilation.

## Dead-Space Ventilation

Sudden changes in dead space may occur with rapidly deteriorating CO, large pulmonary emboli, lung compliance change resulting from or related to acute lung injury, or the institution of mechanical ventilation. When dead-space ventilation increases, alveolar ventilation needs to be increased to maintain alveolar $P_{CO_2}$ constant. Normal dead space volume is 2 mL/kg.

## Minute Volume Ventilation and $PaCO_2$

Increasing minute volume ventilation without decreasing $PaCO_2$ should raise the possibility of increased dead space as a possible explanation. Another possibility is a defective lime filter in an anesthesia ventilator circuit, which could raise inspired $CO_2$ levels and thereby the alveolar and the arterial $CO_2$. Conversely, an exaggerated $PaCO_2$ decrease for a relatively small increase in minute volume ventilation suggests decreased $CO_2$ output or depleted $CO_2$ stores. Because $CO_2$ is produced in the body, is water soluble, and dissociates relatively rapidly, $CO_2$ stores are large (120 L in adult), and changes in $PaCO_2$ will take 20 to 30 minutes to reach steady state. Steady state is reached faster in high-perfusion tissues than in low-perfusion tissues such as bone and fat.

## Arterial End-Tidal $P_{CO_2}$ Gradient

Normally, the arterial to end-tidal $CO_2$ difference is 6 mm Hg. It increases mainly in obstructive lung disease and in severe cardiac dysfunction. In lung disease with slow alveolar emptying, the end-tidal $CO_2$ increases but does not reach a plateau at the end of exhalation. In cardiac disease, poor pulmonary perfusion (but a normal emptying pattern) produces a normal end-tidal flat-top curve, but with a larger than normal gradient.

## Acute Respiratory Failure

Acute respiratory failure with an increasing $PaCO_2$ from 40 to 80 mm Hg results in a corresponding decrease in pH from 7.40 to 7.20. In general, blood gas analysis from this type of patient shows a $P_{CO_2}$ greater than 45 mm Hg, a pH of less than 7.35, and $HCO_3^-$ and BE within the normal range. This finding is the typical picture of acute respiratory acidosis. The reason for this condition can vary from drug-induced hypoventilation to acute neurologic conditions to pulmonary or cardiac dysfunction. Hypoxemia varies with the underlying cause. Symptoms depend on the presentation and on the degree of hypoxemia and hypercapnia. The typical presentation of hypoxemic respiratory failure is severe dyspnea with accessory muscle use, tachycardia, hypertension, diaphoresis, and mental status changes. Worsening status and arterial blood gases are often interpreted as impending ventilatory failure. Options for ventilatory support should be considered on an emergency basis.

Hyperventilation can occur in response to hypoxemia, but it is also seen without hypoxemia in pronounced metabolic acidosis (Kussmaul's breathing in diabetes) and in intracranial dysfunction. This condition leads to respiratory alkalosis with a pH greater than 7.45 and a $PaCO_2$ lower than 35 mm Hg. Additionally, the anxious or painful patient may show signs of treatable hyperventilation. Confounding clinical situations can be associated with tissue hypoxia related to a low amount of transported $O_2$, such as in methemoglobinemia, carbon monoxide poisoning, and severe anemia. In chronic hyperventilation, pH normalizes over time as a result of renal compensation, but $PaCO_2$ remains lower than 35 mm Hg.

## Chronic Carbon Dioxide Retainer

Renal compensation of respiratory acidosis is by increased urinary excretion of hydrogen ions and resorption of $HCO_3^-$. This relatively slow process occurs over several days. Slowly, pH reaches low normal values, but $HCO_3^-$ levels and BE are increased. This is the situation of the patient with chronic respiratory failure. Pulmonary patients usually have chronic obstructive pulmonary disease or restrictive pulmonary disease, or they are morbidly obese. Increased $CO_2$ stores are the rule, and the normal respiratory drive to $PaCO_2$ is obtunded. This group of patients is sensitive to $O_2$ supplementation because respiratory drive is predominantly determined by hypoxemia. Patients with a $PaO_2$ in the mid-50s and a $PaCO_2$ at the same level usually receive home $O_2$ treatment, initially at night to reduce pulmonary hypertension and to relieve dyspnea. When the chronic $CO_2$ retainer develops an acute respiratory problem and pH levels fall to less than 7.20, noninvasive ventilatory assistance is usually indicated.

## Extreme Exposure

At extreme altitude, hypoxemia-induced hyperventilation ($PaO_2 < 52$) reduces $PaCO_2$ significantly, and consequently $PaO_2$ will increase according to the alveolar gas equation (see earlier). For example, at the peak of Mt. Everest (28,028 ft), the barometric pressure is 253 mm Hg, but the water vapor pressure remains constant at 47 mm Hg. Because of extreme hyperventilation, $PaCO_2$ is 7.5 mm Hg, inspired $PO_2$ is 43 mm Hg (calculated $PaO_2$ should be 33.6), and measured $PaO_2$ is 28 mm Hg, whereas $SaO_2$ is higher than expected at 70%, as a result of severe respiratory alkalosis and left shift of the hemoglobin-$O_2$ association curve. Given time, renal compensation will correct some of the alkalosis. Hultgren provides a more in-depth discussion of this topic.[14]

## ARTERIAL BLOOD GAS ASSESSMENT IN RESUSCITATION

In a resuscitation situation, pulmonary blood flow determines oxygenation and $CO_2$ excretion, and the normal arteriovenous $PCO_2$ gradient is 3 to 10 times larger than normal, which is 5 to 8 mm Hg. Thus, respiratory acidosis is common in these patients. Inadequate tissue perfusion leads to lactic acidosis after 10 to 15 minutes of resuscitation, particularly if the liver is underperfused and unable to metabolize lactate to $CO_2$. An $HCO_3^-$ deficit develops parallel to metabolic acidosis. A pH lower than 7.20 is a poor prognostic sign. Mixed venous blood may be the most appropriate mirror of the acid-base status in this situation. $PaO_2$ is usually high because 100% $O_2$ is generally used for resuscitation; however, it can be low in patients with significant shunting or dead-space ventilation. Right main stem intubation or pneumothorax or hematothorax may be present to explain this latter situation. Massive aspiration pneumonia usually does not develop until 1 or 2 days after aspiration and rarely explains the acute, severe shunting, except when large food particles obstruct a bronchial lumen. In these situations, $PCO_2$ may also be elevated, and chest radiography can be helpful.

## PERMISSIVE HYPERCAPNIA

To date, there are no randomized controlled trials that support improved clinical outcomes using permissive hypercapnia. However, in several smaller trials of lung-protective strategy using small tidal volumes, permissive hypercapnia was a direct consequence of the approach,[37,38] and it was part of the treatment strategy. In the trial sponsored by the Acute Respiratory Distress Syndrome Network of the National Institutes of Health, permissive hypercapnia was not used, however.[39] Animal models showed that the protective effect may include inhibition of xanthine oxidase, known to produce $O_2$ free radicals.[40] Furthermore, buffering of hypercapnic acidosis worsens acute lung injury.[41] It appears that pH greater than 7.25 and $PaCO_2$ in the range of 50 to 60 mm Hg range are well tolerated by most patients, with the possible exception of patients with high intracranial pressure.

## TEMPERATURE CORRECTION OF ARTERIAL BLOOD GAS

When a blood gas sample from a hypothermic patient is analyzed at 37°C, pH rises at 0.015/°C, whereas $PCO_2$ falls 4.5%/°C. Measurements of ventricular irritability and myocardial contractility suggest that the heart is safe at high pH and low $PCO_2$. Investigations in poikilothermic animals showed that normal pH increased 0.015/°C with falling body temperatures. Why the ratio of OH- to hydrogen ions remains constant at 16:1 across the temperature range is not well understood,[42] but investigators have proposed that the charge affects protein dissociation (in particular the peptide-linked histidine imidazole groups).[43] Historically, two approaches have been used to manage the hypothermic patient under cardiopulmonary bypass. The *alpha-stat* approach lets pH rise to alkalosis for the foregoing reasons, whereas the *pH-stat* approach tries to keep pH stable by adding more $CO_2$

and thus avoiding the effect of too much hyperventilation on cerebral perfusion. This area is controversial, and data in support of either approach are limited (see also Chapter 14). pH-stat management has been associated with decreased myocardial contractility during rewarming while presumedly better preserving cerebral perfusion.

In addition, lower temperature increases $O_2$ solubility in plasma as well as hemoglobin $O_2$ affinity, as characterized by a left shift of the hemoglobin-$O_2$ dissociation curve. The combined effect is to decrease $Po_2$ but not the $O_2$ content. In the blood gas machine, all analyses are conducted at 37°C. At present, no data appear to suggest that temperature-corrected values are more useful than 37°C values, partly because acid-base balance is best judged at 37°C,[44] and partly because oxygenation is also best evaluated at normal temperature. It also addresses the issues of erroneous patient temperature and of confusion about whether values are temperature corrected.

## REFERENCES

1. Astrup P, Severinghaus JW: The History of Blood Gases, Acids and Bases. Copenhagen: Munksgaard, 1986.
2. West JB: A century of pulmonary gas exchange. Am J Respir Crit Care Med 2004;169:897–902.
3. Hürter: Untersuchungen am arteriellen menschlichen Blute. Deutsch Arch Klin Med 1912;108:1–34.
4. Magnus HG: Über die im blute enthaltene Gase, Sauerstoffe, Stickstoff und Kohlensäure. Ann Phys Chem (Leipzig) 1837;12:583–606.
5. Krogh A: On the oxygen-metabolism of the blood. Scand Arch Physiol 1910;23:192–199.
6. Van Slyke DD, Neill, JM: The determination of blood gases in blood and other solutions by vacuum extraction and manometric measurement. J Biol Chem 1924;61:523–573.
7. Berthelsen PG, Cronqvist M: The first intensive care unit in the world: Copenhagen 1953. Acta Anaesthesiol Scand 2003;47:1190–1195.
8. Ibsen B, Kvittingen TD: Arbejdet pa en anaesthesiologisk observationsafdelning. Nord Med 1958;38:1349–1355.
9. Siggaard-Andersen O, Engel K, Jørgensen K, et al: A micro method for determination of pH, carbon dioxide tension, base excess and standard bicarbonate in capillary blood. Scand J Clin Lab Invest 1960;12:172–176.
10. Clark LC Jr, Wolf R, Granger D, Taylor Z: Continuous recording of blood oxygen tension by polarography. J Appl Physiol 1953;6:189–193.
11. Severinghaus JW, Bradley AF: Electrodes of blood $Po_2$ and $Pco_2$ determination. J Appl Physiol 1958;13:515–520.
12. Menzel M, Soukup J, Henze D, et al: Experiences with continuous intra-arterial blood gas monitoring: Precision and drift of a pure optode-system. Intensive Care Med 2003;29:2180–2186.
13. Aoyagi T: Pulse oximetry: Its invention, theory and future. J Anesth 2003;17:259–266.
14. Hultgren H: High Altitude Medicine. San Francisco: Hultgren Publications, 1997.
15. Brubakk AO, Neuman T: Bennett and Elliott's Physiology and Medicine of Diving, 5th ed. London: WB Saunders, 2002.
16. Bates DV, Boucot NG, Dormer AE: Pulmonary diffusing capacity in normal subjects. J Physiol (Lond) 1955;129:237–252.
17. Wagner PD Saltzman HA, West JB: Measurement of continuous distribution of ventilation-perfusion ratios: Theory. J Appl Physiol 1974;36:533–537.
18. Marshall BE, Wyche MQ Jr: Hypoxemia during and after anesthesia. Anesthesiology 1972;37:178–209.
19. Gilbert R, Auchincloss JH Jr, Kubbinger M, et al: Stability of the arterial/alveolar oxygen partial pressure ratio: Effects of low ventilation/perfusion regions. Crit Care Med 1979;7:267–272.
20. Covelli HD, Nessan VJ, Tuttle WK: Oxygen derived variables in acute respiratory failure. Crit Care Med 1983;11:646–649.
21. Sganga G, Siegel JA, Coleman B, et al: The physiologic meaning of the respiratory index in various types of critical illness. Circ Shock 1985;17:179–193.
22. Gregory IC: The oxygen and carbon monoxide capacities of fetal and adult blood. J Physiol (Lond) 1974;236:625–634.
23. Barcroft J: The Respiratory Function of the Blood. Cambridge: Cambridge University Press, 1914.
24. Perutz MF: Stereochemistry of cooperative effects in haemoglobin. Nature 1970;228:726–739.
25. Christiansen J, Douglas CJ, Haldane JS: The adsorption and dissociation of carbon dioxide by human blood. J Physiol (Lond) 1914;48:244–271.
26. Benesch R, Benesch RE: The effect of organic phosphate from human erythrocyte on the allosteric properties of hemoglobin. Biochem Biophys Res Commun 1967;26:162–167.
27. Chanutin A, Curnish RR: Effect of organic and inorganic phosphates on the oxygen equilibrium of human erythrocytes. Arch Biochem Biophys 1967;121:96–102.
28. MacDonald R: 2,3-diphosphoglycerate and oxygen affinity. Anaesthesia 1977;32:544–553.
29. Shappell SD, Lenfant CJ: Adaptive, genetic and iatrogenic alterations of the oxyhemoglobin-dissociation curve. Anesthesiology 1972;32:127–139.
30. Heaton A, Keegan T, Holme S: In vivo regeneration of red blood cell 2,3-diphosphoglycerate following transfusion of DPG-depleted AS-1, AS-3 and CPDA-1 red cells. Br J Haematol 1989;71:131–136.
31. Kelman GR, Nunn JF: Nomograms for correction of blood $Po_2$, $Pco_2$, pH and base excess for time and temperature. J Appl Physiol 1996;21:1484.
32. Rivers E, Nguyen B, Havstad S, et al: Early goal-directed therapy in the treatment of severe sepsis and septic shock. N Engl J Med 2001;345:1368–1377.
33. Lundsgaard C, Van Slyke D: Cyanosis. Baltimore: Williams & Wilkins, 1923.
34. Goss GA, Hayes JA, Burdon JGW: Deoxyhaemoglobin in the detection of central cyanosis. Thorax 1988;43:212–213.
35. Swartz HM, Dunn JF: Measurements of oxygen in tissues: Overview and perspectives on methods. Adv Exp Med Biol 2003;530:1–12.
36. Connett RJ, Honig CR, Gayeski TEJ, et al: Defining hypoxia: A systems review of $Vo_2$, glycolysis, energetics and intracellular $Po_2$. J Appl Physiol 1990;68:833–842.
37. Amato MBP, Barbas CS, Medeiros DM, et al: Effect of a protective-ventilation strategy on mortality in the acute respiratory distress syndrome. N Engl J Med 1998;338:347–354.
38. Hickling KG, Henderson S, Jackson R: Low mortality with low volume pressure limited ventilation with permissive hypercapnia in severe adult respiratory distress syndrome. Intensive Care Med 1990;16:372–377.
39. Acute Respiratory Distress Syndrome Network: Ventilation with lower tidal volumes as compared with traditional tidal volumes for acute lung injury and acute respiratory distress syndrome. N Engl J Med 2000;342:1301–1308.

40. Shibata K, Cregg N, Engelberts D, et al: Hypercapnic acidosis may attenuate acute lung injury by inhibition of endogenous xanthine oxidase. Am J Respir Crit Care Med 1998;158:1578–1584.

41. Laffey JG, Engleberts D, Kavanagh BP: Buffering hypercapnic acidosis worsens acute lung injury. Am J Respir Crit Care Med 2000;161:141–146.

42. Robin ED: Relationship between temperature and plasma pH and carbon dioxide tension in the turtle. Nature 1962;195:249–251.

43. Reeves RB: An imidazole alphastat hypothesis of vertebrate acid-base regulation: Tissue carbondioxide and body temperature in bull frogs. Respir Physiol 1972;14:219–236.

44. Rahn H, Reeves RB, Howell BJ: Hydrogen ion regulation, temperature, and evolution. Am Rev Respir Dis 1975;112:165–172.

# CHAPTER 41

# Hemodynamic Monitoring

Rahul Nanchal and Robert W. Taylor

To wedge or not to wedge: that is the question. Over the past few decades, the belief that intensive monitoring of critically ill patients leads to better outcomes has gained tremendous support and popularity. From this belief stemmed the era of intensive care units (ICUs). However, no randomized control trials exist to prove that even noninvasive measurement of common vital signs is beneficial. In fact, no such trials are likely ever to be conducted. It is sobering to reflect on the paucity of high-quality validation of commonly used hemodynamic monitoring tools.

In simple terms, *hemodynamic monitoring* consists of the measurement and analysis of biologic signals from the cardiovascular system. Therapies based on these biologic signals are then titrated, and the physiologic response is monitored. Although important, hemodynamic monitoring, thus defined, is only one piece of the puzzle. Ideally, intensive monitoring of the critically ill patient should involve a holistic approach. Tissue perfusion, oxygen delivery ($DO_2$), and cellular health should be assessed at both regional and global levels. Although this objective is easy to articulate, our current ability to monitor patients in this fashion remains limited.

Hemodynamic monitors today present raw data without much intelligent integration. Convincing evidence suggests that significant lacunae exist in many clinicians' understanding of the basic concepts of hemodynamic monitoring. No consensus exists among experts regarding the proper therapeutic strategy for a given set of hemodynamic parameters. Furthermore, little evidence is available to suggest that hemodynamic monitoring improves patient outcome, that the tools we use are the correct ones, or that even the signals we monitor are appropriate.

The rationale for hemodynamic monitoring stems from two basic assumptions: first, the clinician's understanding of the patient's underlying pathophysiologic condition is important; and second, monitoring and responding to derangements encountered will either prevent the disease from progressing or change the outcome for the better. Monitoring is not therapy, however. Not only is our understanding of the pathophysiology and fundamental derangements of the majority of the critical care disease states rudimentary, but also we are limited in our ability to alter the course of many of these illnesses. To expect a monitoring system to improve outcome in a disease state for which no effective therapy exists is simply unrealistic.

Given the paucity of high-quality information documenting improved patient outcomes with current hemodynamic monitoring tools, skepticism on the part of the clinician is warranted. Shall we conclude that neither the tools nor the data collected are clinically useful? Shall we call for a moratorium on the use of monitoring equipment and technology? Common sense teaches us otherwise. Much of the monitoring in the ICU today represents an integration of technology with physiology. As technology is improving, the focus is now shifting toward more noninvasive monitoring. The task that lies ahead includes refinement in our understanding of just what variables to measure. We must learn to measure them correctly and to institute effective therapies, where available. Finally, all of this must be done at low cost with minimum to no risk to the patient.

The following sections discuss physiologic principles on which hemodynamic monitoring is based, the variables measured, and the instrumentation and technologies in current use. Both invasive and noninvasive devices are discussed.

In conclusion, a course for future direction in hemodynamic monitoring is charted.

## PHYSIOLOGIC PRINCIPLES

Adequate oxygenation at the cellular level is a fundamental goal of resuscitation. Manipulation of physiologic variables as a consequence of monitoring is therefore directed toward this end. Outside of experimental technologies, it is not possible to monitor cellular hypoxia. The indices of $DO_2$ and oxygen consumption ($VO_2$) are described in the following sections.

### Oxygen Delivery

$VO_2$ varies among tissue beds and changes depending on many regional and systemic variables. Our ability to access regional tissue $DO_2$ and $VO_2$ accurately is limited. Global $DO_2$ equals the product of cardiac output (CO) arterial content of $O_2$ ($CaO_2$):

$$DO_2 \text{ (mL } O_2/\text{minute)} = CO \text{ (L/minute)} \times CaO_2 \text{ (mL } O_2/\text{dL)} \times 10$$

Normal $DO_2$ is approximately 1000 mL $O_2$/minute but varies widely in critical illness. CO is the product of heart rate (HR) and stroke volume (SV):

$$CO \text{ (L/minute)} = HR \text{ (beats/minute)} \times SV \text{ (L/beat)}$$

The determinants of SV are preload, afterload, and cardiac contractility. The determinants of $CaO_2$ are hemoglobin (Hb), $O_2$ saturation of Hb ($SaO_2$) in arterial blood, and $O_2$ dissolved in arterial blood. Because $DO_2$ depends largely on $SaO_2$ rather than on partial pressure, little benefit is derived by increasing the arterial partial pressure of $O_2$ ($PaO_2$) to more than 80 mm Hg, because of the sigmoid nature of the oxyhemoglobin dissociation curve (Fig. 41.1):

$$CaO_2 \text{ (mL } O_2/\text{dL)} = [1.34 \times (Hb) \text{ (g/dL)} \times SaO_2] + [0.003 \times PaO_2 \text{ mm Hg}]$$

$VO_2$ is the difference between $O_2$ delivered to the tissues and $O_2$ returned to the right side of the heart. The determinants of mixed venous $O_2$ content ($CvO_2$) (mL/dL) are Hb, $O_2$ saturation of Hb in mixed venous blood ($SvO_2$), and $O_2$ dissolved in mixed venous blood:

$$CvO_2 \text{ (mL } O_2/\text{dL)} = [1.34 \times (Hb) \text{ (g/dL)} \times SvO_2] + [0.003 \times PvO_2 \text{ mm Hg}]$$

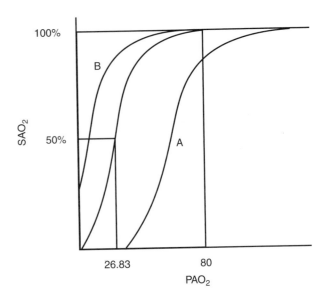

**Figure 41.1** Oxyhemoglobin dissociation curve. *A*, Rightward curve shift by increase in partial pressure of carbon dioxide ($Pco_2$) (Haldane effect), increase in 2,3-diphosphoglycerate (2,3-DPG) or decrease in pH. *B*, Leftward curve shift by decrease in $Pco_2$, decrease in 2,3-DPG, or increase in pH.

$VO_2$ is calculated as follows:

$$VO_2 \text{ (mL } O_2/\text{minute)} = CO \times (CaO_2 - CvO_2) \times 10$$

The $O_2$ extraction ratio is calculated as:

$$VO_2/DO_2$$

$VO_2$ is usually 250 mL $O_2$/minute in a physiologically normal, 70-kg adult performing routine activities, but this value varies widely in critical illness. Under normal circumstances, only 25% of the $O_2$ delivered is consumed ($O_2$ extraction ratio, 25%), thus leaving a significant reserve.

### Determinants of Cardiac Performance

Ernest Starling and Otto Frank defined basic principles of cardiac function almost 100 years ago. These principles (Starling's law of the heart) still provide the foundation for current understanding of cardiac performance. Starling stated that ". . . the mechanical energy set free on passage from the resting to the contracted state depends on the area of chemically active surfaces, i.e. on the length of the muscle fibers."[1] Starling described the relationship between end-diastolic volume and systolic pressure generated in the heart (Fig. 41.2). This principle is a manifestation of the length-tension relationship, which today has been shown to be the result of length-dependent changes in calcium release from the

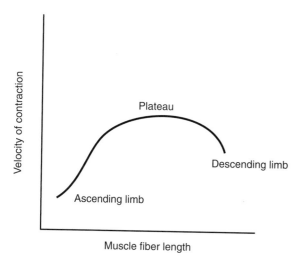

**Figure 41.2** Frank-Starling curve.

sarcolemma, as well as length-dependent changes in sensitivity of the contractile proteins to calcium. In the clinical setting, the heart operates on the ascending as opposed to the descending limb of the Starling curve. Operating on the descending limb would set up a vicious cycle whereby increases in filling would decrease emptying. On the curve's plateau, further augmentation of venous return has no effect on CO. The plateau of the ventricular function curve occurs at a much lower pressure in the right ventricle than in the left.

The right and left ventricles are coupled at three levels. They are inexorably linked by the pericardium and the interventricular septum, as well as by the fact that the output of the two ventricles must match over any extended period of time. Collectively, these phenomena are known as *ventricular interdependence*. Thus, an increase in right ventricular end-diastolic volume (RVEDV) can occur only at the expense of space devoted to the left ventricle. A stiff pericardium and a shift of the interventricular septum are responsible for this effect. Consequently, this manifests as increased left ventricular (LV) distending pressure, whereas the LV end-diastolic volume (LVEDV) may actually decrease. Hence, clinical assessment of cardiac function should include both the ventricles and the phenomenon of ventricular interdependence.

SV is the difference between the volume of ventricular blood at end-diastole and that at end-systole. End-diastolic volume or preload is determined by venous return, end-systolic volume, and lusitropy (ability of the heart to fill). End-systolic volume is determined by inotropy or ventricular contractility, aortic impedance or afterload, and end-diastolic volume.

*Preload* (end-diastolic fiber length or volume) is the load before contraction. In the absence of valvular disease, pulmonary vascular disease, intracardiac shunt, or cardiac tamponade, central venous pressure (CVP), and pulmonary artery occlusion pressure (PAOP) have been used as surrogates for RVEDV and LVEDV, respectively.

*Afterload* is the load or impedance against which the ventricles work during contraction. There are many determinants of afterload, including blood viscosity and characteristics of the arterial tree.

Systemic vascular resistance (SVR) is a reasonable surrogate of LV afterload.

$$SVR \text{ dynes/sec} = [\text{mean arterial pressure (MAP)} - CVP]/CO \times 80$$

Pulmonary vascular resistance (PVR) is a reasonable surrogate of RV afterload.

$$PVR \text{ dynes/sec} = [\text{mean pulmonary arterial pressure} (PAP) - PAOP]/CO \times 80$$

*Myocardial contractility*, simply stated, is the ability of the heart to do work. It represents the interplay among various factors that influence interactions between contractile proteins. In contrast to the Starling relationship, which influences beat-to-beat adjustment in cardiac performance, contractility is important in more sustained changes (e.g., changes in response to inotropic drugs).

*Lusitropic properties* primarily determine cardiac filling during diastole. Many structural and physiologic mechanisms can modify ventricular filling (e.g., tachycardia, valvular stenosis). Changes in ventricular compliance are the most frequent cause of alteration in ventricular filling in critical illness.

Pressure is often used as a surrogate for volume. However, pressures and volumes in the heart are linked by the ventricle's lusitropic properties of compliance (Figs. 41.3 and 41.4). Ventricular compliance often changes with hemodynamic instability, thus altering the pressure-volume relationship. In addition, airway pressures affect vascular pressures and therefore make these assumptions tenuous at best in critically ill patients receiving positive pressure mechanical ventilation. Multiple investigators have documented that in critically ill patients, CVP poorly reflects RVEDV, and PAOP poorly reflects LVEDV. Trend analysis of pressures is more valuable than single pressure measurements, but it is also fraught with difficulty.

In truth, it is difficult to separate preload, afterload, and cardiac contractility as independent variables because a change in one often intimately affects the other. Nevertheless, it is important to understand how manipulating a single variable in theory influences CO and the other variables. This interplay among venous return, preload, afterload, contractility, lusitropy, and CO is shown schematically in Figures 41.5 and 41.6.

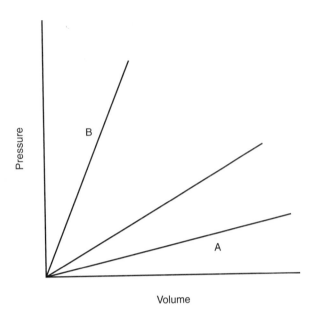

**Figure 41.3** Effect of decreasing compliance on pressure-volume relationship. *A*, Increased compliance. *B*, Decreased compliance.

## COMMONLY USED HEMODYNAMIC MONITORS

### Electrocardiographic Monitoring

The electrocardiogram (ECG), although not mentioned routinely as a part of a monograph on hemodynamic monitoring, is perhaps the most ideal monitor.

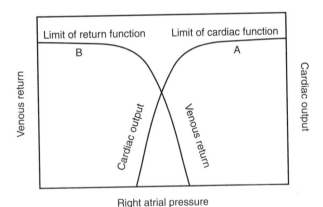

**Figure 41.4** Venous return, cardiac output, and the concept of limits. *A*, Limit of cardiac function. Increasing venous return and right atrial pressure does not increase cardiac output. *B*, Limit of venous return. Lowering right atrial pressure does not increase venous return because the veins act as Starling resistors and collapse. *C*, Cardiac output determined by intersection of venous return function and cardiac function.

It is noninvasive and is easy to comprehend. Sophisticated computerized interpretation of the signal provides relatively reliable warnings about cardiac rhythm disturbances and myocardial ischemia.

### Automated Blood Pressure Devices

Automated blood pressure devices are used in most ICUs to obtain intermittent or continuous blood pressure measurements. The methodology applied is auscultatory, oscillometric, or both. Also available is a photo-oscillometric technique. These devices are advantageous because they cycle over a set frequency, and an alarm is sounded if a preset limit is exceeded.

The auscultatory devices rely on Korotkoff's sounds. They measure systolic and diastolic pressure and calculate MAP. The cuff with the acoustic sensor is very sensitive to placement over the artery in the arm. These devices are not reliable when they are used on the calf or forearm because Korotkoff's sounds are less audible in these areas.

The oscillometric technique is most often used. These devices can be placed on all extremities and even on the digits if the correct cuff size is used. The devices cycle periodically and assess cuff pressure and minute pressure oscillations within the cuff. The initial cuff inflation just exceeds systolic pressure. Then, during graded cuff deflation, systolic pressure is recorded when the oscillations first increase in amplitude. MAP is measured at the point of maximal oscillation, and diastolic pressure is measured when the oscillations rapidly diminish or disappear. The most accurate measurement is MAP, and the least accurate is diastolic pressure.

The volume unloading technique, or the volume clamp method, is another means to measure systolic and diastolic blood pressures and MAP from beat to beat. The device consists of an inflatable finger cuff that is equipped with an infrared photoplethysmograph, which measures the finger artery blood volume under the cuff. The thumb is most commonly used because of its greater vascular supply and tissue mass. Cuff inflation is maintained at the point where the blood volume of the digit, as determined by the photoplethysmograph, is held constant. This is usually set at about two thirds of the maximal artery volume because this value corresponds to a point at which the arterial wall is considered unloaded or, in simple terms, the inside pressure equals outside pressure. The arterial pressure waveform is tracked to every beat. Although attractive, this device is rarely used in clinical practice because of its unreliability and inaccuracy in states of hypoperfusion and peripheral vasoconstriction.

The arterial applanation tonometry technique based on the Imbert-Fick law is a relatively new method that uses piezoelectric elements to assess the radial pulse and to determine blood pressure. This technique has not been validated in clinical trials.

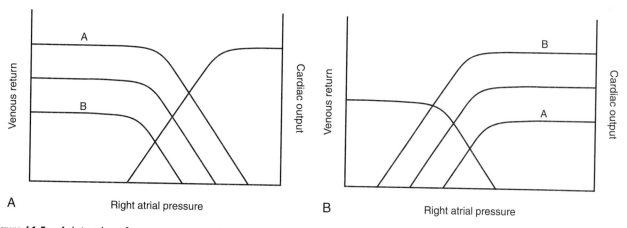

**Figure 41.5** *A*, Interplay of venous return and cardiac output. Within limits, increasing venous return increases cardiac output, and vice versa: increased venous return (A) and decreased venous return (B). *B*, Interplay of cardiac output and contractility. With a constant venous return, increasing contractility increases cardiac output and vice versa: decreased contractility (A) and increased contractility (B).

## Intravascular Pressure Measurements

The clinician must possess a sound knowledge of the principles of intravascular pressure monitoring to interpret hemodynamic data reliably. Clinicians should be familiar with all aspects of the pressure monitoring system, including the intravascular catheter, stopcocks, pressure tubing, flush device, transducer, and monitor. The basic principles are the same for systemic arterial pressure, CVP, RV pressure, PAP, and PAOP.

For accurate measurement of intravascular pressure, a reference pressure has to be established as ambient from which all vascular pressure measurements will be made. By standard convention, this reference point is at the level of the right atrium (phlebostatic axis). In supine patients, this is most commonly the midaxillary line. The procedure is called *zeroing the transducer*. An appropriate stopcock is opened to atmosphere, and the resulting air-fluid interface is aligned to the phlebostatic axis. It is not essential to keep the transducer at the midaxillary line. If kept lower or higher than this line, a positive or negative hydrostatic pressure, which is equal to the height of the water column above or below the transducer, will be added or subtracted once the stopcock is opened. On electronically zeroing the system, the appropriate pressure will be added or subtracted to set the system to zero. Once the system is zeroed, the stopcock is closed to atmospheric pressure, and the waveform is displayed. After zeroing, care should be taken to keep the transducer at the reference point at which it was zeroed.

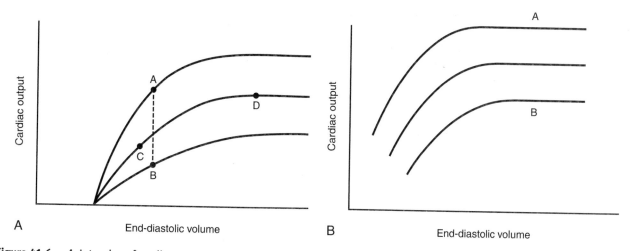

**Figure 41.6** *A*, Interplay of cardiac output, venous return, and contractility: increased contractility (A), decreased contractility (B), decreased venous return (C), and increased venous return (D). *B*, Cardiac output and afterload: decreased afterload (A) and increased afterload (B).

Subsequent transducer movement above or below the reference point is a common source of error in pressure measurements. Modern disposable pressure transducers are calibrated by the manufacturers to within ±3%. There is therefore no need to calibrate the monitoring system at the bedside.

Intravascular pressure measurement systems are underdamped, second-order dynamic systems. The natural frequency of a system is the frequency at which it oscillates maximally. A fluid-filled catheter/transducer system oscillates because of the pressure waves reflecting back and forth between the transducer membrane and the distal end of the catheter. When the transducer membrane is repeatedly stimulated at the same frequency as the reflected waves, the oscillations become amplified, the pulse pressure widens, the systolic pressure is overestimated, and the diastolic pressure is underestimated. Ideally, the natural frequency of a pressure monitoring system should be sufficiently higher than that of the waveform being measured. Shorter and stiffer pressure monitoring tubing is associated with a higher natural frequency.

The damping coefficient determines how quickly an oscillating system comes to rest. Some amount of damping is necessary so that characteristics of the recorded waveforms near the natural frequency of the system are not amplified. The natural frequency and damping coefficient of the system determine its dynamic characteristics. Overdamping of the system diminishes waveform transmission and is often caused by air bubbles, blood clots, compliant tubing, or kinking of the pressure tubing. Underdamping accentuates waveform transmission and is often caused by excessively long pressure tubing or numerous in-line stopcocks.

A fast-flush technique or square wave test is used to determine damping of the system and to optimize its dynamic response and performance. This technique involves opening and then rapidly closing the valve of the flush device. This maneuver produces a square pressure tracing (Fig. 41.7). In optimally damped systems, one small undershoot and one small overshoot (bounce) are seen, followed by a return to the normal waveform. Systems that are overdamped demonstrate an absence of

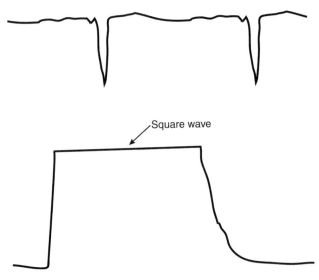

**Figure 41.8** Overdamped system.

bounces with a slurring of the square wave downstroke (Fig. 41.8). An underdamped system is characterized by multiple accentuated bounces (Fig. 41.9). In the case of inadequacy of the dynamic characteristics of the system, the problem is corrected by removing air or blood clots, replacing kinked tubing, reducing the length of the tubing, or removing unnecessary stopcocks.

## Arterial Pressure Measurement

Indications for arterial cannulation are the need for reliable beat-to-beat measurement of blood pressure (e.g., during administration of vasoactive drugs) or frequent arterial blood sampling and an inability to measure blood pressure noninvasively. Common insertion sites include the radial, femoral, axillary, and dorsalis pedis arteries. The indwelling arterial catheter allows the measurement of systolic and diastolic pressures as well as MAP. Renewed interest has arisen in the respiratory variation in arterial pressure as an index of fluid responsiveness and pulse-contour analysis for continuous measurement of SV (discussed later).

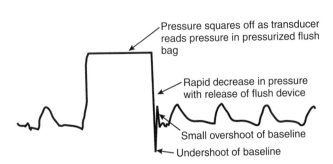

**Figure 41.7** Square wave test.

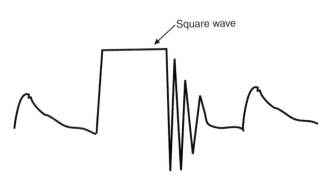

**Figure 41.9** Underdamped system.

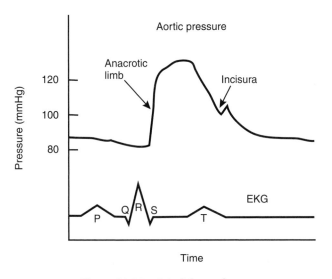

**Figure 41.10**    Arterial waveform.

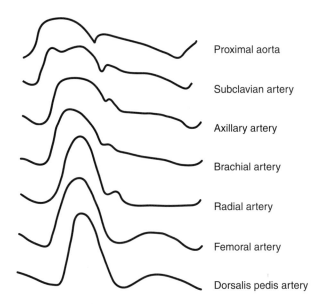

**Figure 41.11**    Arterial waveforms at different sites of the arterial tree.

Arterial cannulation is relatively safe. Bleeding diatheses and anticoagulant therapy increase the risk of hemorrhagic complications. Severe occlusive arterial disease with distal ischemia, the presence of a vascular prosthesis, and local infection are contraindications to specific sites of cannulation. Complications include hemorrhage, hematoma formation, arterial thrombosis, proximal or distal embolization, arterial pseudoaneurysm, and infection.

The arterial pressure waveform is generated by LV ejection and the subsequent peripheral runoff (Fig. 41.10). The waveform begins with the opening of the aortic valve during the ejection phase of the left ventricle. Aortic pressure rises early because the rate at which blood enters the aorta is initially faster than peripheral runoff. This rapid pressure upstroke is known as the *anacrotic limb.* A slight pressure overshoot may be seen because many monitoring systems in clinical practice are slightly underdamped. The anacrotic limb is rounded and reaches a plateau because the ejection rate is rather constant and peripheral runoff gradually increases as the aortic pressure increases. At the waveform summit, runoff equals ejection. As the rate of ejection then diminishes, peripheral runoff remains high, and aortic pressure gradually falls. End-systole and the beginning of isovolumic relaxation are marked by the closure of the aortic valve, which is inscribed as the incisura in the aortic pressure waveform tracing. The subsequent smaller, secondary positive wave is caused by elastic aortic recoil and the reflection of waves from the distal arteries. The aortic pressure decreases again as further runoff continues.

The morphology of the arterial pressure waveform changes at different sites in the arterial tree. As the waveform moves distally from the aorta, the systolic peak becomes steeper and higher, a slightly later dicrotic notch replaces the incisura, the diastolic limb becomes more prominent, and the end-diastolic pressure becomes lower. This is caused by harmonic resonance, differences in impedance, and pulse wave reflection. This phenomenon of distal pulse amplification causes the systolic pressure to be higher, the diastolic pressure to be lower, and the pulse pressure to be magnified peripherally. The MAP in the periphery, however, remains close to the mean pressure in the aortic arch (Fig. 41.11).

## Respiratory Variation of Arterial Pressure

Positive pressure ventilation decreases venous return during inspiration by increasing intrathoracic pressure and CVP. This temporarily decreases RVEDV, which becomes minimal at the end of the positive pressure breath. This inspiratory reduction in RVEDV leads to a decrease in LVEDV after a lag phase of a few heartbeats caused by the pulmonary vascular transit time. This reduction in LVEDV manifests as a decrease in SV during the expiration phase. The diminished SV induces a reduction in systolic blood pressure that is minimum during expiration. Conversely, during positive pressure ventilation, the highest systolic pressure is seen during inspiration and is a reflection of increased RVEDV a few beats earlier during expiration. Thus, systolic arterial pressure varies cyclically during a positive pressure mechanical breath; it is maximal during inspiration and minimal at expiration. *Systolic pressure variation* is defined as the difference between maximal inspiratory and minimal expiratory systolic pressures. It is further characterized by dUp, which is the increase of pressure from baseline, and dDown, which is the decrease in pressure from baseline (Fig. 41.12).

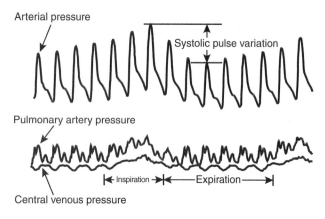

**Figure 41.12** Cyclic variation of respiratory pressures affecting vascular pressures.

| Table 41-1 | Normal Hemodynamic Values |
|---|---|
| Mixed venous oxygen saturation | 60%–75% |
| Stroke volume | 50–100 mL |
| Stroke index | 25–45 mL/m² |
| Cardiac output | 4–8 L/min |
| Cardiac index | 2.5–4.0 L/min/m² |
| Mean arterial pressure | 60–100 mm Hg |
| Central venous pressure | 2–6 mm Hg |
| Pulmonary arterial pressure: systolic | 20–30 mm Hg |
| Pulmonary arterial pressure: diastolic | 5–15 mm Hg |
| Pulmonary artery occlusion pressure | 8–12 mm hg |
| Systemic vascular resistance | 900–1300 dynes/sec |

*Systolic pulse pressure variation* is defined as the difference between the maximum pulse pressure (PPmax) and the minimum pulse pressure (PPmin). Systolic pressure variation, dDown, and pulse pressure variations have all been found to be accurate predictors of response to volume loading. The greater the pressure variation, the greater will be the expected increase in SV with volume expansion. Fluid responsiveness does not automatically imply that fluids are needed or that CO is inadequate. Furthermore, these parameters depend on positive pressure ventilation and are tidal volume dependent. In addition, this technique is difficult to use in the presence of cardiac arrhythmias, especially atrial fibrillation, in which LV SV changes with every beat.

## Pulmonary Artery Catheter

Since its introduction into clinical use by Swan and colleagues in 1970,[2] the pulmonary artery catheter (PAC) has been the subject of great controversy and discussion. Even so, the fact remains that the use of this catheter is still widespread throughout the world in the ICU. CVP and PAP are monitored continuously. PAOP, thermodilution CO, and SvO₂ are measured intermittently. Some catheters have the ability to monitor SvO₂ and CO continuously. Volumetric PACs have the ability to measure RVEDV but suffer the error of mathematical coupling through CO. Normal hemodynamic values are shown in Table 41.1.

The assessment and management of shock are among the most frequent indications for insertion of a PAC. Shock may be classified as cardiogenic, hypovolemic, obstructive, distributive, or cytopathic. Critically ill patients often exhibit elements of more than one shock classification.

*Cardiogenic shock* generally implies a deranged functioning of the myocardium. The problem may lie with the right ventricle, the left ventricle, or both. It is manifested by decreased SV and CO. Congestive heart failure resulting from acute LV infarction is the prototype of cardiogenic shock. In this circumstance, CO is low, and PAOP, PAP (systolic and diastolic), and CVP are high. Therapies are aimed at improving the contractile performance of the heart.

*Hypovolemic shock* implies an absolute or relative intravascular volume deficiency. Hemorrhage associated with trauma is a common cause of hypovolemic shock. In this case, CO, PAOP, PAP (systolic and diastolic), and CVP are usually low. Therapies are aimed at rapidly restoring intravascular volume.

*Obstructive shock* implies some type of physical obstruction to blood flow in the cardiovascular system. Massive pulmonary embolism obstructs blood flow through the pulmonary vascular beds and thereby impedes LV filling. CO and PAOP are low, with elevations of PAP (systolic and diastolic) and CVP. Intravascular volume expansion is typically employed. Pericardial tamponade is another cause of obstructive shock. The CVP waveform demonstrates a prominent x descent but an absent y descent. CVP, PAP (systolic and diastolic), and PAOP are elevated. An equalization of diastolic pressures is seen from the CVP to the PAP diastolic and the PAOP. CO is reduced. Definitive therapy is emergency pericardial drainage, and volume expansion is employed in the interim.

*Distributive shock* implies loss of circulatory control with widespread maldistribution of blood flow. Septic shock, anaphylactic shock, and spinal shock are examples of this type of distributive abnormality. Patients with septic shock may, in fact, have multiple defects in addition to maldistribution of blood flow. Because of alteration in capillary permeability associated with severe sepsis, significant intravascular volume may be lost to the extravascular space. In addition, cardiac contractility is impaired (cardiogenic shock) secondary to circulating myocardial depressant substances (cytokines and other molecules). Widespread microvascular clotting may obstruct blood flow (obstructive shock), and circulating humoral factors may cause cellular dysoxia (cytopathic shock). The precise hemodynamic profile is difficult to predict. Arterial blood pressure is usually low. The CVP, PAP, and PAOP may be low, normal, or high. Typically, the CO is elevated (secondary to tachycardia), but this depends on the underlying cardiovascular status and what prior therapeutic interventions have been introduced. SVR is usually low as a result of widespread cytokine-mediated arteriolar dilation. The hemodynamic strategy usually involves expansion of the intravascular volume, augmentation of myocardial performance (inotropes), and improvement in arteriolar tone (vasoconstrictors) to maintain a reasonable MAP (60 to 70 mm Hg). Treatment with drotrecogin alfa activated may improve organ perfusion and outcome by preventing microvascular clot formation and thus improving blood flow obstruction.

## Waveform Analysis

Reading pressures directly from the monitor frequently leads to misinterpretation. Because intracardiac pressure waveforms cannot be interpreted without the aid of a single-lead ECG tracing, a two-channel physiologic recorder is essential. The pressure waveform is recorded simultaneously with the single-lead ECG, normally at a paper speed of approximately 25 mm/second. Because the electrical activity of the heart governs all mechanical activity, rhythm analysis before waveform interpretation is essential. It is best to include several respiratory cycles on the tracing so that all pressures can be recorded at end-expiration. The various waveforms are then interpreted in correlation with the ECG.

The CVP is dependent on right atrial blood volume, right atrial compliance, the functioning of the tricuspid valve, and RV compliance. The waveform comprises three positive waves (a, c, and v) and two negative descents (x and y) (Fig. 41.13). The a wave is the dominant wave and denotes atrial systole. Its peak occurs approximately 80 milliseconds after the peak of the P wave on the ECG. This is because of the inherent electromechanical delay and the delay in transmission

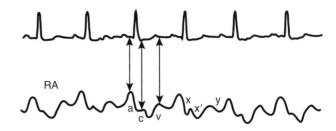

**Figure 41.13**  Central venous waveform.

through the fluid-filled system. The c wave denotes closure of the tricuspid valve at the onset of RV systole. It occurs immediately after the QRS complex and follows the a wave with a period equal to the PR interval. The v wave is caused by passive filling of the atrium during ventricular systole. It occurs after the T wave on the ECG. The x descent is the result of atrial relaxation during ventricular systole, and the y descent is caused by rapid flow of blood from the atrium to the ventricle at the time of tricuspid valve opening. Usually, CVP is measured by averaging the a wave.

The RV waveform is characterized by a rapid upstroke to peak systole, a rapid downstroke, and a small terminal rise at end-diastole. The peak-systolic pressure is found after the QRS complex but before the peak of the T wave. End-diastole is found near the end of the QRS complex (Fig. 41.14). The RV waveform is usually not monitored. The CVP is often used to estimate RV end-diastolic pressure, and the PAP systolic is used to estimate RV systolic pressure.

As the PAC is advanced through the pulmonic valve into the PA, the waveform changes. Peak systole of the right atrium and PA are similar. The characteristic change is a rise in diastolic pressure (Fig. 41.15).

A rapid upstroke reflecting the onset of RV ejection, a dicrotic notch resulting from closure of the pulmonic valve, and a smooth progressive diastolic runoff characterize the PAP waveform (Fig. 41.16). Peak systole is found after the QRS complex but before the peak of the T wave. End-diastole is found near the end of the QRS complex (Fig. 41.17). Distinguishing the PAP waveform from that of a v wave can sometimes be difficult. The key difference lies in timing. The peak PA occurs before the

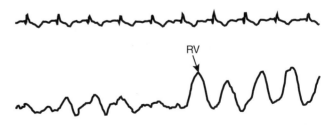

**Figure 41.14**  Right ventricular waveform.

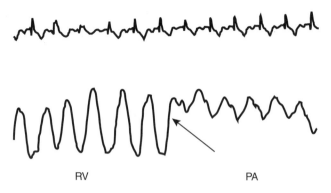

**Figure 41.15** Transition from right ventricular to pulmonary artery waveform.

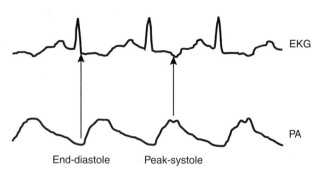

**Figure 41.17** Timing of pulmonary artery systole and diastole with the electrocardiogram.

peak of the T wave, whereas the v wave peak occurs after the T wave (see later). If the PVR and mitral valve are normal, then PAP diastolic is a reasonable estimate of left atrial pressure and left ventricular end-diastolic (LVEDP). In this case, PAP diastolic can be substituted for PAOP, thus minimizing the risk of PA injury from balloon inflation.

The PAOP, like the CVP, contains three positive (a, c, and v) and two negative (x and y) waves (Fig. 41.18). The a wave is typically the most prominent, and the c wave is often not visible secondary to damping. The a wave occurs with atrial contraction, the c wave occurs with closure of the mitral valve, and the v wave occurs with left atrial filling. The x descent denotes atrial relaxation, and the y descent is caused by exit of blood from the left atrium at the time of mitral valve opening. The y descent marks the onset of ventricular diastole. The PAOP is determined by averaging the a wave. The a wave in the PAOP tracing occurs approximately 200 milliseconds after the ECG P wave. The time delay in the PAOP a wave compared with the CVP a wave is caused by the longer distance the pressure wave travels through the pulmonary circulation and monitoring catheter to the transducer in the PAOP waveform compared with the CVP waveform. In the PAOP waveform, the v wave occurs after the T wave and occurs significantly later than the PAP systolic wave.

When obtaining a PAOP waveform, the balloon should be inflated with no more than 1.5 cc of air. Air should not be aspirated from the balloon but allowed to exit passively. Fluid should not be injected into the balloon, and balloon inflation should be limited to a maximum of 15 seconds.

The PAOP accurately reflects pulmonary capillary pressure in patients with normal lungs and minimal pulmonary venous resistance. However, in critically ill patients, hypoxia, inflammatory mediators, and other factors influence arteriolar and venous resistance to varying degrees. Thus, the PAOP does not accurately reflect pulmonary capillary pressure in disease states such as sepsis and the acute respiratory distress syndrome. The pulmonary capillary pressure, not the PAOP, is the driving pressure behind fluid permeating into the lungs in these conditions.

Mitral regurgitation and tricuspid regurgitation cause the appearance of giant v waves on PAOP and CVP tracings, respectively. As previously mentioned, a large v wave occurring in the PAOP tracing may be mistaken for a PAP waveform. These waves can be differentiated using the ECG. Peak-systole in the PAP waveform occurs before the T wave, whereas the v wave occurs after the T wave (Fig. 41.19). When reading the PAOP in the presence of a large v wave, the a wave is averaged (Fig. 41.20).

Large a waves may occur with valvular stenosis, ventricular noncompliance, and loss of atrioventricular

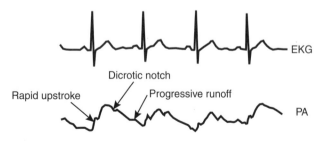

**Figure 41.16** Pulmonary artery waveform.

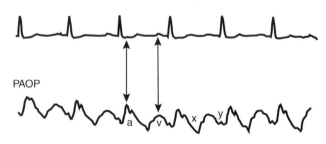

**Figure 41.18** Pulmonary artery occlusion waveform.

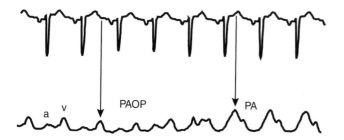

**Figure 41.19** Large v wave in a pulmonary artery occlusion waveform.

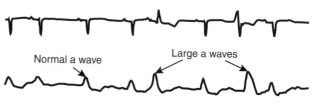

**Figure 41.21** Large a waves.

synchrony (Fig. 41.21). The pressure reading in this circumstance is made by finding a normal a wave and taking the average of the peak and trough values. Alternatively, the pressure may be read at the end of the QRS complex (Z point). The absence of a waves occurs in atrial fibrillation and in ventricular, junctional, or paced rhythms. The Z point technique is also helpful in the case of absent a waves.

Atrial pressure usually decreases with inspiration during spontaneous ventilation. In the case of a diseased pericardium or a noncompliant atrium, the atrial pressure may increase with inspiration, a condition called *Kussmaul's sign.*

## Hemodynamic Effects of Respiration

Positive pressure mechanical ventilation affects cardiovascular performance by altering lung volume and intrathoracic pressure. As intrathoracic pressure decreases during spontaneous inspiration, lung volume increases. Thus, volume and pressure move in opposite directions. During positive pressure inspiration, however, intrathoracic pressure increases, and lung volume increases. Pressure and volume under these conditions therefore change in similar directions.

Lung inflation and an increase in intrathoracic pressure, although seemingly related, are in reality quite dissociated and have important effects on the cardiovascular system. Lung inflation causes a decrease in vagal tone

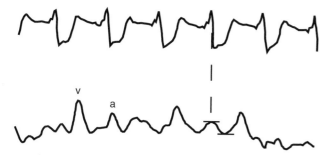

**Figure 41.20** Determining the pulmonary artery occlusion pressure in the presence of a large v wave.

and an increase in HR. This cyclic variation in HR is known as respiratory sinus arrhythmia. However, inflation with large tidal volumes (>10 mL/kg) causes a decrease in sympathetic tone that results in slowing of the HR and vasodilation.

The pulmonary circulation is unique because it is exposed to two pressures: intrathoracic pressure in the extra-alveolar vessels and alveolar pressure in the alveolar vessels. Therefore, any deviation of lung volume from functional residual capacity potentially causes an increase in PVR. Smaller lung volumes may be associated with hypoxic vasoconstriction and collapse of extra-alveolar vessels by loss of radial traction. Hyperinflation tends to compress the alveolar vessels and to decrease pulmonary circulatory cross-sectional area thereby increasing PVR. If the pulmonary vasculature is compromised, then further increases in PVR may precipitate acute cor pulmonale.

An increase in intrathoracic pressure raises CVP and diminishes the pressure gradient for venous return. This change is manifested as a decrease in RV filling, lower RV end-diastolic pressure, and diminished RV SV. This decrease in SV is manifested a few beats later as diminished LV preload resulting from the series connection of the two ventricles, and hence LV SV is reduced.

Laplace's law states that wall tension is proportional to the product of developed pressure and the radius of curvature. In the absence of aortic valve or LV outflow tract disease, arterial pressure is used as a surrogate for maximal ventricular systolic pressure or afterload. An increase in intrathoracic pressure decreases afterload by reducing transmural arterial pressure. This is the basis of the improved ventricular performance and resolution of pulmonary edema in patients with congestive heart failure when mechanical ventilation is instituted.

The effect of respiration, whether spontaneous or mechanical, should always be considered when measuring intracardiac pressures. Intrathoracic pressure is transmitted to the heart and affects intracardiac pressure measurement. True distending or transmural pressure is intracardiac pressure minus intrathoracic pressure. At the bedside, it is very difficult to measure intrathoracic pressure; however, it approaches zero at end-expiration in the absence of significant lung disease or application of large amounts of positive end-expiratory pressure (PEEP). Thus, all pressures in spontaneously breathing and

Spontaneous breathing

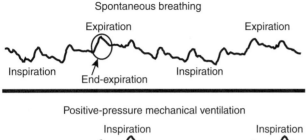

Positive-pressure mechanical ventilation

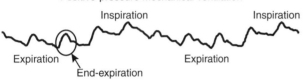

**Figure 41.22** Impact of breathing on vascular pressures.

mechanically ventilated patients should be made at end-expiration when the excursions in intrathoracic pressures are minimal (Fig. 41.22). For an accurate measurement of the PAOP, a patent blood-filled column must exist between the catheter tip and the left atrium. This occurs when the catheter tip is located in a lung segment in which pulmonary venous pressure exceeds alveolar pressure. Based on the relationship between pulmonary vascular and alveolar pressure, three physiologic zones, known as *West zones*, have been described in the lung (Fig. 41.23). Because of the balloon flotation nature of the PAC, its tip is directed by blood flow. The bulk of pulmonary blood flow goes to gravity-dependent regions of the lung (zone III). Therefore, the tip of the PAC most often resides in zone III. If alveolar pressure exceeds pulmonary venous pressure (zone II), then the PAOP reflects both vascular and alveolar pressure. This often results in a loss of a and v waves on the PAOP tracing. If alveolar pressure exceeds both pulmonary venous and arterial pressure (zone I), the resultant PAOP is largely a reflection of alveolar pressure. PEEP

complicates hemodynamic measurements, because it is often associated with alveolar pressures that exceed pulmonary venous pressures (zones I and II). The degree to which airway pressures are transmitted to the heart is difficult to determine in an individual patient. Hence determining the precise impact of PEEP on vascular pressure is difficult. The practice of simply subtracting the level of PEEP or some fraction thereof from vascular pressure measurement is fraught with error and is discouraged. Discontinuation of PEEP for the purpose of vascular pressure measurement may be associated with alveolar collapse and dangerous hypoxemia. In addition, alteration in airway pressure also changes cardiac physiology and creates a totally different hemodynamic paradigm. This practice is therefore not recommended. In these situations, it is best to tailor therapy according to other clinical variables. Complications associated with PAC use are shown in Table 41.1.

## Cardiac Output Measurement

### Thermodilution Cardiac Output

The thermodilution method for CO determination was introduced by Fegler in 1954. Ganz and co-workers introduced the technique into clinical practice in 1971. It is a form of the indicator dilution technique and involves the administration of cold saline solution into the proximal port of the PAC. The resultant temperature drop is measured by a thermistor near the catheter tip. A thermodilution curve is then generated, and the area under the curve is inversely proportional to CO. This method is accurate and has also been validated with room temperature saline. However it is highly operator dependent. The accuracy of CO measurements is reduced in the setting of poor technique, sensor malfunction, tricuspid regurgitation, septal defects, and very-low-CO states.

### Other Minimally Invasive Techniques for Cardiac Output Determination

**Transpulmonary Cardiac Output**  A cold injectate is introduced into the venous circulation through a central venous catheter. The resultant temperature change is measured in the arterial circulation through a thermistor-tipped arterial catheter. CO is estimated using the Stewart-Hamilton equation. In contrast to the PAC, which measures right-sided output, left-sided output is measured by this technique. Compared with PAC-determined CO, the correlation coefficient is 0.72 to 0.96.

**Pulse Contour Analysis Cardiac Output**  Provided the compliance, impedance, and inertance variables of the arterial tree and aorta remain constant, then the shape of the arterial waveform is dependent only on LV SV. Arterial pulse-contour analysis under these circumstances

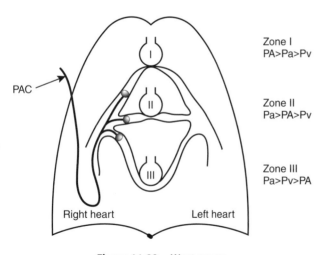

**Figure 41.23** West zones.

can be used to estimate continuous CO on a beat-to-beat basis. Wesseling and colleagues first developed the algorithm for this technique in 1983. However, for calibration, CO must be measured by an alternative technique such as transpulmonary or lithium dilution CO, and impedance needs to be calculated. This measurement of CO at the least requires the placement of arterial and central venous catheters. Variations in pulse contour-derived estimates of SV are used to predict response to volume expansion. However, this method is unreliable in the presence of changing arterial tone. Frequent recalibration is required in critically ill patients with hemodynamic instability or vasopressor use. Compared with PAC-determined CO, the correlation coefficient is 0.88 to 0.91. A commercial device is currently available and measures global end-diastolic volume, intrathoracic blood volume, and extravascular lung water.

**Lithium Dilution Cardiac Output** Isotonic lithium chloride is used as an indicator and is injected as a small bolus either centrally or peripherally. A concentration time curve is then generated by an arterial ion selective electrode attached to the arterial line manometer system. CO is calculated by the lithium dose and the area under the concentration time curve before recirculation. The dose of lithium is too small to cause pharmacologic effects. The advantage of this technique is that it there is no absolute need for central venous cannulation. However, it cannot be used in patients receiving lithium therapy and is inaccurate in the presence of arteriovenous shunts with the use of muscle relaxant infusions.

**Esophageal Doppler Cardiac Output** This technique uses a Doppler probe approximately the size of a nasogastric tube. The probe is placed in the esophagus in close proximity to the descending aorta. The velocity time integral is then calculated as the area under the curve based on the principle of Doppler shift of signals from the aorta. SV is obtained by multiplying the cross-sectional area of the descending aorta with the velocity time integral. A correction factor is required because not all of the CO enters the descending aorta. This technique also provides indirect measures of preload and contractility. Peak flow velocity is an indicator of contractility, and LV ejection time or flow time is an index of preload. Patient movement, the shape of the aorta, turbulent flow, tachycardia, and aortic valvular disease affect measurements. This technique is very operator dependent, and accurate positioning of the probe is required. Compared with PAC-determined CO, the correlation coefficient is 0.60 to 0.95.

## Thoracic Electrical Bioimpedance Cardiac Output

This technique is based on Ohm's law, which states that voltage drop is equal to the product of impedance and current. This principle is applied to the thorax, which is viewed as a volume conductor, and impedance is measured continuously across the thorax to a continuously applied high-frequency, low-magnitude alternating current. Changes in blood velocity are reflected as changes in impedance, and estimates of SV and contractility are indirectly provided systolic time intervals. Compared with PAC-determined CO, the correlation coefficient is 0.67 to 0.93.

## Monitoring Tissue Perfusion and Microcirculation

### Mixed Venous Saturation Monitoring

Shock represents an imbalance between $DO_2$ and $VO_2$ wherein either the supply is inadequate to meet tissue demands or $O_2$ extraction or utilization is impaired. $SvO_2$ has been used as a surrogate for the adequacy of $DO_2$. $SvO_2$ can be altered by changes in CO, Hb, arterial Hb saturation, or $VO_2$ (Fig. 41.24). As $DO_2$ decreases, $O_2$ extraction by the tissues increases, so $VO_2$ is relatively constant. Blood returning to the heart therefore has a reduced $O_2$ content and low $SvO_2$. A reduced $SvO_2$ is thus indicative of global hypoxia and $O_2$ debt. This debt leads to anaerobic metabolism and lactate production and is associated with increased mortality. Indicative as it is of global hypoxia, a low $SvO_2$ does not allow any inference about the cause of diminished global $DO_2$. Rather, it is an early sign that something is amiss and forces the clinician to evaluate all the aspects of reduced $DO_2$ or increased $VO_2$. $SvO_2$ is usually measured intermittently by withdrawing blood from the pulmonary port of the PAC. Catheters using the technology of infrared oximetry based on reflection spectrophotometry have the ability to monitor $SvO_2$ continuously. Although a low $SvO_2$ value is associated with $O_2$ debt, a normal or elevated $SvO_2$ value is not always indicative of well-being. Patients with severe sepsis or hepatic failure,

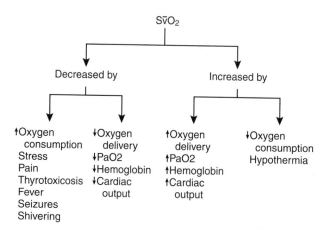

**Figure 41.24** Causes of changes in mixed venous oxygen saturation.

for example, may have cellular or microvascular dysfunction and are unable to use $O_2$ properly even if $DO_2$ is adequate. In these cases, $DO_2$ is often elevated, whereas $O_2$ extraction is reduced. Thus, the $SvO_2$ is often normal or high. Monitoring of $SvO_2$ gives the clinician global information about $DO_2$ and $O_2$ extraction. It does not provide information about the adequacy of regional $DO_2$ or $O_2$ extraction.

Monitoring of $SvO_2$ requires the placement of a PAC, which may not always be possible or desirable. Monitoring of venous saturation in the superior vena cava ($ScvO_2$) as a surrogate for $SvO_2$ was used in a study of early goal directed therapy in patients with septic shock.[3]

## Tissue Perfusion

Transport of $O_2$ to the various tissues of the body is the primary function of the circulatory system. $O_2$ is finally delivered to the cell by passive diffusion across the capillary system. Blood flow at the microcirculatory level is regulated locally according to metabolic needs. This process, controlled by vascular smooth muscle, endothelial cells, and nerve cells, is referred to as *metabolic, neurohormonal, and myogenic regulation.*

Our ability to monitor the microcirculation and tissue perfusion is limited. At present, we cannot tell when hypoxia, ischemia, dysoxia, dysfunctional energy use, frank energy failure, or disruption of cellular integrity is occurring in tissue beds. Lactate and lactate/pyruvate ratios have been used as a surrogate for tissue hypoperfusion. Unfortunately, these are global rather than regional indicators that become elevated relatively late in the stages of tissue dysoxia.

Gastric tonometry has been suggested as a method to monitor mesenteric perfusion. The device detects tissue carbon dioxide ($CO_2$) that diffuses from the gastric mucosa into a saline-filled balloon. The saline is then aspirated after allowing time for equilibration of gastric $CO_2$ to the $CO_2$ in the saline. The partial pressure of $CO_2$ ($PCO_2$) is measured, and pHi (gastric intramucosal pH) is calculated from a modified Henderson-Hasselbalch equation. It is assumed that mesenteric ischemia leads to increased hydrogen ion ($H^+$) production as a result of anaerobic metabolism. The increased $H^+$ combines with bicarbonate to produce increased $PCO_2$. However, this technique assumes that gastric bicarbonate is the same as serum bicarbonate, which may not be the case. Accumulation of $CO_2$ resulting from hypoperfusion states may also give rise to errors. Moreover, no trial has ever documented the benefit of correcting pHi to normal values, although sufficient data support the view that lower pHi portends a poor prognosis, especially in trauma victims.

Sublingual capnometry involves placing a sublingual $CO_2$ sensor under the tongue, facing the sublingual mucosa. The technique may prove to be an early indicator of systemic perfusion failure in critically ill patients. One study, by Weil and colleagues, demonstrated that when sublingual pressure of $CO_2$ ($PslCO_2$) exceeded a value of 70 mm Hg, physical signs of circulatory shock were present in all patients.[4] By contrast, patients with $PslCO_2$ lower than 70 mm Hg had a 93% survival rate. The technology looks promising as a noninvasive early monitor of tissue hypoperfusion, but further studies are clearly warranted.

Near-infrared spectroscopy and nuclear magnetic resonance spectroscopy are newer technologies that are currently used only for research purposes. However, they have the potential one day to give us noninvasive, accurate information about cellular energetics and metabolism, as well as cellular dysoxia.

## The Pulmonary Artery Catheter: On the Horns of a Dilemma

Since its introduction in clinical practice, the use of the PAC remains shrouded in controversy. Some investigators called for a moratorium on its use following the study reported by Conners and associates that suggested an increased mortality, hospital stay, and hospital costs with PAC use. However, there was no mention about the way in which the hemodynamic data were obtained or used in this study. More recently, a randomized controlled trial investigating PAC use in high-risk surgical patients was published by Sandham and associates.[5] This study randomized high-risk surgical patients to either receive or not to receive a PAC. The study demonstrated no difference in mortality between the two groups. The group that received the PAC had a greater incidence of pulmonary embolism. Despite absolute lack of proof of efficacy, it appears to many investigators that, in expert hands, the PAC remains an important diagnostic tool that provides physiologic measurements that are difficult or impossible to obtain by other means. Nevertheless, nonexpert, indiscriminate use of PAC is ill advised. Adequate training should be provided to medical and nursing personnel about the appropriate use of this catheter. Trials are ongoing using the PAC in specialized group of patients such as those with acute lung injury. Perhaps these trials will improve our understanding about the appropriate use of this technology.

## THE FUTURE OF HEMODYNAMIC MONITORING

Hemodynamic monitoring systems currently exist to guide therapies designed to support the cardiovascular system during times of circulatory instability. Today, these monitors present rather raw data without much intelligent integration. Many of the monitoring technologies discussed in this chapter are promising and will likely help to direct our care over the next few decades. As we look toward the future, however, it is clear that hemodynamic monitoring is only one piece of the puzzle. The patient does not benefit by careful monitoring and optimizing of hemodynamic variables if the fundamental problem is the inability of mitochondria to use $O_2$ in production of adenosine triphosphate. We must learn to think in terms of the entire organism. Our ability to monitor and treat effectively will improve as our knowledge about critical illness is refined.

We should therefore be designing and testing integrated, closed-loop systems that monitor at the macroscopic, microscopic, and molecular levels. These systems should give us real-time, accurate, and relevant information. They should be user-friendly and should do no harm. When derangements are detected, effective therapies should be immediately and precisely titrated.

Technologic advances in miniaturization, biosensors, and computer processing coupled with an improved understanding of critical illness at the molecular level will lead to development of new monitoring systems that will integrate physiologic and biochemical information in a relatively noninvasive manner. When coupled with more effective therapies, these integrated, closed-loop systems promise to help improve outcome in critically ill patients.

## REFERENCES

1. Starling EH: The Linacre Lecture on the Law of the Heart. Presented at Cambridge. 1915. London: Longmans, Green, 1918.
2. Swan HJC, Ganz W, Forrester J, et al: Catheterization of the heart in man with the use of a flow directed balloon tipped catheter. N Engl J Med 1970;283:447–451.
3. Rivers E, Nguyen B, Havstad S, et al: Early goal-directed therapy in the treatment of severe sepsis and septic shock. N Engl J Med 2001;345:1368–1377.
4. Weil MH, Nakagawa Y, Tang W, et al: Sublingual capnometry: A new noninvasive measurement for diagnosis and quantitation of circulatory shock. Crit Care Med 1999;27:1225–1229.
5. Sandham JD, Hull RD, Brant RF, et al: A randomized, controlled trial of the use of pulmonary artery catheters in high-risk surgical patients. N Engl J Med 2003;348:5–15.

## SUGGESTED READINGS

Allen DG, Kentish JC: The cellular basis of length tension relationship in cardiac muscle. J Mol Cell Cardiol 1985;17:821–840.
Alonso-Gonales J, Olsen DB, Saltin B: Erythrocyte and the regulation of human skeletal muscle blood flow and oxygen delivery: Role of circulation ATP. Circ Res 2002;91:1046–1057.
Bakker J, Gris P, Coffernils M, et al: Serial blood lactate levels can predict development of multi organ failure following septic shock. Am J Surg 1996;171:221–226.

Beilman GJ, Cerra FB: The future: Monitoring cellular energetics. Crit Care Clin 1996;12:1031–1042.
Bove AA, Santamore WP: Ventricular interdependence. Prog Cardiovasc Dis 1981;23:365–388.
Bruner JMR, Krenis CJ, Kunsman JM, Sherman AP: Comparison of direct and indirect methods of measuring arterial blood pressure. Part III. Med Instrum 1981;15:182–188.
Buda AJ, Pinsky MR, Ingles NB: Effect of intrathoracic pressure on left ventricular performance. N Engl J Med 1979;301:453–459.
Chaney JC, Derdak S: Minimally invasive hemodynamic monitoring for the intensivist: Current and emerging technology. Crit Care Med 2002;30:2338–2345.
Chiara O, Pelusi P, Segala M, et al: Mesenteric and renal oxygen transport during hemorrhage and reperfusion: Evaluation of optimal goals for resuscitation. J Trauma 2001;51:356–362.
Dabrowski GP, Steinberg SM, Ferrara JJ, et al: A critical assessment of end points of shock resuscitation. Surg Clin North Am 2000;80:825–844.
Dellinger RP, Carlet JM, Masur H, et al: Surviving Sepsis Campaign guidelines for management of severe sepsis and septic shock. Crit Care Med 2004;32:858–873.
Fessler HE, Brower RG, Wise RA, Permutt S: Effect of positive end expiratory pressure on the gradient for venous return. Am Rev Respir Dis 191;146:4–10.
Fink MP: Cytopathic hypoxia. Crit Care Clin 2002;18:165–175.
Gardner RM: Invasive pressure monitoring. In Civetta JM, Taylor RW, Kirby RR (eds): Critical Care, 3rd ed. Philadelphia: Lippincott-Raven, 1997, pp 839–845.
Gomersall, CD, Joynt GM, Freebairn RC, et al: Resuscitation of critically ill patients based on the results of gastric tonometry: A prospective, randomized, controlled trial. Crit Care Med 2000;28:607–614.
Hotchkiss RS, Karl IE: The pathophysiology and treatment of sepsis. N Engl J Med 2003;348:138–150.
Hsia CC: Respiratory functions of hemoglobin. N Engl J Med 1998;338:239–248.
Ivatury RR, Simon RJ, Islam S, et al: A prospective randomized study of end points of resuscitation after major trauma: Global oxygen transport indices versus organ-specific gastric mucosal pH. J Am Coll Surg 1996;183:145–154.
Jardin F, Genevray B, Brun-Ney D, et al: Influence of lung and chest wall compliances on the transmission of airway pressure to the pleural space in critically ill patients. Chest 1985;86:653–658.
Kandel G, Aberman A: Mixed venous oxygen saturation: Its role in the assessment of the critically ill patient: Arch Intern Med 1983;143:1400–1402.
Kemmotsu O, Ueda M, Otsuka H, et al: Arterial tonometry for non invasive, continuous blood pressure monitoring during anesthesia. Anesthesiology 1991;75:333–340.
Laupland KB, Bands CJ: Utility of esophageal Doppler as a minimally invasive hemodynamic monitor: A review. Can J Anaesth 2002;49:393–401.
Linton R, Band O, O'Brien T: Lithium dilution cardiac output measurement: A comparison with thermodilution. Crit Care Med 1997;25:1796–1800.
Marini JJ, O'Quinn R, Culver BW, et al: Estimation of transmural cardiac pressures during ventilation with PEEP. J Appl Physiol 1982;53:384–391.
Michard F, Boussat S, Chelma D, et al: Relation between respiratory changes in arterial pulse pressure and fluid responsiveness in septic patients with acute circulatory failure. Am J Respir Crit Care Med 2000;162:134–138.
Michard F, Chelma D, Richard C, et al: Clinical use of respiratory changes in arterial pulse pressure to monitor the hemodynamic effects of PEEP. Am J Respir Crit Care Med 1999;159:935–939.

Nelson L: The new pulmonary artery catheter: Continuous venous oximetry—Right ventricular ejection fraction and continuous cardiac output. New Horiz 1997;5:251–258.

Nguyen HB, Rivers EP, Knoblich BP, et al: Early lactate clearance is associated with improved outcomes in severe sepsis and septic shock. Crit Care Med 2004;32:1637–1642.

Pinsky MR, Summer WR, Wise WA, et al: Augmentation of cardiac function by elevation of intrathoracic pressure. J Appl Physiol 1983;54:950–955.

Pinsky MR: Clinical significance of the pulmonary artery occlusion pressure. Intensive Care Med 2003;29:175–178.

Pinsky MR: Pulmonary artery occlusion pressure. Intensive Care Med 2003;29:19–22.

Quebbeman EJ, Dawson CA: Influence of inflation and atelectasis on hypoxic pressure response in isolated dog lung lobes. Cardiovasc Res 1976;10:672–677.

Reuter DA, Felbinger TW, Kilger E, et al: Stroke volume variations for assessment of cardiac responsiveness to volume loading in mechanically ventilated patients after cardiac surgery. Intensive Care Med 2002;28:392–398.

Reuter DA, Felbinger TW, Schmidt C, et al: Stroke volume variations for assessment of cardiac responsiveness to volume loading in mechanically ventilated patients after cardiac surgery. Intensive Care Med 2002;28:392–398.

Ronco JJ, Fenwick JC, Tweeddale MG, et al: Identification of critical oxygen delivery for anaerobic metabolism in critically ill septic and non septic humans. JAMA 1993;270:1724–1730.

Roopa KS, Oropello JM: The future of bedside monitoring. Crit Care Clin 2000;16:557–578.

Rosenberg P, Clyde WY: Non invasive assessment of hemodynamics: An emphasis on bioimpedance cardiography. Curr Opin Cardiol 2000;15:151–155.

Shoemaker WC, Appel PL, Kram HB: Role of oxygen debt in development of organ failure, sepsis and death in high risk surgical patients. Chest 1992;102:208–225.

Stez CW, Miller RG, Kelly GE, et al: Reliability of the thermodilution method in determination of cardiac output in clinical practice. Am Rev Respir Dis 1982;126:1001–1004.

Takala J: Pulmonary capillary pressure. Intensive Care Med 2003;29:890–893.

Tanaka H, Thulesius O, Yamaguchi H, et al: Continuous non invasive finger blood pressure monitoring in children. Acta Paediatr 1994;83:646–652.

Taylor RW, Ahrens TA, Beilin Y, et al: Pulmonary artery catheter consensus conference: Consensus statement. Crit Care Med 1997;25:910–925.

Taylor RW: Controversies in pulmonary artery catheterization. New Horiz 1997;5:1–296.

Trottier SJ, Taylor RW: Physicians' attitudes toward and knowledge of the pulmonary artery catheter: Society of Critical Care Medicine Membership survey. New Horiz 1997;5: 201–206.

Vincent JL, De Backer D: Oxygen uptake/oxygen supply dependency: Fact or fiction. Acta Anaesthesiol Scand Suppl 1995;107:229–237.

West JB, Dollery CT, Naimark A: Distribution of pulmonary blood flow in isolated lung: Relation to vascular and alveolar pressures. J Appl Physiol 1964;19:713–724.

Whittenberger JL, McGregor M, Berglund E, Borst HG: Influence of the state of inflation of the lung on pulmonary vascular resistance. J Appl Physiol 1960;15:878–882.

Wilson DF, Erecinska M, Brown C, et al: The oxygen dependence of cellular energy metabolism. Arch Biochem Biophys 1979; 14S:485.

# CHAPTER 42

# In-Line Blood Gas Monitoring

Bala Venkatesh

The ability to measure arterial blood gases and pH became a clinical reality in the 1950s. The results provide valuable information concerning the state of the patient's oxygenation, gas exchange, ventilation, and acid-base homeostasis. Modern blood gas analyzers (BGAs) incorporate a glass electrode for the measurement of pH,[1] a Stow-Severinghaus electrode for the measurement of partial pressure of carbon dioxide ($Pco_2$),[2,3] and a Clark electrode[4] for the measurement of partial pressure of oxygen ($Po_2$). Before 1950, vacuum extraction of gases from blood and volumetric analysis was possible. Although the impetus for the development of modern BGAs is traditionally attributed to the development of mechanical ventilation during the poliomyelitis epidemic in the 1950s, other contemporaneous events also provided momentum. These included recognition of the limitations of volumetric analyses during physiologic research in aviation and diving medicine that flourished during the Second World War, as well as the development of bubble oxygenators, which required a means for accurate efficacy assessment. The scientific milestones culminating in the development of modern BGAs are listed in Box 42.1.[5]

Despite the rapidity of measurement and automation and the need for only small volumes of blood for analysis, current techniques take intermittent measurements and are not without problems (e.g., errors in sampling, storage, and analysis of specimens; Box 42.2).[6] Furthermore, the intermittent nature of the measurement may provide only a snapshot of a continuously changing variable and may therefore potentially miss short-term trends. It is well known that arterial blood gases fluctuate even in stable patients in the intensive care unit (ICU).[7] Often, a blood gas analysis is performed after a critical incident has occurred. Thus, an intermittent measurement may not provide an early warning signal of deteriorating respiratory function.

Advances in technology have shifted the thrust from intermittent analysis to continuous monitoring by the bedside. Pulse oximetry and capnography, routinely used in anesthesia and intensive care, have greatly aided patient management and have increased patient safety, thus reducing the need for frequent blood gas analysis.[8] However, these noninvasive technologies do not replace arterial blood gas and pH analysis. Moreover, the inability of the pulse oximeter to differentiate among the various forms of dyshemoglobinemias, the loss of the oximeter's signal during low-flow states, and the propensity to motion artifacts and measurement errors when $O_2$ saturations are less than 70% reduce the specificity and sensitivity of pulse oximetry in the critically ill patient.[6,9–12]

Continuous noninvasive assessment of blood gas tensions is possible with transcutaneous $Po_2$ and $Pco_2$ monitoring. Available systems incorporate $Po_2$ and $Pco_2$ electrodes with integral thermistors and servo-controlled heaters. $Po_2$ measurement uses the principle of the Clark electrode, whereas the $Pco_2$ device is a pH-sensitive glass electrode. To achieve good correlation with arterial values, the skin is warmed to a temperature of 42°C to 44°C. Transcutaneous monitors generate reliable $Pco_2$ values in adequately perfused patients, but $Po_2$ measurements are used more for trend analysis. Skin warming necessitates frequent site changes to prevent burns, and there is a need for regular recalibration. Monitoring in hemodynamically unstable patients is not recommended. The monitors have a role in the prevention of neonatal hyperoxia, a problem not reliably detected by pulse oximetry.[13]

**BOX 42-1**

### Major Milestones in the Development of Blood Gas Analysis

| | |
|---|---|
| 1909 | Sorensen described a pH unit |
| 1922 | Heyrovsky described measurement of partial pressure of oxygen by using a mercury electrode |
| 1933 | Mcinnes and Belcher described an apparatus for pH measurement |
| 1934 | Kramer described continuous arterial oxygen saturation measurement |
| 1942 | Millikan first described an ear oximeter |
| 1952 | Dubois and colleagues described an infrared technique for measurement of partial pressure of carbon dioxide in expired air |
| 1956 | Clark described his electrode |
| | Astrup developed a new technique for determining the partial pressure of carbon dioxide |
| 1958 | Severinghaus described his electrode |
| | Severinghaus demonstrated a prototype blood gas machine |

The technical challenges confronting the development of a continuous intraarterial blood gas monitoring (CIABGM) system include the following:[14,15] (1) the need to miniaturize sensors for use with conventional intra-arterial cannulas without compromising the ease of simultaneous arterial blood sampling and the fidelity of transduction of the arterial waveform, (2) the ability to

**BOX 42-2**

### Problems Associated with Intermittent Blood Gas Analysis

**Preanalytic Errors**
Inadequate removal of dead-space volume; discard volume should be two to three times the internal volume of the cannula and tubing
Presence of air bubbles in the sample
Incomplete mixing of the specimen
Delay in analysis
Lack of storage in ice during transportation and while awaiting analysis
Pseudohypoxemia: reduction in partial pressure of oxygen induced by leukocyte oxygen consumption resulting from delayed analysis

**Analytic Problems**
Reproducibility and variability (7% to 8%) between analyzers
Inadequate anticoagulation, thus allowing protein deposition on the electrodes

**Miscellaneous Concerns**
Lack of forewarning of a deleterious event
Exposure of personnel to potentially infected blood
Blood loss associated with repeated sampling

produce accurate and reproducible data for a reasonable length of time to make the procedure cost effective, (3) the need to maintain the fluidity of blood, (4) the need for a rapid response time, and (5) the ability to trend blood gases reliably under conditions of varied blood flow.

## SYSTEM CONFIGURATIONS

Although several methods of analyte detection have been adapted, currently available CIABGMs employ two general configurations: fiberoptic and electrochemical.

### Fiberoptic Systems

*Fluorescence* is the emission of light by a substance that is energized by an appropriate light source. *Fiberoptics* transmit light to and from an indicator phase that possesses certain optical properties. The indicator phase interacts chemically with the analyte whose concentration is to be measured. This chemical interaction alters the optical properties of the indicator phase and leads to a modification of the incident light signal. The returning light signal is changed either in intensity with the same wavelength (*absorbance spectrophotometry*) or in both intensity and wavelength (*fluorescence spectrophotometry*). These techniques of spectrophotometry are well-established analytic tools and form the basis of optical sensors.

In *absorbance-based systems*, light is transmitted to an optical dye phase. The absorbance of specific wavelengths by the dye varies in inverse relation to the analyte of interest. The intensity of the returning light signal varies according to the analyte concentration, and this relationship is described by Beer-Lambert's law.

In *fluorescent systems*, the excitation wavelength of the incident light is absorbed by the dye, thus causing electrons to be briefly excited to a higher energy level. When the electrons return to a lower energy level, they emit energy in the form of light (i.e., fluorescence). This fluorescence is inhibited in the presence of $O_2$, and the so-called $O_2$ quenching can be mathematically described by the Stern-Volmer equation.[16] This principle forms the basis of most fiberoptic $O_2$ sensors, which have generally become known as optodes.[17] The term *optode* was coined by Optiz and Lubbers to describe fiberoptic sensors as an analogy to the electrode.

An important feature of the fiberoptic sensor design is the principle of optical compensation. There is a potential for artifacts such as fiber bending or indicator degradation to compromise the integrity of the measurement. The use of a dual-light signal with differing wavelengths, one at the peak absorbance level and one at the isosbestic point, allows the use of the ratio of the intensities at these wavelengths to determine analyte concentration. If both wavelengths are similarly affected by artifacts and

| Table 42-1 | Dye Indicators in Fiberoptic Sensors | |
|---|---|---|
| **Property** | **pH** | **Po$_2$** |
| Absorbance | Phenol red<br>Bromthymol blue<br>Alizarin | |
| Fluorescence | 4-Methylumbelliferone<br>Polyaromatics<br>Pyrenetrisulfonic acid<br>Fluorescein derivatives | Lanthanide<br>Fluorinated porphyrins |

Po$_2$, partial pressure of oxygen.

are dissimilarly affected by the analyte, a compensation algorithm can be derived to eliminate artifact-induced perturbation. Other important aspects of sensor design include selection of nontoxic dyes (Table 42.1), with appropriate absorption and emission wavelength characteristics, ease of attachment to an optical fiber, high-intensity variation in the physiologic range of measurement (i.e., sensitivity), and rapid response time.

## Electrochemical Systems

Electrochemical systems measure voltage (*potentiometric:* a characteristic of the pH and the Pco$_2$ electrodes) or current (*amperometric:* a characteristic of the Po$_2$ electrode). Although potentiometric electrodes have found little application in intravascular sensor technology, the amperometric (Clark) system has been successfully miniaturized in several commercial intravascular devices. The electrodes are poised at a fixed potential and immersed in an electrolyte solution, and the current generated by the reduction of O$_2$ is linearly related to the Po$_2$ in the solution.

Because the output current depends on the diffusion of O$_2$ to the sensor, there can be some sensitivity of the sensor to blood flow, although in most clinical situations this is negligible. The direct relationship between the amplitude of the current generated and the Po$_2$ makes the Clark electrode more sensitive at higher levels of Po$_2$. In contrast, the optodes have an inverse relationship between the luminescence intensity and the Po$_2$ and are therefore potentially more sensitive at a lower Po$_2$.[18] Electrochemical systems for intraarterial measurement of pH and Pco$_2$ are not feasible because the sensing element is the glass electrode.

## Temperature Compensation

Temperature compensation of sensors is essential because all sensor chemistries involve steady states and rate constants that are temperature dependent.

Furthermore, the activities of analytes in biologic fluids are temperature dependent. Conventionally, BGAs measure temperature at 37°C, and corrections must be made for comparisons with data at other temperatures.

## EVOLUTION OF CONTINUOUS MONITORING SYSTEMS: HISTORICAL PERSPECTIVE

### Single-Parameter Systems

#### pH

Continuous measurements of intraarterial pH were accomplished as early as 1927 using antimony electrodes.[19] One of the limitations of electrode use was its large size. Band and Semple measured pH using miniaturized glass electrodes,[20] whereas LeBlanc and colleagues used membrane polymer electrodes.[21,22] Both these electrodes suffered from a degree of inaccuracy in the measurement of pH. In 1981, Nilsson and Edwall revived the use of antimony electrodes, but they utilized monocrystalline antimony.[22] The results were an improvement in accuracy and reduction in electrode size to 0.8 mm. In 1980, Peterson described a fiberoptic pH probe based on spectrophotometric absorption and used phenol red as an indicator in anesthetized sheep.[23] Abraham and associates developed the sensor further and achieved acceptable levels of bias and a high degree of precision in anesthetized dogs.[24] Fluorescence-based intraarterial pH probes were developed by Wolfbeis and colleagues and by Miller and associates.[25,26] Despite their high degree of accuracy, these systems are less commonly used than the absorbance systems.

### Pco$_2$ Sensors

Pco$_2$ sensors are based on the principle of encapsulating a pH electrode in a bicarbonate-filled CO$_2$-permeable membrane. Both forms of fiberoptic Pco$_2$ sensors have been described, absorbance[27] and fluorescence,[28] and varying degrees of accuracy have been reported.

### Po$_2$ Sensors

The development of the Clark electrode in 1956 revolutionized the measurement of O$_2$ in clinical practice.[4] Kreuzer and Nessler, in 1958, were the first to develop a miniaturized polarographic O$_2$ electrode.[29] Several investigators improved on the original design.[30-35] Some of the problems encountered by these investigators included a lack of reliability, excessive drift, flow sensitivity, a large size precluding blood pressure measurement, and cannula occlusion and interference from halothane and nitrous oxide. In 1978, Severinghaus described chloride-free electrodes to reduce excessive drifting.[36] Nilsson and colleagues refined the electrode further by reducing its size to 0.55 mm and coating the external surface with covalently bonded heparin to reduce fibrin deposition and thrombus formation.[37] This electrode was marketed as the Continucath 1000 by Biomedical Sensors (High Wycomb, UK). Pfeifer and colleagues and Rithalia and associates reported problems with cannula occlusion, thrombus formation, and excessive drift with this electrode.[38–40] Optode-based $O_2$ sensors were described by Peterson and associates,[41] Barker and colleagues,[42] and Shapiro and colleagues.[43] Of the single-parameter intravascular sensors, only the Continucath 1000 intravascular $PO_2$ sensor and the Neocath (Biomedical Sensors, High Wycomb, UK) $O_2$ sensor for use in the umbilical artery of neonates became commercially available.

## Multiparameter Systems

### Multiparameter Sensors

Several systems have been developed based on the foregoing theoretical principles. Broadly, these systems can be grouped into pure optode-based systems and hybrid electrode-optode systems. Three devices, based entirely on optode technology, were the CDI 1000 (Cardiovascular Devices, Irvine, CA),[26,44,45] the Optex Biomedical (Woodlands, TX),[46] and the PB3300 (Puritan Bennet, Pleasanton, CA).[47–49] The first-generation Paratrend 7, a product of Diametrics Medical UK, was a hybrid electrode-optode system incorporating a fiberoptic pH and $PCO_2$ sensor with an amperometric $O_2$ sensor and a thermocouple to facilitate temperature compensation.[50–53] The second-generation Paratrend 7 was a pure optode-based system.[54] The PB3300 and the Paratrend 7 systems

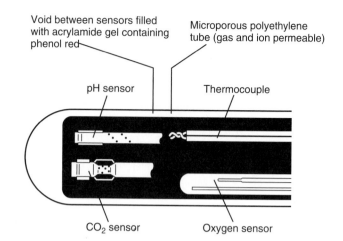

**Figure 42.1** Cross section of the Paratrend 7 sensor tip. (Courtesy Biomedical Sensors, High Wycombe, UK.)

reached commercial availability. A cross section of the Paratrend 7 sensor tip is illustrated in Figure 42.1.

The comparative physical and performance characteristics of the various blood gas monitoring systems are presented in Tables 42.2 and 42.3. Although CIABGM has certain desirable features (Table 42.4), none of the currently available systems meets all the requirements of these systems.

## EVALUATION OF CONTINUOUS BLOOD GAS MONITORING SYSTEMS

CIABGMs are usually evaluated in the following manner: (1) in vitro, in which the sensors are evaluated

**Table 42-2** Data on the Physical Characteristics of the Intravascular Sensors

| Sensor | Type | Measures | Temperature Compensation | Size | 90% in Vitro Response Times (sec) | | | Calibration |
|---|---|---|---|---|---|---|---|---|
| | | | | | pH | $PCO_2$ | $PO_2$ | |
| PB 3300 | Optode | pH, $PCO_2$, and $PO_2$ | Yes | 0.55 mm | 30 | 84 | 48 | In vitro 15 min |
| CDI 3M | Optode | pH, $PCO_2$, and $PO_2$ | Yes | 0.6 mm | N/A | N/A | N/A | In vitro 15 min |
| Optex | Optode | pH, $PCO_2$, and $PO_2$ | Yes | N/A | N/A | N/A | N/A | In vitro |
| Paratrend 7 | Hybrid electrode-optode | pH, $PCO_2$, and $PO_2$ | Yes | 0.5 mm | 78 | 143 | 70 | In vitro 30 min |
| Neotrend | Optode | pH, $PCO_2$, and $PO_2$ | Yes | <0.5 mm | N/A | N/A | N/A | In vitro 35 min |

$PCO_2$, partial pressure of carbon dioxide; $PO_2$, partial pressure of oxygen.

**Table 42-3** Published Data on the Clinical Performance of Intravascular Sensors

| Investigator and Reference | Sensor | Number of Patients | Clinical Setting (Site of Insertion) | pH* Bias ± Precision | Pco₂† Bias ± Precision | Po₂† Bias ± Precision |
|---|---|---|---|---|---|---|
| Barker and Hyatt[45] | CDI-1000 | 14 | OR (radial) | −0.03±0.04 | -0.5±0.62 | −1.2±3.1 |
| Smith et al[99] | Optex Biomedical | 5 | OR (radial) | −0.01±0.02 | 0.42±0.33 | −0.79±1.6 |
| Zimmerman and Dellinger[46] | PB 3300 | 5 | ICU (radial) | −0.02±0.037 | 0.23±0.81 | −0.79±1.76 |
| Larson et al[48] | PB 3300 | 29 | OR/ICU (radial) | 0.01±0.04 | 0.16±0.44 | 0.04±1.2 |
| Venkatesh et al[68] | P7 | 14 | ICU (radial) | 0.02±0.06 | 0.22±0.6 | 0.4±3.4 |
| Venkatesh et al[51] | P7 | 10 | ICU (femoral) | 0.006±0.07 | 0.22±1.65 | 0.8±2.7 |
| Venkatesh et al[53] | P7 | 20 | Cardiopulmonary bypass (radial) | 0.01±0.06 | 0.53±0.33 | 0.5±6 |
| Venkatesh et al[14] | P7 | 10 | OR: hip replacement (radial) | 0.02±0.03 | 0.07±0.24 | 0.16±2.6 |
| Myles et al[76] | P7 | 11 | OR: thoracic anesthesia (radial) | 0.01±0.05 | −0.21±0.78 | −2.93±7.2 |
| Menzel et al[54] | P7: second-generation | 20 | OR: neurosurgery (radial) | −0.02±0.02 | 0.25±0.23 | 0.2±2.04 |
| Weiss et al[100] | P7 | 5 (pediatric) | ICU (femoral) | 0.01±0.02 | −0.1±0.62 | 1.9±17 |
| Morgan et al[101] | Neotrend | 27 (neonatal) | ICU (umbilical) | 0.00±0.02 | 0.26±0.52 | −0.19±0.99 |
| Coule et al[102] | P7 | 50 (pediatric) | ICU (radial/femoral) | 0.00±0.04 | −0.05±0.64 | 0.1±3.3 |

*pH expressed in pH units.
†Pco₂ and Po₂ expressed in kPa.
ICU, intensive care unit; OR, operating room; Pco₂, partial pressure of carbon dioxide; Po₂, partial pressure of oxygen.

**Table 42-4** Bias and Precision of the Paratrend 7 Sensor for Each Insertion Length

| Insertion Length | pH (pH units) | | Pco₂ (kPa) | | Po₂ (kPa) | |
|---|---|---|---|---|---|---|
| | Bias | Precision | Bias | Precision | Bias | Precision |
| 11 cm | −0.03 | 0.03 | 0.25 | 0.5 | 1.1 | 4 |
| 15 cm | 0.02 | 0.03 | 0.25 | 0.5 | −0.3 | 1.6 |
| 22 cm | −0.06 | 0.16 | 0.3 | 0.4 | 1.8 | 3.7 |

Pco₂, partial pressure of carbon dioxide; Po₂, partial pressure of oxygen.

by bubbling a calibration gas containing a known concentration of $O_2$ and $CO_2$ through blood in a bubble tonometer[55] and comparing the data from the sensors with the expected values; and (2) in vivo, in animal models and in human clinical trials, in which the data from the sensors are compared with data from a BGA. The latter are taken as the reference standards.

The degree of agreement between the sensor and the BGA can be quantified in terms of bias and precision.[56] *Bias* is a consistent difference in the measured value of a known variable, whereas *precision* is the reproducibility of the measurements of the variable. Despite encouraging results in vitro and in animal testing, the same degree of bias and of precision has not been achieved consistently with intravascular sensors in clinical trials. Some of the factors that could explain the discrepancy are discussed later.

## Factors Producing a Dissociation between Blood Gas Analyzer and Continuous Intraarterial Blood Gas Monitoring Measurements

### Accuracy of the Blood Gas Analyzer

The BGA is used as the reference standard for evaluation of intraarterial blood gas monitors in clinical trials. Among the limitations of intermittent blood gas analysis listed in Box 42.2,[57-61] interanalyzer variability as a cause of potential discrepancy between BGA and CIABGM merits further discussion. Interanalyzer measurement variability (6% to 8%) on the same blood sample has been reported as a result of differences in calibration techniques, sample chamber design, sample introduction technique, sample size, warming, and electronics.[62-66] BGAs are recalibrated at frequent, predetermined intervals, in contrast to CIABGMs. Although quality control limits exist for bench-top BGAs,[67] no such regulatory measures have been developed for CIABGMs.

### Arterial Blood Flow

Theoretical considerations and experimental data support the notion that blood flow down the artery in which the sensor is placed may affect sensor performance. Blood sampling for blood gas measurement is achieved by aspirating a sample of blood from the arterial line; initially, a sample is aspirated to clear the dead space, and then immediately thereafter another sample is aspirated for blood gas analysis. Removal of the dead-space volume has the effect of drawing a specimen of blood from the central arterial tree. An intraarterial sensor placed in a peripheral artery measures gases in the peripheral arterial blood; theoretically, values should be the same as those of a central arterial sample if there is good peripheral blood flow. In the presence of peripheral circulatory failure, the sensor is in a relatively stagnant pool of blood, and the measurements obtained from the sensor may not agree with those from a conventional arterial sample. Experimental data exist to support this hypothesis.[38,68]

In one of the preliminary trials with a CIABGM, the authors observed large biphasic changes in temperatures (Fig. 42.2), as measured by the thermocouple of the intravascular sensor, during sampling of the blood for arterial blood gases and subsequent flushing with a heparinized saline.[68] This finding suggested that the sensor was not in contact with a continuous flow of blood and that contact with warm core blood during sampling caused the temperature to increase. Similarly, the drop in temperature, owing to the heparin flush following the sampling, would not be of such magnitude in a subject with good peripheral flow. Measurements at these time points were often associated with large offsets in $PO_2$ measurements.

Evidence for the flow hypothesis is also supported by data from another study that reported a trend toward better sensor performance in patients with improved arterial flow. These authors compared three different insertion lengths (11, 15, and 22 cm) of the sensor into the radial artery in critically ill patients and observed that the 15-cm insertion provided the most accurate data (see Table 42.4). Too long an insertion length into the artery resulted in flow changes, whereas too short an insertion length increased the potential for the flush effect (see later).

### Wall Effect

Mahutte and colleagues observed sudden unexplained decreases in sensor $PO_2$ readings that were overcome by alteration of wrist position or retraction of the sensor into the cannula.[44] The decreases in arterial $PO_2$ ($PaO_2$), termed the *wall effect*, were thought to result from contact between the sensor and the arterial wall and hence reading some average of blood $PO_2$ (~12 to 13 kPa) and tissue $PO_2$ values (~5.5 kPa). Circumferential distribution of the $PO_2$ sensing chamber within the optode was thought to minimize the wall effect. Hybrid probes such as the Paratrend 7 are thought to be less susceptible to

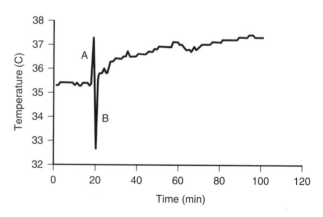

**Figure 42.2** Temperature changes in the radial artery during blood sampling and heparinized saline flushing. *A,* Temperature rise with sampling. *B,* Temperature drop with flushing.

the wall effect because the Clark electrode has a larger surface area. This phenomenon should be considered when the $Po_2$ sensor tends to underread.

## Flush Effect

The continuous heparinized saline flush used to maintain the patency of arterial cannulas can potentially affect sensor data. The flush solution, at room temperature, contains dissolved $O_2$ and $CO_2$ at partial pressures similar to that of the atmosphere. If the sensing elements of the device are not inserted to an adequate distance past the tip of the arterial cannula, then they may measure the blood gases in the flush solution, with resulting erroneous blood gas measurements. The effect of the flush is twofold: (1) to alter the local gas tensions and (2) to induce a change in temperature of the blood flowing past the sensor. Although the significance of this phenomenon in clinical practice is not clear, Venkatesh et al has observed that a longer insertion length of the sensor past the tip of the cannula often results in improved sensor performance.

## Impact of Wrist Position

The radial artery is the most commonly used site for arterial cannulation in intensive care practice. An intraarterial sensor placed in the radial artery may be prone to wrist movement artifacts (Fig. 42.3). Bending of the wrist may interfere with light transmission to and from the optodes to varying degrees. This effect is clinically relevant because patients in the ICU who are restless may not always maintain their wrists in a neutral position.

## Stability of Sensor Values

It is important to compare measurements between the sensor and the BGA, when the sensor demonstrates stable trends in arterial blood gas values. Sensor instability has many potential causes. Any of these factors, either singly or in combination, may contribute to unstable sensor data. Vessel wall *spasm*, either momentary or prolonged, may lead to fluctuations in blood flow. These fluctuations may result in temperature changes locally that will then alter the thermocouple reading and thereby affect the blood gases measured by the sensor. *Diminished peripheral blood flow, shock,* and *catecholamine-induced vasoconstriction* can produce similar effects. Another reason for unstable sensor data is the time period of response of the sensor (inherent to all sensors) to changes in arterial blood gases. Comparisons during these periods of instability may show a poor degree of agreement between the sensor and the BGA.

## Failed Thermocouple

Blood gases are measured at the patient's temperature, and a nomogram is applied for correction to 37°C. This approach facilitates comparison with laboratory analyzers, which conventionally measure gases at 37°C. The indicator

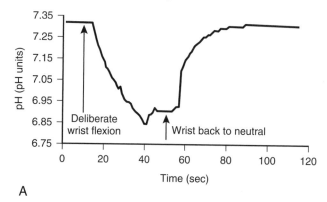

EFFECT OF FLEXION OF THE WRIST ON SENSOR pH MEASUREMENTS

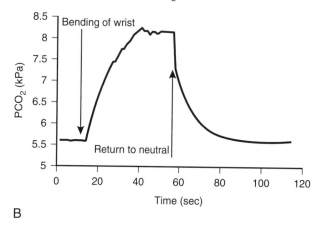

EFFECT OF WRIST FLEXION ON SENSOR $PCO_2$ MEASUREMENT

**Figure 42.3** Aberrant pH (*A*) and partial pressure of carbon dioxide ($Pco_2$) (*B*) data resulting from bending of the wrist.

chemistry is also temperature dependent, and, therefore, correction factors must be applied for changes in temperature. Alterations in cardiac output and peripheral blood flow produce changes in peripheral temperature, and accurate measurement of blood gases in peripheral blood requires proper detection of the shifts in the peripheral blood temperature. A malfunctioning thermocouple leads to erroneous measurement of temperature that results in incorrect and inappropriate temperature compensation of blood gases.

## Limitations and Problems of Indwelling Sensors

The technology has been developed, by necessity, in the laboratory, where the sample containing the analyte is in a static environment with a fixed volume. In clinical practice, it is a dynamic environment of undetermined volume, and there is an associated body response to the sensor. Potential reasons for in vivo malfunction include the position of the sensor in relation to the arterial wall, thrombus formation, a constantly changing environment, and host reaction to the sensor. The interface between the sensor and the analyte can be fouled by protein adsorption and cellular attachment. Macrophage accumulation around sensors has been documented.[70] Thrombogenicity is a well-recognized problem with all commercially available intravascular catheters. The use of heparin flushing and heparin bonding of sensors has minimized these problems. The incorporation of nitric oxide–releasing compounds as polymers into the coating of the sensor has been shown to reduce thrombogenicity and to improve $PO_2$ measurement accuracy in canine models.[71] Another problem may be that, with the passage of time, the reactive species may be depleted. The process of conduction of signal from sensor to monitor may fail, and finally the process of sterilization and shipping, in which the sensor is stored at cold temperatures for prolonged periods, may produce structural alterations in the sensor that may lead to sensor failure. Finally, interference with arterial waveform and sampling of blood from the arterial line are other potential problems that may arise during use of these monitors.

Certain design features have been developed to increase the robustness of intraarterial sensors and sensor longevity without causing arterial occlusion or interference with waveform or blood sampling. These features include the use of flexible fiberoptics, employment of glass (Puritan Bennet, Optex) and plastic fibers (Paratrend 7) to minimize size (yielding sensor diameters between 0.5 and 0.62 mm), and support of the fibers with Kevlar strips. Despite the foregoing design characteristics, if sufficient care is not taken, the sensors will be prone to damage during medical and nursing maneuvers.

## CLINICAL APPLICATIONS OF CONTINUOUS INTRAARTERIAL BLOOD GAS MONITORING

The proposed advantages of CIABGM over intermittent measurements include the availability of continuous data, a decrease in the laboratory turnaround time, a decrease in the amount of blood lost through sampling, reduced exposure of personnel to potentially infected blood, a reduction in infection risk, alarm availability, and a decrease in therapeutic decision time (Box 42.3). However, none of these proposed advantages has been proven by controlled outcome studies.

### Intensive Care

Although most of the published data on CIABGMs testify to the accuracy of these systems in various clinical groups, few published data exist on their usefulness in the management of critically ill patients. The evidence for the latter is largely anecdotal[52,72–75] (Figs. 42.4).

---

**BOX 42-3**

**Advantages of a Continuous Intraarterial Blood Gas Monitoring System over Intermittent Blood Gas Analysis**

1. Availability of continuous data
2. Earlier detection of deleterious events
3. Potential for trend analysis
4. Decrease in blood loss
5. Decrease in laboratory turnaround time
6. Decrease in exposure of staff to potentially infected blood

---

The ability to trend arterial blood gases with CIABGM should potentially facilitate management of patients with severe acute respiratory distress syndrome and other forms of respiratory failure, requiring high levels of inspired $O_2$, positive end-expiratory pressure, and other adjunctive therapy (e.g., nitric oxide, prone positioning, surfactant therapy, prostacyclin therapy, liquid ventilation, and tracheal gas insufflation). The trending ability of CIABGMs would alert the clinician to any evolving deleterious changes in respiratory function not otherwise detected by intermittent blood gas analysis and would therefore enhance therapeutic decision making. From a practical point of view, a case can be made for using CIABGM in patients in whom pulse oximetry monitoring is either technically difficult (e.g., severe burn injury) or unreliable (e.g., severe circulatory failure).

### Anesthesia

Anecdotally, the use of CIABGM during major surgical procedures such as hip replacement,[69] cardiac bypass,[76] thoracic surgery[77] and one-lung anesthesia,[78] major laparotomies,[79] and transplantation[80] has been demonstrated to lead to earlier detection and treatment of severe derangements in acid-base balance and arterial blood gases. The use of these monitors during total hip replacement has allowed the elucidation of $PaO_2$ changes during cement implantation (Figure 42.5).[69] Elective monitoring of the blood gas status on a continuous basis in high-risk patients may also facilitate patient management during the postoperative period.

### Pediatric and Neonatal Intensive Care

CIABGMs have been validated for use in the pediatric population, and published data are available relating to their use in anesthesia and intensive care.[81] A multiparameter sensor for use in the umbilical artery of neonates has been developed (Neotrend-L, Diametrics Medical, Ltd., High Wycombe, UK). It can be inserted into a 3.7-Fr catheter. Blood gas data comparing the Neotrend with BGA have shown an acceptable degree of accuracy

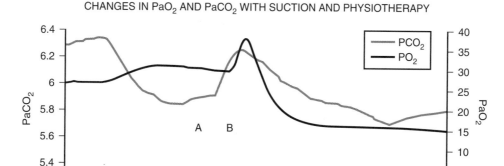

CHANGES IN PaO$_2$ AND PaCO$_2$ WITH SUCTION AND PHYSIOTHERAPY

**Figure 42.4** An illustrative example of changes in arterial partial pressure of oxygen (Pao$_2$) (in kPa) during total hip replacement. Time points A and B correspond to times of acetabular and femoral cement implantation, respectively.

in critically ill neonates and during extracorporeal membrane oxygenation.[82,83]

## EXTRACORPOREAL ON-DEMAND BLOOD GAS MONITOR

Some of the problems encountered with intraarterial sensors, particularly the effects of flow and position, have prompted the development of continuous extracorporeal monitors. The CDI-2000 blood gas monitoring system (CDI-3M Healthcare, Tustin, CA) is an example of an extracorporeal, optode-based, on-demand blood gas monitor, and results from a four-center trial demonstrated a consistent level of accuracy equivalent to that of a BGA.[84,85] The Sensicath (Optical Sensors, Minneapolis, MN) system is another example of an optode-based, in-line, on-demand monitor; data during cardiopulmonary bypass and in postoperative cardiovascular surgical patients were demonstrated to be accurate, with an acceptable degree of bias and precision.[86] The VIA-LVM showed promise in two trials in pediatric patients. In an initial validation study, the VIA LVM monitor (VIA Medical, San Diego, CA) was shown to have an acceptable level of accuracy.[87] A subsequent,

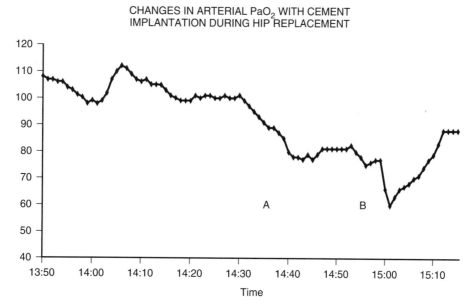

CHANGES IN ARTERIAL PaO$_2$ WITH CEMENT IMPLANTATION DURING HIP REPLACEMENT

**Figure 42.5** An illustrative example of changes in arterial partial pressure of oxygen and carbon dioxide (Pao$_2$ and Paco$_2$, respectively) (in kPa) during suction and physiotherapy. Time points A and B correspond to times of preoxygenation and suction, respectively.

randomized two-center study demonstrated that the use of this monitor in preterm infants was associated with a reduction in red blood cell transfusions.[88]

Although the use of these devices produces immediate bedside data, the need for personnel to initiate an analysis makes it similar to a conventional BGA in terms of operation. However, obviation of the need to sample blood and minimization of exposure of staff to potentially infected blood are significant advantages. The study by Widness and associates was the first demonstration of the usefulness of these devices in a controlled trial.

## CONTINUOUS EXTRACORPOREAL BLOOD GAS MONITORING SYSTEMS

Other examples of extracorporeal blood gas monitoring systems include those designed for use in the extracorporeal circuit during cardiopulmonary bypass (Gas STAT [Cardiovasular Devices Inc., USA], Cardiomet 4000 [Biomedical Sensors, High Wycombe, UK]).[89,90] Although these systems provide reliable trend monitoring, the bias and precision data are not consistent when compared with continuous intravascular blood gas systems.[53] This problem, combined with the need for anticoagulation with the use of extracorporeal systems, limits their role in ICU patients.

## CENTRAL VENOUS SATURATION

The incorporation of reflectance spectrophotometry methodology into a central venous catheter design has allowed the continuous measurement of central venous $O_2$ saturation ($ScvO_2$). $ScvO_2$ is normally 2% to 3% lower than mixed venous $O_2$ saturation ($SvO_2$). In an influential single-center study of the early hypodynamic phase of severe sepsis and septic shock, resuscitation guided by an $ScvO_2$ target of greater than 0.7, as well as by central venous pressure and mean arterial pressure values, appeared to reduce 28-day and 60-day mortality and duration of hospitalization.[91] It remains to be seen whether this success can be replicated in larger trials and, if so, whether intermittent sampling is of equivalent benefit. Nevertheless, $ScvO_2$ currently has equal billing with $SvO_2$ in the management guidelines of the Surviving Sepsis Campaign.

## APPLICATIONS OF CONTINUOUS BLOOD GAS MONITORING SYSTEMS

Although these systems were initially designed for continuous blood gas monitoring, they have found greater application in the continuous monitoring of tissue oxygenation and tissue perfusion. The authors demonstrated the usefulness of these sensors for the measurement of subcutaneous and gut oxygenation in animal models of hemorrhagic and endotoxic shock.[92,93] The usefulness of continuous gut luminal $PCO_2$ measurements as a sensitive indicator of splanchnic ischemia was also validated.[94] These systems have also been adapted for monitoring cerebral oxygenation.[95,96] Although only one published study examined the usefulness of continuous arterial-end tidal $CO_2$ gradient as a trend of continuous cardiac output in the presence of stable ventilatory parameters and found a poor correlation,[76] this measurement offers a novel method of titrating inotropic therapy with minimally invasive technology.

## FUTURE OF CONTINUOUS BLOOD GAS MONITORING

Further refinements to this technology and data on cost effectiveness are required before it will have widespread application in intensive care practice. Physiologic studies to define the interaction between the probe and the host environment will enable us to develop and apply this exciting technology further. Extracorporeal in-line, on-demand systems have shown promise in preliminary trials. A major factor determining the widespread acceptance of these technologies is the issue of cost effectiveness, particularly in the current climate of escalating health care costs. The cost of disposable devices for a CIABGM in the United States is approximately $300 to $400 for the single use sensor. The cost of blood gas analysis has been reported to be between $25 and $150 in a North American ICU. In contrast, most European and Australasian ICUs possess their own BGAs, thus significantly decreasing the cost of an individual blood gas analysis. Although an argument may be made on the savings made by the reduced number of conventional blood gas analyses performed, a significant reduction in costs is not achieved in most ICU patients because at least two blood gas analyses per day are required to perform in vivo calibration of the CIABGM every 12 hours. There is also a significant capital cost to purchase the equipment. In addition, most modern BGAs also measure hemoglobin, sodium, potassium, glucose, ionized calcium, and lactate and thus provide significant additional information.

The other important issue to examine is whether the regular use of these in-line systems would lead to an improvement in patient outcome in terms of a reduction in the number of adverse events, ventilator days, or duration of weaning. Data are currently nonexistent and would be difficult and costly to provide. To decipher the exact contribution of one monitoring system within a plethora of monitoring modalities, together with the numerous variables that influence patient outcome, would be a very complex task. Cost effectiveness data do not exist for many of the standard monitoring techniques used in the ICU despite their widespread use in clinical practice (e.g., pulse oximetry, pulmonary artery catheterization). Two trials of the usefulness of pulse oximetry produced conflicting results. A study examining the impact of pulse oximetry in surgical patients on reducing ICU admissions demonstrated that routine monitoring did not reduce transfer to ICU, mortality, or overall estimated cost of hospitalization.[97] One multicenter trial showed that the use of intrapartum fetal pulse oximetry in the presence of a nonreassuring fetal heart rate pattern was associated with a reduction in operative interventions.[98] It is likely that the wholesale acceptance of CIABGM will ultimately be determined by outcome studies.

## REFERENCES

1. Mcinnes D, Belcher D: A durable glass electrode. Industrial Eng Chem 1933;5:199–200.
2. Stow R, Randall B: Electrical measurement of the $P_{CO_2}$ of blood. Am J Physiol 1954;179:678–681.
3. Severinghaus JW, Bradley AK: Electrodes for blood $P_{O_2}$ and $P_{CO_2}$ determination. J Appl Physiol 1958;13:515–520.
4. Clark LC: Monitor and control of blood and tissue oxygen measurements. Trans Am Soc Artif Intern Organs 1956;2:41–48.
5. Severinghaus JW, Astrup PB: History of blood gas analysis. Int Anesthesiol Clin 1987;25:11–15.
6. Morgan T, Venkatesh B: Monitoring oxygenation. In Bersten AD, Soni N (eds): Oh's Intensive Care Manual, 5th ed. Sydney: Butterworth-Heinemann, 2003, pp 95–106.
7. Thorson SH, Marini JJ, Pierson DJ, Hudson LD: Variability in arterial blood gas values in stable patients in the ICU. Chest 1983;84:14–18.
8. Roizen MF, Schreider B, Austin W, et al: Pulse oximetry, capnography, and blood gas measurements: Reducing cost and improving the quality of care with technology. J Clin Monit 1993;9:237–240.
9. Ralston AC, Webb RK, Runciman WB, et al: Potential errors in pulse oximetry. I. Pulse oximetry evaluation. Anaesthesia 1991; 46:202–206.
10. Ralston AC, Webb RK, Runciman WB, et al: Potential errors in pulse oximetry. III. Pulse oximetry evaluation. Anaesthesia 1991; 46:291–295.
11. Webb RK, Ralston AC, Runciman WB: Potential errors in pulse oximetry. II. Pulse oximetry evaluation. Anaesthesia 1991;46: 207–212.
12. McMorrow RC, Mythen MG: Pulse oximetry. Curr Opin Crit Care 2006;12:269-271.
13. Rudiger M, Topfer K, Hammer H, et al: A survey of transcutaneous blood gas monitoring among European neonatal intensive care units. BMC Pediatr 2005;5:30.
14. Venkatesh B, Hendry SP: Continuous intra-arterial blood gas monitoring. Intensive Care Medicine 1996;22:818–828.
15. Venkatesh B: Continuous intra-arterial blood gas monitoring. Crit Care Resus 1999;1:150.
16. Kautsky H: Quenching of luminescence by oxygen. Trans Faraday Soc 1939;35:216–219.
17. Opitz N, Lubbers DW: Theory and development of fluorescence-based optochemical oxygen sensors: Oxygen optodes. Int Anesthesiol Clin 1987;25:177–197.
18. Tremper KK, Barker SJ: The optode: Next generation in blood gas measurement. Crit Care Med 1989;17:481–482.
19. Buytendijk F: The use of the antinomy electrode in the determination of pH in vivo. Arch Neerland Physiol 1927; 12:319.
20. Band D, Semple S: Continuous measurement of blood pH with an indwelling arterial glass electrode. J Appl Physiol 1967;22: 854.
21. LeBlanc O, Brown J, Klebe JF, et al: Polymer membrane sensors for continuous intravascular monitoring of blood pH. J Appl Physiol 1976;40:644–647.
22. Nilsson E, Edwall E: Continuous intra-arterial pH-monitoring using monocrystalline antimony as sensor. Scand J Clin Lab Invest 1981;41:333–338.
23. Peterson JI, Goldstein S, Fitzgerald PF: Fiber Optic PH probe for physiological use. Anal Chem 1980;52:864–869.
24. Abraham E, Markle D, Fink S, et al: Continuous measurement of intravascular pH with a fiber optic sensor. Anesth Analg 1985;64:731–736.
25. Wolfbeis O, Furlinger E, Kroneis H, et al: Fluorometric analysis 1: A study on fluorescent indicators for measuring near neutral (physiological) pH values. J Anal Chem 1983;314:119–124.
26. Miller WW, Yafuso M, Yan CF, et al: Performance of an in-vivo, continuous blood-gas monitor with disposable probe. Clin Chem 1987;33:538–542.
27. Vurek G, Feustel P, Severinghaus JW: A fiber optic $P_{CO_2}$ sensor. Ann Biomed Eng 1983;11:499–510.
28. Gehrich JL, Lubbers DW, Opitz N, et al: Optical fluorescence and its application to an intravascular blood gas monitoring system. IEEE Trans Biomed Eng 1986;33:117–132.
29. Kreuzer F, Nessler C: Method of polarographic in vivo continuous recording of blood oxygen tension. Science 1958;128: 1005–1006.
30. Charlton G, Read D, Read J: Continuous intra-arterial $P_{O_2}$ in normal man using a flexible microelectrode. J Appl Physiol 1963;18:1247–1251.
31. Parker D, Key A, Davies R, et al: A disposable catheter-tip transducer for continuous measurement of blood oxygen tension in vivo. Biomed Eng 1971;6:313–317.
32. Mindt W: Sauerstoffsensor fur in vivo Messung. Proc Jahrestag Ges Biomed Techn Erlangen 1973;29–33.
33. Armstrong R, Hutchinson J, Lincoln C, et al: Continuous measurement of arterial oxygen tension during one-lung anaesthesia. Br J Anaesth 1976;48:1005–1010.
34. Eberhard P, Fehlmann W, Mindt W: An electrochemical sensor for continuous intravascular oxygen monitoring. Biotelem Patient Monit 1979;6:16–31.
35. Bratanow N, Polk K, Bland R, et al: Continuous polarographic monitoring of intra-arterial oxygen in the perioperative period. Crit Care Med 1985;13:859–861.
36. Severinghaus JW: Alkaline chloride-free oxygen electrodes. Acta Anaesthiol Scand 1978;68(Suppl):73–75.
37. Nilsson E, Alme B, Edwall G et al: Continuous Intra-arterial $P_{O_2}$ Registrations with Conventional and Surface Heparinised Catheter Electrodes. In: Kimmich, Nijmegen (eds): Monitoring of vital parameters during extra-corporeal circulation. Basel: S. Karger, 1981.
38. Rithalia SVS, Bennet PJ, Tinker J: The performance characteristics of an intra-arterial oxygen electrode. Intensive Care Med 1981;7:305–307.
39. Pfeifer PM, Pearson DT, Clayton RH: Clinical trial of the Continucath intra-arterial oxygen monitor: A comparison with

intermittent arterial blood gas analysis. Anaesthesia 1988;43:
677–682.

40. Rithalia S, Edwards D, Doran BRH, et al: Performance
characteristics of an intra-arterial oxygen electrode in critically ill
adult patients. Br J Intensive Care 1992;2:29–33.

41. Peterson J, Fitzgerald R, Buckhol DK: Fibre optic probe for
in vivo measurement of oxygen partial pressure. Anal Chem
1984;56:62–67.

42. Barker SJ, Tremper KK, Hyatt J, et al: Continuous fiberoptic
arterial oxygen tension measurements in dogs. J Clin Monit
1987;3:48–52.

43. Shapiro BA, Cane RD, Chomka CM, et al: Preliminary evaluation of an intra-arterial blood gas system in dogs and humans.
Crit Care Med 1989;17:455–460.

44. Mahutte CK, Sassoon CS, Muro JR, et al: Progress in the development of a fluorescent intravascular blood gas system in man.
J Clin Monit 1990;6:147–157.

45. Barker SJ, Hyatt J: Continuous measurement of intraarterial
pHa, Pco₂, and Pao₂ in the operating room. Anesth Analg
1991;73:43–48.

46. Zimmerman J, Dellinger R: Initial evaluation of a new intra-
arterial blood gas system in humans. Crit Care Med
1993;21:495–500.

47. Haller M, Kilger E, Briegel J, et al: Continuous intra-arterial
blood gas and pH monitoring in critically ill patients with severe
respiratory failure: A prospective, criterion standard study. Crit
Care Med 1994;22:580–587.

48. Larson CP, Vender J, Seiver A: Multisite evaluation of a continuous intraarterial blood gas monitoring system. Anesthesiology
1994;81:543–552.

49. Roupie EE, Brochard L, Lemaire FJ: Clinical evaluation of a
continuous intra-arterial blood gas system in critically ill patients.
Intensive Care Med 1996;22:1162–1168.

50. Clutton-Brock, TH, Fink S, Luthra AJ, et al: The evaluation of a
new intravascular monitoring system in the pig. J Clin Monit
1994;10:387–391.

51. Venkatesh B, Clutton-Brock TH, Hendry SP: Continuous measurement of blood gases using a combined electrochemical and
spectrophotometric sensor. J Med Eng Technol
1994;18:165–168.

52. Venkatesh B, Clutton-Brock TH, Hendry SP: Continuous
intra-arterial blood gas monitoring during cardiopulmonary
resuscitation. Resuscitation 1995;29:135–138.

53. Venkatesh B, Clutton-Brock TH, Hendry SP: Evaluation of the
Paratrend 7 intravascular blood gas monitor during cardiac
surgery: Comparison with an in-line blood gas monitor during
cardiopulmonary bypass. J Cardiothor Vasc Anesth 1995;9:412–419.

54. Menzel M, Henze D, Soukup J, et al: Experiences with continuous intra-arterial blood gas monitoring. Minerva Anestesiol
2001;67:325–331.

55. Adams AP, Morgan-Hughes JO: Determination of the blood gas
factor of the oxygen electrode using a new tonometer.
Br J Anaesth 1967;39:107–113.

56. Bland JM, Altman DG: Statistical methods for assessing
agreement between two methods of clinical measurement.
Lancet 1986;1:307–310.

57. Jalavisto E: Oxygen consumption of blood and plasma and the
percentage of reticulocytes. Acta Physiol Scand 1959;46:
244–251.

58. Adams AP, Morgan-Hughes JO, Sykes MK: pH and blood gas
analysis: Methods of measurement and sources of error using
electrode systems. Part 1. Anaesthesia 1967;22:575–597.

59. Adams, AP, Morgan-Hughes JO, Sykes MK: pH and blood gas
analysis. Methods of measurement and sources of error using
electrode systems. Part 2 Measurement of Carbon dioxide
tension and acid base. Anasthesia 1968;23:47–64.

60. Scott PV, Horton JN, Mapleson WW: Leakage of oxygen from
blood and water samples stored in plastic and glass syringes. BMJ
1971;3:512–516.

61. Hess EC, Nichols AB, Hunt WB, Suratt PM: Pseudohypoxemia
secondary to leukemia and thrombocytosis. N Engl J Med
1979;301:361–363.

62. Metzger LF, Stauffer WB, Krupinski AV, et al: Detecting errors
in blood gas measurements by analysis with two instruments.
Clin Chem 1987;33:512–517.

63. Hansen J, Casaburi R, Crapo RO, Jensen RL: Assessing precision
and accuracy in blood gas proficiency testing. Am Rev Respir Dis
1990;141:1190–1193.

64. MacGregor DA, Scuderi PE, Bowton DL, et al: A side by side
comparison of four blood gas analyzers using tonometered
human blood. Chest 1990;98(Suppl):33S.

65. Kampelmacher MJ, van Kesteren RG, Winckers EK:
Instrumental variability of respiratory blood gases among
different blood gas analysers in different laboratories. Eur Respir
J 1997;10:1341–1344.

66. Hansen JE, Casaburi R: Patterns of dissimilarities among
instrument models in measuring Po₂, Pco₂, and pH in blood gas
laboratories. Chest 1998;113:780–787.

67. HCFA/CLIA: Proficiency testing requirements for analytical
quality. Fed Regist 1992;40:70002.

68. Venkatesh B, Clutton-Brock TH, Hendry SP: A multiparameter
sensor for continuous intra-arterial blood gas monitoring:
A prospective evaluation. Crit Care Med 1994;22:588–594.

69. Venkatesh B, Pigott DW, Fernandez A, Hendry S: Continuous
measurement of arterial blood gas status during total hip
replacement: A prospective study. Anaesth Intensive Care
1996;24:334–341.

70. Anderson JM, Miller KM: Biomaterial biocompatibility and the
macrophage. Biomaterials 19845:5–10.

71. Schoenfisch MH, Zhang H, Frost MC, Meyerhoff ME: Nitric
oxide–releasing fluorescence-based oxygen sensing polymeric
films. Anal Chem 2002;74:5937–5941.

72. Greenblott G, Barker SJ, Tremper KK, et al: Detection of venous
air embolism by continuous intra-arterial oxygen monitoring.
J Clin Monit 1990;6:53–56.

73. Bein T, Pfeifer M, Riegger GA, Taeger K: Continuous intraarterial measurement of oxygenation during aerosolized prostacyclin
administration in severe respiratory failure [letter]. N Engl J Med
1994;331:335–336.

74. Pappert D, Rossaint R, Gerlach H, Falke K: Continuous monitoring of blood gases during hypercapnia in a patient with severe
acute lung failure. Intensive Care Med 1994;20:210–211.

75. Benson J, Venkatesh B, Patla V: Misleading information from a
pulse oximeter and the usefulness of a continuous intra-arterial
blood gas monitor in a post cardiac surgical patient. Intensive
Care Med 1995;21:437–439.

76. Myles PS, Story DA, Higgs MA, Buckland MR: Continuous measurement of arterial and end-tidal carbon dioxide during cardiac surgery: Pa-ETCO₂ gradient. Anaesth Intensive Care 1997;25:459–463.

77. Ganter MT, Hofer CK, Zollinger A, et al: Accuracy and
performance of a modified continuous intravascular blood gas
monitoring device during thoracoscopic surgery. J Cardiothorac
Vasc Anesth 2004;18:587–591.

78. Aschkenasy SV, Hofer CK, Zalunardo MP, et al: Patterns of
changes in arterial Po₂ during one-lung ventilation: A comparison between patients with severe pulmonary emphysema and
patients with preserved lung function. J Cardiothorac Vasc
Anesth 2005;19:479–484.

79. Pavlidis T, Papaziogas B, Vretzakis G, et al: Continuous monitoring of arterial blood gases and pH during laparoscopic cholecystectomy using a Paratrend sensor. Minerva Chir
2002;57:17–22.

80. Myles PS, Buckland MR, Weeks AM, et al: Continuous arterial blood gas monitoring during bilateral sequential lung transplantation. J Cardiothorac Vasc Anesth 1999;13:253–257.

81. Hatherill M, Tibby SM, Durward A, et al: Continuous intra-arterial blood-gas monitoring in infants and children with cyanotic heart disease. Br J Anaesth 1997;79:665–667.

82. Rais-Bahrami K, Rivera O, Mikesell GT, et al: Continuous blood gas monitoring using an in-dwelling optode method: Clinical evaluation of the Neotrend sensor using a Luer stub adaptor to access the umbilical artery catheter. J Perinatol 2002;22:367–369.

83. Rais-Bahrami K, Rivera O, Mikesell GT, et al: Continuous blood gas monitoring using an in-dwelling optode method: Comparison to intermittent arterial blood gas sampling in ECMO patients. J Perinatol 2002;22:472–474.

84. Shapiro B, Mahutte C, Cane RD, Gilmour IJ: Clinical performance of a blood gas monitor: A prospective, multicenter trial. Crit Care Med 1993;21:487–494.

85. Mahutte CK, Sasse SA, Chen PA, Holody M: Performance of a patient-dedicated, on-demand blood gas monitor in medical ICU patients. Am J Respir Crit Care Med 1994;150:865–869.

86. Myklejord DJ, Pritzker MR, Nicoloff DM, et al: Clinical evaluation of the in-line Sensicath blood gas monitoring system. Heart Surg Forum 1998;1:60–64.

87. Billman GF, Hughes AB, Dudell GG, et al: Clinical performance of an in-line, ex vivo point-of-care monitor: A multicenter study. Clin Chem 2002;48:2030–2043.

88. Widness JA, Madan A, Grindeanu LA, et al: Reduction in red blood cell transfusions among preterm infants: Results of a randomized trial with an in-line blood gas and chemistry monitor. Pediatrics 2005;115:1299–1306.

89. Gothgen IH, Siggaard-Andersen O, Rasmussen JP, et al: Fiber-optic chemical sensors (Gas-Stat) for blood gas monitoring during hypothermic extracorporeal circulation. Scand J Clin Lab Invest 1987;188(Suppl):27–29.

90. Clark JI, Pearson DT, Stone T, et al: An in vitro evaluation of the IL 1312, Gas-Stat and Cardiomet 4000 systems for blood gas analysis. Perfusionist 1990:7–10.

91. Rivers E, Nguyen B, Havstad S, et al: Early goal-directed therapy in the treatment of severe sepsis and septic shock. N Engl J Med 2001;345:1368–1377.

92. Venkatesh B, Morgan TJ, Lipman J: Subcutaneous oxygen tensions provide similar information to ileal luminal $CO_2$

93. tensions in an animal model of haemorrhagic shock. Intensive Care Med 2000;26:592–600.

93. Venkatesh B, Morgan TJ, Hall J, et al: Subcutaneous gas tensions closely track ileal mucosal gas tensions in a model of endotoxaemia without anaerobism. Intensive Care Med 2005;31:447–453.

94. Morgan TJ, Venkatesh B, Endre ZH: Continuous measurement of gut luminal $P_{CO_2}$ in the rat: Responses to transient episodes of graded aortic hypotension. Crit Care Med 1997;25:1575–1578.

95. Zauner A, Bullock R, Di X, Young HF: Brain oxygen, $CO_2$, pH and temperature monitoring: Evaluation in the feline brain. Neurosurgery 1995;37:19.

96. Hoffman WE, Charbel FT, Edelman G, et al: Brain tissue oxygen pressure, carbon dioxide pressure and pH during ischemia. Neurol Res 1996;18:54–56.

97. Ochroch EA, Russell MW, Hanson WC 3rd, et al: The impact of continuous pulse oximetry monitoring on intensive care unit admissions from a postsurgical care floor. Anesth Analg 2006;102:868–875.

98. East CE, Brennecke SP, King JF, et al: The effect of intrapartum fetal pulse oximetry, in the presence of a nonreassuring fetal heart rate pattern, on operative delivery rates: A multicenter, randomized, controlled trial (the FOREMOST trial). Am J Obstet Gynecol 2006;194:606.e1–606.e16.

## SUGGESTED READING

Coule LW, Truemper EJ, Steinhart CM, Lutin WA: Accuracy and utility of a continuous intra-arterial blood gas monitoring system in pediatric patients. Crit Care Med 2001;29:420–426.

Morgan C, Newell SJ, Ducker DA, et al: Continuous neonatal blood gas monitoring using a multiparameter intra-arterial sensor. Arch Dis Child Fetal Neonatal Ed 1999;80:F93–F98.

Smith BE, King PH, Schlain L: Clinical evaluation: Continuous real-time intra-arterial blood gas monitoring during anesthesia and surgery by fiber optic sensor. Int J Clin Monit Comput 1992;9:45–52.

Weiss IK, Fink S, Edmunds S, et al: Continuous arterial gas monitoring: Initial experience with the Paratrend 7 in children. Intensive Care Med 1996;22:1414–1417.

SECTION 7

# FUTURE THERAPY

# CHAPTER 43

# Cytokine Modulation Therapy in Acute Respiratory Failure and ARDS

Jean-Louis Vincent, Gustavo Buchele, and Gustavo A. Ospina-Tascón

Cytokine modulation therapy in sepsis has been extensively researched. Multiple potential agents are in development, and many of these agents are in clinical trials. In acute respiratory distress syndrome (ARDS), however, the potential benefits of immunomodulatory therapy are less commonly discussed. Yet is ARDS so different from sepsis? Indeed, ARDS is one component of the multiple organ failure that complicates severe sepsis, and some 80% of patients with ARDS will die of multiple organ failure and not of respiratory failure per se.[1] The same mediators (e.g., tumor necrosis factor-$\alpha$ [TNF-$\alpha$] and interleukin-1 [IL-1]) and inflammatory cells that participate in the initiation and maintenance of the septic response to infection are involved in the development and continuation of ARDS[2] regardless of the underlying cause. ARDS is a respiratory disease, but it is also part of a much bigger picture. Therapeutic strategies targeting only the lung are unlikely to be effective in enhancing outcomes even if they provide temporary improvement in lung function. To date, no cytokine modulation therapy has been shown to improve outcomes specifically in patients with ARDS, but research is ongoing. In this chapter, we discuss some of the key agents currently undergoing investigation and those that hold promise for the future.

## NONSPECIFIC MEASURES THAT MAY INFLUENCE CYTOKINE RELEASE OR ACTIVATION

### Low–Tidal Volume Ventilation

Overstretching the lungs may increase the inflammatory response. The results of the ARDS Network trial, published in 2000, demonstrated that, in patients with acute lung injury (ALI) and ARDS, mechanical ventilation with lower tidal volumes (6 mL/kg) than traditionally used (12 mL/kg) decreased mortality rates and increased the number of days without ventilator use.[3] By day 3, the 6 mL/kg strategy was associated with a greater decrease in IL-6 and IL-8 levels, with a 26% reduction in IL-6 levels (95% confidence interval, 12% to 37%) and a 12% reduction in IL-8 levels (95% confidence interval, 1% to 23%) in the 6 mL/kg group compared with the 12 mL/kg group.[4] This finding suggested that lower–tidal volume ventilation was associated with a more rapid attenuation of the inflammatory response.[4] Hence, tidal volume should be limited in all patients with ALI/ARDS, especially when the airway pressures exceed 30 cmH$_2$O. It may even be worthwhile to limit tidal volumes in patients with severe sepsis, even in the absence of ALI/ARDS.[5] Accordingly, the Surviving Sepsis Campaign guidelines for the management of severe sepsis recommend that high tidal volumes should be avoided in patients with ALI/ARDS, and tidal volumes of 6 mL/kg should be the target.[6]

## Liquid Ventilation

Partial liquid ventilation, in which the lungs are partially filled with perfluorocarbons (PFCs), has been suggested as an approach to the treatment of patients with ARDS. The theory is that, in ARDS, PFCs improve gas exchange by recruiting dependent lung regions, by clearing retained secretions, and by redistributing blood flow to ventilated regions. PFCs have also been reported to have anti-inflammatory properties.[7] Animal models have demonstrated improved oxygenation and reduced histologic evidence of lung injury with partial liquid ventilation,[8] and a post hoc analysis of a phase II trial of partial liquid ventilation versus conventional ventilation demonstrated faster discontinuation of mechanical ventilation and a trend to decreased mortality in PFC-treated patients who were less than 55 years old.[9] However, in a randomized controlled trial of 311 patients with ARDS, partial liquid ventilation, at two doses, was not associated with reduced duration of ventilation or reduced mortality, and it was linked to increased adverse events including pneumothorax and hypoxic and hypotensive episodes.[10] Hence partial liquid ventilation cannot be recommended for patients with ARDS.

## Surfactant

Pulmonary surfactant lines the gas-exchanging surface of the pulmonary epithelium and forms a key part of the body's defense against infection.[11] In ARDS, surfactant is decreased in quantity and is also functionally abnormal. Animal studies and small clinical studies have shown that exogenous surfactant instillation can improve gas exchange and lung mechanics in ALI/ARDS.[12–14] One study reported reduced IL-6 levels in patients treated with surfactant, a finding that suggested an anti-inflammatory effect.[15] Despite the results of several early studies suggesting that surfactant administration may be associated with improved survival,[12,13] two phase III studies were unable to demonstrate any beneficial effect of surfactant administration on outcome in adult patients with ARDS.[16,17] In pediatric patients with ALI, however, intratracheal instillation of surfactant did seem to improve oxygenation and reduce mortality rates.[18] The reasons behind the discrepancies in results between phase II and phase III trials and between children and adults may be related to the different surfactant preparations used, the method of administration (e.g., bronchoscopic or intratracheal instillation, aerosolization), and

the dose.[19] Surfactant appears to have the potential to improve pulmonary function in ALI and ARDS, and it is possible that future studies will demonstrate improved outcomes once questions have been answered regarding type of surfactant preparation, dose, and method of administration.[20]

## Nitric Oxide

Nitric oxide (NO) is synthesized by the vascular endothelium from L-arginine. NO acts as a natural local vasodilator, relaxing muscular arteries and veins by activating guanylate cyclase and increasing cyclic guanosine 3′,5′-monophosphate. ARDS is characterized by intrapulmonary shunting that results in arterial hypoxemia and by acute pulmonary arterial hypertension secondary to vasoconstriction and widespread occlusion of the pulmonary microvasculature. Inhaled NO has therefore been proposed as a means of improving the perfusion of ventilated regions, with the objective of potentially improving oxygenation and lowering pulmonary vascular resistance. Inhaled NO may also have immunomodulatory effects. In animal models administration of NO is associated with reduced sequestration of polymorphonuclear leukocytes,[21] a key modulator of lung injury in ARDS. However, the effects of NO on the immune system are complex and poorly understood. Clinical trials using inhaled NO in patients with ARDS have demonstrated transiently improved oxygenation in treated patients, but no increase in survival rates.[22–24] Guidelines currently recommend that inhaled NO be reserved for use as a rescue treatment in patients with severe refractory hypoxemia.[25]

## SPECIFIC CYTOKINE-MODULATING AGENTS

### Neutrophil Elastase Inhibitors

Neutrophils and neutrophil elastase are important in the endothelial injury characteristics of ARDS.[26,27] Although neutrophil elastase has certain beneficial effects, including antimicrobial actions and enhancement of tissue repair, excess neutrophil elastase is associated with cell and tissue injury. Neutrophil elastase can promote microvascular injury leading to increased permeability and interstitial edema.[27] Neutrophil elastase also increases the release of IL-8, a potent neutrophil chemoattractant and activator, thus potentiating the inflammatory response.[28] Raised levels of neutrophil elastase have been found in the bronchoalveolar fluid and blood of patients with ARDS, and serum levels have correlated with the degree of subsequent lung injury and ARDS.[29] In animal models, neutrophil elastase knockout mice were resistant to the lethal effects of endotoxin,[30] and neutrophil elastase inhibition attenuated lung injury.[31–33] These encouraging results were followed by clinical trials. A phase III study in Japan showed pulmonary function improvement and reduced intensive care unit stay, along with trends toward reduced mortality and duration of mechanical ventilation.[34] However, a multicenter randomized controlled trial of sivelestat (ONO-5046) was unable to confirm these results and reported no effect on pulmonary function, ventilator-free days, or 28-day mortality.[35]

## Anticoagulants

Local tissue factor–dependent activation of coagulation and concomitant inhibition of fibrinolysis are pathophysiologic features of ARDS, and alveolar and interstitial fibrin deposition are the hallmarks of early-phase ALI.[36] Animal studies suggested improved lung function with various anticoagulant agents in models of ALI and ARDS.[37–39] Therefore, several anticoagulant agents have now been evaluated as potential therapies in patients with sepsis and ARDS.

In a phase II study, recombinant tissue factor pathway inhibitor (rTFPI) was evaluated in 210 patients with severe sepsis.[40] Patients treated with rTFPI had a nonsignificant reduction in 28-day mortality and an improvement in lung and composite organ dysfunction scores. In the subgroups of patients with ARDS, rTFPI treatment was associated with improved pulmonary function and a trend toward reduced mortality. However, in a phase III study, which included 1955 patients with severe sepsis,[41] treatment with rTFPI had no effect on all-cause mortality in patients with severe sepsis, including those with ARDS. rTFPI administration was associated with an increased risk of bleeding.

In a small-scale study involving 42 subjects with severe sepsis, Eisele and associates showed that antithrombin treatment improved lung function.[42] However, in 40 trauma patients who were randomized either to antithrombin or to placebo, Waydhas and colleagues reported no differences in mortality, incidence of respiratory failure, or duration of mechanical ventilation between the two groups.[43] In a large randomized controlled trial involving 2314 patients with severe sepsis or septic shock, Warren and associates showed that antithrombin therapy had no effect on 28-day mortality.[44] The incidence of bleeding complications was significantly higher with antithrombin therapy than with placebo. Although the study did not specifically consider patients with ALI at baseline, antithrombin administration was associated with a lower prevalence of new pulmonary dysfunction compared with placebo (22.5% versus 26.6%).

FFR-rFVIIa is a modified recombinant factor VIIa in which the catalytic site is irreversibly blocked by a synthetic ketone. The result is an enzymatically inactive rFVIIa that retains its tissue factor binding capacity. The resultant inactive tissue factor–FFR-rFVIIa complexes block the tissue factor/FVII-induced activation of the coagulation cascade,[45] and its other intracellular activities. In a baboon model of sepsis-induced ALI, FFR-rFVIIa limited the development of ALI, protected gas exchange and lung compliance, prevented lung edema and pulmonary hypertension, and preserved renal function. Treatment also decreased systemic proinflammatory cytokine responses.[46,47] However, in a phase II study reported in 2005 of patients with recent-onset ALI/ARDS, treatment with FFR-rFVIIa had no effect on the inflammatory response, hemodynamic and ventilator parameters, or outcome.[48]

Activated protein C is an endogenous protein that promotes fibrinolysis and inhibits thrombosis and inflammation. Plasma protein C levels were reported to be lower in patients with ALI/ARDS than in patients with hydrostatic pulmonary edema resulting from acute myocardial infarction, congestive heart failure, or volume overload.[49] Lower levels of protein C were associated with worse clinical outcomes, including death, fewer ventilator-free days, and more cases of nonpulmonary organ failure, even in patients with noninfectious causes of ARDS. Drotrecogin alfa (activated), a recombinant form of activated protein C, was shown to reduce absolute mortality rates from 30% to 24% in patients with severe sepsis, but this agent has not been evaluated specifically in patients with ALI/ARDS. Drotrecogin alfa (activated) has anti-inflammatory effects in addition to its anticoagulant properties,[50] and these properties may explain in part the agent's success where other anticoagulant agents have failed. A phase II randomized controlled trial of drotrecogin alfa (activated) in patients with ALI/ARDS is ongoing.

## Granulocyte-Macrophage Colony-Stimulating Factor

Granulocyte-macrophage colony-stimulating factor (GM-CSF) is a naturally occurring cytokine that is involved in the normal maturation and functioning of alveolar macrophages, cells involved in host defense to infection, and inflammation. GM-CSF also promotes proliferation of epithelial cells and limits epithelial cell death, key features in the pathogenesis of ARDS. GM-CSF has been shown to protect animals against ALI and to be protective against pulmonary fibrosis following ALI.[51] In a phase II study in patients with severe sepsis and respiratory dysfunction, low-dose GM-CSF was associated with restoration or preservation of blood and alveolar leukocyte phagocytic function and with improved gas exchange without pulmonary neutrophil infiltration.[52] The investigators noted no effect on mortality rates compared with placebo. A larger phase II study comparing GM-CSF with placebo in adult patients with ARDS is currently ongoing.

## High-Mobility Group Box 1 Protein Inhibitors

High-mobility group box 1 protein (HMGB1) is a DNA binding protein involved in maintenance of nucleosome structure and regulation of gene transcription. It also functions as a late-acting cytokine in sepsis, and raised HMGB1 levels are correlated with poor survival in patients with sepsis.[53] Unlike other proinflammatory cytokines, such as IL-1 and TNF-α, which are produced within minutes of recognition of an infectious insult, HMGB1 is a late-appearing inflammatory cytokine that is released several hours after endotoxin exposure.[53] This late onset of action has raised considerable interest because it provides a wider time frame for clinical intervention against progressive inflammatory disorders. Ethyl pyruvate, a stable aliphatic ester derived from pyruvic acid, has been shown to inhibit HMGB1 release from human macrophages in a concentration-dependent fashion. Administration of ethyl pyruvate improved survival in mice subjected to cecal ligation and puncture, even when it was given 1 day after the onset of disease.[54] In a sheep model of septic shock, ethyl pyruvate prolonged the time to develop organ dysfunction and markedly prolonged survival.[55]

In the lungs, HMGB1 can cause an acute pulmonary inflammatory response, manifested by neutrophil accumulation, interstitial edema, and increased production of proinflammatory cytokines.[56] Administration of anti-HMGB1 antibodies decreased neutrophil accumulation and edema formation and improved survival in a mouse model of ALI.[56] In a rabbit model of ventilator-induced lung injury, blockade of HMGB1 improved oxygenation, limited microvascular permeability and neutrophil influx into the alveolar lumen, and decreased concentrations of TNF-α in bronchoalveolar lavage fluid.[57] Although plasma HMGB1 levels were raised in patients with ALI/ARDS compared with control patients who did not have ALI/ARDS, pulmonary epithelial lining fluid HMGB1 levels were raised in both groups of patients, a finding suggesting an important physiologic role for HMGB1 in the lung.[58] Clearly, HMGB1 is involved in the pathogenesis of ALI/ARDS, but its precise roles in disease and health remain to be elucidated before clinical trials can be conducted.

## Continuous Renal Replacement Therapy

Because the pathophysiology of sepsis and ARDS is associated with high circulating levels of inflammatory cytokines, strategies to remove these cytokines, such as hemofiltration, have been investigated as providing a means of limiting the inflammatory response, by a global reduction in mediators rather than focusing on the blockade on any one cytokine. Several studies using animal models of ALI showed improved hemodynamics and lung function with various hemofiltration strategies.[59-61] Some clinical studies also showed that continuous renal replacement therapy (CRRT) improved oxygenation in patients with respiratory failure,[62,63] whereas other studies have reported no effect of CRRT on respiratory function in patients with ALI.[64] Further study is required to determine whether this strategy has a place in the management of patients with ARDS and, if so, to define optimal timing and choice of CRRT strategy.[65]

## CONCLUSION

Despite advances in our understanding of the pathogenesis of ARDS and improvements in supportive strategies including mechanical ventilation, mortality rates from ARDS remain high. Currently, management relies on identifying and controlling the underlying cause, ensuring hemodynamic stabilization, providing appropriate organ support, and minimizing further damage, such as by using low–tidal volume ventilation. Because ARDS is part of a larger systemic picture, strategies that target only the lung are unlikely to be effective. Cytokine modulation is an exciting area of ongoing research. Although we have touched just the surface, new studies appear on an almost weekly basis, and investigators detail potential new therapies that may either directly or indirectly influence cytokine release and activity. Eventually, some of these interventions will be shown convincingly to improve outcomes in patients with ARDS. The challenge then will to determine which patients will benefit most from which treatments and when.

## REFERENCES

1. Vincent JL, Sakr Y, Ranieri VM: Epidemiology and outcome of acute respiratory failure in intensive care unit patients. Crit Care Med 2003;31:S296–S299.
2. Bhatia M, Moochhala S: Role of inflammatory mediators in the pathophysiology of acute respiratory distress syndrome. J Pathol 2004;202:145–156.
3. ARDS Network: Ventilation with lower tidal volumes as compared with traditional tidal volumes for acute lung injury and the acute respiratory distress syndrome. N Engl J Med 2000;342: 1301–1308.
4. Parsons PE, Eisner MD, Thompson BT, et al: Lower tidal volume ventilation and plasma cytokine markers of inflammation in patients with acute lung injury. Crit Care Med 2005;33:1–6.
5. Su F, Nguyen ND, Creteur J, et al: Use of low tidal volume in septic shock may decrease severity of subsequent acute lung injury. Shock 2004;22:145–150.
6. Dellinger RP, Carlet JM, Masur H, et al: Surviving Sepsis Campaign guidelines for management of severe sepsis and septic shock. Crit Care Med 2004;32:858–873.

7. Thomassen MJ, Buhrow LT, Wiedemann HP: Perflubron decreases inflammatory cytokine production by human alveolar macrophages. Crit Care Med 1997;25:2045–2047.

8. Hirschl RB, Parent A, Tooley R, et al: Liquid ventilation improves pulmonary function, gas exchange, and lung injury in a model of respiratory failure. Ann Surg 1995;221:79–88.

9. Hirschl RB, Croce M, Gore D, et al: Prospective, randomized, controlled pilot study of partial liquid ventilation in adult acute respiratory distress syndrome. Am J Respir Crit Care Med 2002;165:781–787.

10. Kacmarek RM, Wiedemann HP, Lavin PT, et al: Partial liquid ventilation in adult patients with acute respiratory distress syndrome. Am J Respir Crit Care Med 2006;173:882–889.

11. McCormack FX, Whitsett JA: The pulmonary collectins, SP-A and SP-D, orchestrate innate immunity in the lung. J Clin Invest 2002;109:707–712.

12. Gregory TJ, Steinberg KP, Spragg R, et al: Bovine surfactant therapy for patients with acute respiratory distress syndrome. Am J Respir Crit Care Med 1997;155:1309–1315.

13. Walmrath D, Grimminger F, Pappert D, et al: Bronchoscopic administration of bovine natural surfactant in ARDS and septic shock: Impact on gas exchange and haemodynamics. Eur Respir J 2002;19:805–810.

14. Walmrath D, Günther A, Ghofani HA, et al: Bronchoscopic surfactant administration in patients with severe adult respiratory distress syndrome and sepsis. Am J Respir Crit Care Med 1996;154:57–62.

15. Spragg RG, Lewis JF, Wurst W, et al: Treatment of acute respiratory distress syndrome with recombinant surfactant protein C surfactant. Am J Respir Crit Care Med 2003;167:1562–1566.

16. Anzueto A, Baughmann RP, Guntupalli KK, et al: Aerosolized surfactant in adults with sepsis-induced acute respiratory distress syndrome. N Engl J Med 1996;334:1417–1421.

17. Spragg RG, Lewis JF, Walmrath HD, et al: Effect of recombinant surfactant protein C–based surfactant on the acute respiratory distress syndrome. N Engl J Med 2004;351:884–892.

18. Willson DF, Thomas NJ, Markovitz BP, et al: Effect of exogenous surfactant (calfactant) in pediatric acute lung injury: A randomized controlled trial. JAMA 2005;293:470–476.

19. Kesecioglu J, Haitsma JJ: Surfactant therapy in adults with acute lung injury/acute respiratory distress syndrome. Curr Opin Crit Care 2006;12:55–60.

20. Westphal M, Traber DL: Exogenous surfactant in acute lung injury: No longer a question? Crit Care Med 2005;33:2431–2433.

21. Sato Y, Walley KR, Klut ME, et al: Nitric oxide reduces the sequestration of polymorphonuclear leukocytes in lung by changing deformability and CD18 expression. Am J Respir Crit Care Med 1999;159:1469–1476.

22. Dellinger RP, Zimmerman JL, Taylor RW, et al: Effects of inhaled nitric oxide in patients with acute respiratory distress syndrome: Results of a randomized phase II trial. Crit Care Med 1998;26:15–23.

23. Lundin S, Mang H, Smithies M, et al: Inhalation of nitric oxide in acute lung injury: Results of a European multicentre study. The European Study Group of Inhaled Nitric Oxide. Intensive Care Med 1999;25:911–919.

24. Taylor RW, Zimmerman JL, Dellinger RP, et al: Low-dose inhaled nitric oxide in patients with acute lung injury: A randomized controlled trial. JAMA 2004;291:1603–1609.

25. Germann P, Braschi A, Della RG, et al: Inhaled nitric oxide therapy in adults: European expert recommendations. Intensive Care Med 2005;31:1029–1041.

26. Carden D, Xiao F, Moak C, et al: Neutrophil elastase promotes lung microvascular injury and proteolysis of endothelial cadherins. Am J Physiol 1998;275:H385–H392.

27. Moraes TJ, Chow CW, Downey GP: Proteases and lung injury. Crit Care Med 2003;31:S189–S194.

28. Chen HC, Lin HC, Liu CY, et al: Neutrophil elastase induces IL-8 synthesis by lung epithelial cells via the mitogen-activated protein kinase pathway. J Biomed Sci 2004;11:49–58.

29. Donnelly SC, MacGregor I, Zamani A, et al: Plasma elastase levels and the development of the adult respiratory distress syndrome. Am J Respir Crit Care Med 1995;151:1428–1433.

30. Tkalcevic J, Novelli M, Phylactides M, et al: Impaired immunity and enhanced resistance to endotoxin in the absence of neutrophil elastase and cathepsin G. Immunity 2000;12:201–210.

31. Delacourt C, Herigault S, Delclaux C, et al: Protection against acute lung injury by intravenous or intratracheal pretreatment with EPI-HNE-4, a new potent neutrophil elastase inhibitor. Am J Respir Cell Mol Biol 2002;26:290–297.

32. Miyazaki Y, Inoue T, Kyi M, et al: Effects of a neutrophil elastase inhibitor (ONO-5046) on acute pulmonary injury induced by tumor necrosis factor alpha (TNFα) and activated neutrophils in isolated perfused rabbit lungs. Am J Respir Crit Care Med 1998;157:89–94.

33. Tremblay GM, Vachon E, Larouche C, et al: Inhibition of human neutrophil elastase-induced acute lung injury in hamsters by recombinant human pre-elafin (trappin-2). Chest 2002;121:582–588.

34. Tamakuma S, Shiba T, Hirasawa H, et al: [A phase III clinical study of neutrophil elastase inhibitor ONO-5046 Na in SIRS patients.] J Clin Ther Med 1998;14:289–318.

35. Zeiher BG, Artigas A, Vincent JL, et al: Neutrophil elastase inhibition in acute lung injury: Results of the STRIVE study. Crit Care Med 2004;32:1695–1702.

36. Laterre PF, Wittebole X, Dhainaut JF: Anticoagulant therapy in acute lung injury. Crit Care Med 2003;31(Suppl):S329–S336.

37. Enkhbaatar P, Okajima K, Murakami K, et al: Recombinant tissue factor pathway inhibitor reduces lipopolysaccharide-induced pulmonary vascular injury by inhibiting leukocyte activation. Am J Respir Crit Care Med 2000;162:1752–1759.

38. Miller DL, Welty-Wolf K, Carraway MS, et al: Extrinsic coagulation blockade attenuates lung injury and proinflammatory cytokine release after intratracheal lipopolysaccharide. Am J Respir Cell Mol Biol 2002;26:650–658.

39. Uchiba M, Okajima K, Murakami K: Effects of various doses of antithrombin III on endotoxin-induced endothelial cell injury and coagulation abnormalities in rats. Thromb Res 1998;89:233–241.

40. Abraham E, Reinhart K, Svoboda P, et al: Assessment of the safety of recombinant tissue factor pathway inhibitor in patients with severe sepsis: A multicenter, randomized, placebo-controlled, single-blind, dose escalation study. Crit Care Med 2001;29:2081–2089.

41. Abraham E, Reinhart K, Opal S, et al: Efficacy and safety of tifacogin (recombinant tissue factor pathway inhibitor) in severe sepsis: A randomized controlled trial. JAMA 2003;290:238–247.

42. Eisele B, Lamy M, Thijs LG, et al: Antithrombin III in patients with severe sepsis: A randomized, placebo-controlled, double-blind multicenter trial plus a meta-analysis on all randomized, placebo-controlled, double-blind trials with antithrombin III in severe sepsis. Intensive Care Med 1998;24:663–672

43. Waydhas C, Nast-Kolb D, Gippner-Steppert C, et al: High-dose antithrombin III treatment of severely injured patients: Results of a prospective study. J Trauma 1998;45:931–940.

44. Warren BL, Eid A, Singer P, et al: Caring for the critically ill patient: High-dose antithrombin III in severe sepsis: A randomized controlled trial. JAMA 2001;286:1869–1878.

45. Kjalke M, Monroe DM, Hoffman M, et al: The effects of activated factor VII in a cell-based model for tissue factor-initiated coagulation. Blood Coagul Fibrinolysis 1998;9(Suppl 1):S21–S25.

46. Carraway MS, Welty-Wolf KE, Miller DL, et al: Blockade of tissue factor: Treatment for organ injury in established sepsis. Am J Respir Crit Care Med 2003;167:1200–1209.

47. Welty-Wolf KE, Carraway MS, Miller DL, et al: Coagulation blockade prevents sepsis-induced respiratory and renal failure in baboons. Am J Respir Crit Care Med 2001;164:1988–1996.

48. Vincent JL, Artigas A, Lundin S, et al: Multicenter, randomized study of ASIS in patients with ALI/ARDS (abstract). Intensive Care Med 2005;31:S5.

49. Ware LB, Fang X, Matthay MA: Protein C and thrombomodulin in human acute lung injury. Am J Physiol 2003;285:L514–L521.

50. Macias WL, Yan SB, Williams MD, et al: New insights into the protein C pathway: Potential implications for the biological activities of drotrecogin alfa (activated). Crit Care 2005;9 (Suppl 4):S38–S45.

51. Paine R III, Wilcoxen SE, Morris SB, et al: Transgenic overexpression of granulocyte macrophage-colony stimulating factor in the lung prevents hyperoxic lung injury. Am J Pathol 2003;163:2397–2406.

52. Presneill JJ, Harris T, Stewart AG, et al: A randomized phase II trial of granulocyte-macrophage colony-stimulating factor therapy in severe sepsis with respiratory dysfunction. Am J Respir Crit Care Med 2002;166:138–143.

53. Wang H, Bloom O, Zhang M, et al: HMG-1 as a late mediator of endotoxin lethality in mice. Science 1999;285:248–251.

54. Ulloa L, Ochani M, Yang H, et al: Ethyl pyruvate prevents lethality in mice with established lethal sepsis and systemic inflammation. Proc Natl Acad Sci U S A 2002;99:12351–12356.

55. Abraham E, Arcaroli J, Carmody A, et al: HMG-1 as a mediator of acute lung inflammation. J Immunol 2002;165:2950–2954.

56. Su F, Wang Z, Cai Y, et al: Beneficial effects of ethyl pyruvate in septic shock due to peritonitis. Arch Surg 2007;142:166–171.

57. Ogawa EN, Ishizaka A, Tasaka S, et al: Contribution of high mobility group box-1 to the development of ventilator-induced lung injury. Am J Respir Crit Care Med 2006;174:400–407.

58. Ueno H, Matsuda T, Hashimoto S, et al: Contributions of high mobility group box protein in experimental and clinical acute lung injury. Am J Respir Crit Care Med 2004;170:1310–1316.

59. Su X, Bai C, Hong Q, et al: Effect of continuous hemofiltration on hemodynamics, lung inflammation and pulmonary edema in a canine model of acute lung injury. Intensive Care Med 2003;29:2034–2042.

60. Ullrich R, Roeder G, Lorber C, et al: Continuous venovenous hemofiltration improves arterial oxygenation in endotoxin-induced lung injury in pigs. Anesthesiology 2001;95:428–436.

61. Yan XW, Li WQ, Wang H, et al: Effects of high-volume continuous hemofiltration on experimental pancreatitis associated lung injury in pigs. Int J Artif Organs 2006;29:293–302.

62. Bagshaw ON, Anaes FR, Hutchinson A: Continuous arteriovenous haemofiltration and respiratory function in multiple organ systems failure. Intensive Care Med 1992;18:334–338.

63. Garzia F, Todor R, Scalea T: Continuous arteriovenous hemofiltration countercurrent dialysis (CAVH-D) in acute respiratory failure (ARDS). J Trauma 1991;31:1277–1285.

64. Hoste EA, Vanholder RC, Lameire NH, et al: No early respiratory benefit with CVVHDF in patients with acute renal failure and acute lung injury. Nephrol Dial Transplant 2002;17:2153–2158.

65. Venkataraman R, Subramanian S, Kellum JA: Clinical review: Extracorporeal blood purification in severe sepsis. Crit Care 2003;7:139–145.

# CHAPTER 44

# Gene Transfer in the Lung

Terence R. Flotte

The susceptibility to lung diseases depends to varying extents on host cell gene expression. In certain situations, lung disease can be directly caused by the absence of a single functional copy of one particular gene, as in cystic fibrosis. In other conditions, however, such as acute respiratory distress syndrome (ARDS), numerous different genetic and environmental factors interact to predispose patients to disease. Gene transfer to the lung has the potential to provide a therapeutic effect either in single-gene diseases or in multifactorial diseases, if safe and effective means of gene expression can be achieved. In many instances, the specific therapeutic gene to be augmented has been elucidated by studies in the modern era of molecular research. In those instances, the only remaining limitation is the presence of an appropriate vector for gene delivery.

A limited repertoire of viral and nonviral gene transfer vectors currently exists, and the properties of these vectors have been fairly well defined (Table 44.1). As outlined in Table 44.1, the properties of viral gene transfer vectors generally mimic those of the virus on which each vector is based. Furthermore, knowledge of the molecular virology of each of these viruses forms the basis for understanding the features of recombinant vectors that do differ somewhat from their respective parental viruses. Nonviral vectors are less clearly understood, but they have the potential to incorporate synthetic elements of a variety of types (protein, DNA, chemical) that may produce predicted effects based on known cellular mechanisms.

The apparent efficacy of each vector system can further be considered in the context of the specific lung compartment that contains the target cell for gene transfer. The pathobiology of each specific disease and the properties of the transgene product determine the compartmental localization.

## COMPARTMENTAL TARGETS FOR GENE TRANSFER

The proximal goal of any gene transfer is to deliver genetic material to the nucleus of a cell, thus increasing (or decreasing in some cases) the expression of a protein of interest. The first question to be addressed in the approach to any gene transfer therapy is "What is the gene/protein?" For a single-gene disease such as cystic fibrosis (CF), the answer is usually obvious, whereas for a multifactorial disease such as asthma, it may not be. The second question to be addressed is "Which cell?" This question must further be broken down into two parts. The first subquestion concerns the location where the protein of interest has to be active, and the second concerns the area where the protein should or could be produced. The answer to these latter two questions may or may not be the same.

For instance, CF is a disease of the conducting airways in which the transgene product is an integral membrane protein that is unable to spread to other compartments once it is expressed within the target cells. This situation mandates that the airway compartment must necessarily be the compartment targeted for gene transfer. In contrast, $\alpha_1$-antitrypsin (AAT) deficiency (A1AD) is a disease in which lung injury may occur within the interstitium and perhaps also in the airways. However, the gene product in this case is secreted into the extracellular space and therefore can be delivered to its site of

**Table 44-1    Vectors Available for Gene Transfer to the Lungs**

| Vector Class | Advantages | Disadvantages |
|---|---|---|
| Adenovirus | Highly efficient | Transient, proinflammatory |
| Adeno-associated virus | Persistent, safe | Small packaging capacity |
| Lentivirus | Stable integration | Long-term safety? |
| Nonviral | High packaging capacity | Transient, proinflammatory |
| Other (herpes, simian virus 40) | Potential high efficiency | Not well characterized |

**BOX 44-1**

**Components of the Lung**

- Conducting airways
  - Surface epithelium
  - Smooth muscle
  - Submucosal glands
- Alveoli (airspaces)
- Alveolar interstitium
- Vascular structures
  - Pulmonary circulation
  - Endothelium
  - Arterial smooth muscle
  - Bronchial circulation
  - Lymphatic vessels
- Pleura
- Extrapulmonary compartment

action from any of several different producer cells. Thus, a broad range of intrapulmonary and extrapulmonary compartments may be considered as targets for gene therapy of A1AD.

As illustrated in this example, the likelihood of success in gene therapy entirely depends on the state of scientific knowledge about the site of action of the therapeutic protein and the distribution properties of that protein. Therefore, as we move forward with this analysis, we incur the risk that faulty assumptions with regard to the pathobiology of the disease in question or with regard to the therapeutic protein could prove to be fatal flaws in the process. In fact, in some situations, gene transfer itself may potentially represent the definitive means of answering the question whether the expression of a certain protein within a certain cell is necessary for prevention of disease.

Having acknowledged that possibility, there is clearly a broad base of knowledge from which to proceed. Finally, one must concede that the categorical assignment of compartments is inherently an oversimplification. When we speak of an airway compartment, we lump together numerous diverse cell types resident within the airways and arbitrarily exclude adjacent vascular structures. Nonetheless, as a first approximation, cells within a given compartment do differ quite significantly from cells in other compartments in terms of the optimal choice of vector class and route of delivery.

For the purposes of this discussion, the lung may be viewed as consisting of the compartments shown in Box 44.1. This classification is obviously arbitrary and is meant to be functional with regard to potential gene transfer targets, rather than comprehensive in the context of pulmonary anatomy. In that regard, one begins to consider individual disease states in terms of which compartment or compartments must serve as targets for gene transfer.

## DISEASES OF THE CONDUCTING AIRWAYS

The diseases of the conducting airways that may be amenable to gene therapy are listed in Table 44.2. CF is the prototype, but other diseases that could be approached in this manner may include asthma, primary ciliary dyskinesias, and infectious diseases. Even within this list, one must consider subcompartments within the conducting airways in the analysis. In CF, there is consensus in favor of targeting the surface epithelium, but clear evidence also indicates that the serous cells of the submucosal glands represent a focus of native *CFTR* gene expression. Does that mean that submucosal gland expression of *CFTR* will be required for clinical efficacy? The answer is currently unknown.

### Cystic Fibrosis Gene Therapy

Various gene transfer approaches have been attempted for CF, the most notable of which have been trials of recombinant adeno-associated virus (rAAV) and recombinant adenovirus (rAd). The rAd-CFTR trials were initiated

**Table 44-2    Diseases of the Conducting Airways That May Be Amenable to Gene Therapy**

| Genetic | Inflammatory | Infectious | Neoplastic |
|---|---|---|---|
| Cystic fibrosis | Asthma | Respiratory syncytial viral infection | Carcinoma |
| Primary ciliary dyskinesias | | Influenza | |

2 years earlier and quickly generated data demonstrating the feasibility of gene expression.[1] However, gene transfer was short term and was associated with an immediate cytokine-mediated inflammatory response, which limited the dose.[2–4] Early studies seemed to indicate that correction of the transepithelial potential difference abnormalities in CF could be feasible with rAd-CFTR,[5] but later studies with a control vector indicated that vector-mediated cytotoxicity could have confounded those earlier results.[6]

Nonviral gene transfer has also been studied in the context of CF. A series of studies with cationic liposomes indicated that short-term gene transfer was feasible in the upper airways.[7–11] One such study used a naked DNA control for cationic liposome gene transfer. This study indicated that naked DNA itself may have some biologic activity for gene transfer.[12] Although these studies were quite encouraging, a subsequent study of aerosol inhalation of cationic liposome-DNA complexes indicated that these complexes elicited a flulike syndrome in experimental subjects when the agent was delivered as an aerosol.[13]

Trials of rAAV-CFTR have progressed further. Preclinical[14–18] and phase I trials showed a very favorable safety profile in the nose,[19] segmental bronchus,[19] and the maxillary sinus,[20,21] as well as after generalized airway delivery by inhaled aerosol.[22] Gene transfer was demonstrated in these trials to occur, to be dose-dependent, and to be free of any vector-related adverse effects. Two phase II trials have been completed, one in the sinus and the other in the lower respiratory tract. These trials have shown definite indications of clinical efficacy, including a decline in the proinflammatory cytokine interleukin-8 and improvement in the transepithelial potential difference in the sinuses, as well as an increase in forced expiratory volume in 1 second after aerosol delivery (Fig. 44.1).[23] Unfortunately, the effects after aerosol delivery have lasted for only 30 days, perhaps reflecting the rate of turnover of the surface epithelium in the CF-affected lung, which is thought to be more rapid than in the normal lung. A phase IIb trial of aerosol delivery is currently ongoing.

Certain key limitations to rAAV-CFTR gene transfer have been defined. These limitations include extracellular barriers, such as partial inactivation of vector by inflammatory byproducts in CF airway secretions and the effects of neutralizing antibodies. The receptors for the common rAAV serotype 2 vector have also been defined, and these receptors are apparently in low abundance on the apical surface of human respiratory epithelium. Finally, postentry blockades to rAAV-CFTR activation have been defined, including proteosome-mediated degradation of rAAV genomes and inhibition of conversion of rAAV DNA to its transcriptionally active double-stranded form by a host protein, FKBP52. rAAV also has an intrinsic limitation owing to the small net packaging capacity of this virion (4.7 kb) relative to the size of the CFTR coding sequence (4.43 kb).[18,24,25]

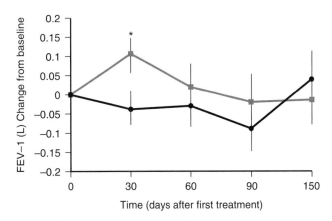

**Figure 44.1** Short-term efficacy of recombinant serotype 2 vector adeno-associated virus (rAAV2)-CFTR gene therapy in a prospective, double-blind, placebo-controlled trial. Plotted are the changes from baseline in forced expiratory volume in 1 second (FEV₁) in liters, in vector-treated (N = 20) and placebo-treated controls (N = 17, *closed circles*). The *asterisk* indicates a significant difference at $P < .04$.

Numerous approaches have been introduced in an attempt to overcome the limitations to rAAV transduction (Table 44.3). These approaches include the introduction of new rAAV serotypes and capsid mutants capable of targeting other receptors that may be present in greater abundance on the apical surface of airway cells.[26–31] Postentry blockades also may be amenable to intervention. For instance, proteosome inhibitors have been shown to accentuate the efficacy of rAAV-CFTR gene transfer greatly in a number of in vitro models.[32] Some of these agents are already approved for use in humans in other conditions and so could be incorporated fairly readily into future gene therapy trials. Finally, there is also an indication that tyrosine kinase inhibitors could

**Table 44-3** Limitations of Recombinant Adeno-Associated Virus Transduction and Strategies to Overcome Those Limitations

| Limitation | Strategy to Circumvent |
|---|---|
| Extracellular barriers (DNA, enzymes, mucus) | Airway clearance, anti-inflammatory, antiprotease pretreatments |
| Paucity of receptors | Alternate serotypes, targeted capsid mutants |
| Proteosome-mediated degradation | Proteosome inhibitors (tripeptides, anthracyclines) |
| Inhibition of second-strand synthesis | Tyrosine kinase inhibitors |

maximize the transcriptional activity of rAAV vectors by inhibiting the phosphorylation of FKBP52.

Lentiviral vectors have also been extensively studied for gene transfer to the conducting airways in the context of potential gene therapy for CF.[33–35] This system, which can integrate its genome into nondividing cells, has strong potential. The greatest efficiency to date has been reported with lentiviral vectors that are pseudotyped with other envelope glycoproteins, such as those from vesicular stomatitis virus (VSV-G) or from filoviruses such as Ebola.[36] The latter class may enter the apical surface of respiratory epithelial cells either through the folate receptor or through an alternative pathway.[37]

## Gene Therapy for Asthma and Other Airway Diseases

The potential for gene therapy for asthma and other diseases of the airways has also been investigated in preclinical models. In particular, some studies showed that the expression of cytokines that bias the immune response toward a T-helper cell-1 (Th1) predominance decreased the severity of asthmatic inflammation in ovalbumin-sensitized mice.[38–43] Other studies focused on blockade of the effector arm of the Th2-predominant asthmatic response.[44] The list of genes that may potentially be therapeutic for asthma is growing (Table 44.4).

The finding that plasmid DNA with CpG sequence motifs elicits cytokine responses on its own regardless of the primary DNA sequence is an observation that was contributed to, in part, by early nonviral gene transfer attempts.[45] It is now known that CpG DNA interacts with a subtype of Toll-like receptors and triggers an innate immune response that itself biases toward a Th1 phenotype. In that context, naked DNA could be particularly well suited for asthma gene therapy.

## DISEASES OF THE ALVEOLI

Diseases of the alveoli that may be amenable to gene therapy include those with a primary genetic cause, such

**Table 44-4  Genes with Potential for Efficacy in Asthma**

| T-Helper Cell-1 Biasing | Inhibitors of Effector Response |
|---|---|
| Interferon-γ | Interleukin-13 inhibitor (soluble receptor fusion) |
| Interleukin-2 | Dominant negative mutant interleukin-4 |
| Interleukin-12 | Interleukin-10 |
| CpG oligonucleotides | Galectin-3 |
| Interleukin-18 | |

as surfactant protein-B (SP-B) deficiency and SP-C deficiency, or acquired diseases in which gene augmentation may ameliorate underlying pathogenic mechanisms. In the latter category are diseases such as ARDS and various infectious diseases (Table 44.5).[46–50]

In the case of ARDS, proof-of-concept studies have already been performed with rAd vectors for transient expression of some potentially biologically active molecules. Examples of these include sodium adenosine triphosphatase, which promotes reabsorption of alveolar fluid,[51,52] as well as antioxidants or anti-inflammatory cytokines that may block propagation of the cytokine storm associated with ARDS and the systemic inflammatory response syndrome.[53,54]

## DISEASES OF THE ALVEOLAR INTERSTITIUM

The primary example of a disease of the alveolar interstitium that may be amenable to gene therapy is A1AD. In this disease, a genetic lack of function of AAT results in gradual degradation of interstitial elastin owing to the unopposed action of neutrophil elastase and other neutrophil-derived products, including the serine proteases (cathepsin-G, proteinase-3), neutrophil defensins,

**Table 44-5  Alveolar and Interstitial Diseases That May Be Amenable to Gene Therapy**

| Genetic | Inflammatory | Infectious |
|---|---|---|
| $\alpha_1$-Antitrypsin deficiency | Acute respiratory distress syndrome | Pneumocystis carinii pneumonia |
| Surfactant protein deficiency (SP-B, SP-C) | Idiopathic interstitial pulmonary fibrosis | Bacterial pneumonia |
| Alveolar proteinosis | Interstitial pneumonitis | Tuberculosis |

and some other metalloproteases. The multifaceted action of AAT probably means that optimal therapy for this disease cannot be achieved without resupplying the protein itself. More selective neutrophil elastase inhibitors have failed to produce any definite benefits.

Several protein transfer approaches have been developed for A1AD. These include two licensed intravenous protein replacement products, the $\alpha_1$-proteinase inhibitors Prolastin and Aralast. Each of these products was approved based on a biomarker approach, in which replacement of serum AAT levels and some changes in inflammatory markers in the lung were deemed to be sufficiently indicative of efficacy to warrant licensure. Neither product has, strictly speaking, been proved efficacious for prevention of lung disease in a prospective manner, but retrospective data definitely suggest a beneficial effect. This concept is also supported by the original genotype-phenotype data, which established the therapeutic threshold level of AAT at 11 μM (512 to 800 μg/mL in serum).[55] Intravenous protein replacement therapy has been remarkably safe. In fact, it is one of the few types of protein replacement products that have not been found to elicit an immune response. The likely reason is the relative genetic homogeneity of this A1AD population, of whom approximately 96% have one particular missense mutant allele, the so-called PiZ allele.

The safety and apparent efficacy of protein replacement in A1AD provide much of the proof-of-concept support for gene therapy. In fact, gene therapy in this context can be conceived of as a form of sustained-release protein replacement. Because AAT appears to be secreted efficiently from numerous different sites, including the liver (its natural site of production), the skeletal muscle, the airway, the pleura, and the peritoneum, any of these sites could potentially be chosen for a gene augmentation strategy for patients with A1AD lung disease. The few patients with A1AD-associated liver disease are thought to suffer from hepatotoxicity resulting from a toxic gain of function from the mutant protein. Thus, gene transfer of normal AAT would not likely be therapeutic in that context unless gene transfer directly to hepatocytes were accompanied by downregulation of the mutant protein.

In the case of augmentation of AAT levels to treat A1AD lung disease, many different approaches were studied initially. A strong body of preclinical data was generated in support of intramuscular administration of rAAV-AAT gene therapy, including mouse, rabbit, and baboon data demonstrating safety and bioactivity of the product.[56-59] In fact, a phase I clinical trial has been initiated in patients with A1AD.[60]

Gene therapy for disorders directly affecting the interstitium, such as the various interstitial pneumonitides and idiopathic pulmonary fibrosis, has been studied much less thoroughly. However, as the body of knowledge regarding cytokine aberrations in these diseases grows, it seems likely that gene transfer approaches will emerge.

## DISEASES OF THE PULMONARY VASCULATURE

The identification of the basic mechanisms underlying pulmonary hypertension set the stage for potential gene therapy of this disorder. Most approaches have focused either on the prostacyclin synthase pathway (for generation of prostacyclin) or on the nitric oxide synthase pathway (for the generation of nitric oxide). The efficacy of epoprostenol (Flolan) by continuous infusion demonstrated the clinical importance of the former pathway, whereas observations of both inhaled nitric oxide and systemic sildenafil therapy demonstrated the efficacy of strategies to increase nitric oxide. Gene transfer could potentially provide a means for sustained delivery of either of these agents. The emergence of new information implicating mutations in the bone morphogenic protein receptor type 2 (*BMP-R-II*) gene as the cause of familial cases of primary pulmonary hypertension has opened the possibility of considering that molecule as another therapeutic target for gene therapy.[61,62]

## DISEASES OF THE PLEURA

Gene therapy for pleural disease has been less thoroughly studied than gene delivery to other compartments within the lung. However, several studies of cancer gene therapy approaches have been developed for treatment of mesothelioma in both the pleura and the peritoneum.[63-68] These approaches have progressed to later-phase clinical trials.

## PROSPECTS FOR FUTURE GENE THERAPY IN THE LUNG

Numerous potential gene therapies are progressing through preclinical and clinical trials for classic genetic diseases such as CF and A1AD, as well as for acquired disorders such as ARDS. The repertoire of gene therapy vectors has been greatly expanded, particularly by the emergence of vectors based on alternate AAV serotypes that have greater efficiency of gene transfer to certain cell types within the various intrapulmonary and extrapulmonary compartments. The ultimate niche for which gene therapy will prove to be optimal is yet to be determined. However, it seems very likely that gene therapy will soon take its place among the multiple classes of therapeutic approaches available to practicing clinicians.

## ACKNOWLEDGMENTS

This work was supported in part by grants from the National Center for Research Resources (RR00082, RR16586), the National Heart, Lung and Blood Institute (HL69877, HL51811, HL59412), the National Institute of Diabetes and Digestive and Kidney Diseases (DK583237), the National Eye Institute (EY13729), the Alpha One Foundation, and the Cystic Fibrosis Foundation.

## REFERENCES

1. Rosenfeld MA, Yoshimura K, Trapnell BC, et al: In vivo transfer of the human cystic fibrosis transmembrane conductance regulator gene to the airway epithelium. Cell 1992;68:143–155.
2. Crystal RG, McElvaney NG, Rosenfeld MA, et al: Administration of an adenovirus containing the human CFTR cDNA to the respiratory tract of individuals with cystic fibrosis. Nat Genet 1994;8:42–51.
3. Brody SL, Metzger M, Danel C, et al: Acute responses of non-human primates to airway delivery of an adenovirus vector containing the human cystic fibrosis transmembrane conductance regulator cDNA. Hum Gene Ther 1994;5:821–836.
4. Ben-Gary H, McKinney RL, Rosengart T, et al: Systemic interleukin-6 responses following administration of adenovirus gene transfer vectors to humans by different routes. Mol Ther 2002;6:287–297.
5. Zabner J, Couture LA, Gregory RJ, et al: Adenovirus-mediated gene transfer transiently corrects the chloride transport defect in nasal epithelia of patients with cystic fibrosis. Cell 1993;75:207–216.
6. Knowles MR, Hohneker KW, Zhou Z, et al: A controlled study of adenoviral-vector–mediated gene transfer in the nasal epithelium of patients with cystic fibrosis. N Engl J Med 1995;333:823–831.
7. Hyde SC, Southern KW, Gileadi U, et al: Repeat administration of DNA/liposomes to the nasal epithelium of patients with cystic fibrosis. Gene Ther 2000;7:1156–1165.
8. Porteous DJ, Dorin JR, McLachlan G, et al: Evidence for safety and efficacy of DOTAP cationic liposome mediated CFTR gene transfer to the nasal epithelium of patients with cystic fibrosis. Gene Ther 1997;4:210–218.
9. Caplen NJ, Alton EW, Middleton PG, et al: Liposome-mediated CFTR gene transfer to the nasal epithelium of patients with cystic fibrosis [published erratum appears in Nat Med 1995;1:272]. Nat Med 1995;1:39–46.
10. Alton EW, Middleton PG, Caplen NJ, et al: Non-invasive liposome-mediated gene delivery can correct the ion transport defect in cystic fibrosis mutant mice [published erratum appears in Nat Genet 1993;5:312]. Nat Genet 1993;5:135–142.
11. Knowles MR, Noone PG, Hohneker K, et al: A double-blind, placebo controlled, dose ranging study to evaluate the safety and biological efficacy of the lipid-DNA complex GR213487B in the nasal epithelium of adult patients with cystic fibrosis. Hum Gene Ther 1998;9:249–269.
12. Zabner J, Cheng SH, Meeker D, et al: Comparison of DNA-lipid complexes and DNA alone for gene transfer to cystic fibrosis airway epithelia in vivo. J Clin Invest 1997;100:1529–1537.
13. Ruiz FE, Clancy JP, Perricone MA, et al: A clinical inflammatory syndrome attributable to aerosolized lipid-DNA administration in cystic fibrosis. Hum Gene Ther 2001;12:751–761.
14. Afione SA, Conrad CK, Kearns WG, et al: In vivo model of adeno-associated virus vector persistence and rescue. J Virol 1996;70:3235–3241.
15. Beck SE, Laube BL, Barberena CI, et al: Deposition and expression of aerosolized rAAV vectors in the lungs of rhesus macaques. Mol Ther 2002;6:546–554.
16. Conrad CK, Allen SS, Afione SA, et al: Safety of single-dose administration of an adeno-associated virus (AAV)-CFTR vector in the primate lung. Gene Ther 1996;3:658–668.
17. Flotte TR, Afione SA, Conrad C, et al: Stable in vivo expression of the cystic fibrosis transmembrane conductance regulator with an adeno-associated virus vector. Proc Natl Acad Sci U S A 1993;90:10613–10617.
18. Flotte TR, Afione SA, Solow R, et al: Expression of the cystic fibrosis transmembrane conductance regulator from a novel adeno-associated virus promoter. J Biol Chem 1993;268:3781–3790.
19. Flotte TR, Zeitlin PL, Reynolds TC, et al: Phase I trial of intranasal and endobronchial administration of a recombinant adeno-associated virus serotype 2 (rAAV2)-CFTR vector in adult cystic fibrosis patients: A two-part clinical study. Hum Gene Ther 2003;14:1079–1088.
20. Wagner JA, Reynolds T, Moran ML, et al: Efficient and persistent gene transfer of AAV-CFTR in maxillary sinus. Lancet 1998;351:1702–1703.
21. Wagner JA, Messner AH, Moran ML, et al: Safety and biological efficacy of an adeno-associated virus vector-cystic fibrosis transmembrane conductance regulator (AAV-CFTR) in the cystic fibrosis maxillary sinus. Laryngoscope 1999;109:266–274.
22. Aitken ML, Moss RB, Waltz DA, et al: A phase I study of aerosolized administration of tgAAVCF to cystic fibrosis subjects with mild lung disease. Hum Gene Ther 2001;12:1907–1916.
23. Moss RB, Rodman D, Spencer LT, et al: Repeated adeno-associated virus serotype 2 aerosol-mediated cystic fibrosis transmembrane regulator gene transfer to the lungs of patients with cystic fibrosis: A multicenter, double-blind, placebo-controlled trial. Chest 2004;125:509–521.
24. Duan D, Yue Y, Engelhardt JF: Expanding AAV packaging capacity with trans-splicing or overlapping vectors: A quantitative comparison. Mol Ther 2001;4:383–391.
25. Duan D, Yue Y, Yan Z, Engelhardt JF: A new dual-vector approach to enhance recombinant adeno-associated virus-mediated gene expression through intermolecular cis activation. Nat Med 2000;6:595–598.
26. Zabner J, Seiler M, Walters R, et al: Adeno-associated virus type 5 (AAV5) but not AAV2 binds to the apical surfaces of airway epithelia and facilitates gene transfer. J Virol 2000;74:3852–3858.
27. Gao G, Alvira MR, Somanathan S, et al: Adeno-associated viruses undergo substantial evolution in primates during natural infections. Proc Natl Acad Sci U S A 2003;100:6081–6086.
28. Gao GP, Alvira MR, Wang L, et al: Novel adeno-associated viruses from rhesus monkeys as vectors for human gene therapy. Proc Natl Acad Sci U S A 2002;99:11854–11859.
29. Wu P, Xiao W, Conlon T, et al: Mutational analysis of the adeno-associated virus type 2 (AAV2) capsid gene and construction of AAV2 vectors with altered tropism. J Virol 2000;74:8635–8647.
30. Bartlett JS, Kleinschmidt J, Boucher RC, Samulski RJ: Targeted adeno-associated virus vector transduction of nonpermissive cells mediated by a bispecific F(ab'gamma)2 antibody. Nat Biotechnol 1999;17:181–186.
31. Loiler SA, Conlon TJ, Song S, et al: Targeting recombinant adeno-associated virus vectors to enhance gene transfer to pancreatic islets and liver. Gene Ther 2003;10:1551–1558.

32. Yan Z, Zak R, Luxton GW, et al: Ubiquitination of both adeno-associated virus type 2 and 5 capsid proteins affects the transduction efficiency of recombinant vectors. J Virol 2002;76:2043–2053.

33. Goldman MJ, Lee PS, Yang JS, Wilson JM: Lentiviral vectors for gene therapy of cystic fibrosis. Hum Gene Ther 1997;8:2261–2268.

34. Limberis M, Anson DS, Fuller M, Parsons DW: Recovery of airway cystic fibrosis transmembrane conductance regulator function in mice with cystic fibrosis after single-dose lentivirus-mediated gene transfer. Hum Gene Ther 2002;13:1961–1970.

35. Wang G, Sinn PL, McCray PB Jr: Development of retroviral vectors for gene transfer to airway epithelia. Curr Opin Mol Ther 2000;2:497–506.

36. Lim FY, Kobinger GP, Weiner DJ, et al: Human fetal trachea-SCID mouse xenografts: Efficacy of vesicular stomatitis virus-G pseudotyped lentiviral-mediated gene transfer. J Pediatr Surg 2003;38:834–839.

37. Sinn PL, Hickey MA, Staber PD, et al: Lentivirus vectors pseudotyped with filoviral envelope glycoproteins transduce airway epithelia from the apical surface independently of folate receptor alpha. J Virol 2003;77:5902–5910.

38. Kumar M, Kong X, Behera AK, et al: Chitosan IFN-gamma-pDNA nanoparticle (CIN) therapy for allergic asthma. Genet Vaccines Ther 2003;1:3.

39. Zavorotinskaya T, Tomkinson A, Murphy JE: Treatment of experimental asthma by long-term gene therapy directed against IL-4 and IL-13. Mol Ther 2003;7:155–162.

40. Nishikubo K, Murata Y, Tamaki S, et al: A single administration of interleukin-4 antagonistic mutant DNA inhibits allergic airway inflammation in a mouse model of asthma. Gene Ther 2003;10:2119–2125.

41. Kline JN: DNA therapy for asthma. Curr Opin Allergy Clin Immunol 2002;2:69–73.

42. Walter DM, Wong CP, DeKruyff RH, et al: Il-18 gene transfer by adenovirus prevents the development of and reverses established allergen-induced airway hyperreactivity. J Immunol 2001;166:6392–6398.

43. Kumar M, Behera AK, Matsuse H, et al: Intranasal IFN-gamma gene transfer protects BALB/c mice against respiratory syncytial virus infection. Vaccine 1999;18:558–567.

44. del Pozo V, Rojo M, Rubio ML, et al: Gene therapy with galectin-3 inhibits bronchial obstruction and inflammation in antigen-challenged rats through interleukin-5 gene downregulation. Am J Respir Crit Care Med 2002;166:732–737.

45. McLachlan G, Stevenson BJ, Davidson DJ, Porteous DJ: Bacterial DNA is implicated in the inflammatory response to delivery of DNA/DOTAP to mouse lungs. Gene Ther 2000;7:384–392.

46. Cheers C, Janas M, Ramsay A, Ramshaw I: Use of recombinant viruses to deliver cytokines influencing the course of experimental bacterial infection. Immunol Cell Biol 1999;77:324–330.

47. Kolls JK, Lei D, Stoltz D, et al: Adenoviral-mediated interferon-gamma gene therapy augments pulmonary host defense of ethanol-treated rats. Alcohol Clin Exp Res 1998;22:157–162.

48. Kolls JK, Lei D, Nelson S, et al: Pulmonary cytokine gene therapy: Adenoviral-mediated murine interferon gene transfer compartmentally activates alveolar macrophages and enhances bacterial clearance. Chest 1997;111:104S.

49. Ruan S, Tate C, Lee JJ, et al: Local delivery of the viral interleukin-10 gene suppresses tissue inflammation in murine *Pneumocystis carinii* infection. Infect Immun 2002;70:6107–6113.

50. Kolls JK, Ye P, Shellito JE: Gene therapy to modify pulmonary host defenses. Semin Respir Infect 2001;16:18–26.

51. Factor P, Dumasius V, Saldias F, Sznajder JI: Adenoviral-mediated overexpression of the NA,K-ATPase beta1 subunit gene increases lung edema clearance and improves survival during acute hyperoxic lung injury in rats. Chest 1999;116(Suppl):24S–25S.

52. Sartori C, Matthay MA: Alveolar epithelial fluid transport in acute lung injury: New insights. Eur Respir J 2002;20:1299–1313.

53. Dumasius V, Mendez M, Mutlu GM, Factor P: Acute lung injury does not impair adenoviral-mediated gene transfer to the alveolar epithelium. Chest 2002;121(Suppl):33S–34S.

54. Van Laethem JL, Eskinazi R, Louis H, et al: Multisystemic production of interleukin 10 limits the severity of acute pancreatitis in mice. Gut 1998;43:408–413.

55. Crystal RG: Alpha 1-antitrypsin deficiency, emphysema, and liver disease: Genetic basis and strategies for therapy. J Clin Invest 1990;85:1343–1352.

56. Song S, Morgan M, Ellis T, et al: Sustained secretion of human alpha-1-antitrypsin from murine muscle transduced with adeno-associated virus vectors. Proc Natl Acad Sci U S A 1998;95:14384–14388.

57. Song S, Laipis PJ, Berns KI, Flotte TR: Effect of DNA-dependent protein kinase on the molecular fate of the rAAV2 genome in skeletal muscle. Proc Natl Acad Sci U S A 2001;98:4084–4088.

58. Song S, Scott-Jorgensen M, Wang J, et al: Intramuscular administration of recombinant adeno-associated virus 2 alpha-1 antitrypsin (rAAV-SERPINA1) vectors in a nonhuman primate model: Safety and immunologic aspects. Mol Ther 2002;6:329–335.

59. Poirier A, Campbell-Thompson M, et al: Toxicology and biodistribution studies of a recombinant adeno-associated virus 2-alpha-1 antitrypsin vector. Preclinica 2004;2:43–51.

60. Flotte TR, Brantly ML, Spencer LT, et al: Phase I trial of intramuscular injection of a recombinant adeno-associated virus alpha 1-antitrypsin (rAAV2-CB-hAAT) gene vector to AAT-deficient adults. Hum Gene Ther 2004;15:93–128.

61. Morse JH: Bone morphogenetic protein receptor 2 mutations in pulmonary hypertension. Chest 2002;121(Suppl):50S–53S.

62. Eddahibi S, Morrell N, d'Ortho MP, et al: Pathobiology of pulmonary arterial hypertension. Eur Respir J 2002;20:1559–1572.

63. Friedlander PL, Delaune CL, Abadie JM, et al: Efficacy of CD40 ligand gene therapy in malignant mesothelioma. Am J Respir Cell Mol Biol 2003;29:321–330.

64. Schwarzenberger P, Harrison L, Weinacker A, et al: The treatment of malignant mesothelioma with a gene modified cancer cell line: A phase I study. Hum Gene Ther 1998;9:2641–2649.

65. Schwarzenberger P, Harrison L, Weinacker A, et al: Gene therapy for malignant mesothelioma: A novel approach for an incurable cancer with increased incidence in Louisiana. J La State Med Soc 1998;150:168–174.

66. Sterman DH, Treat J, Litzky LA, et al: Adenovirus-mediated herpes simplex virus thymidine kinase/ganciclovir gene therapy in patients with localized malignancy: Results of a phase I clinical trial in malignant mesothelioma. Hum Gene Ther 1998;9:1083–1092.

67. Elshami AA, Kucharczuk JC, Zhang HB, et al: Treatment of pleural mesothelioma in an immunocompetent rat model utilizing adenoviral transfer of the herpes simplex virus thymidine kinase gene. Hum Gene Ther 1996;7:141–148.

68. Albelda SM, Wiewrodt R, Sterman DH: Gene therapy for lung neoplasms. Clin Chest Med 2002;23:265–277.

# SECTION 8

## WEANING

# CHAPTER 45

# Weaning through Noninvasive Ventilation

Stefano Nava and Annalisa Carlucci

## FACTORS PREVENTING WEANING

Endotracheal intubation and invasive mechanical ventilation are lifesaving procedures in the management of critically ill patients. However, these techniques are often accompanied by complications that carry their own morbidity and mortality. Nosocomial infections and ventilator-associated pneumonia, in particular, are associated with a longer hospital stay and an increased risk of death. Torres and co-workers showed that the presence of chronic airway obstruction and an endotracheal tube in situ for more than 3 days were significantly associated with an increased risk of nosocomial pneumonia.[1] These findings were confirmed by other investigators,[2] in particular by Fagon and associates,[3] who showed that this risk increased by 1% per day of invasive mechanical ventilation. An endotracheal tube can predispose patients to the development of pneumonia by impairing cough and mucociliary clearance either because contaminated secretions can accumulate above the cuff and can leak around the cuff or because bacterial binding to the surface of bronchial epithelium is increased. Invasive ventilatory support also increases the risk of aspiration of food. Elpern and associates showed that approximately 50% of tracheotomized patients receiving prolonged ventilation aspirated food.[4]

Kollef and colleagues showed that the use of continuous intravenous sedation was associated with prolonged mechanical ventilation.[5] Moreover, the possible need for heavy sedation or curarization during the first days of ventilation may lead to generalized myopathy,[6] another important complication of prolonged mechanical ventilation. Latronico and associates showed that critically ill patients with sepsis and multiple organ failure are at great risk of developing both late myopathy and neuropathy, which may be responsible for neuromuscular respiratory failure after resolution of respiratory and cardiac dysfunction.[7] Long-term sequelae may develop after complications directly related to intubation,[8] such as laryngeal or tracheal injury,[9] with the development of false airways, stenosis, and granulomatosis.[8] The improper use of controlled mechanical ventilation may also lead to the development of selective diaphragmatic atrophy after only 48 hours, as shown in a laboratory study performed on rats.[10]

The incidence of all these complications, directly or indirectly resulting from invasive mechanical ventilation, may explain why patients who need prolonged invasive mechanical ventilation have such a poor prognosis. Therefore, the clinician should try to reduce the duration of invasive ventilation when it is not possible to avoid this approach. Minimizing the duration of invasive ventilation should be the most important goal, especially in selected populations such as patients with chronic obstructive pulmonary disease (COPD).

## WEANING FROM MECHANICAL VENTILATION

In the majority of cases, withdrawal of mechanical ventilation and extubation are possible immediately after resolution of underlying problems responsible for acute respiratory failure. However, some ventilated patients require a gradual and longer withdrawal of respiratory support.[11] As reported in one Spanish survey,[12] 41% of the total time of mechanical ventilation was devoted to weaning, and large differences were noted among patients with different diseases. In this survey, the percentage of the total duration of mechanical ventilation that was spent on weaning was close to 50%, or even higher, in patients affected by COPD, cardiac failure, and neurologic disorders. Further, in a prospective cohort study of 289 patients who underwent a trial of extubation, Epstein and colleagues showed that weaning failure had a significant independent association with increased risk for death, prolonged intensive care unit (ICU) stay, and transfer to a long-term care or rehabilitation facility.[13] Relevant differences in the weaning failure rate reported in the literature may depend on the case mix and the specifics of individual ICUs.[14] In fact, as Brochard and colleagues stated, "the length of weaning is first explained by etiology of the diseases, with patients with COPD being the most difficult to separate from the ventilator."[11] Two published studies, one carried out in North America[15] and the other in Europe,[16] were specifically aimed at assessing the survival rates of patients with COPD who did or did not require prolonged mechanical ventilation. These investigators found a very important difference in mortality rate at 1 year between the group successfully weaned (23% to 54%) and the group of patients who could not reach respiratory autonomy (62% to 87%).

## WEANING PROTOCOLS

The finding that the use of standardized protocols to wean patients from mechanical ventilation gives better results in terms of outcome and costs less than the traditional practice of physician-directed weaning was emphasized by two important articles.[17,18] In an editorial in response to this finding, Ely concluded that "the new challenge is to effect the necessary changes in physicians' practice styles."[19]

Several studies were performed in an attempt to assess the best ventilatory methods to use for discontinuing ventilatory support at the earliest possible time. Two important multicenter trials were performed in the mid-1990s, by Brochard and co-workers[11] and by Esteban and colleagues.[20] Both studies compared the following methods: intermittent T-piece breathing, pressure support ventilation (PSV), and spontaneous intermittent mandatory ventilation. The former study, performed on 456 medical and surgical patients, concluded that the outcome of weaning was influenced by ventilatory strategy and also noted that the use of PSV (reductions of pressure support by 2 to 4 cm $H_2O$ twice a day until pressure support was 8 cm $H_2O$) resulted in significantly faster weaning than the other

two techniques. Conversely, the latter study found that a once-daily trial of spontaneous breathing with a T-piece, of gradually increasing duration, led to extubation three times more quickly than spontaneous intermittent mandatory ventilation and twice as quickly as PSV. In this study, the minimum target pressure support level before extubation was 5 cm $H_2O$. The explanation for these contrasting results is that the method employed is probably less important than the patient's pathologic condition in determining the duration of mechanical ventilation.

Confidence and familiarity with the technique adopted are likely to be more important than the chosen method. Certainly, the rate of failure following extubation was similar after T-piece weaning and PSV, a finding suggesting that either approach is acceptable during weaning from mechanical ventilation. In both studies, weaning trials were performed only in those patients who had first failed a 2-hour T-piece trial. These patients represented about 25% of all patients who had reached the criteria for weaning. Accordingly, most patients judged "weanable" (75%), according to the foregoing criteria, were safely extubated after a single brief trial of spontaneous breathing. Later, Esteban and colleagues demonstrated that successful extubation could be achieved using a shorter trial period (30 minutes) of spontaneous breathing.[21]

## NONINVASIVE VENTILATION TO AVOID INTUBATION

Investigators demonstrated that NIV significantly reduced the need for intubation and consequently decreased intubation-related short-term and long-term complications, in a selected group of patients affected by acute hypercapnic respiratory failure.[22] To investigate whether these benefits translated into clinical practice, Girou and colleagues performed a retrospective matched case-control study conducted in a French medical ICU, to compare outcomes for similar patients admitted for acute exacerbation of COPD or severe cardiogenic pulmonary edema and treated by NIV or conventional mechanical ventilation during a period of 3 years.[23] These investigators found that, when compared with conventional mechanical ventilation, NIV significantly reduced the rate of nosocomial infections, particularly nosocomial pneumonia, and this likely benefit contributed to the reduced mortality rate in this group of patients. In a retrospective observational cohort study, these same authors showed that increased use of NIV in their ICU in the same critically ill patients through an 8-year period was associated with significant reductions in nosocomial infections and mortality rate.[24]

## Rationale for Use

Weaning failure frequently results from an imbalance between respiratory muscle capacity and load that may be not always detected during a 2-hour T-piece trial. Another important mechanism is represented by left ventricular dysfunction caused by the large negative deflection of intrathoracic pressure and the consequent increase in venous return. Finally, the extubation process per se may lead to upper airway obstruction or an inability to manage respiratory secretions. Definitive weaning from mechanical ventilation may be difficult when these two conditions occur. Patients may develop hypoxemia and hypercapnia secondary to a slower and deeper breathing pattern.

NIV is theoretically able to counteract several of the foregoing physiologic mechanisms associated with weaning failure or difficulties. Evidence indicates that NIV is responsible for a reduction in work of breathing, a decrease in negative deflections of intrathoracic pressure,[25] and an improvement of hypoxemia and hypercapnia secondary to a slower and deeper breathing pattern, even if no effect on ventilation/perfusion mismatch is demonstrated.[26] Indeed, investigators showed that in patients with COPD who were not capable of totally spontaneous autonomous breathing, both invasive and noninvasive pressure support methods were effective in reducing the diaphragmatic efforts and in improving arterial blood gas values. This study highlighted the possibility that, in clinically stable patients, NIV may be attempted as an alternative to invasive ventilation, with the goal of shortening the duration of intubation.[27]

## Noninvasive Ventilation as a Weaning Technique

In light of this knowledge, the first application of NIV in the weaning process was to substitute at the endotracheal tube with NIV by face mask or nasal mask, with the aim of shortening the duration of intubation. The technique was first used in the Royal Brompton Hospital in London, where Udwadia and co-workers studied 22 consecutive patients referred to their hospital for weaning difficulties.[28] Nine patients had chest wall defects, six had neuromuscular disorders, and seven had primary cardiac disease. Most of the patients had hypercapnic respiratory insufficiency. All had undergone at least one conventional weaning attempt, including the use of PSV. The decision to attempt weaning through NIV was taken only when the patients met the following criteria: (1) intact bulbar function with preserved cough reflex, (2) minimal airway secretion, (3) the ability to breathe spontaneously for 10 to 15 minutes, (4) low requirement of oxygen supplementation, (5) cardiac stability, and (6) the presence of a functioning gastrointestinal tract.

In the patients in the foregoing report,[28] weaning was performed using either volume-cycled ventilation or PSV combined with continuous positive airway pressure. Mechanical ventilation was continued for 16 to 20 hours/day in the first few days and was then gradually decreased to nocturnal use, depending on the rate of progress of the individual patient. Twenty of the 22 patients were successfully stabilized on NIV, and all these patients were transferred from the ICU to a step-down unit or a general ward. Only two patients did not tolerate NIV, and both were affected by "pure" hypoxemic respiratory failure resulting from pulmonary fibrosis after acute respiratory distress syndrome and cryptogenic pulmonary fibrosis. Weaning from invasive mechanical ventilation was successful in all 20 patients, although after discharge from the hospital, two patients died of complications after reintubation.

The duration of mechanical ventilation was not reported by Udwadia and colleagues,[28] but it was presumably shorter than the time spent in the hospital, which averaged 11 days. The duration of NIV was approximately 10% of that of invasive ventilation. Follow-up (median, 21 months) showed that 16 patients in the report were still alive and well. This study has the scientific limitation of not being randomized or controlled, but it was extremely important from a clinical point of view because it was the first to describe the feasibility and utility of this method of weaning. Indeed, it clearly demonstrated that the technique is possible only in a selected population of patients, based not only on the disease (failure of the two patients with pulmonary fibrosis), but also on the clinical status and stability of the patients (see the exclusion criteria). The same year, Goodemberger and associates published the case reports of two patients affected by neuromuscular diseases in whom nocturnal invasive ventilation was fully substituted by night-time NIV through a nasal mask allowing the tracheostomy to be removed.[29]

Restrick and co-workers in the London Chest Hospital reported later on their experience of weaning patients through NIV.[30] These investigators enrolled 14 patients, 8 of whom had COPD and 4 of whom had restrictive disease. The patients were also at different points in the weaning process, thus making interpretation of the data somewhat difficult. These investigators showed that 13 of 14 patients were successfully weaned with the new technique, whereas only 1 patient died in the ICU. The most striking result of this report was that in 5 of 14 patients, trials with NIV were started within 1 week of intubation, and in 3 of these patients, NIV was performed within the first 24 hours. This experience introduced the idea that the switch from intubation to NIV could be carried out earlier than normal even in patients considered by the attending physician to be "individuals in whom weaning from ventilation was predicted to be difficult."

Some other preliminary results also encouraged the use of NIV as a weaning technique. In Germany, Laier Groeneveld and associates demonstrated that all but 1 of their 35 patients, affected by chronic hypercapnic respiratory failure and considered unweanable by the attending physicians after $66\pm44$ days of mechanical ventilation, had their tracheostomies removed after they were switched to NIV.[31] Most of the patients continued to receive nocturnal ventilatory assistance. All these studies were clinically very promising, but in the era of the evidence-based medicine, only randomized controlled trials could change the attitude of physicians toward the controversial problem of weaning.

In the late 1990s, two European randomized-controlled studies were conducted in patients intubated for an episode of acute hypercapnic respiratory failure. The first study was performed by Nava and associates in three Italian respiratory ICUs that were limited to severely ill COPD patients.[32] After intubation, in response to emergency situations (i.e., gasping for air or respiratory arrest) or initial failure of NIV, 68 patients were sedated, many of them were paralyzed, and they were frequently suctioned for the first 6 to 12 hours after intubation. For the next 24 to 36 hours, PSV was used. Forty-eight hours after intubation, a T-piece trial was performed, but only when the patients were hemodynamically stable and had a normal temperature, an acceptable neurologic status, and no signs of pneumonia. Strict criteria were used to consider the T-piece trial a failure. Only patients in whom this trial failed (a total of 50) were randomized, after having been reconnected to the ventilator until previous arterial blood gas levels were reached, to either extubation with immediate application of NIV or continued weaning with the endotracheal tube in place. Both groups were weaned by daily reductions in the level of PSV and spontaneous breathing trials at least twice a day. By 60 days, 22 of 25 (88%) patients who had NIV had been successfully weaned, as opposed to 17 of 25 (68%) patients ventilated invasively. The mean duration of mechanical ventilation was significantly different: $10\pm6$ days versus $16\pm11$, respectively. The probability of success (survival and weaning) during ventilation was found to be significantly higher and the ICU stay was significantly shorter in the group receiving NIV. Survival rates at 60 days were also statistically different. None of the patients weaned with NIV developed nosocomial pneumonia, whereas 7 (28%) of those treated invasively did. Overall, this study showed that the likelihood of weaning success increases, whereas the duration of mechanical ventilation and ICU stay decreases, when NIV is used as a weaning technique.

The other randomized controlled study, performed by a French group in a single ICU, was conducted in patients intubated for an episode of acute respiratory failure resulting from COPD or other restrictive disease.[33] Thirty-three patients in whom a 2-hour T-piece weaning trial failed were randomized to receive "traditional" weaning with invasive PSV (IPSV) or the same modality delivered noninvasively by face mask or nasal mask. The following weaning strategies were used in the two groups. In the NIV-treated group, intermittent periods initially lasting from 2 to 4 hours were separated by periods of spontaneous breathing that were gradually increased throughout the day to achieve a nocturnal period of exclusive NIV, followed by the withdrawal of NIV whenever possible. In the IPSV-treated group, the initial pressure support level was gradually decreased by 3 to 5 cm $H_2O$, with each level assessed for at least 2 hours. Extubation was performed when the pressure support level reached 8 cm $H_2O$. Successful weaning in both groups was defined as the absence of reintubation within 5 days after extubation, whereas failure was defined as the need to reintubate the patients within 5 days after extubation in both groups or when extubation was impossible 5 days after the start of weaning in the IPSV-treated group.

The French investigators confirmed the finding of shorter duration of invasive mechanical ventilation in the groups weaned with NIV.[33] However, no differences were found in length of ICU and hospital stays as well as in 3-month survival in the two groups. Moreover, even when the mean period of daily ventilatory support in the NIV-treated group was significantly shorter than in the IPSV-treated group, the total duration of mechanical ventilation was found to be longer in the same group. This apparently contradictory result may be explained by the different definition of weaning in the two studies. In the Italian study, weaning was defined as an all or none phenomenon, to make a real comparison with extubation.[32] In contrast, the French study reflected a more clinical attitude by ventilating patients, once extubated, for a few hours a day to provide further ventilatory support, even in the absence of any sign of postextubation failure.[33]

In a randomized controlled trial, Ferrer and colleagues studied the efficacy of NIV in patients with "persistent" weaning failure regardless of their underlying disease.[34] These investigators enrolled all patients in whom a consecutive 3-day spontaneous breathing trial had failed and randomized them to be extubated and receive NIV or to remain intubated following a conventional weaning approach. The conventional weaning process was performed by daily spontaneous breathing trials until patients could be extubated. In the NIV-treated group, ventilation was gradually withdrawn until the patients could permanently sustain spontaneous breathing. The study was stopped after inclusion of 50% (n.43) of the estimated patients because a planned interim analysis showed a significant reduction of duration of mechanical ventilation in the NIV-treated group

(9.5±8.3 for the NIV group and 20.1±13.1 for the conventional weaning group). ICU and hospital stays were also significantly shorter in the NIV-treated group. There were no significant differences in the incidence of reintubation between the two groups. However, patients treated by NIV had a minor incidence of serious complications (nosocomial pneumonia and septic shock) and a better ICU and 90-day survival.

In the study by Nava and co-workers as well as in the study by Ferrer and associates, NIV was continuously delivered immediately after extubation for as long as possible, whereas in the study by Girault and colleagues, NIV was used intermittently. This distinction could explain the differences in the incidence of complications and outcomes in the study by Girault and associates. Moreover, the study by Ferrer and colleagues was planned to enroll only patients who were difficult to wean regardless of the underlying disease, and almost 80% of recruited patients were affected by chronic pulmonary disorders. The likelihood of prolonged ventilation is higher in this subset of patients. Further studies are clearly needed to assess the benefits of NIV for weaning in other forms of respiratory failure, such as acute respiratory distress syndrome, postsurgical complications, and cardiac impairment.

A clinical and physiologic study, which was not randomized, of patients affected by hypoxemic respiratory failure was performed by Gregoretti and co-workers.[35] The primary aim of the study was to compare blood gases, tidal volume, and respiratory rate at equal pressure values delivered invasively or noninvasively, but some important clinical data were obtained from the follow-up. Twenty-two trauma patients underwent a T-piece trial of at least 15 minutes, after a median period of 4±2 days of invasive ventilation, and were then switched to NIV. Nine patients (41%) were reintubated after approximately 2 days because of clinical deterioration, intolerance to the mask, or an inability to clear the airways, and six of these patients died while still being ventilated.

In 1999, Kilger and associates investigated the effects of NIV on gas exchange, breathing pattern, oxygen consumption, and resting energy expenditure in patients who did not have COPD but who had persistent acute respiratory failure after early extubation.[36] Fifteen patients were enrolled after very early extubation, compared with usual practice (i.e., arterial oxygen tension, 46±4 mm Hg; tidal volume, 4±1 mL/kg; and respiratory rate, 29±6 breaths/minute, during unsupported breathing). Two modes of NIV were applied: continuous positive airway pressure, 5 cm $H_2O$ alone, or with the addition of 15 cm $H_2O$ of inspiratory pressure. The latter modality significantly improved arterial blood gases, corrected the rapid shallow breathing pattern, and reduced resting energy expenditure. From a clinical point of view, only 2 of 15 patients needed to be reintubated for "nonrespiratory" reasons.

Even though the foregoing two studies were not controlled and were not specifically aimed at assessing the feasibility of using of NIV as a weaning technique, they were the first to show that this approach could be used in patients other than those with COPD or restrictive thoracic disease. The probability of success was lower than in these latter groups, however, a finding once again highlighting the possible important difference in outcome according to the underlying disease.

## Noninvasive Ventilation for Postextubation Failure

Postextubation failure remains one of the major clinical problems in ICUs. Investigators have reported that the incidence of postextubation failure in patients ventilated in ICUs is relatively high,[37] although values ranging from 3.3% to 23.5% have been quoted.[13] The prognosis of these patients is very poor because their hospital mortality exceeds 30% to 40%; the cause of extubation failure (i.e., problems unrelated to airway disorders) and the time to reintubation are independent predictors of outcome in these patients.[38] Because clinical evidence suggests that the act of reintubation itself is an insufficient explanation for the high mortality rate, it has been claimed that clinical deterioration occurring during unsupported ventilation allows the development of multiple organ failure, which leads to poor prognosis. This period of unsupported ventilation may, in some cases, be unduly protracted because physicians avoid new intubation for the following reasons: the severity of the patient's disease; the belief that the patient has a very poor chance of survival; or concerns about worsening the patient's clinical status as a result of the well-known complications of intubation. Bearing in mind the importance of this time factor, early institution of a noninvasive form of mechanical ventilation in patients who show signs of "incipient" respiratory failure, or even the sequential use of this technique right from the time of extubation, may be attractive strategies that deserve future study.

The so-called sequential use of NIV is an interesting application described by Hilbert and co-workers.[39] It consists of periods of NIV, delivered by home care ventilators, lasting at least 30 minutes every 3 hours; between periods of ventilation, patients can be systematically returned to being ventilated if their arterial oxygen saturation is less than 85% or their respiratory rate is greater than 30 breaths/minute. This sequential use has been successfully employed in the management of patients with acute exacerbations of COPD, and it may be applied to all patients identified as being at risk of postextubation failure. These same investigators also demonstrated that NIV delivered in this fashion improved the outcome of patients with COPD and postextubation hypercapnic respiratory failure by reducing the need for endotracheal intubation, the mean duration of ventilatory assistance, and the length of ICU stay when compared with matched subjects treated conventionally.[40] No statistically significant effects were found on mortality, although mortality was three times higher in the group treated conventionally, a finding suggesting that a larger study could possibly show a significant difference in survival. This study also demonstrated a lower incidence of pneumonia in the group treated noninvasively (7% versus 20%). The study presents the obvious limitation that it used historically matched controls, but the two groups seem to have been well matched because the investigators followed strict parameters.

In a more recent randomized controlled trial, NIV was applied to patients who developed acute respiratory distress within 48 hours after extubation and compared with standard medical therapy (oxygen, diuretics, bronchodilators, and aggressive physiotherapy).[41] Respiratory distress was defined as a respiratory rate greater than 30/minute, an increase in respiratory rate of more than 50% from baseline, or the use of accessory muscles of respiration or abdominal paradox. Eighty-one consecutive patients developed respiratory distress after extubation and were randomized, 42 to standard therapy and 39 to NIV. These investigators did not find any difference in reintubation rate (69% in the standard therapy group versus 72% in the NIV group) or in ICU (24% versus 15%) and hospital mortality rate (31% versus 31%) between patients receiving standard therapy and the NIV-treated group. Moreover, the length of ICU and hospital stay did not differ between the two groups, although a trend toward shorter ICU stays was noted in the NIV-treated group. Because of the relatively small sample size and the study's single-center basis, the extent to which these results can be generalized has been questioned.

In 2004, Esteban and associates conducted a large multicenter, randomized trial to evaluate the effect of NIV on mortality in this clinical setting.[42] Patients in 37 different ICUs who were electively extubated after at least 2 days of invasive ventilation and who had respiratory failure within the subsequent 48 hours were randomly assigned to either NIV (114 patients) or standard medical therapy (107 patients). The study was stopped early after an ad interim analysis. There was no difference between the two groups in the need for reintubation, whereas the rate of death was higher in the NIV-treated group (25% versus 14%; relative risk, 1.78), and the median time from respiratory failure to reintubation was longer again in the NIV group. These authors concluded that NIV does not prevent the need for reintubation or reduce mortality in unselected patients who have respiratory failure after extubation. However they

also stated that some selected patients (i.e., those with hypercapnic postextubation failure) may benefit from this therapy, so this hypothesis should be tested prospectively.

One problem with the studies dealing with NIV and postextubation failure may be related to the finding that when this event occurs, it may be too late and patients may be too sick to undergo a trial of NIV to prevent reintubation. It has already been demonstrated, in fact, that mortality increased with the duration of time between extubation and reintubation, a finding suggesting a possible role of a clinical deterioration occurring during the time of unsupported ventilation.[38] Moreover, the same authors showed that the presence of comorbidities, increased work of breathing at the time of extubation, and upper airway obstruction are independent factors influencing the need for reintubation.[13,38] Therefore, subsets of patients at risk may be identified beforehand. In the light of these results, it has been questioned whether "early" application of NIV, immediately after extubation, may decrease the rate of postextubation failure. Jiang and associates conducted a prospective study on 93 patients randomized to receive NIV or unassisted oxygen therapy after planned or unplanned extubation; 7 of 46 patients in the oxygen-treated group and 13 of 47 in the NIV-treated group required reintubation, and this difference was not statistically significant.[43] Patients with excessive bronchial secretions and intolerance to ventilation were found to be poor candidates for NIV. Therefore, these investigators concluded that the early application of NIV was not associated with a more favorable extubation outcome. The limitation of the study was the indiscriminate use of NIV in all the patients being extubated, whereas Epstein and colleagues had clearly shown that a certain subset of patients has clinical characteristics at the time of extubation that may predict a high probability of reintubation.[38]

Two randomized controlled studies were recently performed in Europe to assess the hypothesis that NIV may be used to prevent the occurrence of postextubation failure in patients at risk of developing this complication.[44,45] The two trials adopted similar criteria to define the category of patients at potential risk (i.e., persistent weaning failure, postextubation hypercapnia, age, weak cough reflex, or preexisting cardiac disease) and similar design (i.e., sequential use of NIV in the first 48 hours). In the first trial,[44] 97 patients were randomly assigned to receive SMT or NIV. The use of NIV determined a 16% reduction in the risk for reintubation (P = .027), whereas the protective effect on ICU mortality (−12%) was close to achieving statistical significance (P = .064). Moreover, the need for reintubation was associated with a 60% increase in the risk of ICU mortality (P < .01). Patients needing reintubation had a statistically higher ICU length of stay compared with those who did not

(23.89±29.51 versus 8.64±5.19, P < .001). These investigators concluded that the preventive application of NIV in a subset of patients at risk of postextubation failure who pass a spontaneous breathing trial may reduce the need for reintubation. The latter was associated with a higher risk of ICU mortality, and the use of NIV resulted in a reduction of risk of ICU mortality, mediated by the reduction for the need of reintubation.

Similar results were found in the second randomized trial, by Ferrer and associates.[45] Unlike in the previous study, in this trial, NIV was also used as rescue therapy in patients from the two groups in case of respiratory failure after extubation without needing immediate reintubation. In 162 patients, these investigators found that NIV significantly reduced the incidence of respiratory failure after extubation, but the differences between the two groups in the reintubation rate failed to be significant. This finding was the result of the efficacy of NIV as rescue therapy, which prevented reintubation in 9 of 19 patients in the SMT group and in 4 of 4 patients in the NIV-treated group. Moreover, although reintubation after rescue therapy with NIV occurred later than direct reintubation, the time from extubation to reintubation did not influence mortality. However, the beneficial effects of NIV on survival appear restricted to patients with chronic respiratory disorders and hypercapnia during the spontaneous breathing trial.

In conclusion, we have solid evidence that NIV may be used in the weaning process in selected patients with stable hypercapnia to shorten the length of invasive mechanical ventilation. The role of NIV in all other conditions (i.e., hypoxic patients, postsurgical patients) still remains to be elucidated. Randomized controlled studies have also demonstrated that NIV may be even harmful when treating an "overt" episode of postextubation respiratory failure, whereas promising results were obtaining when NIV was used to prevent reintubation in the subset of patients considered at risk.

## REFERENCES

1. Torres A, Aznar R, Gatell JM, et al: Incidence, risk, and prognosis factors of nosocomial pneumonia in mechanically ventilated patients. Am Rev Respir Dis 1990;142:523–528.
2. Craven DE, Kunches LM, Kilinsky V, et al: Risk factors for pneumonia and fatality in patients receiving continuous mechanical ventilation. Am Rev Respir Dis 1986;133:792–796.
3. Fagon JY, Chastre J, Domart Y, et al: Nosocomial pneumonia in patients receiving continuous mechanical ventilation: Prospective analysis of 52 episodes with use of protected specimen brush and quantitative culture techniques. Am Rev Respir Dis 1989;139:877–884.
4. Elpern EH, Scott MG, Petro L, Ries MH: Pulmonary aspiration in mechanically ventilated patients with tracheostomies. Chest 1994;105:563–566.
5. Kollef MH, Levy NT, Ahrens TS, et al: The use of continuous IV sedation is associated with prolongation of mechanical ventilation. Chest 1998;114:541–548.
6. Berek K, Margreiter J, Willeit J, et al: Polyneuropathies in critically ill patients: A prospective evaluation. Intensive Care Med 1996;22:849–855.
7. Latronico N, Fenzi F, Recupero D, et al: Critical illness myopathy and neuropathy. Lancet 1996;347:1579–1582.
8. Stauffer JL: Complications of translaryngeal intubation. In Tobin M (ed): Principles and Practice of Mechanical Ventilation. New York: McGraw-Hill, 1994, pp 711–747.
9. Belson TP: Cuff induced tracheal injury in dogs following prolonged intubation. Laryngoscope 1983;93:549–555.
10. Le Bourdelles G, Vires N, Bockzowki J, et al: Effects of mechanical ventilation on diaphragmatic contractile properties in rats. Am J Respir Crit Care Med 1994;149:1539–1544.
11. Brochard L, Rauss A, Benito S, et al: Comparison of three methods of gradual withdrawal from ventilatory support during weaning from mechanical ventilation. Am J Respir Crit Care Med 1994;150:896–903.
12. Esteban A, Alia I, Ibanez J, et al: Modes of mechanical ventilation and weaning: A national survey of Spanish hospitals. Chest 1994;106:1188–1193.
13. Epstein SK, Ciubataru RL, Wong JB: Effect of failed extubation on the outcome of mechanical ventilation. Chest 1997; 112:186–192.
14. Manthous C, Schmidt GA, Hall J: Liberation from mechanical ventilation: A decade of progress. Chest 1998;114:886–901.
15. Menzies R, Gibbons W, Goldberg P: Determinants of weaning and survival among patients with COPD who require mechanical ventilation for acute respiratory failure. Chest 1989;95:398–405.
16. Nava S, Rubini F, Zanotti E, et al: Survival and prediction of successful ventilator weaning in COPD patients requiring mechanical ventilation for more than 21 days. Eur Respir J 1994;7:1645–1652.
17. Ely WE, Baker AM, Dunagan DP, et al: Effect on the duration of mechanical ventilation of identifying patients capable of breathing spontaneously. N Engl J Med 1996;335:1864–1869.
18. Kollef MH, Shapiro SD, Silver P, et al: A randomized, controlled trial of protocol-directed versus physician-directed weaning from mechanical ventilation. Crit Care Med 1997;25:567–574.
19. Ely EW: Challenges encountered in changing physicians' practice styles: The ventilator weaning experience [editorial]. Intensive Care Med 1998;24:539–541.
20. Esteban A, Frutos F, Tobin MJ, et al: A comparison of four methods of weaning from mechanical ventilation: Spanish Lung Failure Collaborative Group. N Engl J Med 1995;332:345–350.
21. Esteban A, Alia I, Tobin MJ, et al: Effect of spontaneous breathing trial duration on outcome of attempts to discontinue mechanical ventilation: Spanish Lung Failure Collaborative Groupe. AJRCCM 1999;159:512–518.
22. Keenan SP, Kernerman PD, Cook DJ, et al: Effect of noninvasive positive pressure ventilation on mortality in patients admitted with acute respiratory failure: A meta-analysis. Crit Care Med 1997;25:1685–1692.
23. Girou E, Schortgen F, Delclaux C, et al: Association of noninvasive ventilation with nosocomial infections and survival in critically ill patients. JAMA 2000;284:2361–2367.
24. Girou E, Brun-Buisson C, Taille S, et al: Secular trends in nosocomial infections and mortality associated with noninvasive ventilation in patients with exacerbation of COPD and pulmonary edema. JAMA 2003;290:2985–2991.
25. Appendini L, Patessio A, Zanaboni S, et al: Physiologic effects of positive end-expiratory pressure and mask pressure support during exacerbations of chronic obstructive pulmonary disease. Am J Respir Crit Care Med 1994;149:1069–1076.

26. Diaz O, Iglesia R, Ferrer M, et al: Effects of noninvasive ventilation on pulmonary gas exchange and hemodynamics during acute hypercapnic exacerbations of chronic obstructive pulmonary disease. Am J Respir Crit Care Med 1997;156:1840–1845.

27. Vitacca M, Ambrosino N, Clini E, et al: Physiological response to pressure support ventilation delivered before and after extubation in patients not capable of totally spontaneous autonomous breathing. Am J Respir Crit Care Med 2001;164:638–641.

28. Udwadia ZF, Santis GK, Steven MH, Simonds AK: Nasal ventilation to facilitate weaning in patients with chronic respiratory insufficiency. Thorax 1992;47:715–718.

29. Goodenberger DM, Couser J, May JJ: Successful discontinuation of ventilation via tracheostomy by substitution of nasal positive pressure ventilation. Chest 1992;102:1277–1279.

30. Restrick LJ, Scott AD, Ward EM, et al: Nasal intermittent positive-pressure ventilation in weaning intubated patients with chronic respiratory disease from assisted intermittent, positive-pressure ventilation. Respir Med 1993;87:199–204.

31. Laier-Groeneveld G, Kupfer J, Huttemann U, Criee CP: Weaning from invasive mechanical ventilation. Am Rev Respir Dis 1992;145:A518.

32. Nava S, Ambrosino N, Clini E, et al: Noninvasive mechanical ventilation in the weaning of patients with respiratory failure due to chronic obstructive pulmonary disease. A randomized, controlled trial. Ann Intern Med 1998;128:721–728.

33. Girault C, Daudenthun I, Chevron V, et al: Noninvasive ventilation as a systematic extubation and weaning technique in acute-on-chronic respiratory failure: A prospective, randomized controlled study. Am J Respir Crit Care Med 1999;160:86–92.

34. Ferrer M, Esqinas A, Arancibia F, et al: Noninvasive ventilation during persistent weaning failure. Am J Respir Crit Care Med 2003;168:70–76.

35. Gregoretti C, Beltrame F, Lucangelo U, et al: Physiologic evaluation of non-invasive pressure support ventilation in trauma patients with acute respiratory failure. Intensive Care Med 1998;24:785–790.

36. Kilger E, Briegel J, Haller M, et al: Effects of noninvasive positive pressure ventilatory support in non-COPD patients with acute respiratory insufficiency after early extubation. Intensive Care Med 1999;25:1374–1380.

37. Torres A, Gatell JM, Aznar E, et al: Re-intubation increases the risk of nosocomial pneumonia in patients needing mechanical ventilation. Am J Respir Crit Care Med 1995;152:137–141.

38. Espstein SK, Ciubotaru RL: Independent effects of etiology of failure and time to reintubation on outcome for patients failing extubation. Am J Respir Crit Care Med 1998;158:489–493.

39. Hilbert G, Gruson D, Gbikpi-Benissan G, Cardinaud JP: Sequential use of noninvasive pressure support ventilation for acute exacerbations of COPD. Intensive Care Med 1997;23:955–961.

40. Hilbert G, Gruson D, Portel L, et al: Noninvasive pressure support ventilation in COPD patients with postextubation hypercapnic respiratory insufficiency. Eur Respir J 1998;11:1349–1353.

41. Keenan SP, Powers C, McCormack DG, et al: Noninvasive positive-pressure ventilation for postextubation respiratory distress. JAMA 2002;287:3238–3244.

42. Esteban A, Frutos-Vivar F, Ferguson ND, et al: Non-invasive positive pressure ventilation for respiratory failure after extubation. N Engl J Med 2004;350:2452–2460.

43. Jiang JS, Kao SJ, Wang SN: Effect of early application of biphasic positive airway pressure on the outcome of extubation in ventilator weaning. Respirology 1999;4:161–165.

44. Nava S, Gregoretti C, Fanfulla F, et al: Noninvasive ventilation to prevent respiratory failure after extubation in high-risk patients. Crit Care Med 2005;33:2465–2470.

45. Ferrer M, Valencia M, Nicolas JM, et al: Early noninvasive ventilation averts extubation failure in patients at risk: A randomized trial. Am J Respir Crit Care Med 2006;173:164–170.

# SECTION 9

# NEONATAL AND PEDIATRIC VENTILATION

# CHAPTER 46

# Neonatal Mechanical Ventilation

A.H.L.C. van Kaam

## INTRODUCTION

Neonatal respiratory failure is a common and serious clinical problem associated with high morbidity and mortality.[1] A majority of newborn infants with respiratory failure will require mechanical ventilation, which has successfully lowered mortality after its introduction in the 1960s.[2] Unfortunately, in its goal to correct gas exchange, mechanical ventilation often results in secondary lung damage also referred to as ventilator-induced lung injury (VILI).[3] VILI is considered one of the major risk factors for development of chronic pulmonary morbidity in newborn infants, i.e., bronchopulmonary dysplasia (BPD).[4] Over the last two decades several new ventilation modes and strategies have been introduced in an attempt to reduce VILI and subsequently the incidence of BPD. This chapter will summarize the most common causes of neonatal respiratory failure and the different modes of respiratory support, including adjunctive therapies.

## NEONATAL RESPIRATORY FAILURE

### Neonatal Respiratory Distress Syndrome (nRDS)

This is the most common cause of respiratory failure in neonates. The incidence of nRDS is strongly related to the gestational age, with an overall incidence of 50%–70% in infants born with a birth weight below 1500 g.[5,6] In addition to gestational age and birth weight, several other risk factors for the development of nRDS have been identified, including male sex, twin gestation and delivery by cesarean section.[7] Besides structural immaturities, the key feature of nRDS is surfactant deficiency resulting in alveolar/saccular collapse.[8,9] These changes will result in deteriorating lung mechanics and gas exchange, explaining the typical clinical picture of nRDS consisting of tachypnea and dyspnea with cyanosis in room air.[10,11] The chest radiographic picture shows reduced lung inflation and an opacity that ranges from diffuse granularity to a ground glass appearance. Although typical for nRDS, these radiographic changes may also be visible during group B streptococcal pneumonia.[12]

Nowadays, the three cornerstones for prevention and treatment of nRDS are antenatal glucocorticoids, exogenous surfactant therapy, and respiratory support. There is ample human evidence that glucocorticoids administered to pregnant women prior to preterm delivery result in a decreased infant mortality and a decreased incidence of nRDS.[13a] Based on this convincing evidence the use of antenatal glucocorticoids has increased steadily over the last 15 years to more than 70% of all preterm deliveries.[6] The role of exogenous surfactant and respiratory support in the treatment of nRDS will be discussed in more detail elsewhere in this chapter. The overall mortality of infants with nRDS is approximately 20%–25%, showing a strong inverse correlation with gestational age.[7,11]

### Transient Tachypnea of the Newborn (TTN)

This condition, also referred to as "wet lung," typically affects (near) term infants. The reported incidence of TTN varies between 3.5/1000 and 9.3/1000 live births.[7,13b] Some of the reported risk factors for TTN are male sex and delivery by cesarean section.[7,14] Many feel TTN is caused by a delayed resorption of fetal lung fluid, which could also explain the association with delivery by cesarean section.[15] The clinical presentation of TTN is characterized by respiratory distress with tachypnea, retractions and oxygen requirement. However, in contrast to nRDS, these symptoms are usually not progressive but instead resolve within the first 24–48 hrs.[16] The chest roentgenogram shows hyperaeriation of the lungs, perihilar streaking, and fluid in the interlobar fissures.[15,17] Treatment consists mainly of respiratory support and the clinical course is usually benign with an overall mortality of approximately 1%.[7]

## Meconium Aspiration Syndrome (MAS)

About 15% of all pregnancies will be complicated by meconium-stained amniotic fluid. Approximately 5% of these infants will develop meconium aspiration syndrome (MAS), and 30% of these infants will develop severe ARF.[18] MAS is encountered mainly in term infants and some of the reported risk factors are increasing gestational age and male sex.[19,20]

The pathophysiology of MAS is complex and includes airway obstruction, surfactant inactivation, inflammation, and altered pulmonary vascular resistance.[21–24] These changes will result in atelectasis, increased ventilation-perfusion mismatch, and persistent pulmonary hypertension of the newborn, leading to severe hypoxia due to increased intra- and extrapulmonary shunt.[24,25]

The clinical presentation is one of severe cyanosis with respiratory distress, although the latter may not always be apparent at birth due to birth asphyxia which is often associated with meconium-stained amniotic fluid.[26]

The first step in the treatment of severe MAS is to restore lung function and gas exchange, using both mechanical ventilation and exogenous surfactant.[27] If the subsequent improvement in gas exchange is insufficient to lower pulmonary hypertension and reverse the extrapulmonary right-to-left shunt, inhaled nitric oxide (iNO) and extracorporeal membrane oxygenation (ECMO) may be successful in achieving this goal, as discussed later in this chapter. Mortality is reported to be approximately 4% of all infants presenting with MAS.[25]

## Pneumonia

The incidence of neonatal pneumonia has been estimated at 1% in term and at least 10% in preterm infants.[28] Neonatal pneumonia can be classified as perinatal pneumonia, presenting within the first 24 hrs after birth or as nosocomial pneumonia presenting several days after birth.

Perinatal pneumonia often occurs as a result of an ascending infection via the maternal genital tract. Risk factors are prematurity, prolonged rupture of membranes, and signs of intraamniotic infection.[29] The most common cause of perinatal pneumonia is group B streptococcus followed by gram-negative organisms like Escherichia Coli and Klebsiella.[30,31] Infants usually present with signs of respiratory distress which can clinically and radiologically be indistinguishable from nRDS.[32]

Organisms responsible for nosocomial pneumonia are transmitted to the infants after birth, and constitute mainly of Staphylococci, Pseudomonas, Enterobacter, and Klebsiella.[33] The most important risk factors for nosocomial pneumonia are prematurity and mechanical ventilation.[34,35] Again clinical symptoms can be aspecific, with signs of respiratory distress accompanied by failure to improve or even deterioration during mechanical ventilation.[16] The most common radiographic findings are bilateral alveolar densities, although these may also be present in noninfectious disease.[36]

Both perinatal and nosocomial pneumonia are often associated with sepsis and some have suggested that the lung is an important entry site for systemic bacterial infection.[30,37,38]

Besides treatment with antibiotics neonates suffering from pneumonia will frequently require mechanical ventilation. In addition, some have suggested a beneficial effect of exogenous surfactant.[39–41] Despite these treatment options, the reported mortality of both perinatal and nosocomial pneumonia is still high, ranging from 20%–50%.[28,30,42]

## Congenital Malformations

This group is diverse and includes malformation of both the upper and lower respiratory tract. Compared to other causes of neonatal respiratory failure, as described above, most of these conditions are rare and only described as case reports or series.

One of the most important congenital anomalies that leads to acute respiratory failure is congenital diaphragmatic hernia (CDH). The reported incidence of CDH is 1 in approximately 3000 live births.[43] CDH is characterized by a protusion of abdominal viscera in the chest via a (often left sided) diaphragmatic defect and failure of both alveolar and pulmonary vascular development.[44] Pulmonary hypoplasia and pulmonary hypertension are the key features leading to severe deterioration of gas exchange. Management emphasis is on stabilizing the patient's hemodynamic and pulmonary condition, followed by (often delayed) surgical repair.[44] Mechanical ventilation, iNO, and ECMO are some of the therapeutic options in this management, and will be discussed in more detail elsewhere in this chapter. Recent outcome data have reported a 75% survival of infants with CDH.[45]

Risk factors for adverse outcome are other congenital anomalies and severe pulmonary hypoplasia.

Besides CDH, several other congenital anomalies or pregnancy complications may result in secondary pulmonary hypoplasia.[46] The estimated incidence of pulmonary hypoplasia is 1 per 1000 live births.[47] Morphometric and biochemical studies on hypoplastic lung have reported arrested lung growth, impairment of lung maturation, and disturbances in the development of the pulmonary vessels including an increased size of the pulmonary arterial smooth muscle.[48–50] The latter forms the morphologic basis for the increased pulmonary vascular resistance often encountered in infants with pulmonary hypoplasia. Most infants with moderate to severe pulmonary hypoplasia present with acute respiratory failure immediately after birth, with no signs of atelectasis on the chest radiograph. The latter often shows air leaks due to the high pressure ventilation needed to treat the hypercapnia and hypoxia. In addition, a bell-shaped chest contour may be found in almost 60% of the cases of pulmonary hypoplasia.[51] Treatment consists of mechanical ventilation and reducing the degree of the pulmonary hypertension. Depending on the cause and severity of pulmonary hypoplasia, almost all outcome reports show a mortality rate of more than 50%.[52]

## VENTILATOR-INDUCED LUNG INJURY

The initial goal of mechanical ventilation was to correct or prevent impaired oxygenation and hypercapnia.[53] However, animal experiments conducted over the last 25 years have shown that mechanical ventilation itself may also inflict damage to the injured lung. This so-called ventilator-induced lung injury (VILI) often presents itself as subtle physiologic and morphologic alterations, such as pulmonary edema due to epithelial permeability changes.[54,55] These animal experiments have also provided insight into the pathophysiological mechanisms responsible for VILI. Several key risk factors for the development of VILI have thus been identified.

### Volutrauma

As early as 1974, Webb and Tierney showed that the application of high inflation pressures, leading to high tidal volumes, resulted in alveolar and perivascular edema, deteriorating lung mechanics, and ultimately death in healthy rats.[54] One of the issues following this report was the separate contributions of high inflation pressures (barotrauma) on the one hand and high tidal volumes (volutrauma) on the other hand. Several experiments have shown that application of high inflation pressures will only damage the lung if the thorax can freely expand and volume can enter the lungs. Preventing this expansion by thoracic strapping (low volume, high pressure) will protect the lung against VILI.[56,57] Based on these experiments it is nowadays believed that volutrauma and not barotrauma is one of the main determinants in the development of VILI.

Volutrauma is often thought to be equivalent to high tidal volume ventilation. Although this is true in most cases it is important to realize that even low tidal volumes can induce volutrauma if superimposed on a high functional residual capacity (FRC), thereby exceeding total lung capacity.[58] This is why some authors feel that end-inspiratory lung volume and not tidal volume is the main determinant in volutrauma.

Experiments in preterm animal models also showed that volutrauma induces VILI and that only 5 large breaths administered immediately after birth are sufficient to trigger the cascade of VILI.[59,60] The latter suggests a higher susceptibility of newborns for volutrauma as also suggested by others.[61]

### Atelectrauma

Although neonatal and adult respiratory failure have different causes, surfactant deficiency or inactivation resulting in alveolar collapse, atelectasis, and increased intrapulmonary shunt is a common feature independent of the underlying disease. As lung injury develops over time, the process becomes nonuniform, resulting in uneven distribution of ventilation. Roughly three zones can be identified: (1) alveoli which remain open during the entire respiratory cycle; (2) alveoli that are recruitable during the inspiration phase, but collapse during expiration; and (3) non-recruitable alveoli.[62] Alveoli in zone (2) will be subjected to repetitive opening and collapse during conventional ventilation with insufficient positive end-expiratory pressure (PEEP). Animal experiments in both adult and preterm models have shown that this condition is injurious in the diseased lung.[63–65] As alveoli in zone (3) do not participate in tidal ventilation, the tidal volume is redistributed over the alveoli in the other two zones, which may increase the risk of regional overdistension (volutrauma).[66] Finally, co-existence of atelectatic and open alveoli may results in shear forces that exceed transpulmonary pressures, increasing the risk of structural damage to the alveolar unit.[67]

### Biotrauma

Besides structural damage to the alveolar unit and permeability changes resulting in edema, volutrauma and atelectrauma will also induce an inflammatory response in the lung which can further aggravate VILI. In vitro studies have shown that cyclic stretch of both alveolar epithelial cells and alveolar macrophages stimulates the production of inflammatory cytokines like tumor necrosis factor alpha (TNF-α) and interleukin-8 (IL-8).[68,69]

These findings have also been confirmed using both ex vivo and in vivo animal models.[70–73] During recent years, numerous cytokines have been identified as players in the inflammatory process in VILI. However to date, it remains unclear how these cytokines interact and at what time their role changes from physiological to pathological.

One of the changes induced by the production of inflammatory mediators like IL-8 is the recruitment of PMN cells in the lung.[74,75] PMN can inflict tissue damage through the release of proteases, the production of reactive oxygen species, and the release of cytokines.[76] The importance of PMN in the development of VILI has been shown by Kawano et al., who found little evidence of VILI in rabbits depleted of granulocytes prior to initiation of injurious conventional ventilation.[77]

Besides upregulation of local inflammation in the lung there is now also evidence from both experimental and human data that injurious ventilation will also lead to a decompartmentalization of inflammatory mediators into the systemic circulation, possibly leading to multiple organ failure.[72,78–80]

In the neonatal population there is additional evidence for the important role of biotrauma in the development of secondary lung injury and subsequent respiratory morbidity (BPD). Based on human observational data, it has been postulated that BPD is in part mediated by an inflammatory process starting prior to birth.[81] This has been substantiated by clear associations between chorio-amnionitis on the one hand, and preterm delivery and the risk for developing BPD on the other hand.[82–84] After birth several observational studies in ventilated preterm infants with nRDS have shown that progression to BPD is accompanied by an enhanced inflammatory response consisting of a persisting neutrophil influx and upregulation of inflammatory mediators in the lung.[85–87]

## Oxygen Toxicity

Ventilation with high fractions of inspiratory oxygen concentrations can result in excessive production of oxygen radicals overwhelming the normal antioxidant-detoxifying capacity of the cell. Data mainly from experimental studies have shown that free oxygen radicals can damage the lung in several ways. First of all there is a direct cytotoxic effect on alveolar endothelial and epithelial cells, leading to pulmonary edema and hemorrhage.[88–90] There is a loss of pulmonary vascular reactivity, which may increase ventilation/perfusion mismatch during hypoxia.[91] Hyperoxia results in both inactivation and decreased synthesis of pulmonary surfactant, resulting in a deterioration of lung mechanics.[92,93]

Pulmonary inflammation is upregulated as hyperoxia stimulates neutrophil migration into the alveoli and enhances inflammatory cytokine response of alveolar macrophages.[90,94,95] Besides lung damage, prolonged exposure to high oxygen concentrations will also have an inhibitory effect on lung development, resulting in decreased alveolarization.[96,97]

Both animal and human studies have indicated that prematurity impairs the ability to increase antioxidant enzymes in response to hyperoxia, making this group of patients extremely vulnerable to oxidative stress often present after premature birth.[98,99]

## The Role of Surfactant

Although many of the diseases responsible for neonatal ARF are characterized by either primary surfactant deficiency or secondary surfactant inactivation, the surfactant system of the lung is also subjected to secondary changes due to mechanical ventilation. Several of these mechanisms have been identified.

*Protein-induced surfactant inactivation.* As previously mentioned, animal studies have shown that injurious ventilation using high tidal volumes will change the permeability of both the endothelial and epithelial barrier, promoting influx of plasma proteins in the alveolar space.[100,101] It has been shown that this alveolar protein influx results in a dose-dependent inhibition of surfactant.[102,103]

*Surfactant conversion.* Studies investigating the alveolar metabolism of pulmonary surfactant have shown that surfactant exists in different subfractions.[104] The two major subfractions of surfactant obtained from lung lavage material are large aggregates (LA) and small aggregates (SA).[105] LA surfactant is able to lower alveolar surface tension, but SA surfactant is not surface active and is the metabolic product of the LA fraction.[106] Animal experiments have shown that the conversion from LA to SA surfactant is increased when high tidal volumes are applied during ventilation of the injured lung.[107,108] The increased conversion of surfactant has also been documented in newborn and adult patients with acute lung injury.[109,110]

*Loss of surfactant in small airways.* Animal experiments have shown that ventilation can enhance the secretion of endogenous surfactant by the type II cells.[111,112] This surfactant can subsequently be squeezed out the alveolar space into the small airways as a result of compression of the surfactant film when the surface of the alveolus becomes smaller. Ex vivo experiments in rat lungs showed that this movement of surfactant into the airways is directly related to the tidal volume and inversely related to the end-expiratory pressure.[113]

These changes will induce a vicious circle of surfactant inhibition, as illustrated by Figure 46.1. Secondary surfactant inactivation due to injurious ventilation will

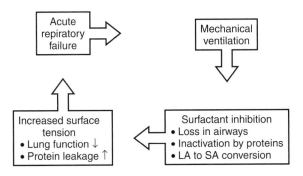

**Figure 46.1** Schematic pathway of the vicious circle leading to surfactant inactivation during mechanical ventilation.

lead to deteriorating lung mechanics and increased permeability of the alveolar-capillary barrier.[114,115] This will lead to more aggressive ventilation which in turn will lead to further inactivation of surfactant. This phenomenon is even further enhanced by the fact that surfactant dysfunction will increase the susceptibility of the lung for both volutrauma and atelectrauma.[63,116]

## LUNG PROTECTIVE VENTILATION

In 1967 Northway and colleagues introduced the term bronchopulmonary dysplasia (BPD) to describe a condition encountered in preterm infants who were mechanically ventilated for nRDS.[117] Lung histology of these infants showed airway injury, fibrosis, and emphysema. With the introduction of new therapies like antenatal corticosteroids and exogenous surfactant, this classical form of BPD is nowadays much less common. It has instead been replaced by a new condition also referred to as the "new BPD" or chronic lung disease of prematurity.[4] The pathological findings show an arrest in alveolar and microvascular development, with much less fibrosis and airway injury as compared with classical BPD.[118] And although it is now clear that the development of BPD is a multifactorial process, mechanical ventilation and high levels of supplemental oxygen are still considered important risk factors for the development of BPD.[4,119] Experimental studies have confirmed that both hyperoxia and mechanical ventilation are able to arrest the alveolarization process in preterm animals.[96,120–122] Based on these findings development of lung protective ventilation strategies remains a priority for improving respiratory outcome in newborn infants.

Besides improving our knowledge on the pathogenesis of VILI, experimental studies have also provided us the tools to develop so-called lung protective ventilation

strategies. The basic goal of lung protective ventilation is to establish an acceptable level of gas exchange while minimizing VILI as much as possible.

The cornerstones of lung protective ventilation strategies are prevention of both alveolar overdistension and collapse (atelectasis). The strategies are also referred to as "optimal volume strategy" or "open lung ventilation."[123,124] Numerous animal studies have shown that reducing alveolar overdistension by limiting tidal volumes during mechanical ventilation will attenuate VILI assessed by pulmonary edema and inflammation.[56,59,60,70,125] The same is true for preventing alveolar collapse by using higher levels of PEEP.[54,65,70,126,127]

### Recruitment

It is essential to realize that in a diseased lung the reduction of atelectasis is based on two principles. First of all, already collapsed alveoli need to be recruited by applying sufficient airway pressures. Secondly, after recruitment sufficient end-expiratory pressure should be applied in order to prevent subsequent collapse during expiration.[124] Figure 46.2 shows the pressure-volume (P/V) relationship of an individual alveolus. Staub and colleagues proposed that the behavior of alveoli is quantal in nature.[128] After a critical opening pressure is reached the collapsed alveolus pops open, immediately resulting

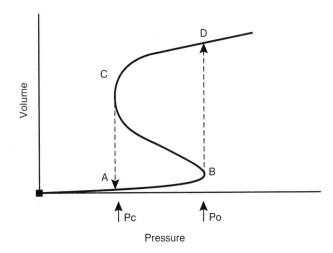

**Figure 46.2** Schematic drawing of the pressure-volume relationship of a single alveolus during inspiration and expiration (*solid line*). At the start of the inspiration (**A**) the alveolus is collapsed. At point **B**, the pressure increase has reached the critical opening pressure (**Po**), leading to an immediate volume increase (*dashed line*) as the alveolus is recruited (**D**). As the pressure is slowly decreased there is little volume loss until the critical closing pressure (**Pc**) is reached at point **C**. The alveolus immediately collapses to point A. Note that **Pc** is lower than **Po** due to the law of Laplace.

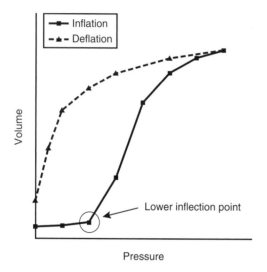

**Figure 46.3** Pressure-volume relationship of the lung showing the inflation (*solid line*) and the deflation limb (*dashed line*). Note the clear difference in lung volume between both limbs at identical pressures (*hysteresis*).

in a large volume increase. As follows by the law of Laplace, which states that the pressure (P) necessary to keep a spherical structure opened is two times the surface tension (γ) divided by the radius (r), the critical closing pressure of the alveolus will be lower than the opening pressure.

The pressure volume curve of the entire lung, as shown in Figure 46.3, will be the cumulative relationship of all alveoli of the lung, each with a different degree of injury. The inflation limb of the P/V curve shows the changes in lung volume during incremental airway pressures and usually contains a so-called lower inflection point above which lung volume suddenly increases in a linear fashion. As lung volume approaches total lung capacity (TLC) the inflation limb flattens off. The deflation limb represents the changes in lung volume during decremental airway pressures starting at TLC. Again, as explained by the law of Laplace, lung volume is initially maintained as pressures are lowered (*hysteresis*) but eventually decreases due to progressive alveolar collapse. This P/V relationship has been shown in both newborns and adults.[10,129]

It was initially assumed that lung recruitment occurred primarily around the lower inflection point of the P/V curve. However, recent observations in adults have indicated that recruitment occurs along the entire inflation limb of the P/V curve.[129,130] Although sometimes stated differently, the *inspiratory* pressures or volumes and not PEEP are responsible for alveolar recruitment during conventional ventilation.[129,131,132] PEEP is an expiratory phenomenon and its main purpose is to stabilize the previously opened alveoli and

thereby prevent subsequent collapse during expiration.[130,132] Failing to recruit the lung prior to increasing PEEP will not prevent VILI.[65,133] On the other hand, recruiting the lung but applying insufficient PEEP in order to prevent subsequent collapse will augment rather than reduce lung injury.[134]

Initially it was believed that the optimal PEEP levels preventing alveolar collapse should be above the lower inflection point of the P/V curve.[64,135] However, recent experimental and human data have shown that the critical closing pressure of the lung is not related to the lower inflection point.[133,136,137] It is important to realize that animal and human data have shown that, besides PEEP, derecruitment is also influenced by tidal volumes and ventilatory rate.[138,139]

Both mathematical models and animal experiments have shown that adequate recruitment of collapsed alveoli, followed by optimal stabilization with adequate levels of PEEP, will place ventilation on the deflation limb of the P/V curve.[132,140] This position will improve compliance and reduce VILI compared to ventilation on or close to the inspiration limb of the P/V curve.

As most underlying lung diseases during ARF are inhomogeneous, regional overdistension of relatively healthy lung parts has been a major concern during recruitment. Although this concern seems valid, there is little evidence that recruitment maneuvers actually damage the lung if accompanied by sufficient PEEP. More importantly, to date most experiments have indicated that derecruitment is more injurious than recruitment.[141–143] Experimental studies have indicated a possible role for partial liquid ventilation as a means to achieve optimal recruitment at lower airway pressures.[144,145]

## Practical Issues on Optimizing Lung Volume

One of the difficulties of the practical implementation of open lung ventilation is the lack of a standardized definition of optimal lung volume. A compilation of several suggested definitions for optimal lung volume could be the volume resulting in optimal dynamic compliance and gas exchange at the lowest possible pressure level and $FiO_2$, without compromising hemodynamics.[140,146,147]

Although both dynamic compliance and oxygenation can be measured bedside, the latter is most often used in newborn infants to optimize lung volume. Figure 46.4 shows a schematic overview of how we use oxygenation in our clinic as a tool to optimize lung volume during high frequency ventilation (HFV) in patients with nRDS. The basic principle in this approach is the assumption that optimal lung recruitment reduces ventilation-perfusion mismatch to less than 10%, making it possible to ventilate patients with an inspired oxygen fraction ($FiO_2$) of less than 25%. Animal studies have confirmed this correlation between oxygenation and

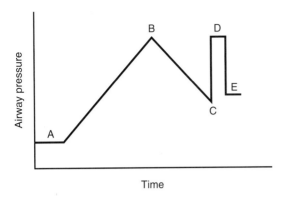

**Figure 46.4** Schematic presentation using oxygenation to optimize lung volume in preterm infants with nRDS. At the start **(A)** airway pressures are low and $Fio_2$ is high indicating a high degree of atelectasis and intrapulmonary shunt. Over time, airway pressures are stepwise increased resulting in alveolar recruitment, a reduction in intrapulmonary shunt, and an improvement in oxygenation. The latter will allow a stepwise reduction in $Fio_2$, thus preventing hyperoxia. Airway pressures are increased until $Fio_2$ is below 25% or oxygenation no longer improves **(B)**. The pressure level at point B is called the opening pressure (Po). Airway pressures are stepwise reduced until $Fio_2$ starts to increase indicating alveolar derecruitment **(C)**. This pressure level is called the closing pressure (Pc). After re-opening collapsed alveoli with the known Po **(D)**, airway pressure is set 2 $cmH_2O$ above Pc to ensure a stabilization of lung volume **(E)**.

lung volume.[148] As shown in Figure 46.4, the airway pressure during the recruitment process is stepwise increased until oxygenation no longer improves or $FiO_2$ is weaned to 25% or less. To make sure the lowest possible pressures are used to maintain alveolar patency, airway pressures are stepwise reduced until oxygenation deteriorates indicating increased ventilation-perfusion mismatch due to alveolar collapse. We recently showed that this approach is feasible in the majority of preterm infants.[149] Failure to achieve an $FiO_2$ below 25% is in our experience most often caused by extrapulmonary right-to-left shunt (pulmonary hypertension) or recruitment of non-functional alveoli filled with debris (pneumonia).

Direct measurement of changes in lung volume (FRC) using wash-out techniques is an alternative and more direct method to optimize lung volume during ventilation. Unfortunately, these techniques are not easy to apply bedside. In addition, patients ventilated with HFV need to be switched back to conventional tidal ventilation.[150] Alternative methods of measuring lung volume like respiratory inductive plethysmography are currently under investigation and look promising.[151] The main disadvantage of techniques that measure changes in total lung volumes is the inability to differentiate volume increments caused by alveolar *recruitment* (which is the aim

of volume optimization) and those caused by alveolar *distension* (of already open alveoli). Only oxygenation is able to make this distinction.[152]

Computer tomography assessment of recruitment and derecruitment has mainly been used in the adult population.[153] Disadvantages like transporting critically ill patients and exposure to radiation have prevented its use in ventilated newborn infants. Newer imaging techniques, such as electrical impedance tomography, which monitors regional changes in lung volume, are now under investigation and might prove useful in the process of volume optimization in newborn infants.[154]

## Experimental Data on Open Lung Ventilation

The majority of animal studies investigating lung protective ventilation explored the effect of changing one or two ventilator settings (e.g., PEEP and/or tidal volume) on the amount of VILI. Relatively few studies explored the concept of open lung ventilation, including all factors of lung protective ventilation, i.e., preventing alveolar overdistension and collapse. As discussed above, the latter should include a recruitment maneuver and sufficient airway pressure to stabilize opened alveoli.

High-frequency ventilation (HFV) was the initial ventilation mode used to explore the effect of open lung ventilation on VILI. Several studies reported that the low tidal volumes applied during HFV combined with optimization of lung volume attenuates VILI compared with more conventional ventilation modes (172,170). More recent reports have shown that open lung ventilation is also possible using more conventional ventilation modes and ventilators.[73,155] More importantly, these reports showed that the attenuation of VILI during open lung ventilation was comparable during both HFV and positive pressure ventilation (PPV). These reports emphasize that the ventilation strategy (open lung ventilation) is more important than the ventilator or ventilation mode (HFV or PPV).

## CONTINUOUS POSITIVE AIRWAY PRESSURE (CPAP)

In 1971, Gregory et al. first reported the use of CPAP in the treatment of nRDS.[156] Although initially administered via head box or endotracheal tube, nasal CPAP was introduced several years later and is nowadays the most common route for CPAP treatment.[157] Nasal masks, nasal cannula, and single and binasal tubes/prongs of varying lengths have been used as nasal interfaces. Positive pressure in the CPAP circuit is generated by using variable or constant gas flow, the latter combined with varying resistance to exhalation using either a valve or a column of water (bubble CPAP).[158]

## Physiological Effects

A variety of physiological effects of CPAP have been described in the literature. The absence or presence of these effects depends on the underlying pulmonary pathology. CPAP is believed to recruit collapsed alveoli and thereby increase FRC.[159] This effect will improve oxygenation as intrapulmonary shunt decreases. In addition, CPAP will reduce inspiratory resistance possibly by splinting of the upper airways.[159,160]

Data on the optimal level of CPAP to achieve these physiological effects are scarce. There is some evidence that pressure levels >4 cm water are more effective than nasal CPAP at lower pressures, although direct comparison has not been made.[161] Others have reported the use of pressures up to 10 cmH$_2$O.[162] Future trials will have to explore these unresolved issues.

### The Use of CPAP in nRDS

Following its introduction in the early 1970s, several randomized controlled trials (RCTs) have compared CPAP to the standard of care treatment for nRDS at that time. A meta-analysis of these RCTs showed a reduction in respiratory failure and mortality in the CPAP arm.[163] This was especially true for infants with a birth weight >1500 g. The fact that standard care for nRDS has changed significantly (surfactant, antenatal steroids), makes it difficult to extrapolate these results to the current time frame.

The fact that nasal CPAP is able to restore FRC and improve gas exchange without positive pressure ventilation (PPV) might potentially reduce VILI and subsequent BPD. A recent study in preterm baboons showed that nasal CPAP instituted after 24 h of life was well tolerated and did not arrest alveolar maturation, as seen in BPD.[164]

Several observational studies in humans also showed that early nasal CPAP reduced the need for mechanical ventilation and lowered the incidence of BPD.[165] However, two recent RCTs combining early nasal CPAP and exogenous surfactant could not confirm the latter showing no differences in the incidence of BPD.[166,167] Still, CPAP has been increasingly used as a primary mode of support in preterm infants with mild to moderate respiratory failure due to nRDS.

### The Use of CPAP in Other Causes of Respiratory Failure

Another important indication for nasal CPAP is apnea of prematurity. Observational studies have shown that CPAP is an effective treatment for obstructive or mixed apnea.[168] In accordance with these observations, a meta-analysis on the use of nasal CPAP following extubation from mechanical ventilation, showed a reduction in the occurrence of apnea needing additional ventilatory support.[161]

CPAP may be a useful adjunct in several other causes of neonatal respiratory failure although evidence for long-term benefits is usually lacking.[169]

### Complications of CPAP

Although less invasive as mechanical ventilation, nasal CPAP is not free of complications.[162] Applying too much pressure may result in pulmonary overdistension. This may lead to hypercapnia, possible air leaks, and increased work of breathing. Increasing pulmonary pressures with nasal CPAP may also compromise cardiac output and induce venous pooling. Other reported adverse effects are gastric distension and damage to the nasal septal mucosa or the skin.

## CONVENTIONAL MECHANICAL VENTILATION

Conventional mechanical ventilation is a nonspecific description for different ventilation modalities used in the treatment of (neonatal) respiratory failure. The word "conventional" indicates that these ventilation modalities are considered standard of care and have been used over a longer period of time. The word "conventional" may also refer to the ventilation settings or strategy used during mechanical ventilation. Sometimes the word "mechanical" is replaced with "positive pressure," in order to differentiate these ventilation modalities from negative pressure ventilation.

Despite the introduction of new ventilation modes like HFV, conventional ventilation is still the primary mode of ventilation applied in almost 75% of the newborn infants.[6,170]

### Pressure Limited Ventilation

Conventional mechanical ventilation can be roughly classified in either volume-controlled or pressure-controlled ventilation. Both modalities are usually time-cycled, meaning that an electrical timer initiates and terminates the inspiratory phase. During volume-controlled ventilation a preset tidal volume is delivered during each mechanical breath, using a constant inspiratory flow. The inspiratory pressure accompanying this volume delivery usually differs between breaths and depends on the compliance of the respiratory system. Volume-controlled ventilation is the primary ventilation mode in adult and pediatric patients.[171] During pressure controlled ventilation the lung of the patient is inflated until a preset pressure level is reached. The actual delivered tidal volume varies and is dependent on the compliance of the respiratory system. Because in the early days of mechanical ventilation, micro-processors were not available to control inspiration and expiration time (time-cycled), inspiration was terminated when the preset pressure limit was reached, also referred to as pressure limited ventilation. Nowadays, the term pressure limited ventilation is used to describe positive pressure ventilation using a continuous flow pattern, resulting in a relatively slow pressure built up during inspiration. This is in contrast to the rapid increase in pressure during pressure controlled ventilation using a decelerating flow pattern. The latter might improve gas distribution resulting in short-term benefits like improved oxygenation, carbon dioxide removal, and lung compliance, as shown in adult respiratory failure.[172] However, there are no comparative studies in the neonatal population, where pressure limited ventilation seems to be the primary mode of ventilation. Manually increasing the continuous flow during pressure limited ventilation will also result in a rapid pressure increase during inspiration and a (semi) decelerating flow pattern measured at the Y-piece.

To date only two small controlled trials compared volume controlled to pressure limited ventilation in newborn infants.[173,174] Although volume controlled ventilation appeared safe and effective, it did not offer major advantages compared to pressure limited ventilation. Hence, many neonatologists continued to use the ventilator modality they were familiar with, being in most cases pressure limited ventilation.

## Patient Triggered Ventilation

Initially time-cycled pressure limited ventilators delivered a mechanical breath at preset intervals, irrespective of the spontaneous ventilatory efforts of the infant (intermittent mandatory ventilation). These infants often experienced asynchronous breathing, during which their own spontaneous breaths were out of phase with the mechanical delivered breaths. Advances in microprocessor technology and ventilator design have allowed the introduction of patient triggered ventilation (PTV) in newborn infants. During PTV, both spontaneous and mechanical breaths are synchronized, as the latter is delivered in response to a signal derived from the patient representing spontaneous respiratory effort. The most commonly used modes of PTV are synchronized intermittent mandatory ventilation (SIMV) and assist/control (A/C) ventilation. During SIMV the mechanically delivered breaths are synchronized with the patient's efforts, allowing spontaneous (non-supported) breathing between mechanical breaths. During A/C control mechanical breaths are delivered in response to every spontaneous effort of the patient. Still both modes do not allow the patient to control timing of inspiration, which can still result in partial asynchrony.

Several cross-over trials in newborn infants showed that PTV improved tidal volume delivery, improved oxygenation, and reduced the work of breathing.[175,176] Unfortunately, a meta-analysis reviewing synchronized modes of mechanical ventilation for respiratory support in newborn infants failed to show clear advantages of PTV concerning important long-term outcome parameters like BPD.[177]

## Conventional Mechanical Ventilation in nRDS

As mentioned previously, conventional mechanical ventilation is still the primary ventilation modality in preterm infants.[6] However, data on which mode of conventional mechanical ventilation is most often used are scarce. The same goes for ventilator settings and strategies. Based on recent RCTs on high-frequency ventilation, most preterm infants seems to be ventilated with time-cycled pressure limited mode.[178–181] These trials also show that PEEP levels are usually below 6 cmH$_2$O and ventilatory rates below 60 breaths/min. The ventilation strategy often used during conventional mechanical ventilation in preterm infants is to lower PIP as soon as possible in order to prevent alveolar overdistension. Some report the use of tidal volume below 7 mL/kg.[180]

This low volume pressure limited ventilation has also been explored in recent animal studies using baboons and preterm lambs.[121,122] Despite the use of low tidal volumes these studies showed pathological lesions comparable to human BPD. However, these animals were chronically ventilated for up to 28 days, which is not in accordance with the 7 days (median) reported in human preterm infants.[180] Furthermore, the high FiO$_2$ (50%) levels required in the initial days of ventilation indicate that lung volume was not optimized. Indeed, these experimental studies did not apply a recruitment maneuver and used relatively low levels of PEEP.

Two recent RCTs exploring the effect of using minimal ventilation combined with permissive hypercapnia in preterm infants with nRDS on the incidence of BPD also failed to show a clear benefit.[182,183] This finding might be explained by the fact that the tidal volume was comparable in both groups. In addition, the focus of this RCT was only on one aspect of lung protective ventilation, i.e., reducing peak inspiratory pressures, thus aiming to reduce alveolar overdistension (but potentially increasing the risk of alveolar collapse!). No attempts were made in this RCT to reduce atelectrauma by recruitment and stabilization of collapsed alveoli, which is considered an important aspect of lung protective ventilation. We recently reported in short-term experiments in lavaged newborn piglets, that such an approach is able to attenuate several parameters of VILI during positive pressure ventilation.[73,155] To date the open lung strategy during positive pressure ventilation has not been tested in newborn infants.

## Conventional Mechanical Ventilation in MAS

Comparable to nRDS, the majority of infants with MAS are ventilated with conventional mechanical ventilation.[170,184] Little is know, however, on the optimal modality and/or ventilation strategy. As meconium inactivates pulmonary surfactant, leading to alveolar collapse, some have advocated the use of PEEP during conventional mechanical ventilation. Both animal and observational human studies conducted in the late 1970s and early 1980s reported a beneficial effect of PEEP on oxygenation.[185,186] Others, however, have warned about the possible air trapping due to increased FRC following PEEP.[23,187] We have recently shown in a piglet model of MAS that applying high levels of PEEP following a recruitment procedure (open lung strategy) during positive pressure ventilation was able to optimize gas exchange and attenuate VILI compared to conventional positive pressure ventilation.[188]

In an attempt to lower the often increased pulmonary vascular resistance during MAS, some clinicians use a ventilation strategy aiming at hyperventilation. A recent prospective observational study in newborn infants with persistent pulmonary hypertension (41% caused by MAS) showed that this was the case in 66% of the patients.[184] Hyperventilation did not change overall mortality but was associated with a decrease in ECMO use. The drawback of such an approach is the possible increase in lung injury due the use of relatively high PIP levels necessary to reduce $PaCO_2$. Almost opposite to this approach is the gentle ventilation strategy advocated by Wung and co-workers, which is discussed in more detail below.[189]

Despite the animal data and observational data in humans, we are still awaiting a randomized controlled trial to determine which ventilation strategy during conventional mechanical ventilation is best applied in newborn infants with MAS.

## Conventional Mechanical Ventilation in Pneumonia

Although there are no data available to substantiate this, it is reasonable to assume that, in accordance with nRDS and MAS, most infants are treated with the time-cycled pressure limited ventilation mode using a comparable ventilation strategy. However, there are no RCTs comparing different modalities or ventilation strategies. Experiments in healthy adult animals have shown that injurious conventional mechanical ventilation using low PEEP and high tidal volume promotes bacterial growth in the lung and bacterial translocation from the lung into the blood stream.[190–192] We recently showed that in the surfactant-deficient lung, as often encountered in newborn infants, ventilator settings nowadays considered noninjurious (PEEP 5 $cmH_2O$, tidal volume 7 mL/kg) still promote bacterial growth in the lung and translocation into the bloodstream.[193] Reversing atelectasis by applying a recruitment maneuver and sufficient PEEP (open lung ventilation) attenuated both bacterial growth and translocation.

## Conventional Mechanical Ventilation in CDH and Pulmonary Hypoplasia

Reports on ventilation modalities and strategies are mainly published in relation to CDH. However, due to the similarities and overlap between these two disease entities the findings are probably also applicable to patients with pulmonary hypoplasia. Most reports are cohort studies comparing changes in treatment regimes over a period of time. Time-cycled pressure limited ventilation with or without synchronization, seems to be the most often used mode of conventional mechanical ventilation.[189,194] The initial ventilatory strategy consisted of an aggressive approach, using high PIP to correct hypoxia and lower $PaCO_2$ (hyperventilation), the latter with the intention to lower pulmonary vascular resistance.[184] In 1985 Wung and co-workers published their experiences with more "gentle ventilation" in newborn infants with PPHN.[195] Others have adopted this ventilation strategy and reported improved survival in patients with CDH.[194,196] During "gentle ventilation" PIP is set at the lowest possible pressure levels which ensures a preductal $SaO_2 > 85\%$ and allows $PaCO_2$ to rise up to 60 mm Hg (permissive hypercapnia). PIP is maximized at 25 $cmH_2O$ and if necessary ventilatory rates are increased up to 100 breaths/min.[44,189] Unfortunately, no RCT has substantiated the results from these observational reports. This seems especially important in the light of many other changes in the management of CDH (NO, ECMO, timing of surgery) which could also have influenced the reported outcome parameters.

## Complications of Conventional Mechanical Ventilation

The most important complication of conventional mechanical ventilation is ventilator-induced lung injury (VILI) and subsequent development of bronchopulmonary dysplasia (BPD), as previously described in this chapter. Besides long-term complications like BPD, VILI may also result in more acute pulmonary complications like pneumothorax and pulmonary interstitial emphysema (air leaks).[197] As mentioned previously, mechanical ventilation is also considered one of the major risk factors for ventilator-associated pneumonia.[34,35] The presence of an endotracheal tube may result in airway injury like subglottic stenosis and tracheobronchitis.[198,199]

Finally, airway pressures applied during mechanical ventilation may compromise hemodynamics.[200]

# HIGH-FREQUENCY VENTILATION (HFV)

Comparable to conventional mechanical ventilation, high-frequency ventilation (HFV) also consists of different modalities. Although similar in the basic principles of ventilation, each HFV modality has its own characteristics. An extensive review on the mechanisms of gas transport and the different HFV modalities is beyond the scope of this chapter but we will discuss these items briefly and thereafter focus on the clinical application of HFV during the different causes of neonatal respiratory failure.

## Mechanisms of Gas Transport during High-Frequency Ventilation

The most striking phenomena of HFV is its ability to achieve adequate gas exchange while delivering tidal volumes equal or less than the anatomic dead space. As bulk flow is greatly reduced during HFV, other mechanisms of convection like coaxial flow, asymmetric velocity profiles, and the pendelluft effect, will deliver fresh gas to the alveolar level. At this level the gas is further "transported" by molecular diffusion. Furthermore, a combination of these two mechanisms (convection and diffusion) will further enhance gas transfer during HFV (Taylor dispersion). For more details on gas transport during HFV, the reader is referred to the available literature.[201]

## High-Frequency Ventilation Modalities

*High-frequency oscillatory ventilation (HFOV).* During HFOV the gas within the airways is moved inwards and outwards by an in-line piston or diaphragm, usually in a frequency of 10–15 Hz. This means that during HFOV both the inspiration and expiration are active. The so-called bias flow provides a continuous flow of fresh air. The pressure swings generated by the oscillator are superimposed on a constant mean airway pressure or continuous distending pressure, which maintains lung volume.

*High-frequency jet ventilation (HFJV).* Using a special endotracheal tube containing an HFJV injector port, HFJV delivers short pulses of pressurized gas directly into the upper airway at frequencies up to 10 Hz. In contrast to HFOV, exhalation is always passive. The mean airway pressure is in part generated by applying positive end-expiratory pressure, sometimes combined with low rate conventional mechanical ventilation.

*High-frequency flow interruption (HFFI).* This modality is usually delivered by hybrid machines, also capable of delivering conventional mechanical ventilation.

Using (software) modification, the flow and/or expiration valve generated short bursts of gas delivered into the ventilatory circuit proximal from the endotracheal tube. Although a Venturi system on the exhalation valve facilitates the expiration, the latter is still considered passive. This is debatable in the latest generation of hybrid ventilators that use high flows or negative pressures to "suck" air away from the patient during the expiration phase and therefore claim an active expiration comparable to HFOV. The mean airway pressure is mostly generated by applying continuous positive airway pressure.

## High Frequency Ventilation in nRDS

The fact that HFV uses a much lower tidal volume than conventional mechanical ventilation stimulated several investigators to explore a possible reduction in alveolar overdistension (volutrauma) during HFV. Animal studies confirmed this hypothesis and showed a clear reduction in VILI during HFV, but only if combined with an optimal lung volume strategy.[202,203] Unfortunately, these initial experiments were conducted over a relatively short period of time and used rather injurious settings during conventional mechanical ventilation, applying high peak inflation pressures combined with a relatively low ventilatory rate. However, more recent long-term experiments (28 days) in preterm baboons comparing HFOV to low tidal volume positive pressure ventilation once again showed that HFOV attenuated VILI and, more importantly, also improved long-term pulmonary outcome.[204] This improvement consisted of lower alveolar levels of interleukin-8 and macrophages, improved pulmonary mechanics, and improvement in the histopathological appearance of the lung.

Based on these encouraging results HFV was also investigated in preterm infants with nRDS. The HIFI study, conducted in 1989, was the first large multicenter randomized controlled trial comparing HFV to conventional positive pressure ventilation in preterm infants.[205] This trial showed that HFV did not reduce mortality nor the incidence of BPD, compared to conventional positive pressure ventilation. In addition, HFV seemed to increase barotrauma, intracranial hemorrhage, and perventricular leucomalacia. Although at first glance, the similar incidence in BPD after HFV and conventional ventilation seems contradictory to the early animal experiments, further analysis of the ventilation strategy used during HFV in the HIFI trial makes this finding consistent with experimental data. As mentioned previously, HFV will only result in an attenuation of VILI if lung volume is optimized.[203] During the HIFI trial airway pressures were preferentially lowered before reducing $Fio_2$, i.e., a low lung volume ventilation strategy. So this initial trial once again emphasized the importance of applying an open lung ventilation strategy during HFV.

Following the HIFI trial several randomized controlled trials over an almost 15 year period have tried to answer the crucial question: does HFV reduce the incidence of BPD? Up to now the answer remains unclear, as some trials reported no differences and others showed a reduction in the incidence of BPD in favor of HFV.[180,206] This is also reflected in the different meta-analyses in this same time period, showing a modest but inconsistent reduction in the incidence of BPD in the HFV arm.[207] Factors that might explain these inconsistencies on the incidence of BPD are large differences in the gestational age of included infants, the introduction of prenatal steroids and exogenous surfactant, different HFV modalities, and, most importantly, differences in ventilation strategies during both HFV and conventional ventilation. As mentioned previously, conventional ventilation has evolved over time from a high pressure low rate to a low pressure high rate ventilation strategy, which might in part explain the reduced risk difference for BPD between HFV and conventional ventilation over time. On the other hand, many trials that claimed to have used an open lung strategy during HFV probably failed, based on the oxygen requirements reported during HFV.[180,206] Future trials should therefore clearly define the criteria for an open lung strategy, preferably by using a $PaO_2/FiO_2$ ratio, and report the pressures used to obtain and preserve this preset goal.

Despite the uncertainty on the effect of HFV on the incidence of BPD, recent large randomized controlled trials in extremely low birth weight infants did show that HFV was not associated with increased intracranial hemorrhage or periventricular malacia.[180,181]

Several studies have tried to determine the effect of HFV on long-term pulmonary and developmental outcome, again showing inconsistent results. A recent cohort study of infants with BPD showed improved lung mechanics at the age of 12 months.[208] Data on neurodevelopmental outcome at the age of 2 and 6 years from some of the early HFV trials showed no differences between infants treated with HFV and conventional ventilation.[209,210] This is in contrast to improved neurodevelopmental outcome at 2 years of age after HFV treatment in a more recent trial.[211]

Although HFV has been widely implemented as a rescue treatment in preterm infants with nRDS failing conventional mechanical ventilation, the inconsistent findings as described above have prevented its use as the primary ventilation mode in nRDS. According to the latest Vermont Oxford database report 25% of the infants with a birth weight below 1500 g are nowadays treated with HFV.[6]

## High Frequency Ventilation in MAS

In contrast to the RDS animal model, most reports on the use of HFV in experimental MAS showed little or no benefits on gas exchange and VILI compared to conventional mechanical ventilation.[212–215] However, none of these reports used an open lung approach during HFV. We recently showed that when combined with an open lung strategy, HFV improves gas exchange and attenuated VILI compared to conventional mechanical ventilation in an animal model of MAS.[188]

To date there is only one multicenter randomized controlled trial which compared HFV to conventional mechanical ventilation in newborns who were candidates for extracorporeal membrane oxygenation, mostly infants with MAS.[216] This study showed that HFOV was an effective mode of ventilation especially when conventional mechanical ventilation failed. However, mortality and significant long-term morbidity did not differ between the groups. The latter may have been influenced by the relatively advanced age at randomization (40 h) and the high cross-over rate in each treatment arm (>50%). Another randomized controlled trial investigating the use of HFOV and/or inhaled nitric oxide also showed improved oxygenation when switching from conventional ventilation to HFOV in the treatment of MAS.[217] Furthermore, combining inhaled nitric oxide with HFOV was superior compared to a combination with conventional mechanical ventilation. Although these reports indicate that HFOV is safe and effective in the treatment of MAS, a large randomized controlled trial including infants with a wide range of disease severity needs to confirm this assumption and more importantly investigate long-term pulmonary and neurodevelopmental morbidity.

## High Frequency Ventilation in Pneumonia

Although several animal studies have shown that the ventilation strategy can affect the course of pneumonia and its complications, there are no animal or human studies that have evaluated the role of HFV in neonatal pneumonia.[190,192,193] The design of such studies is often complicated by the fact that perinatal pneumonia can often not be differentiated from nRDS. In addition, there are no clear and conclusive diagnostic tests available to diagnose nosocomial pneumonia. Like MAS, some randomized trials exploring HFV and/or inhaled nitric oxide in the treatment of persistent pulmonary hypertension also included (near) term infants with pneumonia, but the small number of patients makes definite conclusions impossible.[216,217]

## High Frequency Ventilation in CDH and Lung Hypoplasia

Although animal data on the use of HFV in CDH are scarce, there is a considerable amount of human case reports and case series published. Most of these reports described an improved survival after adopting HFV in the management of CDH mostly compared to historical controls.[44,218–220] Due to the fact that CDH is not characterized by alveolar collapse (like nRDS or MAS), lung recruitment and subsequent stabilization are often achieved at low mean airway pressures, thus minimizing volutrauma during the ventilation period. Reports that showed no benefit from HFV often used this ventilation mode as a rescue therapy, applying it to those patients that failed (high pressure) conventional mechanical ventilation, thus subjecting their lungs to volutrauma for a considerable period of time.[194,221] This in contrast to primary HFV instituted as soon as possible after birth, thereby limiting volutrauma as much as possible.

To date, no randomized controlled trials have confirmed these apparently beneficial effects of HFV and its impact on long-term outcome parameters.

### Complications of HFV

Possible complications of HFV have been an issue of concern ever since the first randomized controlled trial in 1989. It is probably one of the most important reasons why HFV has not been implemented as a primary mode of ventilation in preterm infants with nRDS. One of the major concerns was the increased incidence of intraventricular hemorrhages (grades 3 and 4) and periventricular leucomalecia during HFV, as reported in several randomized controlled trials.[205,206] One of the suggested mechanisms for this observation was a compromising effect of the higher mean airway pressures during HFV on hemodynamics. Several observational cross-over studies have shown a reduced venous return with subsequent lower left ventricular output (but not mean arterial blood pressure) during HFV compared to conventional mechanical ventilation.[222,223] However, these observations have not been substantiated by a recent randomized controlled trial showing no significant adverse hemodynamic effect of HFV compared to conventional mechanical ventilation in very preterm infants during the first 24 h of life.[224] Two recent large randomized controlled trials in (high risk) extremely low birth weight infants have shown conclusively that HFV does not increase the risk for major cerebral adverse effects.[180,181]

A second reported complication of HFV is an increase in the incidence of barotrauma.[178,205] This despite early reports, that showed HFV to be an effective treatment for barotrauma caused by conventional mechanical ventilation.[225] Although the mechanism for this increase in barotrauma remains unclear, this complication was not observed in two recent large randomized controlled trials.[180,181]

Finally, several animal studies reported increased inflammation of the tracheal and bronchial mucosa (necrotizing tracheobronchitis) after HFV, which can cause airway and endotracheal tube obstructions.[226,227] However, human data on this complication are scarce and to date its clinical relevance remains unclear.

## NEW MODES OF VENTILATION

Although most newborn infants are treated with time-cycled pressure limited synchronized ventilation and high frequency ventilation, new modalities and techniques are currently under investigation. The (often combined) aims of these new modes of ventilation are: (1) achieving and maintaining adequate gas exchange; (2) reducing VILI and subsequent long-term pulmonary morbidity, and; (3) reducing the work of breathing and improving patient comfort. We will discuss some of these new techniques or modifications briefly.

### Volume Guaranteed Ventilation

As mentioned earlier, one of the disadvantages of pressure limited ventilation is the possible variation in delivered tidal volume due to changes in pulmonary compliance and resistance. These changes may result in atelectasis when tidal volume is too low and alveolar overdistension when the tidal volume is too high. In theory this may impair gas exchange and enhance VILI. Volume guaranteed ventilation tries to solve this problem by measuring the tidal volume delivered during each pressure-limited breath and adjusting the peak inspiratory pressure during the following breaths if the tidal volume delivered does not correspond to the preset tidal volume. Several cross-over trials in preterm infants showed that adding a volume guarantee to several modes of pressure limited ventilation enabled a reduction in airway pressures without compromising gas exchange.[228,229] In addition some of these trials showed less variability in the delivered tidal volume during volume guaranteed ventilation.[229,230] The latter might reduce the duration and severity of hypoxemic episodes often encountered in ventilated preterm infants with BPD due to forced expiration efforts.[231,232] Unfortunately there are no large randomized controlled trials that have evaluated the effect of volume guaranteed ventilation on important long-term outcome parameters like BPD and neurodevelopment. One small randomized controlled trial reported a reduction in ventilation days and a lower incidence of severe intraventricular hemorrhages in favor of volume guaranteed ventilation.[233] However, besides the contrast of volume guaranteed ventilation, there were additional differences in ventilation style between the two treatment arms, which makes interpretation of these results difficult.

## Pressure Support Ventilation

Although used for many years in the adult and pediatric population, pressure support ventilation has only recently become available for newborn infants. During pressure support ventilation, each patient-triggered breath is supported by a preset inspiratory pressure and the patient controls the onset of the inspiration and the expiration, thus controlling inspiration time. Pressure support ventilation can also be combined with synchronized intermittent mandatory ventilation and volume guaranteed ventilation. During the latter the inspiratory pressure support and/or inspiration time is adjusted in order to deliver the preset tidal volume. Studies in adults and children have shown that pressure support ventilation reduces the work of breathing during the weaning phase.[234,235] A cross-over trial in relatively mature preterm infants compared pressure support ventilation to synchronized intermittent mandatory ventilation and reported a tendency to shorter inspiration times and lower peak inspiratory pressures.[230] When combined with volume guarantee, pressure support ventilation also reduced mean airway pressure, although the latter was not confirmed in a second cross-over trial.[236]

To date, only one small randomized controlled trial in extremely low birth weight infants compared synchronized intermittent mandatory ventilation with and without pressure support ventilation during the weaning phase of mechanical ventilation.[237] The authors reported a reduction in the mean duration of mechanical ventilation in the pressure support group, although the incidence of BPD was not significantly different between the groups. Larger randomized controlled trials will need to determine the place of pressure support ventilation in newborn infants.

## Proportional Assist Ventilation

Proportional assist ventilation is a new mode of assisted ventilation which aims to fully compensate disease-related changes in respiratory system compliance and resistance by using so-called elastic and resistive unloading. During unloading, airway pressures are servo controlled throughout each spontaneous breath, depending on the tidal volume and inspiratory airflow generated by the patient. In contrast to other modes of mechanical ventilation, proportional assist ventilation allows the patient to fully control frequency, timing, and the amplitude of lung inflation. This might improve patient-ventilator synchronization, reduce ventilatory pressure, and work of breathing. Only one small cross-over trial in preterm infants with mild to moderate lung disease evaluated several short-term physiological variables and safety of proportional assist ventilation to assist control and intermittent mandatory ventilation.[238] Proportional assist ventilation resulted in a (small) reduction in peak and mean airway pressures while gas exchange remained similar in all groups. Future randomized controlled trials will have to investigate the benefits on long-term outcome parameters like BPD.

## Tracheal Gas Insufflation

The relatively large dead space volume created by the endotracheal tube and flow sensors is a significant problem in neonatal ventilation. This problem is mainly solved by increasing the tidal volume during ventilation, thus increasing the risk of alveolar overdistension. Tracheal gas insufflation is an alternative way to approach the dead space problem during neonatal ventilation. Using a pump and a multichannel endotracheal tube containing several capillary tubes within its wall, oxygenated, heated, and humidified gas is injected directly into the trachea at the end of the tube during regular conventional mechanical ventilation. This flow of fresh gas clears expired $CO_2$ from the instrumental dead space during expiration. Cross-over trials in preterm infants have shown that this $CO_2$ wash-out decreased $PaCO_2$ and enabled a significant reduction in pressure amplitude during conventional mechanical ventilation.[239] This was also confirmed by a small randomized controlled trial in preterm infants, which also showed a shorter duration of ventilation when combining conventional mechanical ventilation with continuous tracheal gas insufflation.[240] However, there were no differences in BPD. Again, larger randomized controlled trials are needed to determine the long-term benefits of this intriguing adjunct for mechanical ventilation.

## Liquid Ventilation

The concept of liquid ventilation has been investigated for more than 40 years. The basic principle of liquid ventilation is to fill the lung with perfluorocarbon up to a volume equivalent to functional residual capacity. Perfluorocarbon has an excellent oxygen and carbon dioxide carrying capacity and a low surface tension. Following this first step, the lung is ventilated using either perfluorocarbon (*total* liquid ventilation) or gas (*partial* liquid ventilation). Animal studies have shown that compared to conventional mechanical ventilation, liquid ventilation improves gas exchange and pulmonary compliance, and attenuates secondary lung injury.[145,241,242] One of the suggested mechanisms is the recruitment of atelectatic and consolidated (dependent) lung regions, thereby reducing intrapulmonary shunt.[243]

For technical reasons clinical application of liquid ventilation has mainly focused on partial liquid ventilation. Despite the promising animal data, studies in adults, children, and newborns have failed to show clear benefits of partial liquid ventilation compared to conventional mechanical ventilation.[244,245] Based on these results several ongoing trials have been stopped and placed on hold. It is unclear if and when trials in newborn infants will be continued.

Despite these disappointing results partial liquid ventilation is also investigated for other purposes. As previously mentioned in this chapter, it may play a future role as an adjunctive therapy for open lung ventilation, facilitating recruitment of atelectatic lung regions.[144,145] Secondly, animal and human data have proposed a role for partial liquid ventilation for the induction of lung growth in congenital diaphragmatic hernia.[246–248]

Total liquid ventilation is still in the preclinical phase, but as some of the technical aspects of device design and technique are refined, we can expect this mode of ventilation to enter the clinical arena in the near future.

## SUPPORTIVE THERAPIES

Besides respiratory support several supportive therapies can be used to further optimize gas exchange and reduce possible VILI. Although not the primary focus of this chapter we will discuss the most important supportive therapies briefly.

### Exogenous Surfactant

As previously mentioned most causes of neonatal respiratory failure are accompanied by surfactant deficiency or inhibition. Secondly, the remaining surfactant function is often compromised by mechanical ventilation. From this point of view the introduction of surfactant replacement therapy in 1980 was a logical step and is nowadays widely implemented in the treatment of neonatal respiratory failure.

*Surfactant in nRDS.* Numerous randomized controlled trials combined in several meta-analyses have shown that treatment of nRDS with exogenous surfactant optimizes gas exchange, reduces barotrauma, and, most importantly, reduces mortality.[249] In addition, these studies showed that natural surfactant is superior to a synthetic product, two surfactant doses are more effective than one, and early treatment (prophylactic or within 2 h after birth) is more effective than late rescue treatment (>2 h after birth).[250–253] It is important to realize that the primary mode of ventilation during most surfactant trials has been conventional mechanical ventilation. Little is known on the interaction between new ventilation modes like HFV or different ventilation strategies like open lung ventilation. Previous animals studies have shown that changes in ventilation strategies can indeed change the surfactant treatment response.[59,60,254] We recently showed in an animal model of RDS that, in contrast to conventional mechanical ventilation, open lung ventilation, using either HFV or positive pressure ventilation, improved gas exchange and attenuated VILI

independent of the surfactant dose.[255] Furthermore, applying open lung ventilation also preserved the surfactant response after delayed treatment.[256]

*Surfactant in other causes of respiratory failure.* Exogenous surfactant is nowadays increasingly used in the treatment of MAS, following two human RCTs which showed that a bolus of exogenous surfactant significantly reduced the number of patients with MAS that required extracorporeal membrane oxygenation (ECMO).[170,257] A different technique using surfactant lavage is currently under investigation and the first preliminary result looks promising.[258] Although, animal data showed that exogenous surfactant might be beneficial in reducing bacterial growth and translocation during pneumonia, human data are scarce consisting mainly of case series.[193,259] The same is true for CDH where animal studies showed signs of surfactant deficiency in experimental CDH.[260] However, human studies are inconclusive, some showing no surfactant abnormalities and others showing an abnormal turnover and reduced surfactant pool size, although the latter could also be caused by reduced lung size and/or differences in ventilatory support.[261,262] A small randomized controlled trial on the use of exogenous surfactant in patients with CDH on ECMO failed to show any improvement in pulmonary outcome parameters.[263] Future large randomized controlled trials will hopefully answer these unresolved issues concerning surfactant therapy during pneumonia and CDH.

### Inhaled Nitric Oxide

Many of the above mentioned causes of neonatal respiratory failure are often complicated by increased pulmonary vascular resistance leading persistent pulmonary hypertension (PPHN). The subsequent extrapulmonary right-to-left shunt via the foramen oval and the ductus arteriosus will result in severe hypoxia, often refractory to mechanical ventilation and/or exogenous surfactant. Nitric oxide (NO) is one of the most important regulators of pulmonary vascular muscle tone and has therefore been explored as a potential treatment for PPHN. Several randomized controlled trials combined in a recent meta-analysis have shown that inhaled NO significantly improves oxygenation and more importantly reduces the need for extracorporeal membrane oxygenation (ECMO).[264] However, it does not reduce mortality. Although highly effective in MAS and pneumonia, inhaled NO showed little or no benefit in patients with CDH.[265–267] Using a higher dose (up to 80 ppm) in those infants showing no or only a partial response to 20 ppm, does not seem to be very effective.[265] Although initiating inhaled NO in infants with less severe lung disease (OI < 25) improves oxygenation compared to the regular criteria (OI > 25), this approach did not improve long-term outcome parameters.[268] As mentioned previously, inhaled NO seems to be more effective in infants treated with HFV, especially if PPHN is caused by recruitable lung disease.[269,270]

Besides regulating vascular tone, NO also plays an important role in normal lung development and inhibits the pulmonary inflammatory response often seen in the development of BPD. From this point of view, several randomized controlled trials have investigated the use of inhaled NO in preterm infants at risk for BPD. The latest trial showed that inhaled NO administered in a dose of 5–10 ppm during the first week of life significantly decreases the incidence of BPD or death in preterm infants. In addition, inhaled NO also decreased the incidence of severe intraventricular hemorrhages and periventricular leucomalacia.[271] Data on long-term follow-up are needed before implementing this treatment in daily clinical practice.

## Extracorporeal Membrane Oxygenation (ECMO)

The basic aim of ECMO is to support the function of the lung and/or the heart using an external artificial organ. In the strict sense of the word ECMO is not a treatment, but mainly serves as a means of temporary support in order to buy time while the reversible disease of heart/lung responds to other therapeutic interventions.

For (near) term newborn infants with severe respiratory failure (MAS, pneumonia) often complicated by PPHN, ECMO has, in contrast to all other supportive therapies, significantly lowered mortality.[272] However, the efficacy of ECMO in CDH still remains unclear. Some feel that combined treatment of all other supportive therapies like HFOV, surfactant, and inhaled NO, is as effective as ECMO.[44]

Most infants are subjected to so-called resting ventilation during ECMO. During resting ventilation the ventilation pressures and rate are lowered in order to allow the lung to heal without inflicting more damage due to aggressive ventilation. The chest radiograph usually shows general opacification within 24 hours after initiating ECMO, indicating either fluid accumulation and/or alveolar collapse.[273] As discussed previously, the latter may increase rather than decrease secondary lung damage. In accordance with this hypothesis a randomized controlled trial showed that preventing atelectasis during resting ventilation on ECMO by applying high levels of PEEP shortened ECMO duration compared to infants ventilated with low PEEP levels.[274]

## REFERENCES

1. Angus DC, Linde-Zwirble WT, Clermont G et al: Epidemiology of neonatal respiratory failure in the United States: projections from California and New York. Am J Respir Crit Care Med 2001;164:1154–1160.

2. Henderson-Smart DJ, Wilkinson A, Raynes-Greenow CH: Mechanical ventilation for newborn infants with respiratory failure due to pulmonary disease. Cochrane Database Syst Rev 2002.

3. Dreyfuss D, Saumon G: Ventilator-induced lung injury: lessons from experimental studies. Am J Respir Crit Care Med 1998;157:294–323.

4. Jobe AH, Bancalari E: Bronchopulmonary dysplasia. Am J Respir Crit Care Med 2001;163:1723–1729.

5. Lemons JA, Bauer CR, Oh W et al: Very low birth weight outcomes of the National Institute of Child health and human development neonatal research network, January 1995 through December 1996. NICHD Neonatal Research Network. Pediatrics 2001;107:E1.

6. Horbar JD, Badger GJ, Carpenter JH et al: Trends in mortality and morbidity for very low birth weight infants, 1991–1999. Pediatrics 2002;110:143–151.

7. Dani C, Reali MF, Bertini G et al: Risk factors for the development of respiratory distress syndrome and transient tachypnoea in newborn infants. Italian Group of Neonatal Pneumology. Eur Respir J 1999;14:155–159.

8. Hodson WA, Bancalari E: Normal and abnormal structural development of the lung. In Polin RA, Fox WW (eds): Fetal and Neonatal Physiology. Philadelphia: WB Saunders, 1998, pp 1033–1046.

9. Avery ME, Mead J: Surface properties in relation to atelectasis and hyaline membrane disease. Am J Dis Child 1959;97: 517–523.

10. Gribetz I, Frank NR, Avery ME: Static volume-pressure relations of excised lungs of infants with hyaline membrane disease, newborn and stillborn infants. J Clin Invest 1959;38: 2168–2175.

11. Verma RP: Respiratory distress syndrome of the newborn infant. Obstet Gynecol Surv 1995;50:542–555.

12. Ablow RC, Gross I, Effmann EL et al: The radiographic features of early onset Group B streptococcal neonatal sepsis. Radiology 1977;124:771–777.

13a. Crowley P: Prophylactic corticosteroids for preterm birth. Cochrane Database Syst Rev 2000.

13b. Field DJ, Milner AD, Hopkin IE et al: Changing patterns in neonatal respiratory diseases. Pediatr Pulmonol 1987; 3:231–235.

14. Rawlings JS, Smith FR: Transient tachypnea of the newborn. An analysis of neonatal and obstetric risk factors. Am J Dis Child 1984;138:869–871.

15. Avery ME, Gatewood OB, Brumley G: Transient tachypnea of newborn. Possible delayed resorption of fluid at birth. Am J Dis Child 1966;111:380–385.

16. Bohin S, Field DJ: The epidemiology of neonatal respiratory disease. Early Hum Dev 1994;37:73–90.

17. Miller MJ, Fanaroff AA, Martin RJ: The respiratory system. In Fanaroff AA, Martin RJ (eds): Neonatal-Perinatal Medicine. St. Louis: Mosby-Year Book, Inc., 1992, pp 834–861.

18. Wiswell TE, Tuggle JM, Turner BS: Meconium aspiration syndrome: have we made a difference? Pediatrics 1990;85: 715–721.

19. Knox GE, Huddleston JF, Flowers CE, Jr: Management of prolonged pregnancy: results of a prospective randomized trial. Am J Obstet Gynecol 1979;134:376–384.

20. Coltart TM, Byrne DL, Bates SA: Meconium aspiration syndrome: a 6-year retrospective study. Br J Obstet Gynaecol 1989;96:411–414.

21. Sun B, Curstedt T, Robertson B: Surfactant inhibition in experimental meconium aspiration. Acta Paediatr 1993;82:182–189.

22. Davey AM, Becker JD, Davis JM: Meconium aspiration syndrome: physiological and inflammatory changes in a newborn piglet model. Pediatr Pulmonol 1993;16:101–108.

23. Tran N, Lowe C, Sivieri EM et al: Sequential effects of acute meconium obstruction on pulmonary function. Pediatr Res 1980;14:34–38.

24. Tyler DC, Murphy J, Cheney FW: Mechanical and chemical damage to lung tissue caused by meconium aspiration. Pediatrics 1978;62:454–459.

25. Cleary GM, Wiswell TE: Meconium-stained amniotic fluid and the meconium aspiration syndrome. An update. Pediatr Clin North Am 1998;45:511–529.

26. Starks GC: Correlation of meconium-stained amniotic fluid, early intrapartum fetal pH, and Apgar scores as predictors of perinatal outcome. Obstet Gynecol 1980;56:604–609.

27. Soll RF, Dargaville P: Surfactant for meconium aspiration syndrome in full term infants. Cochrane Database Syst Rev 2000.

28. Campbell JR: Neonatal pneumonia. Semin Respir Infect 1996;11:155–162.

29. Davies JK, Gibbs RS: Obstetric factors associated with infections of fetus and newborn infant. In Remington JS, Klein JO (eds): Infectious diseases of the fetus and newborn infant. Philadelphia: WB Saunders, 2001, pp 1345–1370.

30. Webber S, Wilkinson AR, Lindsell D et al: Neonatal pneumonia. Arch Dis Child 1990;65:207–211.

31. Barnett ED, Klein JO: Bacterial infections of the respiratory tract. In Remington JS, Klein JO (eds): Infectious diseases of the fetus and newborn infant. Philadelphia: WB Saunders, 2001, pp 999–1018.

32. Ablow RC, Driscoll SG, Effmann EL et al: A comparison of early-onset group B steptococcal neonatal infection and the respiratory-distress syndrome of the newborn. N Engl J Med 1976;294:65–70.

33. Gaynes RP, Edwards JR, Jarvis WR et al: Nosocomial infections among neonates in high-risk nurseries in the United States. National Nosocomial Infections Surveillance System. Pediatrics 1996;98:357–361.

34. Nagata E, Brito AS, Matsuo T: Nosocomial infections in a neonatal intensive care unit: incidence and risk factors. Am J Infect Control 2002;30:26–31.

35. Kawagoe JY, Segre CA, Pereira CR et al: Risk factors for nosocomial infections in critically ill newborns: a 5–year prospective cohort study. Am J Infect Control 2001;29:109–114.

36. Haney PJ, Bohlman M, Sun CC: Radiographic findings in neonatal pneumonia. AJR Am J Roentgenol 1984;143:23–26.

37. Cordero L, Ayers LW, Miller RR et al: Surveillance of ventilator-associated pneumonia in very-low-birth-weight infants. Am J Infect Control 2002;30:32–39.

38. Harris H, Wirtschafter D, Cassady G: Endotracheal intubation and its relationship to bacterial colonization and systemic infection of newborn infants. Pediatrics 1976;58:816–823.

39. Auten RL, Notter RH, Kendig JW et al: Surfactant treatment of full-term newborns with respiratory failure. Pediatrics 1991;87:101–107.

40. Herting E, Moller O, Schiffmann JH et al: Surfactant improves oxygenation in infants and children with pneumonia and acute respiratory distress syndrome. Acta Paediatr 2002; 91:1174–1178.

41. Herting E, Gefeller O, Land M et al: Surfactant treatment of neonates with respiratory failure and group B streptococcal infection. Members of the Collaborative European Multicenter Study Group. Pediatrics 2000;106:957–964.

42. Apisarnthanarak A, Holzmann-Pazgal G, Hamvas A et al: Ventilator-associated pneumonia in extremely preterm neonates in a neonatal intensive care unit: characteristics, risk factors, and outcomes. Pediatrics 2003;112:1283–1289.

43. Langham MR, Jr., Kays DW, Ledbetter DJ et al: Congenital diaphragmatic hernia. Epidemiology and outcome. Clin Perinatol 1996;23:671–688.

44. Bohn D: Congenital diaphragmatic hernia. Am J Respir Crit Care Med 2002;166:911–915.

45. Boloker J, Bateman DA, Wung JT et al: Congenital diaphragmatic hernia in 120 infants treated consecutively with permissive hypercapnea/spontaneous respiration/elective repair. J Pediatr Surg 2002;37:357–366.

46. Laudy JA, Wladimiroff JW: The fetal lung. 2: Pulmonary hypoplasia. Ultrasound Obstet Gynecol 2000;16:482–494.

47. Knox WF, Barson AJ: Pulmonary hypoplasia in a regional perinatal unit. Early Hum Dev 1986;14:33–42.

48. Wigglesworth JS, Hislop AA, Desai R: Biochemical and morphometric analyses in hypoplastic lungs. Pediatr Pathol 1991;11:537–549.

49. Nakamura Y, Yamamoto I, Funatsu Y et al: Decreased surfactant level in the lung with oligohydramnios: a morphometric and biochemical study. J Pediatr 1988;112:471–474.

50. Barth PJ, Ruschoff J: Morphometric study on pulmonary arterial thickness in pulmonary hypoplasia. Pediatr Pathol 1992;12:653–663.

51. Leonidas JC, Bhan I, Beatty EC: Radiographic chest contour and pulmonary air leaks in oligohydramnios-related pulmonary hypoplasia (Potter's syndrome). Invest Radiol 1982;17:6–10.

52. Winn HN, Chen M, Amon E et al: Neonatal pulmonary hypoplasia and perinatal mortality in patients with midtrimester rupture of amniotic membranes—a critical analysis. Am J Obstet Gynecol 2000;182:1638–1644.

53. Bendixen HH, Hedley-Whyte J, Laver MB: Impaired oxygenation in surgical patients during general anesthesia with controlled ventilation. N Engl J Med 1963;269:991–996.

54. Webb HH, Tierney DF: Experimental pulmonary edema due to intermittent positive pressure ventilation with high inflation pressures. Protection by positive end-expiratory pressure. Am Rev Respir Dis 1974;110:556–565.

55. Egan EA, Nelson RM, Olver RE: Lung inflation and alveolar permeability to non-electrolytes in the adult sheep in vivo. J Physiol 1976;260:409–424.

56. Dreyfuss D, Soler P, Basset G et al: High inflation pressure pulmonary edema. Respective effects of high airway pressure, high tidal volume, and positive end-expiratory pressure. Am Rev Respir Dis 1988;137:1159–1164.

57. Hernandez LA, Peevy KJ, Moise AA et al: Chest wall restriction limits high airway pressure-induced lung injury in young rabbits. J Appl Physiol 1989;66:2364–2368.

58. Dreyfuss D, Saumon G: Role of tidal volume, FRC, and end-inspiratory volume in the development of pulmonary edema following mechanical ventilation. Am Rev Respir Dis 1993;148: 1194–1203.

59. Wada K, Jobe AH, Ikegami M: Tidal volume effects on surfactant treatment responses with the initiation of ventilation in preterm lambs. J Appl Physiol 1997;83:1054–1061.

60. Bjorklund LJ, Ingimarsson J, Curstedt T et al: Manual ventilation with a few large breaths at birth compromises the therapeutic effect of subsequent surfactant replacement in immature lambs. Pediatr Res 1997;42:348–355.

61. Jobe AH, Ikegami M: Mechanisms initiating lung injury in the preterm. Early Hum Dev 1998;53:81–94.

62. Gattinoni L, Pesenti A, Avalli L et al: Pressure-volume curve of total respiratory system in acute respiratory failure. Computed tomographic scan study. Am Rev Respir Dis 1987;136:730–736.

63. Taskar V, John J, Evander E et al: Surfactant dysfunction makes lungs vulnerable to repetitive collapse and reexpansion. Am J Respir Crit Care Med 1997;155:313–320.

64. Muscedere JG, Mullen JB, Gan K et al: Tidal ventilation at low airway pressures can augment lung injury. Am J Respir Crit Care Med 1994;149:1327–1334.

65. Naik AS, Kallapur SG, Bachurski CJ et al: Effects of ventilation with different positive end-expiratory pressures on cytokine expression in the preterm lamb lung. Am J Respir Crit Care Med 2001;164:494–498.

66. Tsuchida S, Engelberts D, Peltekova V et al: Atelectasis causes alveolar injury in nonatelectatic lung regions. Am J Respir Crit Care Med 2006;174:279–289.

67. Mead J, Takishima T, Leith D: Stress distribution in lungs: a model of pulmonary elasticity. J Appl Physiol 1970;28:596–608.

68. Vlahakis NE, Schroeder MA, Limper AH et al: Stretch induces cytokine release by alveolar epithelial cells in vitro. Am J Physiol 1999;277:L167–L173.

69. Pugin J, Dunn I, Jolliet P et al: Activation of human macrophages by mechanical ventilation in vitro. Am J Physiol 1998;275:L1040–L1050.

70. Tremblay L, Valenza F, Ribeiro SP et al: Injurious ventilatory strategies increase cytokines and c-fos m-RNA expression in an isolated rat lung model. J Clin Invest 1997;99:944–952.

71. von Bethmann AN, Brasch F, Nusing R et al: Hyperventilation induces release of cytokines from perfused mouse lung. Am J Respir Crit Care Med 1998;157:263–272.

72. Chiumello D, Pristine G, Slutsky AS: Mechanical ventilation affects local and systemic cytokines in an animal model of acute respiratory distress syndrome. Am J Respir Crit Care Med 1999;160:109–116.

73. van Kaam AH, Dik WA, Haitsma JJ et al: Application of the open-lung concept during positive-pressure ventilation reduces pulmonary inflammation in newborn piglets. Biol Neonate 2003;83:273–280.

74. Imanaka H, Shimaoka M, Matsuura N et al: Ventilator-induced lung injury is associated with neutrophil infiltration, macrophage activation, and TGF-beta 1 mRNA upregulation in rat lungs. Anesth Analg 2001;92:428–436.

75. Sugiura M, McCulloch PR, Wren S et al: Ventilator pattern influences neutrophil influx and activation in atelectasis-prone rabbit lung. J Appl Physiol 1994;77:1355–1365.

76. Papoff P: Infection, neutrophils, and hematopoietic growth factors in the pathogenesis of neonatal chronic lung disease. Clin Perinatol 2000;27:717–731.

77. Kawano T, Mori S, Cybulsky M et al: Effect of granulocyte depletion in a ventilated surfactant-depleted lung. J Appl Physiol 1987;62:27–33.

78. Haitsma JJ, Uhlig S, Goggel R et al: Ventilator-induced lung injury leads to loss of alveolar and systemic compartmentalization of tumor necrosis factor-alpha. Intensive Care Med 2000; 26:1515–1522.

79. Imai Y, Parodo J, Kajikawa O et al: Injurious mechanical ventilation and end-organ epithelial cell apoptosis and organ dysfunction in an experimental model of acute respiratory distress syndrome. JAMA 2003;289:2104–2112.

80. Ranieri VM, Suter PM, Tortorella C et al: Effect of mechanical ventilation on inflammatory mediators in patients with acute respiratory distress syndrome: a randomized controlled trial. JAMA 1999;282:54–61.

81. Jobe AH: Antenatal factors and the development of bronchopulmonary dysplasia. Semin Neonatol 2003;8:9–17.

82. Goldenberg RL, Hauth JC, Andrews WW: Intrauterine infection and preterm delivery. N Engl J Med 2000;342:1500–1507.

83. Yoon BH, Romero R, Jun JK et al: Amniotic fluid cytokines (interleukin-6, tumor necrosis factor-alpha, interleukin-1 beta, and interleukin-8) and the risk for the development of bronchopulmonary dysplasia. Am J Obstet Gynecol 1997; 177:825–830.

84. Watterberg KL, Demers LM, Scott SM et al: Chorioamnionitis and early lung inflammation in infants in whom bronchopulmonary dysplasia develops. Pediatrics 1996;97:210–215.

85. Jonsson B, Tullus K, Brauner A et al: Early increase of TNF alpha and IL-6 in tracheobronchial aspirate fluid indicator of subsequent chronic lung disease in preterm infants. Arch Dis Child Fetal Neonatal Ed 1997;77:F198–F201.

86. Kotecha S, Chan B, Azam N et al: Increase in interleukin-8 and soluble intercellular adhesion molecule-1 in bronchoalveolar lavage fluid from premature infants who develop chronic lung disease. Arch Dis Child Fetal Neonatal Ed 1995;72:F90–F96.

87. Groneck P, Gotze-Speer B, Oppermann M et al: Association of pulmonary inflammation and increased microvascular permeability during the development of bronchopulmonary dysplasia: a sequential analysis of inflammatory mediators in respiratory fluids of high-risk preterm neonates. Pediatrics 1994;93:712–718.

88. Crapo JD, Barry BE, Foscue HA et al: Structural and biochemical changes in rat lungs occurring during exposures to lethal and adaptive doses of oxygen. Am Rev Respir Dis 1980;122:123–143.

89. Davis JM, Dickerson B, Metlay L et al: Differential effects of oxygen and barotrauma on lung injury in the neonatal piglet. Pediatr Pulmonol 1991;10:157–163.

90. Quinn DA, Moufarrej RK, Volokhov A et al: Interactions of lung stretch, hyperoxia, and MIP-2 production in ventilator-induced lung injury. J Appl Physiol 2002;93:517–525.

91. Newman JH, Loyd JE, English DK et al: Effects of 100% oxygen on lung vascular function in awake sheep. J Appl Physiol 1983;54:1379–1386.

92. Holm BA, Notter RH, Siegle J et al: Pulmonary physiological and surfactant changes during injury and recovery from hyperoxia. J Appl Physiol 1985;59:1402–1409.

93. Holm BA, Matalon S, Finkelstein JN et al: Type II pneumocyte changes during hyperoxic lung injury and recovery. J Appl Physiol 1988;65:2672–2678.

94. Horinouchi H, Wang CC, Shepherd KE et al: TNF alpha gene and protein expression in alveolar macrophages in acute and chronic hyperoxia-induced lung injury. Am J Respir Cell Mol Biol 1996;14:548–555.

95. Rozycki HJ, Comber PG, Huff TF: Cytokines and oxygen radicals after hyperoxia in preterm and term alveolar macrophages. Am J Physiol Lung Cell Mol Physiol 2002;282:L1222–L1228.

96. Warner BB, Stuart LA, Papes RA et al: Functional and pathological effects of prolonged hyperoxia in neonatal mice. Am J Physiol 1998;275:L110–L117.

97. Dauger S, Ferkdadji L, Saumon G et al: Neonatal exposure to 65% oxygen durably impairs lung architecture and breathing pattern in adult mice. Chest 2003;123:530–538.

98. Frank L, Sosenko IR: Failure of premature rabbits to increase antioxidant enzymes during hyperoxic exposure: increased susceptibility to pulmonary oxygen toxicity compared with term rabbits. Pediatr Res 1991;29:292–296.

99. Georgeson GD, Szony BJ, Streitman K et al: Antioxidant enzyme activities are decreased in preterm infants and in neonates born via caesarean section. Eur J Obstet Gynecol Reprod Biol 2002;103:136–139.

100. Dreyfuss D, Basset G, Soler P et al: Intermittent positive-pressure hyperventilation with high inflation pressures produces pulmonary microvascular injury in rats. Am Rev Respir Dis 1985;132:880–884.

101. Parker JC, Hernandez LA, Longenecker GL et al: Lung edema caused by high peak inspiratory pressures in dogs. Role of increased microvascular filtration pressure and permeability. Am Rev Respir Dis 1990;142:321–328.

102. Lachmann B, Eijking EP, So KL et al: In vivo evaluation of the inhibitory capacity of human plasma on exogenous surfactant function. Intensive Care Med 1994;20:6–11.

103. Kobayashi T, Nitta K, Ganzuka M et al: Inactivation of exogenous surfactant by pulmonary edema fluid. Pediatr Res 1991;29:353–356.

104. Magoon MW, Wright JR, Baritussio A et al: Subfractionation of lung surfactant. Implications for metabolism and surface activity. Biochim Biophys Acta 1983;750:18–31.

105. Lewis JF, Ikegami M, Jobe AH: Altered surfactant function and metabolism in rabbits with acute lung injury. J Appl Physiol 1990;69:2303–2310.

106. Yamada T, Ikegami M, Jobe AH: Effects of surfactant subfractions on preterm rabbit lung function. Pediatr Res 1990;27:592–598.

107. Ito Y, Veldhuizen RA, Yao LJ et al: Ventilation strategies affect surfactant aggregate conversion in acute lung injury. Am J Respir Crit Care Med 1997;155:493–499.

108. Veldhuizen RA, Marcou J, Yao LJ et al: Alveolar surfactant aggregate conversion in ventilated normal and injured rabbits. Am J Physiol 1996;270:L152–L158.

109. Griese M, Westerburg B, Potz C et al: Respiratory support, surface activity and protein content during nosocomial infection in preterm neonates. Biol Neonate 1996;70:271–279.

110. Gunther A, Siebert C, Schmidt R et al: Surfactant alterations in severe pneumonia, acute respiratory distress syndrome, and cardiogenic lung edema. Am J Respir Crit Care Med 1996;153:176–184.

111. Faridy EE: Effect of distension on release of surfactant in excised dogs' lungs. Respir Physiol 1976;27:99–114.

112. Massaro GD, Massaro D: Morphologic evidence that large inflations of the lung stimulate secretion of surfactant. Am Rev Respir Dis 1983;127:235–236.

113. Faridy EE: Effect of ventilation on movement of surfactant in airways. Respir Physiol 1976;27:323–334.

114. Bos JA, Wollmer P, Bakker W et al: Clearance of 99mTc-DTPA and experimentally increased alveolar surfactant content. J Appl Physiol 1992;72:1413–1417.

115. Jobe A, Ikegami M, Jacobs H et al: Permeability of premature lamb lungs to protein and the effect of surfactant on that permeability. J Appl Physiol 1983;55:169–176.

116. Coker PJ, Hernandez LA, Peevy KJ et al: Increased sensitivity to mechanical ventilation after surfactant inactivation in young rabbit lungs. Crit Care Med 1992;20:635–640.

117. Northway WH, Jr., Rosan RC, Porter DY: Pulmonary disease following respirator therapy of hyaline-membrane disease. Bronchopulmonary dysplasia. N Engl J Med 1967;276:357–368.

118. Husain AN, Siddiqui NH, Stocker JT: Pathology of arrested acinar development in postsurfactant bronchopulmonary dysplasia. Hum Pathol 1998;29:710–717.

119. Van Marter LJ, Dammann O, Allred EN et al: Chorioamnionitis, mechanical ventilation, and postnatal sepsis as modulators of chronic lung disease in preterm infants. J Pediatr 2002;140:171–176.

120. Coalson JJ, Winter V, Delemos RA: Decreased alveolarization in baboon survivors with bronchopulmonary dysplasia. Am J Respir Crit Care Med 1995;152:640–646.

121. Coalson JJ, Winter VT, Siler-Khodr T et al: Neonatal chronic lung disease in extremely immature baboons. Am J Respir Crit Care Med 1999;160:1333–1346.

122. Albertine KH, Jones GP, Starcher BC et al: Chronic lung injury in preterm lambs. Disordered respiratory tract development. Am J Respir Crit Care Med 1999;159:945–958.

123. Clark RH, Gerstmann DR, Jobe AH et al: Lung injury in neonates: causes, strategies for prevention, and long-term consequences. J Pediatr 2001;139:478–486.

124. Lachmann B: Open up the lung and keep the lung open. Intensive Care Med 1992;18:319–321.

125. Carlton DP, Cummings JJ, Scheerer RG et al: Lung overexpansion increases pulmonary microvascular protein permeability in young lambs. J Appl Physiol 1990;69:577–583.

126. Sandhar BK, Niblett DJ, Argiras EP et al: Effects of positive end-expiratory pressure on hyaline membrane formation in a rabbit model of the neonatal respiratory distress syndrome. Intensive Care Med 1988;14:538–546.

127. Michna J, Jobe AH, Ikegami M: Positive end-expiratory pressure preserves surfactant function in preterm lambs. Am J Respir Crit Care Med 1999;160:634–639.

128. Staub NC, Nagano H, Pearce ML: Pulmonary edema in dogs, especially the sequence of fluid accumulation in lungs. J Appl Physiol 1967;22:227–240.

129. Crotti S, Mascheroni D, Caironi P et al: Recruitment and derecruitment during acute respiratory failure: a clinical study. Am J Respir Crit Care Med 2001;164:131–140.

130. Jonson B, Richard JC, Straus C et al: Pressure-volume curves and compliance in acute lung injury: evidence of recruitment above the lower inflection point. Am J Respir Crit Care Med 1999;159:1172–1178.

131. Vogel J: Analyse der Atemmechanik. Bad Oeynhausener Gespräche I. Springer Verlag Berlin, Göttingen, Heidelberg 1957;41–44.

132. Rimensberger PC, Cox PN, Frndova H et al: The open lung during small tidal volume ventilation: concepts of recruitment and "optimal" positive end-expiratory pressure. Crit Care Med 1999;27:1946–1952.

133. Rimensberger PC, Pristine G, Mullen BM et al: Lung recruitment during small tidal volume ventilation allows minimal positive end-expiratory pressure without augmenting lung injury. Crit Care Med 1999;27:1940–1945.

134. Halter JM, Steinberg JM, Schiller HJ et al: Positive end-expiratory pressure after a recruitment maneuver prevents both alveolar collapse and recruitment/derecruitment. Am J Respir Crit Care Med 2003;167:1620–1626.

135. Amato MB, Barbas CS, Medeiros DM et al: Effect of a protective-ventilation strategy on mortality in the acute respiratory distress syndrome. N Engl J Med 1998;338:347–354.

136. Ingimarsson J, Bjorklund LJ, Larsson A et al: The pressure at the lower inflexion point has no relation to airway collapse in surfactant-treated premature lambs. Acta Anaesthesiologica Scandinavica 2001;45:690–695.

137. Maggiore SM, Jonson B, Richard JC et al: Alveolar derecruitment at decremental positive end-expiratory pressure levels in acute lung injury: comparison with the lower inflection point, oxygenation, and compliance. Am J Respir Crit Care Med 2001;164:795–801.

138. Baumgardner JE, Markstaller K, Pfeiffer B et al: Effects of respiratory rate, plateau pressure, and positive end-expiratory pressure on PaO$_2$ oscillations after saline lavage. Am J Respir Crit Care Med 2002;166:1556–1562.

139. Richard JC, Maggiore SM, Jonson B et al: Influence of tidal volume on alveolar recruitment. Respective role of PEEP and a recruitment maneuver. Am J Respir Crit Care Med 2001;163:1609–1613.

140. Hickling KG: Best compliance during a decremental, but not incremental, positive end-expiratory pressure trial is related to open-lung positive end-expiratory pressure: a mathematical model of acute respiratory distress syndrome lungs. Am J Respir Crit Care Med 2001;163:69–78.

141. Bond DM, Froese AB: Volume recruitment maneuvers are less deleterious than persistent low lung volumes in the atelectasis-prone rabbit lung during high-frequency oscillation. Crit Care Med 1993;21:402–412.

142. Fujino Y, Goddon S, Dolhnikoff M et al: Repetitive high-pressure recruitment maneuvers required to maximally recruit lung in a sheep model of acute respiratory distress syndrome. Crit Care Med 2001;29:1579–1586.

143. Suh GY, Koh Y, Chung MP et al: Repeated derecruitments accentuate lung injury during mechanical ventilation. Crit Care Med 2002;30:1848–1853.

144. Sukumar M, Bommaraju M, Fisher JE et al: High-frequency partial liquid ventilation in respiratory distress syndrome: hemodynamics and gas exchange. J Appl Physiol 1998;84: 327–334.

145. Kinsella JP, Parker TA, Galan H et al: Independent and combined effects of inhaled nitric oxide, liquid perfluorochemical, and high-frequency oscillatory ventilation in premature lambs with respiratory distress syndrome. Am J Respir Crit Care Med 1999;159:1220–1227.

146. Suter PM, Fairley B, Isenberg MD: Optimum end-expiratory airway pressure in patients with acute pulmonary failure. N Engl J Med 1975;292:284–289.

147. Lachmann B, Jonson B, Lindroth M et al: Modes of artificial ventilation in severe respiratory distress syndrome. Lung function and morphology in rabbits after wash-out of alveolar surfactant. Crit Care Med 1982;10:724–732.

148. Suzuki H, Papazoglou K, Bryan AC: Relationship between $PaO_2$ and lung volume during high frequency oscillatory ventilation. Acta Paediatr Jpn 1992;34:494–500.

149. De Jaegere A, van Veenendaal MB, Michiels A et al: Lung recruitment using oxygenation during open lung high-frequency ventilation in preterm infants. Am J Respir Crit Care Med 2006;174:639–645.

150. Thome U, Topfer A, Schaller P et al: Effects of mean airway pressure on lung volume during high-frequency oscillatory ventilation of preterm infants. Am J Respir Crit Care Med 1998;157:1213–1218.

151. Brazelton TB, Watson KF, Murphy M et al: Identification of optimal lung volume during high-frequency oscillatory ventilation using respiratory inductive plethysmography. Crit Care Med 2001;29:2349–2359.

152. van Kaam AH, van Veenendaal MB: Oxygenation as an indicator for the optimal lung volume in ventilated newborn infants: useful or useless? Am J Respir Crit Care Med 2006;174: 229–230.

153. Gattinoni L, Caironi P, Pelosi P et al: What has computed tomography taught us about the acute respiratory distress syndrome? Am J Respir Crit Care Med 2001;164:1701–1711.

154. Hinz J, Neumann P, Dudykevych T et al: Regional ventilation by electrical impedance tomography: a comparison with ventilation scintigraphy in pigs. Chest 2003;124:314–322.

155. van Kaam AH, De Jaegere A, Haitsma JJ et al: Positive pressure ventilation with the open lung concept optimizes gas exchange and reduces ventilator-induced lung injury in newborn piglets. Pediatr Res 2003;53:245–253.

156. Gregory GA, Kitterman JA, Phibbs RH et al: Treatment of the idiopathic respiratory-distress syndrome with continuous positive airway pressure. N Engl J Med 1971;284:1333–1340.

157. Caliumi-Pellegrini G, Agostino R, Orzalesi M et al: Twin nasal cannula for administration of continuous positive airway pressure to newborn infants. Arch Dis Child 1974;49:228–230.

158. Polin RA, Sahni R: Newer experience with CPAP. Semin Neonatol 2002;7:379–389.

159. Saunders RA, Milner AD, Hopkin IE: The effects of continuous positive airway pressure on lung mechanics and lung volumes in the neonate. Biol Neonate 1976;29:178–186.

160. Miller MJ, DiFiore JM, Strohl KP et al: Effects of nasal CPAP on supraglottic and total pulmonary resistance in preterm infants. J Appl Physiol 1990;68:141–146.

161. Davis PG, Henderson-Smart DJ: Nasal continuous positive airways pressure immediately after extubation for preventing morbidity in preterm infants. Cochrane Database Syst Rev 2003.

162. Morley C: Continuous distending pressure. Arch Dis Child Fetal Neonatal Ed 1999;81:F152–F156.

163. Ho JJ, Subramaniam P, Henderson-Smart DJ et al: Continuous distending pressure for respiratory distress syndrome in preterm infants. Cochrane Database Syst Rev 2002.

164. Thomson MA, Yoder BA, Winter VT et al: Treatment of immature baboons for 28 days with early nasal continuous positive airway pressure. Am J Respir Crit Care Med 2004;169:1054–1062.

165. De Klerk AM, De Klerk RK: Nasal continuous positive airway pressure and outcomes of preterm infants. J Paediatr Child Health 2001;37:161–167.

166. Verder H, Albertsen P, Ebbesen F et al: Nasal continuous positive airway pressure and early surfactant therapy for respiratory distress syndrome in newborns of less than 30 weeks' gestation. Pediatrics 1999;103:E24.

167. Thomson MA: Continuous positive airway pressure and surfactant; combined data from animal experiments and clinical trials. Biol Neonate 2002; 81 Suppl 1:16–19.

168. Miller MJ, Carlo WA, Martin RJ: Continuous positive airway pressure selectively reduces obstructive apnea in preterm infants. J Pediatr 1985;106:91–94.

169. Ahumada CA, Goldsmith JP: Continuous distending pressure. In Goldsmith JP, Karotkin EH (eds): Assisted Ventilation of the Neonate. Philadelphia: WB Saunders, 1996, pp 151–165.

170. Lotze A, Mitchell BR, Bulas DI et al: Multicenter study of surfactant (beractant) use in the treatment of term infants with severe respiratory failure. Survanta in Term Infants Study Group. J Pediatr 1998;132:40–47.

171. Esteban A, Anzueto A, Alia I et al: How is mechanical ventilation employed in the intensive care unit? An international utilization review. Am J Respir Crit Care Med 2000;161:1450–1458.

172. Rappaport SH, Shpiner R, Yoshihara G et al: Randomized, prospective trial of pressure-limited versus volume-controlled ventilation in severe respiratory failure. Crit Care Med 1994;22:22–32.

173. Boros SJ, Orgill AA: Mortality and morbidity associated with pressure- and volume-limited infant ventilators. Am J Dis Child 1978;132:865–869.

174. Sinha SK, Donn SM, Gavey J et al: Randomised trial of volume controlled versus time cycled, pressure limited ventilation in preterm infants with respiratory distress syndrome. Arch Dis Child Fetal Neonatal Ed 1997;77:F202–F205.

175. Cleary JP, Bernstein G, Mannino FL et al: Improved oxygenation during synchronized intermittent mandatory ventilation in neonates with respiratory distress syndrome: a randomized, crossover study. J Pediatr 1995;126:407–411.

176. Jarreau PH, Moriette G, Mussat P et al: Patient-triggered ventilation decreases the work of breathing in neonates. Am J Respir Crit Care Med 1996;153:1176–1181.

177. Greenough A, Milner AD, Dimitriou G: Synchronized mechanical ventilation for respiratory support in newborn infants. Cochrane Database Syst Rev 2001.

178. Thome U, Kossel H, Lipowsky G et al: Randomized comparison of high-frequency ventilation with high-rate intermittent positive pressure ventilation in preterm infants with respiratory failure. J Pediatr 1999;135:39–46.

179. Plavka R, Kopecky P, Sebron V et al: A prospective randomized comparison of conventional mechanical ventilation and very early high frequency oscillatory ventilation in extremely premature newborns with respiratory distress syndrome. Intensive Care Med 1999;25:68–75.

180. Johnson AH, Peacock JL, Greenough A et al: High-frequency oscillatory ventilation for the prevention of chronic lung disease of prematurity. N Engl J Med 2002;347:633–642.

181. Courtney SE, Durand DJ, Asselin JM et al: High-frequency oscillatory ventilation versus conventional mechanical ventilation

for very-low-birth-weight infants. N Engl J Med 2002;347:
643–652.

182. Mariani G, Cifuentes J, Carlo WA: Randomized trial of permissive hypercapnia in preterm infants. Pediatrics 1999;104:
1082–1088.

183. Carlo WA, Stark AR, Wright LL et al: Minimal ventilation to prevent bronchopulmonary dysplasia in extremely-low-birth-weight infants. J Pediatr 2002;141:370–374.

184. Walsh-Sukys MC, Tyson JE, Wright LL et al: Persistent pulmonary hypertension of the newborn in the era before nitric oxide: practice variation and outcomes. Pediatrics 2000;105:
14–20.

185. Truog WE, Lyrene RK, Standaert TA et al: Effects of PEEP and tolazoline infusion on respiratory and inert gas exchange in experimental meconium aspiration. J Pediatr 1982;100:
284–290.

186. Fox WW, Berman LS, Downes JJ, Jr. et al: The therapeutic application of end-expiratory pressure in the meconium aspiration syndrome. Pediatrics 1975;56:214–217.

187. Yeh TF, Lilien LD, Barathi A et al: Lung volume, dynamic lung compliance, and blood gases during the first 3 days of postnatal life in infants with meconium aspiration syndrome. Crit Care Med 1982;10:588–592.

188. van Kaam AH, Haitsma JJ, De Jaegere A et al: Open lung ventilation improves gas exchange and attenuates secondary lung injury in a piglet model of meconium aspiration. Crit Care Med 2004;32:443–449.

189. Gupta A, Rastogi S, Sahni R et al: Inhaled nitric oxide and gentle ventilation in the treatment of pulmonary hypertension of the newborn—a single-center, 5-year experience. J Perinatol 2002;22:435–441.

190. Verbrugge SJ, Sorm V, van 't Veen A et al: Lung overinflation without positive end-expiratory pressure promotes bacteremia after experimental *Klebsiella pneumoniae* inoculation. Intensive Care Med 1998;24:172–177.

191. Nahum A, Hoyt J, Schmitz L et al: Effect of mechanical ventilation strategy on dissemination of intratracheally instilled Escherichia coli in dogs. Crit Care Med 1997;25:1733–1743.

192. Lin CY, Zhang H, Cheng KC et al: Mechanical ventilation may increase susceptibility to the development of bacteremia. Crit Care Med 2003;31:1429–1434.

193. van Kaam AH, Lachmann RA, Herting E et al: Reducing atelectasis attenuates bacterial growth and translocation in experimental pneumonia. Am J Respir Crit Care Med 2004;169:1046–1053.

194. Bagolan P, Casaccia G, Crescenzi F et al: Impact of a current treatment protocol on outcome of high-risk congenital diaphragmatic hernia. J Pediatr Surg 2004;39:313–318.

195. Wung JT, James LS, Kilchevsky E et al: Management of infants with severe respiratory failure and persistence of the fetal circulation, without hyperventilation. Pediatrics 1985;76:
488–494.

196. Kays DW, Langham MR, Jr., Ledbetter DJ et al: Detrimental effects of standard medical therapy in congenital diaphragmatic hernia. Ann Surg 1999;230:340–348.

197. Rivera R, Tibballs J: Complications of endotracheal intubation and mechanical ventilation in infants and children. Crit Care Med 1992;20:193–199.

198. Kolatat T, Aunganon K, Yosthiem P: Airway complications in neonates who received mechanical ventilation. J Med Assoc Thai 2002;85 Suppl 2:S455–S462.

199. Hwang WS, Boras V, Trevenen CL et al: The histopathology of the upper airway in the neonate following mechanical ventilation. J Pathol 1988;156:189–195.

200. Maayan C, Eyal F, Mandelberg A et al: Effect of mechanical ventilation and volume loading on left ventricular performance

201. dos Santos CC, Slutsky AS: Overview of high-frequency ventilation modes, clinical rationale, and gas transport mechanisms. Respir Care Clin N Am 2001;7:549–575.

202. Meredith KS, Delemos RA, Coalson JJ et al: Role of lung injury in the pathogenesis of hyaline membrane disease in premature baboons. J Appl Physiol 1989;66:2150–2158.

203. McCulloch PR, Forkert PG, Froese AB: Lung volume maintenance prevents lung injury during high frequency oscillatory ventilation in surfactant-deficient rabbits. Am Rev Respir Dis 1988;137:1185–1192.

204. Yoder BA, Siler-Khodr T, Winter VT et al: High-frequency oscillatory ventilation: effects on lung function, mechanics, and airway cytokines in the immature baboon model for neonatal chronic lung disease. Am J Respir Crit Care Med 2000;162:1867–1876.

205. The HIFI Study Group: High-frequency oscillatory ventilation compared with conventional mechanical ventilation in the treatment of respiratory failure in preterm infants. N Engl J Med 1989;320:88–93.

206. Moriette G, Paris-Llado J, Walti H et al: Prospective randomized multicenter comparison of high-frequency oscillatory ventilation and conventional ventilation in preterm infants of less than 30 weeks with respiratory distress syndrome. Pediatrics 2001;107:363–372.

207. Henderson-Smart DJ, Bhuta T, Cools F et al: Elective high frequency oscillatory ventilation versus conventional ventilation for acute pulmonary dysfunction in preterm infants. Cochrane Database Syst Rev 2003.

208. Hofhuis W, Huysman MW, van der Wiel EC et al: Worsening of V'maxFRC in infants with chronic lung disease in the first year of life: a more favorable outcome after high-frequency oscillation ventilation. Am J Respir Crit Care Med 2002;166:1539–1543.

209. The HIFI Study Group: High-frequency oscillatory ventilation compared with conventional intermittent mechanical ventilation in the treatment of respiratory failure in preterm infants: neurodevelopmental status at 16 to 24 months of postterm age. J Pediatr 1990;117:939–946.

210. Gerstmann DR, Wood K, Miller A et al: Childhood outcome after early high-frequency oscillatory ventilation for neonatal respiratory distress syndrome. Pediatrics 2001;108:617–623.

211. Moriette G, Paris-Llado J, Escande B et al: Outcome at 2 years of age in preterm infants less than 30 weeks gestational age randomized to receive high-frequency oscillatory ventilation of conventional ventilation for treatment of RDS. Pediatr Res 2004;55:466A.

212. Mammel MC, Gordon MJ, Connett JE et al: Comparison of high-frequency jet ventilation and conventional mechanical ventilation in a meconium aspiration model. J Pediatr 1983;103:630–634.

213. Trindade O, Goldberg RN, Bancalari E et al: Conventional vs high-frequency jet ventilation in a piglet model of meconium aspiration: comparison of pulmonary and hemodynamic effects. J Pediatr 1985;107:115–120.

214. Wiswell TE, Foster NH, Slayter MV et al: Management of a piglet model of the meconium aspiration syndrome with high-frequency or conventional ventilation. Am J Dis Child 1992;146:1287–1293.

215. Hachey WE, Eyal FG, Curtet-Eyal NL et al: High-frequency oscillatory ventilation versus conventional ventilation in a piglet model of early meconium aspiration. Crit Care Med 1998;
26:556–561.

216. Clark RH, Yoder BA, Sell MS: Prospective, randomized comparison of high-frequency oscillation and conventional ventilation

in premature infants with respiratory distress syndrome. Crit Care Med 1986;14:858–860.

in candidates for extracorporeal membrane oxygenation. J Pediatr 1994;124:447–454.

217. Kinsella JP, Truog WE, Walsh WF et al: Randomized, multicenter trial of inhaled nitric oxide and high-frequency oscillatory ventilation in severe, persistent pulmonary hypertension of the newborn. J Pediatr 1997;131:55–62.

218. Somaschini M, Locatelli G, Salvoni L et al: Impact of new treatments for respiratory failure on outcome of infants with congenital diaphragmatic hernia. Eur J Pediatr 1999;158: 780–784.

219. Desfrere L, Jarreau PH, Dommergues M et al: Impact of delayed repair and elective high-frequency oscillatory ventilation on survival of antenatally diagnosed congenital diaphragmatic hernia: first application of these strategies in the more "severe" subgroup of antenatally diagnosed newborns. Intensive Care Med 2000;26:934–941.

220. Cacciari A, Ruggeri G, Mordenti M et al: High-frequency oscillatory ventilation versus conventional mechanical ventilation in congenital diaphragmatic hernia. Eur J Pediatr Surg 2001;11:3–7.

221. Azarow K, Messineo A, Pearl R et al: Congenital diaphragmatic hernia—a tale of two cities: the Toronto experience. J Pediatr Surg 1997;32:395–400.

222. Laubscher B, van Melle G, Fawer CL et al: Haemodynamic changes during high frequency oscillation for respiratory distress syndrome. Arch Dis Child Fetal Neonatal Ed 1996;74:F172–F176.

223. Simma B, Fritz M, Fink C et al: Conventional ventilation versus high-frequency oscillation: hemodynamic effects in newborn babies. Crit Care Med 2000;28:227–231.

224. Osborn DA, Evans N: Randomized trial of high-frequency oscillatory ventilation versus conventional ventilation: effect on systemic blood flow in very preterm infants. J Pediatr 2003;143:192–198.

225. Clark RH, Gerstmann DR, Null DM et al: Pulmonary interstitial emphysema treated by high-frequency oscillatory ventilation. Crit Care Med 1986;14:926–930.

226. Mammel MC, Ophoven JP, Lewallen PK et al: High-frequency ventilation and tracheal injuries. Pediatrics 1986;77:608–613.

227. Wiswell TE, Clark RH, Null DM et al: Tracheal and bronchial injury in high-frequency oscillatory ventilation and high-frequency flow interruption compared with conventional positive-pressure ventilation. J Pediatr 1988;112:249–256.

228. Cheema IU, Ahluwalia JS: Feasibility of tidal volume-guided ventilation in newborn infants: a randomized, crossover trial using the volume guarantee modality. Pediatrics 2001;107: 1323–1328.

229. Herrera CM, Gerhardt T, Claure N et al: Effects of volume-guaranteed synchronized intermittent mandatory ventilation in preterm infants recovering from respiratory failure. Pediatrics 2002;110:529–533.

230. Abubakar KM, Keszler M: Patient-ventilator interactions in new modes of patient-triggered ventilation. Pediatr Pulmonol 2001;32:71–75.

231. Polimeni V, Claure N, D'Ugard C et al: Efficacy of volume guarantee ventilation in reducing hypoxemic episodes in preterm infants. Pediatr Res 2004;55:508A.

232. Keszler M, Abubakar KM: Volume guarantee accelerates recovery from forced exhalation episodes. Pediatr Res 2004;55:545A.

233. Piotrowski A, Sobala W, Kawczynski P: Patient-initiated, pressure-regulated, volume-controlled ventilation compared with intermittent mandatory ventilation in neonates: a prospective, randomised study. Intensive Care Med 1997;23:975–981.

234. Mancebo J, Amaro P, Mollo JL et al: Comparison of the effects of pressure support ventilation delivered by three different ventilators during weaning from mechanical ventilation. Intensive Care Med 1995;21:913–919.

235. Tokioka H, Kinjo M, Hirakawa M: The effectiveness of pressure support ventilation for mechanical ventilatory support in children. Anesthesiology 1993;78:880–884.

236. Olsen SL, Thibeault DW, Truog WE: Crossover trial comparing pressure support with synchronized intermittent mandatory ventilation. J Perinatol 2002;22:461–466.

237. Reyes Z, Tauscher M, Claure N et al: Randomized, controlled trial comparing pressure support (PS) + synchronized intermittent mandatory ventilation (SIMV) with SIMV in preterm infants. Pediatr Res 2004;55:466A.

238. Schulze A, Gerhardt T, Musante G et al: Proportional assist ventilation in low birth weight infants with acute respiratory disease: A comparison to assist/control and conventional mechanical ventilation. J Pediatr 1999;135: 339–344.

239. Dassieu G, Brochard L, Agudze E et al: Continuous tracheal gas insufflation enables a volume reduction strategy in hyaline membrane disease: technical aspects and clinical results. Intensive Care Med 1998;24:1076–1082.

240. Dassieu G, Brochard L, Benani M et al: Continuous tracheal gas insufflation in preterm infants with hyaline membrane disease. A prospective randomized trial. Am J Respir Crit Care Med 2000;162:826–831.

241. Leach CL, Holm B, Morin FC, III et al: Partial liquid ventilation in premature lambs with respiratory distress syndrome: efficacy and compatibility with exogenous surfactant. J Pediatr 1995;126:412–420.

242. Wolfson MR, Greenspan JS, Deoras KS et al: Comparison of gas and liquid ventilation: clinical, physiological, and histological correlates. J Appl Physiol 1992;72:1024–1031.

243. Gauger PG, Overbeck MC, Chambers SD et al: Partial liquid ventilation improves gas exchange and increases EELV in acute lung injury. J Appl Physiol 1998;84:1566–1572.

244. Hirschl RB: Current experience with liquid ventilation. Paediatr Respir Rev 2004; 5 Suppl A:S339–S345.

245. Hirschl RB, Croce M, Gore D et al: Prospective, randomized, controlled pilot study of partial liquid ventilation in adult acute respiratory distress syndrome. Am J Respir Crit Care Med 2002;165:781–787.

246. Nobuhara KK, Fauza DO, DiFiore JW et al: Continuous intrapulmonary distension with perfluorocarbon accelerates neonatal (but not adult) lung growth. J Pediatr Surg 1998;33:292–298.

247. Fauza DO, Hirschl RB, Wilson JM: Continuous intrapulmonary distension with perfluorocarbon accelerates lung growth in infants with congenital diaphragmatic hernia: initial experience. J Pediatr Surg 2001;36:1237–1240.

248. Hirschl RB, Philip WF, Glick L et al: A prospective, randomized pilot trial of perfluorocarbon-induced lung growth in newborns with congenital diaphragmatic hernia. J Pediatr Surg 2003;38:283–289.

249. Soll RF: Prophylactic natural surfactant extract for preventing morbidity and mortality in preterm infants. Cochrane Database Syst Rev 2000.

250. Soll RF, Blanco F: Natural surfactant extract versus synthetic surfactant for neonatal respiratory distress syndrome. Cochrane Database Syst Rev 2001.

251. Soll RF: Multiple versus single dose natural surfactant extract for severe neonatal respiratory distress syndrome. Cochrane Database Syst Rev 2000.

252. Soll RF, Morley CJ: Prophylactic versus selective use of surfactant in preventing morbidity and mortality in preterm infants. Cochrane Database Syst Rev 2001.

253. Yost CC, Soll RF: Early versus delayed selective surfactant treatment for neonatal respiratory distress syndrome. Cochrane Database Syst Rev 2000.

254. Rider ED, Jobe AH, Ikegami M et al: Different ventilation strategies alter surfactant responses in preterm rabbits. J Appl Physiol 1992;73:2089–2096.

255. van Kaam AH, Haitsma JJ, Dik WA et al: Response to exogenous surfactant is different during open lung and conventional ventilation. Crit Care Med 2004;32:774–780.

256. van Veenendaal MB, van Kaam AH, Haitsma JJ et al: Open lung ventilation preserves the response to delayed surfactant treatment in surfactant-deficient newborn piglets. Crit Care Med 2006;34:2827–2834.

257. Findlay RD, Taeusch HW, Walther FJ: Surfactant replacement therapy for meconium aspiration syndrome. Pediatrics 1996;97:48–52.

258. Wiswell TE, Knight GR, Finer NN et al: A multicenter, randomized, controlled trial comparing Surfaxin (lucinactant) lavage with standard care for treatment of meconium aspiration syndrome. Pediatrics 2002;109:1081–1087.

259. Herting E, Jarstrand C, Rasool O et al: Experimental neonatal group B streptococcal pneumonia: effect of a modified porcine surfactant on bacterial proliferation in ventilated near-term rabbits. Pediatr Res 1994;36:784–791.

260. Glick PL, Stannard VA, Leach CL et al: Pathophysiology of congenital diaphragmatic hernia II: the fetal lamb CDH model is surfactant deficient. J Pediatr Surg 1992;27:382–387.

261. IJsselstijn H, Zimmermann LJ, Bunt JE et al: Prospective evaluation of surfactant composition in bronchoalveolar lavage fluid of infants with congenital diaphragmatic hernia and of age-matched controls. Crit Care Med 1998;26:573–580.

262. Cogo PE, Zimmermann LJ, Rosso F et al: Surfactant synthesis and kinetics in infants with congenital diaphragmatic hernia. Am J Respir Crit Care Med 2002;166:154–158.

263. Lotze A, Knight GR, Anderson KD et al: Surfactant (beractant) therapy for infants with congenital diaphragmatic hernia on ECMO: evidence of persistent surfactant deficiency. J Pediatr Surg 1994;29:407–412.

264. Finer NN, Barrington KJ: Nitric oxide for respiratory failure in infants born at or near term. Cochrane Database Syst Rev 2001.

265. The Neonatal Inhaled Nitric Oxide Study Group: Inhaled nitric oxide in full-term and nearly full-term infants with hypoxic respiratory failure. N Engl J Med 1997;336:597–604.

266. The Neonatal Inhaled Nitric Oxide Study Group (NINOS): Inhaled nitric oxide and hypoxic respiratory failure in infants with congenital diaphragmatic hernia. Pediatrics 1997;99: 838–845.

267. Clark RH, Kueser TJ, Walker MW et al: Low-dose nitric oxide therapy for persistent pulmonary hypertension of the newborn. Clinical Inhaled Nitric Oxide Research Group. N Engl J Med 2000;342:469–474.

268. Konduri GG, Solimano A, Sokol GM et al: A randomized trial of early versus standard inhaled nitric oxide therapy in term and near-term newborn infants with hypoxic respiratory failure. Pediatrics 2004;113:559–564.

269. Kinsella JP, Abman SH: High-frequency oscillatory ventilation augments the response to inhaled nitric oxide in persistent pulmonary hypertension of the newborn: Nitric Oxide Study Group. Chest 1998;114:100S.

270. Christou H, Van Marter LJ, Wessel DL et al: Inhaled nitric oxide reduces the need for extracorporeal membrane oxygenation in infants with persistent pulmonary hypertension of the newborn. Crit Care Med 2000;28: 3722–3727.

271. Schreiber MD, Gin-Mestan K, Marks JD et al: Inhaled nitric oxide in premature infants with the respiratory distress syndrome. N Engl J Med 2003;349:2099–2107.

272. Elbourne D, Field D, Mugford M: Extracorporeal membrane oxygenation for severe respiratory failure in newborn infants. Cochrane Database Syst Rev 2002.

273. Taylor GA, Lotze A, Kapur S et al: Diffuse pulmonary opacification in infants undergoing extracorporeal membrane oxygenation: clinical and pathologic correlation. Radiology 1986;161:347–350.

274. Keszler M, Ryckman FC, McDonald JV, Jr. et al: A prospective, multicenter, randomized study of high versus low positive end-expiratory pressure during extracorporeal membrane oxygenation. J Pediatr 1992;120:107–113.

# CHAPTER 47

# Ventilator Management for Congenital Abnormalities

Irwin Reiss, Robert-Jan Houmes, and Dick Tibboel

## CONGENITAL LUNG ABNORMALITIES

Congenital lung anomalies are increasingly discovered on routine prenatal ultrasound or incidentally during postnatal imaging for respiratory insufficiency of unknown origin.[1] Infants born with compromised respiratory status, whether due to immaturity or other conditions such as congenital lung hypoplasia or space-occupying processes including lobar emphysema, often require mechanical ventilation and supplemental oxygen to maintain adequate oxygenation and ventilation. Individually and in combination, oxygen and mechanical ventilation predispose the newborn to ventilator-induced lung injury (VILI).[2] For years, VILI was synonymous with barotrauma/volutrauma.

## VENTILATOR-INDUCED LUNG INJURY OF THE DEVELOPING LUNG

Maturation in the human lung continues well after the newborn period and through childhood. Compared with adults, pediatric patients show a spectrum raging from neonatal to infant and adult stages of lung development.[3] Important differences between infant and adult lungs include a different alveolar structure, matrix composition, and angiogenesis, especially in the phase in which new alveoli are formed and septa differentiate (mainly during the first few years of life).[4-6]

The effect of mechanical ventilation on the developing lung cannot be fully understood without considering the effects of intubation and endotracheal suctioning, which are integral components of the ventilation process. Both interventions contribute to injury to the tracheobronchial tree and damage to the ciliated cells of the tracheal epithelium and mucociliary transport system.[7,8] Disruption of the epithelium results in retained secretions and debris, thus setting the stage for inflammation and pulmonary infection.

In addition to intubation and endotracheal suctioning, high concentrations of oxygen also disrupt the epithelial cells and cilia activity. When the tracheal epithelium is exposed to high concentrations of oxygen, the cilia cavity stops.[9] Initiation of mechanical ventilation with high oxygen concentrations causes injury to the lung through various inflammatory mediators.[10] Pulmonary macrophages are activated and release substances that cause an accumulation of polymorphonuclear cells in the alveolar compartment. These leukocytes contain elastases and collagenases that can further damage the lung connective tissue.[11,12] Elastase is known to play an essential role in the pathogenesis of acute and chronic lung disease in the immature lung. Although still controversial, it is generally accepted that increased production of cytokines, chemokines, and other inflammatory mediators is one of the major mechanisms of VILI in the immature and hypoplastic lung.[13-16] Inflammatory cytokines and other inflammatory mediators appear to influence the severity of lung injury and the risk for chronic lung disease (as has been reviewed by several authors) for the premature lung, the so-called bronchopulmonary dysplasia (BPD).[17,18] The concept of VILI must be regarded much more as a secondary than a primary injury in a structurally immature lung that is fluid filled and hypoplastic. Ongoing exposure to potentially noxious stimuli, such as mechanical forces, infectious agents, or toxic agents, together with the need for endotracheal suctioning, may cause further damage.[19] The individual response and susceptibility to lung injury may vary extensively. Previous lung damage seems to be essential for ventilation to cause an increased systemic inflammatory response in normal humans. However, VILI is not only caused by classic barotraumas (air leaks), but also by more subtle forms of lung injury such as epithelial and endothelial damage leading to fluid and protein leak into airways, alveoli, and interstitium; surfactant disruption and inactivation; and mediator-induced airway and systemic inflammation (*biotrauma*).[2] The process of inflammation is a vital response to injury whereby blood leukocytes recruit into the alveolar compartment, activate tissue macrophages, and produce a series of inflammatory mediators. The inflammatory process may trigger events that lead to cell regeneration and healing, or progression of the inflammatory response, which often lead to progressive organ dysfunction. Schultz et al. demonstrated an association between prolonged mechanical ventilation and pulmonary inflammation in ventilated infants with an immature lung by inducing proinflammatory cytokines and by failing to stimulate the anti-inflammatory cytokine IL-10.[15]

The injury caused by ventilation has been attributed to two major mechanisms: (1) overdistension of terminal airways (*volutrauma*) and (2) shear stress forces on the epithelial layer of small airways and terminal lung units during closing and cyclic reopening of these units (*atelectrauma*).[20-22]

Results of a number of animal studies have shown that peak inspiratory pressure (PIP) above 30 cmH$_2$O can produce injury in normal lungs after relatively short periods of mechanical ventilation. Dreyfuss et al. have shown that ventilation at a PIP of 45 cmH$_2$O, together with a low positive end-expiratory pressure (PEEP), can produce pulmonary edema and protein leakage in about 20 minutes.[23] This ventilation-induced protein leak results in denaturation of surfactant and loss of surfactant functions;[24,25] this pattern may develop early in postnatal life. Bjorklund et al. have shown that as few as five high-peak airway pressure breaths immediately after birth in the premature lamb model are sufficient to cause diffuse alveolar damage and hyaline membrane formation.[26]

Lung injury secondary to mechanical ventilation is certainly one of the major contributors to mortality in cases of lung hypoplasia and is a major risk factor for the bad outcome following acute respiratory failure, particularly in neonates with congenital diaphragmatic hernia (CDH).[27-29] Experimental data have resulted in a trend toward using a lung protective strategy in patients with acute respiratory failure by ventilating with reduced tidal volumes and the introduction of pressure-limited "permissive hypercapnia" ventilation in the treatment of adults and children with acute respiratory failure. This concept of "gentle ventilation" was introduced by Wung et al. and is characterized by preservation of spontaneous breathing, permissive levels of hypercapnia (PaCO$_2$, 60 to 65 mm Hg or 9 kPa), and avoidance of high inspiratory airway pressures.[30] Iatrogenic lung injury is avoided where possible. Retrospective series have shown improved survival in infants with persistent pulmonary hypertension of the newborn (PPHN) when hyperventilation was not used.[27] In addition, improved survival and reduced need for extracorporeal membrane oxygenation (ECMO) support was shown when PIP was limited to 30 cmH$_2$O or less without attempts to correct hypercarbia in infants with lung hypoplasia.[31-33]

## CONGENITAL DIAPHRAGMATIC HERNIA

Over the past 20 years, pulmonary hypoplasia and pulmonary hypertension have been recognized as the two cornerstones of the pathophysiology of CDH, while more recently VILI has been recognized as a contributing iatrogenic factor for the development of chronic lung disease.[34,35]

The degree of pulmonary hypoplasia was initially thought to correlate directly with survival, although this may not be true in most infants. With the advent of neonatal mechanical ventilation in the 1960s, many CDH patients with previously fatal respiratory failure were surviving long enough to undergo surgical repair.[36,37]

Pathologic examination of the hypoplastic lungs from patients with CDH revealed a marked reduction in the number of bronchial branchings, but the development of pulmonary acini and alveoli was relatively less affected. The lung injury secondary to mechanical ventilation in these patients was characterized by hyaline membrane formation, parenchymal hemorrhage pneumothorax, and pulmonary interstitial emphysema. Lung injury in patients with CDH was microscopically more evident in the ipsilateral lung. Regarding the relationship between respiratory measurements and lung injury, a clinical study on barotrauma in lung hypoplasia found evidence of pulmonary hemorrhage in lungs that were ventilated with high peak pressure of 50 cmH$_2$O.[38]

Mechanical ventilation is the initial therapy for infants with respiratory failure due to CDH. In the delivery room, infants with CDH should immediately be intubated to prevent hypoxia-induced pulmonary vasoconstriction.

Because of gastric and abdominal distension and compression of the lung, supply of oxygen by bag-masking must be avoided. To minimize lung injury, the newborn should be ventilated initially with peak pressure below 25 cmH$_2$O.[32,33] Any delay in obtaining an airway can intensify acidosis and hypoxia, which triggers pulmonary hypertension. For decompression of the abdominal contents in the thorax and thus to help the available lung tissue to expand, early use of a nasogastric tube and continuous suctioning of the stomach are warranted. For optimal mechanical ventilation, blood pressure support by isotonic fluid and inotropic drugs such as dopamine and/or dobutamine should be given to maintain arterial mean blood pressure levels at 50 mm Hg and thus to minimize any right to left shunting.

The aim of mechanical ventilation is to administer peak pressure to maintain preductal oxygen saturations above 80% or preductal partial oxygen pressure (PaO$_2$) above 60 mm Hg. Initiation of conventional ventilator management includes pressure-limited ventilation at rates of 30 to 100 breaths per minute at peak pressures of 20 to 25 cmH$_2$O. Peak inspiratory pressures that exceed 28 cmH$_2$O are used only for a short period as a bridge to ECMO. The early institution of high-frequency oscillation (HFO), especially in case of CO$_2$ retention, should be considered. PEEP should be maintained at physiologic levels (3 to 5 cmH$_2$O) whenever possible. Hyperventilation, hypocarbia, and alkalosis may decrease ductal shunting and control pulmonary hypertension in CDH, but do so at the expense of increased barotrauma.[39] Permissive hypercapnia, the so-called gentle ventilation approach, is now commonly used in neonates with CDH, with increased survival compared with hyperventilation and alkalization.[27,28,40,41]

HFO is reserved for neonates who continue to have hypoxia and hypercarbia refractory to conventional ventilation. Although the indications for HFO are not clearly defined, there are observational reports of effective PCO$_2$ reduction and increased survival in neonates with CDH.[42-44] In one such study, the use of HFO avoided hyperventilation as well as the need for ECMO. Although there are no randomized controlled studies (RCTs), HFO may have a role in managing neonates, especially in avoiding the need for ECMO.[45] Clinical studies of HFO and mean airway pressure (MAP) in lung injury found that HFO provides better oxygenation and higher MAP without increasing the incidence of barotrauma. On the other hand, low MAP settings do not allow the alveoli to open in the low-compliance lung, which leads to the development of atelectasis and an increase in the amplitude of swing pressure, resulting in excessive expression of cytokines in the airway. At present, no available RCTs show the benefit of HFO as an initial ventilation modality in CDH.

To adjust the ventilator settings, frequent preductal arterial blood gases are important parameters to be determined.

FiO$_2$ should only be weaned after a period of stabilization and should be done very slowly to prevent (recurrent) pulmonary hypertension. Deep analgosedation and sometimes even the use of muscle paralysis may enhance compliance and reduce vasoconstriction, potentially leading to lower ventilator settings. However, the loss of the spontaneous contribution to minute ventilation increases the third space edema and negates the benefits of paralysis and therefore should be avoided.[46,47] In summary, although the optimal mode of ventilation in CDH remains controversial, clinical data suggest that management strategies designed to limit lung distension and barotrauma result in improved survival.[27,28]

## Surfactant

Studies of different animals models have shown that the lungs of animals with CDH are surfactant deficient. Surfactant phospholipids and apoprotein SP-A were decreased in nitrofen CDH rats.[48,49] However, their synthetic capacity to produce surfactant was equal to that in controls. The administration of surfactant therapy has been suggested in the treatment of infants with CDH.[44,50] A body of data demonstrates that the lungs of infants with CDH are surfactant deficient.[51,52] Whether a primary surfactant deficiency truly exists or whether secondary inactivation of surfactant is the underlying problem is the subject of ongoing debate. A report from the Congenital Diaphragmatic Hernia Registry did not find that surfactant therapy improved outcome.[49] As a consequence, the routine giving of surfactant to infants with CDH initially is not recommended. Using surfactant in neonates with a gestational age of 34 weeks can be considered in the event that clinical radiologic findings of alveolar atelectasis are suggestive of respiratory distress syndrome. Cogo et al. studied the surfactant phosphatidylcholine (PC) kinetics in CDH patients who did not require ECMO by using stable isotopes.[53] Although the amounts of surfactant disaturated surfactant synthesis (DSPC) and SP-A in the tracheal aspirates of CDH patients were reduced, these patients had rates of endogenous surfactant DSPC synthesis comparable to control patients.[54,55] The decreased surfactant PC synthesis in CDH patients who require ECMO could serve as a rationale for the need for ECMO in this particular group and might be a result of lung damage by VILI. Nevertheless, because of several side effects (e.g., bronchus obstruction, hypoxia), surfactant administration should be used with caution in infants with CDH.

## Persistent Pulmonary Hypertension of the Newborn in Lung Hypoplasia

In many neonates with respiratory insufficiency, pulmonary hypertension (PPHN) complicates the clinical presentation.[39] PPHN is defined as failure of the pulmonary circulation to adapt normally to extrauterine life, resulting in unoxygenated blood shunting to the systemic circulation.[56] PPHN remains a significant problem in infants with CDH.[57] Multiple factors, including decreased cross-sectional area of the pulmonary arteries due to lung hypoplasia, increased media thickness of the pulmonary arteries, adventitial thickening, blunted oxygen-induced vasodilatation, and increased endothelin-A receptor expression, are thought to contribute to the pulmonary hypertension seen in CDH.[58] The diagnosis of PPHN should be considered in any infant with CDH and other cases of pulmonary hypertension in which a difference in pre- and postductal saturations exists. The diagnosis of PPHN should be confirmed by cardiac ultrasound.

The management of PPHN in infants with CDH is largely supportive. It is directed toward promoting a progressive decline in the ratio of pulmonary vascular resistance (PVR) to systemic vascular resistance (SVR) to maintain adequate tissue oxygenation until PVR falls. The initial treatment of the newborn with PPHN includes correction of hypothermia, hypoglycemia, hypocalcemia, anemia, hypovolemia, and stress. Although the use of alkalinizing agents is controversial, correction of metabolic acidosis is standard.[39] Because PVR is elevated in PPHN, decreased SVR or poor cardiac output results in decreased mean systemic blood pressure, which can increase right-to-left shunting. Therapy of elevated PVR includes aggressive support of cardiac function and perfusion with volume and inotropic agents to maintain the mean arterial blood pressure at a level that minimizes right-to-left shunting (>50 mm Hg).

## Inhaled Nitric Oxide

Inhaled nitric oxide (iNO) is a selective pulmonary vasodilator and is widely accepted as the gold standard treatment in PPHN.[59,60] Its use has contributed to reduced rates of ECMO. Nitric oxide (NO) is produced in endothelial cells during conversion of L-argine to L-citrulline by NO-synthetase. NO diffuses from endothelial cells into adjacent smooth muscle cells to cause vasodilatation through activation of soluble guanylate cyclase (sGC) and the production of cyclic guanosine monophosphate (cGMP). cGMP stimulates a cGMP-dependent kinase, causing vasodilation through myosin phosphorylation. To date, results of iNO therapy in patients with CDH have been poor. In CDH, iNO does not appear to be of long-term benefit. In the one trial that specifically addressed this issue, 53 infants with CDH and hypoxemic respiratory failure (gestational age, 34 weeks) were randomly assigned to receive either iNO (20 ppm) or 100% oxygen. Death before 120 days or need for ECMO was not significantly different in iNO or control groups.[61] ECMO use occurred significantly more in the iNO group, although the percentage of infants who died was not different. Although a transient improvement occurred in approximately 50% of the infants treated with iNO, it did not consistently improve oxygenation, nor did it decrease the use of ECMO. With the increasing use of iNO and HFO, the absolute number of non-CDH, noncardiac neonates with hypoxemic respiratory failure requiring ECMO has decreased. Initiation of ECMO has become progressively later, likely because of the use of these rescue therapies, but the overall mortality rate remains unchanged despite this delay. Inhaled therapy with NO might be helpful in stabilizing some patients for transport and initiation of ECMO.

## Phosphodiesterase Inhibitors

Approximately 30% of patients with PPHN do not respond to iNO and require alternative treatments. Substances that stimulate the formation of the second messengers cyclic adenosine monophosphate (cAMP) or cGMP have proved useful in the treatment of various forms of precapillary pulmonary hypertension.[62] Milrinone is a bipyridine compound that selectively inhibits phosphodiesterase type 3 (PDE3) and may lead to early and sustained improvements in oxygenation without compromising hemodynamic status. Prospective evaluation of the acute clinical and physiologic effects and long-term outcome of intravenous milrinone therapy as an alternative cardiotrophic agent or as a combination therapy with iNO in neonates with PPHN in lung hypoplasia is required.[63]

Sildenafil (Viagra), a phosphodiesterase type 5 (PDE5) inhibitor, is an oral agent that has been shown to selectively reduce pulmonary vascular resistance in both animal models and adult humans and produced vasodilation by increasing cGMP through inhibition of the phosphodiesterase involved in the degradation of cGMP to guanosine monophosphate. PDE5 is a key regulator of NO-induced vasodilation in the postnatal pulmonary arteries. PDE5 inhibitors were shown to be effective in decreasing pulmonary arterial pressure and pulmonary vascular resistance in several neonatal models of acute pulmonary hypertension. One of the recent adult randomized studies in humans shows that oral sildenafil significantly improves exercise tolerance, cardiac index, and quality of life in adult patients with primary pulmonary hypertension.[64-66]

## Prostacyclin

Prostacyclin ($PGI_2$) stimulates membrane-bound adenylate cyclase, increases cAMP, and inhibits pulmonary artery smooth muscle cell proliferation in vitro.

Although the use of systemic infusions of $PGI_2$ may be limited by the development of systemic hypotension, inhaled $PGI_2$ has been shown to have vasodilator effects limited to the pulmonary circulation. Reports in children have been encouraging, but to date there have been few reports of inhaled $PGI_2$ use in neonates with PPHN. The actions of inhaled $PGI_2$ and iNO appear to be additive in humans and even synergistic in animal studies. Rebound PPHN following withdrawal of iNO has been mitigated by intravenous $PGI_2$ in children with PPHN following CDH.[67]

Ventilatory strategies have changed in the last decade toward use of permissive hypercapnia and gentle ventilation. Partial liquid ventilation has also been tried in individual cases, but without definite advantages.[70] The concept of a liquid tissue interface is still very promising, and phase I clinical trials have recently begun. A decreased response to NO is believed to occur with pulmonary hypertension associated with hypoplasia. Apart from respiratory insufficiency in premature infants, no appropriate RCTs are available that evaluate HFO versus conventional ventilation.[71]

## PULMONARY HYPOPLASIA DUE TO OTHER CAUSES

Pulmonary hypoplasia is part of the spectrum of anomalies characterized by incomplete development of lung tissue. The severity of the lesion depends on the timing of the insult in relation to the stage of lung development and the presence of other anatomic anomalies. The hypoplastic lung consists of a carina, a malformed bronchial stump, and absent or poorly differentiated distal lung tissue. In more than 50% of these cases, coexisting cardiac, gastrointestinal, genitourinary, and skeletal malformations are present, as well as variations in the bronchopulmonary vasculature. Isolated primary pulmonary hypoplasia is rare but in its milder forms can present a diagnostic dilemma. It usually presents at or shortly after delivery of a child in varying degrees of respiratory distress who may require high ventilatory pressures and has noncompliant lungs. There may be a genetic component, but more commonly pulmonary hypoplasia is secondary to an underlying abnormality such as restrictive malformation of the chest wall and decreased fetal breathing (fetal neuromuscular disease), decreased fetal lung fluid (prolonged rupture of membrane, fetal renal dysplasias and obstruction), and decreased vascular supply (tetralogy of Fallot, interrupted pulmonary artery).[68] In cases of premature rupture of membranes at 15 to 28 weeks' gestation, the reported incidence of pulmonary hypoplasia ranges from 9% to 28% (13% in most studies).[69] In different studies, mortality rates of 71% to 95% have been reported during the perinatal period in patients with pulmonary hypoplasia. Even after correction of the underlying abnormality (if possible), the pulmonary hypoplasia may be so severe as to be incompatible with life. Postnatal growth of the lung can occur, but in severely affected children, even newer technologies (such as ECMO) have contributed little to an improved outcome. In milder cases (e.g., certain instances of primary pulmonary hypertension or children who have had maturation arrest due to oligohydramnion following premature rupture of membranes), artificial pulmonary support may maintain oxygenation while alveolar growth occurs.

## CONGENITAL CYSTIC LUNG LESION

Lesions such as congenital cystic adenomatoid malformations (CCAMs), sequestrations, bronchogenic cysts, and congenital lobar emphysema may be asymptomatic at birth or at the time of discovery later in life.[72] Some authors advocate simple observation because of the lack of data regarding the incidence of long-term complications.[72] However, there are very few described cases in which CCAM and intralobar sequestration have remained asymptomatic throughout life; complications eventually develop in nearly all patients. The most common complication is pneumonia, which may respond poorly to medical treatment. Other complications include the development of malignancies (carcinomas and pleuropulmonary blastomas), pneumothorax, and hemoptysis or hemothorax. Because lung resection will be required sooner or later for CCAM, intralobar sequestration, and intrapulmonary bronchogenic cysts, our approach is to not wait until complications occur. For patients diagnosed prenatally, we recommend surgery at 3 to 6 months of life at the latest so that compensatory lung growth may occur. At this age the postoperative course is usually smooth, with a low risk of complicating pulmonary hypertension, and long-term follow-up has shown normal respiratory function. Mediastinal bronchogenic cysts also tend to become symptomatic, and elective resection is recommended. On the other hand, asymptomatic congenital lobar emphysema may regress spontaneously, and observation is justified. The management of small noncommunicating extralobar sequestrations is more controversial; it is known that these lesions can remain asymptomatic throughout life, but complications may develop and they are sometimes difficult to differentiate from neuroblastoma.

Congenital cystic lung lesions (especially CCAM and/or pulmonary sequestration) often present as a benign pulmonary mass in infants and children and are traditionally described as a multicystic lung mass resulting from a proliferation of terminal bronchiolar structures with an associated suppression of alveolar growth. Death in utero or at birth in such fetuses and neonates is often due to hydrops and pulmonary hypoplasia.

Hydrops occurs in 45% of fetuses with CCAM and is reported to be associated with combined fetal and postnatal mortality rates of 68% to 89%. The mortality rate is less than 10% when fetal hydrops is not present.[72,73]

The presentation of congenital cystic lung lesions is variable. Many patients with congenital lung cystic lesions are identified by routine prenatal ultrasound examination. Controversy exists as to the management of newborns with asymptomatic congenital lung cyst lesions. In case of isolated cystic lesions with overt mediastinal shift, drainage during fetal life by placement of a pigtail to guarantee flow of fluid may be considered. In the management of infants with congenital cyst lung lesion, the same therapeutic approach as that in patients with hypoplastic lungs with persistent pulmonary hypertension and poor compliance with increased pulmonary vascular resistance has to be considered. Postnatally some patients with CCAM may even need ECMO, either due to respiratory insufficiency or postsurgically after pneumectomy resulting from increased blood flow to the remaining lung.[74,75]

## CONGENITAL LOBAR EMPHYSEMA

Congenital lobar emphysema (CLE) is a developmental anomaly of the lower respiratory tract that is characterized by overexpansion of a pulmonary lobe with resultant compression of the remaining ipsilateral lung, and it is a potentially reversible cause of respiratory distress in the neonate.[76] Mediastinal shifting away from the increased-volume lung can also compress the contralateral lung. The abnormality is related to a congenital bronchial narrowing. In these cases weakened or absent bronchial cartilage is present, such that there is inspiratory air entry but collapse of the narrow bronchial lumen during expiration. This bronchial defect results in lobar air trapping. In case of congenital extrinsic compression, such as by a large pulmonary artery, affected cartilage rings are malformed, soft, and collapsible as a result of the long-term in utero extrinsic effect.[77]

Emergency surgical lobectomy was once considered the only treatment for CLE, but appropriate care may be nonsurgical in some infants with only moderate respiratory distress. Prevention of endotracheal intubation should be considered to diminish the risk of progressive hyperinflation. Maintaining ventilatory pressures and volume as low as possible avoids producing ventilator-related hyperexpansion of an affected lobe. Management by a more conservative gentle ventilation technique is often successful. Fewer surgeries result because the affected lobe only occasionally continues to expand after diagnosis and initial treatment. Infants with CLE who are not clinically in respiratory distress and who are able to feed and grow do not necessarily need surgery. Lobar emphysema can occur in hypoalveolar (fewer than the expected number of alveoli) and polyalveolar (more than the expected number of alveoli) forms.

## CONGENITAL TRACHEAL OBSTRUCTION

Laryngotracheal stenosis is a congenital or acquired narrowing of the airway that may affect the glottis, subglottis, or trachea. It causes severe symptoms and should be suspected in children less than 1 year of age with either multiple episodes of croup or croup that fails to respond to medical management or requires endotracheal intubation. The trachea and the upper airway, although considered to be relatively rigid conducting airways, do show some changes in caliber during the normal respiratory cycle. There is expansion of the intrathoracic airways along with the expanding lungs, while the extrathoracic airways diminish in caliber due to their intraluminal pressure being lower than atmospheric pressure. The reverse of this process occurs during expiration. If the intrathoracic trachea is soft, the narrowing will accentuate during expiration due to positive intrathoracic pressure. The mechanics of critical tracheal stenosis is such that it would severely compromise delivery of gases beyond the obstruction allowing adequate emptying of the lungs as well. Other obstructive upper airway anomalies (e.g., subglottis stenosis) could be overcome by the use of tracheostomy, but in more distal lesions of the trachea, ventilatory management is more challenging. With conventional ventilator settings in a patient with severe tracheal stenosis, there would be inadequate delivery of gases beyond the site of obstruction, with build-up of proximal pressure resulting in progressive $CO_2$ retention and inadequate lung expansion. Because of inadequate emptying of the lungs during expiration, air trapping occurs, along with a subsequent decrease in cardiac output. In order to ensure adequate delivery of gases beyond the obstruction, it is necessary to prolong the inspiratory time so that adequate lung expansion can be achieved. In view of the markedly increased resistance, the time constant will also be increased, justifying the need for high inspiratory time. For this, the frequency of breaths would have to be kept at a low value in order to allow adequate time for expiration and at the same time avoid progressive air trapping. For patients undergoing surgical repair of the tracheal lesions, ECMO has also been used.[78-81]

## CONGENITAL ALVEOLAR CAPILLARY DYSPLASIA

Congenital alveolar capillary dysplasia (ACD), with or without misalignment of the pulmonary veins, is a rare cause of PPHN.[82] This malformation represents a failure of capillaries to extend into alveolar tissue of the lung and is an unusual cause of pulmonary hypertension, persistent fetal circulation, and respiratory distress in the newborn. Histology shows increased septal connective tissue and pulmonary veins accompanying small arteries in the centers of the acini, rather than occupying their normal position in the interlobular septa. The number of pulmonary arteries is decreased, and they show increased muscularization. Pulmonary lobules are small, and radial alveolar counts may be decreased. Alveoli are decreased in complexity, their walls contain few capillaries, and there is poor contact of capillaries with alveolar epithelium. The primary defect is poorly understood. ACD causes severe and irreversible PPHN with a uniformly fatal outcome. Although most cases are sporadic, a familial predisposition has been reported, and a number of studies have suggested that ACD be considered in any infant with severe respiratory acidosis and PPHN who fails to improve after the application of routine treatment modalities. As Michalsky et al. reported,[83] the usual presentation is that of a term neonate, appropriate for gestational age, who appears to be normal at the time of delivery. Most infants develop progressive respiratory distress and cyanosis with hypoxia, respiratory acidosis, and hypotension within 48 hours of birth. The rapidly progressive nature of this process results in the need for full ventilatory support soon after the onset of symptoms. Associated anomalies have been noted in approximately 50% of infants with ACD.

Initial chest radiographs are often reported to be unremarkable or to show a mild hazy pattern. Radiographic changes associated with barotraumas may develop later in the course of treatment. Because of its lethal outcome, ACD should be diagnosed as early as possible.

Clinicans should have a high suspicion for ACD in a term infant with good Apgar scores who goes on to experience respiratory deterioration within a few hours of age. The patient may have transient response to NO, minimal response to HFOV, and variable response to prostacyclin. Although ECMO is typically used as rescue therapy, resulting in rapid hemodynamic stabilization, open lung biopsy should be considered before initiation of ECMO to prevent the institution of futile and expensive treatment modalities.[83]

## PULMONARY ALVEOLAR PROTEINOSIS AND INTERSTITIAL LUNG DISEASES

A number of genetic and environmental factors have been clearly identified as affecting the severity of neonatal respiratory distress syndromes.[84] Congenital alveolar proteinosis syndromes are characterized by the accumulation of surfactant material in the alveolar space.[85] SP-B deficiency leads to alveolar proteinosis, but it is likely that many other causes may lead to similar pulmonary pathology. Interstitial lung diseases (ILDs) in childhood are a diverse group of conditions primarily involving the alveoli and perialveolar tissues and leading to derangement of gas exchange, restrictive lung physiology, and diffuse infiltrates on radiographs.[86] Childhood ILD is not a disease entity but rather a group of disorders. However, most ILDs share a common pathophysiologic feature: namely, structural remodeling of the distal airspaces, leading to impaired gas exchange. In general, this remodeling has been believed to be the sequela of persistent inflammation; however, more recently the paradigm has shifted away from inflammation to one of tissue injury with aberrant wound healing resulting in collagenous fibrosis.[85] The multiple possible diagnostic entities and lack of RCTs make specific recommendations regarding treatment of childhood ILD impossible. If the process is secondary to an underlying condition, patients should be treated for the underlying disease. The appropriate management depends on the patient's age at presentation, the severity of symptoms, and the anticipated course of the disease. Mechanical ventilation is necessary in children with congenital alveolar proteinosis and in some cases of interstitial lung diseases. No reports show any benefit from the use of HFO or other unconventional forms of mechanical ventilation.

## CONCLUSIONS

VILI is one of the major contributors to mortality and morbidity in patients with congenital lung anomalies. The clinical picture has changed following the application of a lung protective strategy consisting of preservation of spontaneous ventilation, permissive levels of hypercapnia ($PaCO_2$, 60 to 65 mm Hg or 9 kPa), and avoidance of high inspiratory airway pressure (25 to 28 $cmH_2O$), increasingly known as the gentle ventilation concept. More newborns with severe respiratory insufficiency are saved and the amount of pulmonary sequelae (BPD, chronic infections, progressive pulmonary vascular disease) diminished. There is a continuing need for RCTs with enough power to determine the role of HFO compared with conventional ventilation, as new modalities such as liquid ventilation are still experimental at this stage.

## REFERENCES

1. Laberge JM, Puligandla P, Flageole H: Asymptomatic congenital lung malformations. Semin Pediatr Surg 2005;14:16–33.
2. Attar MA, Donn SM: Mechanisms of ventilator-induced lung injury in premature infants. Semin Neonatol 2002;7:353–360.

3. Cardoso WV, Lu J: Regulation of early lung morphogenesis: Questions, facts and controversies. Development 2006;133:1611–1624.

4. Christou H, Brodsky D: Lung injury and bronchopulmonary dysplasia in newborn infants. J Intensive Care Med 2005;20:76–87.

5. Lemaitre V, D'Armiento J: Matrix metalloproteinases in development and disease. Birth Defects Res C Embryo Today 2006;78:1–10.

6. Kotecha S: Lung growth for beginners. Paediatr Respir Rev 2000;1:308–313.

7. Turner BS, Loan LA: Tracheobronchial trauma associated with airway management in neonates. AACN Clin Issues 2000;11:283–299.

8. O'Callaghan C, Smith K, Wilkinson M, et al: Ciliary beat frequency in newborn infants. Arch Dis Child 1991;66:443–444.

9. Konradova V, Janota J, Sulova J, et al: Effects of 90% oxygen exposure on the ultrastructure of the tracheal epithelium in rabbits. Respiration 1988;54:24–32.

10. Ozdemir A, Brown MA, Morgan WJ: Markers and mediators of inflammation in neonatal lung disease. Pediatr Pulmonol 1997;23:292–306.

11. Speer CP: Pulmonary inflammation and bronchopulmonary dysplasia. J Perinatol 2006;26(Suppl 1):S57–S62; discussion S63–S64.

12. Speer CP: Inflammatory mechanisms in neonatal chronic lung disease. Eur J Pediatr 1999;158(Suppl 1):S18–S22.

13. Dreyfuss D, Saumon G: Ventilator-induced lung injury: Lessons from experimental studies. Am J Respir Crit Care Med 1998;157:294–323.

14. Rimensberger PC: Neonatal respiratory failure. Curr Opin Pediatr 2002;14:315–321.

15. Schultz C, Tautz J, Reiss I, et al: Prolonged mechanical ventilation induces pulmonary inflammation in preterm infants. Biol Neonate 2003;84:64–66.

16. Greenspan JS, Shaffer TH: Ventilator-induced airway injury: A critical consideration during mechanical ventilation of the infant. Neonatal Netw 2006;25:159–166.

17. Jobe AH, Bancalari E: Bronchopulmonary dysplasia. Am J Respir Crit Care Med 2001;163:1723–1729.

18. Kinsella JP, Greenough A, Abman SH: Bronchopulmonary dysplasia. Lancet 2006;367:1421–1431.

19. Turner BS, Bradshaw W, Brandon D: Neonatal lung remodeling: Structural, inflammatory, and ventilator-induced injury. J Perinat Neonatal Nurs 2005;19:362–376; quiz 377–378.

20. Sandhar BK, Niblett DJ, Argiras EP, et al: Effects of positive end-expiratory pressure on hyaline membrane formation in a rabbit model of the neonatal respiratory distress syndrome. Intensive Care Med 1988;14:538–546.

21. Muscedere JG, Mullen JB, Gan K, et al: Tidal ventilation at low airway pressures can augment lung injury. Am J Respir Crit Care Med 1994;149:1327–1334.

22. Jobe AH, Ikegami M: Mechanisms initiating lung injury in the preterm. Early Hum Dev 1998;53:81–94.

23. Dreyfuss D, Basset G, Soler P, et al: Intermittent positive-pressure hyperventilation with high inflation pressures produces pulmonary microvascular injury in rats. Am Rev Respir Dis 1985;132:880–884.

24. Parker JC, Hernandez LA, Peevy KJ: Mechanisms of ventilator-induced lung injury. Crit Care Med 1993;21:131–143.

25. Robertson B, Halliday HL: Principles of surfactant replacement. Biochim Biophys Acta 1998;1408:346–361.

26. Bjorklund LJ, Ingimarsson J, Curstedt T, et al: Lung recruitment at birth does not improve lung function in immature lambs receiving surfactant. Acta Anaesthesiol Scand 2001;45:986–993.

27. Wilson JM, Lund DP, Lillehei CW, et al: Congenital diaphragmatic hernia—a tale of two cities: The Boston experience. J Pediatr Surg 1997;32:401–405.

28. Kolobow T, Moretti MP, Fumagalli R, et al: Severe impairment in lung function induced by high peak airway pressure during mechanical ventilation. An experimental study. Am Rev Respir Dis 1987;135:312–315.

29. Dworetz AR, Moya FR, Sabo B, et al: Survival of infants with persistent pulmonary hypertension without extracorporeal membrane oxygenation. Pediatrics 1989;84:1–6.

30. Wung JT, James LS, Kilchevsky E, et al: Management of infants with severe respiratory failure and persistence of the fetal circulation, without hyperventilation. Pediatrics 1985;76:488–494.

31. Boloker J, Bateman DA, Wung JT, et al: Congenital diaphragmatic hernia in 120 infants treated consecutively with permissive hypercapnea/spontaneous respiration/elective repair. J Pediatr Surg 2002;37:357–366.

32. Kays DW, Langham MR Jr, Ledbetter DJ, et al: Detrimental effects of standard medical therapy in congenital diaphragmatic hernia. Ann Surg 1999;230:340–348; discussion 348–351.

33. Wung JT, Sahni R, Moffitt ST, et al: Congenital diaphragmatic hernia: Survival treated with very delayed surgery, spontaneous respiration, and no chest tube. J Pediatr Surg 1995;30:406–409.

34. Conforti AF, Losty PD: Perinatal management of congenital diaphragmatic hernia. Early Hum Dev 2006;82:283–287.

35. Bloss RS, Aranda JV, Beardmore HE: Congenital diaphragmatic hernia: Pathophysiology and pharmacologic support. Surgery 1981;89:518–524.

36. Lally KP: Congenital diaphragmatic hernia. Curr Opin Pediatr 2002;14:486–490.

37. Clark RH, Hardin WD Jr, Hirschl RB, et al: Current surgical management of congenital diaphragmatic hernia: A report from the Congenital Diaphragmatic Hernia Study Group. J Pediatr Surg 1998;33:1004–1009.

38. Sakurai Y, Azarow K, Cutz E, et al: Pulmonary barotrauma in congenital diaphragmatic hernia: A clinicopathological correlation. J Pediatr Surg 1999;34:1813–1817.

39. Walsh-Sukys MC, Tyson JE, Wright LL, et al: Persistent pulmonary hypertension of the newborn in the era before nitric oxide: Practice variation and outcomes. Pediatrics 2000;105:14–20.

40. Drummond WH, Gregory GA, Heymann MA, et al: The independent effects of hyperventilation, tolazoline, and dopamine on infants with persistent pulmonary hypertension. J Pediatr 1981;98:603–611.

41. Reynolds M, Luck SR, Lappen R: The "critical" neonate with diaphragmatic hernia: A 21-year perspective. J Pediatr Surg 1984;19:364–369.

42. Miguet D, Claris O, Lapillonne A, et al: Preoperative stabilization using high-frequency oscillatory ventilation in the management of congenital diaphragmatic hernia. Crit Care Med 1994;22:S77–S82.

43. Reyes C, Chang LK, Waffarn F, et al. Delayed repair of congenital diaphragmatic hernia with early high-frequency oscillatory ventilation during preoperative stabilization. J Pediatr Surg 1998;33:1010–1014; discussion 1014–1016.

44. Somaschini M, Locatelli G, Salvoni L, et al: Impact of new treatments for respiratory failure on outcome of infants with congenital diaphragmatic hernia. Eur J Pediatr 1999;158: 780–784.

45. Cacciari A, Ruggeri G, Mordenti M, et al: High-frequency oscillatory ventilation versus conventional mechanical ventilation in congenital diaphragmatic hernia. Eur J Pediatr Surg 2001;11:3–7.

46. Cools F, Offringa M: Neuromuscular paralysis for newborn infants receiving mechanical ventilation. Cochrane Database Syst Rev 2000;CD002773.

47. Bhutani VK, Abbasi S, Sivieri EM: Continuous skeletal muscle paralysis: Effect on neonatal pulmonary mechanics. Pediatrics 1988;81:419–422.

48. Wilcox DT, Glick PL, Karamanoukian HL, et al: Contributions by individual lungs to the surfactant status in congenital diaphragmatic hernia. Pediatr Res 1997;41:686–691.

49. Mysore MR, Margraf LR, Jaramillo MA, et al: Surfactant protein A is decreased in a rat model of congenital diaphragmatic hernia. Am J Respir Crit Care Med 1998;157:654–657.

50. Finer NN, Tierney A, Etches PC, et al: Congenital diaphragmatic hernia: Developing a protocolized approach. J Pediatr Surg 1998;33:1331–1337.

51. Lotze A, Knight GR, Anderson KD, et al: Surfactant (beractant) therapy for infants with congenital diaphragmatic hernia on ECMO: Evidence of persistent surfactant deficiency. J Pediatr Surg 1994;29:407–412.

52. Moya FR, Thomas VL, Romaguera J, et al: Fetal lung maturation in congenital diaphragmatic hernia. Am J Obstet Gynecol 1995;173:1401–1405.

53. Cogo PE, Toffolo GM, Gucciardi A, et al: Surfactant disaturated phosphatidylcholine kinetics in infants with bronchopulmonary dysplasia measured with stable isotopes and a two-compartment model. J Appl Physiol 2005;99:323–329.

54. Colby CE, Lally KP, Hintz SR, et al: Surfactant replacement therapy on ECMO does not improve outcome in neonates with congenital diaphragmatic hernia. J Pediatr Surg 2004;39:1632–1637.

55. Zimmermann LJ, Janssen DJ, Tibboel D, et al: Surfactant metabolism in the neonate. Biol Neonate 2005;87:296–307.

56. Wojciak-Stothard B, Haworth SG: Perinatal changes in pulmonary vascular endothelial function. Pharmacol Ther 2006;109:78–91.

57. Geggel RL, Murphy JD, Langleben D, et al: Congenital diaphragmatic hernia: Arterial structural changes and persistent pulmonary hypertension after surgical repair. J Pediatr 1985;107:457–464.

58. Greenough A, Khetriwal B: Pulmonary hypertension in the newborn. Paediatr Respir Rev 2005;6:111–116.

59. Barrington KJ, Finer NN: Inhaled nitric oxide for respiratory failure in preterm infants. Cochrane Database Syst Rev 2006;CD000509.

60. The Neonatal Inhaled Nitric Oxide Study Group (NINOS): Inhaled nitric oxide and hypoxic respiratory failure in infants with congenital diaphragmatic hernia. Pediatrics 1997;99:838–845.

61. Konduri GG: New approaches for persistent pulmonary hypertension of newborn. Clin Perinatol 2004;31:591–611.

62. Dakshinamurti S: Pathophysiologic mechanisms of persistent pulmonary hypertension of the newborn. Pediatr Pulmonol 2005;39:492–503.

63. McNamara PJ, Laique F, Muang-In S, et al: Milrinone improves oxygenation in neonates with severe persistent pulmonary hypertension of the newborn. J Crit Care 2006;21:217–222.

64. Karatza AA, Narang I, Rosenthal M, et al: Treatment of primary pulmonary hypertension with oral sildenafil. Respiration 2004;71:192–194.

65. Keller RL, Hamrick SE, Kitterman JA, et al: Treatment of rebound and chronic pulmonary hypertension with oral sildenafil in an infant with congenital diaphragmatic hernia. Pediatr Crit Care Med 2004;5:184–187.

66. Baquero H, Soliz A, Neira F, et al: Oral sildenafil in infants with persistent pulmonary hypertension of the newborn: A pilot randomized blinded study. Pediatrics 2006;117:1077–1083.

67. Golzand E, Bar-Oz B, Arad I: Intravenous prostacyclin in the treatment of persistent pulmonary hypertension of the newborn refractory to inhaled nitric oxide. Isr Med Assoc J 2005;7:408–409.

68. Wallis C: Clinical outcomes of congenital lung abnormalities. Paediatr Respir Rev 2000;1:328–335.

69. Merenstein GB, Weisman LE: Premature rupture of the membranes: Neonatal consequences. Semin Perinatol 1996;20:375–380.

70. Leach CL, Greenspan JS, Rubenstein SD, et al: Partial liquid ventilation with perflubron in premature infants with severe respiratory distress syndrome. The LiquiVent Study Group. N Engl J Med 1996;335:761–767.

71. Henderson-Smart DJ, Bhuta T, Cools F, et al: Elective high frequency oscillatory ventilation versus conventional ventilation for acute pulmonary dysfunction in preterm infants. Cochrane Database Syst Rev 2003;CD000104.

72. Sauvat F, Michel JL, Benachi A, et al: Management of asymptomatic neonatal cystic adenomatoid malformations. J Pediatr Surg 2003;38:548–552.

73. Crombleholme TM, Coleman B, Hedrick H, et al: Cystic adenomatoid malformation volume ratio predicts outcome in prenatally diagnosed cystic adenomatoid malformation of the lung. J Pediatr Surg 2002;37:331–338.

74. Adzick NS: Management of fetal lung lesions. Clin Perinatol 2003;30:481–492.

75. Njinimbam CG, Hebra A, Kicklighter SD, et al: Persistent pulmonary hypertension in a neonate with cystic adenomatoid malformation of the lung following lobectomy: Survival with prolonged extracorporeal membrane oxygenation therapy. J Perinatol 1999;19:64–67.

76. Kravitz RM: Congenital malformations of the lung. Pediatr Clin North Am 1994;41:453–472.

77. Karnak I, Senocak ME, Ciftci AO, et al: Congenital lobar emphysema: Diagnostic and therapeutic considerations. J Pediatr Surg 1999;34:1347–1351.

78. Elliott M, Roebuck D, Noctor C, et al: The management of congenital tracheal stenosis. Int J Pediatr Otorhinolaryngol 2003;67(Suppl 1):S183–S192.

79. Hines MH, Hansell DR: Elective extracorporeal support for complex tracheal reconstruction in neonates. Ann Thorac Surg 2003;76:175–178; discussion 179.

80. Connolly KM, McGuirt WF Jr: Elective extracorporeal membrane oxygenation: An improved perioperative technique in the treatment of tracheal obstruction. Ann Otol Rhinol Laryngol 2001;110:205–209.

81. Angel C, Murillo C, Zwischenberger J, et al: Perioperative extracorporeal membrane oxygenation for tracheal reconstruction in congenital tracheal stenosis. Pediatr Surg Int 2000;16:98–101.

82. Somaschini M, Bellan C, Chinaglia D, et al: Congenital misalignment of pulmonary vessels and alveolar capillary dysplasia: How to manage a neonatal irreversible lung disease? J Perinatol 2000;20:189–192.

83. Michalsky MP, Arca MJ, Groenman F, et al: Alveolar capillary dysplasia: A logical approach to a fatal disease. J Pediatr Surg 2005;40:1100–1105.

84. Clark H, Clark LS: The genetics of neonatal respiratory disease. Semin Fetal Neonatal Med 2005;10:271–282.

85. Ioachimescu OC, Kavuru MS: Pulmonary alveolar proteinosis. Chron Respir Dis 2006;3:149–159.

86. Brasch F, Griese M, Tredano M, et al: Interstitial lung disease in a baby with a de novo mutation in the SFTPC gene. Eur Respir J 2004;24:30–39.

# CHAPTER 48

# Extracorporeal Membrane Oxygenation (ECMO) in Pediatric and Neonatal Patients

Robert-Jan Houmes, Saskia Gischler, and Dick Tibboel

Since the first reported successful use of prolonged cardiopulmonary bypass in neonates in 1976, *extracorporeal membrane oxygenation* (ECMO) has been the principal term used to describe the use of extracorporeal cardiopulmonary support in the ICU. Over the years the use of ECMO has expanded from neonates to adults and consists of pulmonary, cardiac, or combined support. Initially ECMO was applied when patients were on maximal conventional support and were considered to be moribund. The initial results in the neonatal population showed a mortality reduction from the predicted greater than 90% risk of mortality to a greater than 50% survival rate. In 1989 the Extracorporeal Life Support Organization (ELSO) was voluntarily formed to pool data and knowledge from all active ECMO centers. ELSO also started a registry database in which, as of June 2006, 32,905 patients had been recorded from 109 centers in 17 countries. The database offers a benchmark for the individual centers. Annual congresses and discussion web sites all helped to form an international community of ECMO centers.

## GOAL OF ECMO

The goal of ECMO is to ensure sufficient oxygen supply to the body. ECMO does not heal the heart or lungs but gives them time to rest and recover. Establishing a lung-protective ventilation strategy in severe cases of acute respiratory distress syndrome (ARDS) may be incompatible with the goal of maintaining sufficient gas exchange.

The institution of ECMO partly results in the takeover of oxygenation and carbon dioxide removal and thereby may allow ventilator settings to be adjusted to the mechanical and gas exchange properties of the diseased lung. In this way the goals of lung protective mechanical ventilation can be reached, even in severe ARDS.[1,2] In respiratory insufficiency, lung rest can prevent further ventilator-induced lung injury (VILI). It is imperative that lung tissue remains recruited during the ECMO run to avoid shear forces that induce further injury to the lung[3] and to prevent a radiographic picture of consolidation and congestion, referred to as "white-out," in which little or no gas exchange through the native lung is possible.[4] When white-out occurs and the patient is entirely dependent on ECMO, even small periods of 1 to 2 minutes can lead to profound hypoxemia.

After exposure of blood to artificial surfaces, a systemic inflammatory reaction is activated; this reaction is well known after standard cardiopulmonary bypass (CPB). The differences between ECMO and CPB include maintenance of pulmonary blood flow, normothermic perfusion, lack of hemodilution, different priming solutions, and inflammatory stimuli that may be the reason for initiating ECMO. Most patients in need of ECMO are profoundly hypoxic or are in septic shock, resulting in activation of the vascular endothelium, activation of the complement system, and up-regulation of polymorphonuclear neutrophils. This systemic inflammatory response often leads to an increase in vascular permeability.[5] However, long-term ECMO was shown to contribute very little to the inflammatory response.[6–8]

## ECMO TECHNIQUE

Various techniques for ECMO support are currently used worldwide. The basic ECMO setup consists of catheters, tubing, a pump, and a membrane lung. When starting an ECMO procedure the first decision is whether only the lung is to be supported. Improvement of gas exchange can be achieved by oxygenation and $CO_2$ removal of venous blood only. This type of ECMO is called *veno-venous* (VV)-ECMO, as venous blood is drained from the patient and oxygenated externally and is reperfused in the venous circulation. Advantages of VV-ECMO are as follows:

- Possible thromboemboli that may enter the body from the ECMO system are routed first to the pulmonary circulation.
- Cannulation of arteries is not necessary (as the long-term effects into adulthood of ligation of the carotid artery in the newborn are still not known).
- Blood entering the cerebral arterial tree is less highly oxygenated.
- Physiologic pulsatile flow is maintained.

When additional cardiac support is necessary, the drained blood is reperfused in the arterial circulation, thereby bypassing the pulmonary circulation. This type of ECMO is called *veno-arterial* (VA)-ECMO and is the standard procedure in more than 75% of neonatal cases worldwide.

## CANNULAS

The choice of ECMO cannula is an important factor in optimizing ECMO flow. Typical ECMO flows are maintained at 60 to 150 ml/kg/min. The flow-pressure characteristics of a given cannula are determined by a number of geometric factors including length, internal diameter, and side hole placement. The "M number" provides a standardized means for describing the flow-pressure relationships in a variety of vascular access devices to minimize resistance as cannulas that are large as possible are placed. To drain venous blood from the patient, a large, multi-hole cannula is placed in the superior caval vein, with the holes positioned at the right atrial level. Usually the right internal jugular vein is used for this procedure. The drained blood is directed through the ECMO system and is reperfused to the patient. The site of reperfusion depends on the type of ECMO technique. In VV-ECMO, one double-lumen cannula can serve as the source end return site for blood flow, reducing the sites for cannulation to one. In VA-ECMO, the most common site for reperfusion is the right common carotid artery,

with the tip of the cannula at the bifurcation of the right common carotid artery and aortic arch. Insertion too far into the ascending aorta can cause increased afterload to left ventricular outflow and may contribute to left ventricular failure. Insertion too far down the descending aorta can compromise coronary and cerebral oxygenated flow.

## BLADDER

The drained venous blood is directed through tubing toward a reservoir called the *bladder*. The bladder is filled by hydrostatic pressure and prevents the buildup of negative pressure in the patient that could result from the suction from the mechanical pump as the pump is temporarily switched off or its speed is reduced when the bladder volume decreases by a servo-regulated mechanism. Two types of mechanical pumps are used. The first and most widely used pump is an occlusive roller pump, which guarantees the desired output as long as the bladder is full. The second type of pump is a centrifugal pump in which a spinning rotor generates flow and pressure. The main advantage of the roller pump is the delivery of constant flow, in which the output of the centrifugal pump is dependent on changes in preload and afterload. On low-flow settings the centrifugal pump produces more hemolysis, where at higher-flow settings, less mechanical energy is required than with the roller pump.

## MEMBRANE OXYGENATOR

After the pump the blood is oxygenated in a membrane lung. The membrane lung, which is the type most commonly used, consists of two sheets of silicone that are sealed at their edges. Oxygen gas flows through connector tubing segments at opposite ends, which are in continuity with the inside of the silicone envelope. The envelope is wound up on a polycarbonate spool, and blood is distributed, via a manifold, lengthwise through the interstices of the wound-up envelope. Gas exchange takes place across the silicone membrane. Membrane lungs are available from 0.4 to 4.5 $m^2$ in surface area. Oxygenation of blood in the membrane lung is comparable to the natural lung: Size, ventilation-perfusion matching, changes in $Fio_2$, the thickness of the blood film, and the pre-membrane hemoglobin oxygen saturation interact in the performance of the membrane lung. As in the natural lung, the membrane lung can also be subject to pulmonary edema, pulmonary hypertension, or pulmonary embolism. $CO_2$ elimination through a membrane lung depends on gas flow (called *sweep gas flow*) over the membrane lung. This situation is comparable to the minute ventilation in the natural lung. Other variables influencing $CO_2$ exchange are the surface area of the membrane lung and the concentration of $CO_2$ in the sweep gas. $CO_2$ exchange is independent of blood flow through the membrane lung.

## HEAT EXCHANGER

As it passes through the ECMO system, the blood is exposed to a large surface area, resulting in significant heat loss. Therefore all ECMO systems use a heat exchanger. ECMO heat exchangers consist of stainless steel tubes enclosed in a clear, hollow polycarbonate core. The blood runs inside the stainless steel tubes with a hot water counterflow outside the tubes, warming the blood. Simultaneously the heat exchanger serves as a bubble trap to catch any stray air before the blood returns to the patient.

## MONITORING

In addition to the standard intensive care unit (ICU) monitoring, the ECMO system is equipped with additional monitors and safety devices.

### Venous Saturation

Venous blood entering the ECMO system is measured for venous hemoglobin oxygen saturation ($SvO_2$). In VA-ECMO this $SvO_2$ directly reflects the effectiveness of oxygen delivery. The ECMO flow is adjusted to maintain an $SvO_2$ of 60% to 75%. In VV-ECMO, $SvO_2$ provides a measure of recirculation of blood from ECMO to ECMO instead of from ECMO to the patient. Evaluation of the amount of recirculation is sometimes difficult in the clinical setting.

### Pressure Measurements

Measurement of blood pressure in the ECMO system before (pre-membrane) and after the membrane lung (post-membrane) gives an indication of the resistance of the membrane lung. At constant flow, rapidly increasing differences between pre- and post-membrane pressures indicate a rise in resistance that possibly results from thrombosis inside the membrane lung.

### Blood Gas Analysis

Online or intermittent analysis of post-membranous ECMO blood gives an indication of the function of the membrane lung.

## Activated Clotting Time

Activation of coagulation is a normal response of blood to contact with an artificial surface. To reduce coagulability, a continuous infusion of heparin or other anticoagulation therapy is started at the beginning of an ECMO procedure. The dose of heparin is titrated to the activated clotting time (ACT). ACT is a test used to monitor the effectiveness of high-dose heparin therapy. The ACT can be determined at the bedside reference value for the ACT ranges between 70 and 180 seconds; the desired range for anticoagulation depends on the reason for heparinization. During CPB the desired range may exceed 400 to 500 seconds, whereas during ECMO the target values range from 180 to 240 seconds. The ACT lacks correlation with other coagulation tests. In general it is used to demonstrate the inability to coagulate rather than to quantify the ability to clot. Results can be affected by methodology, platelet count and function, hypothermia, hemodilution, and the use of certain drugs such as aprotinin that interfere with coagulation.

As a logical consequence, ECMO has potential intrinsic risks. Thus the application of ECMO should only be done by highly trained staff who perform ECMO on a regular basis.

## NEONATAL ECMO

The rationale for ECMO is mainly based on the U.K. multicenter randomized controlled trial. This trial revealed that ECMO improved survival to 1 year when compared with conventional management (32% versus 59%, respectively).[9] The relative risk was 0.55 (95% confidence interval [CI], 0.39 to 0.77; P = 0.0005), which is equivalent to one extra survivor for every three to four infants allocated ECMO.

### Indications

ECMO is indicated when conventional management of cardiopulmonary disorders fails and the incipient predicted mortality is very high. The criteria for use of ECMO in the neonatal age group continue to evolve.[10] The oxygenation index (OI) is the most commonly used measure of severity of respiratory failure in neonates.[11] OI is equal to the mean airway pressure × inspired oxygen fraction × 100 divided by $PaO_2$. Classically, an OI of 40 has been used as an indication of the need for ECMO.[10] Infants on ECMO with less stringent OI criteria have shorter and less costly hospital stays.[12] In newborns with severe cardiopulmonary disease, the degree of ventilatory support required for maintaining adequate oxygenation determines the mortality risk. Because ECMO is an invasive procedure involving significant risk, it is used only under restricted and well-defined circumstances. Conversely, one should consider that delaying ECMO therapy might cause further deterioration of cardiopulmonary function and increase the threat of cerebral hypoxia.

In the majority of centers, the following inclusion criteria for neonatal respiratory ECMO are as follows:

Gestational age >34 weeks
Weight > 2kg
Mechanical ventilation <14 days
Reversible lung injury
Oxygenation index (OI) >30 to 35
No major congenital heart disease
No lethal malformations or congenital anomalies
No evidence of irreversible brain injury

## Contraindications

Gestational age has been found to be a predictor of intracranial hemorrhage (ICH).[13] Infants younger than 34 weeks were found to have a near 50% incidence of ICH and a lower survival (63% versus 84%; P < .001).[14] Therefore gestational age younger than 34 weeks is considered by most centers to be an exclusion criterion.

Patients weighing less than 2 kg have extremely small vessels for cannulation, thus hindering adequate flow because of limitations from cannula size and subsequent higher resistance to blood flow. A higher rate of ICH and mortality has been documented in this low-birth-weight group.[15] Therefore birth weight less than 2 kg, especially in combination with low gestational age, is an exclusion criterion.

When ICH is already present, most centers will only accept ICH grade 1 for ECMO treatment.

### Congenital Heart Disease

Unstable patients eligible for ECMO should be screened by echocardiogram for major congenital heart disease. Congenital heart disease in itself is not a contraindication for ECMO. However, in patients with total anomalous pulmonary venous return (TAVPR) or transposition of the great arteries (TGA), ECMO is not the solution to the problem. In these cases, primary cardiosurgical correction is indicated in which CPB sometimes needs to be continued mainly because of persistent pulmonary hypertension.

### Irreversible Organ Failure

Irreversible damage to organs is considered a relative contraindication. More than 14 days of mechanical ventilation can induce chronic lung injury that may need more time to heal than ECMO can provide safely. This is one of the major reasons why early consultation with an ECMO center is preferable. Progression of the disease or combinations of clinical problems (e.g., pneumothoraces, sepsis) can be an indication to begin ECMO,[12] even when the patient does not fulfill the entry criteria for respiratory failure in neonates. When no definite improvement is made after 2 to 3 days of optimal conventional treatment, ECMO should again be considered.[10] When these patients are referred to an ECMO center, 60% to 80% will eventually receive ECMO.

Sometimes the definite diagnosis of lethal congenital disease cannot be made without the help of ECMO, especially TAPVR, which is frequently diagnosed following the start of ECMO. In these circumstances, placing the patient on ECMO provides the time for the diagnosis to be confirmed, such as with computed tomography (CT), angiography, or lung biopsy.

## Common Neonatal ECMO Indications

Specific respiratory diseases treated with ECMO include meconium aspiration syndrome (MAS), congenital diaphragmatic hernia (CDH), persistent pulmonary hypertension of the newborn (PPHN), sepsis, pneumonia, airleak syndrome, complex tracheal reconstruction, cystic adenomatoid malformation of the lung (CCAML), and others. Cardiac failure is an increasing indication for neonatal ECMO treatment. This group of patients consists of postoperative cardiac failure after major cardiac surgery; for example, TAPVR, TGA, or atrioventricular septal defect. In addition, cardiomyopathy (e.g., following maternal diabetes) can be a valid reason to start ECMO treatment.

The number of neonates treated annually with ECMO for respiratory failure has shown a steady decline from 1516 neonates in 1992 to 713 patients in 2005. However, in the ELSO Registry, the number of cardiac runs increased from 103 in 1992 to 247 in 2005, although this resulted in a decrease in survival from 78% to 68%, respectively. This decline in survival can be partly explained by the relative increase in the percentage of ECMO patients with CHD and the downward trend for survival in these patients. The overall decrease in neonatal respiratory ECMO runs can be explained by the introduction of new techniques in conventional treatment. A number of studies showed that treatment modalities such as nitric oxide (NO), high-frequency oscillation (HFO), and surfactant improved conventional survival without decreasing ECMO survival.[16–18] Consequently the number of ECMO centers is decreasing as patient selection becomes more and more critical.

## Results

The international cumulative results of neonatal ECMO are shown in Table 48.1.

**Table 48-1  International Summary July 2006 ELSO Registry: Cumulative Neonatal Runs by Diagnosis**

| Diagnosis | Total ECMO Runs | Average Run Time | Survived | % Survived |
|---|---|---|---|---|
| Congenital diaphragmatic hernia | 4983 | 238 | 2590 | 52% |
| Meconium aspiration syndrome | 6969 | 129 | 6538 | 94% |
| Persistent pulmonary hypertension of the newborn | 3227 | 146 | 2519 | 78% |
| Sepsis | 2465 | 139 | 1856 | 75% |
| Pneumonia | 281 | 218 | 164 | 58% |
| Airleak syndrome | 106 | 166 | 77 | 73% |
| Other respiratory | 1446 | 172 | 915 | 63% |
| Congenital cardiac defect | 2487 | 242 | 897 | 36% |
| Cardiac arrest | 29 | 103 | 7 | 24% |
| Cardiogenic shock | 29 | 180 | 12 | 41% |
| Cardiomyopathy | 78 | 211 | 50 | 64% |
| Myocarditis | 32 | 247 | 14 | 44% |
| Other cardiac | 216 | 187 | 91 | 42% |

ECMO, extracorporeal membrane oxygenation; ELSO, Extracorporeal Life Support Organization.

## PEDIATRIC ECMO

The initial success of ECMO and the increased number of ECMO centers in the 1990s resulted in an increased interest in the use of ECMO in pediatric and adult cardiorespiratory failure. The number of pediatric patients receiving ECMO increased from 273 in 1992 to 504 pediatric patients receiving ECMO in 2005. Several studies demonstrated survival rates from 50% to 70%. A total of 3271 pediatric patients have been treated with ECMO for respiratory failure.[19–23]

Due to the variety in etiology and recent improvements in the treatment of respiratory failure, it is difficult for the clinician to know when to start ECMO. Unlike neonatal indications, solid entry criteria are still not available.

When, despite maximal treatment including lung-protective ventilation, recruitment maneuvers, NO, and prone positioning, death of the patient is believed to be nearly certain, ECMO has to be considered. The most difficult decisions are when to consider ECMO and when to transfer patients to an ECMO center. All these dilemmas require an individualized approach. Although in the pediatric population OI has been shown to predict mortality,[24] in the pediatric population OI is not as predictive as in neonates.[25] Each ECMO center has its own set of inclusion and exclusion criteria, which serve more as a guide to make an individualized approach. Over the years positive results have been reported with patients with burns or malignancies and with trauma victims. Therefore when an ECMO treatment is considered (because of the potential reversibility of the disease), each patient must be discussed with the nearest ECMO center, keeping in mind that the chance of successful weaning of ECMO is improved when the patient is ventilated for less than 10 days.[26,27]

ECMO can be continued as long as there is reason to believe lung function can recover and significant ECMO-related complications can be avoided.

### Frequent Pediatric Respiratory ECMO Indications

Viral pneumonia, bacterial pneumonia, ARDS, and aspiration are the most common diagnoses encountered. Many patients have conditions that are rare or difficult to

**Table 48-2**  International Summary July 2006 ELSO Registry: Cumulative Pediatric Respiratory ECMO Runs (<16 years) by Diagnosis

| Diagnosis | Total ECMO Runs | Average Run Time | Survived | % Survived |
|---|---|---|---|---|
| Viral pneumonia | 815 | 319 | 517 | 63% |
| Bacterial pneumonia | 359 | 262 | 203 | 57% |
| Pneumocystis pneumonia | 25 | 363 | 12 | 48% |
| Aspiration pneumonia | 174 | 279 | 116 | 67% |
| ARDS, postoperative/trauma | 84 | 227 | 51 | 61% |
| ARDS, not postoperative/trauma | 317 | 289 | 168 | 53% |
| Acute respiratory failure, non ARDS | 646 | 243 | 315 | 49% |
| Other | 910 | 200 | 479 | 53% |

ARDS, acute respiratory distress syndrome; ECMO, extracorporeal membrane oxygenation; ELSO, Extracorporeal Life Support Organization.

place into diagnostic categories. Consequently, many pediatric patients in the ELSO Registry are reported as having "other" diagnoses. Table 48.2 shows the cumulative results of pediatric respiratory ECMO.

In 2004, approximately half of the pediatric respiratory ECMO cases used VV-ECMO, whereas traditionally VA-ECMO has been predominant.

Alleged disadvantages of VV-ECMO relate to the inability to directly control systemic cardiovascular support and systemic oxygenation. However, improved myocardial oxygen delivery, as provided by direct delivery of highly oxygenated coronary blood with VV-ECMO,[28] would be expected to improve myocardial performance. In one series of 15 infants, echocardiographic indexes of cardiac performance improved with initiation of VV-ECMO, and vasoactive infusions were weaned significantly within 8 hours. In contrast, left ventricular function deteriorated during VA-ECMO[29,30] in association with documented coronary perfusion with desaturated mixed venous blood. Also, in our experience, initiation of VV-ECMO leads to resolution of metabolic acidosis and improvement of myocardial function and hypotension. The use of the vasopressor score revealed that even the use of a combination of vasopressor drugs has no negative effect on the outcome of VV-ECMO. Pettigano and colleagues showed that patients with advanced renal failure (ARF) frequently required vasoactive infusions; they were adequately supported with VV techniques and could be weaned off vasopressors,[21] again underlining the benefits of the primary use of VV-ECMO in pediatric respiratory patients. If myocardial performance is still inadequate, conversion to

VA-ECMO may be necessary. In the ELSO registry, 6% of pediatric patients were converted from VV to VA. VA-ECMO supports both cardiac and pulmonary function; however, the coronary arteries are perfused with blood at low saturation as long as blood is ejected from the left ventricle.

## CARDIAC ECMO

Despite the fact that ECMO was originally developed by cardiothoracic surgeons, its use for the treatment of cardiac problems is far less common than that for acute respiratory failure.[31-34] According to the ELSO Registry, in the neonatal period only 10% of the ECMO patients had a primary cardiac failure, whereas in the pediatric group 50% of the ECMO population was classified as cardiac ECMO. Postoperatively, failure to wean from CPB, cardiogenic shock, or postoperative cardiac arrest is the most frequent indication for ECMO.[35] In preoperative ECMO, the most common problems leading to the use of ECMO are hypoxia and pulmonary hypertension. Nonsurgically related indications are myocarditis, cardiomyopathy, and cardiac arrest. Tables 48.3 and 48.4 show the result of the pediatric cardiac runs in the ESLO Registry as of July 2006.

Postoperative cardiac failure is best treated with early application of ECMO.[36-38] Prolonged periods of low cardiac output result in end organ damage. In principle ECMO is used for "short" periods of cardiac support and should be compared with the introduction of left or

**Table 48-3**  International Summary ELSO Registry July 2005: Pediatric (31 Days and <1 year) Cardiac ECMO Runs by Diagnosis

| Diagnosis | Total ECMO Runs | Average Run Time | Survived | % Survived |
|---|---|---|---|---|
| Congenital defect | 1546 | 144 | 652 | 42% |
| Cardiac arrest | 33 | 133 | 10 | 30% |
| Cardiogenic shock | 14 | 160 | 14 | 29% |
| Cardiomyopathy | 81 | 209 | 42 | 52% |
| Myocarditis | 40 | 231 | 25 | 63% |
| Other | 200 | 159 | 85 | 43% |

ECMO, extracorporeal membrane oxygenation; ELSO, Extracorporeal Life Support Organization.

biventricular assist devices on an individual basis.[39] One of the major complications of direct switch from CPB to ECMO is the excessive mediastinal hemorrhage. The primary hemostasis cannot set in as a result of the continuous presence of heparin. The duration of ECMO has been shown to affect survival. Although some researchers have shown that most patients who survive recover contractile function within 48 to 72 hours,[40,41] others have noted that minimal survival exists after 144 hours.[42] Recent studies advocate a greater use of ECMO, considering improvements of the results in terms of survival.[40,43,44] According to European and American recommendations, centers of congenital heart surgery should have ECMO available.[45,46]

Patients who are not transplant candidates should be considered for support only in carefully selected cases, as any patient placed on ECMO may ultimately require cardiac transplantation for recovery.[47]

## Rapid-Response ECMO for Resuscitation

ECMO has been included as a form of "very advanced life support" in resuscitation for cardiac arrest. Although many remain guarded about the outcomes for patients who receive ECMO in the setting of cardiopulmonary resuscitation (CPR), there are now a number of case series describing promising outcomes if emergency cardiac life support (ECLS) is initiated with sufficient rapidity.[48,49] Rapid deployment of ECMO will most likely produce the best results in terms of minimizing the duration of conventional CPR and the associated risk of permanent myocardial injury and, most important,

**Table 48-4**  International Summary ELSO Registry July 2005: Pediatric (1 Year to <16 Years) Cardiac ECMO Runs by Diagnosis

| Diagnosis | Total ECMO Runs | Average Run Time | Survived | % Survived |
|---|---|---|---|---|
| Congenital defect | 850 | 137 | 349 | 41% |
| Cardiac arrest | 58 | 116 | 24 | 41% |
| Cardiogenic shock | 38 | 111 | 13 | 34% |
| Cardiomyopathy | 249 | 203 | 136 | 55% |
| Myocarditis | 117 | 193 | 72 | 62% |
| Other | 330 | 152 | 148 | 45% |

ECMO, extracorporeal membrane oxygenation; ELSO, Extracorporeal Life Support Organization.

brain injury. Survival without significant neurologic impairment following a witnessed cardiac arrest is approximately 20% in children, and early implementation of ECMO can improve the percentage of survivors to 50%.[50-53]

## Type of Support

Most patients with cardiac disease require a venoarterial mode to provide circulatory as well as respiratory support. However, venovenous ECMO may be underutilized in pediatric cardiac patients, as elimination of hypoxia along with decreased pulmonary vascular resistance may improve right ventricular function.[41,54]

## ECMO FOR PATIENT TRANSPORT

Previously ECMO was believed to be too complex to be used during patient transport. At present, however, numerous patients have been transported worldwide.[55-57] These experiences have included both adult and pediatric patients and involved patients who required support for pulmonary as well as cardiac disease. Further improvement of transport systems can lead to a reduction in the number of ECMO centers, resulting in a higher number of patients per individual center, which could benefit outcome.

## OUTCOME AND FOLLOW-UP

Despite the positive results in survival to discharge, especially in the neonatal respiratory ECMO patients, little is known about the long-term morbidity associated with ECMO. Over the years, the development of high-frequency ventilation, inhaled NO (iNO), and surfactant and changing policies in the delivery room have changed the demographic data of neonates treated with ECMO. From 1988 to 1998, neonates were exposed to an ever-expanding group of new therapies, they appeared to be healthier based on indices of gas exchange, and were cared for at centers that reported fewer cases per year.[17] In neonatal respiratory failure, the main area of concern is neurologic morbidity that is likely to be multifactorial in etiology. This increased use of iNO and HFO has led to an increase in neonatal age at ECMO initiation (from 40.5 hours to 68.5 hours) and an increased length of ECMO run (from 154.7 hours to 174.5 hours) in recent years.[18] Factors that may influence this morbidity are the degree of hypoxemia prior to cannulation, the use of hyperventilation to treat PPHN, the cannulation and ligation of the carotid artery and the internal jugular vein,

the use of systemic heparinization in the near-term or pre-term infant, and the duration of ECMO support. Follow-up studies of neonates treated with ECMO in the United Kingdom and United States showed considerable morbidity with major disability in terms of severe developmental delay or neuromotor disabilities of as much as 20% at 1 to 5 years of age.[58-60] In the U.K. Collaborative Randomized Trial of Neonatal Extracorporeal Membrane Oxygenation, for the follow-up data at age 7 years, 68 of 89 (76%) children showed a cognitive level within the normal range. Learning problems were similar in the ECMO-treated and control groups, but in the ECMO group there were notable difficulties with spatial and processing tasks. A higher respiratory morbidity and increased risk of behavioral problems persisted among children treated conventionally. Progressive sensorineural hearing loss was found in both groups.[61]

Apart from the central nervous system, major factors that determine long-term pulmonary morbidity are preexisting pulmonary morbidity (BPD) and the pulmonary vascular disease and pulmonary hypoplasia such as that seen in congenital diaphragmatic hernia. It remains essential to assess lung function regardless of whether ECMO results in a survival advantage.[62]

We presented a nationwide survey of neurodevelopmental sequelae of 98 VA-ECMO–treated neonates at 5 years of age (87% of all survivors). Neurologic deficits at medical assessment were present in 17% of the children. Another 24 (26%) of the children presented with some kind of motor difficulty, of which 15% had a motor problem and 11% were at risk. Cognitive delay was present in 14% of the children.[63]

In our opinion, a successful follow-up program would have a multidisciplinary character represented by, for example, a pediatrician, a pediatric physiotherapist, a psychologist, and a speech therapist.

Long-term outcome in older children with acute hypoxic respiratory failure is more difficult to determine. Many of these children are being placed on ECMO support for ARDS, which, unlike neonatal respiratory failure, is not a single-system pulmonary disease but more likely is a picture of multiorgan failure. Outcome therefore may not be solely determined by recovery of lung function but may also be influenced by nonpulmonary morbidity. The one potential advantage in this age group is that these patients can frequently be supported by VV-ECMO rather than sacrifice the carotid artery for VA support; therefore long-term neurologic morbidity may be significantly reduced.

## CONCLUSION

After more than 25 years of ECMO treatment, it is now time to reevaluate the situation. We have to keep focusing on new therapies and improvement in materials and techniques and to determine the correct position of the institution (use) of ECMO using treatment algorithms. Especially in the non-neonatal group, an individual approach is warranted because properly designed randomized controlled trials, such as the ARDS trial, will not be possible in the pediatric group. Most of all, we have to shift our goal from survival to discharge to reduction of long-term morbidity only, as most of our patients potentially still have a long life ahead of them.

# REFERENCES

1. Lewandowski K: Extracorporeal membrane oxygenation for severe acute respiratory failure. Crit Care 2000;4:156–168.
2. Alpard SK, Zwischenberger JB: Extracorporeal membrane oxygenation for severe respiratory failure. Chest Surg Clin N Am 2002;12:355–378, vii.
3. Dos Santos CC, Slutsky AS: Invited review: Mechanisms of ventilator-induced lung injury: A perspective. J Appl Physiol 2000;89:1645–1655.
4. Keszler M, Ryckman FC, McDonald JV Jr, et al: A prospective, multicenter, randomized study of high versus low positive end-expiratory pressure during extracorporeal membrane oxygenation. J Pediatr 1992;120:107–113.
5. Peek GJ, Firmin RK: The inflammatory and coagulative response to prolonged extracorporeal membrane oxygenation. Asaio J 1999;45:250–263.
6. Kelly RE Jr, Phillips JD, Foglia RP, et al: Pulmonary edema and fluid mobilization as determinants of the duration of ECMO support. J Pediatr Surg 1991;26:1016–1022.
7. Demling RH, Hicks RE, Edmunds LH Jr: Changes in extravascular lung water during venovenous perfusion. J Thorac Cardiovasc Surg 1976;71:291–294.
8. Kazzi NJ, Schwartz CA, Palder SB, et al: Effect of extracorporeal membrane oxygenation on body water content and distribution in lambs. ASAIO Trans 1990;36:817–820.
9. UK collaborative randomised trial of neonatal extracorporeal membrane oxygenation. UK Collaborative ECMO Trial Group. Lancet 1996;348:75–82.
10. Kossel H, Bauer K, Kewitz G, et al: Do we need new indications for ECMO in neonates pretreated with high-frequency ventilation and/or inhaled nitric oxide? Intensive Care Med 2000;26:1489–1495.
11. Finer N: Neonatal selection criteria for ECMO. In Zwischenberger JB SR, Bartlett RH (eds): ECMO: Extracorporeal Cardiopulmonary Support in Critical Care. Ann Arbor, MI: Extracorporeal Life Support Organization, 2000, pp 357–362.
12. Schumacher RE, Roloff DW, Chapman R, et al: Extracorporeal membrane oxygenation in term newborns. A prospective cost-benefit analysis. Asaio J 1993;39:873–879.
13. Hardart GE, Hardart MK, Arnold JH: Intracranial hemorrhage in premature neonates treated with extracorporeal membrane oxygenation correlates with conceptional age. J Pediatr 2004;145:184–189.
14. Hirschl RB, Schumacher RE, Snedecor SN, et al: The efficacy of extracorporeal life support in premature and low birth weight newborns. J Pediatr Surg 1993;28:1336–1340; discussion 1341.
15. Revenis ME, Glass P, Short BL: Mortality and morbidity rates among lower birth weight infants (2000 to 2500 grams) treated with extracorporeal membrane oxygenation. J Pediatr 1992;121:452–458.
16. Fliman PJ, deRegnier RA, Kinsella JP, et al: Neonatal extracorporeal life support: Impact of new therapies on survival. J Pediatr 2006;148:595–599.
17. Roy BJ, Rycus P, Conrad SA, et al: The changing demographics of neonatal extracorporeal membrane oxygenation patients reported to the Extracorporeal Life Support Organization (ELSO) Registry. Pediatrics 2000;106:1334–1338.
18. Hui TT, Danielson PD, Anderson KD, et al: The impact of changing neonatal respiratory management on extracorporeal membrane oxygenation utilization. J Pediatr Surg 2002;37:703–705.
19. Zahraa JN, Moler FW, Annich GM, et al: Venovenous versus venoarterial extracorporeal life support for pediatric respiratory failure: Are there differences in survival and acute complications? Crit Care Med 2000;28:521–525.
20. Cengiz P, Seidel K, Rycus PT, et al: Central nervous system complications during pediatric extracorporeal life support: Incidence and risk factors. Crit Care Med 2005;33:2817–2824.
21. Pettignano R, Fortenberry JD, Heard ML, et al: Primary use of the venovenous approach for extracorporeal membrane oxygenation in pediatric acute respiratory failure. Pediatr Crit Care Med 2003;4:291–298.
22. Kulik TJ, Moler FW, Palmisano JM, et al: Outcome-associated factors in pediatric patients treated with extracorporeal membrane oxygenator after cardiac surgery. Circulation 1996;94(II):63–68.
23. Green TP, Timmons OD, Fackler JC, et al: The impact of extracorporeal membrane oxygenation on survival in pediatric patients with acute respiratory failure. Pediatric Critical Care Study Group. Crit Care Med 1996;24:323–329.
24. Timmons OD, Havens PL, Fackler JC: Predicting death in pediatric patients with acute respiratory failure. Pediatric Critical Care Study Group. Extracorporeal Life Support Organization. Chest 1995;108:789–797.
25. Peters MJ, Tasker RC, Kiff KM, et al: Acute hypoxemic respiratory failure in children: Case mix and the utility of respiratory severity indices. Intensive Care Med 1998;24:699–705.
26. Moler FW, Palmisano J, Custer JR: Extracorporeal life support for pediatric respiratory failure: Predictors of survival from 220 patients. Crit Care Med 1993;21:1604–1611.
27. Pranikoff T, Hirschl RB, Steimle CN, et al: Mortality is directly related to the duration of mechanical ventilation before the initiation of extracorporeal life support for severe respiratory failure. Crit Care Med 1997;25:28–32.
28. Strieper MJ, Sharma S, Dooley KJ, et al: Effects of venovenous extracorporeal membrane oxygenation on cardiac performance as determined by echocardiographic measurements. J Pediatr 1993;122:950–955.
29. Karr SS, Martin GR, Short BL: Cardiac performance in infants referred for extracorporeal membrane oxygenation. J Pediatr 1991;118:437–442.
30. Kinsella JP, Gerstmann DR, Rosenberg AA: The effect of extracorporeal membrane oxygenation on coronary perfusion and regional blood flow distribution. Pediatr Res 1992;31:80–84.
31. Baffes TG, Fridman JL, Bicoff JP, et al: Extracorporeal circulation for support of palliative cardiac surgery in infants. Ann Thorac Surg 1970;10:354–363.
32. Bartlett RH, Gazzaniga AB, Fong SW, et al: Prolonged extracorporeal cardiopulmonary support in man. J Thorac Cardiovasc Surg 1974;68:918–932.

33. Bartlett RH, Gazzaniga AB, Wetmore N, et al: Extracorporeal membrane oxygenator support for cardiopulmonary failure: Experience in 40 cases. Nippon Kyobu Geka Gakkai Zasshi 1978;26:249–263.

34. Bartlett RH, Gazzaniga AB, Fong SW, et al: Extracorporeal membrane oxygenator support for cardiopulmonary failure. Experience in 28 cases. J Thorac Cardiovasc Surg 1977;73:375–386.

35. Huang SC, Wu ET, Chen YS, et al: Experience with extracorporeal life support in pediatric patients after cardiac surgery. Asaio J 2005;51:517–521.

36. Delius RE, Bove EL, Meliones JN, et al: Use of extracorporeal life support in patients with congenital heart disease. Crit Care Med 1992;20:1216–1222.

37. Raithel SC, Pennington DG, Boegner E, et al: Extracorporeal membrane oxygenation in children after cardiac surgery. Circulation 1992;86(II):305–310.

38. Ghez O, Feier H, Ughetto F, et al: Postoperative extracorporeal life support in pediatric cardiac surgery: Recent results. Asaio J 2005;51:513–516.

39. Hines MH: ECMO and congenital heart disease. Semin Perinatol 2005;29:34–39.

40. Aharon AS, Drinkwater DC Jr, Churchwell KB, et al: Extracorporeal membrane oxygenation in children after repair of congenital cardiac lesions. Ann Thorac Surg 2001;72:2095–2101; discussion 2101–2192.

41. Duncan BW, Hraska V, Jonas RA, et al: Mechanical circulatory support in children with cardiac disease. J Thorac Cardiovasc Surg 1999;117:529–542.

42. Black MD, Coles JG, Williams WG, et al: Determinants of success in pediatric cardiac patients undergoing extracorporeal membrane oxygenation. Ann Thorac Surg 1995;60:133–138.

43. Bennett CC, Johnson A, Field DJ, et al: UK collaborative randomised trial of neonatal extracorporeal membrane oxygenation: Follow-up to age 4 years. Lancet 2001;357:1094–1096.

44. Morris MC, Ittenbach RF, Godinez RI, et al: Risk factors for mortality in 137 pediatric cardiac intensive care unit patients managed with extracorporeal membrane oxygenation. Crit Care Med 2004;32:1061–1069.

45. Guidelines for pediatric cardiovascular centers. Pediatrics 2002;109:544–549.

46. Daenen W, Lacour-Gayet F, Aberg T, et al: Optimal structure of a congenital heart surgery department in Europe. Eur J Cardiothorac Surg 2003;24:343–351.

47. Dalton HJ, Siewers RD, Fuhrman BP, et al: Extracorporeal membrane oxygenation for cardiac rescue in children with severe myocardial dysfunction. Crit Care Med 1993;21:1020–1028.

48. del Nido PJ, Dalton HJ, Thompson AE, et al: Extracorporeal membrane oxygenator rescue in children during cardiac arrest after cardiac surgery. Circulation 1992;86(II):300–304.

49. Morris MC, Wernovsky G, Nadkarni VM: Survival outcomes after extracorporeal cardiopulmonary resuscitation instituted during active chest compressions following refractory in-hospital pediatric cardiac arrest. Pediatr Crit Care Med 2004;5:440–446.

50. Mair P, Hoermann C, Moertl M, et al: Percutaneous venoarterial extracorporeal membrane oxygenation for emergency mechanical circulatory support. Resuscitation 1996;33:29–34.

51. Patel H, Pagani FD: Extracorporeal mechanical circulatory assist. Cardiol Clin 2003;21:29–41.

52. von Segesser LK: Cardiopulmonary support and extracorporeal membrane oxygenation for cardiac assist. Ann Thorac Surg 1999;68:672–677.

53. Younger JG, Schreiner RJ, Swaniker F, et al: Extracorporeal resuscitation of cardiac arrest. Acad Emerg Med 1999;6:700–707.

54. Trittenwein G, Furst G, Golej J, et al: Preoperative ECMO in congenital cyanotic heart disease using the AREC system. Ann Thorac Surg 1997;63:1298–1302.

55. Foley DS, Pranikoff T, Younger JG, et al: A review of 100 patients transported on extracorporeal life support. Asaio J 2002;48:612–619.

56. Heulitt MJ, Taylor BJ, Faulkner SC, et al: Inter-hospital transport of neonatal patients on extracorporeal membrane oxygenation: Mobile-ECMO. Pediatrics 1995;95:562–566.

57. Linden V, Palmer K, Reinhard J, et al: Inter-hospital transportation of patients with severe acute respiratory failure on extracorporeal membrane oxygenation—national and international experience. Intensive Care Med 2001;27:1643–1648.

58. The collaborative UK ECMO (Extracorporeal Membrane Oxygenation) trial: Follow-up to 1 year of age. Pediatrics 1998;101:E1.

59. Glass P, Miller M, Short B: Morbidity for survivors of extracorporeal membrane oxygenation: Neurodevelopmental outcome at 1 year of age. Pediatrics 1989;83:72–78.

60. Glass P, Wagner AE, Papero PH, et al: Neurodevelopmental status at age five years of neonates treated with extracorporeal membrane oxygenation. J Pediatr 1995;127:447–457.

61. McNally H, Bennett CC, Elbourne D, et al: United Kingdom collaborative randomized trial of neonatal extracorporeal membrane oxygenation: Follow-up to age 7 years. Pediatrics 2006;117:e845–e854.

62. Bohn D: ECMO—long term follow-up. Paediatr Respir Rev 2006;7(Suppl 1):S194–S195.

63. Hanekamp M, Mazer P, van der Cammen M, et al: Follow-up of newborns treated with Extracorporeal Membrane Oxygenation; a nationwide evaluation at 5 years of age. Crit Care 2006;10(5):R127.

# CHAPTER 49

# Noninvasive Ventilation in Children

Brigitte Fauroux and Frédéric Lofaso

Noninvasive positive pressure ventilation (NIPPV) represents a promising technique in children. First, a number of diseases leading to chronic respiratory failure in childhood—such as neuromuscular diseases; abnormalities of the airways, the chest wall, and/or the lungs; or disorders of ventilatory control—are primarily disorders that lead to alveolar hypoventilation, which can be improved by a ventilatory assistance. As such, oxygen therapy *alone* is not only usually ineffective in relieving symptoms but also has been shown to be dangerous and may lead to a marked acceleration of carbon dioxide ($CO_2$) retention.[1-3] Second, by definition, NIPPV is a noninvasive technique that can be applied on demand and preferentially at night, causing much less morbidity, discomfort, and social life and family disruption than a tracheostomy.

NIPPV is probably underused in children because this technique is more difficult technically to apply in infants and young children. Few physiologic studies have been performed in this age group, the optimal ventilatory mode and setting for each medical condition has not been defined, and the criteria that justify the initiation of NIPPV are most often based on consensus reports focused on neuromuscular diseases.[4-6] However, several recent physiologic studies provide a rationale for NIPPV in some pediatric diseases responsible for alveolar hypoventilation.[7,8]

This chapter focuses on noninvasive ventilator management of infants and children. It examines the diagnoses requiring ventilatory assistance for infants and children, the physiologic effects of ventilatory assistance in children, the special considerations for infants and children concerning ventilation techniques and how they are used in the different pediatric disorders, ventilation equipment, and use.

## PEDIATRIC CONDITIONS THAT CAN BE IMPROVED BY NIPPV

The ability to sustain spontaneous ventilation can be viewed as a balance between neurologic mechanisms controlling ventilation, together with ventilatory muscle power on one side, and the respiratory load, determined by lung, thoracic, and airway mechanics, on the other (Fig. 49.1). Significant dysfunction of any of these three components of the respiratory system may impair the ability to have spontaneously efficacious breaths. In normal children, central respiratory drive and ventilatory muscle power exceed the respiratory load, and these children are thus able to sustain adequate spontaneous ventilation. However, if the respiratory load is too high and/or ventilatory muscle power or central respiratory drive is too low, ventilation may be inadequate, resulting in hypercapnia. Chronic ventilatory failure thus is the result of an uncorrectable imbalance in the respiratory system, in which ventilatory muscle power and central respiratory drive are inadequate to overcome the respiratory load. If these abnormalities cannot be corrected with medical treatment, the child will benefit from long-term ventilatory support.

Some specific issues deserve particular concern when chronic respiratory insufficiency develops in pediatric patients. Successful management of the ventilator-assisted pediatric patient requires close persistent attention to the changing anatomy and physiology of the developing respiratory system. In most adolescents, respiratory system function is similar to that of adults, but in normal infants and young children, the respiratory system is immature, unstable, and subject to dysfunction

PHYSIOPATHOLOGY OF RESPIRATORY FAILURE

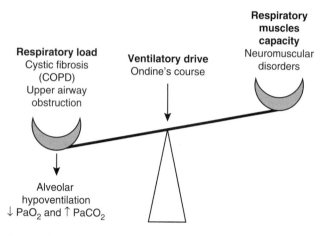

**Figure 49.1** Spontaneous ventilation is the result of a balance among neurologic mechanisms controlling ventilation together with ventilatory muscle power on one side and the respiratory load, determined by lung, thoracic, and airway mechanics, on the other side. If the respiratory load is too high and/or ventilatory muscle power or central respiratory drive is too low, ventilation may be inadequate, resulting in alveolar hypoventilation with hypercapnia and hypoxemia.

as well as constant changes through growth and development. Because of pulmonary and chest wall mechanics, normal respiratory load is higher in children than in adults, there are fewer alveoli, and therefore less surface area is available for gas exchange and less elastic support for intrapulmonary structures. This predisposes the infant to manifest lung disease such as atelectasis, airway obstruction, increased pulmonary vascular resistance, and pulmonary edema due to developmental immaturity of pulmonary mechanics. Less ventilatory muscle strength and endurance increase the infant's susceptibility to respiratory fatigue.[9,10] In addition, neurologic control of breathing in the infant is an intrinsically unstable system, which predisposes to apnea and hypoventilation. As the child grows, the balance among these factors is continuously changing. Furthermore, infants and young children are also subject to external factors that influence the function of the respiratory system, such as frequent respiratory tract infections in early childhood and environmental irritants such as tobacco smoke and other respiratory pollutants. These external factors can precipitate respiratory failure in this age group.

## Disorders Characterized by a Ventilatory Muscle Weakness

Most often, the respiratory muscles are not spared in patients with a neuromuscular disease. In neuromuscular disorders, elastic load and respiratory muscle weakness are responsible for a rapid shallow breathing, leading to

chronic $CO_2$ retention.[11] Ventilatory muscle weakness may be present at birth (spinal muscular atrophy [SMA]), develop later in the course of the disease (Duchenne muscular dystrophy), or be acquired (myopathy, spinal cord injury). Generally, respiratory muscle weakness associates with inspiratory muscle weakness, which results in inability to inspire fully with the consequent hypoventilation, leading to inadequate gas exchange. Expiratory muscle weakness is frequently observed, causing inability to cough and predisposing to pulmonary infection and recurrent atelectasis. Some comorbidities can precipitate alveolar hypoventilation or respiratory failure. Indeed, in individuals in whom vertebral and respiratory muscle weakness is present before spinal growth is complete, a thoracic scoliosis often complicates the clinical picture. These children with ventilatory muscle weakness often do not have patent parenchymal lung disease and thus are good candidates for home NIPPV.

The SMAs are inherited as autosomal recessive disorders of anterior horn cells with the genetic defect at chromosome 5q13.[12] Gene deletions are detectable in 98% of patients. The incidence is about 1 per 5000 live births. Severity is inversely proportional to the amount of survival motoneuron protein in the anterior horn cell. SMA ranges from essentially total paralysis and need for ventilatory support from birth to the relatively mild muscle weakness that presents in the young adult. The diaphragm strength is generally preserved and respiratory muscle weakness predominates on the other inspiratory muscles and the expiratory muscles, predisposing these patients to recurrent lung infections. The pediatric SMAs have been arbitrarily divided into three types, based on clinical severity: type 1, Werdnig Hoffman disease, is defined by never attaining the ability to sit independently; in type 2, patients at least temporarily attain the ability to sit unsupported but usually develop respiratory failure during childhood; in type 3, patients at least attain the ability to walk; type 4 is adult onset. The diagnosis of type 1 has been reported to be uniformly fatal by 2 years of age with 50% mortality by 7 months and 80% mortality by 12 months. However, some highly experienced groups have been able to manage these patients successfully with NIPPV.[13,14] Yet a tracheostomy is often necessary after a variable period, an issue that requires a prior ethical discussion with the parents and the medical team. The use of home NIPPV is clearly less problematic in the other SMA types, where it counteracts hypoventilation and is associated with prolonged life and improved quality of life.

Duchenne muscular dystrophy is currently the most common myopathy that produces respiratory failure in childhood. This is a progressive disorder, and ventilatory failure is inevitable in the course of the disease, although the time course of its progression varies among individuals.[15,16] Home NIPPV counteracts the hypoventilation and can improve the length and the quality of life.[17,18] Respiratory failure is less frequent in other muscular dystrophies, such as Becker, limb-girdle, and facioscapulohumeral dystrophies. However, successful management of chronic respiratory failure by bilevel NIPPV of two brothers with limb-girdle muscular dystrophy has been reported.[19] Congenital myopathies are often static. However, the conditions of children will deteriorate functionally with growth because weakened muscles are unable to cope with increasing body mass. Static motor neuropathies can also cause chronic respiratory failure. Even though the neurologic lesion does not progress, children will often become ventilator dependent at or near the pubertal growth spurt. This occurs because the ventilatory muscles do not increase in strength as increased body mass places an increased functional demand on these muscles.

The importance of respiratory failure associated with spinal cord injury depends on the level of the injury. High spinal cord injury above the third vertebra causes diaphragm paralysis. This nearly always causes respiratory failure in infants and young children. NIPPV can be tried in older children who have a sufficient respiratory autonomy for at least 8 to 10 hours per day. In patients with lower cervical cord injury, expiratory muscle function is severely compromised and thus cough is defective and the clearance of bronchial sections is greatly impaired. As a result, retention of secretion leading to atelectasis and bronchopneumonia frequently occurs in such patients and may require short periods of NIPPV during these episodes of acute respiratory failure.

## Disorders Characterized by an Increase in Respiratory Load

Upper or lower airway obstruction and chest wall deformity are pediatric diseases that cause an increase in respiratory load. Obstructive sleep apnea (OSA) is less common in children than in adults. The pathophysiology is also different, with the predominant role of enlarged tonsils and adenoids.[20] Most often, airway obstruction is relieved after adenotonsillectomy,[21] and the persistence of sleep disturbance after surgery is observed in less than 20% of the patients. Other causes of upper airway obstruction can cause severe alveolar hypoventilation in young children such as laryngomalacia, tracheomalacia, Pierre Robin syndrome, cystic lymphangioma, or some rare congenital disorders of the face such as picnodysostosis.[7] In these infants, alveolar hypoventilation can persist after adenotonsillectomy, especially during sleep. Indeed, because of small lung volumes and the progressive maturation of sleep stages, infants are particularly susceptible to cardiovascular consequences of increased upper airway resistance during sleep. We have shown that the respiratory effort, assessed by the esophageal (PTPes)

and diaphragmatic pressure time product (PTPdi), of young children with upper airway obstruction was greatly increased during wakefulness.[7] NIPPV successfully relieved the additional load imposed on the respiratory muscles, as reflected by the significant reduction in PTPdi, from a mean value of $541.0\pm196.6$ cmH$_2$O.s.min$^{-1}$ during spontaneous breathing to $214.8\pm116.0$ cmH$_2$O.s.min$^{-1}$ during NIPPV (P = .04). This translated into a significant increase in tidal volume, a decrease in respiratory rate, and a significant improvement in diurnal and nocturnal gas exchange.[7]

Children with achondroplasia, because of the abnormalities of the chest, often have sleep-related respiratory disturbances, primarily hypoxemia.[22] A substantial minority of them also have obstructive or central apnea, which has been linked to brain stem compression.[22] If tonsillectomy and adenoidectomy are not able to relieve upper airway obstruction, then NIPPV can be proposed as a first therapeutic option.[22,23]

Cystic fibrosis (CF) represents the most common genetic disease in the Caucasian population. Most of the morbidity and mortality is due to the involvement of the lungs, which is characterized by progressive airflow obstruction, due to mucus plugging and inflammation within the bronchial walls, and destruction of the lung parenchyma secondary to bronchiectasis. In children and young adults with advanced stable pulmonary CF disease, as lung disease progresses, as assessed by a fall in the forced expiratory volume in 1 second (FEV$_1$), there is an increase in the respiratory muscle load, as assessed by the increases in PTPes, PTPdi, and the elastic work of breathing.[24] As a result the patients develop a compensatory mechanism of rapid shallow breathing pattern in an attempt to reduce the increase in load. Although this breathing strategy maintains the level of ventilation, partial arterial carbon dioxide pressure (PaCO$_2$) rises, and thus the efficiency of the respiratory muscle pump to clear CO$_2$ decreases. NIPPV, by unloading the respiratory muscles, improves alveolar hypoventilation and thus gas exchange. This explains why NIPPV is as effective as oxygen therapy to improve arterial oxygenation but significantly more effective than oxygen therapy to decrease PaCO$_2$.[3,25]

Restrictive parenchymal lung diseases are difficult to manage with long-term NIPPV. Experience of NIPPV in this group of patients is poor. Infants with hypoplastic lungs may be candidates for long-term mechanical ventilation but, because of their age and poor prognosis, they are most often ventilated with a tracheostomy.

Chest wall abnormalities such as severe scoliosis, kyphosis, or thoracic dystrophy are among the chest wall abnormalities that may cause restrictive disease severe enough to require long-term NIPPV.[16] The prognosis of these children depends on the severity, type, and evolution of the disease. In some children, the chest wall abnormalities will cause progressive restrictive pulmonary disease, ultimately resulting in death even with mechanical ventilation. Other children appear to improve clinically, even in the absence of changes in the chest wall anomaly, due to a certain degree of catch-up because of the physiologic growth.

## Disorders Characterized by a Failure of the Neurologic Control of Ventilation

Disorders of neurologic control of breathing that are severe enough to cause chronic respiratory failure are uncommon to rare. Congenital central hypoventilation syndrome (Ondine's curse) is the most common presentation in childhood and is characterized by failure of autonomic control of breathing.[26] Hypoxia and hypercapnia worsen during sleep. NIPPV has been tried in older children who sustain adequate ventilation during wakefulness but require ventilatory assistance only during sleep.[27–29] Failure of NIPPV requires ventilatory support via a tracheostomy.

A recent study reported the experience with domiciliary NIPPV in children in France.[30] An anonymous cross-sectional national study was performed using a postal questionnaire sent to all specialist centers using domiciliary NIPPV for chronic respiratory failure. Patients aged younger than18 years and receiving long-term home NIPPV were included in the study. Detailed information was obtained from 102 patients from 15 centers; 4 of 15 centers cared for 84% of patients. Seven percent of patients were less than 3 years old, 35% were between 4 and 11 years, and 58% were older than 12 years. Underlying diagnoses included neuromuscular disease (34%), OSA and/or craniofacial abnormalities (30%), cystic fibrosis (17%), congenital hypoventilation (9%), scoliosis (8%), and other disorders (2%) (Fig. 49.2). NIPPV was started because of nocturnal hypoventilation (67%), acute exacerbation (28%), and/or a failure to thrive (21%). This observational study showed the relative low number of pediatric patients receiving home NIPPV in a country with a great experience in this technique, supporting the fact that this technique is probably underused in this age group.

## CRITERIA TO INITIATE NIPPV

The best accepted indication for NIPPV is diurnal hypercapnia.[6] NIPPV is also indicated when acute exacerbations caused by bronchitis or pneumonia precipitate the patient in acute respiratory failure.[6] Ideally, however, NIPPV should be initiated before an acute exacerbation, which does not represent an optimal physiologic and psychologic situation to start such a treatment. There is

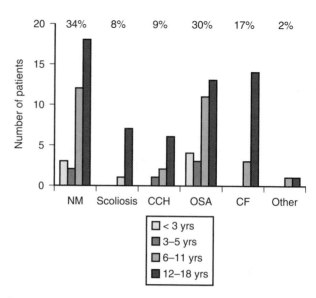

**Figure 49.2** Diagnostic categories of the 102 children (<18 years) on long-term domiciliary, noninvasive mechanical ventilation in France in 2001 (CCH, congenital central hypoventilation; CF, cystic fibrosis; NM, neuromuscular disease; OSA, obstructive sleep apnea; other, other diagnoses). (From Fauroux B, Boffa C, Desguerre I, et al: Long-term noninvasive mechanical ventilation for children at home: A national survey. Pediatr Pulmonol 2003;35:119–125.)

also a wide agreement to consider that clinical symptoms attributable to nocturnal hypoventilation such as sleep disruption, daytime hypersomnolence, excessive fatigue, and morning headache are most important for the decision of NIPPV. They warrant a polysomnographic sleep study to document nocturnal hypoventilation. In addition, when NIPPV is decided, its effect on diurnal $Paco_2$, sleep, growth, and neuropsychologic development such as improvements in alertness, attention/concentration, and behavior/temperament are crucial factors in children that should merit further investigation.[31,32]

Current guidelines have been published, but precise criteria for starting NIPPV are only available for patients with Duchenne myopathy.[4,5] A recent study suggested that arterial blood gases should be performed in patients with Duchenne myopathy when $FEV_1$ falls below 40% of the predicted value and that polysomnography should be considered when $Paco_2 = 45$ mm Hg.[31] $Paco_2$ correlated inversely with survival,[33] and ventilatory support should be considered in Duchenne myopathy when daytime $Paco_2$ exceeds 6.0 kPa (45 mm Hg).[5] NIPPV administered during sleep is associated with a decrease in awake $Paco_2$ despite a further decline in ventilatory capacity (VC).[31] Raphaël and co-workers have demonstrated, in a randomized trial of 70 cases of NIPPV in Duchenne muscular dystrophy (mean age, 15.5 years) free of daytime respiratory failure and a VC between 20%

and 50% of predicted values, that this preventive NIPPV did not improve respiratory handicap and reduced survival of these patients.[34] Thus it appears reasonable to consider NIPPV in Duchenne muscular dystrophy only when patients develop daytime hypercapnia or symptomatic nocturnal hypercapnia.[5] The average age for developing ventilatory failure in Duchenne myopathy is approximately 20 years, but in a recent pediatric series, the average age at which NIPPV was started was 13.9 years.[16] The severity of the respiratory involvement can thus vary among patients.

For patients with OSA and CF, no guidelines or recommendations have been published. For both groups of patients, diurnal hypercapnia represents a reasonable indication for NIPPV. When diurnal hypercapnia is not present, a sleep study is recommended in case of failure to thrive or excessive fatigue because clinical symptoms of nocturnal hypoventilation can be subtle, especially in infants.

## CONTRAINDICATIONS, SIDE EFFECTS, AND LIMITS OF NIPPV

The general point of view is that NIPPV is preferred over invasive mechanical ventilation as the first therapy of chronic respiratory failure. However, NIPPV is contraindicated in some circumstances[35] (Box 49.1). NIPPV is also contraindicated in cases of recent pneumothorax, which can occur in patients with advanced cystic fibrosis lung disease. In this population, nasal polyps are common and should be treated before the initiating of NIPPV.

Side effects are common. They are caused by the interface and the delivery of a positive pressure. In our experience, skin injury—from transient erythema to permanent skin necrosis due to the nasal mask—has been observed in 53% of the 40 patients during their routine 6-month follow-up in our department. In young children there is also a potential risk of facial deformity, such as facial flattening and maxilla retrusion (Fig. 49.3), caused by the pressure applied by the mask on growing facial structures. These potential side effects justify the systematic follow-up of children receiving NIPPV by a pediatric maxillofacial specialist. Abdominal distension is an uncommon problem that can be lessened by switching to a PS ventilator or decreasing the $V_T$ on a volume-targeted ventilator.[21] One exceptional case of a cerebral air embolism complicating a bilevel PPV has been reported in a 13-year-old boy presenting with post–bone marrow transplant pneumonitis.[36]

NIPPV is not always successful in adequately relieving hypoventilation. One study of 325 ventilated neuromuscular patients observed persistent hypercapnia in more than 20% of the study population.[37] Air leaks have been shown to be an important cause of persistent hypercapnia

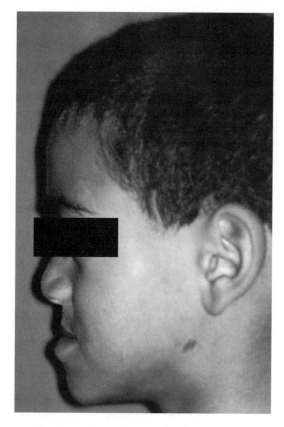

**Figure 49.3** Facial flattening and maxilla retrusion in a 3-year-old after 2.5 years of noninvasive positive pressure ventilation (NIPPV) for severe laryngomalacia. This facial deformity regressed completely 6 months after the withdrawal of NIPPV.

---

**BOX 49-1**

**Contraindications for NIPPV**

**Relative Contraindications**
Severe swallowing impairment
Inadequate family/caregiver support
Need for full-time ventilatory assistance

**Absolute Contraindications**
Upper airway obstruction
Uncontrollable secretion retention
Inability to cooperate
Inability to achieve adequate peak cough flow, even with assistance
Inadequate financial resource
Inability to fit mask

*NIPPV, noninvasive positive pressure ventilation.*
*From Hill NS: Ventilator management for neuromuscular disease. Semin Respir Crit Care Med 2002;23:293–305.*

in both invasively and noninvasively ventilated neuro-muscular patients.[38] In these patients, simple practical measures such as changing the mask, using a chin strap, increasing minute ventilation, and changing the type of ventilator were able to reduce the volume of air leaks and improve the efficacy of ventilation.[38] However, despite these measures, a tracheotomy will become necessary at a certain moment in progressive diseases such as some neuromuscular diseases. Close monitoring of the patient's physiologic status and disease progression, together with clear information from the family, are essential. Technical problems, especially regarding the nasal mask and the ventilator equipment, frequently limit the use of NIPPV in infants. Because noninvasive ventilation leaves airway protection, those patients with copious secretions or severe swallowing dysfunction may respond poorly, requiring the discussion of a tracheostomy with the patient and his or her family.

## VENTILATORY MODES AND INTERFACES FOR CHILDREN

### Ventilatory Modes

The ventilatory mode and the ventilator settings that are most appropriate for each specific condition remain a matter of debate. Moreover, the specific equipment available for therapy evolves more rapidly with industry capability rather than with clear indications available from scientific trials.

Since the original publication by Sullivan and co-workers,[39] nasal continuous positive airway pressure (CPAP) has become the treatment of choice for the treatment of obstructive events during sleep.[21,40] Upper airway patency is maintained with nasal CPAP by a pneumatic splinting effect. In addition, it has been demonstrated that CPAP reduces the work of breathing in patients with flow limitation. In such patients, CPAP overcomes the inspiratory threshold imposed by intrinsic positive end-expiratory pressure (PEEPi) and pneumatically splints the airways to prevent dynamic collapse during exhalation. Thus, if the main indication of CPAP is OSA, it is also advocated in obstructive lung disease, when PEEPi increases the work of breathing. In this way, this ventilatory mode has proved its efficacy in increasing exercise tolerance in patients with CF, with a positive correlation between the efficacy of the CPAP and the severity of the lung disease assessed by the percentage of decrease in $FEV_1$.[41] However, because upper airway loading with complete or partial obstruction and PEEPO are not the sole mechanisms of hypoventilation, CPAP should be insufficient in patients with respiratory function abnormalities.

Volume-targeted ventilation is characterized by the delivery of a fixed, predetermined $V_T$. Thus the main advantage of assist control/volume-targeted (AC/$V_T$) ventilation is that a guaranteed minimal $V_T$ is delivered, but this can result in detrimentally high inspiratory airway pressures, causing discomfort and poor tolerability. Despite the lack of leak compensation mechanisms in many of the volume-targeted ventilators, this mode is suited for patients with neuromuscular diseases where the ventilator acts as a substitute for the weakened respiratory muscles, which are unable to trigger the ventilator. However, a relatively high back-up rate (2 to 3 breaths lower than the spontaneous respiratory rate of the patient) is required to avoid nocturnal desaturations, and consequently many patients adopt a controlled mode without triggering the ventilator. Also, the inspiratory triggers of these ventilators are not very sensitive, which is another factor justifying the use of a relatively high back-up rate.[42] The recommendation of a high back-up rate is also supported by the fact that on most of the ventilators, the inspiratory/expiratory ratio is adjusted based on the back-up rate of the ventilator and not on the patient's respiratory rate. Initial studies with long-term NIPPV in children with neuromuscular disease and CF have used volume-targeted devices.[43,44] The generally recommended settings are a $V_T$ of 10 to 15 mL/kg and a frequency that is 2 or 3 rates below the spontaneous breathing rate of the child.[6] These ventilators, which are designed for home use, are relatively portable. They are not as technologically sophisticated as hospital ventilators. Another limitation of AC/$V_T$ devices is that when infants and children acquire super-added infection, these ventilators may not be able to adequately ventilate the child. Furthermore, few of them are capable to operate within certain limits (i.e., $V_T < 50$ to 100 mL).

Pressure support (PS) is a more recent mode of ventilation. This ventilatory mode is pressure-targeted, and each breath is triggered and terminated by the patient and supported by the ventilator; the patient can control his or her respiratory rate, inspiratory duration (TI), and $V_T$.[45] This explains the relative ease in adapting to and the greater comfort and synchrony of this mode. In contrast to volume-targeted ventilation, in this mode $V_T$ is not predetermined but depends on the level of PS, the inspiratory effort of the patient, and the mechanical properties of the patient's respiratory system. During this mode, because there are no mandatory breaths present, a built-in, low-frequency back-up rate is used to prevent episodes of apnea. Furthermore, because the breaths are triggered by the patient, the sensitivity of the trigger is crucial. The sensitivity of the inspiratory triggers of the different ventilators designed for the home is variable, but some are as sensitive as those of intensive care devices.[46] Because inspiratory muscle activity may influence respiratory frequency and VT during PS, this ventilatory mode is generally proposed in patients who can breathe spontaneously for substantial periods of time and require mainly nocturnal ventilation.

Bilevel PPV is the combination of PS and PEEP, permitting an independent adjustment of expiratory positive airway pressure (EPAP) and inspiratory positive airway pressure (IPAP). In this condition, upper airway obstruction and/or the work of breathing induced by PEEPi is prevented by EPAP, and thus PS can be triggered easily by the patient. This ventilatory mode has been used in children with OSA, CF,[47,48] and neuromuscular disease.[19,47,49]

Proportional assist ventilation (PAV) is a patient-guided mode of synchronized partial assistance in which the ventilator pressure output is proportional to the instantaneous effort of the patient. In this mode, there is thus automatic synchrony between the patient's effort and the ventilator cycle. With PAV, the level of pressure delivered to the patient increases and decreases according to the demand of the patient, so responsibility for the level and pattern of ventilatory assistance depends entirely upon the patient. A short-term, noninvasive study reported a physiologic and symptomatic improvement with PS and PAV in adult patients with CF.[50] However, despite a relative long experience with this mode, its use in practice remains sparse.

## Ventilatory Mode Preferences According to the Disorder

CPAP represents the most simple and classical ventilatory mode for patients with OSA,[21,40,51] but bilevel PS has been used in older children.[7] These modes have not been compared in pediatric patients, either with regard to the physiologic advantages or to the long-term outcome. However, a recent physiologic study demonstrated that the trigger systems of the bilevel PS ventilators available for the home are insufficiently sensitive for young infants, with important patient-ventilator dyssynchrony during bilevel PS ventilation.[52] In these very young patients, CPAP thus remains the preferred mode.

In patients with neuromuscular disease, volume-targeted ventilators, used in the assist-controlled mode, predominate. This seems logical due to the respiratory muscle weakness and the low VT in these patients. This mode was the first mode used for NIPPV and proved to be very efficient.[53] CPAP has been used initially in some patients with Duchenne myopathy in whom obstructive apneas and hypopneas precede or accompany nocturnal hypoventilation[16,54] and in whom PaCO2 remains within the normal range. However, careful $CO_2$ monitoring is required in order to switch to another ventilatory mode in case of nocturnal hypercapnia. PS or bilevel PS ventilation can then be used, but AC/VT ventilation offers the best security because of the guarantee of a minimal VT and minute ventilation in the absence of leaks.

All the different ventilatory modes have been used in patients with CF. Volume-targeted devices were used initially,[43,44] but in actuality PS and bilevel positive pressure ventilation are used by the majority of the patients because of the better comfort and the security with regard to the inspiratory pressures.[3,8,25,47,55] Several short-term studies demonstrated the benefit of CPAP and bilevel positive pressure ventilation in patients with CF to improve nocturnal hypoventilation[3,25] and exercise tolerance.[41] The efficacy of AC/VT and PS ventilation in reducing the work of breathing (WOB) has been evaluated in 8 children with stable, severe respiratory insufficiency.[8] Eight children (11 to 17 years) were ventilated with PS and AC/VT ventilation in a random order. The two NIPPV sessions significantly improved blood gas variables, and increased VT with no change in respiratory rate. Indices of respiratory effort (PTPes, PTPdi, and WOB) decreased about 60% to 75% during the two modes of NIPPV compared with spontaneous breathing, but in terms of comfort, 6 of the 8 patients preferred the PS to the AC/VT ventilation (Fig. 49.4). A recent short-term physiologic study compared the unloading of the respiratory muscles in 12 adult patients with CF during PS and PAV.[50] The unloading of the respiratory muscles was evaluated on the change in surface diaphragmatic electromyography. On average, both

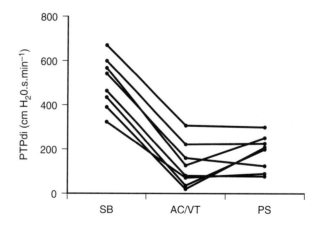

**Figure 49.4** Individual variations of diaphragmatic pressure-time product per minute (PTPdi/min) in 8 patients with cystic fibrosis (11 to 17 years) and chronic respiratory failure (pH, 7.4±0.0; PaO2, 57.5±7.5 mm Hg; PaCO2, 46.1±2.5 mm Hg), during assist control/volume targeted (AC/VT) and pressure support (PS) ventilation, compared with the spontaneous breathing (SB). The two ventilatory modes were associated with a significant reduction in PTPdi/min in all the patients. (See ref. 8)

PS and PAV improved ventilation (+30%), $V_T$ (+30%), and $Ptc_{CO_2}$ (−7%) while reducing diaphragmatic activity (−30% with PS and −20% with PAV). PS remains thus the preferred mode for domiciliary ventilation in these patients because PAV is more difficult to implement and no ventilators delivering PAV are presently available for the home.

NIPPV is preferentially administered during sleep because of the increased risk of alveolar hypoventilation during this period. Moreover, disruption of daily life by NIPPV is less important during nighttime. However, it is also important that NIPPV respects sleep architecture. Indeed, NIPPV is used to improve gas exchange and achieve respiratory muscle rest. To achieve this goal, it is important that the patient does not make respiratory efforts out of synchrony with the cycling of the ventilator. PS predisposes to an abnormal breathing pattern, specifically central apneas with consequent hyperpnea. Unlike PS, $AC/V_T$ ventilation delivers a fixed $V_T$ on every breath and the back-up rate will prevent the development of apneas. A polysomnographic study on 11 critically ill adult patients revealed that sleep fragmentation, measured as the number of arousals and awakenings, was significantly greater during PS than during $AC/V_T$ ventilation ($79\pm7$ versus $54\pm7$ events per hour; $P = .02$).[56] Thus PS can cause hypocapnia, which, combined with the lack of back-up rate and wakefulness drive, can lead to the central apneas and sleep fragmentation. This observation thus justifies a polysomnographic control in every patient who is started on NIPPV.

## Ventilatory Settings

The ventilatory settings should be adjusted to relieve the symptoms associated with alveolar hypoventilation. In clinical practice, these settings are generally adapted according to noninvasive clinical parameters such as $SaO_2$, blood gases, and sleep analysis. The analysis of more invasive parameters of respiratory effort, such as the PTPes and PTPdi, have been rarely used in children.[7,8] We demonstrated a correlation between the unloading of the respiratory muscles evaluated on decrease of the PTPes, PTPdi, and WOB and the subjective impression of comfort during NIPPV in children with CF receiving a PS or $AC/V_T$ ventilation by a nasal mask (8). This observation led us to compare two methods of prescribing noninvasive PS ventilation: a clinical setting ($PS_{Clin}$) based on breathing pattern, gas exchange, and comfort rate, and a physiologic setting ($PS_{Phys}$) based on the maximum decrease in esophageal (Pes) and transdiaphragmatic pressure (Pdi) swings. Both methods improved breathing pattern and $SaO_2$ and reduced diaphragmatic pressure time product per minute, from $398\pm69$ during SB to $71\pm51$ and $72\pm46$ $cmH_2O.s.min^{-1}$ during $PS_{Clin}$ and

$PS_{Phys}$, respectively ($P < .0001$). But patient-ventilator synchrony and patient comfort ($P = .003$) were better during $PS_{Phys}$. In conclusion, in patients with CF, PS ventilation is effective, independent of whether the ventilator settings are determined by the patient's breathing pattern and comfort or by an invasive evaluation of the patient's respiratory effort. Although a standard clinical method to set up the ventilator is satisfactory in the majority of patients with CF, more invasive measurements could improve patient–ventilator synchrony.

For all ventilatory modes, alarms must be correctly set. When positive pressure ventilators are used, low pressure or disconnect alarms are classically present. Alarms for high pressure, incorrect timing, and power failure are also frequently present. The alarm of a minimal $V_T$ is very useful in children. A back-up frequency is generally set on the ventilator. All these alarms must be carefully checked before the home discharge of the patient.

## Interfaces

The necessity of an interface specifically designed for children represents an important technical limitation of NIPPV in pediatric patients. In adults, four different types of interfaces are used: full face masks (enclosing the mouth and nose), nasal masks, nasal pillows or plugs (inserted directly into the nostrils), and mouthpieces. Nasal pillows and plugs are too large for children, and mouthpieces require a good cooperation and are difficult to use in neuromuscular patients. In young children, nasal masks are preferred because they have less static dead space, are less claustrophobic, and allow communication and expectoration more easily than full face masks. However, few industrial masks are available for children. This shortcoming is even more important for infants. Most often, NIPPV is thus restrained to some highly specialized pediatric centers that have the possibility to manufacture custom-made masks for infants and children who cannot use industrial masks (Fig. 49.5).

The nasal interface represents a crucial determinant of the success of NIPPV. The patient will be unable to tolerate and accept NIPPV in case of facial discomfort, skin injury, or significant air leaks. The evaluation of the short-term tolerance of the nasal mask is thus an essential component of NIPPV. Moreover, NIPPV is generally used during sleep, which can represent the major part of the day in young infants. In these young patients, there is thus a potential risk of skin injury and facial deformity, such as facial flattening and maxilla retrusion (Fig. 49.3), caused by the pressure applied by the mask on growing facial structures. These potential side effects justify the systematic follow-up of children receiving NIPPV by a pediatric maxillofacial specialist.

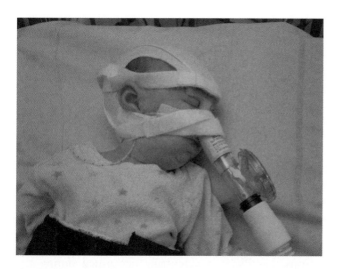

**Figure 49.5** Example of a custom-made mask for a 2-month-old boy who presented with a severe upper airway obstruction due to Pierre Robin syndrome.

## BENEFITS OF NIPPV

### Improvement of Survival

The major benefit of NIPPV is the improved survival, although this has only been demonstrated in patients with neuromuscular diseases. Indeed, a recent study evaluated the effect of NIPPV on the survival of patients with Duchenne muscular dystrophy in Denmark between 1977 and 2001.[57] Although overall incidence remained stable at 2.0 per $10^5$, prevalence rose from 3.1 to 5.5 per $10^5$, mortality fell from 4.7 to 2.6 per 100 years at risk, and the prevalence of ventilator users rose from 0.9 to 43.4 per 100. Ventilator use is probably the main reason for this dramatic increase in survival.

The improvement of survival has not been demonstrated in lung diseases such as CF or in patients with OSA.

### Improvement of Nocturnal Hypoventilation

The effect that is the most obvious in the pediatric population is the correction of nocturnal hypoventilation. During sleep, certain key alterations in respiratory and upper airway function and ventilatory responses lead to a degree of nocturnal hypoventilation even in normal subjects, causing a rise in $PaCO_2$ of upto 3 mm Hg (0.4 kPa) in adults (Fig. 49.6).[58] For example, it has been demonstrated in adolescents that the decrease of minute ventilation during non-rapid eye movement (NREM) sleep was accompanied by a paradoxical increase of inspiratory muscle activity above the waking level, probably due to an increase in upper airway resistance.[59] This may explain why patients with chronic respiratory failure are vulnerable during NREM sleep.

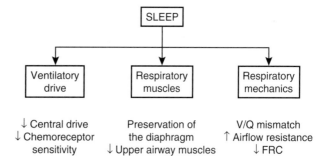

**Figure 49.6** Physiologic alterations during sleep, explaining the worsening or respiratory failure during sleep.

Vulnerability of the respiratory function can also increase during REM sleep in patients with diaphragmatic dysfunction considering that in normal adolescents, ventilation relies heavily on the diaphragm because of a reduced activity of the intercostal muscles.[59] In addition, while diaphragmatic electromyographic activity increases during REM sleep, transdiaphragmatic pressure (Pdi) gradients decrease, indicating a clear decrease in inspiratory efficiency.[60] If this has no clinical significance in healthy subjects, it may explain the considerable hypoventilation during REM sleep observed in some neuromuscular patients such as those with limb girdle dystrophy[61] or Duchenne muscular dystrophy.[33]

Nocturnal respiratory abnormalities can present as two different aspects. First, some children can present with obstructive sleep apnea due to upper airway abnormalities. Obstructive apneas and desaturations will characterize their sleep, with moderate hypercapnia.[21,40] The major role of NIPPV is to maintain a sufficient airway patency during this risky period. On the other hand, the major hallmark of the sleep of children with respiratory muscle weakness is central events such as central alveolar hypoventilation and prolonged central hypopneas or apneas, particularly during REM sleep, leading to marked hypercapnia with moderate or no desaturations. This has been clearly shown recently in adults.[11] In this situation, the role of NIPPV is to maintain sufficient alveolar ventilation.

The efficacy of NIPPV in relieving nocturnal hypoventilation in infants and children with various causes of chronic respiratory insufficiency has been demonstrated in several studies.

Sleep-related disturbances are common in teenagers and adults with Duchenne muscular dystrophy, especially when diurnal arterial hypoxemia is present.[62] In these patients, arterial blood gases should be performed once the $FEV_1$ falls below 40% of the predicted value,[31] and polysomnography should be considered when the $PaCO_2$ = 45 mm Hg, particularly if the base excess = 4 mmol/L. Indeed, survival correlates inversely to $PaCO_2$ and positively with nocturnal $SaO_2$ and VC.[33] NIPPV has been proved to be a very efficient method of correcting nocturnal hypoventilation in these patients because it increases minute ventilation[63] and stabilizes the oropharyngeal airway.[53]

Nasal CPAP has been used by some experienced teams in young children with OSA for nearly 15 years.[51] Therapy with nasal CPAP eliminated the signs of OSA in 90% of the 80 children (mean age, $5.7\pm0.5$ years) in whom this treatment was tried because of the persistence of the symptoms after adenotonsillectomy.[40] We showed also that NIPPV was associated with a significant improvement in nocturnal gas exchange in 12 children with laryngomalacia.[7] Indeed, mean nocturnal pulse oximetry ($SaO_2$) improved significantly from $91.7\pm2.3\%$ before to $96.2\pm2.0\%$ during NIPPV (P = .03). The percentage of nighttime spent with an $SaO_2 < 90\%$ fell from $29.5\pm19.6\%$ before NIPPV to $0.5\pm0.8\%$ while on NIPPV (P = .03). Nasal CPAP has also demonstrated its efficacy in children in facilitating tracheal extubation after laryngotracheal reconstruction.[64]

The benefit of NIPPV in improving nocturnal alveolar hypoventilation has also been demonstrated in patients with CF. These patients have periods of oxyhemoglobin desaturation during sleep that are most marked during REM sleep.[65] A study including 7 adults with CF showed that, compared with a control night without noninvasive CPAP ventilation, CPAP resulted in a significant improvement in $SaO_2$ during both REM and NREM sleep.[65] However, transcutaneous $CO_2$ ($PtcCO_2$) measurements were not significantly different among the control and the CPAP nights. Another interesting study compared the gas exchange and the quality of sleep in adults with CF during 3 nights, a control night, a night with oxygen, and a night with NIPPV.[3] Similar significant improvements of $SaO_2$ and time spent in REM sleep were observed during the nights with oxygen and NIPPV. But most importantly, the night with oxygen was associated with a significant increase in $PtcCO_2$, whereas NIPPV resulted in a significant decrease in $PtcCO_2$. A third study showed that noninvasive bilevel positive airway pressure ventilation was able to maintain a sufficient $V_T$ and thus a minute ventilation during sleep, whereas this was not observed during a control night, with or without oxygen.[25] A major limitation of these studies is their duration, as only 2 or 3 consecutive nights were compared. Further studies that confirm these results on a long-term basis in different diagnostic groups are clearly needed.

This improvement of nocturnal alveolar hypoventilation by NIPPV translates to a decrease of diurnal hypercapnia. This has been demonstrated in adults with OSA as early as 48 hours following the institution of CPAP therapy.[66] Annane and co-workers found that the improvement in diurnal $PaCO_2$ due to nocturnal NIPPV correlated with the improvement in the slope of the ventilatory response to $CO_2$ in patients with neuromuscular disease and chest wall deformity.[67] The benefits of NIPPV may be due to combined effects of several interrelated processes. The increase in respiratory drive is probably due to a reduction in cerebrospinal fluid bicarbonate concentration, which resets the ventilatory response to $CO_2$, and to an improvement in sleep quality, which influences the ventilatory response to $CO_2$ and respiratory muscle endurance.[68] In addition, NIPPV may be responsible for a persistent decrease in WOB during spontaneous ventilation after the periods of NIPPV as a result of an increase in chest wall and lung compliance due to the increase in respiratory movements during NIPPV.

Because sleep is an at-risk period in patients with chronic respiratory insufficiency, and also for practical reasons, NIPPV is preferentially performed during the night, but daytime mechanical ventilation in awake adult patients was reported to be as effective in reversing chronic hypercapnia as nocturnal mechanical ventilation.[69]

## Improvement in Respiratory Muscle Performance

NIPPV has been associated with an improvement in respiratory muscle performance in patients with CF. Piper and co-workers reported an increase in maximal expiratory (PEmax) and inspiratory pressure (PImax) in 4 adults with CF after 1 month of NIPPV.[70] However, improvement due to a learning effect or a better motivation cannot be excluded because of the volitional nature of these tests. We have observed a significant decrease in PImax and PEmax in 19 children with CF after a 20-minute physiotherapy session.[71] When the physiotherapy session was performed with PS ventilation administered by a nasal mask, a significant increase of these parameters was observed. The improvement of PImax after the PS session suggests that PS may "rest" the inspiratory muscles during chest physiotherapy. The improvement of PEmax after the PS ventilation session could be explained by the increase in $V_T$ during this ventilatory assistance. During PS, the $V_T$ tends to the total lung capacity. This allows a larger amount of energy to accumulate, thereby facilitating expiration and decreasing the work of the expiratory muscles. This beneficial effect of NIPPV on the respiratory muscles has not been demonstrated in other pediatric diseases.

## Improvement in Exercise Tolerance

Noninvasive CPAP ventilation has been associated with an improvement in exercise tolerance in 33 patients with cystic fibrosis.[41] Indeed, a 5-$cmH_2O$ CPAP ventilation resulted in decreases in oxygen consumption, respiratory effort assessed by Pdi, and dyspnea score. These beneficial effects during exercise were the most important in patients with severe lung disease in whom the positive end-expiratory pressure (PEEPi) is favorably counteracted by the CPAP.

## Faster Recovery of an Acute Exacerbation

Very few studies on NIPPV in the intensive care beyond the neonatal period have been performed in children. Noninvasive bilevel PPV was effective in improving gas exchange in 28 children (mean age, 8 years) admitted to the pediatric intensive care unit (ICU) for an acute hypoxemic respiratory failure.[72] The most common primary diagnosis was pneumonia. NIPPV was associated with a rapid (within 1 hour) improvement in respiratory rate and gas exchange. Only 3 of the 28 patients required an intubation, which demonstrates the interest of this technique in patients with an acute hypoxemic respiratory failure in whom the underlying condition warrants avoidance of intubation. Two children, aged 12 years, were successfully managed with bilevel NIPPV for an acute pulmonary edema.[73]

NIPPV is also classically used for acute exacerbations in patients with neuromuscular disease. For most groups, such a severe respiratory event represents an indication to start long-term home NIPPV.[16]

Few studies have analyzed the benefits of NIPPV in patients with CF. Bilevel PAP ventilation was successfully used in 9 adult patients with end-stage CF.[48] Respiratory status improved rapidly, with inspiratory (IPAP) and expiratory airway pressures (EPAP) of 14 to 18 cmH$_2$O and 4 to 8 cmH$_2$O for IPAP and EPAP, respectively. All the patients survived the ICU stay, and 6 underwent successful lung transplantation. The outcome of 76 patients with CF who had 136 ICU admissions for a respiratory exacerbation was reported by Sood and co-workers.[74] Eighteen episodes occurring in 12 patients were managed with NIPPV. During these 18 episodes, 4 patients died and 14 survived, which represented a better outcome than those who required endotracheal ventilation. However, this difference in outcome is explained by the difference in severity between the two groups.

## Change in Pulmonary Mechanics

The physiologic changes in the compliance of the lungs and the chest wall play a crucial role in the normal development of the lung. In infancy, the chest wall is nearly three times as compliant as the lung.[75] By the end of the second year of life, chest wall stiffness increases to the point that the chest wall and lung are nearly equally compliant, as in adulthood. Stiffening of the chest wall plays a major role in developmental changes in respiratory system function, such as the ability to passively maintain resting lung volume and improved ventilatory efficiency afforded by reduced rib cage distortion. An important point would be to know whether long-term

NIPPV in infants and young children can preserve a nearly normal chest wall compliance, both in children with a too-stiff chest (e.g., due to chest deformity) and those with neuromuscular disease, who are exposed to ankylosis in the costosternal and costovertebral joints and to gradual stiffening of the rib cage because of breathing at smaller V$_T$ and greater respiratory frequency.

Chronic hypoventilation can alter the dynamic or static compliance of the lung. The majority of observations in patients with neuromuscular disease have shown a significant reduction in pulmonary compliance. The measurements of these patients were of dynamic compliance, reflecting abnormalities in airways rather than a true change in the elastic properties of the lungs. Specific compliance, relating static expiratory compliance to total lung capacity, is normal in patients with respiratory muscle weakness. Atelectasis could explain the hypoxemia due to the ventilation–perfusion mismatching.

A major concern in pediatric patients is the effect of chronic hypoventilation on lung growth, and, as a logical consequence, the effect of NIPPV in promoting or preserving physiologic lung and chest wall growth in the developing child. To our knowledge, this has not been studied in children.

## Effect of NIPPV on Quality of Life

Every "new" long-term treatment should be associated with a significant improvement of quality of life in patients with a chronic disease. Most surprisingly, very few studies have evaluated the effect of NIPPV on quality of life. A recent French study evaluated the social and psychologic impact of invasive and noninvasive home mechanical ventilation in 52 adult patients (mean age, 25±5 years) with Duchenne muscular dystrophy. Although the patient group was not compared with a control group, the self-estimated quality of life of these patients was good and was higher than expected by the health care givers. In pediatric patients, the impact of NIPPV on the quality of life and organization of the family is also an important aspect. Such studies are clearly warranted in the future.

## ORGANIZATION OF HOME CARE

### Requisites for Home Care

The major advantage of NIPPV is that it can be applied at home, combining greater potential for psychosocial development and family function with lower cost. The use of home NIPPV requires appropriate diagnostic procedures, appropriate titration of the ventilator, cooperative and educated families, and a careful, well-organized follow-up. Prior to discharge, the patient's respiratory status should be stable on the actual ventilator and circuit the child will use at home, at least for several days. The settings on a home ventilator do not provide the same ventilation in the child as the same settings on a hospital ventilator, and the efficacy of home equipment must be evaluated in each child prior to discharge.

Once the child is at home and as the child grows, ventilator settings must be evaluated to ensure adequate gas exchange ($SaO_2$, $PtcO_2$, and $PtcCO_2$) on a regular basis. Although the optimal frequency for these evaluations has not been determined, these evaluations generally should be performed more frequently in infants and small children with rapid growth. Polysomnographic evaluations are recommended as a diagnostic tool before the initiating of NIPPV, then as a control test of the efficacy of NIPPV before discharge with the ventilator, and finally as a surveillance test during an overnight hospital admission during the follow-up. Careful extrapolation should be made from a polysomnographic evaluation performed during daytime naps because such naps do not always reflect what happens during the night.

Routine and emergency service must be available. Providers or home care equipment technicians and nurses should make home visits at least every month to perform preventive maintenance and checks on ventilator function. $V_T$ rate, oxygen concentration (if necessary), pressures, and alarms should be calibrated and their function checked. Evaluation of compliance should be systematically checked by counters on the equipment to determine the amount of time the ventilator is effectively used and not merely turned on.

## Additional Therapies

### Oxygen Therapy

Oxygen therapy at home must be justified on the basis of an individual-based medical necessity, as determined by appropriate physiologic monitoring, such as $SaO_2$ during periods of sleep, wakefulness, feeding and physical activity, and arterial blood gases. $CO_2$ should be minimized first by ventilator use before considering oxygen therapy, especially for patients with neuromuscular disorders and OSA. It is important to remember that supplemental oxygen is *not* a replacement for assisted ventilation in patients who hypoventilate.

### Humidification

Systematic humidification of the ventilator gas is not necessary for NIPPV because of the respect of the upper airway. However, nasal intolerance due to excessive dryness can resolve after humidification of the ventilator gas.

### Nutritional Support

Children are frequently undernourished when starting NIPPV. Adequate nutrition is critical for growth and development of the lungs and the chest wall. Nutritional support, via a nasogastric tube, is frequently necessary during the first weeks or months. This can be performed by fashioning a port in a custom-made nasal mask if gastrostomy feeding is not planned. In infants, discoordination of swallowing mechanisms is common, and swallowing function should be evaluated to assess pulmonary aspiration risks. Many patients have also associated gastroesophageal reflux, which may require surgical correction. This can be combined with a gastrostomy if necessary.

## Psychologic Considerations

It is essential that the child (age permitting) and the parents have the opportunity to discuss the NIPPV therapy in advance. Discussion should start far enough before the anticipated need to allow the child and the family to evaluate options thoroughly and to discuss their feelings. NIPPV has here an essential first place as a noninvasive therapy but still represents an objective element that reflects a further step in the severity of a disease. It is crucial to determine short-term and intermediate-term goals of NIPPV with the child and the family in order to explain the principles of NIPPV and to underline the fact that NIPPV will adapt to the child and vice versa. A wide range of ventilators and masks are available, and great care will be taken to choose the most appropriate equipment and settings. The final objective is that NIPPV translates into well-being and a better quality of life, with a total adherence of the child and his or her family.

In conclusion, NIPPV is increasingly used in children and infants. Unfortunately, in this age group, this therapy is generally used on an empiric basis. Pediatricians, physiologists, nurses, physiotherapists, and technicians should combine their efforts to determine more accurately the physiologic effects of NIPPV, especially on the respiratory muscles, the respiratory compliance and growth, and the central drive; the appropriate timing of initiating; and most importantly, the benefits in terms of psychoneurologic development and quality of life.

## REFERENCES

1. Masa J, Celli B, Riesco J, et al: Noninvasive positive pressure ventilation and not oxygen may prevent overt ventilatory failure in patients with chest wall disease. Chest 1997;112:207–213.
2. Gay P, Edmonds L: Severe hypercapnia after low-flow oxygen therapy in patients with neuromuscular disease and diaphragmatic dysfunction. Mayo Clin Proc 1995;70:327–330.
3. Gozal D: Nocturnal ventilatory support in patients with cystic fibrosis: Comparison with supplemental oxygen. Eur Resp J 1997;10:1999–2003.
4. Robert D, Willig TN, Paulus J: Long-term nasal ventilation in neuromuscular disorders: Report of a Consensus Conference. Eur Respir J 1993;6:599–606.

5. Rutgers M, Lucassen H, Kesteren RV, et al: Respiratory insufficiency and ventilatory support. 39th European Neuromuscular Centre International workshop. Neuromusc Disord 1996;6:431–435.

6. Management of pediatric patients requiring long-term ventilation. Chest 1998;113:322S–336S.

7. Fauroux B, Pigeot J, Polkey MI, et al: Chronic stridor caused by laryngomalacia in children. Work of breathing and effects of noninvasive ventilatory assistance. Am J Respir Crit Care Med 2001;164:1874–1878.

8. Fauroux B, Pigeot J, Polkey MI, Isabey D, Clément A, Lofaso F: In vivo physiologic comparison of two ventilators used for domiciliary ventilation in children with cystic fibrosis. Crit Care Med 2001;29(11):2097–2105.

9. Keens TG, Bryan AC, Levison H, et al: Developmental pattern of muscle fiber types in human ventilatory muscles. J Appl Physiol 1978;44:909–913.

10. Scott CB, Nickerson BG, Sargent CW, et al: Developmental pattern of maximal transdiaphragmatic pressure in infants during crying. Pediatr Res 1983;17:707–709.

11. Misuri G, Lannini B, Gigliotti F, et al: Mechanism of $CO_2$ retention in patients with neuromuscular disease. Chest 2000;117:447–453.

12. Innaccone ST: Spinal muscular atrophy. Semin Neurol 1998;18:19–26.

13. Bach JR, Niranjan V: Spinal muscular atrophy type I: A noninvasive respiratory management approach. Chest 2000;117:1100–1105.

14. Bach JR, Baird JS, Plosky D, et al: Spinal muscular atrophy type 1: Management and outcomes. Pediatr Pulmonol 2002;34:16–22.

15. Simonds A, Ward S, Heather S, et al: Outcome of domiciliary nocturnal non-invasive mask ventilation in paediatric neuromuscul-skeletal disease. Thorax 1998;53:A10.

16. Simonds AK, Ward S, Heather S, et al: Outcome of paediatric domiciliary mask ventilation in neuromuscular and skeletal disease. Eur Respir J 2000;16:476–481.

17. Vianello A, Bevilacqua M, Salvador V, et al: Long-term nasal intermittent positive pressure ventilation in advanced Duchenne's muscular dystrophy. Chest 1994;105:445–448.

18. Simonds A, Muntoni F, Heather S, et al: Impact of nasal ventilation on survival in hypercapnic Duchenne muscular dystrophy. Thorax 1998;53:949–952.

19. Robertson PL, Roloff DW: Chronic respiratory failure in limb-girdle muscular dystrophy: Successful long-term therapy with nasal bilevel positive airway pressure. Pediatr Neurol 1994;10:328–331.

20. Croft CB, Brockbank MJ, Wright A, et al: Obstructive sleep apnea in children undergoing routine tonsillectomy and adenoidectomy. Clin Otolaryngol 1990;15:307–314.

21. Guilleminault C, Pelayo R, Clerk A, et al: Home nasal continuous positive airway pressure in infants with sleep-disordered breathing. J Pediatr 1995;127:905–912.

22. Mogayzel PJ, Carroll JL, Loughlin GM, et al: Sleep-disordered breathing in children with achondroplasia. J Pediatr 1998;131:667–671.

23. Waters KA, Everett F, Sillence DO, et al: Treatment of obstructive sleep apnea in achondroplasia: Evaluation of sleep, breathing, and somatosensory-evoked potentials. Am J Med Genet 1995;59:460–466.

24. Hart N, Polkey MI, Clément A, et al: Changes in pulmonary mechanics with increasing disease severity in children and young adults with cystic fibrosis. Am J Respir Crit Care Med 2002;166:61–66.

25. Milross MA, Piper AJ, Norman M, et al: Low-flow oxygen and bilevel ventilatory support. Effects on ventilation during sleep in cystic fibrosis. Am J Respir Crit Care Med 2001;163:129–134.

26. Gozal D: Congenital central hypoventilation syndrome: An update. Pediatr Pulmonol 1998;26:273–282.

27. Ellis ER, McCauley VB, Mellis C, et al: Treatment of alveolar hypoventilation in a six-year-old girl with intermittent positive pressure ventilation through a nose mask. Am Rev Resp Dis 1987;136:188–191.

28. Nielson DW, Black PG: Mask ventilation in congenital central alveolar hypoventilation syndrome. Pediatr Pulmonol 1990;9:44–45.

29. Zaccaria S, Braghiroli A, Sacco C, et al: Central hypoventilation in a seven year old boy. Long-term treatment by nasal mask ventilation. Monaldi Arch Chest Dis 1993;48:37–38.

30. Fauroux B, Boffa C, Desguerre I, et al: Long-term noninvasive mechanical ventilation for children at home: A national survey. Pediatr Pulmonol 2003;35:119–125.

31. Hukins CA, Hillman DR: Daytime predictors of sleep hypoventilation in Duchenne muscular dystrophy. Am J Respir Crit Care Med 2000;161:166–170.

32. Rains JC: Treatment of obstructive sleep apnea in pediatric patients. Clin Pediatr 1995;34:535–541.

33. Phillips M, Smith P, Carrol N, et al: Nocturnal oxygenation and prognosis in Duchenne muscular dystrophy. Am J Respir Crit Care Med 1999;160:198–202.

34. Raphael J, Chevret S, Chastang C, et al: Randomised trial of preventive nasal ventilation in Duchenne muscular dystrophy. Lancet 1994;343:1600–1604.

35. Hill NS: Ventilator management for neuromuscular disease. Semin Respir Crit Care Med 2002;23:293–305.

36. Hung SC, Hsu HC, Chang SC: Cerebral air embolism complicating bilevel positive airway pressure therapy. Eur Resp J 1998;12:235–237.

37. Sharshar T, Chevret S, Fitting JW, et al: Ventilation à domicile (VAD) dans les pathologies neuromusculaires: Une étude prospective et multicentrique de cohorte. Reanimation Soins Intensifs Medecine Urgence 2000;9:88.

38. Gonzalez J, Sharshar T, Hart N, et al: Air leak during mechanical ventilation as a cause of persistent hypercapnia in neuromuscular disorders. Intensive Care Med 2003;29:596–602.

39. Sullivan CE, Issa FG, Berthon-Jones M, et al: Reversal of obstructive sleep apnea by continuous positive airway pressure applied through the nares. Lancet 1981;1:862–865.

40. Waters WA, Everett FM, Bruderer JW, et al: Obstructive sleep apnea: The use of nasal CPAP in 80 children. Am J Respir Crit Care Med 1995;152:780–785.

41. Henke KG, Regnis JA, Bye PTP: Benefits of continuous positive airway pressure during exercise in cystic fibrosis and relationship to disease severity. Am Rev Resp Dis 1993;148:1272–1276.

42. Fauroux B, Louis B, Hart N, et al: The effect of back-up rate during non-invasive ventilation in young patients with cystic fibrosis. Intensive Care Med 2004;30:673–681.

43. Hodson ME, Madden BP, Steven MH, et al: Non-invasive mechanical ventilation for cystic fibrosis patients—a potential bridge to transplantation. Eur Resp J 1991;4:524–527.

44. Bellon G, Mounier M, Guidicelli J, et al: Nasal intermittent positive ventilation in cystic fibrosis. Eur Resp J 1992;2:357–359.

45. Brochard L, Pluskwa F, Lemaire F: Improved efficacy of spontaneous breathing with inspiratory pressure support. Am Rev Resp Dis 1987;136:411–415.

46. Lofaso F, Brochard L, Hang T, et al: Home versus intensive care pressure support devices. Experimental and clinical comparison. Am J Respir Crit Care Med 1996;153:1591–1599.

47. Padman R, Lawless S, Von Nessen S: Use of BiPAP by nasal mask in the treatment of respiratory insufficiency in pediatric

patients: Preliminary investigation. Pediatr Pulmonol 1994;17:119–123.

48. Caronia CG, Silver P, Nimkoff L, et al: Use of bilevel positive airway pressure (BIPAP) in end-stage patients with cystic fibrosis awaiting lung transplantation. Clin Pediatr 1998;37:555–559.

49. Guilleminault C, Philip P, Robinson A: Sleep and neuromuscular disease: Bilevel positive airway pressure by nasal mask as a treatment for sleep disordered breathing in patients with neuromuscular disease. J Neurol Neurosurg Psychiatr 1998;65:225–232.

50. Serra A, Polese G, Braggion C, et al: Non-invasive proportional assist and pressure support ventilation in patients with cystic fibrosis and chronic respiratory failure. Thorax 2002;57:50–54.

51. Guilleminault C, Nino-Murcia G, Heldt G, et al: Alternative treatment to tracheostomy in obstructive sleep apnea syndrome: Nasal continuous positive airway pressure in young children. Pediatrics 1986;78:797–802.

52. Essouri S, Nicot F, Clément A, Garabedian EN, Roger G, Lofaso F, Fauroux B: Noninvasive positive pressure ventilation in infants with upper airway obstruction: Comparison of continous and bilevel positive pressure. Intensive Care Med 2005;31(4)574–580.

53. Ellis ER, Bye PTP, Bruderer JW, et al: Treatment of respiratory failure during sleep in patients with neuromuscular disease. Positive-pressure ventilation through a nasal mask. Am Rev Respir Dis 1987;135:148–152.

54. Khan Y, Heckmatt JZ: Obstructive apnoeas in Duchenne muscular dystrophy. Thorax 1994;49:157–161.

55. Padman R, Nadkarni VM, Von Nessen S, et al: Noninvasive positive pressure ventilation in end-stage cystic fibrosis: A report of seven cases. Respir Care 1994;39:736–739.

56. Parthasarathy S, Tobin MJ: Effect of ventilator mode on sleep quality in critically ill patients. Am J Respir Crit Care Med 2002;166:1423–1429.

57. Jeppesen J, Green A, Steffensen BF, et al: The Duchenne muscular dystrophy population in Denmark, 1977-2001: Prevalence, incidence and survival in relation to the introduction of ventilator use. Neuromuscular Disorders 2003;13:804–812.

58. Gothe B, Altose MD, Goldman MD, et al: Effect of quiet sleep on resting and $CO_2$ stimulated breathing in humans. J Appl Physiol 1981;50:724–730.

59. Tabachnik E, Muller NL, Bryan AC, et al: Changes in ventilation and chest wall mechanics during sleep in normal adolescents. J Appl Physiol 1981;51:557–564.

60. Lopes J, Tabachnik E, Muller N, et al: Total airway resistance and respiratory muscle activity during sleep. J Appl Physiol 1983;54:773–777.

61. Skatrud J, Iber C, McHugh W, et al: Determinants of hypoventilation during wakefulness and sleep in diaphragmatic paralysis. Am Rev Resp Dis 1980;121:587–593.

62. Barbé F, Quera-Salva MA, McCann C, et al: Sleep-related respiratory disturbances in patients with Duchenne muscular dystrophy. Eur Respir J 1994;7:1403–1408.

63. Heckmatt JZ, Loh L, Dubowitz V: Night-time nasal ventilation in neuromuscular disease. Lancet 1990;335:579–582.

64. Hertzog JH, Siegel LB, Hauser GJ, et al: Noninvasive positive-pressure ventilation facilitates tracheal extubation after laryngotracheal reconstruction in children. Chest 1999;116:260–263.

65. Regnis JA, Piper AJ, Henke KG, et al: Benefits of nocturnal nasal CPAP in patients with cystic fibrosis. Chest 1994;106:1717–1724.

66. Berthon-Jones M, Sullivan CE: Time course of change in ventilatory response to $CO_2$ with long-term CPAP therapy for obstructive sleep apnea. Am Rev Resp Dis 1987;135:144–147.

67. Annane D, Quera-Silva MA, Lofaso F, et al: Mechanisms underlying effects of nocturnal ventilation on daytime blood gases in neuromuscular disease. Eur Respir J 1999;13: 157–162.

68. White D, Douglas N, Pickett C, et al: Sleep deprivation and the control of ventilation. Am Rev Respir Dis 1983;128: 984–986.

69. Schönhofer B, Geibel M, Sonneborn M, et al: Daytime mechanical ventilation in chronic respiratory insufficiency. Eur Resp J 1997;10:2840–2846.

70. Piper AJ, Parker S, Torzillo PJ, et al: Nocturnal nasal IPPV stabilizes patients with cystic fibrosis and hypercapnic respiratory failure. Chest 1992;102:846–850.

71. Fauroux B, Boulé M, Lofaso F, et al: Chest physiotherapy in cystic fibrosis: Improved tolerance with nasal pressure support ventilation. Pediatrics 1999;103:e32–e40.

72. Fortenberry JD, Del Toro J, Jefferson LS, et al: Management of pediatric acute hypoxemic respiratory insufficiency with bilevel positive pressure (BiPAP) nasal mask ventilation. Chest 1995;108:1059–1064.

73. Akingbola OA, Servant GM, Custer JR, et al: Noninvasive bi-level positive pressure ventilation: Managment of two pediatric patients. Resp Care 1993;38:1092–1098.

74. Sood N, Paradowski LJ, Yankaskas JR: Outcomes of intensive care unit care in adults with cystic fibrosis. Am J Respir Crit Care Med 2001;163:335–338.

75. Papastamelos C, Panitch HB, England SE, et al: Developmental changes in chest wall compliance in infancy and early childhood. J Appl Physiol 1995;78:179–184.

# SECTION 10

## ETHICAL AND ECONOMIC ISSUES

# CHAPTER 50

# Ethical Issues in the Termination of Ventilator Treatment

Jens Ingemann Jensen

The decision to terminate or to not initiate life support can be one of the most difficult and challenging that a physician makes; it conflicts with every physician's desire to preserve life and to do more good than harm as expressed in the Hippocratic oath. Thus, to assist physicians, the bodies governing medicine, and the public, The American College of Chest Physicians (ACCP) and the Society of Critical Care Medicine (SCCM) published one set of guidelines in 1990,[1] and the American Thoracic Society (ATS) published their guidelines in 1991.[2] Outside of the United States, similar guidelines have been established (f.ex).[3] However, the continuing medical progress as well as demographic, social, and cultural changes keep this problem ever more challenging, and thus the debate continues.

The question of whether to terminate life support arises when intensive care appears to have reached an impasse—when there is no apparent change in the situation of the patient for a certain period. Life supportive treatment can also be considered to have failed if the worsening cannot be reversed.

The decision to terminate ventilatory support in the patient with pulmonary or ventilatory failure naturally takes place in the intensive care unit (ICU). Therefore the intensivist becomes the central person, not only as the initiator of the decision-making process but also as the decision maker, either alone or with input from other specialists. On the other hand, the decision not to initiate life supportive therapy will most often be made outside the ICU. Physicians from other specialties will therefore in these situations often initiate the process. In most cases, however, input from the intensivist will be sought due to his or her experience and expertise, and he or she often provides *the* decisive input. Thus, even if the intensivist is generally the central person in making the decision, doctors in many specialties cannot escape having to deal with the problem, either alone or (more often) together with colleagues from within their own specialty or as part of a multispecialty group.

Many factors have contributed to the increase in the difficulties and challenges. One factor is the steady emergence of new therapeutic options for patients at all stages of life and covering the whole spectrum of diseases. Thus more patients and expanding patient groups will be subjected to interventions that directly involve intensive care; one such example is the expansion of the age brackets for valve replacements over the last decennia. Other emerging therapies may involve intensive care only indirectly, such as when complications occur, bringing the patients into situations where they become dependent upon intensive care and thereby expose them to risk of its failure. An example of this is the increasing number of joint replacement procedures being performed on patients of an increasing age range.

In other cases, continued medical progress has at least eased the burden of intensive life supportive therapy and made it more unlikely for certain patient groups to become dependent upon it. Although this does not eliminate all of the dilemma, it reduces the number of instances and changes the factors that have to be considered in the decision-making process. A good example of this is the application of noninvasive ventilation, which has decreased the number of patients with chronic obstructive pulmonary disease who need ventilator support.[4]

Because noninvasive ventilation is not associated with the risk of ventilator-associated pneumonia, it reduces mortality and morbidity of exacerbations. It can also safely be applied outside of the ICU and thus is associated with a significant reduction of the burden of therapy for respiratory failure. Another example is the substitution of medical for surgical therapies; this has caused a dramatic reduction in the number of patients needing life supportive therapy for upper gastrointestinal bleeding and has caused a similarly dramatic reduction in the number of these complications to other diseases and conditions.

The continued expansion of therapeutic possibilities and their application to expanding age groups contribute to the ever-increasing complexity of decisions to terminate life supportive therapy, as patients with more comorbidity will present with a need for intensive care. For many of the progresses in surgical therapy, this is a function of improvement in anesthetic technique allowing more patients than ever before to survive the insult of anesthesia and surgery.

Along with these changes to medical therapy, other societal changes contribute to the continuing development of new dilemmas in the decision making to terminate life support. The demography in developed nations is changing, with an increasing percentage of older people who, as already mentioned, will present with more comorbidities and have higher risks associated with treatments, changing the spectrum of patients in the ICU. Not only is the population aging, but the increasing prevalence of overweight and obese patients also contributes to this trend.

At the same time, increased population mobility, both nationally and internationally, causes patients of different languages, ethnic, cultural, and religious backgrounds to present with the ethical dilemmas of terminating life supportive therapy. Furthermore, trends that were already present when the ACCP/SCCM and ATS guidelines were published have strengthened. Such trends are the increase in the expectations of the patients and their relatives; with the changes in the legal aspects of medicine, the emphasis on and the requirement of written informed consent; and increased patient input into decision making, the latter reflected in the increasing number of patients who have living wills and established health care proxies.

## MEDICAL ASPECT OF DECISION MAKING

Making the decision to terminate ventilator support has two parts: (1) assessment of the clinical situation and the underlying pathophysiology necessary for making a prognosis (establishing the odds for a recovery) based on the available evidence, and (2) consideration of the moral and ethical aspects. Although it makes no difference to the fundamental ethical issues, differences do exist depending on whether the patient is competent and, if not, whether the patient has a guardian (for children), a health care proxy, or living will. Problems may also differ between a public health care system and a privately financed system, between wealthy and poor societies, and between war-torn and peaceful environments. The latter is particularly relevant for doctors who work for humanitarian rather than for pecuniary or other reasons.

The medical part of the decision making is the more tangible part of the process and is to some extent independent of the patient. It consists of making the diagnosis and ranking the diagnoses, pathophysiological processes, and the patient's age according to his or her respective importance for the outlook. This part mainly depends on the competence and experience of the practitioner, as well as his or her knowledge of the relevant current evidence from the literature. However, with the previously mentioned changes in the ICU patient populations, the complexity of the individual cases may increase. One consequence of this is that the assessment becomes increasingly more difficult and consequently increasingly more difficult to convey to the patient and/or to relatives or the health proxy or to reconcile the outlook with the text of the living will. Along with this comes the difficulty of explaining the side effects of increasingly complex treatments, the extent and invasiveness of the procedures necessary to cause a possible cure (i.e., the burden of treatment), and the time horizon for it to happen. This may be further complicated by the uncertainty of the functional and cognitive condition of the final state. Apparently, a relatively large proportion (11.2%) of patients would reject treatment options causing a heavy burden on them even if the outlook was reestablishment of complete health. Perhaps surprisingly, even treatments causing light burden would be rejected by more than 70% of patients, unless the outlook was complete recovery, reflecting a pronounced dread of invalidity,[3] factors of which the decision-making physicians need to be aware. Without doubting the validity of the study, the data seem difficult to reconcile with the common experience that points of view are very heavily influenced by the current environment and change as reality changes. For example, patients with progressive invalidating diseases do not as a general rule commit suicide, but invariably try to make the best of the situation once impairment has set in, however scary the outlook may have been before the onset of symptoms, even if suicide requires action rather than laissez-faire; in addition, suicide is associated with cultural and religious taboos. One is continually surprised how well patients can adapt to situations that appear impossible for therapists or healthy individuals and require burdensome treatments either to improve quality of life or prolong life.

Establishing the odds for recovery is central to the medical aspect of making the decision to terminate life supportive treatment. This has two components. The first involves assessing the odds for recovery with and without life supportive therapy. The only guidance, aside from the personal experience of the individual physician, is to compare the actual case with reports in the literature investigating the outcomes under similar circumstances. This, however, is not without problems. In prospective studies the outcomes are calculated for patients assigned to groups according to qualitative rather than quantitative criteria. This leaves little room for grading the severity of the individual diagnoses or the specifics thereof, such as f.ex., which organism causes sepsis; in some cases it may not be possible to find studies that match the individual case. The odds found in these studies represent the average outcome, and a priori the average will always be the best prediction. There is, however, no way of telling whether one particular patient could be the one who beats the odds. Physicians also differ in their capacity for critical evaluation of the studies relevant to a particular case. Clinicians with research experience will have an advantage here, demonstrating the importance of research activity and an academic approach to everyday clinical practice. Taking a multidisciplinary approach (i.e., having input from colleagues with different experiences and backgrounds) will also help prevent the pitfalls associated with uncritical acceptance of studies.

Another problem is that the weight given to evidence in the literature and that given to personal experience varies among doctors. Few doctors may claim not to be affected deeply by cases that either came out surprisingly well and against the odds or by cases that against all odds and intentions turned out disastrous. Unfortunately, the bias introduced by personal experiences may be more pervasive than the individual doctor is aware of and much more so than he or she is willing to admit. Many doctors may also fail to recognize that when they decide to terminate life supportive treatment before natural death occurs, they actually confirm and add to their experience and perception of which circumstances and conditions make continued life supportive treatment futile.

Another medical aspect of the decision making is the assessment of the extent to which the decision-making ability of the patient is affected in the actual situation. First and foremost, the disease itself may affect cognition, reasoning, and memory, as would obviously be the case in neurologic disorders but which may also be significant in other diseases, such as hepatic and metabolic encephalopathy. Secondly, more likely than not, necessary sedation and pain relief will affect the mental capabilities of the patient, as may other therapeutic interventions. This can be a nearly impossible task. Nevertheless, a proper assessment of the extent to which the faculties of the patient have been affected takes on an increasingly important role in an age with increased patient participation in medical decision making.

## NONMEDICAL ASPECTS OF DECISION MAKING

The nonmedical aspects of the decision to terminate life support therapy challenge the communicative skills and the ethical standards of the involved physicians as well as their capacity for empathy.

The basic tenet, which must always be kept in mind, is of course the doctor's obligation to the patient and not to the relatives or the society. This basic tenet becomes challenged in situations where continued life supportive therapy takes up resources, preventing other patients from receiving therapy that would either preserve life or improve quality of life. Such considerations are already implicit in many ethical decisions made in health systems, irrespective of whether they are publicly or privately funded. In both systems, health care delivery is detached from the allocation of resources, and every announcement of medical progress contributes to increased expectations of patients. Therefore the challenges to this tenet are bound to keep increasing as the gap between what can be done and what the available resources allow to be done keeps increasing.

In poor societies and war situations, this has been an ever-present problem. Under such circumstances the individual doctor only has his or her moral and ethical compass to rely upon to decide at which level of resources he or she must consider his primary responsibility to be to a group of people, or society on a larger scale, rather than to the individual. There are no guidelines to help with this kind of ethical dilemma. The ethical instincts of any doctor will reflect upon the community and the society in which he or she has been raised and in which his or her training took place. Many poor societies are marked by internal strife, if not war, and lie on the margins of or outside of the western cultural spheres. Doctors working in these societies are therefore likely to meet with different ethical and moral standards and a scarcity of resources. The ensuing conflict of ethical and moral standards and its concomitant may be striking and incapacitating but ideally will be eased when the doctor becomes familiar with the mainstream attitudes of the particular community or society. In such situations, further conflict may easily arise if a doctor is met with a demand for preferential treatment based on rank or place in society. This runs contrary to the Judeo-Christian or western code of ethics, even if it is not entirely unknown in these societies. The dilemma may be exacerbated by threats against the life and health of the physician. In such a case, making the decision may be as easy as the moral scruples may be tormenting.

It goes without saying that the quality of decisions made regarding the termination of life supporting treatments depends on the relationship between the patient and the physicians. As the intensivist will only have a previous patient/doctor relationship in a minority of cases, he or she must rely on input from colleagues who have known the patient and the patient's family and environment for an extended time. In most cases this will be the primary care physician or internist. At least in some health systems the primary care physician or internist will not be involved in the decision-making process, so the intensivist must rely on the input from the living will, the relatives, the health care proxy, or other care providers.

According to the guidelines and many health care proxy statements, discontinuation of life supportive therapy can be considered when the outlook for continued treatment is "futile." As mentioned previously, *chance* and *futility* are other words for "odds." Unfortunately, nearly each individual views odds differently depending on the context. For example, in the case of smoking, no one can doubt that it is associated with major health risks after more than 40 years of anti-smoking campaigns and with the more recent recognition of its highly addictive nature. The actual odds of contracting a possibly debilitating and/or life-shortening disease are worse than 1:4, yet about one in four individuals is a smoker. On the other hand, the risk of being a victim of terrorist acts must be infinitely small, yet it is a major political issue causing major changes in society and life patterns. The prominence of the terrorism issue in the minds of the population is in stark contrast to that of smoking cessation, which would save many more lives. Also to be considered is the long-established norm in science: that we consider outcomes that have an a priori likelihood to be less than 1:20 to be not due to chance (i.e., considered significant), despite the absence of a rational foundation. Likewise, considering that most traffic accidents happen within a rather short distance from home, we seldom think twice of driving to pick up items from the supermarket, despite the danger to our health. Therefore informing a patient or the relatives that the odds of recovery with continued life supportive treatment are such and such may in fact not convey much meaning, neither to the doctor nor to the patient. At best, rather vague impressions are created and acted upon, even if the concept of odds for the patient and the decision makers should happen to coincide.

The concepts of futility of medical treatment may not even exist in some cultures. Thus in fundamentalist Muslim countries, most patients and relatives will accept death as an act of God as long as everything humanly possible has been done up to that point, making it futile to consider termination of life supportive treatment.

Of course, the odds for recovery are not the only factors entering into the decision-making process. The burden to the patient of continued therapy must also be considered. However, in the ICU setting the means available to mitigate the suffering both physically and mentally are widely used; thus in many instances it is hard for physicians and relatives to deny that their own discomfort at watching the patient never enters into the decisions. Often invoked in decision making is the concept of degradation of dignity; however, in the unconscious patient it is debatable whether that is felt, and rather it must often be a sentiment felt by health care providers and relatives. Thus a major emphasis need only be placed on this aspect in the (rare) case in which the patient has expressed orally or in writing that a course of more than a certain number of days in a state of impaired cognition and reasoning, heavily instrumented, and on life supportive therapy violates his or her sense of dignity. Outside of the Judeo-Christian spheres the concept of dignity may not even be an issue. Again, in fundamentalist Muslim cultures the concept of dignity does not exist for the same reason that futility of medical treatment does not exist.

Thus in order to make the decisions that most closely reflect the attitudes of the patient, extraordinary demands are placed on every physician's ability to communicate both verbally and, perhaps more importantly, nonverbally. It is a common experience of practicing physicians that the longer the duration of the patient–doctor relationship, the better the communication. This is due to the simple fact that the better the patient can convey his or her concerns, the more likely is either a satisfactory explanation or treatment. It follows that patient–doctor relationships without good mutual rapport tend to terminate.

The ability to communicate varies from practitioner to practitioner, and in many cases it is a product of the attitudes of the individual practitioner, but it is something that can be trained. One prominent aspect of good communication is patience, which requires time. This is becoming a limiting resource in modern practice, mostly for financial reasons and probably because of the lack of understanding that shortness of time becomes counterproductive at a certain point. A second prominent aspect of good communication is the ability (and patience) to listen without preconception, improving the chances that the communication takes place on the patient's terms, which is essential. A third prominent aspect of good communication is economy with words, because only few patients are able to follow long sentences, as is evident by noticing the writing style, or readability index, of the tabloid newspapers. The vocabulary of many patients is limited, so the words must be chosen carefully for this reason and so that ideally the right connotations will be invoked in the mind of the patient.

Finally, the good communicator is also able to discern when the patient has stopped listening.

To the conscientious health care provider, the lack of indisputable markers that signify futility is a constant strain, and to help patients and health care providers reach the decisions which according to some criteria are the most "satisfactory," some institutions have hired consultant ethicists, who in the personal experience of the author are very helpful. They serve as a third party in consultations with patients and/or relatives; their effectiveness is once again a function of their communication skills, providing a "third ear" that can help keep the conversation on a purposeful track. They also can have separate discussions with the health care provider, the patient, and/or relatives or proxy, helping them to arrive at a solution that appears to all parties to be the best one. This is particularly valuable when the request of the patient/relatives/proxy runs against the best medical advice of the health care provider or where there may be deep cultural differences between the two sides. Situations exist in which the patient's wishes or requests collide not only with the medical knowledge of the provider but also run contrary to the provider's code of ethics. In the setting where another provider cannot take over the care, the dilemma can be very painful for the provider, who can only resort to careful conversations with the patients and/or relatives or proxy using his or her knowledge and capacity for empathy to reach a common ground. In such situations it is imperative that the autonomy of the patient is constantly respected.

Another way of attempting to help relieve the strain of ethical dilemmas and also provide some consistency to the decisions is to establish institutional ethics committees. By nature these committees make decisions on behalf of the patient population of the institution in question. Depending on the criteria for their selection, they may not be representative of the community, and their authority may be questionable. Such committees are likely to include both health care providers, legal and administrative advisors, and ideally lay people. As a hospital committee, it is most likely to be a resource for the health care providers but cannot be directly involved in the patient/relative/proxy communication.

## CONCLUSIONS

The need for decisions regarding the initiation or termination of life supportive treatment, along with their associated ethical dilemmas, is a common occurrence in everyday hospital life. The two sets of North American guidelines are very thorough and complete, yet as guidelines they do not provide answers to specific questions.

This chapter has outlined the reasons why ethical dilemmas inherent in the decisions to terminate life supportive treatment continue to challenge the medical professions. It has also outlined the two main components in the decision making: the medical, more tangible, and the ethical, more ephemeral, aspects. Some of these aspects have been the subjects of commentary. Through these comments the chapter has attempted to help the health care provider better understand the many pitfalls on both sides of the patient/relative/proxy and health care provider equation. The higher the awareness of these pitfalls, the better the quality of the decisions is likely to be. If this chapter has helped fuel awareness of, reflection upon, and discussion of the raised issues, it will have served its intended purpose.

## REFERENCES

1. Bone R, Rackow EC, Weg JC, et al: Ethical and moral guidelines for the initiation, continuation, and withdrawal of intensive care. Chest 1990;97:949–958.
2. Official Statement of the American Thoracic Society: Withholding and withdrawing life-sustaining therapy. Am Rev Resp Crit Care Med 1991;144:726–731.
3. British Medical Association: Withholding and withdrawing life prolonging medical treatment: Guidance for decision making. BMJ Publishing Group, 1999.
4. Fried TR, Bradley E, Towle VR: Understanding the treatment preferences of seriously ill patients. N Engl J Med 2002;346:1061–1066.

# CHAPTER 51

# Economics of Ventilator Care

Werner Kuckelt

Artificial mechanical ventilation (AMV) is a well-established mode of treatment in the intensive care unit (ICU). It is used worldwide to support pulmonary function in critically ill patients.[1,2] At present, most patients treated by AMV are elderly. The frequency of AMV use for these patients has increased rapidly over the past 40 years.[3-5] Hospital costs and ICU mortality rates for patients with any need for AMV are much higher in contrast to patients admitted to an ICU without indication for any ventilatory support.[6,7] It is reported that older patients show a higher hospital mortality rate compared with younger patients receiving AMV,[9-12] and there is a clear impact of age, severity of illness, functional status, and comorbidities on long-term outcomes.

Economic evaluations are increasingly common in the critical care literature, although approaches to their conduct are not standardized. Costs of intensive care may be 20% of all hospital costs.[13] However, population aging likely increases the demand for intensive care services and further increases the financial burden. The financial limitations of modern health care are well established. Therefore data about costs of intensive care and use of ICU resources are needed.

True costs in health care industries and their highly demanding professional environments (ICU, operating room, emergency department, etc.) are difficult to determine and to compare because they include factors such as medications, equipment, personnel, furniture, lighting, and telephones. Therefore in most circumstances we have to use surrogate markers, such as unit costs or hospital charges in the European community.

Data on the ICU effectiveness interventions are often lacking. ICU cases are complex, with multiple concurrent problems and interventions, and most ICU therapies including AMV are only supportive. Therefore these interventions may not result in improved outcome for many individual patients. Accurate cost data are not commonly available and are difficult to obtain, and there is no standardized approach for measuring or valuing costs among different populations and countries.

At present, most known cost studies are retrospective "bottom-up" studies in which data have been extracted from bills of the hospital accounts system, with the problem of imperfect registration of resource usage and activity. The "bottom-up" approach involves recording costs at a cost-object level and multiplies units of resource use with unit costs. This approach measures only indirect costs, and direct costs must be apportioned. To perform this retrospectively requires very accurate patient files or resource use registrations and is very costly by itself.

Furthermore, in the area of unit costs, one of the simple but major problems with costing ICU patients is that it is difficult to obtain the true cost, such as of a lab test, medical service–invested cost for equipment, and many others. This problem has not yet been resolved. Another method commonly used is to multiply the average bed price from the hospital ledger by the number of days of stay.

Most cost-evaluating methods do not represent patient-specific resource usage. Some hospital patients become acutely ill, deteriorate, and are admitted to the ICU where they quickly respond to therapy. Their treatment is very expensive in the first 48 hours. After this time, however, the costs wane.

Other patients continue to worsen after their ICU admission and, as the disease progresses, their treatment becomes more and more expensive (e.g., prolonged antibiotic use, dialysis costs, treatment of complications, mechanical cardiocirculatory support, invasive diagnostic tests, patient positioning, prolonged artificial ventilation). Intensive care patients are also both different from ordinary ward patients and different from each other.[14,15]

To understand to handle the problem of ICU costing, especially to evaluate the costs for patients ventilated artificially, it is useful to look at the working process in hospitals and the working process in the ICU.

The treatment process in the ICU represents a typical working process similar to that in other highly demanding professional environments such as air traffic control centers, nuclear power plants, and aircraft carriers.

The ICU working process has three main components: input, process of treatment, and output. The process of treatment is influenced by at least four main factors: methods used, defined standards, applied equipment, and level of training. The whole process can be translated into consumptive monetary units describing the permanent costs to keep the system running (Fig. 51.1).

The input includes the following:

- Patients classified by diagnosis, severity of the illness (Acute Physiology and Chronic Health Evaluation II [APACHE II], SAPS, SOFA, or other scoring system data), comorbidities, risk factors, and lifestyle- and culture-dependent factors
- Manpower represented by potency of present alert medical personnel, nurses, ward secretaries, technicians, clerks, and others
- Costly organizational structures such as three-shift performance of the working process realized for all professions

The output includes the following:

- Patient outcome
- Measurement of performed therapeutic interventions (Therapeutic Intervention Scoring System [TISS] 72, TISS 28, Nine Equivalent of Nursing Manpower use Score (NEMS)[16]
- Exhaustion of manpower
- Amount of consumed resources

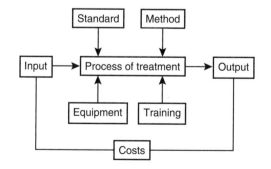

**Figure 51.1** Process of treatment in the ICU.

The applied methods, the used standards, the quality and quantity of the equipment, the training level, and of course the availability of all the necessary medical product resources have a costly impact on the treatment process.

Furthermore, the cost of performing an ICU procedure includes not only direct costs, such as personnel time, but also indirect costs, such as some portion of the administrative costs required to run the ICU.

Direct, variable costs are most easily traced to a new therapy, whereas indirect and fixed costs may be harder to track. A costing system that fails to distinguish between these components may therefore be inaccurate.

All direct measures of resource use and its cost must use a therapeutic intervention scoring system,[17] an activity-based costing method,[18] or a weighted length-of-stay module,[19] but these measures require cost calibration (i.e., a Euro value must be assigned to each TISS point or to each day).

On the other hand, the work that must be done to determine the relative contributions to cost of each component is tremendous, and there is continuous debate regarding the optimal method for doing this.

Another important aspect is that evidence for the effectiveness of critical care interventions is often lacking. The impact of many measures (e.g., pharmacologic substances, technological procedures, and routinely used interventions in the ICU) is not established. Approximately 85% of what is done in the ICU has not really been evaluated in terms of its cost effectiveness.[20] Only 21% of all health technologies used today are evidence based.[21] Therefore their effects on many ICU measures are often estimated or presumed, rather than known, and some concepts accepted as effective simply assume that a patient not receiving this kind of therapy would have died.[22]

Because therapy in the ICU for most patients is supportive rather than curative, the goals of many ICU procedures are aimed at stabilizing and supporting any failing organ system (e.g., mechanical ventilation, hemofiltration, left heart assist devices, catecholamines) rather than curing or improving an underlying condition. However, the therapeutic concepts to treat the underlying disease and support any failing organ are ongoing at the same time.

Under such conditions, isolating the clinical and economic consequences of individual interventions can be difficult. Furthermore, decision-making errors and management errors occur because seven may be the maximum number of simple variables that can be handled by an individual in an effective decision-making process.[23] All this influences dynamics of cost and the cost-effectiveness ratio and cannot be identified by accounting the numbers in any bill.

Critical illness is a complex process that can occur in varied, very heterogeneous patient groups. Therapy in

ICU is often used for critically ill patients with different underlying comorbidities and different initial risk of death. ICU patients can also develop many complications, which can then result in multiorgan failure. Determining the effect of a particular therapy (including artificial mechanical ventilation) in such situations is difficult, which complicates both clinical evaluation and cost analysis.

To evaluate costs, ICU outcome measurements are often used. However, physiologic parameters (arterial oxygenation, level of analgesia-sedation, oxygen uptake, or cardiac ejection fraction) or intermediate outcomes (ventilator-free days) are not very helpful, and the relationships of these endpoints to patient-centered outcomes, such as survival or quality of life, are not clear. Although survival is often used in ICU studies, the time horizon is usually too short (e.g., 28 days). Such short follow-up complicates estimation of the long-term benefits (e.g., years of life gained) of many ICU therapies and their real costs.

Data regarding the ICU costs and individual and or special ICU procedures are often derived from sources with different practice patterns and cost structures. This creates some significant problems. Different health care systems are structured differently, in part due to differences in the relative costs of different aspects of care (Europe versus North America, Australia, and many other countries). Specific interventions can change the use of other health care system resources (introduction of other financing systems, such as Diagnosis Related Groups [DRG]), and the cost of that change can vary depending on the structure of the health care system. Measuring costs in a consistent and uniform way among different health care systems and countries seems to be very difficult.

The goal of any cost analysis in ICU environment is to evaluate the true cost of the process of treatment, the distribution of cost among different classes of patients, the diagnosis of underlying disease, the relationship of effort with outcome, and quality control. With the corresponding information at hand, one may try to provide the optimal outcome at a minimum of effort and cost.

Figure 51.2 represents possible output from an analysis of a cost-output (outcome) model of a particular intervention, demonstrating a cost-output space. Any new intervention, method, standard, or medication can be better, less, or similarly acceptable and equally, more or less costly in comparison with the standard of the literature or a currently used ICU therapy.

Given baseline assumptions, the new therapy is compared with current therapy, and a specific cost-output ratio is estimated (e.g., standardized mortality rate [SMR]). Repetitive evaluations of the model can be constructed with different estimates of the various parameters that are used as inputs.

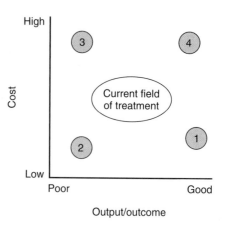

**Figure 51.2** Cost and output/outcome in the ICU as markers of quality of care. The goal of any cost analysis in an ICU environment is to evaluate the true cost to provide the optimal outcome at a minimum of effort and cost. Current field of treatment represents the ongoing status of an ICU. Field 1: New intervention is both more effective and less expensive. Field 2: New intervention is less effective and less costly. Field 3: A new intervention is both less effective and more costly. Field 4: A new intervention is more effective but more costly.

As a result of cost analysis in the ICU, we can answer questions such as the following:

*What were the costs and effects of our performance strategy and how can we describe the proportions and distribution of costs?*

In Fig. 51.2, we can identify the region of the current field of therapy (e.g., artificial mechanical ventilation or others), as follows:

Region 1: A new intervention (e.g., other types of ventilators, other strategies [Pressure Support Ventilation (PSV) versus continuous positive airway pressure (CPAP)]) is both more effective and less expensive. It is strongly dominant. Further evaluation is not necessary.

Region 2: A new intervention is less effective and less costly. This may be cost effective, but it would require evaluation of more outcome data because the SMR is to be found greater than previously.

Region 3: A new intervention is both less effective and more costly. It is clear that no further evaluation is necessary to waste this poor option.

Region 4: A new intervention is more effective and more costly. This is weakly dominant. Strategic evaluations and fundamental decisions are necessary to obtain a consent decision to change the therapeutic concepts and to stabilize hospital economics.

AMV is the most important aspect of life support for patients with respiratory failure. However, AMV interferes with normal physiologic processes. The clinician is often applying levels and patterns of pressure, tidal volume, concentration of inspired oxygen, and ventilatory rate well beyond the level that normal lung usually experiences, making AMV a potentially dangerous tool.

Evidence from experimental studies suggests that AMV can cause or aggravate lung injury.[24] Referred to as *ventilator-induced lung injury* (VILI), this condition resembles acute lung injury and is difficult to identify in critically ill patients because its appearance overlaps the underlying disease.[25]

The concept of VILI supports the hypothesis that acute lung injury may be partly a result of ICU treatment rather than any component of the progressing underlying disease. This in turn supports the assumption that AMV is not an absolute life-saving measure but also extends the severity of preexisting lung injury, and protective ventilatory strategies could prevent this.[26,27]

In the author's ICU, for more than 10 years the AMV-standard includes lower tidal volume (450 to 750 mL), pressure-controlled ventilatory mode, positive end-expiratory pressure (PEEP) $\geq 10$ cm W, and the lowest possible $FiO_2$.

Because the quality control program (Riyadh ICU program, Medical Associated Software House Ltd., London) has been used in this ICU since 1997, no effect of this is seen in the currently available Riyadh data, in contrast to other AMV modes used before.

All patients admitted to the 31-bed ICU at the author's hospital between January 1, 1997, and December 31, 2003, are included in the Riyadh database. Daily physiologic and treatment data were analyzed.

Severity of illness (APACHE II points),[28] the Organ Failure Score points (OFS),[29] and the Therapeutic Intervention Scoring System points (TISS)[30] are measured and calculated.

All the primary data, together with demographic data and patients' hospital outcome, were entered daily to the computer by a team of specifically trained nurses, doctors, and secretaries.

The sensitivity of the information from the daily APACHE II and TISS data is very high. It can be seen that changes in the protocols for the working process correlate with the productivity data of the unit (Fig. 51.3).

The introduction of a new or the revision of an older standard correlates quite well with changes in the average number of TISS points per patient, especially in those treated by AMV for $\geq 7$ days.

When discussing the cost of AMV, it is important to understand that artificially ventilated patients are quite different and any population in different bands of age, comorbidities, diagnoses, and other factors are very heterogeneous.

By classifying the patients at admission according to the underlying disease, risk factors, and severity of illness, it is possible to see that patients artificially ventilated for $\leq 2$ days show a lower APACHE II score at admission than those artificially ventilated for $\geq 7$ days (Fig. 51.4).

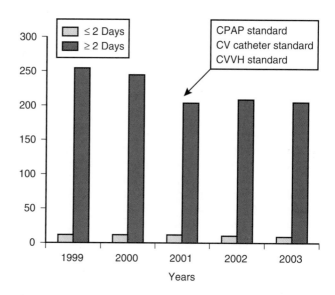

**Figure 51.3** Analysis of TISS point data in 16,863 ICU patients (January 1, 1999, to December 31, 2003). The mean TISS points in patients with short time in ward stay ($\leq 2$ days) are remarkably homogeneous and different from those in patients with longer stay ($\geq 2$ days), and the possible impact of changes in procedural standards can be identified. (Data from Annual ICU Audit, 1999–2003, Riyadh ICU program; Klinikum Links der Weser Bremen.)

A similar effect can be seen if one looks at the data of survivors and nonsurvivors at admission (Fig. 51.5). Survivors show lower APACHE II values than do nonsurvivors. The risk of death at day 1 for survivors is three times lower than that for nonsurvivors.

Any analysis of cost has to take into account that patient populations are changing with time. It must be realized that patients in the ICU are older now than in previous years (Fig. 51.6). We have seen a decrease in the number of treated patients in the age bands less than 45 years to 55 to 65 years but a remarkable increase in the age bands 65 to 75 years and $\geq 75$ years. These changes influence productivity and outcome data for every ICU.

However, to draw the correct conclusions from such information, it is necessary to have data on the performance of the ICU over the years (Table 51.1). The decrease in ICU mortality as well as hospital mortality indicates an acceptable performance of the working process in the department, especially when the standardized mortality rate (SMR) as a marker of efficiency is lower than 1. Any SMR >1 indicates that our prediction assumes a better outcome than the observed output realizes.

An additional but very important aspect is that the incidence of organ failure and multiple organ failure increases and the percentage of patients requiring AMV rises as well (Table 51.2).

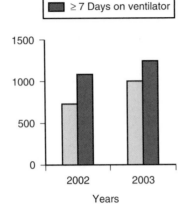

| | ≤ 2 Days | ≥ 7 Days |
|---|---|---|
| 2003 | 1392 pts. | 125 pts. |
| APACHE II (SD) | 11.6 (4.3) | 16.8 (7.2) |
| On vent days | 723 | 1088 |
| 2003 | 1342 pts. | 129 pts. |
| APACHE II (SD) | 11.7 (4.4) | 16.4 (19.7) |
| On vent days | 1007 | 1246 |

**Figure 51.4** Analysis of on ventilator–day data in ICU patients (January 1, 2002, to December 31, 2003). On ventilator–days ≤2 days are compared with those ≥7 days. The number of patients and day 1 APACHE II data as well as the risk of death (ROD) at day 1 is the same for both years. But the on ventilator–days increase in 2003. (Data from Annual ICU Audit, 1999–2003, Riyadh ICU program; Klinikum Links der Weser Bremen.)

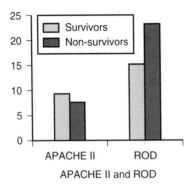

| | Survivors | Non-survivors |
|---|---|---|
| Patients | 2928 | 215 |
| APACHE II (SD) | 9.4 (5.3) | 15.2 (9.1) |
| 95% CI | 9.2–9.6 | 14.1–16.5 |
| ROD (%) | 7.7 (8.1) | 23.2 (22.2) |
| 95% | 7.3–7.9 | 24.3–31.1 |

**Figure 51.5** Analysis of APACHE II and risk of death (ROD) data in ICU patients (January 1, 2003, to December 31, 2003). Differences in mean day 1 APACHE II score and ROD in survivors and nonsurvivors. The day 1 APACHE II as well as the ROD data in survivors and nonsurvivors are different. (Data from Annual ICU Audit, 2003, Riyadh ICU program; Klinikum Links der Weser Bremen.)

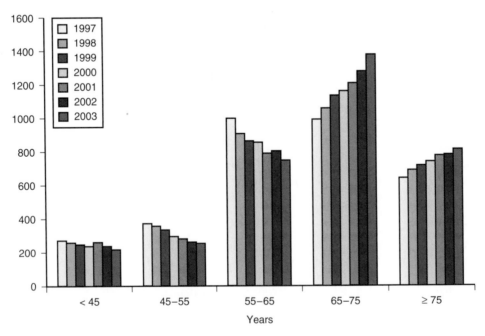

**Figure 51.6** Distribution of patients according to APACHE II age bands in the ICU. Data were collected between January 1, 1997, and December 31, 2003. The age bands <45, 45 to 55, and 55 to 65 are characterized by a decrease in the number of patients treated. The age bands 65 to 75 and ≥75 show a permanent increase in the number of patients treated over the years. (Data from Annual ICU Audit, 1997–2003, Riyadh ICU program; Klinikum Links der Weser Bremen.)

**Table 51-1** Outcome and SMR data of all ICU patients between January 1, 1997, and December 31, 2003 (23.646 ICU patients)

|  | 1997 | 1998 | 1999 | 2000 | 2001 | 2002 | 2003 |
|---|---|---|---|---|---|---|---|
| Patients admitted to ICU (n) | 3398 | 3385 | 3204 | 3254 | 3288 | 3593 | 3524 |
| Patients died in ICU (n) | 254 | 244 | 178 | 174 | 152 | 139 | 153 |
| ICU mortality (%) | 7.5 | 7.2 | 5.5 | 5.3 | 4.6 | 4.2 | 4.1 |
| Patients died in ward post ICU (n) | 59 | 61 | 89 | 80 | 69 | 75 | 62 |
| Total hospital death (n) | 312 | 305 | 267 | 254 | 221 | 214 | 215 |
| Total in hospital mortality (%) | 9.2 | 9.0 | 8.3 | 7.8 | 6.7 | 6.5 | 6.3 |
| SMR | 0.97 | 0.91 | 0.85 | 0.82 | 0.75 | 0.73 | 0.79 |

The ICU mortality and the hospital mortality rate of patients treated in the ICU decreased continuously between 1997 and 2003. The ICU standardized mortality rate remained in the same range (0,7–1,0).
Data source: Annual ICU Audit (1997–2003), Riyadh ICU program; Klinikum Links der Weser Bremen.

From 1997 to 1999, data were analyzed to extrapolate information about AMV and multiple organ failure (Fig. 51.7). During this time, 3740 of 5726 patients were identified as suffering from organ failures and present episodes of AMV. The need for AMV increased with the number of failing organs.

Approximately 10% (347) of the patients were ventilated artificially for ≥7 days, covering a total number of 6835 patient-days. Depending on the number of failing organ systems, the mortality ranged from 8.3% in patients with one organ failure to 21.9% (two organs), 52.4% (three organs), 72.1% (four organs), and 86.2% in patients with five failing organ systems (Fig. 51.8). In the era of large tidal volume ventilation, the same findings were reported 30 years ago.[31]

As of 2003, the mortality of organ system failure has changed dramatically (Fig. 51.9). The mortality ranged in 2003 from 2.3% in patients with one organ failure to 9.0% (two organs), 25.3% (three organs), 48.5% (four organs), and 84.6% in patients with five failing organ systems.

However, this reduction of mortality in organ system failures has its price. During the observation period between January 1, 1998, and December 31, 2003, the productivity rate increased (Table 51.3). In 1998 a total of 330,205 TISS points were registered. In 2003, 398,710 TISS points were counted. The difference of 68,505 TISS points equals a performance activity of 2.5 months or 1824 hours in 1998.

Mortality in ICU is also correlated with patient age (Table 51.4). For all patients according to the Riyadh

**Table 51-2** Frequency of Organ Failure in the ICU (23.646 ICU patients) between January 1, 1997, and December 31, 2003

|  | 1997 | 1998 | 1999 | 2000 | 2001 | 2002 | 2003 |
|---|---|---|---|---|---|---|---|
| Patients | 3398 | 3385 | 3204 | 3254 | 3288 | 3593 | 3524 |
| Organ Failure (%) | 46.7 | 59.3 | 65.4 | 69.9 | 60.4 | 57.8 | 56.2 |
| ≥2 Organ Failure (%) | 14.3 | 19.7 | 23.4 | 28.3 | 20.9 | 21.2 | 23.3 |
| Patients ventilated artificially (%) | 49.4 | 53.0 | 56.0 | 55.2 | 54.4 | 53.1 | 54.4 |

The incidence of Organ Failure and the need for artificial ventilation increased between 1997 and 2003.
Data source: Annual ICU Audit (1997-2003), Riyadh ICU program; Klinikum Links der Weser Bremen.

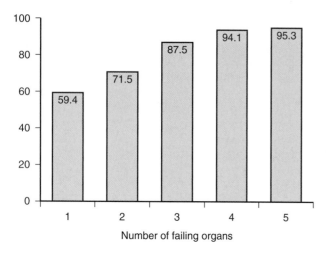

**Figure 51.7** Patients with organ failure (OF) who required artificial mechanical ventilation (AMV) (3740 patients of 5726 patients) between January 1, 1997, and December 31, 1999. Approximately 59.5% to 95.3% of the patients in the OF bands had a need for AMV. (Data from Annual ICU Audit, 1997–1999, Riyadh ICU program; Klinikum Links der Weser Bremen.)

age bands, there is an age-dependent difference in severity of the critical illness (4.6±5.7 APACHE II points in age band ≤45 years to 11.8±5.5 APACHE II points in age band ≥75 years) at the day of admission with a corresponding percent risk of death (ROD) (6.4±10.5% ROD in age band ≤45 years to 11.1±11.6% ROD in age band ≥75 years). This is mirrored by the ICU mortality as well (2.2% mortality in age band ≤45 years to 11.2% mortality in age band ≥75 years).

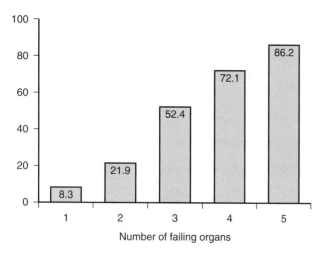

**Figure 51.8** Analysis of ICU mortality in 347 patients ventilated artificially ≥7 days covering 6835 patient-days between January 1, 1997, and December 31, 1999. (Data from Annual ICU Audit, 1997–1999, Riyadh ICU program; Klinikum Links der Weser Bremen.)

To analyze the duration of AMV in critically ill patients, evaluate the cost in patients on artificial ventilation, and establish stable and powerful reference values, we have pooled corresponding Riyadh data from 5255 ICU patients with 16,909 patient-days collected between January 1, 1997, and December 31, 1999 (Table 51.5).

It is important to realize that patients with AMV of ≤2 days are different from those who need AMV for ≥7 days with day 1 in the ICU. At the day of admission, the mean APACHE II points in the age band ≤2 days were found to be lower than in patients in the age band ≥7 days (12.2±4.7 APACHE II points versus 17.2±6.6 APACHE II points), and the mean ROD was 7.5±10.2% versus 24.9±21.2%.

A further important aspect is that 4110 ICU patients in the age band ≤2 days cover 6576 patient-days (38.9% of 16,909), and 347 patients in the age band ≥7 days occupy 6835 (40.4% of all) patient-days. This results in similar total costs: €9,367,445 versus €9,736,388.

In this background, a great difference exists between costs per survivor (€1910 versus €37,519), cost per nonsurvivor (€2267 versus €33,996), and effective cost per survivor (€2012 versus €66,946).

On the 1997–1999 3-year basis reference, the next data for the following years prove the validity and coherency of the cost data, especially for the ICU patients with the need for AMV (Tables 51.6 to 51.8). The cost per survivor (CPS) in patients with AMV ≥7 days increased by 28.7% from 2001 to 2003 (€34,889 versus €44,916), but the effective cost per survivor (ECPS) increased by 15.8%, mainly caused by a decrease in the mortality in these patients (Fig. 51.10).

However, looking at the TISS point data (Fig. 51.11), we have to realize that the decrease in the mortality is only the result of a higher productivity rate, as the number of medical and nursing personnel was not changed during these years. The total number of invested TISS points per survivor increased in the patients with AMV ≥7 days from 1368 to 2245.

AMV has been of enormous value in improving outcome and survival in many critically ill patients around the world. However, the lifesaving value of AMV has never been proven by a prospective, randomized, and controlled study, and to conduct such a study trial entails major ethical problems.

Furthermore, the use of AMV also has adverse effects because the method itself can cause direct damage to the lungs.[25,32,33] This results often via a second-hit pathway[34] to multiple organ failure with dubious outcome and produces a prolonged, resource-engulfing, manpower-consuming, and very costly process.

Patients who need intensive care treatment suffer from a complex disturbance of their whole body function, which has lost the normal synergistic coherency of

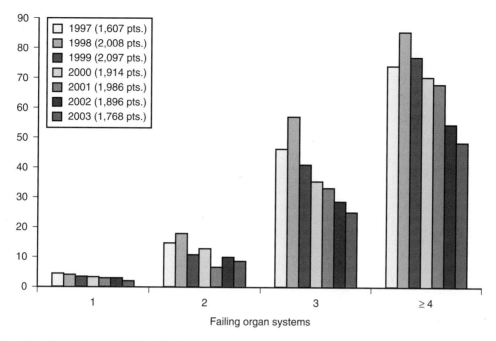

**Figure 51.9** Mortality of organ system failure in the ICU. Data were collected between January 1, 1997, and December 31, 2003. The mortality decreased over the years. (Data from Annual ICU Audit, 1997–2003, Riyadh ICU program; Klinikum Links der Weser Bremen.)

most organ functions. If there is any need for AMV in a patient with complex organ system failures mostly this is a consequence of this multiple organ failure and not only the consequence of an impaired pulmonary gas exchange in a diseased lung.

Intensive care medicine and ICUs provide advanced technical support, multiple pharmacologic treatment, and expensive life support. Health care workers in this specialty have to handle a lot of data to perform any decision-making process. They are burdened by the problem of human error, wrong decision making, and management error.[35]

Until now, in most cases the costs of intensive therapy have been unknown. Although more or less precise estimates of the total costs of running an ICU can be provided through hospital accounts, it is quite difficult

**Table 51-3** Outcome and SMR data of all ICU patients (3.143) in different age bands admitted between January 1, 2003, and December 31, 2003

| Age bands (years) | <45 | 45–55 | 55–65 | 65–75 | ≥75 |
|---|---|---|---|---|---|
| Patients (%) | 219 (6.2) | 330 (9.4) | 747 (21.2) | 1082 (30.7) | 765 (21.7) |
| Mean age (years) | 34.4 | 50.4 | 60.6 | 69.6 | 79.7 |
| Mean APACHE II (SD) | 4.6 (5.7) | 6.6 (4.9) | 9.0 (5.3) | 11.0 (5.4) | 11.8 (5.5) |
| % Risk of death (SD) | 6.4 (10.5) | 5.9 (8.2) | 7.5 (9.9) | 9.2 (11.0) | 11.1 (11.6) |
| ICU mortality (%) | 1.8 | 3.6 | 3.7 | 4.9 | 7.3 |
| Hospital mortality (%) | 2.2 | 3.9 | 4.9 | 6.8 | 11.2 |
| SMR | 0.35 | 0.66 | 0.65 | 0.74 | 1.01 |

The risk of death (ROD), the ICU and hospital mortality increase with age. During the year of 2003 59,9 % of all treated patients were older than 65 years. Every 5th patient was older than 75 years (21.7% of all). The ICU standardized mortality rate (SMR) was extreme low only in the age band <45 years. The SMR rate was quite acceptable between 0,6 and 1,0 for the other age bands.
Data source: Annual ICU Audit (2003), Riyadh ICU program; Klinikum Links der Weser Bremen.

**Table 51-4** Analysis of productivity in the ICU between January 1, 1998, and December 31, 2003

| | TISS Points | | | | | |
|---|---|---|---|---|---|---|
| Years | 1998 | 1999 | 2000 | 2001 | 2002 | 2003 |
| Anesthesiology | 37.268 | 47.628 | 46.359 | 47.116 | 33.456 | 43.825 |
| Surgery | 38.268 | 37.252 | 42.932 | 33.608 | 37.383 | 38.325 |
| Cardiac Surgery | 170.898 | 173.930 | 177.121 | 173.743 | 185.073 | 210.909 |
| Medical | 83.771 | 81.140 | 108.075 | 112.31 | 115.436 | 105.651 |
| All TISS points | 330.205 | 339.953 | 374.487 | 366.777 | 371.348 | 398.710 |
| Total Cost* (Million €) | 8.42 | 8.67 | 9.55 | 9.36 | 9.47 | 10.17 |

*One TISS point equals €25,50
The number of TISS points for the special fields increased each year during the 5 years. All TISS points increased in an amount of 68.505 points. This can be translated into a monetary equivalent of €1.75 Mill..
Data source: Annual ICU Audit (1998–2003), Riyadh ICU program; Klinikum Links der Weser Bremen.

**Table 51-5** Analysis of cost of treatment in the ICU between January 1, 1997, and December 31, 1999

| On ventilator day bands | ≤2 | ≥2 to ≤4 | ≥4 to ≤7 | ≤7 |
|---|---|---|---|---|
| Patients (n) | 4110 | 563 | 245 | 347 |
| Patient days (% of all treatment days) | 6576 (38.9) | 1857 (11.0) | 1641 (9.7) | 6835 (40.4) |
| Mean APACHE II points (SD) | 12.2 (4.7) | 15.6 (7.0) | 17.8 (6.7) | 17.2 (6.6) |
| Mean % Risk of death (SD) | 7.5 (10.2) | 18.9 (20.4) | 25.5 (22.0) | 24.9 (21.2) |
| % Mortality | 4.3 | 22.4 | 45.3 | 46.4 |
| SMR | 0.6 | 1.2 | 1.8 | 1.9 |
| Total Cost (€) | 9,367,445 | 2,645,278 | 12,541,646 | 9,736,388 |
| Cost per survivor (€) | 1,910 | 5,217 | 12,482 | 37,519 |
| Cost per non-survivor (€) | 2,267 | 5,263 | 10,453 | 33,996 |
| Effective cost per survivor (€) | 2,012 | 6,734 | 21,651 | 66,946 |

The data of 5.255 ICU patients with 16.909 patient days were pooled to get a valid reference for the following years. Cost for each classified field were calculated from yearly unit costs, evaluated TISS points, and duration of artificial mechanical ventilation. Mean APACHE II points and mean Risk of death were taken from the corresponding data of day one on ventilator.
Data source: Annual ICU Audit (1997–1999), Riyadh ICU program; Klinikum Links der Weser Bremen.

**Table 51-6   Analysis of cost of treatment in the ICU between January 1, 2001, and December 31, 2001**

| On ventilator day bands | ≤2 | ≥2 to ≤4 | ≥4 to ≤7 | ≥7 |
|---|---|---|---|---|
| Patients (n) | 1435 | 151 | 77 | 126 |
| Patient days (% of all treatment days) | 2296 (41.6) | 558 (10.1) | 477 (8.6) | 2192 (39.7) |
| Mean APACHE II points (SD) | 11.9 (4.4) | 15.3 (6.2) | 14.6 (6.2) | 16.2 (6.5) |
| Mean % Risk of death (SD) | 7.0 (9.6) | 18.7 (18.9) | 17.5 (16.6) | 25.0 (21.3) |
| % Mortality | 3.6 | 19.8 | 23.3 | 40.4 |
| SMR | 0.5 | 1.1 | 1.3 | 1.6 |
| Total Cost (€) | 3,668,952 | 1,152,340 | 1,088,141 | 4,292,756 |
| Cost per survivor (€) | 2,517 | 8,043 | 14,667 | 34,889 |
| Cost per non-survivor (€) | 3,598 | 5,966 | 12,374 | 32,862 |
| Effective cost per survivor (€) | 2,652 | 9,523 | 18,443 | 57,236 |

The data of 3.288 ICU patients with 5.523 patient days were analyzed. Cost for each classified field were calculated from yearly unit costs, evaluated TISS points, and duration of artificial mechanical ventilation. Mean APACHE II points and mean Risk of death were taken from the corresponding data of day one on ventilator. In the category ≥7126 patients cover 2.192 patient days with total costs of €4.292.756 but in the category ≤21.435 patients cover 2.296 patient days with total costs of €3.668.952.
Data source: Annual ICU Audit (2001), Riyadh ICU program; Klinikum Links der Weser Bremen.

**Table 51-7   Analysis of cost of treatment in the ICU between January 1, 2002, and December 31, 2002**

| On ventilator day bands | ≤2 | ≥2 to ≤4 | ≥4 to ≤7 | ≥7 |
|---|---|---|---|---|
| Patients (n) | 1392 | 147 | 75 | 125 |
| Patient days (% of all treatment days) | 2784 (43.0) | 617 (9.3) | 435 (6.5) | 2700 (40.5) |
| Mean APACHE II points (SD) | 11.6 (4.3) | 14.2 (5.2) | 16.5 (7.7) | 16.8 (6.5) |
| Mean % Risk of death (SD) | 6.6 (9.8) | 16.0 (17.1) | 24.0 (23.6) | 22.9 (19.4) |
| % Mortality | 3.2 | 19.7 | 33.3 | 40.8 |
| SMR | 0.5 | 1.2 | 1.4 | 1.8 |
| Total Cost (€) | 3,698,551 | 1,177,030 | 1,036,927 | 4,451,991 |
| Cost per survivor (€) | 2,634 | 8,152 | 15,295 | 38,572 |
| Cost per non-survivor (€) | 3,330 | 7,413 | 10,886 | 31,324 |
| Effective cost per survivor (€) | 2,745 | 9,974 | 20,738 | 60,162 |

The data of 3.276 ICU patients with 6.536 patient days were analyzed. Cost for each classified field were calculated from yearly unit costs, evaluated TISS points, and duration of artificial mechanical ventilation. Mean APACHE II points and mean Risk of death were taken from the corresponding data of day one on ventilator. In the category ≥7125 patients cover 2.700 patient days with total costs of €4.451.991 but in the category ≤21.392 patients cover 2.784 patient days with total costs of €3.698.551.
Data source: Annual ICU Audit (2002), Riyadh ICU program; Klinikum Links der Weser Bremen.

**Table 51-8**  Analysis of cost of treatment in the ICU between January 1, 2003, and December 31, 2003

| On ventilator day bands | ≤2 | ≥2 to ≤4 | ≥4 to ≤7 | ≥7 |
|---|---|---|---|---|
| Patients (n) | 1342 | 173 | 66 | 129 |
| Patient days (% of all treatment days) | 3891 (50.6) | 726 (9.4) | 382 (5.0) | 2786 (36.2) |
| Mean APACHE II points (SD) | 11.7 (4.4) | 15.2 (6.5) | 16.7 (6.9) | 16.4 (6.8) |
| Mean % Risk of death (SD) | 6.2 (8.1) | 18.1 (18.8) | 23.4 (21.3) | 22.5 (19.7) |
| % Mortality | 2.4 | 22.0 | 31.8 | 34.1 |
| SMR | 0.4 | 1.2 | 1.4 | 1.5 |
| Total Cost (€) | 3,778,174 | 1,404,623 | 977,976 | 5,635,770 |
| Cost per survivor (€) | 2,749 | 8,204 | 16,182 | 44,916 |
| Cost per non-survivor (€) | 5,494 | 7,813 | 11,894 | 42,970 |
| Effective cost per survivor (€) | 2,884 | 10,404 | 21,732 | 66,303 |

The data of 3.143 ICU patients with 6.785 patient days were analyzed. Cost for each classified field were calculated from yearly unit costs, evaluated TISS points, and duration of artificial mechanical ventilation. Mean APACHE II points and mean Risk of death were taken from the corresponding data of day one on ventilator. In the category ≥7129 patients cover 2.786 patient days with total costs of €5.635.770 but in the category ≥21.334 patients cover 3.891 patient days with total costs of €3.778.174.
Data source: Annual ICU Audit (2003), Riyadh ICU program; Klinikum Links der Weser Bremen.

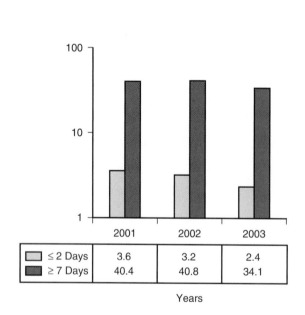

| | 2001 | 2002 | 2003 |
|---|---|---|---|
| ☐ ≤ 2 Days | 3.6 | 3.2 | 2.4 |
| ■ ≥ 7 Days | 40.4 | 40.8 | 34.1 |

Years

**Figure 51.10**  Mean mortality in patients with ≤2 days of AMV decreases slightly, but the mortality in patients with ≥7 days of AMV decreased within 3 years by 6.3%. (Data from Annual ICU Audit, 2001–2003, Riyadh ICU program; Klinikum Links der Weser Bremen.)

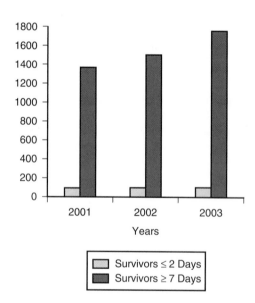

**Figure 51.11**  Analysis of TISS point data in survivors (January 1, 2001, to December 31, 2003). The mean TISS points in patients with ≤2 days of AMV are different from those in patients with ≥7 days of AMV, but there is a continuous increase in cost of survivors in the patient group with ≥7 days of AMV. (Data from Annual ICU Audit, 2001–2003, Riyadh ICU program; Klinikum Links der Weser Bremen.)

to relate these costs to activity and patients and to obtain sufficient information on treatment, resources, patient groups, and productivity of the unit.

On the other hand, it is impossible to evaluate the costs of a single procedure such as AMV in an individual patient and to compare these costs with those costs for any other patient treated in another ICU. AMV as a single measure in a healthy young man suffering from single persistent segmental atelectasis after pneumococcal pneumonia, sufficiently treated with penicillin, is quite different than that for an elderly patient suffering from multiple organ failure after Coronary Artery Bypass Grafting (CABG) and nosocomial pneumonia.

Costing in ICU and patients treated with AMV is necessary to understand the dynamics of the unit's working process, productivity, and efficiency. The aim of costing is not to save money but rather to enable a better utilization of resources. ICU resources are scarce and demand is high, and we need information on how to best use the available resources.

Increasing performance within the confines of the unit budget or other constraints is a common request that requires one to reflect on outcome, costs, and ICU performance.

Every long-term ICU cost study provides information about cost structure of the unit and how these costs can be related to the categories of input, output, efficiency, diagnosis, severity of illness, and performed procedures. Costing serves as a powerful tool for quality control.

## REFERENCES

1. Snider GL: Historical perspective on mechanical ventilation: From simple life support to ethical dilemma. Am Rev Respir Dis 1989;140:S2–S7.
2. Esteban A, Anzueto A, Frutos F, et al: Characteristics and outcomes in adult patients receiving mechanical ventilation. A 28-day international study. JAMA 2002;287:345–355.
3. Behrendt CE: Acute respiratory failure in the United States. Incidence and 31-day survival. Chest 2000;118:1100–1105.
4. Swinburne AJ, Fedullo AJ, Bixby K, et al: Respiratory failure in the elderly: Analysis of outcome after treatment with mechanical ventilation. Arch Intern Med 1993;153:1657–1662.
5. Lubitz J, Greenberg LG, Gorina Y, et al: Three decades of health care use by the elderly, 1965-1998. Health Affairs 2001;20:19–32.
6. Wagner DP: Economics of prolonged mechanical ventilation. Am Rev Respir Dis 1989;140:S14–S18.
7. Chelluri L, Grenvik A, Silverman M: Intensive care for critically ill elderly: Mortality, costs, and quality of life. Arch Intern Med 1995;155:1013–1022.
9. Pesau B, Falger S, Berger E, et al: Influence of age on outcome of mechanically ventilated patients in an intensive care unit. Crit Care Med 1992;20:489–492.
10. Zilberberg MD, Epstein SK: Acute lung injury in the medical ICU. Comorbid conditions, age, etiology, and hospital outcome. Am J Respir Crit Care Med 1998;157:1159–1164.

11. Kurek CJ, Dewar D, Lambrinos J, et al: Clinical and economic outcome of mechanically ventilated patients in New York State during 1993. Analysis of 10,473 cases under DRG 475. Chest 1998;114:214–222.
12. Cohen IL, Lambrinos J: Investigating the impact of age on outcome of mechanical ventilation using a population of 41,848 patients from a statewide database. Chest 1995;107:1673–1680.
13. Parviainen I, Herranen A, Holm A, et al. Results and costs of intensive care in a tertiary university hospital from 1996-2000. Acta Anaesthesiol Scand 2004;48:55–60.
14. Gyldmark M: A review of cost studies of intensive care units: Problems with the cost concept. Crit Care Med 1995;23:964–972.
15. Heyland DK, Konopad E, Noseworthy T, et al: Is it "worthwhile" to continue treating patients with a prolonged stay (>14 days) in the ICU? An economic analysis. Chest 1998;114:192–198.
16. Miranda DR, Moreno R, Iapichino G: Nine equivalents of nursing manpower use score (NEMS). Intensive Care Med 1997;23:760–765.
17. Keene AR, Cullen DJ: Therapeutic Intervention Scoring System: Update 1983. Crit Care Med 1983;11:1–3.
18. Edbrooke DL, Stevens VG, Hibbert CL, et al: A new method of accurately identifying costs of individual patients in intensive care: The initial results. Intensive Care Med 1997;23:645–650.
19. Rapoport J, Teres D, Lemeshow S, et al: A method for assessing the clinical performance and cost-effectiveness of intensive care units: A multicenter inception cohort study. Crit Care Med 1994;22:1385–1391.
20. Shoemaker WC: Critical care research in the 1990s: How our perceptions affect creativity. Crit Care Med 1994;22:1040–1043.
21. Dubinsky M, Ferguson JH: Analysis of the National Institutes of Health Medicare coverage assessment. Int J Technol Assess Health Care 1990;6:480–488.
22. Hamel MB, Phillips RS, Davis RB, et al: Outcomes and cost-effectiveness of initiating dialysis and continuing aggressive care in seriously ill hospitalized adults. SUPPORT Investigators. Study to Understand Prognoses and Preferences for Outcomes and Risks of Treatments. Ann Intern Med 1997;127: 195–202.
23. Miller G: The marginal number seven, plus or minus two: Some limits on our capacity for processing information. Psychol Rev 1956;63:81–97.
24. Dreyfuss D, Saumon G: Ventilator-induced lung injury: Lessons from experimental studies. Am J Respir Crit Care Med 1998;157:294–323.
25. Pinhu L, Withehead T, Evans T, et al: Ventilator-associated lung injury. Lancet 2003;361:332–340.
26. Amato MB, Barbas CS, Medeiros DM, et al: Effect of a protective-ventilation strategy on morality in the acute respiratory distress syndrome. N Engl J Med 1998;338:347–354.
27. The Acute Respiratory Distress Syndrome Network: Ventilation with lower tidal voumes for acute lung injury and the acute respiratory distress syndrome. N Engl J Med 2000;342:1301–1308.
28. Knaus WA, Draper EA, Wagner WP, et al: APACHE II: A severity of disease classification system. Crit Care Med 1985;13:818–882.
29. Chang RWS, Jacobs S, Lee B: Predicting outcome of intensive care unit patients using computerised trend analysis of daily APACHE II scores corrected for organ system failure. Intensive Care Med 1988;14:558–566.

30. Cullen DJ, Keene R, Waternaux C, et al: Results, charges and benefits of intensive care for critically ill patients: Update. Crit Care Med 1984;12:102–106.

31. National Heart, Lung, and Blood Institute, Division of Lung Diseases: Extracorporeal Support for Respiratory Insufficiency: A collaborative study. Bethesda, MD: National Institutes for Health, 1979.

32. Ricard JD, Dreyfuss D, Saumon G: Ventilator-induced lung injury. Eur Respir J 2003;22:2s–9s.

33. Gattinioni L, Carlesso E, Cadringher P, et al: Physical and biochemical triggers of ventilator-induced lung injury and its prevention. Eur Respir J 2003;22:15s–25s.

34. Botha AJ, Moore FA, Moore EE: Postinjury neutrophil priming and active states: Therapeutic challenges. Shock 1995;3:157–162.

35. Kohn LT, Corrigan JM, Donaldson MS (eds): To Err Is Human. Building a Safer Health System. Washington, DC: National Academy Press, 1999.

# CHAPTER 52

# Ventilator Care in the Developing World

Iqbal Mustafa and David J. Baker

Artificial ventilation in both hospital and prehospital practice is a long-established part of emergency and critical care. A wide variety of techniques and devices exist, but for the most part these have been developed for the specific requirements of medicine and surgery in countries that are financially secure and technically well supported. In earlier days anesthetic and intensive care techniques in developed nations were relatively simple and could be transported to more remote and less privileged regions of the world without problems. However, the increasing sophistication and cost of equipment used in the richer nations has widened the gap between potential health care provision compared with other parts of the world. This is true in many areas of practice, including the provision of ventilatory care, which in the developed nations has become almost oversophisticated in many situations due to accelerated electronic advances and competitive commercial pressure from manufacturers. This chapter considers some of the medicoeconomic problems of developing nations and possible solutions for the particular problems they face in terms of ventilation equipment requirements, skill levels, and training.

## PROBLEMS OF MEDICAL CARE IN DEVELOPING NATIONS

As the term implies, *developing nations* (DNs) may be regarded as those that are in a state of socioeconomic progression toward the accepted "developed" model of Western society in terms of utilization of resources and the distribution of gross domestic product (GDP) into a social infrastructure that includes a health care system. In practice there are considerable differences in nations classified in this way, particularly among Asian and African models. Many DNs are not necessarily financially deprived, but there may exist a far wider gap between the rich and poor than is the case in developed countries. This may be evident in terms of wealth but also in terms of the proportion of the GDP that is placed into health care systems. Western notions of state-funded care with a high proportion of GDP entering health care may not be applicable or feasible. The main features of developing nations include the following: a limited proportion of GDP put into a health care system, limited financial resources, large dependent populations who may be unevenly distributed into dense urban masses or spread over large land masses, limited prehospital emergency care systems, uneven provision of referral hospital care, and a limited supply of trained medical and nursing personnel.

An example of the diversity among DNs is found in the Far East, where countries including Singapore, Hong Kong, Taiwan, Thailand, Malaysia, Indonesia, and China have economies that have grown rapidly in the past decade. The resultant increase in affluence in some part of those countries has led to a better quality of medical care, increasing number of hospitals beds, creation of highly specialized tertiary care hospitals, and purchase of the latest technology in many parts of Asia.[1] Many DNs have a widely spread and poorly sustained administrative and technical infrastructure, and physical communication over large distances may be difficult (e.g., in China and Indonesia). As a result, health care can be of widely differing standards depending on location. Although large urban areas may benefit from teaching and regional hospitals that are of the Western standard, the rural areas do not, and the care and equipment available become increasingly limited with distance away from the major centers.

In common with the rest of the world, however, pressures are starting to mount in Asia because of increasing health costs and the rising expectations of the consumer. This has led to moves in several countries to rationalize health resources and to make hospitals accountable for the way these resources are used. In addition, in common with other rapidly developing and industrializing countries, they have begun to experience changes in the pattern of disease and illness. Part of the incidence of disease is attributable to successful economic development and delivery of appropriate health services that have increased life expectancy, exposing people to modern disease characteristic of developing nations. The increasing number of motor vehicle accidents (associated with the proliferation of highways in big cities) in some countries also puts demands on high-cost services including ambulances, emergency rooms, and communications systems.

## EMERGENCY AND CRITICAL CARE SERVICES IN DEVELOPING NATIONS

Intermittent positive pressure ventilation (IPPV) is used in both emergency and critical care management. Ventilation is required in prehospital emergency care and also when transporting a critically ill patient inside the hospital or from one hospital to another.[2,3] In most Western countries there is a degree of standardization in the provision of emergency and hospital critical care. This applies to both equipment and training. Thus in France the state ambulance service (SAMU) provides nationwide standards in the quality and type of emergency care provided, including ventilation.[2] However, in most DNs emergency and critical care overall lags behind the models created by the West. The reasons for this are related to both economics and the scale of the distances involved.

In Southeast Asia there are variable standards in the provision of ventilation in prehospital care. Emergency care may be only a transport system to emergency departments within the regional hospital. Inside the hospital, most of the best intensive care units (ICUs) in each of the countries of the region are in the capital city and have affiliations with the medical school of the state university. They are usually well staffed by medical school departments. In Singapore, Taiwan, and Hong Kong, these units are well equipped and have enough qualified nurses (certified in intensive care). However, in China and most of the Association of South East Asian Nations (ASEAN)

countries, units are not as well equipped and most nurses are not certified in intensive care.[4]

## Cultural Variations

In some DNs the practice of intensive care medicine is often made more difficult by the increased awareness of the general public of advances in organ-sustaining and life-sustaining technology and pharmaceutical advances. This often leads to high expectations for recovery that may not be justified in the presence of multiple organ failure. Stopping treatment is very often impossible because of the difficulty the public has in accepting brain death, even though this has already been accepted by the medical community in some countries. Thus in some countries local custom requires continued ventilation of braindead patients until the "official" death occurs.

## Costs

As a consequence of economic progress, health system development, improved living standards, education, increased life expectancy, and modern diseases, there have been increasing demands for highly technical and expensive medical care by the public, especially among medium- and high-income groups. The total cost of care in an ICU per day in a big hospital in Jakarta is approximately 300 U.S. dollars (USD) to 500 USD. In Indonesia, which has great heterogeneity among provinces and variations in terms of population density, the proportion of those with insurance was estimated at only 14% of the total population. This in turn causes difficulties for prolonged intensive care treatment. The ICU expenses are three times or more than those of an ordinary ward in most countries. Health expenditure as a proportion of the gross domestic product is well below the target of 5% set by the World Health Organization. With budget reallocation and managed care, the limited financial resources will certainly make the development of intensive care based on new high technology in every hospital or district in each country impossible.[1]

A possible solution is to refer patients to hospitals with good intensive care (regionalization of critical care medicine). In university hospitals where the budget is allocated among various clinical departments, funding of intensive care can become even more difficult. In private hospitals and in other public hospitals, the ICU represents a unit of the hospital that is funded by the hospital's budget. As a consequence, hospital administrations often find the ICU is not a profitable unit and are very reluctant to increase its budget. In DNs, health economics play a major role in the provision of care and equipment. Thus individual governments and international aid organizations have to look at the money available in terms of providing the greatest care for the greatest number.

## SPECIFIC PROBLEMS CONCERNING VENTILATION IN DEVELOPING NATIONS

There have been few specific studies of the provision of ventilatory care in DNs. Fieselmann and his colleagues[5] have published a detailed study of mechanical ventilation in rural ICUs, but the setting was in the United States. From a study of morbidity the authors found considerable differences between rural referral and rural hospitals, even in a developed country, indicating the importance of a tertiary referral center. Given the problems of distance and communication in DNs, this concept may be difficult to achieve, and thus specific ventilatory care must be maximized at the rural level.

Factors governing the provision of IPPV in DN include the following:

1. Equipment provision and cost
2. Equipment suitability for the area where it is used
3. Servicing
4. Power supplies
5. Bottled gas supplies
6. Training and experience of medical and nursing staff

Although developed nations work according to models of prehospital and hospital health care that define uniform standards of ventilator care, no such models are appropriate for widely spread and heavily populated countries where regional rather than central government is the controlling force in local health care. Selection of ventilation equipment, at least in the state medical systems, may have to follow this dictum, and therefore careful consideration of where and how the ventilators are to be used is necessary, together with who is to use them and how the users are to be trained.

## LOCATIONS FOR VENTILATORY CARE

As in the developed nations, DN hospital care requires ventilation in all areas of clinical practice. The machines used will depend on the role of the hospital, but the locations may be divided into specialist and general hospital centers. Operating theater and intensive care provide the greatest concentration of ventilators, but there is also expansion in providing IPPV in the emergency room and other parts of the hospital using portable devices.

### Prehospital Care

In prehospital care, emergency services in DNs are usually very limited compared with the developed nations. Many emergency service ambulances are no more than a means of transporting the patient to a hospital with an ER, and onboard equipment is very basic. With the growing incidence of trauma as a world problem, however, many countries are considering how to improve their prehospital emergency services, both in terms of staffing and equipment.

### Regional Hospital Care

In rural areas, hospital services may be limited in scope, and anesthetic and intensive care techniques are therefore more basic. Accordingly, ventilators may be provided that are old and relatively simple in their operation. Often, however, aid agencies and other bodies may provide machines that are inappropriate for the location in terms of being dependent on power supplies and requiring detailed servicing by engineers who may be based many hundreds or even thousands of miles away. China provides a good example of the overall problems of sustaining ventilatory care.

Most of the ventilators used in China, including those in rural areas (if available), are imported. Domestic ventilators are currently of limited quality and have very little market share in China. Hospitals in China are categorized as Grade I, II, or III. Grade III is the top level. Usually only above Grade II do hospitals have the capacity to use and maintain ventilators. The emergency system seldom uses ventilators because its job is simply to transport patients. The knowledge and training of ventilator use among health care workers is limited. Only respiratory specialists and ICU staff have any specific knowledge.[6]

## HIGH TECHNOLOGY VERSUS LOW TECHNOLOGY IN AUTOMATIC VENTILATION

In DNs, ventilators should be suitable for the location, available skills, and infrastructure. For much of the developing world, this implies simple basic ventilators that can be operated and sustained locally.

However, many national doctors returning to DNs have trained in Western hospitals with sophisticated equipment and naturally wish to use such devices in their homeland. Few Western training programs now use simple equipment that is appropriate for developing nations, and thus overseas training programs in anesthesia and critical care may be of limited relevance. In several DN countries such as Indonesia, the National Society of Anesthesiologists working together with the World Federation of Society of Anesthesiologists, although using technically advanced equipment, still operate courses designed to prepare anesthetists and intensivists for conditions in remote areas. It is essential that original basic anesthetic and critical care skills are not lost and that simple reliable and familiar equipment is not discarded simply because it is old or unfashionable.

In broad terms, ventilators and monitors are required that provide a high standard of care in difficult locations while being cheaper and simpler to operate than the current range of ventilators common in developed nations, which are significantly overcomplicated. Many of the computer-controlled modes of pressure support ventilation found on modern ventilators are not essential for basic respiratory care and have developed as part of commercial and technical pressures.

## COMMERCIAL ISSUES

Few DNs produce their own ventilators, and manufacturers in the developed nations produce machines that are primarily designed for use in their own country or other developed nations. Manufacturers may target DNs as recipient customers for ultrasophisticated ventilators that have large profit margins. This may be particularly true when external aid funds are available for capital equipment purchase. The process may also be aided by local agents whose commission depends on the total value of sale. There is often therefore little commercial incentive to sell lower-priced basic equipment for ventilation.

Competitive pressures in the industrialized nations have led to the production of ventilators that are almost all of sophisticated design. This has left a void of simple nonelectronic equipment on the market that is suitable for DN use. Several decades ago, the technical gap between equipment used in the developed and developing worlds was narrower. Simple ventilators, mostly pneumatic in operation, were the rule and were also suitable for use in DNs. Few ventilator manufacturers now use what might be called "sustainable technology"; in other words, ventilators and anesthetic equipment that can be operated and maintained in the often difficult conditions of DNs. Despite this, there is still a pool of equipment produced in the West that does fall into this classification, such as pneumatically operated ventilators.[7,8]

## IDEAL VENTILATOR CHARACTERISTICS FOR USE IN THE WIDEST POSSIBLE RANGE OF HEALTH CARE FACILITIES IN DEVELOPING NATIONS

The provision of equipment must strike a balance among the qualities of desirability, feasibility, practicability, and sustainability, as follows:

1. The characteristics of a basic DN ventilator may be defined by the most taxing environment where it will be used. This is usually in a rural setting.

2. Thus the DN standard ventilator should be of simple reliable function and rugged construction. It should be reasonably priced and able to operate within the limitations of the available electric power and gas supply.

3. Ideally it should be manufactured in the country of use and have servicing facilities close at hand. It should be capable of basic ventilatory modes such as conventional mechanical ventilation (CMV), SIMV, and AC and be able to provide PEEP. It should be capable of both adult and pediatric use.

4. It should be capable for use by a wide range of clinicians and nurses who may have received only a limited amount of critical care training.

5. It should have safety and monitoring features that are compatible with normal standards in developed nations (and often with certain specialized units that may exist with the DN itself).

6. The ventilator may have to perform many tasks and the DN setting.

## VENTILATOR OPTIONS FOR USE IN DEVELOPING NATIONS

The following ventilator options are available:

1. *Servo ventilators* are used widely around the world but developed primarily for developed nation use. They require a reliable mains power and compressed gas supply.

2. *Simpler electromagnetic turbine ventilators* have been developed for a wide range of transport and high-dependency unit operations. Examples include the T Bird (Viays Health Care, Conshohocken, PA) and the Elysee (Saime SA RES MED, Poway, CA). They are of mains/battery operation and do not require a compressed gas supply. Oxygen is used only for gas enrichment and could be replaced by an oxygen concentrator.

3. *Pneumatically operated transport and emergency ventilators* could be used in a basic ICU role. Examples include Pneupac Ventipac (Smiths Medical International, Ltd., Kent, UK) and Drager Oxylog 2000 (Drager Siemens, Luebeck, Germany).

4. *Mixed pneumatic and electric ventilators* require a compressed gas and a mains/battery supply. Examples include the Drager 3000 and Osiris 2 (Taema SA, Cedex, France).

5. *Autonomous transport ventilators* were originally designed for military use. Only the Pneupac CompPac 200 (Smith Medical International, Ltd., Kent, UK) fulfills this role at present. It has a wide range of power options including mains/external DC supply/internal battery, which drives an internal compressor. This ventilator has been used in a variety of DN

operations including transport and disaster medicine and in use with field anesthesia.[9]

6. *Simple and tried bellows ventilators* are gas-driven minute volume dividers. An example is the traditional Manley (Penlon, Ltd., Oxfordshire, UK) ventilator, which is still manufactured and used worldwide.

7. *Bellows-type ventilator* driven by a gas engine is another option. The driving gas can be either compressed air or oxygen of nonmedical quality because the driving engine is separate from the patient circuit. An example is the Oxford Nuffield Ventilator (Penlon, Ltd.).

## MONITORING EQUIPMENT SUITABLE FOR GENERAL USE IN DEVELOPING NATIONS

Safety in providing IPPV depends on good clinical practice aided by the provision of monitoring equipment. In parallel with the development of ventilators in Western nations, there has been a development of sometimes sophisticated monitoring equipment. Much of this may not be appropriate for use in DNS, but many techniques are applicable, portable, and feasible.

Therefore although there may be limited availability of blood gas analysis in rural areas of DNs, monitoring can be achieved using pulse oximetry and capnography analysis, which are technologically sustainable.

In addition, many of the sustainable ventilators mentioned previously have built-in monitoring devices.

The essentials for monitoring are as follows:

1. Monitoring the ventilator. Essential monitoring includes:
   Bottled gas supply pressure alarm
   Mains power failure alarm
   High inflation pressure alarm
   Low inflation pressure (disconnection) alarm
   Tidal and minute volume monitoring
   Inflation pressure and PEEP monitoring
   Inspired $Fio_2$ monitor
2. Monitoring the patient: Any ventilated patient should never be left unattended, and monitoring should include:
   Clinical observation
   Pulse oximetry
   Capnography
   Electrocardiography (ECG)

## OXYGEN SUPPLIES

The provision of piped or bottled oxygen is a facility that is often taken for granted in hospitals in developed nations.

The same may not be true of facilities in other parts of the world. Although the provision of bottled oxygen from a central supply is well within the technical capability of DNs, the transport infrastructure may make delivery difficult. Thus the supply cannot be relied upon in many cases.

The development of pressure-swing oxygen concentrators has provided a useful source of oxygen enrichment for patients being ventilated with air. The development of these devices has been accelerated by home use in developed nations, and there are now multiple bed models that provide supplies of 3 to 5 L/min from a mains- or battery-operated supply.

## TRAINING FOR VENTILATION IN DEVELOPING NATIONS

In several countries in the Southeast Asia region, including Indonesia, Singapore, Malaysia, Taiwan, and Hong Kong, working together with the Society of Critical Care Medicine (USA), the respective national societies have organized a Fundamental Critical Care Course that contains lectures and several workshops on respiratory failure and mechanical ventilation. In Indonesia, under the auspices of the Indonesian Society of Intensive Care Medicine, there has been a regular basic mechanical ventilation course and a 3-day advanced mechanical ventilation course.

## THE NEED FOR STANDARDIZATION

Standardization is required in the provision of hospital organization, care, and training, both medical and nursing, and in the provision of equipment that is familiar.

### Organization

Provision of ventilation care may be defined in terms of levels, as follows:

- Level 1: A basic rural facility capable of providing intraoperative and immediate postoperative care. This should also include prehospital emergency care, which is often linked with the hospital emergency room in such areas. This level should also include prehospital emergency and transportation ventilatory care.
- Level 2: Intermediate hospital facilities. This level covers general surgical and medical care with high-dependency beds capable of providing longer-term ventilator and other ICU care backed by basic laboratory facilities such as blood gas analysis.

- Level 3: Referral center care at a regional level that has full general district hospital care including essential ICU care.
- Level 4: Specialized referral care in major cities (e.g., cardiothoracic, neurosurgical). In many DNs, such as Indonesia, there are only one or two such centers for the whole country.

## NEED FOR CONTINUOUS QUALITY IMPROVEMENT

As noted previously, there is a wide variety in the services and potential resources of DNs. Some have rapidly developing technical and administrative infrastructures that are changing the country quickly. Other DNs are locked into a cycle of poverty and local deprivation through warfare and mass starvation, making any internal progression difficult without substantial foreign help.

The responsibility for quality improvement must be driven from the following:

- Internal national resources
- External agencies (e.g., World Health Organization)
- International professional bodies (e.g., World Federation of Societies of Anaesthesia)

### Priorities

Priorities may be summarized as follows:

1. The provision of equipment suitable for the surroundings and the medical infrastructure
2. Determination of the essential modes of ventilatory support required and avoidance of technological "overkill"
3. Development of a structure that allows transport of critically ill patients from rural facilities to larger, centralized care units

### Publication of Standards

Definition of the minimal safety requirements for airway and ventilation management in all areas of practice in DNs is essential. Transport ventilation safety requirements from EMS services in developed nations may be relevant in this area.[3] Although DNs may have limited resources, this does not necessarily mean that that they cannot be among the leaders in setting standards. The Second Asia Consensus Conference on the management of acute lung injuries[10] provides an example of a collaboration among experts from developed nations and from DNs in providing quality evidence-based guidelines for good ventilatory practice.

## CONCLUSIONS

Given the rapid economic, scientific, and technological development in DNs, it is certain that the development of health care and critical care medicine will be affected. Even with the problems that have to be faced, the future of critical care medicine in East Asia looks promising. Global economic markets and the forthcoming free trade region agreed to by the Asian Pacific Economic Cooperation countries will accelerate the process. In other less stable parts of the world, the problems of providing a stable infrastructure are more severe. Many DNs show signs of becoming poorer and will be less able to procure and use equipment.

The leaders of emergency and critical care medicine in each country, however, should identify the model of emergency and critical care practice that is the most appropriate for their country. There is a great need for simple, inexpensive equipment and methods for monitoring critically ill patients that can be shown to be effective. Efficient systems for transporting critical patients are also needed.

Simple ventilators with inexpensive monitors (capable of monitoring ECG, continuous oxygen saturation, continuous central venous pressure, and continuous invasive blood pressure) and defibrillators are the technology that is most needed and that could have a great impact on the mortality and morbidity of critically ill patients in many units, even in rural areas.

Good referral systems (transportation and communication) and a few high-standard ICUs with good facilities for education and training should be organized on a regional basis in each country. Two or three centers with good research facilities and capabilities, helped by various international or regional joint cooperative initiatives, should be started to conduct cutting-edge research in intensive and critical care medicine.

There should be continued exchange between developed and developing nations to help with training and organization of ventilatory care. The use of technology that is sustainable within the DN infrastructure, together with the development of quality control in equipment and its operation, will lead to significant improvements.

## REFERENCES

1. Mustafa I, Tai HY: Critical care in East Asia: Little dragons and sleeping giants. In Kvetan V (ed): Critical Care Clinics, vol 13. Philadelphia: Saunders, 1997, pp 287–298.
2. Baker DJ, Tillant D, Carli PA: Emergency ventilation. Int J Intensive Care 2000;7:229–232.
3. Tillant D, Baker DJ, Carli PA: Mechanical ventilation during transport of critically-ill patients. Int J Intensive Care 2000;7:59–67.

4. Hillman K: Intensive care in developing countries. Intensive Care World 1995;2:34.

5. Fieselmann JF, Bock M Jeanne, Hendryx MS, et al: Mechanical ventilation in rural ICUs. Crit Care 1999;3:23–31.

6. Xi- Zhao A: Personal communication. Beijing: World Health Organization Regional Office, Feb 2004.

7. Nolan JP, Baskett PJ: Gas-powered and portable ventilators: An evaluation of six models. Prehosp Disaster Med 1992;7:25–34.

8. McCluskey A, Gwinnutt CL: Evaluation of the pneuPac Ventilpac portable ventilator; comparison of performance in mechanical lung and anaesthetised patients. Br J Anaesthesia 1995;75:645–650.

9. Bell G: The use of the CompPac ventilator: Experience in Nepal. Milit Med 2003;168;827–829.

10. The 2nd Asia Pacific Consensus Conference on Acute Lung Injury. Crit Care Shock 1999;3:119–133.

# CHAPTER 53

# Ventilator-Induced Lung Injury

Jack J. Haitsma and Arthur S. Slutsky

At the dawn of the new millennium, the National Institutes of Health (NIH)-sponsored Acute Respiratory Distress Syndrome (ARDS) Network showed unequivocally that the specific ventilatory strategy used influences patient outcome.[1] They compared two ventilation strategies; the first strategy used traditional tidal volume (12 mL/kg predicted body weight (PBW), corresponding to about 10 mL/kg body weight (BW) and a plateau pressure of 50 cmH$_2$O, and the second strategy used reduced tidal volumes (6 mL/kg PBW, corresponding to about 5 mL/kg BW); plateau pressures were limited to 30 cmH$_2$O, which was deemed protective (Fig. 53.1). Using the protective strategy, the ARDS Network reduced mortality to 31% compared with 40% in the traditionally ventilated group.[1]

This study of 861 patients demonstrated that ventilator-induced lung injury (VILI) has an attributable mortality of at least 9%. What is VILI, how does it happen, and what can we do to minimize it?

## ARDS, ALI, VALI, VILI

Every year, millions of patients worldwide receive ventilator support for a number of indications including respiratory failure and during surgery procedures. Mechanical ventilation has become an important therapy in the treatment of patients with impaired pulmonary function and particularly in patients suffering from ARDS. Several terms require definition (Box 53.1). The definition of acute lung injury (ALI) according to the American-European Consensus Conference on ALI/ARDS is as follows: acute onset; PaO$_2$/FiO$_2$ <300 mm Hg; bilateral infiltrates seen on a frontal chest radiograph; and pulmonary artery wedge pressure <18 mm Hg or no clinical evidence of left atrial hypertension.[2] ARDS is simply ALI with greater hypoxemia; the criteria are the same except that PaO$_2$/FiO$_2$ <200 mm Hg. VILI is defined by the international consensus conference on ventilator-associated lung injury (VALI) in ARDS as acute lung injury directly induced by mechanical ventilation in animal models.[3] Because VILI is usually indistinguishable morphologically, physiologically, and

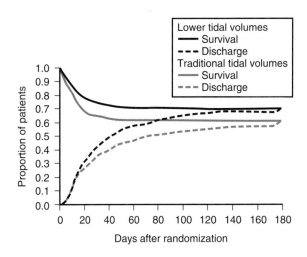

**Figure 53.1** Plot from the ARDS Network trial showing the probability of survival and of being discharged home and breathing without assistance during the first 180 days after randomization to patients either with ALI and ARDS (used with permission (3)). Patients were randomized to either traditional tidal volume (12 mL/kg predicted body weight [PBW]) and a plateau pressure <50 cmH$_2$O or to lower tidal volume (6 mL/kg PBW) and plateau pressure limited to 30 cmH$_2$O.

**Acute lung injury (ALI)[2]**
Acute onset
$Pao_2/Fio_2$ <300 mm Hg
Bilateral infiltrates seen on a frontal chest radiograph
Pulmonary artery wedge pressure <18 mm Hg or no clinical evidence of left atrial hypertension

**Acute respiratory distress syndrome (ARDS)[2]**
Acute onset
$Pao_2/Fio_2$ <200 mm Hg
Bilateral infiltrates seen on a frontal chest radiograph
Pulmonary artery wedge pressure <18 mm Hg or no clinical evidence of left atrial hypertension

**Ventilator-induced lung injury (VILI)[3]**
Acute lung injury directly induced by mechanical ventilation in animal models

**Ventilator-associated lung injury (VALI)[3]**
Acute lung injury that resembles ARDS in patients receiving mechanical ventilation
VALI may be associated with preexisting lung pathology such as ARDS
VALI is associated only with mechanical ventilation

radiologically from the diffuse alveolar damage of acute lung injury, it can only be discerned definitively in animal models. VALI is defined as lung injury that resembles ARDS and is thought to occur due to mechanical ventilation. VALI may be associated with preexisting lung pathology such as ARDS. However, unlike VILI, one cannot be sure that VALI is caused by mechanical ventilation. Barotrauma is defined as extraalveolar air and most often results from overdistension of alveoli and rupture of their walls down a pressure gradient from air space into the bronchovascular sheath.[4]

ARDS is caused by multiple factors and is characterized by respiratory dysfunction including hypoxemia and decreased lung compliance.[2] It is known that the decrease in lung distensibility is due in part to a disturbed surfactant system resulting in an elevated surface tension. This increase in surface tension leads to instability of alveoli at end-expiration and subsequent[4] collapse, as well as an increase in right-to-left shunt and a decrease in $Pao_2$. Mechanical ventilation can maintain arterial oxygenation and allow ventilation of atelectatic areas by generating airway pressures sufficiently high to overcome the opening pressures needed to open these alveoli. However, mechanical ventilation can also cause adverse effects.

## ARDS

The propensity to injury is partly related to the inhomogeneity in distensibility of the injured lung.[5,6] The open and thus relatively healthy lung parts will be prone to overinflation, whereas the injured lung areas will not be inflated. The progression of the injury to the lung will result in atelectatic lung areas and patches of still-open lung tissue. When this lung is ventilated, even with small tidal volumes, air will go preferentially to these open, still-compliant parts. This phenomenon has been described by Gattinoni as a "baby lung," and the subsequent ventilation even with small tidal volumes will result in overdistension.[3,5] Depending on the amount of collapsed lung tissue, even these small tidal volumes will increase the actual tidal volume delivered to the open lung areas by severalfold.

## Atelectrauma

These potentially pathogenic forces include repetitive (cyclic) strain (stretch) from overdistension and interdependence, as well as shear stress to the epithelial cells as lung units collapse and reopen, so-called atelectrauma.[7] The pioneering work of Mead and colleagues demonstrated that, due to the pulmonary interdependence of the alveoli, the forces acting on the fragile lung tissue in nonuniformly expanded lungs are not only the applied transpulmonary pressures, but also the shear forces that are present in the interstitium between open and closed alveoli.[8] Based on a theoretical analysis, they predicted that a transpulmonary pressure of 30 $cmH_2O$ could result in shear forces of 140 $cmH_2O$.[8] Shear forces, rather than end-inspiratory overstretching, may well be the major reason for epithelial disruption and the loss of barrier function of the alveolar epithelium. In an ARDS lung, alveoli are subjected to opening and closing during ventilation.[3,8,9] Using in vivo video microscopy Steinberg et al. directly assessed alveolar stability in normal and surfactant-deactivated lungs and elegantly showed alveolar instability (atelectrauma) during ventilation.[9]

Important evidence for this mechanism comes from the finding that ventilation even at low lung volumes can augment lung injury.[10,11] Muscedere and colleagues ventilated isolated, nonperfused, lavaged rat lungs with physiologic tidal volumes (5 to 6 mL/kg) at different end-expiratory pressures (above and below Pinf).[10] Lung injury was significantly greater in the groups ventilated with a positive end-expiratory pressure (PEEP) below Pinf, and in these groups the site of injury was dependent on the level of PEEP (Fig. 53.2). Thus, in addition to high airway pressures, end-expiratory lung volume is an important determinant of the degree and site of lung injury during positive pressure ventilation. Therefore the prevention of repeated collapse by stabilizing lung tissue at end-expiration with PEEP can reduce lung injury.[3,12–14]

## Volutrauma

In a classical paper published in 1974, Webb and Tierney demonstrated the critical role that PEEP plays in preventing

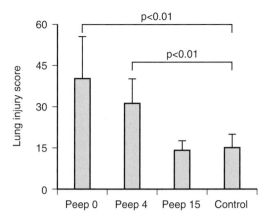

**Figure 53.2** Lung injury scores obtained from isolated nonperfused rat lungs ventilated with identical tidal volumes of 5 to 6 mL/kg body weight, but with different levels of end-expiratory pressures. Lung injury score is a composite of alveolar duct, respiratory bronchiole, and membranous bronchiole injury scored by a pathologist blinded for the samples. (Adapted from Muscedere JG, Mullen JB, Gan K, et al: Tidal ventilation at low airway pressures can augment lung injury. Am J Respir Crit Care Med 1994;149:1327–1334.)

and reducing lung injury.[14] In rats ventilated with 10 cmH$_2$O of PEEP and a peak pressure of 45 cmH$_2$O, little lung injury was present, but if the same peak pressure was used with zero PEEP, the animals developed severe pulmonary edema within 20 minutes.[14] Dreyfuss and colleagues further explored the role of tidal volume and peak inspiratory pressures on lung injury (Fig. 53.3).[15] Using an animal model they applied high inspiratory pressures in combination with high volumes, which resulted in increased alveolar permeability.[15] In a second group, low pressure was combined with high volume (iron lung ventilation), again resulting in increased alveolar permeability.[15] In the third group the effect of high pressures combined with low volume was studied by strapping the chest wall to reduce chest excursions; the permeability of this group (high-pressure, low-volume group) did not differ from the control group.[15] Thus large tidal volume ventilation increases alveolar permeability, whereas peak inspiratory pressures do not influence the development of this type of lung injury. Dreyfuss called this injury *volutrauma* to indicate that it is the distension of the lung, not the pressure at the airway opening, that is important in causing lung injury.[16]

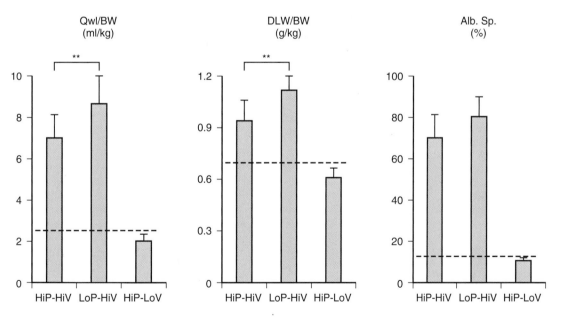

**Figure 53.3** Comparisons of the effects of high-pressure, high-volume ventilation (HiP-HiV) with those of negative inspiratory airway pressure, high tidal volume ventilation (iron lung ventilation = LoP-HiV), and of high-pressure, low-volume ventilation (thoracoabdominal strapping = HiP-LoV). Pulmonary edema was assessed by measuring the extravascular lung water content (Qwl/BW) and changes in permeability by determining the bloodless dry lung weight (DLW/BW) and the distribution space of $^{125}$I-labeled albumin (Alb. Sp) in lungs. Permeability edema occurred in both groups receiving high V$_T$ ventilation. Animals ventilated with a high peak pressure and a normal V$_T$ had no edema. (Reproduced from Dreyfuss D, Soler P, Basset G, et al: High inflation pressure pulmonary edema. Respective effects of high airway pressure, high tidal volume, and positive end-expiratory pressure. Am Rev Respir Dis 1988;137:1159–1164, with permission.)

Similar observations were made in rabbits ventilated with high peak pressures in which thorax excursions were limited by a plaster cast.[17] In injured lungs the effect of higher volumes only aggravated the permeability, as demonstrated in animals in which the surfactant system was inactivated and which were subsequently ventilated with high tidal volumes.[18,19] High transpulmonary pressure has also been demonstrated to lead to much more subtle injury. Ultrastructural abnormalities such as endothelial cell detachment, intracapillary blebs, and disrupted or damaged type I pneumocytes with areas of denuded basement membrane have been described as evidence of volutrauma secondary to alveolar overdistension.[12,20]

## Biotrauma

Recent research has focused on how mechanical stresses caused by mechanical ventilation can affect cellular and molecular processes in the lung, a mechanism that we have called *biotrauma*.[21] It has become clear that during VILI, mechanical ventilation can trigger an inflammatory reaction in the lung and that the degree of inflammation depends on the ventilation strategy.[22,23] Furthermore, this inflammatory reaction may not be limited to the lungs but may also initiate and propagate a systemic inflammatory response, possibly contributing to the onset of multiple organ failure.[24,25] The biotrauma hypothesis proposes that biophysical forces alter normal cellular physiology in the lung, leading to increases in local mediator levels and changes in pulmonary repair, remodeling, and apoptotic mechanisms.[24–26]

Mechanical ventilation will generate pressures on lung tissue and especially on lung cells. Depending on the extent of the physical forces applied, this stress may lead to activation of pulmonary cells through mechanotransduction[27] or to rupture of membranes and tissue destruction.[28] We have demonstrated that VILI can result in loss of the compartmentalized inflammatory response, leading to increased serum levels of inflammatory mediators.[29] In the early stage of inflammation in the lung, the response may be compartmentalized, as observed in community-acquired pneumonia.[30] Steinberg et al. employed in vivo video microscopy to directly assess alveolar stability in normal and surfactant-deactivated lungs and showed that alveolar instability (atelectrauma) caused mechanical injury, which initiated an inflammatory response, finally leading to secondary neutrophil-mediated proteolytic injury.[9] These data suggest that a key inciting event leading to biotrauma is cyclic stretch-induced lung injury (atelectrauma).

## Cytokines, Inflammatory Mediators

Tremblay and colleagues demonstrated that VILI could induce cytokine release.[22] Using an isolated non-perfused rat lung model, they demonstrated that ventilation with high volumes (40 mL/kg BW) and no PEEP resulted in increased levels of TNF-alpha, IL-1 beta, IL-6, MIP-2, IFN gamma, and IL-10.[22] Zero PEEP in combination with high volume ventilation (HVZP) had a synergistic effect on cytokine levels (e.g., 56-fold increase of TNF-alpha versus controls) (Fig. 53.4).

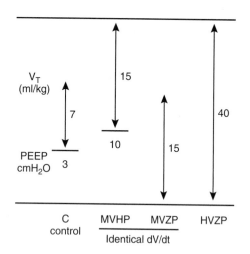

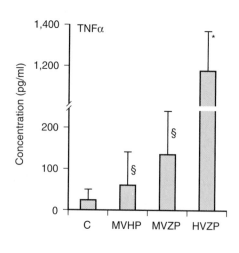

**Figure 53.4** *Left panel:* Schematic diagram of tidal volume and positive end-expiratory pressure (PEEP) levels used in the ex vivo ventilated lung model. The *right panel* demonstrates the values of tumor necrosis factor alpha (TNF-alpha) versus the four different ventilatory strategies shown in the *left panel*. Note that there is a break in the axis at (TNF-alpha) value of about 250 pg/mL. (C, control; HVZP, high volume, zero PEEP; MVHP, medium volume, high PEEP; MVZP, medium volume, zero PEEP.) (From Tremblay L, Valenza F, Ribeiro SP, et al: Injurious ventilatory strategies increase cytokines and c-fos m-RNA expression in an isolated rat lung model. J Clin Invest 1997;99:944–952, with permission.)

Ventilation with equal or higher peak airway pressures but with a PEEP of 10 cmH₂O reduced (MVHP) resulted in only a threefold increase in TNF alpha.[44] Ventilation with a lower volume (15 mL/kg BW; similar to the MVHP) but now without PEEP (MVZP) produced a sixfold increase in lavage TNF alpha, again highlighting the importance of atelectrauma.[22]

See Chapter 19 for a further exploration of the pathways and effects of cytokine release during mechanical ventilation.

## VILI IN CLINICAL TRIALS

The observations that mechanical ventilation influences mediator levels are supported by data from clinical trials.

Ranieri and colleagues randomized patients with ARDS to either a traditional ventilatory strategy or to a lung protective strategy (low tidal volume; high PEEP). The latter resulted in lower levels of inflammatory mediators (Fig. 53.5),[31] which correlated with lower levels of multiple organ failure and improved patient outcome.[32]

In 1990 Hickling and colleagues demonstrated that mechanical ventilation could influence mortality in patients with ARDS.[33] In a retrospective analysis, he demonstrated that 50 patients with ARDS ventilated with a low tidal volume (VT) and permissive hypercapnia had decreased mortality compared with historical controls.[33] The outcome of this study sparked renewed interest in lowering VT in patients with ARDS. Three subsequent controlled trials using low VT strategies were simultaneously started, but all failed to demonstrate improved patient outcomes.[34-36] These studies used a

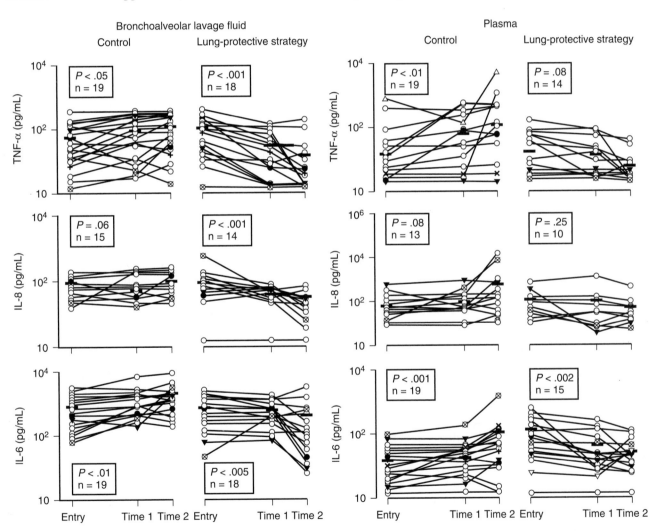

**Figure 53.5** Individual trends of tumor necrosis factor alpha (TNF-alpha), interleukin (IL)-8, and IL-6 in plasma and bronchoalveolar lavage fluid in patients receiving either lung protective ventilation (VT = 8 mL/kg; PEEP = 15 cmH₂O) or control ventilation (VT = 11 mL/kg; PEEP = 7 cmH₂O). Time 1 indicates 24 to 30 hours after study entry; time 2, 36 to 40 hours after study entry. *Horizontal bars* indicate mean values. P values are for repeated measures analysis of variance for time 2 versus entry. (Used with permission of Ranieri VM, Suter PM, Tortorella C, et al: Effect of mechanical ventilation on inflammatory mediators in patients with acute respiratory distress syndrome: A randomized controlled trial. JAMA 1999;282:54–61.)

VT of approximately 7 mL/kg in their low tidal volume arms and a VT of 10 mL/kg in their control arms.[34–36] In contrast, using a VT of 6 mL/kg in their treatment arm and a VT of 12 mL/kg in their control arm (VT calculated using PBW) the ARDS Network was able to reduce mortality.[1] In the ARDS Network study, PBW was approximately 20% lower than measured BW, resulting in a VT of approximately 10 mL/kg measured BW for the control arm.[37]

The explanation given by the ARDS Network trial for the beneficial effect on mortality was the greater difference in tidal volume between the two arms of the study, the power of the study (ARDS Network studied 861 patients, whereas the other three studied a maximum of 120 patients), and the aggressive treatment/prevention of acidosis.[1] Other studies performed since then have demonstrated that higher tidal volumes increase VILI and lead to the development of ALI.[38,39]

The only other randomized controlled trial to show a reduction of mortality in patients with ARDS had been published in 1998. Amato et al. reported that mortality in 53 patients was significantly reduced by applying a protective ventilation strategy.[40] In their study, VT was also reduced to below 6 mL/kg in the low tidal volume group compared with 12 mL/kg VT in the control arm. In contrast to the three negative studies[34–36] the PEEP level in the low tidal volume group of Amato et al.[40] was significantly higher (i.e., almost 17 $cmH_2O$ compared with 8 to 10 $cmH_2O$ PEEP in the studies by Brochard et al.,[34] Brower et al.,[35] and Stewart et al.[36]) Experimental data have shown that ventilation with low tidal volumes by itself does not prevent lung injury and may even worsen lung injury when atelectrauma is not prevented.[10] In the ARDS Network trial the low VT group had a slightly higher set PEEP of 9 $cmH_2O$ compared with a set PEEP of 8 $cmH_2O$ in the control group.[1] However, the increased respiratory rate (to help prevent acidosis) used in the low VT group may have resulted in intrinsic PEEP that contributed to a higher total PEEP (16 $cmH_2O$) in this group[41,42] compared with 12 $cmH_2O$ in the traditional VT group. This higher total PEEP could help explain the decrease in mortality observed in this group, although the data addressing this issue are somewhat contradictory.

In 2004 the ARDS Network published its follow-up study investigating whether increased PEEP levels would decrease mortality.[43] Mean PEEP values on days 1 through 4 were 8.3 $cmH_2O$ in the lower PEEP group and 13.2 $cmH_2O$ in the higher PEEP group. Although in this study no benefit in outcome was observed between the patient groups (the study was stopped early after enrollment of 549 patients), the mortality rate in both study arms was relatively low (24.9% lower PEEP and 27.5% higher PEEP),[43] providing supportive data that adjusting the ventilatory settings decreases mortality

in ARDS/ALI patients. Unfortunately, patients randomized to the higher PEEP group also had at baseline more characteristics that predict a higher mortality; adjustment for these differences in baseline covariates did not alter the final outcome but did favor the higher PEEP group.[43]

A major problem in improving patient care in ARDS is the heterogeneity of the patient population. Recent studies demonstrated that different populations exist among patients with ARDS.[44] Ferguson et al. showed that patients who had transient ARDS (improved oxygenation >200 mm Hg, under standard ventilatory settings, within 30 minutes) had a significant lower mortality of 12.5% versus 52.9% in persistent ARDS.[44] Further stratification of ARDS patient populations should help in improving the power of studies and thus help to identify improved ventilation techniques.

## ROLE OF VILI IN PATIENT OUTCOME

Although ARDS is defined by the $PaO_2/FiO_2$ ratio in the American-European Consensus conference on ARDS,[2] patients do not usually die from hypoxemia but rather die from multiple organ failure.[45,46] Slutsky and Tremblay hypothesized that mediators released in the lung might be translocated into the systemic circulation and lead to the development of multiple organ failure.[21] Ranieri and co-workers demonstrated a linkage between increased levels of serum inflammatory mediators and organ failure in patients with ARDS.[32] These increased serum levels of inflammatory mediators were observed in patients ventilated with conventional ventilation, compared with a lung protective ventilation strategy (high PEEP, low VT) that minimized the inflammatory response and subsequently had a lower incidence of organ failure (Fig. 53.6).[31,32] As discussed previously, ventilation can induce mediator release. Increased levels of cytokines in the serum were also observed in the ARDS Network trial, in which higher levels of IL-6 were observed after 3 days of ventilation in the control arm compared with the reduced tidal volume.[1] An analysis performed later also demonstrated that IL-6, IL-8, and IL-10 correlated with patient outcome.[47] Similarly, the number of days without nonpulmonary organ or system failure (circulatory, coagulation, and renal failure) was significantly higher in the group treated with lower tidal volumes.[1]

The final outcome of patients with ARDS correlates with the magnitude and duration of the host inflammatory response in the serum and is independent of the precipitating cause of ARDS or the occurrence of infections.[48] Similar observation were made in multiple-trauma patients in whom high concentrations of

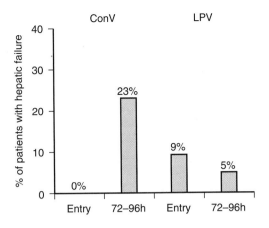

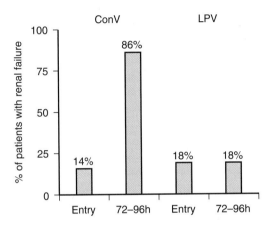

**Figure 53.6** Percentage of hepatic and renal failure in patients receiving either lung protective ventilation (LPV; $V_T = 8$ mL/kg, PEEP = 15 cmH$_2$O) or control ventilation (ConV; $V_T = 11$ mL/kg, PEEP = 7 cmH$_2$O). At time of entry (start of randomization) and 76 to 92 hours after entry. Adapted from Ranieri VM, Giunta F, Suter PM, et al: Mechanical ventilation as a mediator of multisystem organ failure in acute respiratory distress syndrome. JAMA 2000;284:43–44.)

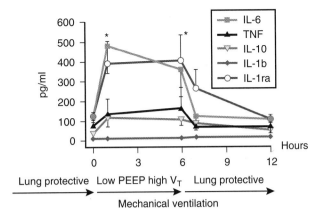

**Figure 53.7** Plot of cytokine levels on the Y axis versus time on the X axis. Patients were ventilated initially with a lung protective strategy, then a low PEEP/high tidal volume (V$_T$) strategy, and then with a lung protective strategy again. Note that when the strategy was changed to the low PEEP/high V$_T$ strategy that levels of most cytokines increased. Similarly, when the ventilatory strategy was changed back to the lung protective strategy, there was a decrease in most cytokines. IL, interleukin; TNF, tumor necrosis factor. (Used with permission of Stüber F, Wrigge H, Schroeder S, et al: Kinetic and reversibility of mechanical ventilation-associated pulmonary and systemic inflammatory response in patients with acute lung injury. Intensive Care Med 2002;28:834–841.)

is reversible and mechanical ventilation has an immediate effect on cytokine release.

Thus in ARDS there is an inflamed lung with increased levels of pro-inflammatory mediators, and ventilation itself can increase the amount of inflammatory mediators produced by the lung. When the barrier function of the alveolar-capillary membrane is disrupted by the underlying disease process or by mechanical ventilation, there may be leakage of mediators into the circulation (decompartmentalization). The subsequent increased levels of these mediators in the circulation correlate with multiple organ failure and finally mortality. Prevention of VILI by the use of lung protective ventilation in both experimental and clinical studies has demonstrated that a reduction in atelectrauma and biotrauma reduces organ failure and mortality.

## REFERENCES

1. ARDS Network: Ventilation with lower tidal volumes as compared with traditional tidal volumes for acute lung injury and the acute respiratory distress syndrome. N Engl J Med 2000;342:1301–1308.
2. Bernard GR, Artigas A, Brigham KL, et al: Report of the American-European Consensus conference on acute respiratory distress syndrome: Definitions, mechanisms, relevant outcomes, and clinical trial coordination. Consensus Committee. J Crit Care 1994;9:72–81.

cytokines correlated with the development of ARDS and finally multiple organ failure.[49]

Adjusting ventilation to reduce VILI can dramatically reduce cytokine release.[50] Stuber et al. demonstrated that this time course of cytokine release due to VILI can be extremely rapid (Fig. 53.7).[50] Patients with ARDS were ventilated with a lung protective strategy, and subsequently the strategy was changed to a less protective approach using higher tidal volumes and zero PEEP for a few hours. An increase in measurable levels of inflammatory cytokines was observed within 1 hour of changing the ventilatory strategy.[50] A decrease in cytokine levels was detected within 1 hour of reversal of the ventilatory strategy back to a protective mode using low tidal volumes. This elegant study demonstrates that VILI

3. International Consensus Conferences in Intensive Care Medicine: Ventilator-associated lung injury in ARDS. Am J Respir Crit Care Med 1999;160:2118–2124.

4. Ricard JD: Barotrauma during mechanical ventilation: Why aren't we seeing any more? Intensive Care Med 2004;30:533–535.

5. Gattinoni L, Pesenti A: The concept of "baby lung." Intensive Care Med 2005;31:776–784.

6. Gattinoni L, Pesenti A, Avalli L, et al: Pressure-volume curve of total respiratory system in acute respiratory failure. Computed tomographic scan study. Am Rev Respir Dis 1987;136:730–736.

7. Slutsky AS: Lung injury caused by mechanical ventilation. Chest 1999;116:9S–15S.

8. Mead J, Takishima T, Leith D: Stress distribution in lungs: A model of pulmonary elasticity. J Appl Physiol 1970;28:596–608.

9. Steinberg JM, Schiller HJ, Halter JM, et al: Alveolar instability causes early ventilator-induced lung injury independent of neutrophils. Am J Respir Crit Care Med 2004;169:57–63.

10. Muscedere JG, Mullen JB, Gan K, et al: Tidal ventilation at low airway pressures can augment lung injury. Am J Respir Crit Care Med 1994;149:1327–1334.

11. Taskar V, John J, Evander E, et al: Surfactant dysfunction makes lungs vulnerable to repetitive collapse and reexpansion. Am J Respir Crit Care Med 1997;155:313–320.

12. Dreyfuss D, Saumon G: Ventilator-induced lung injury: Lessons from experimental studies. Am J Respir Crit Care Med 1998;157:294–323.

13. Verbrugge SJ, Bohm SH, Gommers D, et al: Surfactant impairment after mechanical ventilation with large alveolar surface area changes and effects of positive end-expiratory pressure. Br J Anaesth 1998;80:360–364.

14. Webb HH, Tierney DF: Experimental pulmonary edema due to intermittent positive pressure ventilation with high inflation pressures. Protection by positive end-expiratory pressure. Am Rev Respir Dis 1974;110:556–565.

15. Dreyfuss D, Soler P, Basset G, et al: High inflation pressure pulmonary edema. Respective effects of high airway pressure, high tidal volume, and positive end-expiratory pressure. Am Rev Respir Dis 1988;137:1159–1164.

16. Dreyfuss D, Saumon G: Barotrauma is volutrauma, but which volume is the one responsible? Intensive Care Med 1992;18:139–141.

17. Hernandez LA, Peevy KJ, Moise AA, et al: Chest wall restriction limits high airway pressure-induced lung injury in young rabbits. J Appl Physiol 1989;66:2364–2368.

18. Coker PJ, Hernandez LA, Peevy KJ, et al: Increased sensitivity to mechanical ventilation after surfactant inactivation in young rabbit lungs. Crit Care Med 1992;20:635–640.

19. Dreyfuss D, Soler P, Saumon G: Mechanical ventilation-induced pulmonary edema. Interaction with previous lung alterations. Am J Respir Crit Care Med 1995;151:1568–1575.

20. Vlahakis NE, Hubmayr RD: Cellular stress failure in ventilator-injured lungs. Am J Respir Crit Care Med 2005;171:1328–1342.

21. Tremblay LN, Slutsky AS: Ventilator-induced injury: From barotrauma to biotrauma. Proc Assoc Am Physicians 1998;110:482–488.

22. Tremblay L, Valenza F, Ribeiro SP, et al: Injurious ventilatory strategies increase cytokines and c-fos m-RNA expression in an isolated rat lung model. J Clin Invest 1997;99:944–952.

23. van Kaam AH, Dik WA, Haitsma JJ, et al: Application of the open-lung concept during positive-pressure ventilation reduces pulmonary inflammation in newborn piglets. Biol Neonate 2003;83:273–280.

24. Imai Y, Parodo J, Kajikawa O, et al: Injurious mechanical ventilation and end-organ epithelial cell apoptosis and organ dysfunction in an experimental model of acute respiratory distress syndrome. JAMA 2003;289:2104–2112.

25. Slutsky AS, Tremblay LN: Multiple system organ failure. Is mechanical ventilation a contributing factor? Am J Respir Crit Care Med 1998;157:1721–1725.

26. Dos Santos CC, Slutsky AS: The contribution of biophysical lung injury to the development of biotrauma. Annu Rev Physiol 2006;68:585–618.

27. Dos Santos CC, Slutsky AS: Mechanisms of ventilator-induced lung injury: A perspective. J Appl Physiol 2000;89:1645–1655.

28. Uhlig S: Ventilation-induced lung injury and mechanotransduction: Stretching it too far? Am J Physiol Lung Cell Mol Physiol 2002;282:L892–L896.

29. Haitsma JJ, Uhlig S, Goggel R, et al. Ventilator-induced lung injury leads to loss of alveolar and systemic compartmentalization of tumor necrosis factor-alpha. Intensive Care Med 2000;26:1515–1522.

30. Dehoux MS, Boutten A, Ostinelli J, et al: Compartmentalized cytokine production within the human lung in unilateral pneumonia. Am J Respir Crit Care Med 1994;150:710–716.

31. Ranieri VM, Suter PM, Tortorella C, et al: Effect of mechanical ventilation on inflammatory mediators in patients with acute respiratory distress syndrome: A randomized controlled trial. JAMA 1999;282:54–61.

32. Ranieri VM, Giunta F, Suter PM, et al: Mechanical ventilation as a mediator of multisystem organ failure in acute respiratory distress syndrome. JAMA 2000;284:43–44.

33. Hickling KG, Henderson SJ, Jackson R: Low mortality associated with low volume pressure limited ventilation with permissive hypercapnia in severe adult respiratory distress syndrome. Intensive Care Med 1990;16:372–377.

34. Brochard L, Roudot-Thoraval F, Roupie E, et al: Tidal volume reduction for prevention of ventilator-induced lung injury in acute respiratory distress syndrome. The Multicenter Trial Group on Tidal Volume reduction in ARDS. Am J Respir Crit Care Med 1998;158:1831–1838.

35. Brower RG, Shanholtz CB, Fessler HE, et al: Prospective, randomized, controlled clinical trial comparing traditional versus reduced tidal volume ventilation in acute respiratory distress syndrome patients. Crit Care Med 1999;27:1492–1498.

36. Stewart TE, Meade MO, Cook DJ, et al: Evaluation of a ventilation strategy to prevent barotrauma in patients at high risk for acute respiratory distress syndrome. Pressure- and Volume-Limited Ventilation Strategy Group. N Engl J Med 1998;338:355–361.

37. Brower RG, Matthay M, Schoenfeld D: Meta-analysis of acute lung injury and acute respiratory distress syndrome trials. Am J Respir Crit Care Med 2002;166:1515–1517.

38. Gajic O, Dara SI, Mendez JL, et al: Ventilator-associated lung injury in patients without acute lung injury at the onset of mechanical ventilation. Crit Care Med 2004;32:1817–1824.

39. Gajic O, Frutos-Vivar F, Esteban A, et al: Ventilator settings as a risk factor for acute respiratory distress syndrome in mechanically ventilated patients. Intensive Care Med 2005;31:922–926.

40. Amato MB, Barbas CS, Medeiros DM, et al: Effect of a protective-ventilation strategy on mortality in the acute respiratory distress syndrome. N Engl J Med 1998;338:347–354.

41. De Durante G, Del Turco M, Rustichini L, et al: ARDSNet lower tidal volume ventilatory strategy may generate intrinsic positive end-expiratory pressure in patients with acute respiratory distress syndrome. Am J Respir Crit Care Med 20002;165:1271–1274.

42. Lee CM, Neff MJ, Steinberg KP, et al: Effect of low tidal volume ventilation on intrinsic PEEP in patients with acute lung injury. Am J Respir Crit Care Med 2001;163:A765.

43. Brower RG, Lanken PN, MacIntyre N, et al: Higher versus lower positive end-expiratory pressures in patients with the acute respiratory distress syndrome. N Engl J Med 2004;351:327–336.

44. Ferguson ND, Kacmarek RM, Chiche JD, et al: Screening of ARDS patients using standardized ventilator settings: Influence on enrollment in a clinical trial. Intensive Care Med 2004;30:1111–1116.

45. Esteban A, Anzueto A, Frutos F, et al: Characteristics and outcomes in adult patients receiving mechanical ventilation: A 28-day international study. JAMA 2002;287:345–355.

46. Ferring M, Vincent JL: Is outcome from ARDS related to the severity of respiratory failure? Eur Respir J 1997;10:1297–1300.

47. Parsons PE, Eisner MD, Thompson BT, et al: Lower tidal volume ventilation and plasma cytokine markers of inflammation in patients with acute lung injury. Crit Care Med 2005;33:1–6; discussion 230–232.

48. Headley AS, Tolley E, Meduri GU: Infections and the inflammatory response in acute respiratory distress syndrome. Chest 1997;111:1306–1321.

49. Roumen RM, Hendriks T, van der Ven-Jongekrijg J, et al: Cytokine patterns in patients after major vascular surgery, hemorrhagic shock, and severe blunt trauma. Relation with subsequent adult respiratory distress syndrome and multiple organ failure. Ann Surg 1993;218:769–776.

50. Stüber F, Wrigge H, Schroeder S, et al: Kinetic and reversibility of mechanical ventilation-associated pulmonary and systemic inflammatory response in patients with acute lung injury. Intensive Care Med 2002;28:834–841.

# CHAPTER 54

# Weaning

Michael J. Apostolakos

A 65-year-old, 70-kg, Caucasian male with history of chronic obstructive pulmonary disease, coronary artery disease, and hypertension was admitted 5 days ago to the medical intensive care unit (ICU) with streptococcal pneumonia, respiratory failure, and septic shock. The patients were treated with antibiotics, >15 L of crystalloid, levophed, activated protein-C, stress dose steroids, and mechanical ventilation. Initially the patient required an $FiO_2$ >80% and peak end-expiratory pressure (PEEP) >15 $cmH_2O$ in order to keep oxygen saturation >88%. Chest radiograph (CXR) revealed bilateral disease consistent with acute respiratory distress syndrome (ARDS) (Fig. 54.1). After 2 days the patients were able to come off pressors and intravenous fluids. By day 3, the patient begins to autodiurese. The $FiO_2$ and PEEP are able to be weaned over the next 5 days. On day 7 the patient's $FiO_2$ is 50% with PEEP = 7 $cmH_2O$. He is on VC ventilation with rate set at 12 and TV = 550 mL. The patient is receiving continuous sedation with intravenous lorazepam at 2 mg/hr. The patient is intermittently following commands. He is 8 kg above his dry body weight. The patient is breathing comfortably above the set rate on the ventilator at 14 breaths per minute. His arterial blood gas is pH = 7.37, $Pco_2$ = 41 mm Hg, and $Po_2$ = 110 mm Hg. The patient's CXR reveals mildly increased interstitial markings bilaterally with small pleural effusions (Fig. 54.2).

**Is this patient ready to wean?**

The patient has stable hemodynamics and acid-base balance. The patient meets liberal oxygenation criteria for extubation ($FiO_2$ < 50% and PEEP <8 $cmH_2O$), suggesting that he may be ready to begin weaning trials. He is, however, still fluid overloaded with a significant a-A gradient. The best predictor of readiness for a weaning trial

may be the rapid shallow breathing index described by Tobin and Yang. To obtain this index, the patient is disconnected from the ventilator and attached to a Wright spirometer. The respiratory rate and TV are measured for 1 minute. An f (breaths per minute)/TV (liters) ratio of less than 105 suggests readiness for a weaning trial. A result greater than 105 virtually rules out readiness for weaning. The patient may very well fail the trial, but weaning studies consistently show that patients undergoing daily trials of spontaneous breathing, once they meet oxygenation criteria to extubate, spend less time on mechanical ventilation. Furthermore, studies advocate a team approach to weaning as well as respiratory

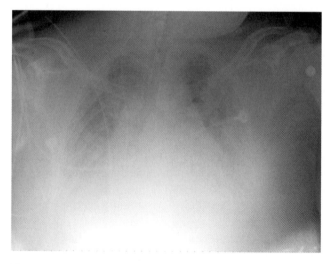

**Figure 54.1** Chest radiograph revealing noncardiogenic pulmonary edema (ARDS).

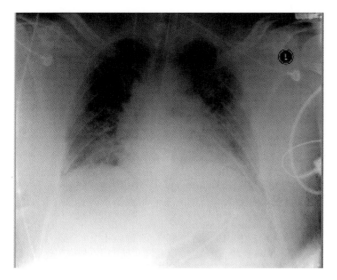

**Figure 54.2**  Chest radiograph revealing mild fluid overload.

BOX 54-1

**Causes of Ventilatory Dependency**

**Hypoxemic Respiratory Failure**
Impaired pulmonary gas exchange
Nonpulmonary shunt
Decreased oxygen content of venous blood
Hypoventilation

**Respiratory Muscle Pump Failure**
Decreased neuromuscular capacity
Increased respiratory pump load

**Psychologic Factors**
Anxiety
Depression
Motivation

*Modified from Tobin MJ: Weaning patients from mechanical ventilation. How to avoid difficulty. Postgrad Med 1991;89:171–178.*

therapist–driven weaning protocols, which assure that this or a similar process occurs.

The patient's level of consciousness may limit extubation but should not limit a weaning trial. He is intermittently following commands. Studies of ICU sedation suggest that daily holding of sedation ("sedation holiday") until the patient follows commands or gets agitated (wakes up) shortens length of mechanical ventilation as well.

**What method of weaning should be chosen?**
Spontaneous breathing trials (SBTs), defined by disconnecting patients from the ventilator and breathing with or without continuous positive airway pressure (CPAP) <5 cmH$_2$O, have been found to consistently lead to patient liberation from the mechanical ventilator in significantly less time than a predefined intermittent mandatory ventilation (IMV) wean. SBTs have also been found to be at least equal, if not superior, to pressure support ventilation (PSV) weaning. Repeating the trial more than once daily has not been shown to shorten time on mechanical ventilation.

The spontaneous breathing trial should last between 30 minutes and 2 hours. Intolerance is judged by tachycardia or bradycardia (>20% increase or decrease from baseline), tachypnea (>35 breaths per minute), hypoxemia (<90% oxygen saturation), hypertension (>180 mm Hg systolic), hypotension (<90 mm Hg systolic), and/or subjective shortness of breath (anxiety, diaphoresis, agitation).

If a patient fails the rapid shallow breathing index or SBT, the patient needs to be reassessed as to why he or she failed and what can be done to correct the problem(s) (Boxes 54.1 and 54.2).

**The patient is given a brief T-piece trial, but his respiratory rate quickly hits 40 breaths per minute and TV drops to 250 mL (f/TV ratio > 105). Should this patient undergo tracheostomy?**
The exact timing of tracheostomy is controversial. Some advocate tracheostomy within 3 days of intubation if mechanical ventilation is believed to be needed for at least another week. Others may wait several weeks before proceeding with tracheostomy. Those advocating early tracheostomy point to better patient tolerance and less need for sedation with tracheostomy as compared with translaryngeal intubation. Those who wait wish to avoid potentially unnecessary surgery or complications and

BOX 54-2

**Steps in Managing Patients Who Have Difficulty Weaning from Mechanical Ventilation**

- Determine cause of ventilatory dependency.
- Rectify correctable problems:
  - Pulmonary gas exchange
  - Fluid balance
  - Mental status
  - Acid-base status
  - Electrolyte disturbance
- Use team approach.
- Use weaning protocol.
- Use daily trials of spontaneous breathing.
- Consider psychologic factors.
- Optimize posture.
- Optimize pulmonary care.
- Ensure adequate nutritional support.
- Optimize general patient care.
- Provide ambulation.

*Modified from Tobin MJ: Weaning patients from mechanical ventilation. How to avoid difficulty. Postgrad Med 1991;89:171–178.*

cost associated with tracheostomy. A reasonable approach is to consider tracheostomy once a patient has undergone translaryngeal intubation for 2 weeks and at least another week is anticipated. Therefore tracheostomy at this point is likely premature.

This patient has comorbidities (COPD and CAD) that make him less likely to be able to tolerate the extra fluid from a cardiopulmonary perspective. Further diuresis is in order.

**The patient is diuresed over the next 48 hours. His weight approaches that of admission. The patient's f/TV ratio is now 40. He tolerates 1 hour of a CPAP 5-cmH$_2$O trial. He is fully alert off sedatives. What is the chance he will tolerate extubation?** Despite meeting the previously established criteria, studies suggest that 4% to 19% of such patients will require reintubation within 48 hours of extubation. Causes of unexpected respiratory failure include laryngeal edema and failure to handle secretions. Respiratory failure occurring more than 48 hours after extubation is generally believed to be due to a new disease process.

## SUGGESTED READINGS

Brook A, Ahrens T, Schaiff R, et al: Effect of a nursing-implemented sedation protocol on the duration of mechanical ventilation. Crit Care Med 1999;27:2609–2615.

Esteban A, Frutos F, Tobin M, et al: A comparison of four methods of weaning patients from mechanical ventilation. N Engl J Med 1995;332:345–350.

Goldstone J: The pulmonary physician in critical care. 10: Difficult weaning. Thorax 2002;57:986–991.

Horst H, Mouro D, Hall-Jenssens, et al: Decrease in ventilation time with a standardized weaning process. Arch Surg 1998;133:483–488.

Kress J, Pohlman A, O'Connor, et al: Daily interruption of sedative infusions in critically ill patients undergoing mechanical ventilation. N Engl J Med 2000;342:1471–1477.

Maziak D, Meade M, Todd T: The timing of tracheostomy: A systematic review. Chest 1998;114:605–609.

Yang K, Tobin M: A prospective study of indexes predicting the outcome of trials of weaning from mechanical ventilation. N Engl J Med 1991;324:1445–1450.

# CHAPTER 55

# Mechanical Ventilation in Severe Chest Trauma

Peter J. Papadakos and Pejman Soheili

In the United States, trauma is the leading cause of death for people under 44 years of age. Trauma deaths have largely evolved from the proliferation of motorized vehicles during the twentieth century. Although injury prevention has controlled the expected increase in trauma deaths, it has not decreased the absolute number of deaths. Furthermore, during the past decade, penetrating injuries such as gunshot wounds have outnumbered motor vehicle deaths in certain states.[1]

Trauma management needs to be guided according to the mechanism of injury, its anatomic involvement, and the staging of the injury. Different actions are needed according to these considerations. Most patients with severe trauma require mechanical ventilation to reduce work of breathing and ensure adequate gas exchange.

Pulmonary contusion is common in patients sustaining multiple traumas, occurring in approximately 17% of patients with multiple injuries. Pulmonary contusions are caused by rapid decelerations and falls as well as shock waves or passage of high-velocity missiles.

Clemedson[2] described the three mechanisms that are important in the etiology of pulmonary contusions. The "spalling effect" is due to bursting that occurs at the gas-liquid interface. The "inertial effect" occurs when low-density alveolar tissue is stripped from heavier hilar structures as they accelerate at different rates. Finally, the "implosion effect" results from overexpansion of gas bubbles after a pressure wave passes. The pulmonary parenchyma can be torn by this excess distension.

Pulmonary contusion typically promotes development of acute lung injury, which may lead to acute respiratory distress syndrome (ARDS). This is due to elevated intrapulmonary shunting, ventilation-perfusion mismatching, increased lung water, pulmonary hemorrhage, loss of lung compliance, and release of cytoactive modulators.[3]

Wagner and Jamieson[4] evaluated pulmonary contusions seen on computed tomography (CT) scans and divided the injuries into four classes based on the type and severity of the lesion. They predicted the need for ventilatory support by the percentage of airspace consolidation. When more than 28% of the airspace was involved, all patients required mechanical ventilation.

Our objective in ventilatory management of patients with severe chest trauma and pulmonary contusions should encompass improvement of gas exchange with the reduction of work of breathing. Furthermore, ventilation-induced lung injury (VILI) should be avoided.

Controversies exist regarding the most appropriate form of mechanical ventilation in patients with pulmonary contusion. We hope to illustrate some of the controversies precipitated by the lack of clinical trials and review some model management scenarios.

This case report describes the use of mechanical ventilation with alveolar recruitment maneuver in the management of a 16-year-old male who sustained a gunshot wound by AK-47, 7.62-mm caliber. Ventilatory therapy of pulmonary contusion and the physiologic grounds for its use are discussed.

## CASE REPORT

A 16-year-old male sustained a gunshot wound to the left shoulder. At the scene, his Glasgow Coma Scale was 6, and his blood pressure was recorded as 218/108 mm Hg;

heart rate, 100 beats per minute; respiratory rate, 32 breaths per minute; and oxygen saturation, 88%. Intravenous access was established, and he was intubated with an 8.0-mm endotracheal tube. He received 1800 mL of crystalloid and remained hemodynamically stable. After helicopter transfer to the Level 1 trauma center, he was started on synchronized intermittent mandatory ventilation; $FiO_2$, 100%; tidal volume, 650 mL (7 mL/kg); positive end-expiratory pressure (PEEP), 10 mm Hg; PS, 5 mm Hg; and rate of 10 breaths per minute.

Breath sounds were diminished over the left chest, and a chest tube was immediately inserted. The left thoracostomy tube drained 500 mL of blood from the chest. A second right-sided thoracostomy tube was also placed, which did not drain any fluid.

Chest radiographic examination revealed a large left-sided pleural effusion (Fig. 55.1).

CT scan of the chest demonstrated blood and air in the mediastinum in addition to moderate pulmonary contusion (Fig. 55.2).

Angiography of great vessels did not show any evidence of injury. Thoracotomy was not performed because the patient was hemodynamic stable with a negative angiography.

During the first 24 hours, the patient received 2 U of packed red cells and 4000 mL of crystalloids to compensate for a loss of 800 mL through the left thoracostomy tube and 2500 mL of urine.

Initially arterial blood gas revealed a pH of 7.20; $PaO_2$, 70 mm Hg; and $PCO_2$, 63 mm Hg. On transfer to the intensive care unit, the ventilatory settings were: SIMV rate, 14; tidal volume ($V_T$), 650 mL; $FiO_2$, 100%,

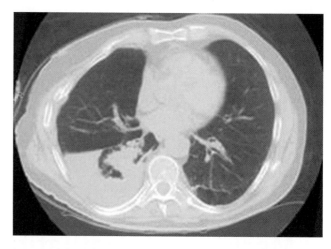

**Figure 55.2** Admission CT scan from Emergency Room Air in Mediastinum and Pulmonary Contusion PS (Pressure Support).

PEEP, 12 mm Hg; PS, 5 mm Hg; and inspiratory flow rate, 60 L/minute. Repeat blood gas analysis revealed a pH of 7.31; $PaO_2$, 70 mm Hg; and $PCO_2$, 40 mm Hg.

During the next 8 hours, his oxygenation continued to deteriorate despite incremental elevation of PEEP (up to 20 mm Hg). The decision was made to switch the SIMV mode to pressure-controlled mode with a decelerating ramp flow waveform due to elevated peak inspiratory pressures as well as elevation of the plateau pressures. The new settings were: pressure control, 45 mm Hg; $FiO_2$, 100%; PEEP, 20 mm Hg; and rate, 14 breaths per minute. Despite the changes, repeat arterial blood gas revealed a pH of 7.51; $PaO_2$, 50 mm Hg; and $PCO_2$, 29 mm Hg.

An alveolar recruitment maneuver was performed in pressure-controlled ventilation by increasing peak inspiratory pressure to 65 mm Hg with inspiratory-to-expiratory (I:E) ratio of 2:1 for 90 seconds. Then peak inspiratory pressure was reduced to 34 mm Hg, and I:E ratio was reduced to 1:2 to avoid barotrauma while PEEP was increased to 22. This maneuver was performed three times in 1 hour.

Thirty minutes after completion of the recruitment maneuver, arterial blood gas analysis was as follows: pH, 7.46; $PaO_2$, 148 mm Hg; and $PCO_2$, 24 mm Hg. Subsequently, the ventilatory mood was switched to: pressure-regulated volume control; $V_T$, 650 mL; $FiO_2$, 60%; rate, 14; and PEEP, 22 mm Hg. Repeat blood gas revealed pH of 7.45; $PaO_2$, 138 mm Hg; and $PCO_2$, 35 mm Hg. Over the next 24 hours we performed three more lung recruitment maneuvers, as described previously, and we were able to decrease the $FiO_2$ gradually to 40%, $V_T$ to 600 mL, and PEEP to 18 mm Hg. The patient did not show any sign of hemodynamic compromise during the recruitment maneuver, and he was successfully extubated on day 5.

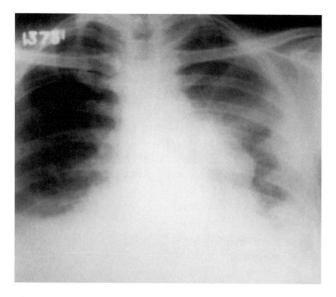

**Figure 55.1** Chest X-ray in Emergency Department left sided effusion.

## DISCUSSION

Many studies have described the physiologic mechanism by which mechanical ventilation may lead to VILI. Predominant factors that contribute to VILI include high distending transalveolar pressure and overdistension of aerated lung units. This is related to high pressures and volumes that occur at the end of inspiration due to excessive stress at the margins between aerated and nonaerated lung units.[5]

Additionally, transalveolar pressure that falls below the critical closing pressure of alveolar units at the end of expiration induces repeated opening and closing of small airways such as alveoli and bronchioles that are atelectatic at end-expiration. This is known as *atelectrauma*, which is an important factor associated with VILI. These processes are associated with increased activation of pulmonary inflammatory mediators, which are released in the lung and systemic circulation and cause histologic lesions that are indistinguishable from ARDS.[6]

Haitsma et al.[7] demonstrated that in VILI there is loss of compartmentalization of cytokines, especially tumor necrosis factor (TNF)-alpha, causing an imbalance in the inflammatory response. These high levels of cytokines can cause severe organ dysfunction. Applied PEEP of 10 $cmH_2O$ significantly diminished this loss of compartmentalization in that animal study.

Both high peak pressures and the absence of PEEP have been shown to increase bacterial translocation from the lung into the systemic circulation in animal models.[8]

D'angelo et al.[9] demonstrated in an animal study that prolonged low-volume ventilation on zero PEEP induced peripheral airway injury, even in normal lungs.

Numerous mechanisms have been proposed to explain the change in lung mechanics in the presence of injury and subsequent edema. Important studies performed by Gattinoni and colleagues[10,11] reinforced the idea that large portions of an injured lung are derecruited and are not aerated during positive pressure ventilation. They also examined the effects of posture and ventilator settings and found that dependent portions of the injured lung are exposed to a compressive pressure and collapse. They attributed dependent atelectasis to the increased weight of edematous lung, moreover, lung injury was determined to be caused by large stresses in the parenchyma surrounding these atelectatic regions.

It has also been postulated that inadequate lung recruitment is a critical factor leading to VILI. Adaptive process to high stress can also initiate collagen deposition and vascular cell proliferation.[12] Recruiting the lung and preventing derecruitment decreases the potential for lung injury by avoiding the repetitive shear stress associated with opening and closing of unstable lung units.[13]

In order to avoid atelectrauma, maximal alveolar aeration and recruitment are needed to minimize shear stresses in the lung tissue during inspiration.

Alveolar recruitment maneuvers should be major goals of mechanical ventilatory support for patients with severe trauma or ARDS.

## RECRUITMENT PRINCIPLES

The only ventilatory strategy that has shown a decrease in ARDS mortality in randomized studies is the use of low tidal volume and limited airway pressure ventilation. Two randomized controlled clinical trials have recently demonstrated that this protective ventilation approach leads to marked improvement in clinical outcome.[14,15] However, it is known that low tidal volumes lead to progressive lung derecruitment that can be detrimental in patients with pulmonary contusions.

Richard and colleagues[16] studied the relationship of decreased $V_T$ on alveolar recruitment and found that reduction of $V_T$ from 10 to 6 mL/kg, while keeping PEEP constant, was responsible for a significant lung volume loss corresponding to alveolar derecruitment.

Cereda and colleagues[17] have shown that low tidal volume ventilation could induce a progressive decrease in compliance, indicating a time-dependent derecruitment, which could be prevented by a higher PEEP level.

The traditional mechanical ventilation approach uses low to moderate levels of PEEP to support oxygenation by preventing or reversing alveolar atelectasis or flooding, as seen in patients with pulmonary contusion. This strategy uses the lowest PEEP that results in acceptable oxygenation.

Halter and colleagues[18] demonstrated that alveoli opened with recruitment maneuver may collapse without adequate PEEP, and most recruited alveoli that do not collapse are unstable. The unstable alveoli are vulnerable to the shear stress–induced damage. Although the recruitment maneuver may improve arterial oxygenation, the recruitment maneuver followed by inadequate PEEP could potentially exacerbate VILI.

Ranieri and colleagues[19] studied the influence of tidal volume on PEEP-related cardiorespiratory effect. These investigators concluded that with high tidal volume, PEEP mainly induced hyperinflation of alveoli already recruited by tidal ventilation, whereas with low tidal volume, PEEP induced alveolar recruitment and counterbalanced low tidal volume–related derecruitment.

Amato and colleagues[14] demonstrated that mechanical lung protection in patients with ARDS resulted in better pulmonary function and higher rate of weaning from the ventilator. Their lung protection was based on maintaining low inspiratory driving pressure with low

VT and preferential use of limited airway pressure, with the simultaneous use of high PEEP to keep end-expiratory pressures above the lower inflection point of the static pressure volume curve of the respiratory system.

Higher PEEP combined with lower VT was also associated with a lower concentration of inflammatory cytokines and mediators in bronchoalveolar lavage fluid and blood in patients with ARDS.[6]

PEEP and VT are interactive variables that determine the extent of lung recruitment. However, controversy still exists over the approach used to set PEEP.

## PEEP SELECTION

Application of PEEP has beneficial effects on lung mechanics, gas exchange, edema formation, and release of inflammation mediators. PEEP plays a fundamental role in the lung protective strategy with the aim of minimizing lung collapse. The extent of end-expiratory collapse mainly depends on two phenomena: the gravitational forces, which are the superimposed pressures that compress the most dependent regions of the lung, and the maximum volume pressure achieved during the previous inspiration.

The findings of Crotti and colleagues[20] suggest that the different lung regions present different opening pressures. The pressure is lowest in the nondependent lung, intermediate in the mid-lung, and highest in the most dependent lung.

The recruitment of the most dependent lung region, where atelectasis was present, occurred at pressures as high as 45 $cmH_2O$. Decreasing the PEEP level from total lung capacity caused progressive collapse of the most dependent regions, which were subjected to the greatest superimposed pressure, therefore causing derecruitment. The authors also reported that collapse maximally occurred between 0 and 15 $cmH_2O$ in patients with acute lung injury or ARDS. Therefore recruited lung units tend to stay open at pressures lower than the initial pressure that opened them.

The lower inflection point (LIP) on the total respiratory system pressure-volume curve is widely used to set PEEP in patients with acute respiratory failure, based on the assumption that a lower inflection point represents alveolar recruitment. The concept is that the lower inflection point on the pressure-volume curve reflects the average critical pressure needed to reopen those regions of the lung that close during expiration. However, only a few studies have specifically addressed the relationship between the lower inflection point and the amount of alveolar recruitment.

Muscedere and co-workers[21] studied saline-lavaged rat lungs that were ventilated with PEEP above and below the lower inflection point of their static pressure-volume curves. Lungs that were ventilated without PEEP showed decreases in compliance and marked histologic damage. The distal airway collapse with resulting shear stress in airway walls caused damage and mediator release. The same mechanism may contribute to VILI in patients with ARDS.

Mergoni and co-workers[22] studied the relationship between LIP and alveolar recruitment and demonstrated that there is a poor relationship between the level of LIP and the amount of the alveolar recruitment determined by application of PEEP. They showed a loose relationship, suggesting that recruitment was occurring also when PEEP was raised above the LIP. In that study, the LIP was <10 $cmH_2O$ in all but four patients. Nonetheless, the recruitment obtained by increasing PEEP to 10 to 15 $cmH_2O$ was only 40% of the whole recruited volume, which suggests that a large amount of lung tissue was still recruitable when the patients were ventilated with a PEEP level slightly above the LIP.

Crotti et al.[20] performed thoracic CT scans at different PEEP levels and plateau pressures (maximum PEEP was 20 $cmH_2O$, and maximum plateau was 45 $cmH_2O$). They also found that alveolar recruitment occurred along the entire pressure-volume curve, independent of lower and upper inflection points. Alveolar recruitment was progressive from nondependent to dependent lung zones.

Based on theses studies, the lower inflection point on the pressure-volume curve should not be further considered as the method of choice to set the value of PEEP. Recruitment occurs along the entire volume-pressure curve, independent of lower and upper inflection points. Therefore a direct measurement of the recruitment obtained when PEEP is applied can be useful in implementing a ventilatory strategy aimed at recruiting most of the collapsed lung units.

It is important to note that PEEP holds unstable alveoli open but does not open them; rather, it is sustained high pressures that open the alveoli and reopen the closed airway. Therefore PEEP should be increased to some degree after the recruitment maneuver to preserve the recruited units.

The normal lung becomes maximally inflated at a transpulmonary pressure of 30 to 35 $cmH_2O$ (pleural pressure is assumed to be close to 0 $cmH_2O$).

Transpulmonary pressure is defined as alveolar pressure minus pleural pressure (or the difference between the plateau pressure and PEEP minus the difference between esophageal pressure at end-inspiration and end-expiration). Transpulmonary pressure, rather than peak inspiratory pressure or plateau pressure, is the most important determinant of alveolar distension.[23]

Respiratory responses of an ARDS lung to ventilatory measures are known to differ according to the etiologic category of diffuse lung injury.[24] ARDS that is associated with indirect lung injury or extrapulmonary ARDS, such as that seen in trauma patients, responds more favorably to ventilatory measures that alter transpulmonary pressure, because reversible or compressive atelectasis (rather than consolidated airspace) is the predominant finding seen in pulmonary ARDS. Therefore the pathogenic pathway that produces lung injury influences the potential for recruitment.

Mead and colleagues[25] demonstrated that the tissue attachments between collapsed units and large aerated units carry a stress that is much greater than the average transpulmonary pressure. Lung overdistension may not occur if pleural pressure is also elevated, such as when there is reduced chest-wall or abdominal compliance, as seen in patients with severe trauma. Instead, in that case for a given plateau pressure, the change in transpulmonary pressure is rather low, and thus there is a high potential for recruitment.

## RECRUITMENT TECHNIQUES

The importance of early lung recruitment with an "open lung" approach has been well documented. The "open lung" concept was first used by Lachmann;[26] it implies little or no atelectasis and an optimal gas exchange. Intrapulmonary shunt ideally should be less than 10%, corresponding to a $PaO_2$ of more than 450 mm Hg, when breathing 100% oxygen at sea level.[27]

This concept has led to an "open lung" procedure in which the lung is opened and kept open to minimize cyclic alveolar opening-closing.

Recruitment maneuvers are characterized by a sustained increase in airway pressure for 30 to 90 seconds or by repeated periodic increases in inspiratory pressure during a short time. Sustained increase in airway pressure usually performs recruitment either via application of continuous positive airway pressure (CPAP) by setting the PEEP to the aimed pressure or via application of pressure-controlled ventilation. On the other hand, periodic increases in inspiratory pressure use increased tidal volume or PEEP such as frequent sighs in which a high airway pressure is imposed on the lung for a short period (60 seconds). Other techniques such as the use of high-frequency oscillatory ventilation have also been described.

Pelosi et al.[28] performed a study of 10 patients with ARDS (5 with pulmonary and 5 with extrapulmonary origin) who were ventilated with protective strategy (low $V_T$ and plateau pressure lower than 35 $cmH_2O$). Their recruitment maneuver was the application of three consecutive sighs per minute for 1 hour at plateau pressure of 45 $cmH_2O$ in volume control mode. The average

PEEP used was 14 $cmH_2O$. After 1 hour of sigh, they reported a marked decrease in intrapulmonary shunt as well as a significant increase in end-expiratory lung volume, which correlated with improvement in arterial oxygenation, as compared with patients who were only ventilated with protective strategy without the use of the recruitment maneuver. Improvements of lung mechanics and oxygenation were seen only in patients with extrapulmonary ARDS.

Lapinsky and colleagues[29] used CPAP mode to apply sustained inflation pressure of 30 to 45 $cmH_2O$ for 20 seconds in 14 patients with hypoxic respiratory failure and bilateral pulmonary infiltrates who had been ventilated less than 72 hours. They found a significantly improved level of oxygen saturation that was maintained in 10 of 14 patients for at least 4 hours. Of the 4 patients without improvement, repeat recruitment maneuvers and institution of higher PEEP caused a sustained improvement in oxygenation in all but 1 patient.

Grasso and co-workers[30] used 40 $cmH_2O$ of CPAP for 40 seconds in 24 patients. They defined the patients as recruitment maneuver responders if their arterial oxygenation increased by >50% from the baseline. This study also showed a significant improvement in arterial oxygenation with the use of recruitment maneuver, but the underlying disease responsible for ARDS did not influence the amount of improvement in arterial oxygenation after application of the recruitment maneuver.

Schreiter and colleagues[31] used intrinsic PEEP by pressure-cycled, high-frequency, inverse-ratio ventilation (80 minutes; I:E ration, 2:1) and maintained the ventilatory strategy for 24 hours in patients with severe chest trauma. They found increased arterial oxygenation and increased total lung volume, whereas the amount of collapsed tissue decreased.

These findings suggest that, regardless of the technique used for recruitment, the strategy remains the same and should fulfill the present concept of lung recruitment.

Our group uses pressure-controlled ventilation with a decelerating ramp flow waveform to achieve sustained increase in airway pressure in recruitment maneuvers.[32] Pressure-controlled ventilation allows the practitioner to control ventilatory pressure throughout the cycle in order to generate the pressure necessary to expand the collapsed alveoli. The pressure needed for alveolar recruitment may reach values of 60 to 70 $cmH_2O$ in patients with severe chest trauma. After recruitment maneuver, peak inspiratory pressure (PIP) is adjusted to the lowest pressure needed to keep the lung open. The ideal pressure is generally 15 to 30 $cmH_2O$ lower than the required recruitment pressure. This lowest pressure is realized when $V_T$ remains stable and the arterial gases are acceptable. We select the appropriate PEEP at which greatest $PaO_2$ improvement is observed without worsening hemodynamics. The set PEEP of 10 to 20 $cmH_2O$ is generally used to avoid alveolar collapse. Arterial blood gas analysis is used as a measurement of recruitment success. We have also periodically used CT scans before and after recruitment maneuvers as further evidence of recruitment success.

Amato and colleagues[14] were the first to demonstrate an improved outcome in patients who had been placed on pressure-controlled ventilation and received the alveolar recruitment maneuver as compared with those using conventional modes. They showed a higher weaning rate as well as improved 28-day mortality based on the mode of ventilation and the use of the recruitment maneuver.

Oczenski et al.[33] performed the only randomized controlled study to evaluate the impact of lung recruitment maneuvers on gas exchange and hemodynamics in patients with early extrapulmonary ARDS. Their recruitment maneuver resulted in only short-term improvement of oxygenation and decrease of venous admixture in patients with early extrapulmonary ARDS who underwent a PEEP trial. Within 30 minutes after the recruitment maneuver, the improved oxygenation and venous admixture returned to baseline values. It is prudent to note (and the authors also agree) that the PEEP applied after the recruitment maneuver may have been insufficient for sustained recruitment. PEEP holds unstable alveoli open, but it does not open them. Rather, it is sustained high pressures that open the alveoli and reopen the closed airways. Therefore PEEP should be increased to some degree after the recruitment maneuver to preserve the recruited units. If sufficient PEEP is not applied after the recruitment maneuver, improvement in lung mechanics and oxygenation is only brief. Alveoli will collapse within seconds after the recruitment maneuver if PEEP does not adequately stabilize the alveoli.[34]

## DERECRUITMENT

Alveolar recruitment can be functionally monitored by measuring $PaO_2$, which reliably correlates with the amount of lung parenchyma taking part in gas exchange.

Keeping the lung open after the recruitment maneuver is especially important for the success of alveolar recruitment. In patients undergoing high levels of PEEP to achieve optimal recruitment, sudden withdrawal of PEEP causes derecruitment and may accentuate further lung injury.

Suh et al.[35] demonstrated that repeated derecruitment accentuated lung injury during mechanical ventilation in animals. They found significant pathologic changes at the bronchiolar level, showing desquamation and necrosis of epithelium, which were associated with profound inflammatory cell infiltration. Enhorning and

Robertson[36] also found desquamation and necrosis of bronchiolar epithelium with cyclic volume changes in the surfactant-deficient lung.

Crotti and colleagues[20] obtained CT scans of patients with ARDS who were ventilated with plateau pressures from 10 to 45 $cmH_2O$ and PEEP of 5 to 20 $cmH_2O$. They concluded that the majority of derecruitment occurred at PEEP values ranging from 0 to 15 $cmH_2O$. They found that decreasing the PEEP level from total lung capacity caused progressive collapse of the most dependent regions. When superimposed gravitational pressure exceeded PEEP, end-expiratory collapse increased.

Sudden derecruitment can occur during suctioning, during aerosol therapy, and also during transport of patients. Furthermore, the influence of composition of inspired gas may play a role on recurrence of atelectasis and in maintaining the recruitment effect, as more rapid derecruitment occurs at higher $FiO_2$.[37]

## LIMITATION

General concerns remain about exploiting high airway pressures and its potential harmful side effects, such as barotrauma and hemodynamic compromise, which may be caused by recruitment maneuvers. Based on recent experimental work and review of literature, it could be deduced that slightly higher transalveolar pressure would be less dangerous than the cyclic opening and closing of recently injured alveoli because the effect of higher transalveolar pressure is markedly attenuated by use of sufficient PEEP.

Elevation of intrathoracic pressure and its effect on preload and cardiac output have also raised some concerns regarding the use of high-PEEP recruitment maneuvers. With the application of PEEP, a decrease in cardiac output may contribute to a reduction in shunt through a preferential distribution of perfusion to functioning lung units. On the other hand, because moderate hypercapnia (caused by limited tidal volume) can induce a reduction in systemic vascular resistance and an elevation of cardiac output, the reduction in cardiac preload induced by the elevation of intrathoracic pressure might be counterbalanced by the systemic effects of hypercapnia. Nevertheless, transient hypotension and desaturation remain the two most frequently observed side effects of recruitment maneuvers.

Grasso et al.[30] reported a 20% to 30% decrease in cardiac output and mean arterial pressure during a recruitment maneuver in patients who did not respond to recruitment maneuvers, whereas no significant hemodynamic changes were detected in responders to recruitment maneuvers.

Use of the recruitment maneuver in unilateral lung injury should be avoided because this would increase lung volume by overdistending the more compliant aerated alveolar units that are already open, rather than recruiting collapsed alveoli. This overdistension would favor capillary collapse in the healthy, more compliant parenchyma and diversion of blood flow into the collapsed areas, causing increased intrapulmonary shunting. Decreased cardiac output, increased pulmonary arterial pressure, severe hypotension, and bradycardia may also occur when recruitment maneuvers cause overdistension.

Bein et al.[38] analyzed the impact of the recruitment maneuver on intercranial pressure (ICP) and cerebral metabolism in patients with acute cerebral injury and respiratory failure. They used progressive peak pressure up to 60 cmH$_2$O, which was maintained for 30 seconds. Increased ICP was found with the resulting decrease in cerebral perfusion pressure (72 mm Hg versus 60 mm Hg). Until further studies are performed, use of recruitment maneuver in patients with cerebral injury should be avoided. Furthermore, alveolar recruitment maneuver should be terminated if any of the following events occur: hypotension (more than 30% decrease in arterial pressure), new arrhythmia, bradycardia, or desaturation of oxygen to <85%. Recruitment maneuvers should be performed with extreme caution in patients who are hypovolemic.

In conclusion, many questions still remain, such as the recommended ventilatory mode or the timing, duration, and monitoring of recruitment maneuvers. Questions regarding the duration of improvement in lung mechanics following recruitment maneuvers have not yet been fully answered. Some studies suggest the immediate improvement in lung mechanics may be transitory, and long-term benefit has yet to be demonstrated.

At this time, the optimal method of performing the recruitment maneuver remains elusive; moreover, no double-blind randomized data are yet available that demonstrate improved survival with recruitment maneuvers. Nonetheless, recruitment maneuvers appear to be warranted and may be life saving for trauma patients who require extremely high levels of PEEP or FiO$_2$ to achieve adequate levels of oxygenation. Further studies are needed to evaluate the potential benefit of the recruitment maneuver in trauma patients.

## REFERENCES

1. National Safety Council: Injury facts. Itasca, IL.: National Safety Council, 2000, pp 1–15.
2. Clemedson CJ: Blast injury. Physiology 1956;36:336.
3. Cohen S: Pulmonary contusion: Review of clinical entity. J Trauma 1997;42:973–979.
4. Wagner RB, Jamieson PM: Pulmonary contusion. Evaluation and classification by computed tomography. Surg Clin North Am 1989;69:31.
5. The Acute Respiratory Distress Syndrome Clinical Trials Network: Effects of recruitment maneuvers in patients with acute lung injury and acute respiratory distress syndrome ventilated with high positive end-expiratory pressure. Crit Care Med 2003;31:2592–2597.
6. Ranieri M, Suter PM, Cosimo T, et al: Effect of mechanical ventilation on inflammatory mediators in patients with acute respiratory distress syndrome. JAMA 1999;282:54–61.
7. Haitsma JJ, Uhlig S, Goggel R, et al: Ventilator-induced lung injury leads to loss of alveolar and systemic compartmentalization of tumor necrosis factor-alpha. Intensive Care Med 2000; 26:1515–1522.
8. Nahum A, Hoyt J, Schmitz L, et al: Effect of mechanical ventilation on dissemination of intratracheally instilled *Escherichia coli* in dogs. Crit Care Med 1997;25:173.
9. D'angelo E, Pecchiari M, Baraggia P, et al: Low-volume ventilation causes peripheral airway injury and increased airway resistance in normal rabbits. J Appl Physiol 2002;92:949–956.
10. Gattioni L, Pelosi P, Crotti S, et al: Effects of positive end-expiratory pressure on regional distribution of tidal volume and recruitment in adult respiratory distress syndrome. Am J Respir Crit Care Med 1995;151:1807–1814.
11. Gattioni L, D'Andrea L, Pelosi P, et al: Regional effects and mechanism of positive end-expiratory pressure in early adult respiratory distress syndrome. JAMA 1993;269:2122–2127.
12. Parker JC, Breen EC, West JB: High vascular and airway pressures increase interstitial protein mRNA expression in isolated rat lung. J Appl Physiol 1997;83:1697–1705.
13. Farias LL, Faffe DS, Xisto DG, et al: Positive end-expiratory pressure prevents lung mechanical stress caused by recruitment/derecruitment. J Appl Physiol 2005;98:43–61.
14. Amato MB, Barbas CS, Medeiros DM, et al: Effect of a protective-ventilation strategy on mortality in acute respiratory distress syndrome. N Engl J Med 1998;338:347–354.
15. Acute Respiratory Distress Syndrome Network: Ventilation with lower tidal volume as compared with traditional tidal volumes for acute lung injury and the acute respiratory distress syndrome. N Engl J Med 2000;342:1301–1308.
16. Richard JC, Maggiore SM, Jonson B, et al: Influence of tidal volume on alveolar recruitment. Respective role of PEEP and a recruitment maneuver. Am J Respir Crit Care Med 2001; 163:1609–1613.
17. Cereda M, Foti G, Musch G, et al: Positive end-expiratory pressure prevents the loss of respiratory compliance during low tidal volume ventilation in acute lung injury patients. Chest 1996; 109:480–485.
18. Halter JM, Steinberg JM, Schiller MD, et al: Positive end-expiratory pressure after a recruitment maneuver prevents both alveolar collapse and recruitment/derecruitment. Am J Respire Crit Care Med 2003;167:1620–1626.
19. Ranieri VM, Mascia L, Fiore T, et al. Cardiorespiratory effects of positive end-expiratory pressure during progressive tidal volume reduction (permissive hypercapnia) in patients with acute respiratory distress syndrome. Anesthesiology 1995;83:710–720.
20. Crotti S, Mascheroni D, Caironi P, et al: Recruitment and derecruitment during acute respiratory failure. Am J Respir Crit Care Med 2001;164:1331–1340.
21. Muscedere JG, Mullen JBM, Gan K, et al: Tidal ventilation at low airway pressures can augment lung injury. Am J Respir Crit Care Med 1994;149:1327–1334.
22. Mergoni M, Volpi A, Bricchi C, et al: Lower inflection point and recruitment with PEEP in ventilated patients with acute respiratory failure. J Appl Physiol 2001;91:441–450.

23. Stewart TE: Establishing an approach to mechanical ventilation. Can Respir J 1996;3:403–408.

24. Gattinoni L, Pelosi P, Suter PM, et al: Acute respiratory distress syndrome caused by pulmonary and extrapulmonary disease: Different syndromes? Am J Respir Crit Care Med 1998; 158:3–11.

25. Mead J, Takishima T, Leith D: Stress distribution in lungs: A model of pulmonary elasticity. J Appl Physiol 1970;28:596–608.

26. Lachmann B: Open up the lung and keep the lung open. Intensive Care Med 1992;18:319–321.

27. Papadakos PJ, Lachmann B: The open lung concept of alveolar recruitment can improve outcome in respiratory failure and ARDS. Mt Sinai J Med 2002;69:73–77.

28. Pelosi P, Cadringher P, Bottino N, et al: Sigh in acute respiratory distress syndrome. Am J Respir Crit Care Med 1999;159:872–880.

29. Lapinsky SE, Abuin M, Mehta S, et al: Safety and efficacy of a sustained inflation for alveolar recruitment in adults with respiratory failure. Intensive Care Med 1999;25:1297–1301.

30. Grasso S, Mascia L, Del Turco M, et al. Effects of recruiting maneuvers in patients with acute respiratory distress syndrome ventilated with protective ventilatory strategy. Anesthesiology 2002;96:795–802.

31. Schreiter D, Reske A, Stichert B, et al: Alveolar recruitment in combination with sufficient positive end-expiratory pressure increases oxygenation and lung aeration in patients with severe chest trauma. Crit Care Med 2004;32:968–975.

32. Papadakos PJ, Lachmann B, Bohem S: Pressure-controlled ventilation: Review and new horizons. Clin Pulm Med 1998;5:120.

33. Oczenski W, Hormann C, Keller C, et al: Recruitment maneuvers after a positive end-expiratory pressure trial do not induce sustained effects in early adult respiratory distress syndrome. Anesthesiology 2004;101:620–625.

34. Lim CM, Jung H, Koh Y, et al: Effect of alveolar recruitment maneuver in early acute respiratory distress syndrome according to antiderecruitment strategy, etiological category of diffuse lung injury, and body position of the patient. Crit Care Med 2003; 31:411–418.

35. Suh GY, Koh Y, Chung MP, et al: Repeated derecruitments accentuate lung injury during mechanical ventilation. Crit Care Med 2002;30:1848–1853.

36. Enhorning G, Robertson B: Lung expansion in the premature rabbit fetus after tracheal deposition of surfactant. Pediatrics 1972;50:58–66.

37. Rothen HU, Sporre B, Engberg G, et al: Influence of gas composition on recurrence of atelectasis after a reexpansion maneuver during general anesthesia. Anesthesiology 1995;82:832–842.

38. Bein T, Kuhr LP, Bele S, et al: Lung recruitment maneuver in patients with cerebral injury: Effects on intracranial pressure and cerebral metabolism. Intensive Care Med 2002;28:554–558.

# CHAPTER 56

# Pneumonia

Jean Chastre, Charles-Edouard Luyt, and Alain Combes

## CASE PRESENTATION

A 75-year-old man with a history of hypertension presents to the emergency department with a 3-day history of a productive cough and fever. He has a temperature of 38.5°C, a blood pressure of 100/55 mm Hg, a respiratory rate of 36 breaths per minute, a heart rate of 128 beats per minute, and oxygen saturation of 88% while breathing room air. Physical examination reveals a mild cyanosis with bibasilar crackles and expiratory wheezes, peripheral signs of skin hypoperfusion, and some degree of confusion. The white cell count is 14,500 per cubic millimeter, and the results of routine chemical tests are normal, except for a blood urea level of 11 mmol/L and a blood lactate level of 3.5 mmol/L. A chest radiograph shows a large infiltrate in the right lower lobe. Blood gas analysis while the patient was receiving 6 L of oxygen by nasal cannula reveals a $PaO_2$ of 55 mm Hg with a $PaCO_2$ of 32 mm Hg and a pH of 7.30. How should this patient be evaluated and treated?

Severe community-acquired pneumonia (CAP) remains a potentially dreadful disease despite modern antibiotics and technology. In industrialized countries, pneumonia is the most common infectious cause of death among patients of all ages and the fifth or the sixth leading cause of death overall.[1,2] Although many of the patients with pneumonia who die have underlying fatal diseases, previously healthy elderly and young persons also die of pneumonia.[3–7] Therefore more-rapid identification of patients with severe pneumonia and those who are at a high risk for a complicated course and accurate selection of appropriate antimicrobial treatment represents important clinical goals in this setting.

The aim of this chapter is to provide current information on these different issues so that an updated approach to diagnosis and management can be rationally formulated. A detailed review of all diagnostic and therapeutic problems of pneumonia in the severely immunocompromised patient is beyond the scope of this issue, and nosocomial infections are not included.

## PROGNOSTIC FACTORS AND PREDICTION RULES FOR DETERMINING DISEASE SEVERITY

*Severe pneumonia* can be defined as pneumonia requiring treatment in the intensive care unit (ICU). In general terms, this definition includes patients with pneumonia who require (1) ventilatory support because of acute respiratory failure, inability to clear secretions, deterioration in gas exchange with hypercapnia, or persisting hypoxemia; (2) circulatory support because of hemodynamic instability and signs of peripheral hypoperfusion; or (3) intensive monitoring and treatment of other organ dysfunctions resulting either from a septic component of pneumonia or the underlying disease. In 1993 the American Thoracic Society adopted a statement on the initial management of patients with CAP in which severe illness was defined by the presence of any one of the following features: an admission respiratory rate of more than 30 per minute, a $PaO_2/FiO_2$ ratio of less than 250, the need for mechanical ventilation, the presence of bilateral or multilobar infiltrates or rapidly expanding infiltrates, shock, a need for vasopressors, oliguria, or acute renal failure.[8] Although this definition was based on factors known to be associated with the need for intensive care, the definition is probably too liberal, and in one study 65% of all patients admitted to the hospital were found to have at least one feature of severe pneumonia present. To improve the specificity of the criteria, one suggestion has been to change the respiratory rate criterion to 35 breaths/min, but it is probable that severe CAP is best defined by patients having at least two of the severe pneumonia criteria mentioned previously. In one more recent study, the nine criteria for severe CAP were divided into five "minor" criteria that could be present on admission and four "major" criteria that could be present on admission or later in the hospital stay.[9] The minor criteria included respiratory rate, 30/min; $PaO_2/FiO_2 < 250$; bilateral pneumonia or multilobar pneumonia; systolic blood pressure (BP), 90 mm Hg; and diastolic BP, 60 mm Hg. The major criteria included a need for mechanical ventilation, an increase in the size of infiltrates by >50% within 48 hours, septic shock or the need for vasopressors for >4 hours, and acute renal failure (urine output <80 mL in 4 hours or serum creatinine >2 mg/dL in the absence of chronic renal failure). In this retrospective study, the need for ICU admission could be defined using a rule that required the presence of either two of three minor criteria (systolic BP, 90 mm Hg; multilobar disease; $PaO_2/FiO_2$ ratio < 250) or one of two major criteria (need for mechanical ventilation or septic shock). When the other criteria for severe illness were evaluated, they did not add to the accuracy of predicting the need for ICU admission. With this rule the sensitivity was 78%, the specificity was 94%, the positive predictive value was 75%, and the negative predictive value was 95%.

In the British Thoracic Society (BTS) study, the authors formulated a simple discriminant rule based on the three variables that were consistently associated with death.[5] The rule was considered positive when at least two of the following three factors were present: respiratory rate of 30/minute or more, diastolic blood pressure of 60 mm Hg or less, and blood urea nitrogen of more than 7 mmol/L. A positive rule was associated with a 21-fold increase in mortality, with a specificity of 79% and a sensitivity of 88%. However, the positive predictive value was low; only 21 patients of the 108 (19%) who met the rule died. A second rule, in which confusion was used instead of blood urea nitrogen, showed even higher specificity but low sensitivity. The BTS rules have now been validated by two studies, one prospective and one retrospective.[10,11] Unfortunately, the positive predictive values of these rules are too low to permit transfer to the ICU of all patients who meet their definition. However, those patients and patients who present with one or more of the other negative prognostic factors have a higher risk for developing severe pneumonia and should be closely monitored for signs of deterioration. This monitoring should include regular checks of vital signs, mental status, fever, and oxygenation, as well as auscultation of the lungs or chest radiography for signs of spread of the pneumonia.[7]

Although the BTS studies attempted to identify patients with a worse prognosis at the time of admission to the hospital so that they could be targeted for special attention in an ICU, the focus of other studies was just the opposite—namely, to identify those patients with pneumonia who are at lower risk of death and do not need hospital care. Based on the analysis of data collected on 14,199 adult inpatients with pneumonia, Fine and colleagues derived a prediction rule that stratifies patients into five classes with respect to the risk of death within 30 days.[12,13] This prediction rule assigns points based on age and the presence of coexisting disease, abnormal physical findings (such as respiratory rate of 30 per minute or temperature of 40°C), and abnormal laboratory findings (such as pH < 7.35, a blood urea nitrogen concentration of 30 mg/dL [11 mmol/L], or a sodium concentration <130 mmol/L) at presentation (Table 56.1). According to this point scoring system, patients 50 years of age or less with none of the five coexisting illnesses and none of the five physical examination abnormalities listed in Table 56.1 are considered class I. Most patient in this class can safely be treated at home, provided they do not have intractable vomiting, a history of noncompliance, or other contraindications to self-care. The prediction rule defines four more treatment classes according to predicted levels of mortality in a logistic regression analysis. Thus physicians can use the rule to estimate the probabilities of death given the presenting clinical features and to suggest where a patient should be treated.[3,7]

## EPIDEMIOLOGY, OUTCOME, AND ETIOLOGY OF SEVERE PNEUMONIA

The case fatality rate in severe CAP requiring ICU management is high, ranging from 17% to more than 50% in some studies.[14] Not surprisingly, patients who were treated with mechanical ventilation had a higher mortality rate in most studies. Several prospective studies have tried to determine which clinical factors immediately after admission and during ICU stay influence outcome.[15–21] In the study by Torres et al., the factors found to be associated with death according to univariate analysis were the presence of a preexisting ultimately fatal disease, inadequate antibiotic treatment, requirement of mechanical ventilation, treatment with positive end-expiratory pressure (PEEP) or an $FiO_2 > 0.6$, adult acute respiratory distress syndrome (ARDS), radiographic spread of infiltrates after admission, bacteremia, septic shock, and *Pseudomonas aeruginosa* pneumonia.[15] Of these, the multivariate evaluation selected radiographic

**Table 56-1** Point Scoring System Assigning Patients with CAP to Different Risk Classes for Mortality*

| Characteristic/ Demographic Factor | Points Assigned† |
|---|---|
| Age | |
| Men | Age (yr) |
| Women | Age (yr) − 10 |
| Nursing home resident | +10 |
| **Coexisting illnesses** | |
| Neoplastic disease | +30 |
| Liver disease | +20 |
| Congestive heart failure | +10 |
| Cerebrovascular disease | +10 |
| Renal disease | +10 |
| **Physical examination findings** | |
| Altered mental status | +20 |
| Respiratory rate >30 per minute | +20 |
| Systolic blood pressure <90 mm Hg | +20 |
| Temperature <35°C or ≥40°C | +15 |
| Pulse >125/min | +10 |
| **Laboratory and radiographic findings** | |
| Arterial pH <7.35 | +30 |
| Blood urea nitrogen >30 mg/dL (11 mmol/L) | +20 |
| Sodium <130 mmol/L | +20 |
| Glucose >250 mg/dL (14 mmol/L) | +10 |
| Hematocrit <30% | +10 |
| Partial pressure of arterial oxygen <60 mm Hg | +10 |
| Pleural effusion | +10 |

*Adapted from Fine MJ, Auble TE, Yealy DM, et al: Prediction rule to identify low-risk patients with community-acquired pneumonia. N Engl J Med 1997;336:243–250.

†A total point score for a given patient is obtained by summing the patient's age in years (age − 10 for women) and the points for each applicable characteristic. Mortalities for patients in risk classes I, II (<70 points), III (71 to 90 points), IV (91 to 130 points), and V (>130 points) were 0.1%, 0.6%, 0.9%, 9.3%, and 27.0%, respectively.

spread, septic shock, and preexisting ultimately fatal disease (in that order) to be independently associated with death.

Intervention-related factors in management of patients with severe CAP have a significant impact on final outcome. In particular, several studies have now reported that if the initial antibiotic regimen is inadequate or delayed in delivery, this was associated with higher mortality.[15,21] In a recent multicenter retrospective cohort study that included 14,069 patients at least 65 years of age who were hospitalized with pneumonia, Meehan et al. demonstrated that a lower 30-day mortality was associated with antibiotic administration within 8 hours of hospital arrival (odds ration [OR], 0.85; 95% confidence interval [CI], 0.75–0.96), even in analyses that adjusted for patient risk factors and performance of other processes of care.[22]

The pathogens most frequently identified among patients with severe CAP include *Streptococcus pneumoniae*, *Legionella* sp., aerobic gram-negative bacilli, *Mycoplasma pneumoniae*, respiratory tract viruses, and a group of miscellaneous pathogens (*Haemophilus influenzae*, *Mycobacterium tuberculosis*, and endemic fungi). Even if its relative importance has decreased, *S. pneumoniae* remains the predominant organism in most recent studies, causing 15% to 60% of cases of acute CAP.[3,5,6,23–28] The BTS's pneumonia research committee concluded after discriminant functional analysis of data on 148 patients with no identifiable pathogens that most of the cases were probably due to *S. pneumoniae*.[29] These data suggest that the true prevalence of *S. pneumoniae* infection is seriously underrepresented in the results of current microbiologic tests. Advanced age, cigarette smoking, dementia, seizures, and the presence of chronic illnesses (e.g., chronic obstructive pulmonary disease, congestive heart failure, splenectomy, cerebrovascular disease) have been identified as significant risk factors for the development of pneumococcal pneumonia.[3,30] In patients with acquired immune deficiency syndrome (AIDS), the incidence of pneumococcal pneumonia is 5.5 to 17.5 times higher than the predicted incidence in general urban populations.[31] The rate of bacteremia is higher than that for patients without human immunodeficiency virus (HIV) infection (60% versus 15% to 30%), but the mortality rate and manifestations of the disease are generally not different from those in patients without HIV infection. Overwhelming pneumococcal sepsis with disseminated intravascular coagulation has been described in asplenic patients and in patients with functional asplenia, such as those with sickle cell anemia.[32] In recent years, antibiotic drug-resistant *S. pneumoniae* (DRSP) has increasingly been identified, with more than 40% of all pneumococci falling into this category by current in vitro definitions of resistance.[3,7] Controversy continues, however, regarding the clinical relevance of in vitro resistance in the absence of meningitis; whether the problem, as currently defined, requires new therapeutic approaches; and whether the presence of resistance influences the outcome of CAP.[3,33–36] The current definitions of resistance include intermediate-level resistance with penicillin minimally inhibitory concentration (MIC) values of 0.12 to 1.0 µg/mL, whereas high-level resistance is defined as MIC values of 2.0 µg/mL.[3,7] When resistance to penicillin is present, there is often in vitro resistance to other agents, including cephalosporins, macrolides, doxycycline, and trimethoprim/sulfamethoxizole. These data underscore the need to test pneumococcal isolates on a routine basis for penicillin susceptibility. Identified risk factors for DRSP include age >65 years (OR, 3.8), alcoholism (OR, 5.2), noninvasive disease (suggesting possibly reduced virulence of resistant organisms) (OR, 4.5), beta-lactam therapy within 3 months (OR, 2.8), multiple medical comorbidities, exposure to children in a day care center, and immunosuppressive illness.[3,36]

*H. influenzae* is now more frequently recognized as an important cause of CAP; it is responsible for an estimated 4% of 15% of all cases.[7] In most studies, *Hemophilus* species are ranked among the top five etiologies. Treatment is complicated by the increasing incidence of ampicillin resistance, which appears to be due to the production of beta-lactamase. The degree of resistance is now estimated to be about 20% in children and 10% in adults. Fortunately, the recently released second- and third-generation cephalosporins are very beta-lactamase stable, and most *Hemophilus* species are exquisitely sensitive.

*S. aureus* accounts for 1% to 10% of cases of acute CAP.[7] The incidence of staphylococcal pneumonia has been reported to be particularly high in elderly patients institutionalized in nursing homes or during outbreaks of viral influenza.[37] In the latter situation, *S. aureus* may be responsible for as much as 20% of the encountered pneumonias, even when pneumococcus remains the most frequent pathogen, accounting for about 46% of the cases in two studies. A small percentage of staphylococcal pneumonia may result from hematogenous embolization to the lungs due to primary extrapulmonary infections, usually in the setting of right-sided endocarditis or venous septic thrombophlebitis in intravenous drug abusers or in patients undergoing hemodialysis or on home intravenous therapy. There are no clinical or radiologic features typical of *S. aureus* pneumonia, except possibly rapid cavitation of a bronchopneumonia and the development of a pleural empyema.

Aerobic gram-negative rods of *Enterobacteriaeceae* and nonfermentative organisms are a relatively uncommon cause of CAP.[5,7] *Klebsiella pneumoniae* is most often considered, but *Escherichia coli, P. aeruginosa, Enterobacter cloacae, Acinetobacter* and *Serratia* spp., *Proteus*, and many other aerobic, gram-negative bacilli may also cause disease. Although these organisms can infect previously healthy patients, they are more likely to cause disease in older patients and patients with chronic underlying disease and prior antibiotic therapy. For example, in the study of Fang et al., pneumonia caused by *P. aeruginosa* was rarely observed except in patients with bronchiectasis or cystic fibrosis.[38] Immunosuppression, defined as hematologic malignancy, solid tumor, neutropenia, and taking corticosteroids, was relatively low (38%), but all deaths in patients with gram-negative pneumonias occurred in immunosuppressed patients.

The importance of *Legionella* spp. in causing CAP varies greatly according to the geographic area. Although incidences as high as 17% to 22% have been reported, many localities report significantly lower rates.[3] Routine testing using selective medium for culture, direct fluorescent antibody labeling, serology (both acute and convalescent), and urinary antigen detection are crucial in uncovering the diagnosis. Community-acquired Legionnaires' disease seems to be more common among males, persons 50 years of age and older, persons requiring renal dialysis or transplantation, smokers, immunosuppressed patients, and persons with a comorbid disease such as chronic bronchitis or diabetes mellitus.[3]

The true incidence of anaerobic etiologies of CAP is uncertain. In some studies using invasive diagnostic methods, anaerobes have been cultured from lower respiratory tract specimens in 20% to 30% of the cases.[39] However, other reports suggest that anaerobic pneumonias account for only 3% to 4% of cases of CAP.

Anaerobic pulmonary infections can usually be recognized by their characteristic clinical and radiographic findings. Commonly the patient's oral hygiene is poor, and he or she may have some underlying disease in which there is prior evidence of altered consciousness, a diminished gag reflex, or an abnormal swallowing mechanism (e.g., epilepsy, alcoholism, esophageal carcinoma, drug overdose). An insidious low-grade fever is typical, and the chest radiography demonstrates segmental involvement of dependent areas of the lung, often with cavitation.

*M. pneumoniae* is a common cause of CAP, accounting for 10% to 20% of infections in some studies.[28,38] Although nearly all infections with this organism are mild, *M. pneumoniae* can also mimic bacterial pneumonia, and some unusual pulmonary manifestations, such as lung abscess, lobar consolidation, or ARDS, have been reported.[40] Most laboratories do not culture *M. pneumoniae*, and the diagnosis is usually made on serologic evidence.

*Chlamydia pneumoniae* is a pulmonary pathogen that has been associated with pneumonia epidemics in teenagers, young adults, and military conscript populations. In the study of Fang et al., this microorganism comprised 6.1% of the pneumonias and was a common etiology for pneumonia in older adults (mean age, 65 years) and patients with chronic underlying illness.[38]

Although much more common in children, viral pneumonia remains a significant problem in adults. Viral pneumonia typically presents subacutely as an upper respiratory tract infection, but it may have an acute onset with severe pulmonary miliary damage and ARDS. Of the viral agents associated with pneumonia in adults, influenza A and B virus and adenovirus are the most common, but respiratory syncytial virus, the predominant respiratory pathogen in infants and children, is now recognized as an etiology of pneumonia in adults.[3] Although the number of cases is small, groups who appear to be at particularly high risk include the elderly and patients who are immunosuppressed. The definitive diagnosis of viral pneumonia requires detection of the virus from sputum, nasopharyngeal swabs, and/or bronchoalveolar lavage fluid. Information based on serology is often not clinically relevant at the time of the acute illness.

The term *SARS* is used to describe outbreaks of pneumonia caused by a novel coronarovirus that were first recognized in Guangdong province in Southern China in late 2002 and that subsequently spread worldwide during March to June 2003.[7,41] As of July 2003, more than 8000 probable cases have been reported from at least 28 countries worldwide. The heaviest concentrations of cases was identified in mainland China, Hong Kong, and Taiwan, with Singapore, Hanoi, and Toronto also experiencing severe outbreaks. In more than 20% of patients, symptoms progress over 2 to 3 weeks to the more severe respiratory distress syndrome, in which patients require intensive care and ventilatory support.[42,43]

Patients with acute tuberculosis (TB) may present with a syndrome indistinguishable from acute CAP, with infiltrates involving primarily the middle and lower lung fields without apical disease.[44] On occasion, patients with TB present with a syndrome reminiscent of ARDS. Therefore TB must be considered in patients with acute respiratory failure and fever who do not respond to the usual antibacterial therapy. This was highlighted by Bobrowitz, who retrospectively identified 20 patients in whom TB was the primary cause of death but was not diagnosed until autopsy.[44]

Finally, it must be stressed that in virtually every clinical series that recorded etiologic agents for CAP, there was a sizable number of cases for which no specific etiology could be determined. This fact is probably largely explained by the increasing use of broad-spectrum antibiotic therapy in the community. Antibiotics given before admission decrease the ability to isolate a specific pathogen and in particular prevent the detection of pneumococcus.[26]

## CLINICAL AND RADIOGRAPHIC EVALUATION

Patients with CAP typically present with chills, cough, sputum production, fever, and pleuritic chest pain. Mental status changes, confusion, or disorientation is also frequently observed and occurs significantly more frequently in elderly patients. Although these clinical manifestations are useful in diagnosing pneumonia, individual symptoms or signs are not specific for defining the etiologic agent. Fang et al. compared the clinical manifestations of the five most common etiologies (pneumococcus, *H. influenzae*, *Legionella* spp., *C. pneumoniae*, and gram-negative bacilli) of CAP found in their study.[38] In contrast to previous studies, they demonstrated that abdominal pain, vomiting, relative bradycardia, neurologic changes, hyponatremia, and abnormal liver function tests did not occur significantly more frequently in pneumonia caused by *Legionella* spp. than in those caused by other microorganisms. However, *Legionella* cases had much more frequently a temperature >40°C and a slightly higher incidence of diarrhea than in pneumonias of other origins. Patients with *Legionella* spp. pneumonias were also more frequently admitted to the ICU.[38]

Studies have also been performed to discover whether radiographic patterns can distinguish between the various causes of pneumonia.[45–47] A panel of six radiologists who had no prior knowledge of the clinical data was only 67% accurate in the identification of 16 bacterial pneumonias and 65% correct in 9 cases of viral etiology; moreover, no consistent pattern was identified in any specific group of pneumonia.[47] In a comparative study of the radiographic features of community-acquired Legionnaires' disease, pneumococcal pneumonia, mycoplasmal pneumonia, and acute psittacosis, investigators found that homogeneous opacities (airspace disease) were more frequent in Legionnaires' disease and pneumococcal infection than in mycoplasmal pneumonia.[46] In both studies, the pattern of mycoplasmal pneumonia could be confused with airspace bacterial pneumonia in at least 50% of the cases.

## NONINVASIVE MICROBIOLOGIC INVESTIGATION

The value of routine microbiological tests in patients with CAP was recently questioned by several experts[3,48] based on the following arguments. First, the bacteriology of this illness is relatively uniform (and therefore predictable), making initial empiric therapy possible. Second, initial broad-spectrum empiric therapy directed at the known spectrum of likely pathogens is associated with an improved outcome, whereas the identification of a specific etiologic pathogen has not been shown to lead to an improved outcome. Presumably this is because the information about etiology becomes known too late in the course of the illness to reverse the effects of the initial inadequate therapy. Third, there are many controversies concerning the diagnostic value of Gram staining and culture of expectorated sputum. Common problems are that 10% to 30% of patients have a nonproductive cough, 15% to 30% have received antibiotic treatment before hospitalization, and negative results are reported for 30% to 65% of cultures of expectorated sputum. Several studies have shown that the yield of fastidious bacteria such as *S. pneumoniae* and *H. influenzae* is zero when nearly any specimen from the respiratory tract is collected after antibiotic therapy.[37,38] Recognizing all these potential drawbacks, the American Thoracic Society in 2001 recommended that an empiric approach, not relying on extensive diagnostic testing, be used for most patients with CAP.[3]

However, the wide spectrum of possible pathogens and the fact that the cause in 20% to 80% of the patients remains unknown suggest the need for a more active attitude toward the establishment of an etiologic diagnosis, especially in patients with severe CAP.[7] The most important function of a positive diagnostic test is to allow for optimization of the initiated empiric treatment as soon as possible after admission. It is also of epidemiologic importance to obtain an etiologic diagnosis. Knowledge of the local epidemiology and resistance situation is necessary for correct treatment decisions. Finally, the possibility of a noninfectious cause for the pneumonia, such as pulmonary embolism, allergic alveolitis, or vasculitis, should always be considered. Of course, the latter becomes increasingly important if an etiologic diagnosis is not obtained despite the use of aggressive methods.

To obtain a proper expectorated sputum specimen, the patient should be carefully instructed and supervised by a physician or a respiratory therapist to obtain secretions resulting from a deep cough. One alternative for some patients who are unable to expectorate anything other than oropharyngeal secretions is to blindly pass a small catheter through the upper respiratory tract into the trachea to directly sample distal secretions. Various criteria based on cytologic characteristics have been suggested for scoring the quality of sputum specimens.[49] In a study in which parallel cytologic and microbiologic analyses of sputa and transtracheal aspirates from patients with pneumonia were performed, Geckler et al.[50] found that the results of sputum culture containing more than 25 squamous epithelial cells per low-power field (magnification ×100) showed poor agreement with those of transtracheal aspiration, regardless of the number of leukocytes that were present. Such samples are therefore nondiagnostic and should be discarded. On the other hand, the presence of fewer than 10 epithelial cells and more than 25 leukocytes per field suggests that the specimen actually represents lower respiratory tract secretions.[49]

Gram-stained smears of acceptable specimens should then be examined under oil immersion (magnification ×1000) to determine whether bacteria of a specific or characteristic morphologic type are present. Neither the fields being examined nor any of the immediately adjacent fields should contain any squamous epithelial cells, but at least several neutrophils or alveolar macrophages should be present. The morphologic and staining characteristics of any bacteria should be recorded, and a semi-quantitative estimate of their number should be made. This method has proved useful for the identification of *S. pneumoniae* in the sputum.[51,52] Rein et al.[53] have suggested that when strict criteria for Gram-stain positivity are used (predominant flora or >10 gram-positive, lancet-shaped diplococci per oil immersion field), the specificity of the technique is 85% with a sensitivity of 62%. Whether this approach is equally useful for the identification of other bacterial causes of pneumonia remains unclear. However, Tillotson and Lerner noted that gram-negative bacilli were seen in smears of all sputum specimens taken from 20 cases of *E. coli* pneumonia.[54] Small gram-negative coccobacillary organisms are characteristic of *H. influenzae*. Staphylococci appear as gram-positive cocci in tetrads and small clusters. In contrast, the failure to detect *S. aureus* or gram-negative bacilli in the pretreatment specimen nearly completely excludes these organisms from diagnostic consideration.[37] Gram-stained smears may also support a diagnosis of atypical pneumonia or Legionnaires' disease when sputum examinations repeatedly show no bacteria in a patient who has received no antimicrobial treatment prior to admission.

The utility of sputum cultures as a means of establishing the agents responsible for pneumonia has been questioned. Patients with bacteremic pneumococcal pneumonia have been reported to have negative sputum cultures in 45% to 50% of the cases, even when large numbers of organisms have been noted on Gram-stained preparations.[37] Similarly, 34% to 47% of sputum cultures are negative with proven *H. influenzae* pneumonia. Furthermore, cultures of expectorated sputum often yield multiple organisms, and it is difficult to tell whether these bacteria are causative or are merely colonizing the upper respiratory tract. For example, contamination with gram-negative bacilli has been noted in more than 30% of sputum cultures.[37] Semiquantitative cultures, washing of sputum samples, and the use of mucolytic agents have been proposed to improve the clinical utility of sputum cultures; however, results have been variable, and the practicality of these techniques for routine use is questionable. In fact, the main role of sputum cultures in clinical practice is to permit definitive identification of the organisms that are present in predominance in the Gram-stained smear and to determine their susceptibility to antibiotics. In other words, results of sputum cultures should always be used as a function of the results of the Gram staining.

## OTHER NONINVASIVE DIAGNOSTIC TECHNIQUES

Approximately 20% to 30% of patients with bacterial pneumonia are bacteremic, and therefore blood cultures should not be overlooked as a means of identifying the bacterial etiology of pneumonia.[37] Pleural fluid cultures, when positive, are also specific for the etiology of the underlying pneumonia.

*L. pneumophila* serogroup I accounts for about 70% of Legionnaire's disease, and the urine antigen test has been shown to be more than 90% specific and about 90% sensitive for this pathogen.[7] The pneumococcal urinary antigen assay is also an acceptable test to augment the standard diagnostic methods of blood culture and sputum Gram stain and culture, with the potential advantage of rapid results similar to those for sputum Gram stain.[7]

Serologic tests are used to diagnose a variety of pulmonary pathogens including *Legionella* species, *M. pneumoniae*, *Chlamydia* spp., and many viruses. Because these tests usually require two blood specimens drawn at a minimum of a 2-week interval, they are of help only in confirming a clinical diagnosis, not for initiating treatment.

## INVASIVE DIAGNOSTIC TECHNIQUES

Bronchoscopy not only enables direct visualization of the endobronchial tree but also affords an opportunity to obtain specimens for culture and histology using various techniques directly from the site of inflammation in the lung. Initial studies concerning the reliability of specimens obtained for culture directly by suction through the inner channel have been disappointing. Bartlett et al.[55] demonstrated that in patients without lower respiratory tract infections, cultures of aspirates obtained during bronchoscopy were frequently contaminated, producing an average of five different bacterial species. Therefore this type of specimen collection has the same potential drawbacks as those observed with expectorated sputum, which underlines the importance of examining a Gram-stained preparation of bronchoscopic secretions before interpreting the results of such cultures.

Bronchoalveolar lavage (BAL), in which a segment of lung is "washed" with sterile saline, has proved to be an excellent means of diagnosing respiratory infections. Lavage is indeed a safe and practical method for obtaining cells and secretions from the lower respiratory tract. This technique samples a relatively large area of the lung (about $10^6$ alveoli). The cells and liquid recovered can be examined microscopically immediately after the procedure and are also suitable for culture and other techniques. Thorpe et al.[56] performed bronchoalveolar lavage with the bronchoscope introduced either transnasally or through an endotracheal tube in a heterogeneous group of 92 hospitalized patients, 15 of whom were thought to have active bacterial pneumonia. Thirteen of the 15 patients with clinically active bacterial pneumonia had a bronchoalveolar lavage culture of more than $10^5$ colony-forming units (CFUs)/mL of bronchoalveolar lavage fluid, whereas none of the other patients, including those with resolving pneumonia or chronic bronchitis, had counts of more than $10^4$ CFUs/mL. Furthermore, Gram staining of cytocentrifuged bronchoalveolar lavage fluid was positive (one or more organisms seen per ×1000 field) only in those patients with active bacterial pneumonia.

Fiberoptic bronchoscopy is regarded as a relatively safe technique with few serious complications. Postbronchoscopy fever with increasing infiltrates may be observed. There is also a 10 to 20 mm Hg decrease in $PaO_2$, which could pose a problem for some patients with severe hypoxemia. Parodoxically, the risk of bronchoscopy is more important in nonventilated patients than in patients receiving mechanical ventilation. Therefore, in a patient already on the verge of needing assisted ventilation, the risk of worsening respiratory failure must be carefully considered. If the potential benefit of the diagnostic procedure is believed to be great, it may be preferable to perform the bronchoscopy after the patient has been safely intubated and ventilated.

In summary, invasive techniques are indicated only in patients with severe CAP, as it has been demonstrated that appropriate initial antibiotic treatment in patients with no signs of severity is associated with good prognosis. If the patient is not receiving mechanical ventilation, the risk of performing bronchoscopy may outweigh the benefit of determining the responsible pathogen(s) in most cases, except in deeply immunosuppressed patients. When patients are receiving mechanical ventilation, bronchoscopy using BAL should probably be performed whenever possible, because this technique permits to safely determine the responsible organisms and therefore to select the appropriate treatment as soon as possible. However, in no case should diagnostic testing lead to delays in the initiation of appropriate antimicrobial therapy (see later discussion).

## TREATMENT

Timely antimicrobial therapy is important for patients who require hospitalization for acute pneumonia. Previous guidelines recommended initial administration within 8 hours after arrival at the hospital. This recommendation was based on a retrospective analysis of 14,000 Medicare hospitalizations for pneumonia in 1994 to 1995.[22] A more recent analysis of Medicare hospitalizations demonstrated an association between initiation of antimicrobial therapy within 4 hours after arrival and improved outcomes.[57] In fact, the time to initiation of antibiotic therapy had a greater influence on patient outcome than did antibiotic selection itself. This study included more than 13,000 patients with pneumonia who were hospitalized in 1998 and 1999 and who had not received antibiotics before admission. Initial therapy within 4 hours after arrival at the hospital was associated with reduced mortality in the hospital (severity-adjusted OR, 0.85; 95% CI, 0.76 to 0.95). Mean length of stay was 0.4 days shorter among patients who received antimicrobials within 4 hours than among those whose initial therapy was given at a later time. Improved outcomes were associated with timely therapy independent of the Pneumonia Severity Index class and the presence of congestive heart failure. These findings are consistent with those of several previous studies.

Initial empiric therapy prior to availability of culture data for a patient ill enough to require admission to a hospital ward can be with a beta-lactam plus macrolide combination or a respiratory fluoroquinolone alone, such as levofloxacin, gatifloxacin, and/or moxifloxacin.[7] If the patient is sufficiently ill to need ICU management and if *Pseudomonas* infection is not a concern, a combination of an intravenous beta-lactam (cefotaxime or ceftriaxone) plus either an advanced intravenous macrolide (azithromycin) or a fluoroquinolone should be used.[3,7]

In patients with a risk factor for *P. aeruginosa*, such as bronchiectasis, corticosteroid therapy (more than 10 mg of prednisone per day), broad-spectrum antibiotic therapy for more than 7 days in the past month, malnutrition, and leukopenic immune suppression, initial therapy should include two antipseudomonal agents and provide coverage for drug-resistant *S. pneumoniae* and *Legionella*.[7] This can be done with selected beta-lactams (cefepime, piperacillin/tazobactam, imipenem, meropenem) plus an antipseudomonal quinolone (ciprofloxacin) or with selected beta-lactams plus an aminoglycoside and either azithromycin or a nonpseudomonal quinolone (levofloxacin, gatifloxacin, and/or moxifloxacin).

Once culture data are available and it is known that the patient has pneumococcal pneumonia with bacteremia without evidence to support infection with a copathogen, treatment will depend on in vitro susceptibility results. If the isolate is penicillin susceptible, a beta-lactam (penicillin G or amoxicillin) alone may be used. If the isolate is penicillin resistant, cefotaxime, ceftriaxone, or a respiratory fluoroquinolone or other agent indicated by in vitro testing may be used.[7]

Several retrospective studies have suggested that dual therapy including a macrolide given empirically may reduce mortality associated with bacteremic pneumococcal pneumonia.[58–62] However, the fact that these studies were neither prospective nor randomized meant that they had significant design limitations. It is important to note that these studies evaluated the effects of initial empiric therapy before the results of blood cultures were known. They did not examine effects of pathogen-specific therapy after the results of blood cultures were available, and many experts believe that the results of these studies do not contradict the principles of pathogen-directed therapy.[7] Two possible explanations for the improved results with a macrolide are the concurrent presence of atypical pathogens (*M. pneumoniae*, *C. pneumoniae*, or *Legionella* species) and the immunomodulating effects of macrolides. A prospective randomized trial is ultimately needed to determine the best regimen without bias or confounding variables distorting the answer.

With respect to the case vignette, the patient should be immediately admitted to an ICU and intubated and mechanically ventilated on the basis of his or her hemodynamic unstability and respiratory condition severity. We would then recommend a urinary antigen test for

*Legionella pneumophilia* serogroup 1, two blood cultures, and a fiberoptic bronchoscopy with BAL if this procedure can be done with no delay. Otherwise, we would recommend to directly suction deep respiratory secretions through the endotracheal tube for Gram staining and cultures. Immediately afterward and without waiting for the results, empiric antimicrobial therapy should be started, combining intravenously a beta-lactam, such as ceftriaxone, plus either an advanced macrolide or a fluoroquinolone, because the patient has no risk factors for *P. aeruginosa*. However, when the presence of gram-negative bacilli is documented by Gram staining, initial antibiotic therapy should be broadened to cover *P. aeruginosa*. Once culture data of deep respiratory secretions are available, treatment should be streamlined based on the susceptibility patterns of the responsible microorganism(s).

## REFERENCES

1. Mortensen EM, Coley CM, Singer DE, et al: Causes of death for patients with community-acquired pneumonia: Results from the Pneumonia Patient Outcomes Research Team cohort study. Arch Intern Med 2002;162:1059–1064.

2. Mortensen EM, Kapoor WN, Chang CC, et al: Assessment of mortality after long-term follow-up of patients with community-acquired pneumonia. Clin Infect Dis 2003;37: 1617–1624.

3. Niederman MS, Mandell LA, Anzueto A, et al: Guidelines for the management of adults with community-acquired pneumonia. Diagnosis, assessment of severity, antimicrobial therapy, and prevention. Am J Respir Crit Care Med 2001;163:1730–1754.

4. ERS Task Force Report: Guidelines for management of adult community-acquired lower respiratory tract infections. European Respiratory Society. Eur Respir J 1998;11:986–991.

5. British Thoracic Society Guidelines for the Management of Community Acquired Pneumonia in Childhood. Thorax 2002;57(Suppl 1):1–24.

6. Mandell LA, Marrie TJ, Grossman RF, et al: Canadian guidelines for the initial management of community-acquired pneumonia: An evidence-based update by the Canadian Infectious Diseases Society and the Canadian Thoracic Society. The Canadian Community-Acquired Pneumonia Working Group. Clin Infect Dis 2000;31:383–421.

7. Mandell LA, Bartlett JG, Dowell SF, et al: Update of practice guidelines for the management of community-acquired pneumonia in immunocompetent adults. Clin Infect Dis 2003;37:1405–1433.

8. Niederman MS, Bass JB Jr, Campbell GD, et al: Guidelines for the initial management of adults with community-acquired pneumonia: Diagnosis, assessment of severity, and initial antimicrobial therapy. American Thoracic Society. Medical Section of the American Lung Association. Am Rev Respir Dis 1993;148:1418–1426.

9. Ewig S, Ruiz M, Mensa J, et al: Severe community-acquired pneumonia. Assessment of severity criteria. Am J Respir Crit Care Med 1998;158:1102–1108.

10. Farr BM, Sloman AJ, Fisch MJ: Predicting death in patients hospitalized for community-acquired pneumonia. Ann Intern Med 1991;115:428–436.

11. Feldman C, Kallenbach JM, Levy H, et al: Community-acquired pneumonia of diverse aetiology: Prognostic features in patients admitted to an intensive care unit and a "severity of illness" core. Intensive Care Med 1989;15:302–307.

12. Fine MJ, Smith MA, Carson CA, et al: Prognosis and outcomes of patients with community-acquired pneumonia. A meta-analysis. JAMA 1996;275:134–141.

13. Fine MJ, Auble TE, Yealy DM, et al: A prediction rule to identify low-risk patients with community-acquired pneumonia. N Engl J Med 1997;336:243–250.

14. Leeper KV Jr: Severe community-acquired pneumonia. Semin Respir Infect 1996;11:96–108.

15. Torres A, Serra-Batlles J, Ferrer A, et al: Severe community-acquired pneumonia. Epidemiology and prognostic factors. Am Rev Respir Dis 1991;144:312–318.

16. Leroy O, Santre C, Beuscart C, et al: A five-year study of severe community-acquired pneumonia with emphasis on prognosis in patients admitted to an intensive care unit. Intensive Care Med 1995;21:24–31.

17. Moine P, Vercken JB, Chevret S, et al: Severe community-acquired pneumococcal pneumonia. The French Study Group of Community-Acquired Pneumonia in ICU. Scand J Infect Dis 1995;27:201–206.

18. el-Ebiary M, Sarmiento X, Torres A, et al: Prognostic factors of severe Legionella pneumonia requiring admission to ICU. Am J Respir Crit Care Med 1997;156:1467–1472.

19. Almirall J, Mesalles E, Klamburg J, et al: Prognostic factors of pneumonia requiring admission to the intensive care unit. Chest 1995;107:511–516.

20. Moine P, Vercken JB, Chevret S, et al: Severe community-acquired pneumonia. Etiology, epidemiology, and prognosis factors. French Study Group for Community-Acquired Pneumonia in the Intensive Care Unit. Chest 1994;105: 1487–1495.

21. Leroy O, Vandenbussche C, Coffinier C, et al: Community-acquired aspiration pneumonia in intensive care units. Epidemiological and prognosis data. Am J Respir Crit Care Med 1997;156:1922–1929.

22. Meehan TP, Fine MJ, Krumholz HM, et al: Quality of care, process, and outcomes in elderly patients with pneumonia. JAMA 1997;278:2080–2084.

23. Lim I, Shaw DR, Stanley DP, et al: A prospective hospital study of the aetiology of community-acquired pneumonia. Med J Aust 1989;151:87–91.

24. Lieberman D, Schlaeffer F, Boldur I, et al: Multiple pathogens in adult patients admitted with community-acquired pneumonia: A 1-year prospective study of 346 consecutive patients. Thorax 1996;51:179–184.

25. Bohte R, van Furth R, van den Broek PJ: Aetiology of community-acquired pneumonia: A prospective study among adults requiring admission to hospital. Thorax 1995;50: 543–547.

26. Woodhead MA, Macfarlane JT, McCracken JS, et al: Prospective study of the aetiology and outcome of pneumonia in the community. Lancet 1987;1:671–674.

27. Lim WS, Macfarlane JT, Boswell TC, et al: Study of community acquired pneumonia aetiology (SCAPA) in adults admitted to hospital: Implications for management guidelines. Thorax 2001;56:296–301.

28. Community-acquired pneumonia in adults in British hospitals in 1982-1983: A survey of aetiology, mortality, prognostic factors and outcome. The British Thoracic Society and the Public Health Laboratory Service. Q J Med 1987;62: 195–220.

29. Farr BM, Kaiser DL, Harrison BD, et al: Prediction of microbial aetiology at admission to hospital for pneumonia from the

presenting clinical features. British Thoracic Society Pneumonia Research Subcommittee. Thorax 1989;44:1031–1035.

30. Lipsky BA, Boyko EJ, Inui TS, et al: Risk factors for acquiring pneumococcal infections. Arch Intern Med 1986;146:2179–2185.

31. Janoff EN, Breiman RF, Daley CL, et al: Pneumococcal disease during HIV infection. Epidemiologic, clinical, and immunologic perspectives. Ann Intern Med 1992;117:314–324.

32. Zarrabi MH, Rosner F: Serious infections in adults following splenectomy for trauma. Arch Intern Med 1984;144:1421–1424.

33. Heffelfinger JD, Dowell SF, Jorgensen JH, et al: Management of community-acquired pneumonia in the era of pneumococcal resistance: A report from the Drug-Resistant *Streptococcus pneumoniae* Therapeutic Working Group. Arch Intern Med 2000;160:1399–1408.

34. Plouffe JF, Breiman RF, Facklam RR: Bacteremia with *Streptococcus pneumoniae*. Implications for therapy and prevention. Franklin County Pneumonia Study Group. JAMA 1996;275:194–198.

35. Pallares R, Linares J, Vadillo M, et al: Resistance to penicillin and cephalosporin and mortality from severe pneumococcal pneumonia in Barcelona, Spain. N Engl J Med 1995;333: 474–480.

36. Feikin DR, Schuchat A, Kolczak M, et al: Mortality from invasive pneumococcal pneumonia in the era of antibiotic resistance, 1995-1997. Am J Public Health 2000;90:223–229.

37. Bartlett JG, Dowell SF, Mandell LA, et al: Practice guidelines for the management of community-acquired pneumonia in adults. Infectious Diseases Society of America. Clin Infect Dis 2000;31:347–382.

38. Fang GD, Fine M, Orloff J, et al: New and emerging etiologies for community-acquired pneumonia with implications for therapy. A prospective multicenter study of 359 cases. Medicine (Baltimore) 1990;69:307–316.

39. Bartlett JG: Anaerobic bacterial infections of the lung. Chest 1987;91:901–909.

40. Ponka A: Clinical and laboratory manifestations in patients with serological evidence of *Mycoplasma pneumoniae* infection. Scand J Infect Dis 1978;10:271–275.

41. From the Centers for Disease Control and Prevention. Update: Severe acute respiratory syndrome—United States, June 11, 2003. JAMA 2003;290:34.

42. Lew TW, Kwek TK, Tai D, et al: Acute respiratory distress syndrome in critically ill patients with severe acute respiratory syndrome. JAMA 2003;290:374–380.

43. Fowler RA, Lapinsky SE, Hallett D, et al: Critically ill patients with severe acute respiratory syndrome. JAMA 2003;290:367–373.

44. Bobrowitz ID: Active tuberculosis undiagnosed until autopsy. Am J Med 1982;72:650–658.

45. Albaum MN, Hill LC, Murphy M, et al: Interobserver reliability of the chest radiograph in community-acquired pneumonia. PORT Investigators. Chest 1996;110:343–350.

46. Macfarlane JT, Miller AC, Roderick Smith WH, et al: Comparative radiographic features of community acquired Legionnaires' disease, pneumococcal pneumonia, mycoplasma pneumonia, and psittacosis. Thorax 1984;39:28–33.

47. Tew J, Calenoff L, Berlin BS: Bacterial or nonbacterial pneumonia: Accuracy of radiographic diagnosis. Radiology 1977;124:607–612.

48. Garcia-Vazquez E, Marcos MA, Mensa J, et al: Assessment of the usefulness of sputum culture for diagnosis of community-acquired pneumonia using the PORT predictive scoring system. Arch Intern Med 2004;164:1807–1811.

49. Murray PR, Washington JA: Microscopic and bacteriologic analysis of expectorated sputum. Mayo Clin Proc 1975;50:339–344.

50. Geckler RW, Gremillion DH, McAllister CK, et al: Microscopic and bacteriological comparison of paired sputa and transtracheal aspirates. J Clin Microbiol 1977;6:396–399.

51. Musher DM, Montoya R, Wanahita A: Diagnostic value of microscopic examination of Gram-stained sputum and sputum cultures in patients with bacteremic pneumococcal pneumonia. Clin Infect Dis 2004;39:165–169.

52. Cordero E, Pachon J, Rivero A, et al: Usefulness of sputum culture for diagnosis of bacterial pneumonia in HIV-infected patients. Eur J Clin Microbiol Infect Dis 2002;21:362–367.

53. Rein MF, Gwaltney JM Jr, O'Brien WM, et al: Accuracy of Gram's stain in identifying pneumococci in sputum. JAMA 1978;239:2671–2673.

54. Tillotson JR, Lerner AM: Characteristics of pneumonias caused by *Escherichia coli*. N Engl J Med 1967;277:115–122.

55. Bartlett JG, Alexander J, Mayhew J, et al: Should fiberoptic bronchoscopy aspirates be cultured? Am Rev Respir Dis 1976;114:73–78.

56. Thorpe JE, Baughman RP, Frame PT, et al: Bronchoalveolar lavage for diagnosing acute bacterial pneumonia. J Infect Dis 1987;155:855–861.

57. Gleason PP, Meehan TP, Fine JM, et al: Associations between initial antimicrobial therapy and medical outcomes for hospitalized elderly patients with pneumonia. Arch Intern Med 1999;159:2562–2572.

58. Lujan M, Gallego M, Fontanals D, et al: Prospective observational study of bacteremic pneumococcal pneumonia: Effect of discordant therapy on mortality. Crit Care Med 2004;32:625–631.

59. Waterer GW, Somes GW, Wunderink RG: Monotherapy may be suboptimal for severe bacteremic pneumococcal pneumonia. Arch Intern Med 2001;161:1837–1842.

60. Martinez JA, Horcajada JP, Almela M, et al: Addition of a macrolide to a beta-lactam-based empirical antibiotic regimen is associated with lower in-hospital mortality for patients with bacteremic pneumococcal pneumonia. Clin Infect Dis 2003;36:389–395.

61. File TM Jr, Mandell LA. What is optimal antimicrobial therapy for bacteremic pneumococcal pneumonia? Clin Infect Dis 2003;36:396–398.

62. Baddour LM, Yu VL, Klugman KP, et al: Combination antibiotic therapy lowers mortality among severely ill patients with pneumococcal bacteremia. Am J Respir Crit Care Med 2004;170:440–444.

# CHAPTER 57

# Ventilator-Associated Pneumonia

Joan R. Badia and Antoni Torres

Nosocomial pneumonia is a frequent and severe complication during mechanical ventilation. *Ventilator-acquired pneumonia* (VAP) is defined as a hospital-acquired pneumonia occurring after 48 to 72 hours of onset of mechanical ventilation. VAP has a raw incidence ranging from 20% to 25% of all patients ventilated for more than 72 hours and bears a high morbidity and mortality. The mean duration of mechanical ventilation increases in more than 1 week, and adjusted mortality may be as much as 30%. Additionally, treatment costs are increased substantially.

Two cases are presented in this chapter, and diagnostic and treatment options are discussed.

## CASE REPORT 1

A 52-year-old man presented with seizures and loss of consciousness. On arrival to the emergency room, he had a Glasgow coma scale below 5, and he was intubated and mechanically ventilated.

The patient was a heavy smoker with an accumulated dose of 100 packs/year and had also been a heavy drinker in the past. In the past 2 years his alcohol intake was estimated to be below 60 g/day. He had systemic hypertension and was being treated with diet plus a conversion enzyme inhibitor (enalapril 10 mg daily). Three years previously, he had been admitted to the hospital for acute pancreatitis related to his alcohol consumption, and he was positive for hepatitis C virus.

On admission, he was hypertensive at 190/120 mm Hg, his temperature was 37.3°C, and his pulse rate was 88 beats per minute. There were no signs or clinical

information suggesting bronchoaspiration during or prior to intubation. He was mechanically ventilated with 480 mL of tidal volume at a frequency of 18 cycles per minute and an oxygen inspiratory fraction of 0.5. The patient was not initially sedated and presented with an apparent 3/5 palsy affecting the left arm and limb, left Babinsky sign, and right-sided eye deviation. A brain computed tomography (CT) scan disclosed a right basal ganglia hematoma with moderate perilesional edema. At this time point, laboratory studies revealed a serum creatinine of 1.5 mg/dL, glycemia of 146 mg/dL, white cell count of $5.32 \times 10^{10}$ cells/L$^{-1}$, and hematocrit of 48% with a mean corpuscular volume of 98 μm$^3$. Platelets and coagulation were within normal ranges. Arterial blood gas measurements on 50% oxygen were as follows: pH, 7.39; PaO$_2$, 181 mm Hg; and PaCO$_2$, 41 mm Hg. Chest radiography was performed on admission and showed only moderate cardiomegalia with clear lung fields. The patient remained under mechanical ventilation and received intravenous fenitoine, stress ulcer prophylaxis, and enteral feeding via a nasogastric tube. He was situated in bed in a semirecumbent position, and the pressure of the tracheal tube cuff was assessed every 8 hours as standardized in the unit. An oral antiseptic, chlorhexidine, was used for oropharyngeal hygiene every 8 hours also as part of the standard ICU care. APACHE II score on admission was 16 points. On day 3 after intubation, a control chest radiograph disclosed a localized alveolar infiltrate on the right lower lobe, which was not present in the previous examination (Fig. 57.1). The patient did not have fever, the white blood cell count was $7.40 \times 10^{10}$ cells/L$^{-1}$, and pulmonary secretions were only moderately increased and did not seem purulent. Oxygenation had improved,

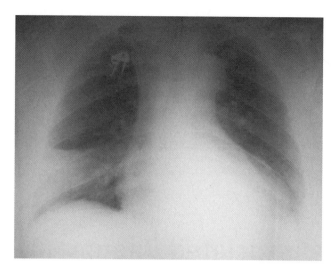

**Figure 57.1** Chest radiograph of Case 1. A new localized pulmonary infiltrate in the right lower lobe can be observed.

and the $PaO_2/FiO_2$ ratio was above 300. Finally, a tracheal bronchoaspirate sample was taken and sent for quantitative culture. A fast Gram stain did not show the presence of pathogenic bacteria. With this clinical situation the decision was taken to treat the patient initially with a quinolone (ciprofloxacin 400 mg IV two times daily) and to reassess the case at the third day. At this time point the patient did not have fever or significant respiratory secretions, white blood cell count was normal, and oxygenation was adequate. The chest radiograph still showed the localized patchy infiltrate, although it was less apparent, and a fast Gram stain of a tracheal aspirate did not show any microorganism. The previous culture was positive for low-count *Proteus mirabillis* ($10^3$ colony-forming units [CFU]/mL). On the basis of all these data, antibiotic treatment was discontinued. The following day, the patient's level of consciousness was appropriate to attempt a T-piece trial that was well tolerated clinically, and blood gases were adequate, so the patient was subsequently weaned from mechanical ventilation. The palsy involving the left arm and limb had recovered only slightly, and a moderate dysarthria was present. After 24 hours the patient was discharged to the neurologic ward. He did not receive further antibiotic treatment, and a chest radiograph taken 3 days later showed clear lung fields.

## CASE REPORT 2

A 78-year-old man was admitted to the ICU for a short postoperative follow-up after elective sigmoidectomy for colorectal neoplasm located at 25 cm of the anal margin. The patient was a mild smoker of 2 to 4 cigarettes

per day, he had an undertreated systemic hypertension, and was dislipemic as main vascular risk factors. He had an ischemic myocardiopathy, and 10 years previously he had required three bypasses and received treatment with aspirin and topic nitrates. There was also a past history of gastric ulcer, and 2 years before admission he presented with an ischemic stroke with right palsy of which he had recovered almost completely. The colorectal tumor had been diagnosed 2 weeks prior to surgery after repeated observation of blood-stained stools. Due to this multiplicity of previous relevant diseases, the surgical team in charge decided to schedule a close follow-up in the ICU after surgery. The patient arrived in spontaneous ventilation and was doing well until 48 hours later. At that time, his situation deteriorated with confusion, fever, hemodynamic instability, and sudden abdominal pain. A gastrografin enema disclosed a surgical dehiscence, and the patient underwent emergency surgery for repair. The patient returned to the ICU under mechanical ventilation through a tracheal tube, and coverage with antibiotics was initiated, with a focus on the treatment of the peritonitis encountered in the surgical procedure. Additionally, parenteral feeding was started and moderate doses of vasoactive agents were required. After 5 days under mechanical ventilation and more than 1 week in the hospital, a patchy infiltrate located in the right lower lobe was observed in the chest radiography and was accompanied by an increase in central body temperature to 38.5°C, abundant and purulent tracheal secretions that required frequent aspiration, and an increase in white blood cell count to $21.32 \times 10^{10}$ cells/L$^{-1}$ with a high count of band forms. This clinical picture was accompanied by a deterioration of blood gas measurements with a decrease of $PaO_2/FiO_2$ ratio to 180. At this point, combination treatment with an antipseudomonic cephalosporin and an aminoglycoside plus vancomycin was started, and a tracheobronchial aspirate was sent to the microbiology laboratory. The Gram stain showed gram-negative bacilli, and the sample proceeded to quantitative culture. *Pseudomonas aeruginosa* was isolated at a count of $6 \times 10^5$ CFU/mL, and the antibiogram showed adequate sensibility to the therapy that had been started. Vancomycin was discontinued. After 3 days another tracheobronchial aspirate was obtained and cultured, showing a substantial decrease of bacterial count to $1 \times 10^3$ CFU/mL. The patient improved initially with disappearance of the fever and improvement in the chest radiograph. The same antibiotic treatment regimen was to be maintained at least 10 days. However, after 7 days the condition of the patient worsened again with an increase in volume and purulence of respiratory secretions, febricula, and worsening oxygenation. Radiography showed persistence of previous infiltrates, although further interpretation was difficult due to moderate transudative pleural effusion. A thoracic scan was ordered, but it could not be performed at that time due to the unstable condition of the patient. Addition of antifungal treatment was considered, and a fiberoptic bronchoscopy with bronchoalveolar lavage (BAL) was carried out. Lavage cell count showed a predominance of polymorphonuclear leukocytes and a moderately inflammatory sample. The Gram stain did not show microorganisms, but the culture isolated colonies of *Candida* spp. and $5 \times 10^4$ CFU/mL of *Stenotrophomonas maltophilia*. This microorganism was resistant to the antibiotics the patient was currently receiving and could only be treated with co-trimoxazole and tobramycin. Another current patient had a previous isolation of this

microorganism with an identical resistance pattern. In addition to intravenous co-trimoxazole and tobramycin, nebulized tobramycin was also implemented in this case. The patient evolved well both clinically and radiologically, although during his ICU stay the chest radiograph did not clear completely. He was extubated on day 16 after the onset of mechanical ventilation and was able to be transferred to a respiratory intermediate care unit 2 days later.

## DISCUSSION

The cases presented here are fully representative of the problems encountered in the diagnosis and treatment of hospital-acquired pneumonia and specifically VAP. Despite many efforts and research in the prevention, diagnosis, and treatment of VAP, the management of this clinical situation remains to some extent controversial. Appropriate diagnosis and initial empiric treatment are critical because these factors have a direct influence on mortality and outcome. Conversely, unnecessary or excessive antibiotic pressure increases costs remarkably and leads directly to the appearance of antibiotic-resistant bacterial strains. Diagnosis is troublesome due to the lack of specificity of clinical signs such as fever, leukocytosis,

---

**BOX 57-1**

**Clinical Pulmonary Infection Score (CPIS)**

**Temperature (° C)**
≥36.5 and ≤38.4 = 0 points
≥38.5 and ≤38.9 = 1 point
≥39 and ≤36 = 2 points

**Blood leukocytes/mm³**
≥4000 and ≤11.000 = 0 point
<4000 or >11.000 = 1 point + band forms ≥ 50% = add 1 point

**Tracheal secretions**
Absence of tracheal secretions = 0 points
Nonpurulent secretions = 1 point
Purulent secretions = 2 points

**Oxygenation $Pao_2/Fio_2$**
>240 or ARDS = 0 points
≤240 and no ARDS = 2 points

**Pulmonary radiography**
No infiltrate = 0 points
Diffuse or patchy infiltrate = 1 point
Localized infiltrate = 2 points

**Progression of pulmonary infiltrate**
No radiographic progression = 0 points
Radiographic progression after CHF and ARDS are
    excluded = 2 points

**Culture of tracheal infiltrates**
Pathogenic bacteria in low counts or no growth = 0 points
Pathogenic bacteria cultured in moderate or heavy
    quantity = 1 point
Same pathogenic bacteria seen on Gram stain =
    add 1 point

*Clinical pulmonary infection score used by Singh et al. as an operational tool to guide antibiotic therapy in suspected ventilator-acquired pneumonia.*
*Modified from Pugin J, Auckenthaler R, Mili N, et al: Diagnosis of ventilator associated pneumonia by bacteriologic analysis of bronchoscopic and non-bronchoscopic "blind" bronchoalveolar lavage fluid. Am Rev Respir Dis 1991;143:1121–1129.*
*ARDS, acute respiratory distress syndrome; CHF, congestive heart failure.*

---

**BOX 57-2**

**Bacteriology of Hospital-Acquired Pneumonia**

**Early-onset pneumonia**
*Streptococcus pneumoniae*
*Haemophilus influenzae*
*Moraxella catarrahlis*
*Staphylococcus aureus**
Aerobic gram-negative bacilli*

**Late-onset pneumonia**
*Pseudomonas aeruginosa*
*Enterobacter* spp
*Acinetobacter* spp.
*Klebsiella pneumoniae*
*Serratia marcescens*
*Escherichia coli*
Other multiresistant gram-negative bacilli
*S. aureus***

**Other**
Anaerobic bacteria
*Legionella* spp.
Influenza A and B
Respiratory virus
Fungi

*\*In patients with risk factors. \*\*Including methicillin-resistant S. aureus.*

or pulmonary infiltrates. A proposed strategy is the use of scoring systems that take into account clinical data, laboratory results, microbiology, and radiology. In our view an interesting model is the clinical pulmonary infection score (CPIS). This score has an acceptable sensitivity (77%) but suboptimal specificity (42%) to establish the diagnosis of pneumonia. However, a modification of this infection score used by Singh et al. appears to be an objective measure to identify those patients with pulmonary infiltrates that can be treated safely with short-course antibiotic monotherapy (Box 57.1). It must be pointed out that if these strategies are applied, early reassessment is mandatory and a new complete evaluation at 2 to 4 days should be performed.

Case 1 is a clear example of the performance of this type of management. This neurologic patient presented with an alveolar localized infiltrate after 4 days of mechanical ventilation that was highly suggestive of early-onset pneumonia. The suspected etiologic agents in this case should include those more frequently responsible of primary endogenous pneumonia (Box 57.2).

However, other signs of infection were not present, and a fast Gram stain was negative. CPIS score was low (3 points), and a short course of antibiotic was started. Most importantly, after 3 days the CPIS score remained low. Therefore antibiotic therapy was discontinued. The key point is that the CPIS score does not assure the clinician with absolute confidence that the patient does not have pneumonia, but it is a tool that helps to identify the patient who may not require prolonged treatment with a combination of antibiotics.

Case 2 is a much more complex situation that is also frequently encountered in routine clinical practice in every ICU. This ventilated patient was receiving broad-spectrum antibiotics to treat another infectious foci and developed pulmonary infiltrates. Clinical and laboratory data were consistent with nosocomial pneumonia. This must be considered initially a late-onset endogenous secondary pneumonia directly associated with a change in oropharyngeal flora. Suspected pathogens are those acquired in the hospital and are potentially drug resistant (see Box 57.2). A tracheobronchial aspirate was taken and empiric therapy initiated. Any clinical strategy

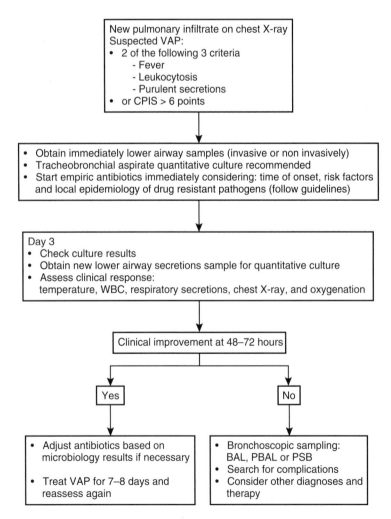

**Figure 57.2** Suggested management algorithm for VAP. BAL, bronchoalveolar lavage; CPIS, clinical pulmonary infection score; PBAL, protected bronchoalveolar lavage; PSB, protected specimen brush; WBC, white blood cell count.

chosen must include prompt initiation of empiric therapy in all cases of suspected VAP. Delayed initiation of appropriate antibiotic therapy has been consistently associated with an increase in mortality. Selection of antibiotic therapy should consider specific risk factors and take into account available information of local patterns of antibiotic resistance and organism prevalence. In this example, tracheobronchial aspirate provided an etiologic diagnosis and antibiotic treatment was adjusted accordingly. Etiologic diagnosis is based on the results of the culture of samples from the lower airways. However, colonization of the trachea and upper airway precedes progression to pneumonia in most cases of VAP. For this reason, positive qualitative cultures may not be able to discriminate between pathogenic infection and colonization. Quantitative cultures are especially valuable in this setting. Endotracheal bronchoaspirates, BAL, or PSB defines pneumonia and the etiologic microorganism. Infection thresholds have been identified for each sampling methodology to the diagnosis of VAP. Growth below the threshold is supposedly due to colonization. A lower respiratory sample for quantitative culture should be collected from all intubated patients when the diagnosis of pneumonia is being considered. Obviously, thresholds are not perfect and their application may be followed both by false-positive and false-negative results. The use of noninvasive techniques versus invasive (mainly bronchoscopic methods) in VAP diagnosis is still a matter of debate. Several randomized trials using quantitative cultures have failed to find differences in outcome when comparing both approaches. In Case 2, a follow-up bronchoaspirate showed a decrease in bacterial count. However—and still under the same antibiotics—the patient worsened. In this case of nonresolving nosocomial pneumonia, bronchoscopic bronchoaspirate and BAL were performed. BAL fluid culture led to isolation of a well-known in-house pathogen with a particular pattern of antibiotic resistance. In our view it seems reasonable to base our current approach on noninvasive sampling, relying on invasive procedures for those cases without improvement of clinical course after rational antibiotic treatment has been implemented. This proposed management algorithm is summarized in Fig. 57.2.

## SUGGESTED READINGS

Fagon JY, Chastre J, Vuagnat A, et al: Nosocomial pneumonia and mortality among patients in intensive care units. JAMA 1996;275:866–869.

Fartoukh M, Maitre B, Honore S, et al: Diagnosing pneumonia during mechanical ventilation: The Clinical Pulmonary Infection Score revisited. Am J Respir Crit Care Med 2003;168: 173–179.

Kollef M: Current concepts: The prevention of ventilator-associated pneumonia. N Engl J Med 1999;340:627–634.

Meduri GU: Diagnosis and differential diagnosis of ventilator-associated pneumonia. Clin Chest Med 1995;16:61–93.

Niederman M, Torres A, Summer W: Invasive diagnostic testing is not needed routinely to manage suspected ventilator-associated pneumonia. Am J Respir Crit Care Med 1994;150:565–569.

Pugin J, Auckenthaler R, Mili N, et al: Diagnosis of ventilator associated pneumonia by bacteriologic analysis of bronchoscopic and non-bronchoscopic "blind" bronchoalveolar lavage fluid. Am Rev Respir Dis 1991; 143:1121–1129.

Singh N, Rogers P, Atwood CHW, et al: Short course empiric therapy for patients with pulmonary infiltrates in the intensive care unit. Am J Respir Crit Care Med 2000; 162:505–511.

Torres A, Aznar R, Gatell JM, et al: Incidence, risk, and prognosis factors of nosocomial pneumonia in mechanically ventilated patients. Am Rev Respir Dis 1990;142:523–528.

Torres A, Ewig S: Diagnosing ventilator-associated pneumonia. N Engl J Med 2004;350:433–435.

# INDEX ••••

Page numbers followed by *b* indicate boxed text. Page numbers followed by *f* indicate figures. Page numbers followed by *t* indicate tables.

## A

Absorbance spectrophotometry, 488
Accelerated silicosis, 6
ACCP. *See* American College of Chest Physicians
ACD. *See* Congenital alveolar capillary dysplasia
ACE. *See* Angiotensin-converting enzyme
Acetaminophen
  as cause of drug-induced lung injury, 23–24
  for use in the intensive care unit, 405*t*
Acetate, effect of replacement fluid composition, 164, 165*f*
Achondroplasia, 573
Acid-base chart, 461
Acidemia, treatment, 168–171
Acidosis, treatment, 168–171
*Acinobacter* spp., 410, 445, 638
Acinus, anatomy, 82–83
Acquired immunodeficiency syndrome (AIDS), flexible bronchoscopy and, 239
ACT. *See* Activated clotting time
ACTH. *See* Adrenocorticotropic hormone
Activated clotting time (ACT), 563
Acute lung injury (ALI). *See also* Acute respiratory distress syndrome
  causes and clinical disorders associated with, 29*t*
  changes in body temperature and, 51–60
    case study, 51–52, 62*f*
    clinical aspects, 55
    general principles, 52–53
    role of heat shock response in, 53–57, 53*f*, 54*f*
  criteria for, 42
  definition, 42, 43*t*, 615, 616*b*
  drug-induced, 18–27
  genetic basis, 207–215
  ventilator-induced, 30, 43
Acute Physiology and Chronic Health Evaluation (APACHE), 63
  economics of ventilator care, 595, 596*f*
Acute renal failure (ARF)
  acid-base balance and, 163–167
  effect of high-volume hemofiltration on acid-base balance, 166–167, 166*f*, 167*f*

Acute renal failure (ARF) *(Continued)*
  effect of renal replacement therapy on acid-base balance, 163–164
  effect of replacement fluid composition, 164–166, 165*f*
  hypothermia and, 56–58
  physiologic effect on lung function, 199–200, 199*f*
Acute respiratory distress syndrome (ARDS), 616
  acute lung injury and, 28–41
  barotrauma, 225, 226*f*
  case study, 624–626
  causes and clinical disorders associated with, 29*t*
  chest radiograph, 225, 227*f*
  clinical presentation and diagnosis, 31–33
    chest radiography, 31–32, 33*f*
    computed tomography, 32–33, 32*f*, 33*f*
    respiratory mechanics, 33
  cytokines
    as inflammatory mediators, 217, 218*f*
    modulation and, 503–508
    release and, 216–224
  death from, 36–37
  definition, 42, 43*t*, 616*b*
  etiology, 28–30
    clinical associations, 29–30, 29*t*
    predispositions, 28–29
    ventilator-induced lung injury, 30
  extracorporeal life support in, 297–303
  exudative, 226, 228*f*
  heart-lung interaction, 180–182
    recruitment and oxygenation, 181
    respiratory elastance, 181
    ventilation strategy, 181–182
  impact of computed tomography on current clinical practice, 228–230
  inreasing airway pressure effect, 230, 230*f*
  long-term findings in survivors of, 230
  lung imaging by computed tomography, 225–235
  lung injury from drugs, 18
  mechanical ventilatory support for, 253*t*
  neutrophils and cytokines, 216–217, 217*f*
  outcome, 36–37
  partial liquid ventilation and, 291, 291*f*
  pathophysiology, 30–31
  proliferative, 228, 229*f*
  pulmonary, 227, 228*f*

Acute respiratory distress syndrome (ARDS) *(Continued)*
  pulmonary infections and, 7–8
  pulmonary versus extrapulmonary, 228
  role of cell types, 217–219, 218*f*
  routine clinical protocols for computed tomography, 230, 230*f*
  treatment, 8, 33–36
    extracorporeal membrane oxygenation, 36
    glucocorticoids, 35
    high-frequency oscillatory ventilation, 34
    liquid ventilation, 36
    lung protective ventilation strategies, 33–34
    open lung approach, 34
    oxygen toxicity avoidance, 34–35
    prone positioning, 35
    of pulmonary hypertension by inhaled nitric oxide, 36
    sedation and paralysis, 35
    surfactant therapy, 35, 140–141
  unexplained, 239–240
Acute Respiratory Distress Syndrome (ARDS) Network, 42, 42*t*, 468, 615
Acute respiratory failure, 467, 566*t*
  cytokine modulation and, 503–508
Acute silicosis, 6
Acute ventilatory failure (AVF), 100
Adrenaline. *See* Epinephrine
Adrenocorticotropic hormone (ACTH), resistive breathing and, 127–128, 128*f*
Adult respiratory distress syndrome (ARDS), ventilator-induced lung injury and, 43
Advanced Life Support (ALS), 308
AECC. *See* American-European Consensus Conference
Aerosol therapy
  antibiotic, 445–446
  respiratory pharmacology and, 428–442. *See also* individual drug names
AFR. *See* Acute renal failure
AG. *See* Anion gap
AIDS. *See* Acquired immunodeficiency syndrome
Aircraft, 310, 310*b*. *See also* Hospitalization
Air embolism
  arterial gas embolism, 366
  cerebral air embolism, 367, 367*f*